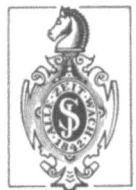

ATHERO-SCLEROSIS IV

Proceedings of the
Fourth International Symposium

Edited by
G. SCHETTLER Y. GOTO Y. HATA G. KLOSE

With 308 Figures and 185 Tables

Springer-Verlag
Berlin Heidelberg New York 1977

Proceedings of the Fourth International Symposium on Atherosclerosis

Held in Tokyo, August 24–28th, 1976

Sponsored by the Japan Atherosclerosis Society, and supported by the Japan Medical Association and the American Heart Association.

ISBN-13: 978-3-642-95310-1   e-ISBN-13: 978-3-642-95308-8
DOI: 10.1007/978-3-642-95308-8

Library of Congress Cataloging in Publication Data. International Symposium on Atherosclerosis, 4th, Tokyo, 1976. Atherosclerosis IV. Bibliography: p. Includes index. 1. Arteriosclerosis – Congresses. I. Schettler, Friedrich Gotthard. II. Title. RC692.I5 1976 616.1'36 77-11091

Softcover reprint of the hardcover 1st edition 1977

EDITORIAL COMMITTEE

G. Schettler, Y. Goto, Y. Hata, G. Klose
H. Greten, G. Middelhoff, R. Mordasini, P. Oster, A. Reinartz, G. Schlierf

EXECUTIVE COMMITTEE

Chairman: K. Oshima
Co-chairmen: G. Schettler, T. Shimamoto
General Secretary: Y. Goto
General Consultants: W. L. Holmes, N. Kimura, M. Murakami, G. Schlierf, R. W. Wissler,
   Y. Yamamura

INTERNATIONAL PROGRAM COMMITTEE

J.-L. Beaumont, H. Buchwald, L. A. Carlson, W. E. Connor, A. J. Day, F. H. Epstein,
Y. Goto, A. M. Gotto, Jr., M. D. Haust, W. L. Holmes, A. N. Klimov, D. Kritchevsky,
K. T. Lee, R. Lovell, H. C. McGill, K. R. Norum, M. F. Oliver, K. Oshima, R. Paoletti,
G. Schlierf, D. Seidel, T. Shimamoto, I. K. Shkhvatsabaya, E. B. Smith, Y. Stein, D. Stein-
berg, J. P. Strong, C. C. S. Toh, N. Werthessen, S. Wolf

THE LOCAL ORGANIZING COMMITTEE

Chairman: K. Oshima
Consultants: J. Hanamura, Y. Mikamo, S. Okinaka, T. Takemi, Y. Tateno
Co-chairmen: T. Aizawa, Y. Goto, N. Kimura, M. Murakami, G. Ooneda, T. Shimamoto,
   K. Tanaka, Y. Yamamura, M. Yoshikawa
Members: J. Fujii, T. Fujinami, T. Fujita, I. Fukui, M. Harasawa, Y. Hata, Y. Hosoda,
   M. Ikeda, Y. Imai, T. Kanazawa, Y. Kaneko, M. Kihata, T. Kimura, F. Kuzuya, J. Mise,
   M. Miyahara, K. Murata, C. Naito, H. Nakamura, M. Nakamura, T. Nakashima, S. Nanbu,
   T. Nasu, K. Nishimori, F. Numano, K. Ogino, R. Okada, T. Omae, K. Ohno, K. Ohta,
   S. Ohtsu, H. Orimo, H. Sekimoto, A. Sumiyoshi, T. Sunaga, Y. Takahashi, N. Takeuchi,
   T. Takeuchi, H. Tauchi, K. Tokita, Y. Ueda, K. Wada, T. Yasugi, Y. Yoshida
Executive Committee: Y. Goto (Chairman)
Local Program Committee: T. Shimamoto (Chairman)
Fund Raising Committee: M. Murakami (Chairman)
Social Program Committee: N. Kimura (Chairman)
Exhibition Committee: G. Ooneda (Chairman)
Secretariat: K. Ogawa, M. Oshima, K. Miyazaki, K. Takakura

ACKNOWLEDGEMENTS

Abbott Australia Pty., Ltd., Kurnell, N.S.W./Australia

Abbott Laboratories, Chicago, IL./USA

Ajinomoto Co., Tokyo/Japan

Astra Chemical Pty., Ltd., Sydney, N.S.W./Australia

Banyu Pharmaceutical Co., Ltd., Tokyo/Japan

Bayer AG, Leverkusen/Germany

Bayer Yakuhin, Ltd., Osaka/Japan

Bene-Chemie GmbH, München/Germany

Best Foods International Inc., Eagle Wood Cliffs, NJ/USA

Boehringer Ingelheim Pty., Ltd., Lane Coven, N.S.W./Australia

Boso Oil Fac. Co., Tokyo/Japan

Bridge Stone Tire Co., Ltd., Kurume/Japan

Burson-Masteller/Fuji, Tokyo/Japan

Chemie Grünenthal GmbH, Stolberg/Germany

Chiba-Gaigy (Japan), Ltd., Osaka/Japan

Chugai Pharmaceutical Co., Ltd., Tokyo/Japan

Cyanamid Australia Pty., Ltd., St. Leonards, N.S.W./Australia

Daido Seiko, Co., Ltd., Tokyo/Japan

Daiichi Seiyaku Co., Ltd., Tokyo/Japan

Dainippon Pharmaceutical Co., Ltd., Tokyo/Japan

Delalande, Arzneimittel GmbH, Köln/Germany

Deutsche Forschungsgemeinschaft, Bonn-Bad Godesberg/Germany

Eisai Co., Ltd., Tokyo/Japan

E. R. Squibb & Sons, Princeton, NJ/USA

Essex Laboratories Pty., Ltd., Baulkham Hills, N.S.W./Australia

Exxon Corporation, New York, NY/USA

Fujisawa Pharmaceutical Co., Ltd., Tokyo/Japan

Fukuda Medical Electron Co., Tokyo/Japan

Fukuoka Broadcasting Corporation, Fukuoka/Japan

G. D. Searl International Co., North Sydney, N.S.W./Australia

Hisamitsu Pharmaceutical Co., Ltd., Saga/Japan

Hoechst Australia Ltd., Melbourne, Victoria/Australia

Hoechst Japan Co., Ltd., Tokyo/Japan

Hoffmann-La Roche AG, Grenzach/Germany

Hoffmann-La Roche Inc., Nutley, NJ/USA

ICI-Pharma Ltd., Osaka/Japan

Idemitsu Kosan Co., Ltd., Tokyo/Japan

Ishihara Pharmaceutical Co., Ltd., Tokyo/Japan

Japan Upjohn, Tokyo/Japan

Kagayama, Akio, Tokyo/Japan

Kaken Chemical Co., Ltd., Tokyo/Japan

Kanebo Medical Supply, Ltd., Tokyo/Japan

Kawasaki Seitetsu, Tokyo/Japan

Kisen Hospital, Tokyo/Japan

Kobe Seikojo (Tokyo), Tokyo/Japan

Kowa Co., Ltd., Tokyo/Japan

Kraftco Corporation, Glenview, IL/USA

Kubota Tekko Ltd., Tokyo/Japan

Kyorin Yakuhin Pharmaceutical Co., Ltd., Tokyo/Japan

Kyowa Hakko Kogyo Co., Ltd., Tokyo/Japan

Kyushu Electric Power, Fukuoka/Japan

Lederle Japan, Tokyo/Japan

Lilly, Eli & Co., Indianapolis, Ia./USA

Maizena-Gesellschaft, Hamburg/Germany

McNeil Laboratories, Inc., Fort Washington, Pa./USA

Mead Johnson, Evansville, IA/USA

Medizinisch-Pharmazeutische Studiengesellschaft, Frankfurt/Germany

Merck AG, Darmstadt/Germany

Merck Sharp & Dohme International, Rahway, NJ/USA

Merckle KG, Blaubeuren/Germany

Midori Juji Pharmaceutical Co., Ltd., Tokyo/Japan

Miles Laboratories Australia Pty., Ltd., Mulgrave Melbourne, Victoria/Australia

Miles Laboratories, Inc., Elkhart, IA/USA
Mitsubishi Seiko, Tokyo/Japan
Mochida Pharmacy Co., Ltd., Tokyo/Japan
Nattermann International GmbH, Köln/Germany
Nihon Shinyaku K. K., Tokyo/Japan
Nippon Abbot K. K., Osaka/Japan
Nippon C. H. Boehringer Sohn Co., Ltd., Osaka/Japan
Nippon Chemiphar Co., Ltd., Tokyo/Japan
Nippon Kokan K. K., Tokyo/Japan
National Livestock & Meat Board, Chicago, IL/USA
Nippon Merck-Banyu Co., Ltd., Tokyo/Japan
Nippon Roche K. K., Tokyo/Japan
Nippon Roussel K. K., Tokyo/Japan
Nippon Sharyo Seizo Kaisha, Ltd., Nagoya/Japan
Nippon Shojikaisha Ltd., Osaka/Japan
Nisshin Steel, Tokyo/Japan
Nordmark-Werke GmbH Hamburg, Uetersen/Germany
Ono Pharmaceutical, Osaka/Japan
Ortho Pharmaceutical Corporation, Raritan, NJ/USA
Osaka Seiko, Tokyo/Japan
Otani Industry Ltd., Tokyo/Japan
Phizer Taito Co., Ltd., Tokyo/Japan
Q. P. Corporation, Tokyo/Japan
Rama Health Information Service, Tokyo/Japan
Richardson-Merrell Pty., Ltd., Villawood, N.S.W./Australia
Roche Products Pty., Ltd., Dee Why, N.S.W./Australia
Roussel Pharmaceuticals Ltd., N.S.W./Australia
Royal Hospital, Tokyo/Japan
Sandoz Ltd., Tokyo/Japan
Sankoy Co., Ltd., Tokyo/Japan
Sanwa Kagaku Kenkyusho, Nagoya/Japan
Searl Laboratories, Chicago, IL/USA
Shimizu Seiyaku K. K., Tokyo/Japan
Shin Nihon Seitetsu, Tokyo/Japan
Shionogi Co., Ltd., Osaka/Japan
Smith Kline & French Laboratories, Philadelphia, PA/USA
Standard Brands Incorporated, New York, NY/USA

Sumitomo Chemical Co., Ltd., Osaka/Japan
Taisho Pharmaceutical Co., Ltd., Tokyo/Japan
Takeda Chemical Industries, Ltd., Osaka/Japan
Tanabe Pharmaceutical Co., Ltd., Tokyo/Japan
Tanaka, Shikibe, Mie/Japan
The Boots Company (Aust) Pty., Ltd., North Rock, N.S.W./Australia
The Commemorative Association for the Japan World Exposition, Tokyo/Japan
The Federation of Electric Power Companies, Tokyo/Japan
The Japan Steel Works Ltd., Tokyo/Japan
The Life Insurance Association of Japan, Tokyo/Japan
The Marine and Fire Insurance Association of Japan, Tokyo/Japan
The Pharmaceutical Manufacture's Association of Osaka, Osaka/Japan
The Pharmaceutical Manufacture's, Association of Tokyo, Tokyo/Japan
The Procter & Gamble Company, Cincinnati, OH/USA
The Tokyo Banker's Association Inc., Tokyo/Japan
The Upjohn Company, Kalamazoo, MI/USA
Tokyo Medical Service Co., Ltd., Tokyo/Japan
Toyota Motor Industry, Aichi/Japan
Tokyo Tanabe Co., Ltd., Tokyo/Japan
Tomita, Kenji, Gunma/Japan
Tomy Seiko Co., Ltd., Tokyo/Japan
Topy Industries Ltd., Tokyo/Japan
Toray Science Foundation, Tokyo/Japan
Ube Industries Ltd., Yamaguchi/Japan
Upjohn GmbH, Heppenheim/Germany
Yamanouchi Pharmaceutical Co., Ltd., Tokyo/Japan
Yamato Tsushin-sha, Tokyo/Japan
Yodogawa Seikojo, Tokyo/Japan
Yoshitomi Pharmaceutical Industries Ltd., Osaka/Japan
William R. Warner & Co., Pty., Ltd., Australia
Wülfing-Bauer, Neuss/Germany

These are the persons who worked hard at the Secretariat of the Symposium:

Miss Kiyoko Ogawa, Miss Kazue Miyazaki, Miss Masako Ohshima, Miss Keiko Yamaguchi, Miss Hajime Esaki, Mrs. Kazuko Takakura.

CONTENTS

Statistical Trend in the Incidence of Cerebrovascular Accidents and Coronary Heart Disease in Japan*

Kenzo Oshima

I would like to heartily welcome all of you who have come from 36 countries of the world to participate in the Fourth International Symposium on Atherosclerosis. The presentations and discussions in this symposium will, we hope, reflect the progress of studies on atherosclerosis and should represent an important contribution to human welfare.

It is regrettable, however, that due to the present difficult economic situation it has not been possible to cover all expenses of speakers in the plenary session and the workshops.

The average human life span has been increasing markedly, and thus the number of old people has increased in every country of the world. Therefore, studies on atherosclerosis, in addition to their scientific interest, are becoming more important to improve the treatment of geriatric diseases. This is reflected in the fact that the higlights of the symposium will be reported in medical weeklies and newspapers.

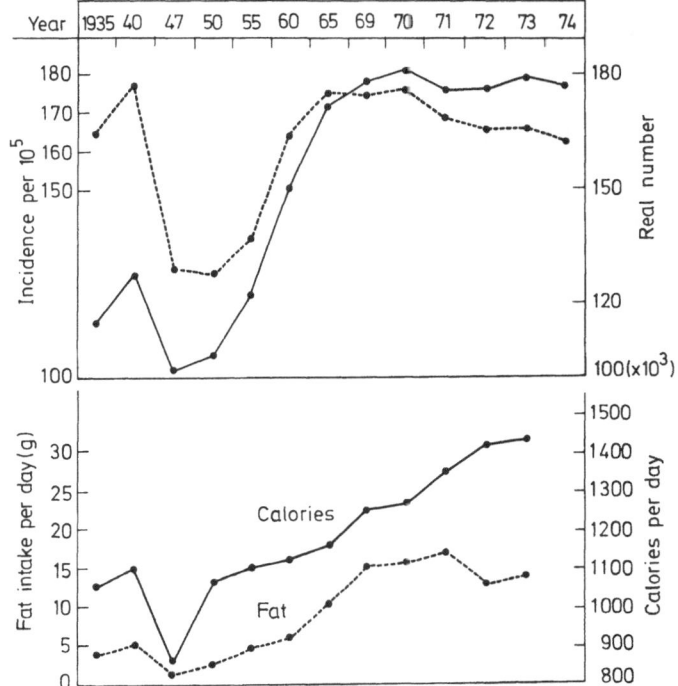

Figure 1. Annual occurence of strokes and average Calorie and fat intakes in Japan

* The data used in this study were based on the Vital Statistics of Japan (in Japanese) edited by Health and Welfare Statistic Department, Ministry of Health and Welfare, Japan.

The Japanese represent an interesting group for the observation of atherosclerotic diseases, in view of their particular eating habits and the fact that now have one on the longest life spans in the world, the male attaining 72, and the female 77 years on average. Hence, as is wellknown, the Japanese are a particulary interesting subject for epidemiological and comparative studies on atherosclerosis. I would, therefore, like to summarize some of the more interesting features. The following data were abstracted from statistics for the whole country.

Figure 1 shows the average calorie and fat intake per day and annual occurence of strokes, which is still the main cause of death in Japan. The food intake was very low during 1945–1948, and the mean calorie intake per person dropped below 1000 calories. It is very interesting that the real number and incidence of strokes dropped sharply at this period. There seems to be little doubt that these sharp drops were due low calorie and fat intake.

From 1950 on, the real number of strokes increased and by 1965 the incidence reached the values seen before the war. This appears to parallel the increase of the calorie intake, but, in fact, it corresponds well to the increase in the number of old people, as can be seen from Figure 2.

Figure 2 shows the incidence of strokes per 100.000 for younger age groups. It can be seen that there has been no increase in the indicende of strokes since 1947. In fact, the incidence has been decreasing since 1960. It is most remarkable in the age group 55–59, since in 1940 the incidence was 562, and this had decreased to 182 by 1974. This decrease in the incidende of strokes is considered to be mainly due to the use of hypotensive drugs, because most Japanese physicians have administered Rauwolfia and chlorothiazide singly or in combination since 1958.

Figure 3 shows the incidence in age groups above 60 years. Here, we can again see a decrease of incidence since 1960 or 1965 in the age groups from 60 to 74 years. There is also a slight increase of incidence in the age group 75–79 and a marked increase in the age group above 80 years. In short, it appears from these data that the incidence of strokes has shifted to a more advanced age group since 1960.

Figure 4 shows the real number of strokes in the groups above 60 years of age. Here, we can see an increase following the sharp drop during 1945–1947. The increase was more marked in more advanced age groups. Thus, the real number and incidence of strokes have both increased overall since 1960, due to the increase of case in advanced age groups. The decrease of incidence in relatively younger groups is due mainly to a decrease of cerebral hemorrhage.

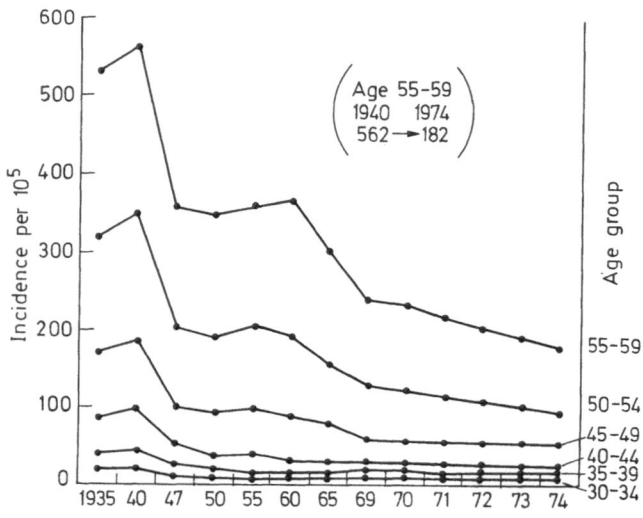

Figure 2. Trends in the incidence of strokes in age groups under 59

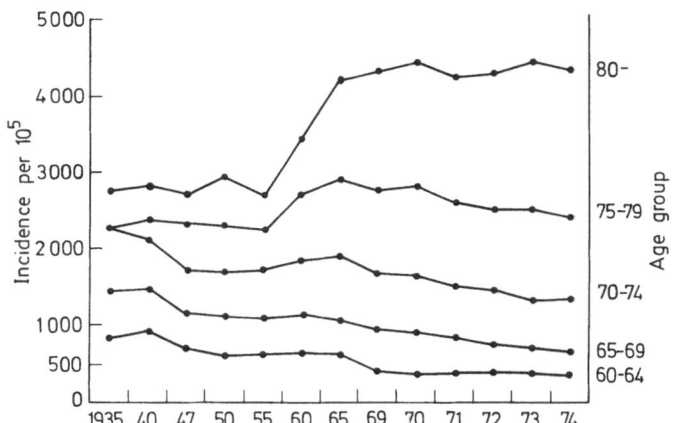

Figure 3. Trends in the incidence of strokes in age groups above 60

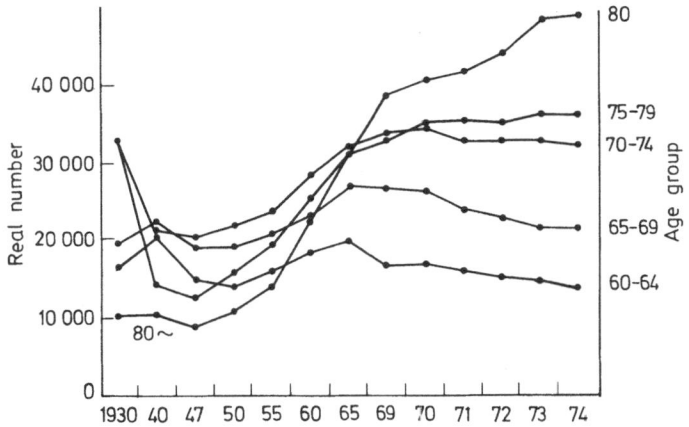

Figure 4. Annual occurence of strokes in age groups above 60

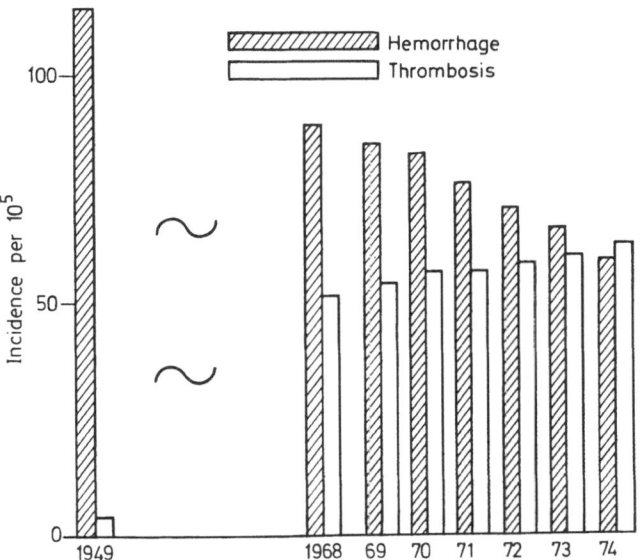

Figure 5. Trends in the ratio of cerebral hemorrhage of thrombosis

XVII

Figure 5 shows this relationship. In 1949, the incidence of cerebral hermorrhage was much higher than that of thrombosis, but it fell steadily, while the incidence of thrombosis increased year by year, and the relationship was reversed in 1974. This does not mean, however, that hemorrhage was replaced by thrombosis. It seems more likely that the incidence of hemorrhage has decreased as a result of improved medical treatment, while that of thrombosis has increased with the increase in the number of older people.

Next, I would like to look at the problem of coronary sclerosis in Japan.

Figure 6 shows the relationship between cardiac death and calorie and fat intake. Since ischemic heart disease was not a separate category in the international classification of causes of death in 1935, but was included in cardiac death, Figure 6 shows cardiac death. As can be seen, the incidence of cardiac death appears to increase with on increase in calorie and fat intake.

However, if we observe the incidence of cardiac death in age groups under 65 years as in Figure 7, it is surprising that the incidence in each case has been decreasing since 1940 or 1947, even though the incidence for the whole population has been increasing year by year. The reason why the indicence of cardiac death is decreasing in the age groups under 65 is not certain, but it must be related to the increase in life span among the Japanese. There can be no doubt that the increase in average life span is largely due to the improvement of general medical care.

Figure 8 shows the results for the age groups above 65. Here, we can see a remarkable increase of incidence in the age group above 80, a marked increase in the age group 75–79, and a slight increase in the age group 70–74. This is why the incidence for the whole population has increased.

Figure 9 shows the incidence of death due to ischemic heart disease in each age group. The full lines show the incidence in 1973, and the dotted lines show that in 1968. During the past 5 years, we can again see a decrease of incidence in age groups under 79 in both sexes.

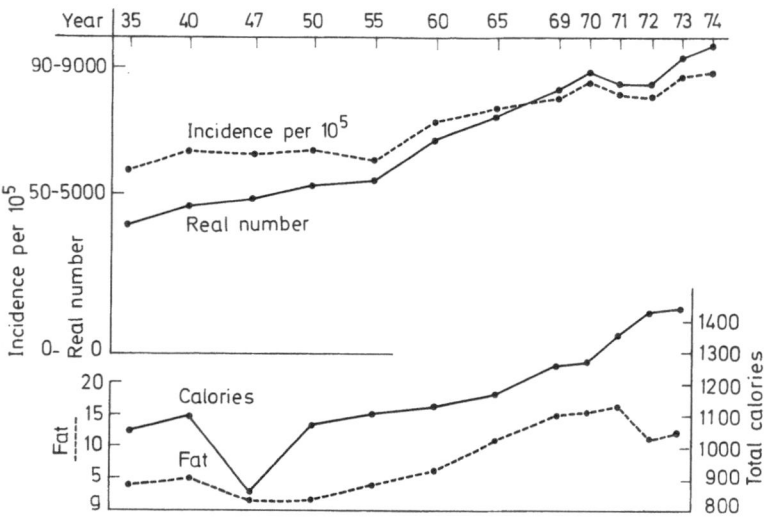

Figure 6. Annual occurence of cardiac death and average Calorie and fat intakes in Japan

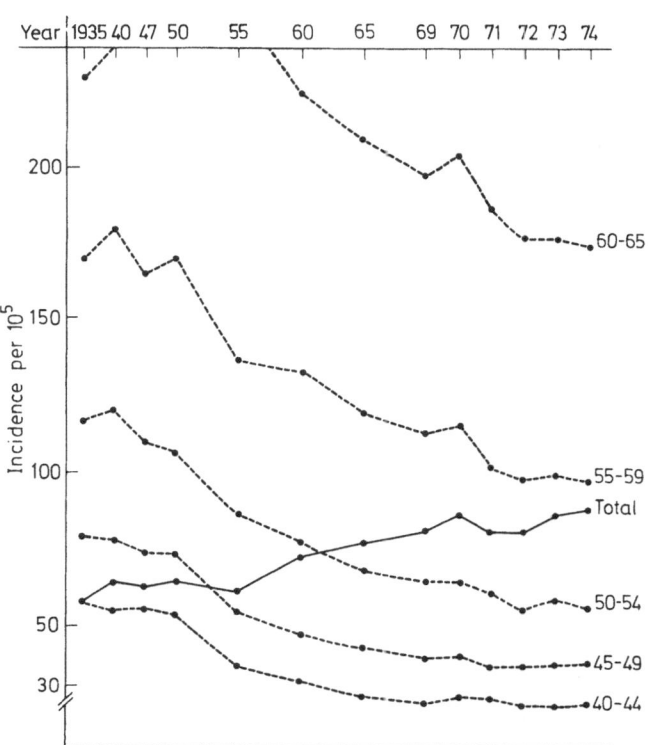

Figure 7. Incidence of cardiac death in age groups under 65

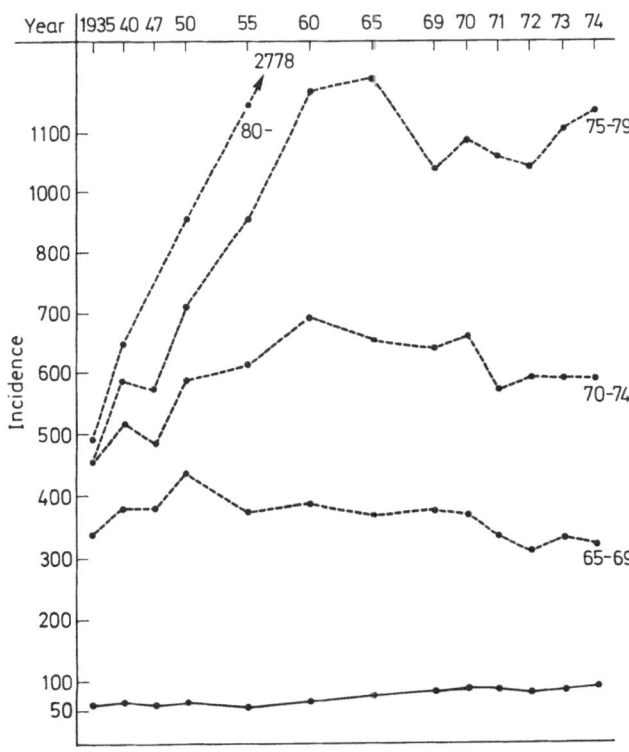

Figure 8. Incidence of cardiac death in age groups above 65

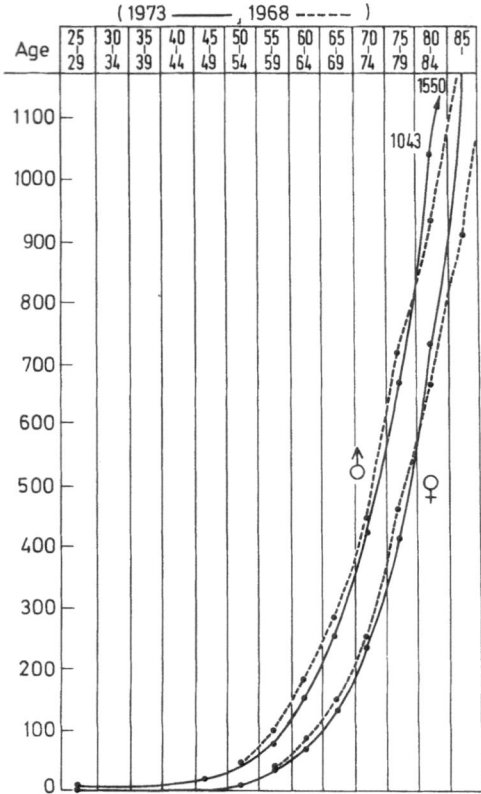

Figure 9. Incidence of ischemic hearth in age groups

These results indicate strongly that modern therapy has decreased the death rate due to atherosclerotic diseases. However, there is still a large number of patients with atherosclerotic diseases. Clearly, research on atherosclerosis contributes not only to the prolongation of human life but also to the health and comfort of old people. Thus, the presentations at this symposium will be of benefit to the whole human race.

KEYNOTE ADDRESS

Atherosclerosis, the Main Problem of the Industrialized Societies

G. Schettler

Atherosclerosis is by far the leading cause of death in the developed countries. More than 50% of all death in the USA are of cardiovascular origin. Indeed, such deaths make up about one-third of all mortalities in the young age groups between 35 and 44. Of course, the percentage rises with increasing age. In the Federal Republic of Germany, we had 120.000 deaths from cardiac infarcts in 1975 alone and a rate of affection by the disease which was approximately three times as high. Sixty percent of the costs of hospital and outpatient treatment are occasioned by illness attributable to atherosclerosis. The resulting explosion in state expenditure is threatening to render the already existing deficit in the financing of public health quite unreasonable. It must be taken into account here that there is a great decline in work productivity and a corresponding rise in social security benefits. In the Federal Republic of Germany, illnesses of vascular origin cost about 10% of the total gross national product, namely 30.000 million marks. If nothing happens, the time will come when the entire national income will be consumed by public health provisions and the payments coming in their wake. In Germany, such a situation will have arisen in about 25 years. It is thus imperative to retard or entirely stop this development. Faint indications of this possibility can be discerned in the latest results in the USA. There are also traces of the same tendencies in other countries, e. g. Sweden.

It is hence no wonder that there has been an extraordinary intensification of research in atherosclerosis in recent decades. There are innumerable individual projects, but unfortunately, only a few rudiments of purposeful, concentrated research. It is exceptionally difficult to disentangle the results of previous research so that specific trends or focal points can be discerned. Irvine Page critically examined atherosclerosis research in 1968. The National Heart and Lung Institute Task Force on atherosclerosis likewise drew up an account balance in 1971 and moreover made recommendations for the desirable points of emphasis in future research. Some of the suggestions made have been partly realized or are in the process of realization; others are illusive.

I would now like to discuss some of the major problems of human atherosclerosis.

Long-Term Studies on th Morbidity and Therapy of Atherosclerosis

Four important papers on long-term studies have recently appeared.

1. A 7-year secondary prevention study of the Coronary Drug Project was able to show that clofibrate and nicotinic acid could not effect any improvement of the cardiovascular mortality or even of the total mortality as compared to the placebo. A slight decrease of the nonfatal myocardial infarctions from 13 to 10% compared to controls was found only in the nicotinic acid group. Because of substantial side-effects, dextrothyroxine and estrogens were

eliminated earlier from the study. A justified objection to the results of this study is that the actual indication for the drugs, namely a reduction in blood lipids, was only achieved to a very slight extent. The reduction of triglycerides was 20–25%, that of serum cholesterol on nicotinic acid was about 10%, and that of cholesterol on clofibrate only 4%. Only half of the test subjects had cholesterol values over 250 mg%. According to the results of epidemiological studies, the cholesterol values attained were still with in a range which furthers the development of atherosclerosis. A significant objection to the results of the study and partially, the conclusions drawn from it is the lack of recording and differentiation of other risk factors for atherosclerosis or myocardial infarction, namely cigarette smoking and arterial hypertension, diabetes, overweight, lack of exercise and training, and finally stress in its various manifestations. If an expression of the protective action of lipid-lowering agents alone is desired, the group under study should have been better selected. Above all, younger test subjects without indication of severe atherosclerosis with substantial combined lesions and partial vessel occlusions should have been included. The study was carried out with great expenditure, with the participation of first-rate institutes; it illustrates how difficult the problem is and how false conclusions can be drawn from such results. There are thousands of studies performed with lipid-lowering agents. Unfortunately, a large proportion have engaged in unadulterated serum cosmetics and do not posess the slightest conclusiveness, due not only to statistical reasons but also faulty methodology.

2. Among long-term studies, that financed by the National Heart and Lung Institut should be mentioned. This is presently being performed at 12 lipid research clinics. Hyperlipoprotein-emias of type II are being investigated in this primary preventive study. All participants receive a cholesterol-lowering diet: the treatment group receives cholestyramine in addition to the diet and a control group receives the diet plus placebo.

3. Another study is concerned with influencing hypertension.

4. The fourth study additionally takes the risk factor, cigarette smoking, into consideration. It is notable that control groups are also established which can be supervised by the family doctor.

Long-term studies which are presently being initiated are concerned with the modification of platelet adhesiveness by aspirin and its possible repercussions on coronary heart diseases. Mention should further be made of a carefully designed primary prevention study with clofibrate which is being undertaken in Edinburgh, Prague, and Budapest.
You will be familiar with the encouraging primary and secondary prevention studies with diets containing polyunsaturated fatty acids by Turpeinen and co-workers (1968) in Finland and Leren (1973) in Oslo.

The Pathogenesis of Atherosclerosis

There ist no doubt that animal studies have made it easier to understand the pathogenesis of atherosclerosis. However, they also often lead in the wrong direction. It is very difficult to simulate the pathogenic factors for human atherosclerosis in animal studies. In particular, the polyetiology creates considerable difficulties.

Since the epoch-making experiments of Ignatowsky (1909), Saltykow (1913), Chalatov and Anitschkow (1913), who personally demonstrated his most recent experiments to me in Leningrad, millions of experimental animals have been sacrificed. A very important step was the inclusing of primates. Newer investigations have given us very significant ideas on the pathogenesis and regression of atherosclerotic lesions.

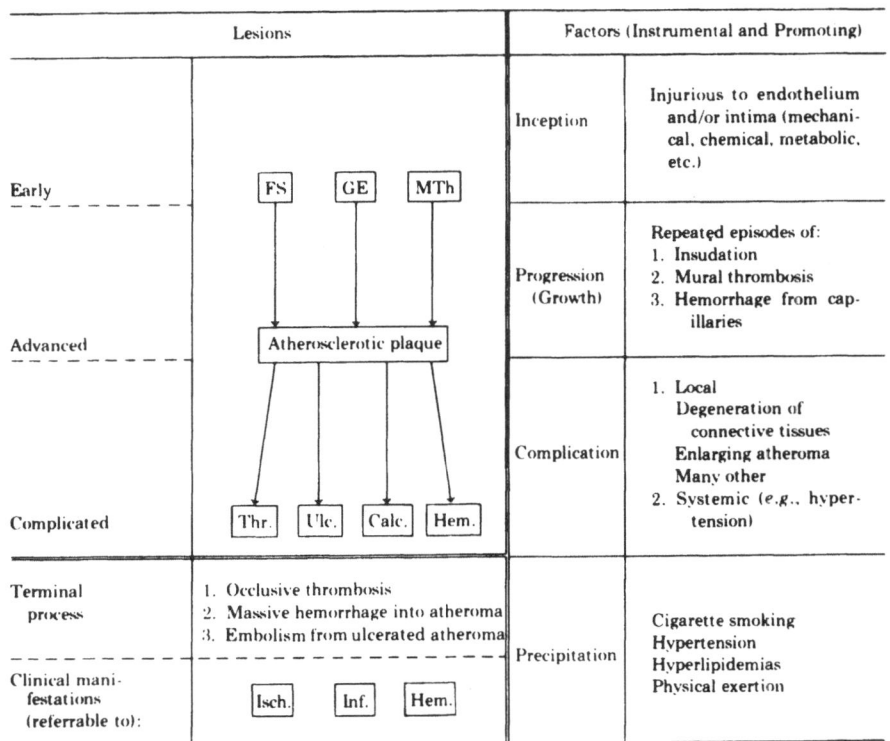

Lesions			Factors (Instrumental and Promoting)	
		Inception	Injurious to endothelium and/or intima (mechanical, chemical, metabolic, etc.)	
Early	FS GE MTh	Progression (Growth)	Repeated episodes of: 1. Insudation 2. Mural thrombosis 3. Hemorrhage from capillaries	
Advanced	Atherosclerotic plaque	Complication	1. Local Degeneration of connective tissues Enlarging atheroma Many other 2. Systemic (e.g., hypertension)	
Complicated	Thr. Ulc. Calc. Hem.			
Terminal process	1. Occlusive thrombosis 2. Massive hemorrhage into atheroma 3. Embolism from ulcerated atheroma	Precipitation	Cigarette smoking Hypertension Hyperlipidemias Physical exertion	
Clinical manifestations (referrable to):	Isch. Inf. Hem.			

Figure 1. Relation of pathogenetic factors to lesions and clinical disease (atherosclerosis)
FS = fatty streaks, GE = gelatinous elevations, MTh = microthrombi, Thr. = thrombosis, Ulc. = ulcerations, Calc. = calcification, Hem. = hemorrhage, Isch. = ischemia, Inf. = infarction

The most important pathogenetic concepts according to Haust and More (1972) are summarized in Figure 1. The early lessions play a key role. *Do they result from a primary vascular alternation or prior plasma changes?*
There is evidence for both from animal experiments and the data of human pathoanatomy. Primary plasma alterations can doubtlessly initiate modifications in the arterial wall. This applies for example to genetically determined hyperlipoproteinemias. On the other hand, arteriopathies caused by purley inflammatory events without additional plasmatic risk factors can initiate the state of vascular sclerosis, loss of elasticity, and narrowing of the lumen which is characteristic of atherosclerosis in man. The barrier function of the endothelium plays a major role in the pathogenetic process between the two possible factors.

Lipids and Lipoproteins

Atherosclerosis is associated with an accumulation of phospholipids, cholesterol, and cholesterol esters within the arterial plaque. Arterial tissue is capable of synthesizing phospholipids in situ.

This synthesis seems to be relatively independent of the influence of the plasma lipids. Unlike the phospholipids, the cholesterol and sterol portions of cholesterol esters that accumulate in arterial plaques are primarily derived from the circulating plasma lipoproteins. This has been strongly suggested in recent years by biochemical, histochemical, immunochemical, and autoradiographic evidence. It may be concluded from in vitro experimental data that his influx of plasma lipids or lipoproteins is governed primarily by a physico chemical process, and that it is probably relatively independent or enzymic or energy-providing mechanisms. Little knowledge is available on the catabolism of the different lipoprotein moieties within the arterial wall, in particular on the catabolism of the apolipoprotein portion, a process which takes place before lipid deposition occurs. It is also unknown whether the presence of lipoproteins in a deseased artery causes plaque formation or whether it results from increased arterial permeability due to the disease. Both mechanisms may independently be relevant. Some important features of normal plasma lipoproteins are given in Figure 2.

Various mechanisms have been proposed to explain the accumulation of lipids in the arterial wall, most of them including high plasma concentrations of β- or pre-β-lipoproteins as an important risk factor for atherosclerosis. For the α-lipoproteins, the major HDL-fraction, the contrary seems to be true. Therefore, hyper-α-lipoproteinemia should not be considered a risk factor, but rather interpreted as an antiatherogenic factor.

Evidence for this hypothesis is provided by genetic, epidemiological, and clinical studies. It seems possible that the positive effect of high HDL concentrations may be due to the particular physico chemical properties of HDL and their role in overall lipoprotein metabolism. This is indicated by in vitro experiments. We have increasing evidence that HDL is capable of mobilizing lipids (particularly cholesterol) from the aterial wall and other body tissues. The clinical picture of Tangier Disease fits into this concept and supports the idea that not only hyperlipoproteinemia but also dyslipoproteinemia may result in an accelerated accumulation of lipids in tissue. Very recently Stein and Stein (1973) have presented strong evidence that high-density lipoproteins inhibit binding, uptake, and degradation of low-density lipoproteins by human endothelial cells grown in culture. If this mechanism holds

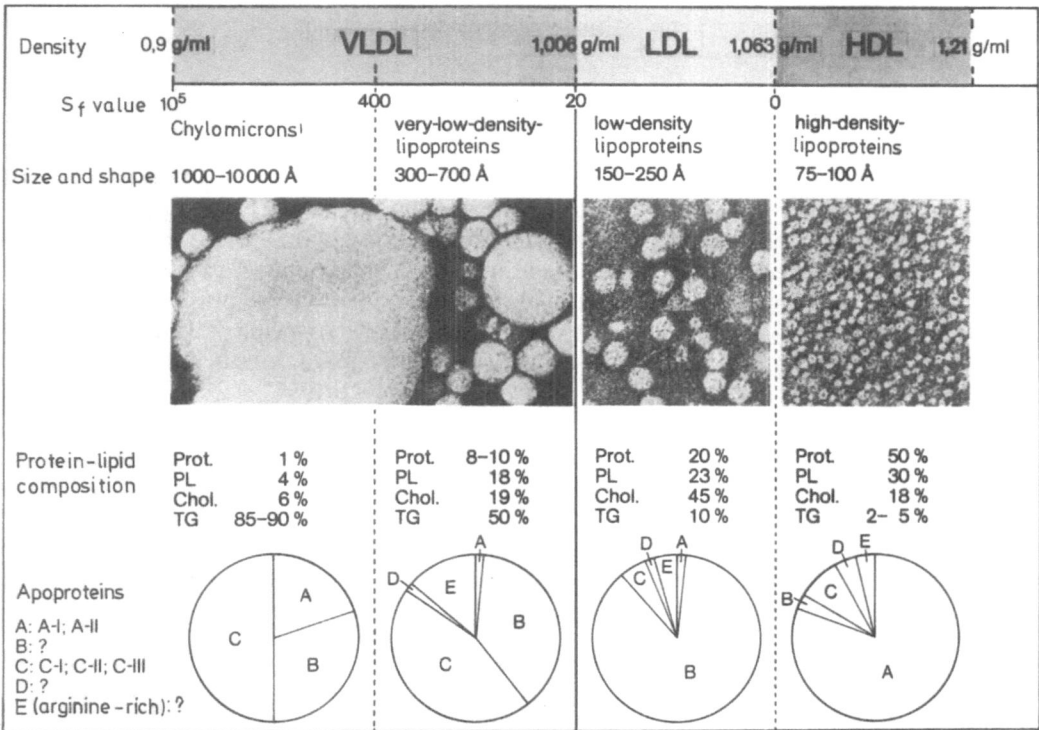

Figure 2. Important features of normal plasma lipoproteins

for intact vessels, the ratio of HDL to LDL and VLDL may turn out to be a most important parameter in determining the role and risk of plasma lipids in the process of atherogenesis. It therefore seems reasonable to anticipate that, in the face of competition between low-density and high-density lipoproteins, high-density lipoproteins might develop a protective action against low-density lipoprotein uptake and accumulation in the arterial wall. In the plasma of women, the ratio of high to low-density lipoprotein, when expressed as particles, is higher than in male. Thus, it is possible that the higher ratio might reduce the transendothelial transport of low-density lipoproteins and hence provide the female with better protection against cholesterol accumulation in the smooth muscle cell of the arterial wall (Stein and Stein, 1973).

In the past years, however, substantial evidence has been accumulated indicating that all different plasma lipoprotein fractions are interrelated in both their protein and lipid portion (see Fig. 3). As a result of lipolysis, pre-β-lipoproteins are converted to β-lipoproteins and postprandial chylomicrons are degraded into "intermediates" or "remnant particles", which are relatively rich in triglycerides and cholesterol. Many of the processes involved in this mechanism are mediated through the activity of various lipolytic enzymes, some of which are affected by apoproteins acting variously as cofactors or inhibitors. Therefore, the metabolic relationship of these conjugated macromolecules seems to depend not only on their lipid portion but also on the apoprotein composition. This fact and the concept that the uptake of plasma lipids by the tissue all depends upon (and is in part regulated by) the protein moiety of the lipoproteins gives reason to study the role of lipids in atherogenesis under dynamic aspects.

On the basis of our present knowledge, Zilversmit (1973) recently proposed a theory of atherogenesis that attributes key roles not only to β- and pre-β-lipoproteins, but also (and in particular) to chylomicrons or to remnants of the latter. In the presence of divalent cations and at physiologic salt concentrations, heparin and other sulphated polysaccharides cause aggregation primarily of chylomicrons, remnants of chylomicrons, and pre-β-lipoproteins. At low ionic strength, β- and pre-β-lipoproteins form insoluble complexes with such compounds. Heparin also binds to lipoprotein lipase and activates lipoprotein lipase. According to Zilversmit's ideas, it is likely that heparin or heparin-like substances may act as a bridge

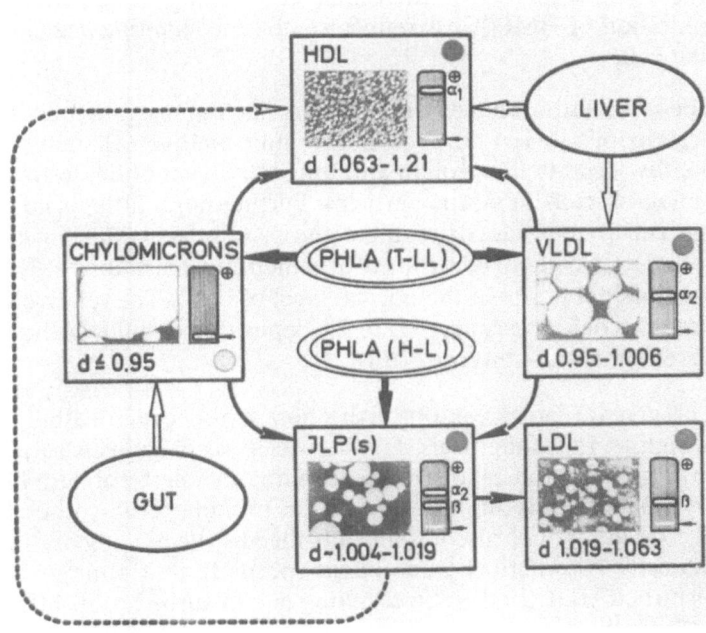

Figure 3. Lipoproteins of human plasma

linking chylomicrons, pre-β-lipoproteins or remnants, and lipoprotein lipase to the vascular endothelium. While adsorbed, the large complexes could be subjected to lipolysis, whereby cholesterol-rich lipoproteins or chylomicron remnants are formed. As the cross-linked effect of heparin and calcium at physiologic salt concentrations is weaker for β-lipoproteins than for chylomicrons, remnants, or pre-β-lipoproteins, much of the newly formed β-lipoprotein may therefore be released into the blood stream. This lipolytic process at the intimal surface might maintain a very high local concentration of cholesterol-rich lipoproteins at the blood-artery interphase and therefore be an important factor fo atherogenesis. In this regard, recent studies by Bierman and Albers (1975) are relevant; it was demonstrated that the uptake to remnant lipoprotein particles by aortic smooth muscle cells in culture far exceeded that of other lipoproteins. Furthermore, those cells which proliferate early in the development of atheroma to become the lipid-filled foam cells have only a limited capacity to catabolize remnants, despite the acceleratd uptake. Of the fasting lipoprotein families, LDL was taken up at the highest rate.

The well-known early manifestation of atherosclerosis in patients with familial type II hyperlipoproteinemia may not only be due to the absolute increase of β-lipoprotein concentration but also to a decrease of the percentage cholesterol esterification in the low-density fraction, to the abnormal tendency of these particles to aggregate (which was earlier demonstrated in our laboratory), and also to the abnormally low HDL/LDL ratio. According to the interesting data provided by Goldstein and Brown (1975), the metabolic nature of hyper-β-lipoproteinemia seems to be an abnormal genetic control of cholesterol metabolism caused by an abnormal apolipoprotein receptor system which is probably found on all cell membranes in the body. The abnormal metabolic pathways due to this effect are rather complicated; for the moment, only the most striking results are important for our purposes.

Goldstein and Brown (1975) have demonstrated (Fig. 4) a receptor for the low-density lipoproteins in normal cells, more specifically, for the apolipoprotein portion of these lipoproteins, which is capable of binding the molecules to the cell. After the lipoprotein is taken up by the cell, it releases cholesterol and the low-density lipoprotein is broken down. The cholesterol is esterified and, in so doing, it controls the synthesis of cholesterol by inhibition of HMG-CoA reductase, the rate-limiting enzyme of cholesterol synthesis within that cell.

The same authors have further shown that homozygous individuals with familial hyper-β-lipo-proteinemia do not have active receptors on their cell membranes (Fig. 5). They cannot bind the low-density lipoprotein and thus these cannot be destroyed. This results in a prolonged biological half-life of the particles. Furthermore, little or no cholesterol is transferred across the cell membrane to regulate the synthesis so that, in homozygotes, synthesis goes on completely without control. At very high concentrations of LDL, synthesis in heterozygotes is controlled, but not at the normal level of LDL. The relatively low HDL/LDL ratio resulting from this defect may accelerate the deposition of lipids in the smooth muscle cell and promote development of atherosclerosis.

This genetic defect resulting in the most severe forms of atherosclerosis raises a question which is highly interesting to us. Is atherosclerosis in subjects suffering from hyper-β-lipoprotein-emia simply or at all due to deposition of cholesterol deriving from serum lipoproteins into arterial wall, or is this lesion in fact due to cholesterol synthesis in the cells themselves going on at a rapid rate because it is uncontrolled by the binding of β-lipoproteins to the membrane of the cell? Alternatively, one might speculate that a major cause of the lesion is due to the disturbed HDL/LDL ratio resulting in a disturbed or insufficient release of cholesterol from such a cell.

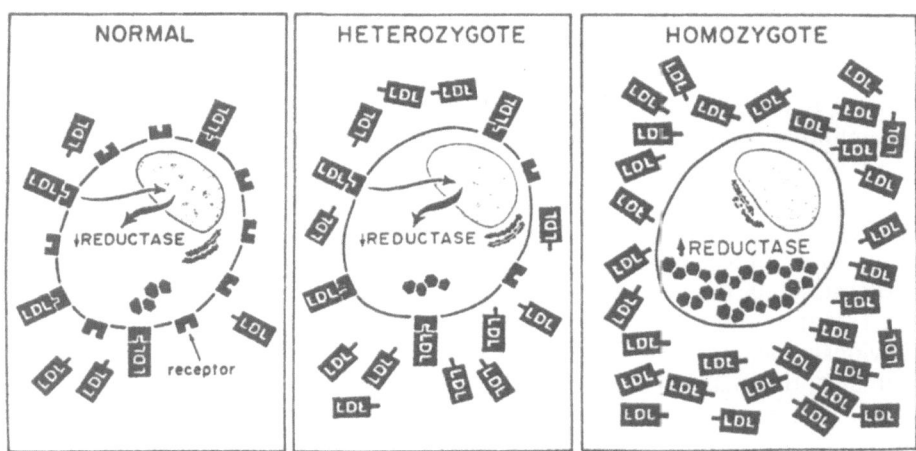

Figure 4

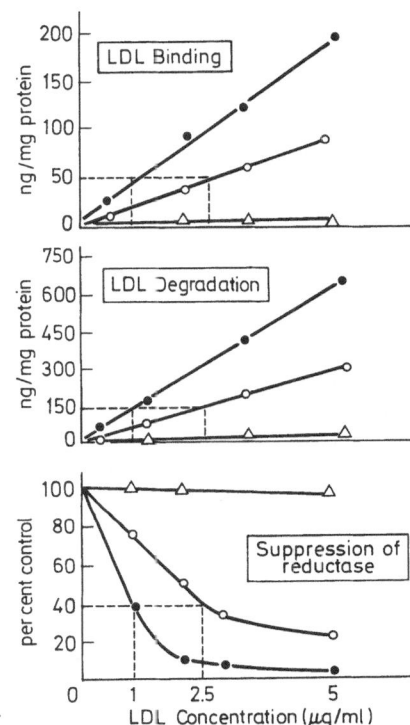

Figure 5. Functions of LDL receptor

Other Dissolved Plasma Components

First of all, hormones are to be mentioned, among them insulin, glucagon, somatotropins, steroids, thyroid hormones. Influences on endothelial function are ascribed. To all these substances some activities being mediated by the lipids and lipoproteins, e. g., activation of lipoprotein lipase by insulin (Fredrickson and co-workers, 1967; Bagdade et al., 1967; Bierman, 1972). Glucagon also acts on lipid metabolism (Stout et al., 1973; Friedman et al., 1971). Time does not permit discussion of the role of the other hormones. However, there are numerous experimental indications for the coincidence between endocrinopathies and premature atherosclerosis. This does not only relate to the epithelial function, but also to the constitution of the ground substance and especially to the mucopolysaccharides (see Hauss et al., 1969).

Among the macromolecules of the blood, fibrin and fibrinogen are especially significant for the atherosclerotic process. The theses of Rokitansky (1852) have been revived by new techniques of investigation. The presence of fibrin in atherosclerosis plaques and the deposition of fibrin on the arterial intima (Duguid, 1949) occasioned a very large number of further studies on the organization of mural thrombi, which are regarded as precursors of atheromas in the arterial wall (Mustard et al., 1974). The plasma lipids play a role here, as made particularly evident in by serial sections of human coronary arteries. Lipoproteins are incorporated in the plaques formed in this way (Scott and Hurley, 1969).

Obviously, platelets should also have significance here. With their phagocytic and contractile elements, the platelets stick to surfaces, aggregate and release enzymes ad vasoactive amines which are important for the formation of thrombi and also affect the vessel wall. Collagen, thrombin, ADP, immune complexes, bacteria, and viruses influence these kind of release reactions, which in turn crucially affect the permeability. ADP, ATP, adrenaline, serotonin, elastase, mucopolysaccharides, as well as lyosomal enzymes are released from the platelets. It could be shown that most of these substances bring about endothelial lesions and thus affect permeability. This may be a significant step in the aggressive action of plasma and plasma components on the vessel wall. In fact, this appears to be a central control point in the atherosclerotic process and in the genesis of the early lesions. It is also remarkable that some of the risk factors which favor the atherosclerotic process as well as cardiac infarction are associated with disturbed platelet function. This applies, e.g., to familial hyperlipoprotein-emia type II, in which an intensified platelet aggregation was found, with increased release of adrenaline, collagen, and ADP (Carvalho et al., 1974). The same study group found close correlations between platelet function and the cholesterol content of the platelets after incubation with cholesterol-rich liposomes; the LDL cholesterol probably has a key function here.

The importance of platelets in the development of atheromatous foci after the endothelial damage was verified by various techniques of investigation. It is still controversial whether the platelets can act aggressively and destructively on intact endothelial surfaces or whether attack must be preceded by an endothelial lesions in every case. The multiplicity of factors which may damage the endothelium and which could be demonstrated in vivo and in vitro confer a secondary importance to this question, however. It is certain that the denuded areas lend particular support to the destructive processes in the vessel wall; the smooth muscle plays an especially active role. In recent years, these smooth muscle cells have also assumed a particular significance in the evaluation of regressive processes. The risk factors which will be outlined later have a considerable role here. We refer you to the literature (Stemerman and Ross, 1972; Ross et al., 1974; Wissler, 1974; Haust, 1975; and others). The morphogenesis of atherosclerotic lesions cannot be discussed further here. The same applies to the effects of rheologic factors on endothelial permeability (see Glagov, 1972). The insudation and perfusion theory of the German School (Doerr, 1963, 1970; Ribbert, 1904; Rössle, 1944) is largely based on these kinds of rheologic factors. They have further significance in arterial lesions caused by hypertension (Lovell and Shaper, 1974; Heath and co-workers, 1960).

Immune Processes and Atherosclerosis

Arterial lesions are produced by antibodies against the vessel wall: a necrotizing arteritis with subsequent changes in the vessel results. The immune complexes IgG and IgM from lymphotoxic serum play an active role here (O'Connell and Mowbray, 1973). Incorporation of cholesterol causes further typical disorders (see Poston and Davies, 1974; Minnick and Murphy, 1974; Hauss et al., 1969). Immunologic processes are also probably involved in human atherosclerosis (for review, see *Lancet* as well as Beaumont and Beaumont, 1973). Autoimmune hyperlipidemias as well as the presence of lipoprotein immune complexes with their IgA- or IgG-specific antibodies were demonstrated in patients with hyperlipemic myelomas, although they are also found in certain hyperlipoproteinemias without myeloma.

A most important concern of further studies will be the role played by these immunologic processes and whether inflammatory processes are found in sudden unexpected cardiac death, especially in the absence of gross atherosclerotic lesions. There are still many open questions here. The same applies to the significance of angiotensin and other vasoactive amines as well as the lyosomes. They are evidently important in the transformation of smooth muscle cells into foam cells (Peters et al., 1973; Goldfischer et al., 1975).

A short comment is called for on the monoclonal theory of Benditt and Benditt (1973) because it was entirely incorrectly interpreted by the lay press in many countries. As you know, Benditt and Benditt assume that the cells of atherosclerotic fibrous plaques derive from a homogenous single cell line. This assumption is based on the observation that cells of benign tumors smooth muscle cells are of monoclonal origin, as shown by measurements of the A and B isoenzymes of the X-linked glucose-6-phosphate dehydrogenase. It was found that samples from normal arterial media and intima consist of mixed cell types, while the fibrous caps over atheromatous plaques consist of cells containing predominantly or exclusively one enzyme type, either A or B. It was concluded from this that human atherosclerotic plaques are of monoclonal origin. In general, monoclonal areas are considered to be neoplasms. The pathogenesis of fibrous plaques may have three phases. In a "subthreshold neoplastic state" produced by various physical, chemical, or viral noxae, a resting phase lasting many years may exist. The process might be activated as a result of further damage by numerous serum factors, giving rise to cellular proliferation with aggressive growth in the vicinity. In the third phase, complicated lesions could then be built up such as those present in advanced neoplasms. Even if one accepts this monoclonal thesis, the significance of the risk factors and further atherosclerosis-promoting factors demonstrated experimentally is not diminished. Hypercholesterolemia, hyperlipoproteinemias, hypertension, cigarette smoking, diabetes, and hyperuricemia thus have the same importance as in the hitherto leading pathogenetic concept of injury and repair in the presence of polyclonal cells.

Risk Factors and Atherosclerosis

What can the practicing physician and the clinician accept from the presently available hypotheses and results? Especial attention should be paid to the results of epidemiological studies. To epidemiology we owe numerous important insights into the pathogenesis, prevention and therapy of atherosclerosis. However, we should not forget to accord due significance to individual observations. Above all, the results of genetic research should be pointed out here. For the time being, it can be assumed that about 60% of all cases in which atherosclerosis is manifested by clinical symptoms are associated with an accumulation (multiplicity) of risk factors. If we examine patients with atherosclerotic manifestations in youth or middle life, the risk frequency is significantly greater than in oulder subjects. This applies in particular to myocardial infarction, sudden unexpected cardiac death, and cerebral infarction.

The most important results of epidemiological research in this sectors will be familiar to you. The assignment of specific types of hyperlipoproteinemia to vascular lesions will not be repeated. It has been shown that hypercholesterolemia and especially type II hyperlipoproteinemia promote premature atherosclerosis, generate early changes, and considerably in crease the risk of coronary heart disease in particular. Myocardial infarction and sudden unexpected cardiac death are already present in children with homozygotically inherited hypercholesterolemia. The vascular lesions are not restricted to the coronary vessel system, but the life expectancy of those affected is largely determined by the raised coronary risk. The pathologic, anatomical, and clinical data are especially enriched by the results of coronary angiography. There are already numerous groups of patients which have been very well studied and which even make it probable that vascular lesions can be made to regress by various preventive measures of a dietetic or drug nature. Our observations in the postwar series strongly support the relation between hypercholesterolemia or hyperlipoproteinemia type II (but also type III and IV according to Fredrickson et al., 1967) and the development of premature atherosclerosis. The global arteriosclerosis and coronary heart disease morbidity and mortality statistics in the starving nations at war show a distinct decline in deaths due to coronary causes. There are also reports from autopsy studies describing a decline in the severe forms of atherosclerosis. However, since the overall statistical material is still quite fragmentary, special significance is doubtless to be accorded to single observations. In the years 1945–1948, we saw no case of myocardial infarction in the clinics and the Pathologic

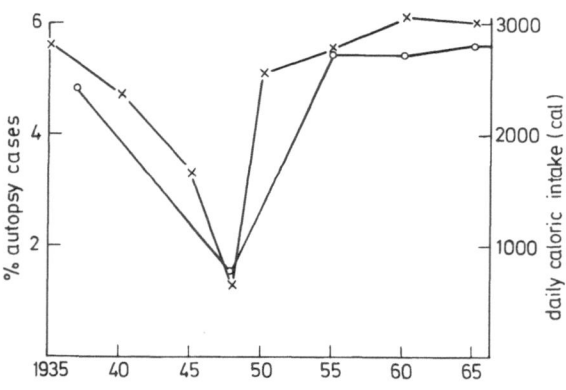

Figure 6. Blood cholesterol (mg%) in normal individuals between 1942 and 1969 (GFR, median of 7 studies) and death from CHD 1932–1972

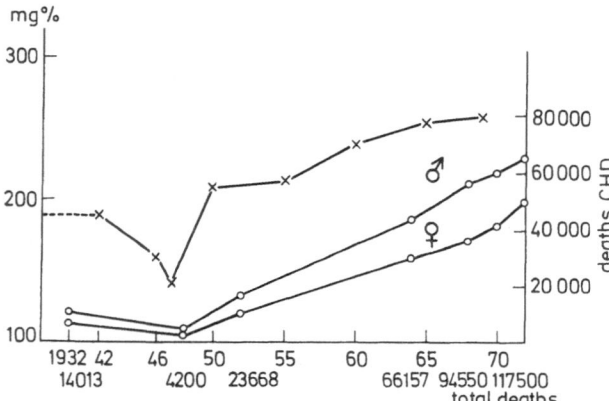

Figure 7. Daily caloric intake and incidence of fatal pulmonary embolism at seven GFR hospitals between 1935 and 1965

Institute of the University of Tübingen, and similar results have also been reported by other University hospitals in this country. Without exception, the nutritional state of the Tübingen population was poor. The average total calorie supply per day was between 600 and 800 kg cal. consisting predominantly of carbohydrates. The daily fat intake was between 10 and 20 g per day and the mean cholesterol values in the serum were about 130 mg%. This is shown in Figure 6.

With normalization of nutrition, there was an increase in weight and a rapid rise of serum cholesterol within a few month. The first cases of coronary deaths were then observed and confirmed by autopsy. Particularly endangered were repatriates who had been prisoners of war and within a few month were again normally fed or overfed. At autopsy, we observed severe forms of fresh atheromatosis with hemorrhages and mural or occlusive coronary thromboses. As documented in Figure 7, the number of thromboembolic events decreased dramatically under the starvation conditions but increased again considerably with normalization of nutrition. Similar observations were also made after the First World War by German, Austrian, and Allied army pathologists. During the first years after nutritional normalization, relatively few atheromatous complications were diagnosed relative to the overall population. However, a steep rise in deaths caused by atherosclerosis (above all, coronary heart diseases followed), especially after 1950. Thereafter, the rate continued to rise up to the year 1976. It is not documented whether the atherosclerotic process itself has been influenced by this in recent decades, but there is no doubt that the atherosclerotic complications increased. Unfortunately, we do not have exact morphologic and clinical data for the years 1936–1945, since the statistics are erroneous.

The most plausible cause to explain this decline in coronary deaths in the post war period is the change in serum cholesterol specified above. Among the first-order risk factors, the smoking habit and the quota of hypertensives have not changed significantly. On the other hand, there was naturally a large reduction in body weight, which roughly paralleled the fall in cholesterol.

We do not have precise data on the behavior of serum uric acid in our group, although there was a general increase in serum uric acid since 1952, and in general, this is doubtlessly reduced under conditions of starvation. In the years 1945–1948, the severe forms of diabetes mellitus, especially acidotic complications, were almost completely absent in our group. They were only seen among the rural population ,which had no nutritional restrictions. Remarkable is the high incidence of ketoacidoses among the diabetics of a cattle-raising area where dairy products constituted the main source of calories. The supply of carbohydrates from other areas agricultural was rendered difficult by the demarcation of certain zones of occupation. The people hence lived, as in comparable animal experiments, on a diet high in fat and cholesterol and poor in carbohydrate.

Other risk factors, such as physical inactivity and the extent of psychic and socioeconomic stress, do not differ in our population in the report years between 1945 and 1952.

If the atherosclerotic complications declined under the conditions of scanty nutrition and greatly increased upon restoration of normal nutrition, this is proof of the pathogenetic significance of the risk factor hypercholesterolemia and also an indication of regressive processes under conditions of undernutrition. There was thus, so to speak, a time lapse in the atherosclerotic process in our population. Furthermore, there is good agreement in time with the animal feeding experiments, especially in primates and minipigs, as well as with animal models of regression.

I believe that the concluding can be drawn from epidemiology and the results just reported that nutrition is an important causal factor in atherosclerosis and its complications and that rational dietetic measures should be recommended for prevention. We thereby follow the experts of the American Medical Association and specialists in Canada, Australia, and the USSR, as well as the Scandinavian countries, who recommend a low-calorie, low-fat diet for prophylaxis of atherosclerosis. Even the Royal College of Physicians has lent its support to these kinds of recommendations. The ideal value for plasma cholesterol probably lies under 200 mg%, though there are evidently regional differences. For example, with comparable cholesterol levels, the infarct risk for Norwegian patients is lower than for American patients. There are doubtless further regional differences. Even if we have no certain data on the course of the atherosclerotic process itself, it is nevertheless justifiable to recommend a prudent diet if there is an increased risk for particular peoples or population groups. There are also well-founded studies on the use of foods rich in polyunsaturated fatty acids and on the atherosclerosis-promoting role of saturated fatty acids.

Cigarette Smoking as a Risk Factor

Cigarette smoking favours the coronary heart diseases and the peripheral aterial occlusive diseases. It has not been proved whether the general vascular process is affected by cigarette smoking. This is connected with the unelucidated mechanism of the action of smoking. Is it due to the carbon monoxide content of inhaled tobacco smoke, the aryl hydrocarbon tar products such as benzpyrene, or to other components? Do the active agents exert their effect via an activation of catecholamines or their metabolism, do they increase platelet adhesiveness or do they alter the coagulation parameters? Do they act on the content of the vessels, on the endothelium, or on the vessel wall itself? It is in any case an established fact that cigarette smoking has an unusually high frequency as a risk factor in juveniles and middle-aged people with coronary infarction. In our group, it is about 90% in men between the 40th and 50th year of life, while in the general population, only 45% of males in their age group were smokers. It is further undisputed that cigarette smokers are also inordinately frequent among women with myocardial infarction, and the increase in heart infarcts in normally menstruating women is primarily attributable to cigarette smoking. The biological protection of normal menstruation is thus broken down by heavy cigarette smoking. It is necessary to study the effect on heart infarct and sudden unexpected cardiac death. Particular attention should be paid to those cases without severe coronary sclerosis and without coronary thrombosis. An action of the components of cigarette smoke on the heart muscle cell itself and on the stimulus conduction

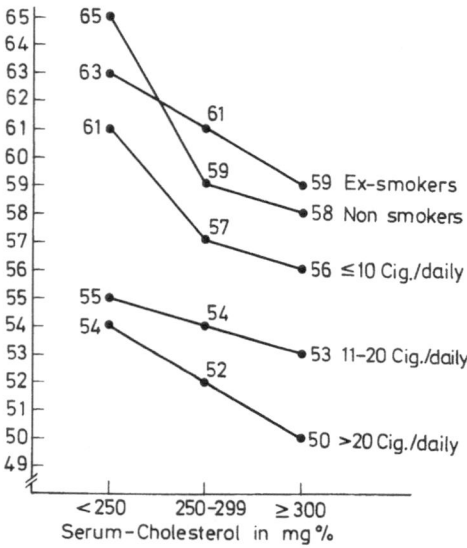

Figure 8. Multicentric myocardial infarction study. Average age, men at first myocardial infarction

system must be thoroughly examined. The epidemiology has pointed out further tasks. It is striking that many peoples and population groups with a very high cigarette consumption exhibit few myocardial infarctions, e. g., countries of the Balkan and Mediterranean regions. It is entirely probable that cigarette smoking effects a risk enhancement in conjunction with other risk factors, e.g., hypercholesterolemia or hyperlipoproteinemia. For example, when Southern Italian and Sicilian workers migrate to the north of the country, there is a steep rise in the cardiac infarct quota even if the same smoking habits are maintained. This may result from a major change in nutrition or from different stress effects. According to our results, cigarette smokers with hypercholesterolemia are in especially great danger of infarction. It can be seen from Figure 8 that the average age of infarct patients with a high cholesterol value and increasing cigarette consumption is advanced by 15 years compared to nonsmokers with low cholesterol. Nonsmokers with a cholesterol value under 250 mg% average 65 years at the onset of the first infarct: men with cholesterol over 300 mg% and smoking more than 20 cigarettes per day have an average age of 50 years (Nüssel and Scola, 1975).

It is evident that preventive measures must be applied here. The possibilities of intervention are unfortunately very limited. We have studied the smoking habits of men after a heart infarct. On the left of Figure 9, you see men with an anamnesis of angina pectoris over many years. In the middle group are men which have only slight prodromal symptoms, and on the right is a group without any prodromal symptoms (Nüssel and Wilcke, 1976). In the angina pectoris group, the quota of smokers is 55%, while in the group without previous complaints, it is 64%. We had thought that few smokers are found among the angina pectoris patients because the ex-smokers are especially numerous here. This was wrong. There are only 26% ex-smokers in the angina pectoris group and 20–23% ex-smokers in the low-complaint and complaint-free groups. The extent of the angina syndrome thus had no effect on the smoking habits.

In Figure 10 you see the smoking behavior after infarction. At the infarct onset, 60% of 1155 patients of all age groups smoked. Three month after infarction, 20% had started smoking again, 1 year after infarct 25%, 2 years after infarct 30%, 3 years after infarct 32% and 4 years

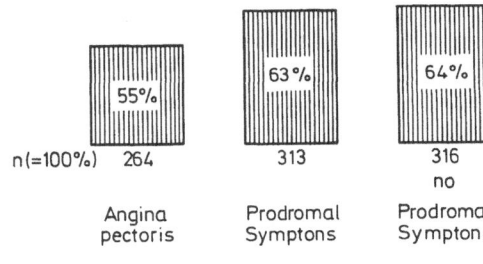

Figure 9. Smoker, men with first myocardial infarction

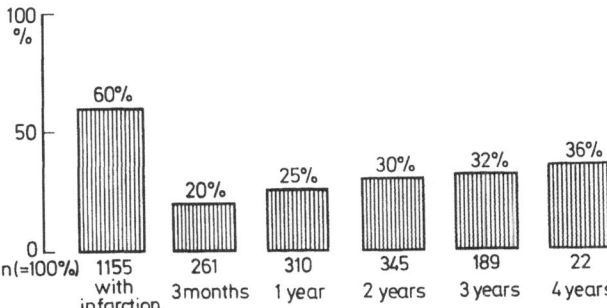

Figure 10. Smoker with/after first myocardial infarction

afterwards 36%. The prodromal symtoms and the angina anamnesis also do not play a role here. In patient who already had angina pectoris before the infarct, 28% of the cases were smoking 2 years after the infarct. Two years later, the figure was 34%. In the group without prior symptoms, there are 28% smokers after 2 years. The finding is remarkable since the angina pectoris group was subjectively and objectively distinctly worse after infarct than the group without prior symptoms, which generally recovered very rapidly after the infarct and remained relatively free of complaints. This supposition that the quota of ex-smokers is especially high in the angina pectoris group is refuted by our findings. It is thus extraordinarily difficult to alter smoking behavior. Appeals to fear, subjective ailments, angina pectoris, or cardiac pains have no effective influence. We are presently engaged in a careful analysis of the psychology of smoker behavior. A further aid could also be the development of a "less harmful" cigarette if people cannot be persuaded, to give up smoking.

Hypertension and Atherosclerosis

Causal relationships have been known for a long time and lead to Virchow's filtration theory of pathogenesis. Individual observations and world-wide statistics leave no doubt as to the existence of these relationships. The hypertensive dies above all from vascular complications. While uremia and massive cerebral hemorrhages are foremost in the most severe forms of hypertension, in the milder forms, kidney failure is declining and the lethal atherosclerotic complications of hypertension are increasing (cerebral infarction with encephalomalacia and cardiac infarction). Patients with values of diastolic blood pressure from 130–150 mm Hg die preferentially of kidney failure. In the category between 110 and 130 mm Hg, cerebral complications are leading causes of death, while it is evidently the mild forms of hypertension which favor genesis of cardiac infraction. Since an antihypertensive therapy which is consistently carried out is able to stop the formation of fibrinoid necroses in the arterioles, and indeed able to bring about regression, a dramatic improvement of the survival chances in the most severe forms of hypertension is thereby attained. Cerebral complications and progressive renal failure are decreasing. More patients thus have the chance of having a heart infarct, as is proved by numerous therapy studies. This is an interesting example of the evaluation of complicated statistical data. If long-term treatment carried out to lower blood pressure improves life expectancy in the most severe forms of hypertension, then heart infarcts in this group do not decrease in number, but increase. This is because massive cerebral hemorrhages and uremia, the formerly predominating causes of death, become more seldom due to the therapy. The patients then survive until the onset of a cardiac infarct or other atherosclerotic complications. Cardiac infarcts are provoked by moderate or mild forms of hypertension. Antihypertensive therapy also improves the survival chances of these cases. Early treatment of mild hypertension is an important preventive measure, especially in men in the fourth and fifth decade of life.

Our hosts have gained fundamental insight into this field, so that the preventive and therapeutic nihilism which is repeatedly expressed today is not justified. It is more difficult to appraise the effect of antihypertensive therapy in angina pectoris. However, remarkable successes have also been achieved here with the introduction of the β-blockers.

The Risk Factor Diabetes Mellitus

Among the second-order risk factors, the atherosclerosis-promoting role of badly regulated diabetes mellitus is epidemiologically ensured. The number of coronary heart conditions as well as peripheral vascular occlusions is higher than in metabolically healthy persons. Cerebral infarcts and strokes are evidently not more frequent in diabetics unless there are further risk factors. The clinician is surprised again and again to discover premature and severe equivalents of atherosclerosis in well-regulated juvenile diabetics. Further studies are unquestionably necessary here to investigate the role of insulin and its concomitant substances, immunologic phenomena, disturbances of permeability or the microcirculation, etc. Just as we came across severe forms of diabetes, acidoses, or coma very rarely in the immediate postwar years, and if at all only in the rural population with normal nutrition, we also did not observe heart infarcts in diabetics in this period. On the other hand, differences in the incidence of stroke were not found. As is well-known, we very often encounter further risk factors such as overweight, hyperlipoproteinemias and hypertension in the diabetic.

Obesity

Even if patients with myocardial infarction are more frequently overweight than underweight, the reasons for this have still not been elucidated. Obesity as a sole risk factor is very rare. According to our results (Nüssel and Buchholz, 1976) in the Eberbach/Wiesloch Study (Fig. 11), risk factors which are dependent on nutrition are rare in subjects with ideal body weight, but already quite frequent in subjects 10–15% above ideal weight. Risk factors are particularly frequent in patients with significant overweight. Overweight does not necessarily entail an increase in blood triglycerides or hypercholesterinemia. Every physician knows of long-lived families with obesity. Such observations even serve as a welcome alibi for epicureans who do not wish to give up the pleasures of the table. The caloric value of alcohol must be mentioned in this connection. In present-day society, there are people who meet 30–40% of their total caloric requirement with alcohol.

Lack of Exercise

The results are also controversial here. The findings of medical epidemiology are highly diverse, and particularly often erroneous and misleading in this area. For example, it is senseless to relate the causes of death of 60-year-old people to their participation in sports at the university. In my keynote address at the Second Conference on Atherosclerosis in Chicago, I gave examples showing that high-performance sportsmen run a particular risk of suffering myocardial infarction and severe premature atherosclerosis after ending their

Prevention-Projekt 1. Invitation			E./W. 1976
MALES 30–59 years	Ideal	Body weight Normal	Over
Blood pressure from 160/95 mm Hg	1%	11%	16%
Cholesterol from 260 mg%	18%	26%	25%
Triglycerides from 200 mg%	5%	11%	23%
Uric acid from 8 mg%	0%	4%	11%
Fasting Blood sugar from 110 mg%	8%	9%	11%

Figure 11

careers if they change their way of life abruptly. I have at my disposal remarkable observations on decathlon competitors, long-distance cyclists, long-distance runners, skiers, and apparatus gymnasts. Even if the epidemiological results are not consonant, I believe that regular physical exercise affords good possibilities for prevention and also for rehabilitation. In my opinion, physical training has an important place in primary and secondary prevention.

Stress as a Possible Risk Factor

This topic is especially problematic since no sure procedure for qualitative or quantitative registration of stress is at present available. All concepts can be found from strict rejection of a risk-enhancing significance to apodictic recognition of stress as the sole or main risk factor. In psychological studies on persons not affected by cardiovascular disease, we found that the attitude of smokers showed less health consciousness than nonsmokers. This was particularly pronounced in patients who smoked up to the time of myocardial infarction. The smoking behavior before and after myocardial infarction just described is in accord with these psychological findings. Certainly, there are already numerous psychological findings which point to suitable ways to change a risky way of life. There is a lack, however, of scientific evidence that there is a causal link between psychological findings and the development of myocardial infarction (Wilcke and Kurz, 1975).

The Risk Factor Hyperuricacidemia and Gout

Gout was formerly a forgotten disease which is again appearing more frequently with increasing prosperity. It evidently intensifies angina pectoris but does not bring about any increase in premature atherosclerosis or coronary heart diseases. Renal complications are not infrequently the sequel of severe vascular changes.

At the present time, epidemiology has yielded fundamental information on the etiology and pathogenesis of atherosclerosis with its complications and forms of clinical development. A certain limit has been reached here and significant insights of a global kind are not to be expected. Of course, detailed studies are still indicated, e.g., of certain risk groups of ethnic, social, or psychological nature. Further results are to be expected form genetic studies and especially research on twins. The time has now come to exploit the significant results of world-wide investigations in prevention and intervention. I consider it extremely dangerous for individual researchers to degenerate into nihilism and negativism. Atherosclerosis and the consequent diseases have today assumed the character of an epidemic which is affecting the life and welfare of all the industrial countries to a highly ominous degree. It is not the conditions of prosperity alone which are increasingly endangering humanity, but the elements of modern life. Nevertheless, we neither wish to abolish prosperity, nor would we be able to. We have a very limited capacity to influence the risks of life in a modern industrial society; as physicians, we are in a most difficult position. However, I believe that medicine in the future must be a science of prevention. This prevention should not be only for the benefit of isolated individuals. Not merely an increase in the average life expectancy should be aimed for, but above all an increment in the years which are worth living. Prevention is consequently not a matter for the geriatrician, but must be instituted as early as possible. Preventive medicine must already be a concern of pediatrics, as has been shown by the results from epidemiology as well as by pathologic anatomy. Our lives course between the milk spots in the infant arteries and the atherosclerotic vascular occlusion or aneurysm. If a man is as old as his arteries, we should attempt to keep our arteries young for as long as possible. J. C. Hufeland described the art of prolonging human life 150 years ago. Today this art is becoming ever more difficult to practice. Rudolf Virchow wrote 100 years ago that epidemics resemble great warning signs in which the true statesman is able to read that the evolution of his nation has been disturbed to a point which even a careless policy is no longer allowed to overlook. This gives a watchword to modern society and the social sciences. It is the same watchword as was spoken by great physicians at the turn of the century. Referring to atherosclerosis, the Tübingen internist Otfried Müller uttered the following prophetic sentences in 1909:

"The first place among the degenerative diseases is held by atherosclerosis, one of the most-feared disorders of our civilized society. Atherosclerosis is responsible for termination of many successful lives by premature death, particularly among the hardest workers, the big businessmen, the civil servants with greatest responsibility, busy physicians and lawyers. There is no doubt that we consume ourselves earlier than our forefathers. There is more competitive struggle, harder work and increased demand by technical progress and there is little we can do about it. We only *seem* to live more comfortably in the age of trains, cars, airplanes, telegraph and telephones but really don't. Peace under arms (sic! — author) may cause more stress for longer periods of time than some of the wars in history. Mankind consumes itself gradually instead of fast destruction. Times are of iron in spite of all humanitarian endeavour. If this trend continues, we must assume a further decrease of the age limit for efficient function. Thus, we have all the reason to create a balance to these factors by prudent habits in our leisure time, to increase recreation and try to keep pace with the fast increase of external culture by the development of an inner culture."

Self-possession instead of excessive diversion, deepening of spiritual values instead of the ever increasing alienation, simplification of the way of life, especially of diet, instead of increasing luxury, restoration of the frequently lost relation to nature and continuous medical supervision are likely to be the most effective weapons in this fight against death.

Wartime and postwar starvation, the conditions of deficient nutrition and undernutrition in the countries of the Third and Fourth World have shown us the path between excess and shortage.

Conclusion

Atherosclerosis is the inevitable fate of all human arteries. For the individual, the crucial point is when it becomes a disease with loss of function. This can be manifested at the vessel wall itself in sclerosis, loss of elasticity, widening or narrowing of the lumen. This has consequences for the organs supplied, especially when there are no collaterals or those present are already damaged. The lethal factors of atherosclerosis include heart infarct, cerebral infarction and hemorrhage, occlusion of the renal arteries, and ruptured aneurysm. These have a predilection for the aged, but are occurring ever earlier and in some cases already appear in childhood or youth. One of the greatest clinical problems is the fact that they cannot be predicted with certainity.

The term atherosclerosis covers very different nosological events. One must be clear about which one is speaking and strictly separate it from pathologic anatomical terms. Angina pectoris, stenocardia, sudden unexpected cardiac death, and stroke are clinical events. They can be (but are not necessarily) caused by coronary occlusion or thrombosis, or by stenosis or occlusion of other arteries.

Our interest should be especially devoted to those clinical cases which have only slight morphologic equivalents. This applies, e.g., to the 10–15% of coronary heart diseases with normal coronary artheriographic findings.
Functional disorders of rheologic nature must be examined carefully.

The risk factors of everyday life have accelerated atherosclerosis in the industrial countries and made it the leading cause of illness and death. This is a challange to the physicians and researchers of the world. Since we must live under the conditions of modern society, it is importang to diminish or eliminate the factors promoting the disease.

The risks of cigarette smoking, acquired hyperlipoproteinemia, obesity, and lack of physical exercise can be manipulated, even if with varying effect. Hypertension, diabetes mellitus, and stress in its various forms can probably also be influenced. Prevention is not a matter of geriatrics but pediatrics. Genetic factors which touch on the defined risk conditions must always be taken into account. The terrible event of the wartime and postwar starvation and the conditions of deficient nutrition and undernutrition in the countries of the Third and Fourth World have shown us the path between excess and shortage.

LIST OF AUTHORS

Ageta, M., see Nanbu, S. *(438)*

Agradi, E., see Sirtori, C. R. *(448)*

Alaupovic, P., Lipoprotein Laboratory, Oklahoma Medical Research Foundation, 825 N. E. 13th Street, Oklahoma City, Oklahoma 73104/USA *(220)*

Albers, J. J. see Chait, A. *(132)*

Arbogast, L. Y., see Rothblat, G. H. *(627)*

Arisue, K., see Fukui, I. *(583)*

Armstrong, M. L., Department of Pathology, College of Medicine, University of Iowa, Iowa City, Iowa 52242/USA *(405)*

Assmann, G., Klinische Chemie, Universität Köln, Joseph-Stelzmann Straße, 5 Köln/GFR *(220, 238)*

Astrup, P., Department of Clinical Chemistry, University of Copenhagen, Rigsholpitalet, Blegdamsvej 9, Copenhagen DK-2100/Denmark *(149, 156)*

Atkinson, D., see Shipley, G. G. *(222)*

Augustyn, J., see Daoud, A. *(642)*

Augustin, J., Klinisches Institut für Herzinfarktforschung, Medizinische Universitätsklinik Heidelberg, Bergheimer Straße 58, 6900 Heidelberg/GFR *(322)*

Avogaro, P., Department of Internal Medicine, Ospidale Regionale Venice, 20100 Venice/Italy *(650, 658)*

Bar-On, H., see Stein, O. *(189)*

Baumgartner, H. R., Department of Experimental Medicine, F. Hoffmann-La Roche & Co., Ltd., Basel 4002/Switzerland *(594, 605)*

Beaumont, J. L., Unite de Recherches sur l'Atherosclerose, Hopital Henri Mondor, 51 Avenue du Tassigny, Creteil 94010/France *(36)*

Beaumont, V., see Beaumont, J. L. *(36)*

Belussi, F., see Avogaro, P. *(658)*

Bengtsson, G., see Olivecrona, T. *(325)*

Berenson, G. S., Department of Medicine, Louisiana State University Medical Center, 1542 Tulane Avenue, New Orleans, Louisiana 70112/USA *(353, 489)*

Bhattacharyya, A. K., Department of Pathology, Louisiana State University Medical Center, 1542 Tulane Avenue, New Orleans, Louisiana 70112/USA *(293)*

Bittolo-Bon, G., see Avogaro, P. *(658)*

Blackwelder, W. C., see Stemmermann, G. N. *(113)*

Blankenhorn, D. H., Department of Medicine, Cardiology Section, University of Southern California, School of Medicine, 2025 Zonal Avenue, Los Angeles, California 90033/USA *(414, 636)*

Blieden, L. C., Tel Aviv University, Sackler School of Medicine, Heart Sheba Medical Center, Tel Hashomer/Israel *(498)*

Bond, M. G., Department of Comparative Medicine, Wake Forest University Bowman Gray, School of Medicine, 300 S. Hawthorne Road, Winston-Salem, North Carolina 27103/USA *(259, 278, 280)*

Borhani, N., see Sodhi, H. S. *(298)*

Bretherton, K. N., see Schwartz, C. J. *(1)*

XL

I

Relation Between Arterial Wall and Risk Factors
for Coronary Heart Disease

Connective Tissue and Immunological Mechanism
on Atherosclerosis

ARTERIAL ENDOTHELIAL PERMEABILITY TO MACROMOLECULES

C.J. Schwartz, R.G. Gerrity, L.J. Lewis, G.M. Chisolm and K.N. Bretherton

Until recent years, arterial endothelium has been considered as little more than a passive barrier to diffusion interposed between the circulating blood and the underlying arterial wall. An ill-defined surface quality described as "nonwettable" has also been attributed to the endothelium to account for its anticoagulant or nonthrombogenic properties. Over the past decade, however, a more precise understanding of the functions of vascular endothelium has emerged. It is now apparent that endothelium exhibits a spectrum of sophisticated functions or properties among which are its more obvious roles in transport and permeability. These are summarized in Table 1. Other properties of potential importance not listed

Table 1. Selected properties or functions of normal vascular endothelium

Property/function	Reference
Regeneration/replication	
In arteries or veins	Poole et al. (1958); Stehbens (1965); Wright (1972); Caplan and Schwartz (1973); Schwartz et al. (1975)
In tissue culture - venous or arterial endothelium	Lewis et al. (1973); Jaffe et al. (1973b); Gimbrone et al. (1974); Booyse et al. (1974); Blose and Chacko (1975); Slater and Sloan (1975)
Contraction/contractile protein	Becker and Murphy (1969); Majno et al. (1969); Joris et al. (1972)
Transport/permeability	Karnovsky (1967); Cotran and Karnovsky (1968); Simionescu et al. (1973, 1975); Schwartz and Benditt (1972); Bell et al. (1974a, 1974b); Majno (1965)
Plasminogen activator/fibrinolysin	Todd (1959); Pugatch et al. (1970)
Tissue thromboplastin	Zeldis et al. (1972); Nemerson et al. (1975)
Factor VIII synthesis	Jaffe et al. (1973a)
Heparin and heparitin sulphate synthesis	Buonassisi and Root (1975)
Platelet inhibitor substance	Saba and Mason (1974)
Collagen/basement membrane synthesis	Howard et al. (1976)
Prostaglandin E, synthesis/release	Gimbrone and Alexander (1975)
Antiotensin conversion	Richardson and Bealnes (1971)
Histamine synthesis	Hollis and Rosen (1972); Markle and Hollis (1975)
Serotonin uptake	Shepro et al. (1975)
Phagocytosis	Welsh et al. (1974)

in Table 1 include the existence and nature of surface receptors to lipoproteins, drugs, and hormones, the presence of endothelial lipoprotein lipase activity, immunologic characteristics, and a possible regulatory control of medial metabolism. Each of these aspects deserves study and clarification. For example, lipoprotein lipase activity on or near the endothelial surface could have important implications not only in the conversion of VLDL to LDL (Fidge and Foxman, 1971), but also in the initial degradation of chylomicrons with resultant small cholesterol-rich remnants (Redgrave, 1970). Such mechanisms, together with the release of potentially membrane-injurious free fatty acids could have relevance to atherogenesis (Zilversmit, 1973). The pharmacologic or physiologic implications of endothelial prostaglandin synthesis (Gimbrone and Alexander, 1975), histamine synthesis (Hollis and Rosen, 1972; Markle and Hollis, 1975), and serotonin transport (Shepro et al., 1975) may be important not only in the maintenance of vascular tone, but also in endothelial transport and platelet endothelial interactions.

Although the various functions or properties of vascular endothelium are of considerable biological interest, this presentation will be focused primarily toward an examination of some aspects of arterial endothelial permeability. Specifically, we shall examine the uptake and transmural gradient distributions of albumin and fibrinogen and the transport of the particulate probe ferritin, as related to endothelial and intimal ultrastructure. In addition, the possible roles of the endothelial glycocalyx will be discussed.

A brief commentary on the background to the subject of endothelial transport and permeability is desirable at this point. Much of the information currently available on vascular endothelial permeability has been obtained from physiologic studies on capillaries, from which the "pore theory" of capillary permeability has evolved (Pappenheimer, 1953; Landis, 1927; Landis and Pappenheimer, 1963). This theory assumes the existence of a two-pore system, one with small pores ($\approx$90 Å diameter) and the other with large pores ($\approx$500 Å diameter). The large pore system has been suggested as the sole passageway for molecules greater than $\approx$90 Å diameter. Morphologically, the "large pore" has long been equated with the plasmalemmal vesicle, mainly on the basis that ferritin (mol wit 500,000, 110 Å diameter), when used as an intravenous particulate tracer, is taken up and transported in capillary endothelium solely by vesicular transport (Hajno, 1965; Bruns and Palade, 1968). More recently, using myoglobin and two heme-peptides of 20 Å and 27 Å diameter, Simionescu et al. (1973, 1975) have demonstrated that these probes cross the endothelium by vesicular transport and have concluded that the vesicle, therefore, is the structural equivalent of both large and small pores, since these molecules are well below the $\approx$90 Å diameter of the physiologists' "small pore".

Karnovsky and colleagues (Karnovsky, 1967, 1970; Cotran and Karnovsky, 1968) on the other hand, using horseradish peroxidase (mol wt 40,000 diameter $\approx$50 Å) as a probe, have concluded that the intercellular junction is the structural equivalent of the small pore, since this probe crosses capillary endothelium primarily via the junctions. Studies in large arteries using horseradish peroxidase (Schwartz and Benditt, 1972; Florey and Sheppard, 1970; Hüttner et al., 1970) have demonstrated that although the junctions are the primary sites of transport, vesicles also contain reaction product. Ferritin enters the endothelium of large arteries solely by vesicular uptake (Hüttner et al., 1970), in keeping with the findings derived from capillaries.

The apparent contradictions between these two mechanisms are not yet resolved, and the extent to which studies on capillary endothelium can be extrapolated to the endothelium of large arteries needs clarification. Capillary endothelium exhibits a high degree of functional morphologic specialization in different organs, as illustrated in Rhodin's (1975) classic work. Similar differences may exist between the endothelium of capillaries and arteries. Alternatively, the differences may reside in the probes themselves, in that horseradish peroxidase may differ from other probes such as myoglobin, ferritin, and the heme-peptides.

In this context, Cotran and Karnovsky (1967) have shown that, at least in the rat, peroxidase releases histamine which could profoundly influence both endothelial structure and transport. Additionally, Stein and Stein (1972) have shown that in the mouse aorta, horseradish peroxidase reaction product appears in both junctions and vesicles following injection of large doses of this probe, but with small doses and short time periods, reaction product is observed primarily in plasmalemmal vesicles. Clearly, the use of horseradish peroxidase as a probe in arterial endothelial permeability studies needs careful reappraisal, and its use should be carefully controlled with respect to time, dosage, and the use of an antihistaminic.

The above-mentioned studies also point out that there are many combinations and permutations of mechanisms theoretically or actually involved in arterial endothelial transport, including vesicular transport and its variations, active or passive diffusion, junctional transport, and combinations of these three. Vesicular transport is a process whereby plasma molecules enter "caveolae intracellulares", or invaginations on the luminal plasma membrane of the endothelial cell. The caveolae bud off into the cytoplasm to form pinocytotic vesicles, ranging in size from 400-1500 Å diameter, which move from the luminal to the abluminal surface of the endothelium. Such movement may be bidirectional, and as has been pointed out, vesicular transport is the major if not exclusive route of ferritin transport in aortic endothelium. From the point of view of molecular size, low-density lipoprotein (≃220 Å diameter) could feasibly move across the normal endothelium in pinocytotic vesicles, a process which would be less likely for the larger VLDL and chylomicrons. A variation on the theme of vesicular transport, recently demonstrated by Simionescu et al. (1975) involves patent transendothelial channels presumably formed by the coalescence of a string of contiguous vesicles. The frequency of such patent channels in the various vascular beds and the magnitude of their contribution to transendothelial transport have yet to be determined.

Diffusion of molecules across the plasmalemmal membrane and through the endothelial cytoplasm may also occur. Such a process could be associated with specific membrane receptor sites and specific enzyme pathways. While the role of diffusion in transendothelial transport has yet to be clarified, if it does occur, it will, in all likelihood be limited to very small molecules such as ions and water.

A controversial route of transport relates to the possible role of intercellular junctions, which under certain circumstances might widen, thus facilitating the passage of macromolecules. This route of transport to a large extent receives its support from earlier peroxidase studies (Karnovsky, 1967, 1970; Cotran and Karnovsky, 1968) and appears to be inextricably confounded with the concept of endothelial contraction. That contraction inducted by vasoactive agents such as 5-hydroxytryptamine, angiotensin II, and the prostaglandins can occur is not in dispute (Majno et al., 1969; Joris et al., 1972). Whether such contractions do result in opening of junctions, however, which then provide functionally patent channels across the endothelium, has not yet been established to our satisfaction. Similarly, the role of junctional complexes, such as tight junctions and gap junctions (Hüttner et al., 1973a, 1973b) in junctional transport is unclear. There is evidence (Reese and Karnovsky, 1967) that tight junctions form a barrier inpenetrable by peroxidase in cerebral vessels that is not found in the aorta (Hüttner et al., 1973b). The possibility exists that at least some junctional complexes are permeable to tracers (Hüttner et al., 1973a), or alternatively, that a combination of vesicular and junctional transport may occur, in which vesicles from either the luminal or junctional surface may discharge their contens into a junctional cleft. In the latter case, this process may serve to by-pass a tight junction.

In the hope of clarifying some of the problems associated with transendothelial transport in large arteries and developing a better understanding of the early biological processes involved in atherogenesis, we have developed and explored the Evans blue model. The protein-binding azo dye Evans blue, after intravenous administration, exhibits a characteristic and consistent focal uptake pattern in vivo in the aortas of the dog, rabbit, and pig (Bell et al., 1974a, 1974b; McGill et al., 1957; Packham et al., 1967). This pattern is dramatically modified by experimental aortic coarctation (Somer et al., 1972), where the extent of blue-ing proximal to the coarctation is enhanced. Moreover, the in vivo patterns can-not be reproduced by in vitro incubations (Bell et al., 1972), suggesting that the in vivo uptake pattern reflects focal differences or disturbances in aortic hemodynamics. It has been shown (Bell et al., 1974a) that the in vivo uptake of ^{131}I-albumin in the aortic arch of the young pig is significantly greater in areas of dye accumulation (blue areas) than in contiguous areas of no dye accumu-lation (white areas). Additionally, uptake in the arch is greater than in either the upper or lower abdominal segments, indicating regional as well as focal dif-ferences in endothelial permeability to albumin. Taking uptake of ^{131}I-albumin in white areas of the aortic arch as 100%, the relative uptakes in areas of dye accumulation in the arch, and in areas of no dye accumulation in the upper and lower abdominal segments are 166.4%, 51% and 55.7%, respectively.

The distribution of radioactivity across the aortic wall in both blue and white areas was found to exhibit a distinct concentration gradient, being greatest in the intima and least in the outer media, suggesting that most albumin has entered the arterial media through the endothelium from the aortic lumen.

Similar focal and regional differences in the uptake and transmural concentration gradients have been observed for ^{131}I-fibrinogen (Bell et al., 1974b), a much larger molecule which because of its configuration probably behaves like a mole-cule of mol wt 1×10^6. Taking the uptake of fibrinogen in areas of no dye accu-mulation in the aortic arch as 100%, the relative uptake was found to be 164.3% for blue areas, and 67.8% and 57.9% for the upper and lower abdominal segments, respectively. It is of interest that the transmural concentration gradient for fibrinogen was found to be steeper than that of albumin, suggesting that the transmural movement of this larger molecule may be subject to greater constraint within the intima and media than the much smaller albumin molecule. It is of in-terest that our preliminary studies show albumin influx into the aortic wall to be significantly enhanced by hypercholesterolemia, a finding consistent with earlier studies by Stefanovich and Gore (1971). The mechanisms responsible for the greater endothelial permeability in hypercholesterolemia are of considerable interest and also of potential significance in atherogenesis. These may relate not only to the induction of endothelial injury (Gerrity, Richardson, and Schwartz, unpublished data), with a concomitant loss of the normal regulatory control of endothelial permeability, but may also reflect changes in the endo-thelial glycocalyx.

Current time-sequence studies at 1, 5, and 15 minutes after injection of intra-venous ferritin, an electron probe with a particle diameter of approximately 110 Å, have shown a significantly greater transendothelial flux of ferritin into the subendothelial space of blue relative to white areas, and moreover, have established that ferritin traverses the endothelium of the pig aorta exclusively via vesicles and vacuoles. An example of ferritin grains traversing the pig aortic endothelium within vesicles is shown in Figure 1, an unstained prepara-tion obtained 5 minutes after the intravenous administration of ferritin. Fer-ritin is present in vesicles within the endothelial cytoplasm, and numerous grains can be seen in the immediately adjacent subendothelial space. No ferritin grains are visible in intercellular junctions. With increasing circulation time (15 min), the amount of ferritin in the subendothelial space increases, the grains become more scattered (Fig. 2) and phagocytosis of ferritin by undiffer-entiated cells in the subendothelial space of blue areas is common (Fig. 2).

Preliminary quantitative studies with ferritin in the Evans blue model, as sum-marized in Table 2, have established that the number of ferritin grains entering the subendothelial space is significantly greater in blue than in white areas at 1, 5 and 15 minutes after the intravenous administration of ferritin. Additional-

4

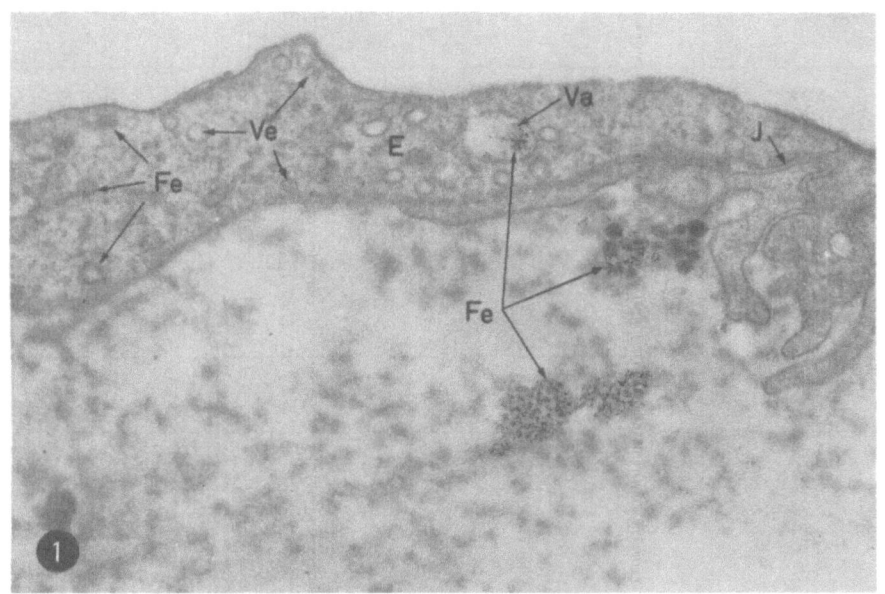

Figure 1. Transmission electron micrograph of an unstained section through the endothelium (E) of a blue area in the pig aorta 5 min after intravenous ferritin injection. Ferritin granules (Fe) are present within vesicles (Ve), vacuoles (Va), and in the subendothelial space (SES) subjacent to the endothelium. Junctions (J) do not contain ferritin. X 51,300

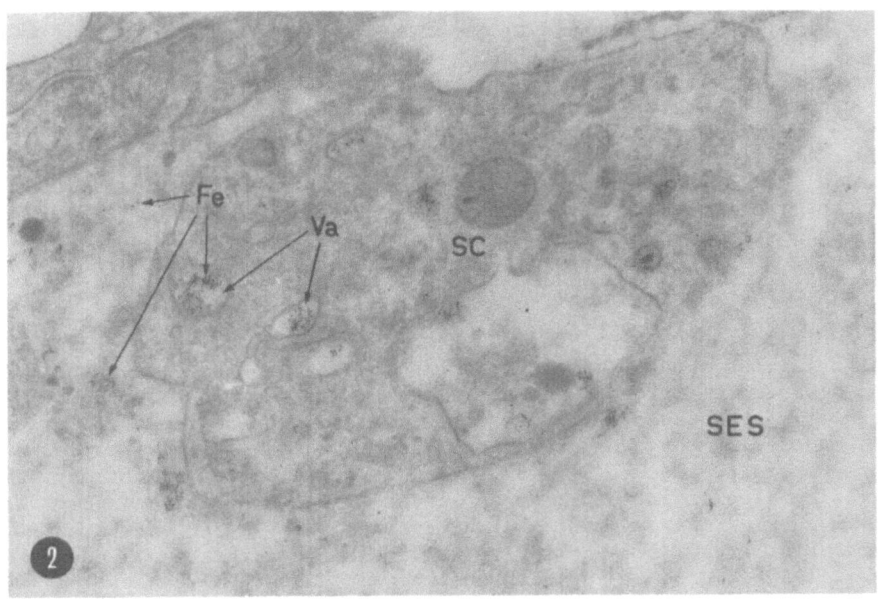

Figure 2. Transmission electron micrograph of an unstained section through the subendothelial space (SES) of pig aortic arch taken 15 min after injection. Numerous ferritin granules (Fe) are visible in the extracellular space and in large vacuoles (Va) in undifferentiated subendothelial cells (SC). X 62,500

Table 2. Uptake of ferritin (Fe) by aortic endothelium in the evans blue model

Time post-injection	Permeability area	Vesicles/μ^2 endothelium[a]	% Vesicles with Fe[b]	Fe grains/ vesicle[a]	Fe grains/ μ^2 SES[b]
1 min	White	39.71	10.26	1.04	0.37
	Blue	25.68	22.10	1.12	7.17
5 min	White	18.73	4.62	2.18	2.44
	Blue	17.91	12.53	2.87	11.75
15 min	White	24.87	12.00	0.87	1.84
	Blue	36.12	21.13	1.26	14.25
Mean	White	27.77	8.96	1.36	1.55
	Blue	26.57	18.59	1.75	11.06

[a]Differences between white and blue areas not significant ($p > 0.05$).
[b]Differences between white and blue areas significant ($p < 0.05$) at each time interval.

ly, at each of the three time periods, the number of ferritin grains per subendo-thelial cell is greater for blue than white areas. These findings confirm the greater endothelial permeability of blue relative to white areas.

Also in Table 2, the areas of spontaneously differing endothelial permeability are compared with respect to the number of vesicles, the percentage of vesicles containing ferritin, and the number of ferritin grains per vesicle. Both the num-bers of vesicles per square micron cross-sectional area of endothelial and the number of ferritin grains per vesicle cross are essentially similar in areas of differ-ing endothelial permeability to proteins, but, as seen in this table, the per-centage of vesicles containing ferritin is significantly greater in blue than in white areas at each of the three time periods studied. This set of observations indicates that in the Evans blue model, the observed permeability differences relate to the number of active vesicles. This concept indicates either that there exists more than one functional type of vesicle, or that the activation of vesicular transport is subject to controlling factors exerted on or by the endo-thelial cells. This concept of active or inactive vesicles as determinants of endothelial transport needs much more development, but at least it will permit us, as a working hypothesis, to ask and explore a series of biologically inter-esting questions relating to the regulation or control of arterial endothelial permeability.

In addition to the preceding observations, areas of greater endothelial perme-ability (blue areas) differ ultrastructurally from contiguous white areas. In the scanning electron microscope, white areas, as shown in Figure 3, exhibit regularly orientated, elongate cells, with a high degree of polarity, whereas the endothelium of blue areas appears more rounded with irregular outlines and less distinctly polar (Fig. 4). Transmission electron microscopy has consistently revealed significant differences in endothelial and intimal morphology (Gerrity et al., 1976) between blue and white areas, only a few of which will be mentioned here. Blue areas, as seen in Figure 5, exhibit a thickened, edematous subendo-thelial space, containing both collagen and elastin elements, and a variable number of undifferentiated cells which have numerous extensions and dense bodies, dispersed in a floccular matrix of low electron density. The endothelial cells of blue areas generally appear cuboid, (Fig. 5) in contrast to those of white areas which are flatter and more elongated, as illustrated in Figure 6, in which edematous thickening of the subendothelial space is absent. The cell present in the subendothelial space in this micrograph contains myofilaments and appears to have the characteristics of a smooth muscle cell.

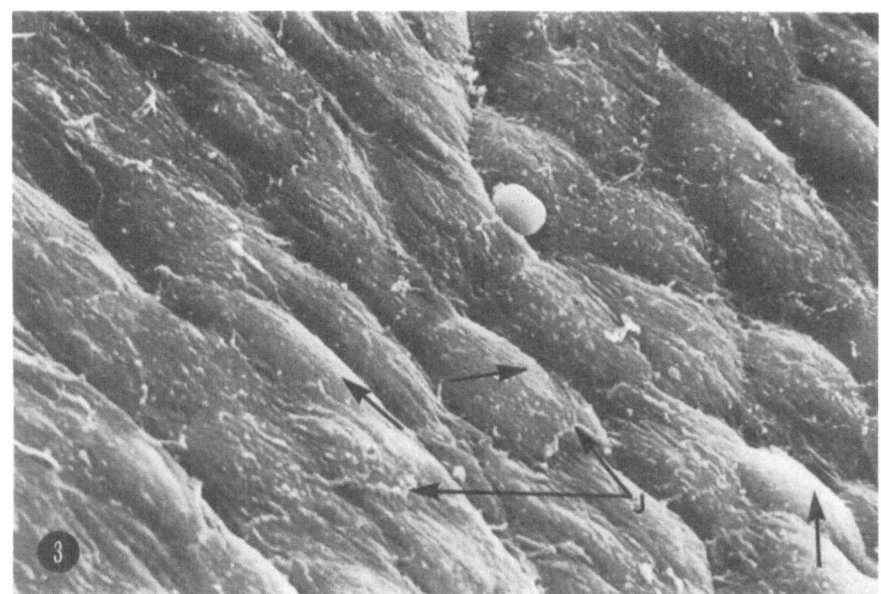

Figure 3. Scanning electron micrograph of endothelial surface from a white area from a perfusion-fixed pig aortic arch. Endothelial cells are elongate with a high degree of polarity, and bulge slightly in the nuclear areas (arrows). Junctions (J) between endothelial cells are visible. X 3100

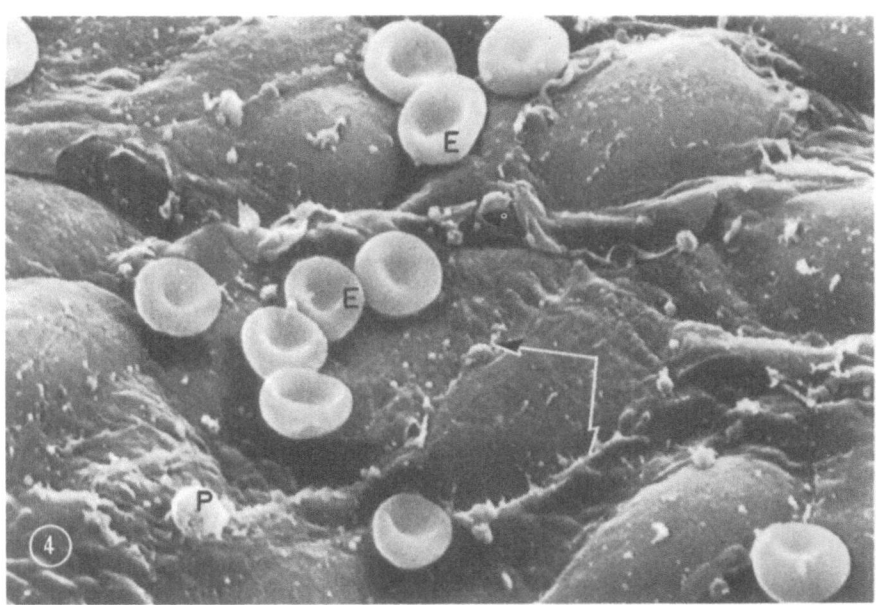

Figure 4. Scanning electron micrograph of endothelial surface from a blue area from a perfusion-fixed pig aortic arch. Endothelial cells are more rounded and irregularly shaped than in white areas, and display less polarity. Erythrocytes (E) and platelet (P) are visible on endothelial surface. Junctions (arrows) between cells are visible. X 7700

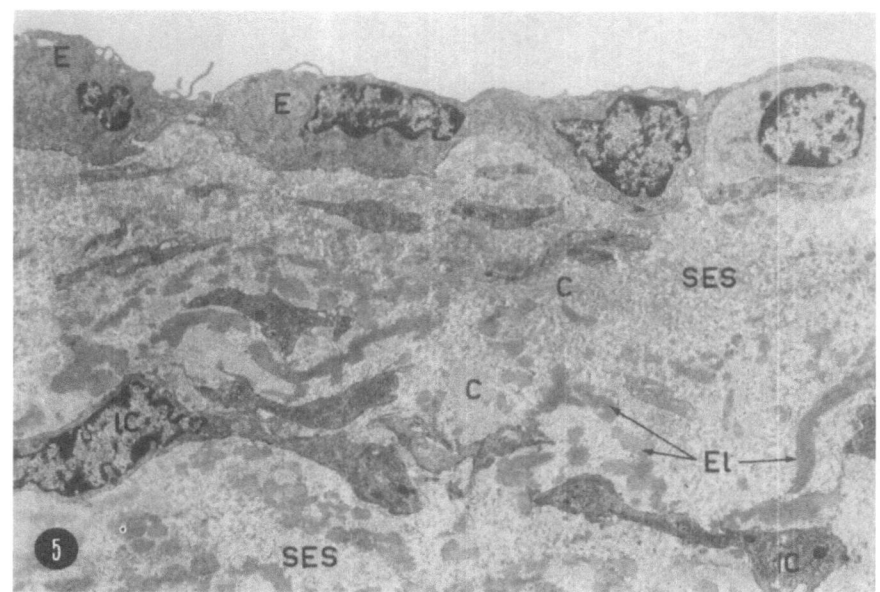

Figure 5. Transmission electron micrograph from a perfusion-fixed pig aorta showing the intima from a blue area. Endothelial cells (E) are cuboid in shape, and adjacent cells meet end to end, with little overlap. The subendothelial space (SES) is thickened and edematous, containing collagen (C) and elastin (El) elements dispersed in a floccular matrix. Undifferentiated intimal cells (IC) have elongate extensions and contain dense lysosomal-like bodies (arrows). X 5700

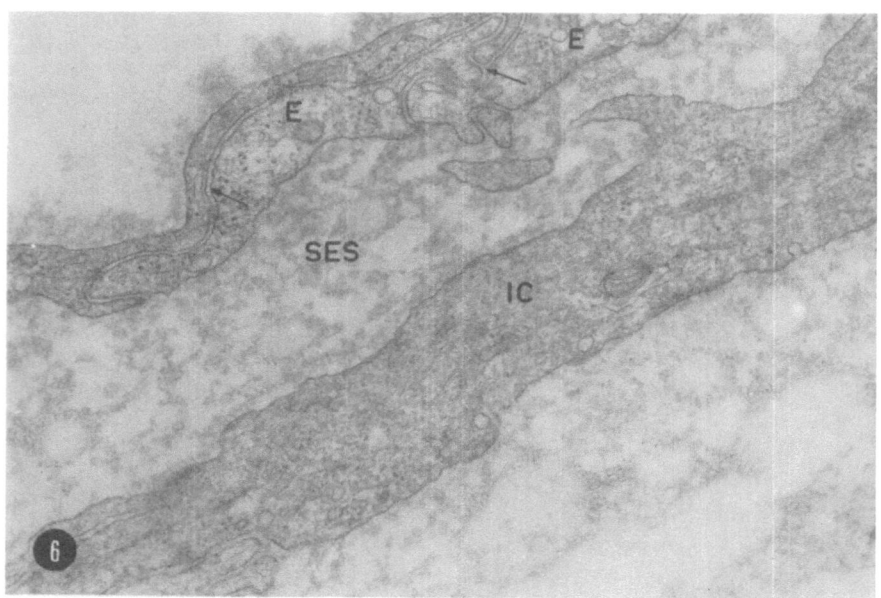

Figure 6. Transmission electron micrograph from a perfusion-fixed pig aorta showing the intima from a white area. Endothelial cells (E) are flat, showing considerable cellular overlap and complex interdigitating junctions (arrows). There is no edema of the subendothelial space (SES), and intimal cells (IC) containing myofilaments are in close proximity to the endothelium. X 45,200

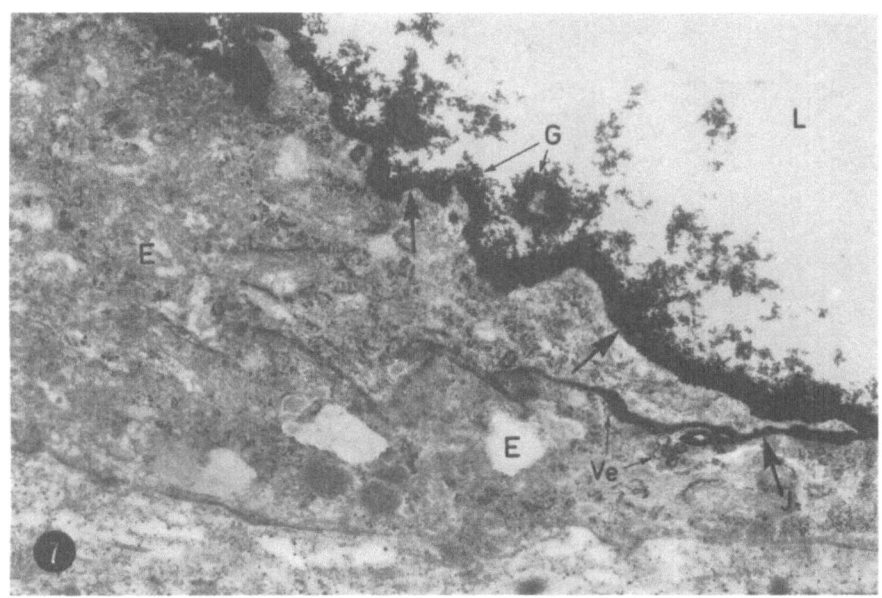

Figure 7. Transmission electron micrograph of endothelium (E) from a white area stained with Ruthenium Red to visualize the glycocalyx (G), which consists of a dense inner lamina (arrows) and a more flocculent, irregular layer extending into the lumen (L). Some vesicles (Ve) also exhibit Ruthenium staining, and intercellular junctions (J) are stained. Compare with Figure 8. X 29,500

The endothelial glycocalyx also differs in blue and white areas. Figure 7, derived from a white area, shows the surface coat or glycocalyx overlying the endothelium. With Ruthenium redstaining, as illustrated in Figure 7, the glycocalyx is more apparent than in preparations not stained with Ruthenium red (Fig. 6). This layer can be seen to consist of a dense lamina closely applied to the plasmalemmal membrane, and superficially, a finely fibrillar mesh of lesser density. Nodular densities, having no discernible periodicity, are also apparent. Note also the presence of Ruthenium staining in some but not all vesicles. Whether the presence or absence of glycocalyx-like, Rutheniumstaining material in pinocytotic vesicles can in any way modulate vesicular transport has yet to be established. By contrast, as illustrated in Figure 8, the glycocalyx layer overlying areas of greater permeability, namely blue areas, is significantly thinner than that observed in white areas (compare with Fig. 7 at identical magnification). This difference has been quantitated using the technique of energy dispersive analysis (Fig. 9), in which the two energy peaks of Ruthenium can be seen. The lower solid computer print-out represents the amount of Ruthenium overlying endothelium from a blue area, and the dotted lines represent the Ruthenium present over the endothelium of a white area, using the same spot size for analysis. With this technique, the endothelial glycocalyx layer has been measured as some two to fivefold thicker over white than contiguous blue areas. While the Ruthenium-staining technique is not chemically specific for acid mucopolysaccarides, as shown by Luft (1971), nevertheless, the amount of Ruthenium present is proportional to the amount of glycocalyx present. The differences observed with this procedure are intriguing, and one might profitably speculate on these findings. It is tempting to suggest that the thicker glycocalyx observed over the endothelium of white areas might partially account for the lesser permeability of these areas, either by limiting access of molecules to surface receptor sites on the plasmalemmal membranes or to plasmalemmal vesicles. It is interesting also to recall that in experimental hypercholsterolemia, a thinning of the endothelial glycocalyx has been described both by Weber et al. (1975) and Balint et al. (1974) and, as mentioned previously, increased permeability to

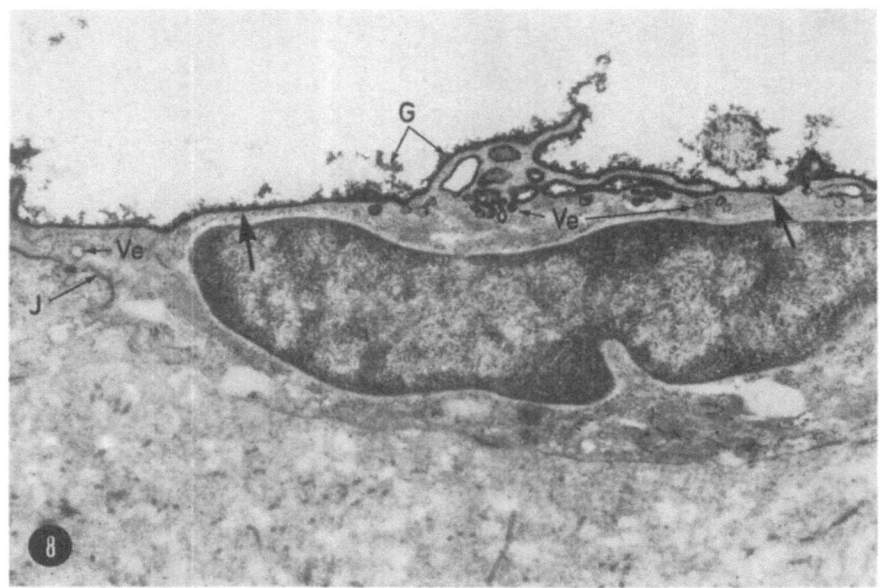

Figure 8. As in Figure 7, but from a blue area. The Ruthenium stained glycocalyx (G) exhibits a dense inner lamina (arrows) and a flocculent layer, but is thinner than that overlying white areas. Some vesicles (Ve) and junctions (J) are also stained. Compare with Figure 7. X 29,500

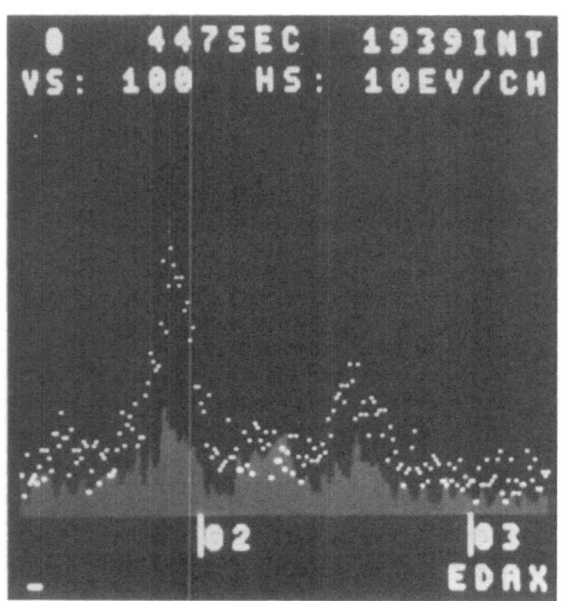

Figure 9. Computer projection of energy dispersive analysis for Ruthenium in the glycocalyx overlying white areas (dotted lines) and blue areas (solid lines) showing the two energy peaks for Ruthenium. Readings from adjacent areas showed a statistically significant two to fivefold greater accumulation of Ruthenium in white as opposed to blue areas

macromolecules also occurs in hypercholesterolemia. The relationship, if any, between these two phenomena requires further explanation.

In summary, we have briefly reviewed some of the background to endothelial permeability and have emphasized the need for caution in extrapolating from capillary to arterial endothelium. Molecules such as albumin and fibrinogen readily cross the arterial endothelium in vivo, and both focal and regional differences in permeability to these macromolecules have been quantitated. Ferritin has also been shown to enter the aortic subendothelial space exclusively by vesicular and vacuolar transport. The concept of active and inactive vesicles, and the regulation of vesicular uptake as possible determinants of endothelial transport has been briefly described. Finally, some features of the endothelial glycocalyx and its possible role in endothelial permeability have been discussed. Apart from the intrinsic biological importance and interest in the factors regulating arterial endothelial permeability, it is probable that this process occupies a key position in the atherogenic sequence.

THE MAINTENANCE OF ENDOTHELIAL INTEGRITY

J.C.F. Poole

It is widely believed among research workers on arterial diseases that breaches in the integrity of arterial endothelium are responsible in part for several aspects of the pathogenesis of atherosclerosis and thrombosis. In the following account, an attempt will be made to distinguish between matters of reasonably well-established fact and matters that are at present conjectural and need further investigation.

The removal of an area of arterial endothelium leads to the adherence of platelets to certain subendothelial structures. Sheppard and French (1971) and Sheppard (1972) studied this phenomenon in some detail in preparations of the lower abdominal aorta of rabbits. The endothelium was removed mechanically or by flushing out with EDTA and selected areas were examined by scanning and transmission electron microscopy. It was found that scattered platelets and occasional leucocytes adhered to the denuded area. The adhesion process seemed to be complete in about 5 minutes and no further changes could be observed at intervals of up to 45 minutes later. An unexpected finding was that platelets did not in general cover the denuded area completely; there were wide spaces between individual platelets and little sign of platelet aggregation. In specimens from which the endothelium had been removed mechanically (but not in those from which it had been removed by EDTA), occasional clumps of platelets were seen with leucocytes adhering to them, i.e. typical early thrombi had formed. Examination of sections through these small thrombi showed that they were always close to regions of obvious gross damage to the underlying internal elastic lamina or smooth muscle or both. It seems, therefore, that removal of endothelium is a necessary but not a sufficient condition for the initiation of thrombosis. It was further demonstrated that endothelial cells apparently had to be destroyed completely before platelet adhesion could occur. Even if only the deep plasma membrane of an endothelial cell remained, platelet adhesion did not occur at that site. Platelets were seen adhering to collagen fibres, microfibrils or endothelial basement membrane. There was no evidence that they could stick to any other structures. While it is conceivable that under certain abnormal conditions platelets can adhere to morphologically intact endothelium, there is at present no clear evidence that this can occur, and existing experimental findings suggest that maintenance of endothelial integrity effectively prevents the initiation of thrombosis.

The technique for removing endothelium mechanically from the distal part of a rabbit's aorta used in the experiments just described had been developed in the course of an earlier study on the regeneration of aortic endothelium (Poole, et al., 1958, 1959). Since the maintenance of endothelial integrity is intimately connected with the capacity of endothelium to regenerate, it will be convenient next to recapitulate briefly the findings of this earlier study. The investigation was undertaken because previous work (reviewed by Altschul, 1954) seemed to suggest that endothelium lining large blood vessels was perennial or very nearly so and not capable of any significant regeneration. This was a most surprising state of affairs if true since there was no dispute about the ability of capillary endothelium to regenerate extensively. Moreover, the question had obvious bearings on many aspects of arterial disease; for example, if Altschul's conclusion had been correct, it would have ruled out any thrombogenic theory of atherosclerosis completely. It seemed therefore necessary to settle the problem clearly one way or the other. Accordingly, endothelium was removed mechanically from the distal 2 cm of rabbit's aortae and the animals were killed at intervals, and the injured parts of the aortae were examined. It was shown that endothelium could indeed regenerate and cover this quite extensive defect in about a year. New endothelial cells were formed by mitosis of surviving endothelial cells near the edge of the denuded area. Since the rate of regeneration was so slow, it was possible to account for earlier negative or equivocal findings on the grounds that previous investigators had not continued their experiments for a sufficient time. The fact that endothelium lining large blood vessels can regenerate and in time cover quite large areas is not now in doubt. Many studies have now been published showing such regeneration in a variety of different vessels in different animal species. For example, Florey et al. (1961, 1962) demonstrated growth of endothelium to line fabric grafts of the aorta in baboons, and Poole et al. (1962) described similar findings in aortic grafts and following endarterectomy in dogs. Though there can be no reasonable doubt that a new endothelial lining can be formed, there has been some controversy about the origin of the newly formed endothelial cells. While the conclusion that they are formed by mitosis of surviving endothelial cells is supported by a considerable body of experimental evidence, there has been some support for the idea that they are formed from precursor cells in the circulating blood. A study by O'Neal et al. (1964) has been widely quoted in support of such an idea but cannot now be regarded as serious evidence, since a later publication from the same laboratory (Ghidoni et al., 1968) effectively retracted the previous claim. The present position seems to be that endothelial regeneration can be accounted for satisfactorily by the observable increased numbers of mitoses to be seen in regenerating endothelium. There is no need to postulate any other mechanism and there is no good evidence that endothelial cells can be derived from blood-borne precursors or from any other type of cell.

The fact that arterial endothelium can regenerate after extensive destruction does not of course provide any information as to whether or not arterial endothelial cells normally divide in the absence of obvious injury. That they do was demonstrated by Poole (1964) in rats injected with ^{3}H-thymidine. Autoradiographs of häutchen preparations were made and numerous labelled nuclei were seen. This finding has been confirmed and extended by later workers and in spite of the formidable technical difficulties of such experiments, increasingly successful quantitative studies are appearing. It is not at present clear if the findings indicate that arterial endothelial cells have a finite life span and are replaced at intervals or that the observed rate of division indicates regeneration following small injuries. These possibilities are not, of course, mutually exclusive.

Gross mechanical injury to endothelium as employed in some of the experiments described above is extremely unlikely to occur in vivo. In recent years, attention has become increasingly centred on experimental treatments that cause minor, diffuse endothelial injury of kinds more likely to correspond to actual in vivo happenings. Constantinides and Robinson (1969a) studied effects of changes in pH, osmolarity and temperature and of anoxia. In another series of experiments (Constantinides and Robinson, 1969b) they studied actions of vasoactive substances, as have Herbertson and Kellaway (1960) and Henniger and Katz (1961). Wright and Giaconcetti (1972) investigated the effects of anaphylactic shock. Gaynor et al. (1968) studied the results of endotoxin treatment. Work along similar lines is at present in progress in a number of centres and promises to yield valuable results.

In considering the maintenance of endothelial integrity, it is important to consider certain properties of newly formed endothelial cells which may be relevant. In the experiments on endothelial regeneration in rabbits' and baboons' aortae described above, numerous polymorphonuclear leucocytes and monocytes were observed in relation to areas of newly formed endothelium, and in a study on the organization of mural thrombi in the rat's aorta (Poole, et al., 1971), leucocytes were actually observed passing through recently regenerated endothelium. Indeed, areas of new endothelial cells have at any rate some properties of inflamed endothelium, and the possibility that permeability may be altered has to be considered and, indeed, is consistent with other evidence, such as that of Caplan and Schwartz (1973).

A further property of newly formed endothelial cells concerns the existence in them of fine filaments resembling those of smooth muscle cells and conceivably having contractile functions. Filaments in endothelial cells have been observed in many electron microscopical studies since the pioneer observations of Palade (1953). The earlier literature was reviewed by French (1966). An important step forward was taken by Phelps and Luft (1969) who studied the endothelium of frog mesenteric arterioles and found that they contained two types of filament (Fl and F2) of about 70 Å and 120 Å diameter, respectively. Both types occurred in parallel bundles. When the vessel contracted Fl filaments remained straight whereas F2 filaments assumed an undulating appearance. This was strong evidence for endothelial contraction in this particular experimental situation. Almost simultaneously, Majno, et al. (1969) produced further electron microscopical evidence for endothelial contraction in a study on histamine-type mediators of the acute inflammatory response; and Becker and Murphy (1969), using immuno-fluorescent techniques, provided evidence for the existence of actomyosin in human endothelial cells. Observations made in the course of the study by Poole et al. (1971) on organizing mural thrombi of the rat's aorta provided the first evidence for the existence in mammalian endothelium of two types of filament similar to those described by Phelps and Luft (1969) in the frog. It was possible to compare the endothelial filaments with those of smooth muscle cells in the organizing thrombus. These also contained two types of filament, corresponding to the "intermediate" and "thin" filaments described by Somlyo and his colleagues (see Somlyo, 1975). In both types of cell, the calibre and spacing of filaments of each kind appeared very similar. Moreover, bundles of the smaller endothelial filaments contained dense bodies closely resembling those seen in smooth muscle cells. In the uninjured rat aorta, most of the endothelial cells did not appear to contain filaments; however, a few isolated cells did, and these may well have been newly formed cells. Although these experiments did not provide any direct evidence that endothelial cells lining the rat aorta are capable of contracting, the possibility deserves serious consideration. If such contraction occurs, it might lead to pulling apart of endothelial cells which could promote passage of materials from the blood into the vessel wall and perhaps initiate thrombosis. Such ideas must at present, however, be regarded as speculative.

Shimamoto and his colleagues in a series of studies (reviewed by Shimamoto, 1974) have examined the filaments of rabbit aortic endothelial cells and have provided evidence that endothelial contraction might be involved in the pathogenosis of the aortic lesions of rabbits fed cholesterol. Endothelial filaments morphologically similar to smooth muscle cell filaments have now been described in a number of different species by various workers and one of the problems that has come to light is that there are substantial species differences. It is therefore necessary to be cautious about drawing general conclusions from observations carried out on animals of any particular species.

Another aspect of arterial endothelial integrity that has interested a number of groups of workers in recent years is its relationship to proliferation of underlying smooth muscle cells. In the course of the experiments by Poole et al. (1958) described above, it was found that removal of endothelium from the rabbit's aorta was followed by extensive intimal thickening. In the longer-term experiments, a layer of smooth muscle cells thicker than the original tunica media was found lying between the newly formed endothelium and the original internal elastic lamina (see Poole, 1975). Other workers have made similar observations in a variety of experimental situations. Björkerud, Bondjers and their co-workers have studied the effects of different types of injury on the rabbit's aorta, using a technique that enabled them to make longitudinal or transverse slits in the tunica intima. Björkerud (1969) found that longitudinal lesions led to intimal thickening which progressed up to about 4 weeks after injury and then regressed. Transverse lesions on the other hand produced intimal thickening that did not regress. Björkerud and Bondjers (1971a) found that the thickened regions following transverse injuries showed increased permeability to various substances. Björkerud and Bondjers (1971b) showed that a deep transverse lesion led to cellular infiltration, calcification and dilatation of the vessel. Using a different technique that produced more extensive destruction of endothelium, Björkerud and Bondjers (1973) found that delayed re-endothelialization was particularly likely to lead to the development of hyperplastic, lipid-containing lesions. The reasons for these interesting variations have yet to be fully worked out. It is to be hoped that further studies along these lines will lead to clarification of the rather confusing information at present available concerning the possibility of regression of arterial intimal thickenings.

It is at present not clear why removal of endothelium causes proliferation of underlying smooth muscle cells. Possibly the presence of endothelium somehow restrains the multiplication of the underlying cells or perhaps into absence exposes these cells to growth-stimulating substances from the blood. But in either case, the importance of endothelium in controlling intimal smooth muscle cell proliferation seems well-established.

ARTERIAL SMOOTH MUSCLE CELLS IN ATHEROGENESIS: BIRTHS, DEATHS AND CLONAL PHENOMENA

W.A. Thomas, J.M. Reiner, R.A. Florentin, K. Janakidevi, and K.J. Lee

It is axiomatic that atherosclerosis is a multifaceted disease. At one extreme, it is a disease of the whole organism in which the victim goes from a state of *ease* to a state of dis-*ease*. At the other extreme, it is a molecular disease and the current star molecules are cholesterol and the lipoproteins. Somewhere in between these extremes it is a cellular disease and the superstar is the arterial smooth muscle cell (SMC).

The arterial SMC presumably starts with the same complement of DNA molecules as all other diploid cells of the whole organism. As in other cells in the process of differentiation, much of the DNA has been "masked" and no longer expresses itself in the metabolic activities of the cell. However, more of the DNA appears to remain unmasked, or is readily demasked, than in most differentiated cells. In addition to its obvious ability to produce functional contractile protein, recent evidence indicates that the cell also produces collagen, elastin, gluco-aminoglycans, and perhaps other elements of the arterial wall (Haust et al., 1960; Jarmolych et al., 1968; Ross, 1971; Wissler et al., 1976). Furthermore, there is evidence indicating that arterial SMC are capable of phagocytizing particulate debris and other undesirable substances that may appear in the arterial wall (Garfield, 1975). All of these "secondary" capabilities appear to be accentuated in the processes of initiation and progression of atherosclerotic lesions.

Thus, the arterial SMC is truly a wonderful cell fully deserving the current attention that it is receiving from workers in the field of atherogenesis. If it is axiomatic that atherosclerosis is a multifaceted disease, it is equally axiomatic that the arterial SMC is a multifaceted cell. In what is to follow, we propose to focus on a few fundamental features of arterial SMC in atherogenesis- births, deaths, and clonal phenomena.

The available information on births, deaths, and clonal phenomena of arterial SMC is sparse. Most is of recent origin and much is derived from studies of experimental animals. Only time can tell whether or not the information obtained from experimental animals is relevant to the human situation. However, at least one important piece of information in regard to one of these phenomena has been obtained recently from studies of human arteries. We shall begin with a brief account of these recent human studies and then shall proceed to summarize a few recent experimental animal studies from our laboratory that we trust will have some relevance for the human condition.

In 1973, the Benditts startled the atherosclerosis research world by reporting some observations from human material that they interpreted as suggesting that each atherosclerotic lesion arose from a single genetically transformed arterial SMC (monoclonal origin) (Benditt and Benditt, 1973). Other atherosclerosis researchers were startled because among the axioms that most had come to accept was that atherosclerosis was an environmental disease in the sense that the environment in the inner wall of arteries was altered in a deleterious fashion by excessive entry of cholesterol and other lipids. In their view, the cellular changes are presumed to be a reaction to the altered cellular environment and multiple cells are involved from the outset.

Of course the monoclonal theory still leaves some room for the environmentalists, as the Benditts were quick to point out. The postulated altered cellular environment in the arterial wall could be such as to favor genetic transformation. Also some factor in the environment could actually cause the alteration in the DNA that is the *sine qua non* of genetic transformation. The Benditts suggested a virus as the possible culprit. Furthermore, whatever the cause of the transformation of the cell, changes in the cellular environment could result in acceleration of the rate of multiplication of the progeny of the transformed cell.

Although the Benditts' theory has the attractiveness of providing a new look at an old problem, many "old-timers" in atherosclerosis research have intuitively shied away from it, even though they may have difficulty at the moment refuting the logic of the Benditts' argument. Perhaps we have seen too many attractive new theories regarding atherosclerosis appear, have their day, and then pass into oblivion. A certain amount of skepticism is healthy in science, and it is in this spirit that the comments to follow are made, not with the intent to denigrate anyone's pet theory. In any event, if the Benditts' theory accomplishes nothing else, it has already stimulated a great deal of interest in the birth and death of arterial SMC; and this is no mean accomplishment.

The observations of the Benditts were made on atherosclerotic lesions from black females who were heterozygous for glucose-6-phosphate dehydrogenase (G-6-PD). The normal arterial and other tissues from these women contain two variants of G-6-PD which can be distinguished by electrophoresis. The two common variants in the USA are referred to as "A" and "B". The gene for G-6-PD is on the X chromosomes; in heterozygotes, the gene for A is on one X and the gene for B is on the other. One or the other X chromosome becomes permanently inactivated early in embryonic life and all subsequent progeny will have either the A or the B type (not both) depending upon which X was inactivated in their ancestor cell. The inactivation is random and the cells of the adult are a mixture of A and B types (mosaicism).

The Benditts observed that the fibrous cap of thick atherosclerotic lesions frequently contained only one of the two G-6-PD variants. Since the normal arterial tissue contained both types, they concluded that the lesions must have arisen from a single type (hence the term monotypism). Since they found both A and B type lesions, they concluded that the observed monotypism in the lesions was not related to "A-ness" or "B-ness". Their explanation then was that each lesion must have arisen from a single cell (hence, they are monoclonal in origin). This quickly led to an analogy with certain neoplasms for which there is truly overwhelming evidence that they arise from a single genetically transformed cell.

The basic observation of the Benditts that the fibrous caps of thick atherosclerotic lesions from black women with G-6-PD mosaicism frequently showed monotypism (only one G-6-PD variant) has been confirmed by Pearson et al. (1975) at Johns Hopkins and by our laboratory at Albany (unpublished observations). The Hopkins group added a new dimension by not only examining thick lesions ("fibrous plaques") but also thin lesions ("fatty streaks"). They found that the latter seldom showed monotypism and the results from our laboratory confirm this. Their interpretation of this difference between fibrous plaques and fatty streaks was that these are different types of lesions and that the former do not arise from the latter. Since we believe on histologic grounds that fatty streaks and fibrous plaques represent successive phases in a continuum, we have offered an alternative explanation. We suggest that the reason that monotypism is seen mainly in thick lesions and seldom in thin ones is because it develops during the progression of the disease and is thus unrelated to origin (i.e., lesions are not monoclonal in origin).

We have thought of two possibilities. Both are based on in vitro studies made by other investigators on cells other than artierial SMC, but we suggest that the conclusions might also apply to arterial SMC.

1. Martin et al. (1974) carried out a series of studies on growth patterns of human diploid fibroblasts. They found by cloning and subcloning that there is marked heterogeneity in cell growth potentials with a continual selection of those cells capable of giving rise to the largest number of progeny. Carried through sufficient generations, this process, if it took place in the atherosclerotic lesion, could in theory result in monoclonal foci which would of course be expected to show monotypism in G-6-PD mosaics.

2. Davidson et al. (1963) cultured fibroblasts from the skin of six (and Gartler and Linder, 1964 from one) black women who were G-6-PD mosaics. After an estimated 15 cell generations, ratios of B:A among multiple clones derived from single cells in Davidson et al. 's study were 8:0, 0:8, 5:0, 8:1, 2:8, 7:7; in Gartler and Linder's study, the B:A ratio was 9:1 as compared to 1:1 from the original biopsy, and eventually the A population disappeared. Gartler and Linder's comment on both sets of data is as follows.

"In the above noted possible discrepancies between the cell culture composition and the parental in vivo tissue makeup, the A:B differences would merely be indicators of selection and not its prime target (i.e., either A or B may predominate in culture). Since, in general, there will be other differences between the two cell types (i.e., between the two X chromosomes) besides the A:B difference, this is not unreasonable."

In the context of the current discussion, we would suggest that the above comment regarding the in vitro situation might also apply to the abnormal environment in the atherosclerotic lesion in vivo.

If our suggestion that G-6-PD monotypism in atherosclerotic lesions of G-6-PD mosaics is a secondary phenomenon arising during development, we would expect that the thicker the lesion, the greater the probability of finding monotypism. To test this hypothesis, we have been taking samples of multiple aortic lesions from G-6-PD mosaics and relating the G-6-PD patterns of these samples to the thickness of the lesions from which they came. Contamination of samples with normal media is checked histologically on all samples used for G-6-PD evaluation and contaminated samples eliminated. The ideal aorta for this purpose is one with multiple discrete lesions of varying degrees of thickness. Only about one-third of black females are mosaic and among these, most have either too many thick lesions (with confluency) or a moderate number of thin lesions. Thus, only an occasional one is suitable for our purpose. We have to date studied only two in depth, and the results are presented in Table 1. It is apparent that in these two aortas presence of G-6-PD monotypism is closely related to the thickness of the lesion. Also, most of the samples showing monotypism from one individual have the A variant of G-6-PD and most from the other individual have B. This is reminiscent of the results obtained by Davidson et al. (1963) and Gartler and Linder (1964) with cultures of human fibroblasts from G-6-PD mosaics carried through 15 or more generation. Since in atherosclerotic lesions in experimental animals we have found SMC going through as many as five generations in 2 months with lesions still as thin as 200 μm, wie would assume that some of the cells in the comparatively very thick human lesions had gone through far more generations than 15.

We do not feel justified in drawing firm conclusions from two human cases. However, if a similar pattern is found in sufficient future cases, it will constitute strong evidence for monotypism appearing during the course of development of atherosclerotic lesions. Further, it will suggest that there is some gene(s) on the X chromosome (other than that for G-6-PD) for which the individual is also heterozygous which provides a selective survival advantage in the abnormal environment of the atherosclerotic lesion for cells with one type X over cells with the other type.

Table 1. Distribution of atherosclerotic lesions in G-6-PD heterozygotes by thickness and frequency among them of one and two G-6-PD variants

Lesion thickness, μ	Black female ≠ 1[a]		Black female ≠ 2[a]	
	1 var.	2 var.	1 var.	2 var.
<200	0	15	1	4
200-299	0	12	0	8
300-399	1	5	3	2
400-499	7	5	3	1
>499	12	2	8	1
Total	20	39	15	16
No. all A	2	-	14	-
No. all B	18	-	1	-

[a] For normal aorta ≠ 1 has 41% A, 59% B; ≠ 2 has 64% A, 36% B.

The remainder of this presentation will deal with studies in experimental animals, particularly swine. One of the most prominent features of early atheroclerosis is excessive focal accumulation of SMC in the arterial intima. This implies either mass migration of SMC from the media or a birthrate of SMC in the intima not counterbalanced by a corresponding death rate or both. We have not devised a satisfactory means for quantifying SMC migration; but we do have quantitative methods for obtaining information on some parameters related to SMC births and deaths. Although births and deaths of arterial SMC are to some extent interlocked, for clarity we shall discuss them separately.

One way to study cell births is to count the number of mitoses that are present. In 1948, McMillan and Duff counted mitoses in rabbit atherosclerosis and found a much higher percentage than in normal media. In 1969 at Albany (Florentin et al., 1969), we broadened the scope of mitotic studies of arteries somewhat by counting mitoses in the aortas of HC diet-fed swine prior to development of overt lesions. We found a significant increase in mitotic activity as compared to controls by 3 days after beginning the HC diet.

A somewhat easier approach to the study of SMC births is to pulse the animal with tritiated thymidine (^{3}HTdR) and to count the number of labeled cells in autoradiographs. All cells in the S (DNA synthesis) phase of the cell cycle will be labeled by the pulse. Since the S period is far longer than the M (mitosis) period, there are more cells to count. We have demonstrated in swine that virtually all cells thus labeled divide within 48 hours or less (Thomas et al., 1971). Using this method, Spraragen et al. (1962) and McMillan and Stary (1968) demonstrated high labeling indices (% of total cells labeled) in rabbit atherosclerotic lesions. Several other laboratories including ours in Albany (Florentin and Nam, 1968; Thomas et al., 1968) have demonstrated similar results for atherosclerotic lesions in several species. In addition, we have demonstrated that, as with mitotic counts, ^{3}HTdR labeling indices rise in the arteries of HC diet-fed swine within a few days after initiating the diet and long before overt lesions appear (Thomas et al., 1971, 1968).

^{3}HTdR labeling studies also can be used to follow cells through several generations. The principle on which the studies are based is that, with each cell division, on the average half the isotope will go with one daughter and half with the other. The halving will continue with each subsequent division. In autoradiographs, the number of grains that one sees in the photographic emulsion is related to the isotopic content. We have devised mathematical means for analyzing grain number counts over nuclei from samples taken at two time points during the course of an experiment (Thomas et al., 1971, 1976). With these mathematical methods, we can determine how many divisions have occurred in the interval by the cells that were observed at the first time point who had surviving progeny at the second time point.

Application of the above approach to an interval starting prior to beginning an HC diet in swine and terminating after either 30 or 60 days on HC diet permitted us to draw conclusions about the SMC involved in the initiation and early development of HC diet-induced atherosclerotic lesions (Thomas et al., 1976). ^{3}HTdR was administered 15 days prior to beginning the HC diet. A baseline group was killed 15 days after injection. The remaining swine were put on an HC diet and killed 30 or 60 days later. Comparisons were made between grain numbers per labeled nucleus found in the pre-HC diet, prelesion period and those found in active atherosclerotic lesions 30 or 60 days later.

In Table 2 are shown the results of our analysis and calculation of the number of divisions made in the lesions over a 60-day period by the cells labeled prior to lesion development. We can draw at least two conclusions. One conclusion is that these HC diet-induced active atherosclerotic lesions in young swine were not monoclonal in origin. Since the results show that many cells labeled before the HC diet had divided multiple times in the lesion, the intimal cellular mass that constitutes the lesion could not consist solely of the progeny of a single cell.

A second conclusion is that there is considerable heterogeneity in the number of divisions made in the development of the lesion by the cells that were involved initially in the process. This heterogeneity is reminiscent of that observed by Martin et al., (1974) in fibroblast cell cultures cited earlier in this report in connection with G-6-PD monotypism. If the heterogeneity observed here were repeated over sufficient generations, one can demonstrate mathematically that regions of monotypism could develop in a G-6-PD mosaic.

Lastly, we shall turn to SMC deaths in atherogenesis. We have devised two approaches for the quantitative study of arterial SMC deaths. The first of these is to count degenerated and dead cells by electron microscopy (Imai et al., 1970, 1976). With this method, we have shown in swine and Rhesus monkeys that even early "proliferative lesions" contain a significant number of dead cells and that the percentage increases as the lesions progress to more advanced stages. Furthermore, we have shown in swine that within 3 days after beginning an HC diet the number of dead cells in normal appearing aortic tissue increases significantly over those found in controls. Thus, SMC births and deaths go hand in hand.

Table 2. Cell births in initiation and early progression of atherosclerotic lesions in HC diet-fed swine. Division pattern of ancestors of atherosclerotic lesion cells expressed as percent of cells labeled at 0 HC diet time that divided 0-5 times in 60 days

Groups	No. of div. 0	1	2	3	4	5	Total 0-5
HC diet only Pearson et al., 1975	28%	10%	41%	12%	9%	0%	100%
HC diet + int. trauma Wissler et al., 1976	8%	27%	7%	26%	24%	8%	100%

Our second approach to the study of SMC deaths is with the use of ^{3}HTdR auto-radiography (Thomas et al., 1976). These studies at the present time are limited to the period at or near the time of mitosis (perimitotic period includes S (DNA synthesis), G_2 (gap between S and mitosis), M (mitosis) and a very small portion of G_1 (period following M and preceding S). The principle underlying the approach is that if cells are labeled prior to mitosis and then allowed to go through mitosis the number of cells with isotope will double if there are no deaths among the labeled cells. The actual number counted will not double because of technical factors, but we can calculate what the observed increase will be with no cell deaths. If there are deaths, the expected increase will be diminisehd accordingly.

We have studied perimitotic SMC deaths in a group of swine with advanced partially necrotic atherosclerotic lesions produced by a combination of balloon intimal trauma and 60 days on an HC diet. The swine were injected with ^{3}HTdR on the 60th HC diet day. We studied the interval starting 2 hours after the pulse (2 hours postinjection of ^{3}HTdR) and continuing until 7 days postpulse which is well after all labeled cells have divided. However, the 7-day period still represented only a relatively small part of the whole cycle as we demonstrated by studying a 30-day post-^{3}HTdR injection group and showing that the arterial SMC in their lesions had not gone through a second division. By analyzing grain number counts and percentage of total cells that were labeled in the group sacrificed 2 hours post-^{3}HTdR compared with the group sacrificed at 7 days, we obtained data on the perimitotic SMC death rate. These data are summarized in Table 3. The calculated expected ^{3}HTdR labeling index (with no deaths) at 7 days for lesions is significantly greater than the actual labeling index that was observed. In contrast, for nonlesion media, calculated and observed values are reasonably close, indicating that the isotope itself did not kill cells. The only plausible explanation for the discrepancy with the lesions is that there were considerable perimitotic SMC deaths. By making the appropriate calculations, we determined that the perimitotic death rate in these labeled cells was approximately 60%. This means that in this particular period in which foci of overt necrosis were beginning to appear, deaths of lesion SMC somewhat exceeded births. In earlier periods of lesion development, the imbalance had to have been in the other direction, or the lesions would otherwise not have attained the large size that was observed. We suspect that during the lifetime of a lesion there are probably many shifts in the direction of imbalance between SMC births and deaths as well as "no-growth" periods when the two are balanced. Further studies at other periods in the "natural history" of lesions produced by various means will be needed before arriving at definitive conclusions on this point.

Table 3. Cell death rates in advanced lesions. Labeling indices observed at 2 h and 7 days compared with labeling indices calculated on 3 bases

	Media		Lesions	
	2 h (n=3)	7 days (n=6)	2 h (n=3)	7 days (n=6)
Observed	0.50%[a]	0.81%	2.05%	1.22%
Predicted				
With zero deaths		0.73%		2.42%
With random deaths		0.73%		2.42%
With 60% perimitotic deaths		0.33%		1.22%

[a]Labeling index.

Summary

The presence of monotypism in thick atherosclerotic lesions of black females
with G-6-PD mosaicism first reported by the Benditts (1973) has been confirmed
in two other laboratories. However, we believe that it is premature to conclude
that the finding of monotypism necessarily indicates monoclonal origin of atherosclerotic lesions. We have suggested two alternative explanations for the observation of monotypism which we believe must be shown to be invalid before accept-
ing monoclonal origin as the only plausible way to account for the observed
G-6-PD monotypism. One of these two alternatives relates to clonal heterogeneity
of cell growth potential, i.e., during the course of progressive growth of a lesion, progeny of one cell may overgrow all others in a portion of the lesion.
The other alternative is that one of the G-6-PD alleles may be linked to genes
that afford a preferential survival characteristic in the abnormal environment
present in atheroscerotic lesions. Thus, cells with one allele may be able to
grow better than cells with the other allele, and this characteristic may be
unrelated to "A-ness" or "B-ness".

We have studied initiation of lesions in HC diet-fed swine and demonstrated that
all active lesions that were studied were of multiple cell origin (not monoclonal). We have studied cell growth patterns in developing atherosclerotic lesions
in HC diet-fed swine and found evidence consistent with clonal heterogeneity in
growth potential of lesion cells. In another swine model in which the HC diet
regimen was combined with balloon intimal trauma to produce advanced thick lesions with foci of necrosis (atheromata), we found a high lesion cell death rate
concentrated near the time of mitosis, i.e., in either S, G_2, M, or early G_1.

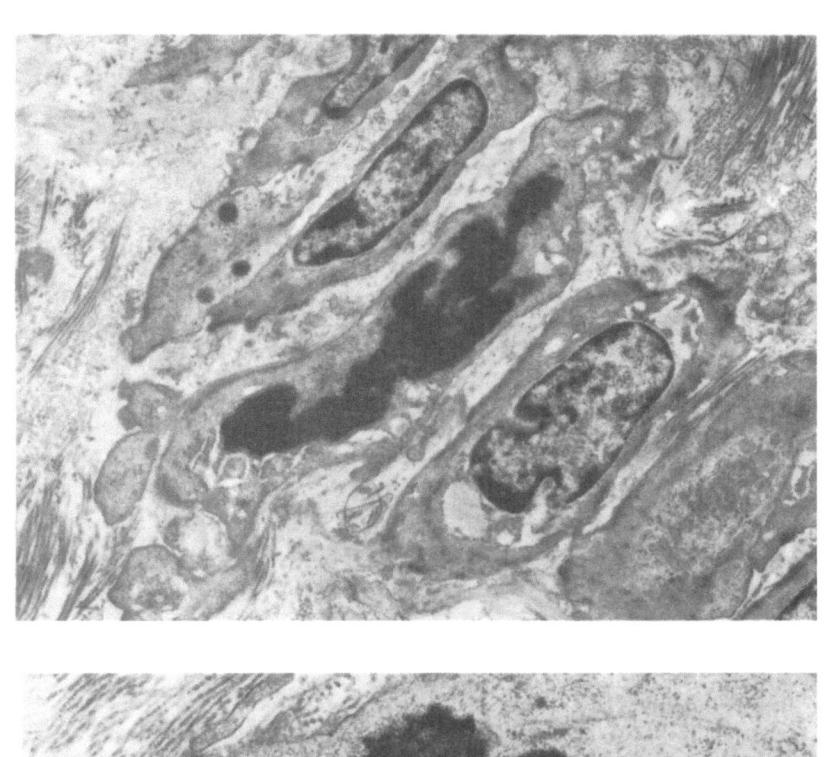

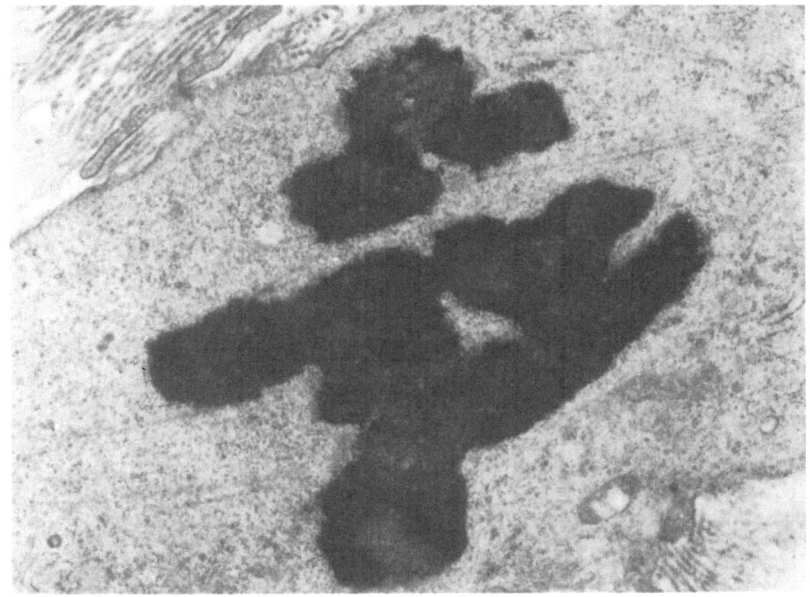

Figures 1 and 2. Electron microscopy views of arterial smooth muscle cells in swine aortas in the mitotic state

LIPOPROTEINS — STEADY STATE ASPECTS*

Elspeth B. Smith

In lesion-free aortic intima from subjects aged 30 years and upwards, the concentration per unit volume of tissue of electrophoretically mobile and immunologically intact low-density lipoprotein (LP) is about the same as the concentration in the patients' plasma, and in gelatinous thickenings, the intimal concentration of LP may be two or three times greater than the plasma concentration. In this talk, I will consider some of the factors that may influence this accumulation, and they are set out schematically in Figure 1. On the left side are factors that are intrinsic to the wall itself — permeability, which has already

Wall factors	'External' factors
	Concentration in plasma
'Permeability'	
'Mobile' LP	Blood pressure
Retention	
'Immobile' LP	
? fibrin	? Plasma fibrinogen
Irreversible destruction	

Figure 1. Some factors influencing the concentration of plasma low density lipoprotein in intima

been discussed by Dr Schwartz, retention within the extracellular matrix, and irreversible destruction of LP either by uptake into the smooth muscle cells or by release of enzymes into the matrix. On the right side are factors that are extrinsic to the wall; two are well-known risk factors, the concentration of LP in plasma and blood pressure level. But blood pressure is not an independent variable because it will interact with the wall to alter permeability, cellularity, and the extracellular matrix. The third, plasma fibrinogen, is not usually regarded as a major risk factor, but it is present in intima in high concentration and appears to be converted to fibrin or some other insoluble derivative of fibrin within the intima (Smith et al., 1976a), and this must again modify the extracellular matrix.

Relation Between Plasma LP, Blood Pressure and Intimal LP

The concentration of LP in intima is very highly correlated with plasma LP levels in normotensive subjects, and is increased significantly in hypertension (Smith and Slater, 1972, 1973). The amount of LP found in normal intima, ex-

*The work reported in this paper was supported by grants from the British Heart Foundation and the Medical Research Council. It was done in collaboration with R.S. Slater, D.C. Crothers, I.B. Massie and K.A. Alexander.

pressed as the volume of the patients' own plasma from which it was derived, was 2303 ± 143 μl/100 mg defatted dry tissue in 11 hypertensive subjects compared with 1193 ± 49 μl in 31 normotensive subjects (p <0.001); serum cholesterol was also higher in the hypertensive group but the difference was not statistically significant — 252 (range 104-426) mg/100 ml in the hypertensive and 212 (range 55-370) in the normotensives.

The effects of blood pressure and serum cholesterol level are additive; Table 1 shows the concentrations of LP in normal intima and the gelatinous thickenings that appear to be the precursors of fibrous plaque (Smith and Slater, 1973) in three patients. LP concentration increased two to threefold in the lesion compared with adjacent normal intima, but combined hypertension and hypercholesterolaemia increased LP concentration in *normal intima* fivefold, so that it was double the level in the *lesion* of the normotensive, normocholesterolaemic patient. This raises the important concept that an increase in the amount of LP in intima (which may result from increased permeability, or increased retention, or both) does not in itself constitute a lesion. The lesion is the response of the intimal cells; from tissue culture experiments, we assume that this response will be influenced by the concentration of plasma constituents (Fisher-Dzoga et al., 1974; Ross, 1975), but no direct correlation has been made in vivo, and it is possible that LP accumulation is secondary, and not an initiating factor.

The relation between intimal LP concentration and age may also be compatible with this idea. From age 30 upwards, the intimal LP concentration is very highly correlated with plasma LP concentration, but in the third decade it is variable, and may be much lower; in the second decade it is about 5% of the expected level, and in the first decade only traces of LP can be detected (Smith and Smith, 1976). By age 25-30 years, normal aortic intima shows well-developed diffuse intimal thickening; in the first decade, the endothelium is separated from the internal elastic lamina by only an occasional smooth muscle cell and a few connective tissue fibrils. Since the endothelium appears to be permeable even in normal young animals (Stein and Stein, 1973; Bell et al., 1974a, 1974b) it seems probable that a sponge layer of subendothelial connective tissue is required for accumulation of LP.

Table 1. Lipoprotein-bound cholesterol in normal intima and early fibrous lesions

Subject sex and age	Serum cholesterol mg/100 ml	Blood pressure	Intimal lipoprotein cholesterol mg/100 mg dry tissue	
			normal	lesion
F.32y	130	$\frac{130}{80}$	1.3	3.2
M.61y	267	$\frac{130}{80}$	3.8	6.2
M.49y	332	$\frac{260}{130} - \frac{220}{120}$	6.4	12.5

Relation Between The Concentration of Electrophoretically Mobile LP and the Concentrations of Other Plasma Proteins

It is probable that all plasma proteins enter the intima and are retained to some extent, and comparison of their concentrations may elucidate some of the factors involved in retention of LP. In normal intima, the concentration of fibrinogen is about half the concentration of LP (Smith et al., 1976a), and in Table 2 it can be seen that LP and fibrinogen change in parallel in lesions, suggesting that their concentrations are influenced by the same factors. The exception is the pool of atheroma lipid under fibrous plaques, where the concentration of fibrinogen becomes greater than the concentration of LP. The significance of this low concentration of mobile LP will be discussed below. If one assumes a precursor-product relationship between LP and the residual cholesterol that is no longer in the form of intact LP, and between fibrinogen and insoluble 'fibrin' (Smith et al., 1976a), the behaviour of the two proteins is again comparable for all samples except the atheroma lipid pool. However, for most of these patients, samples of anticoagulated plasma were not available and the fibrinogen levels were not known, thus the results do not give us precise information on the intimal retention of LP and fibrinogen relative to their concentrations in plasma.

To examine in more detail the retention of LP relative to other proteins, we measured the concentrations in intima of β-LP (mol wt 2×10^6), α_2-macroglobulin (mol wt 820,000), α-lipoprotein (mol wt 200,000) and albumin (mol wt 68,000). Each component was standardized against a sample of the patient's own serum obtained shortly before death (Smith and Crothers, 1975), and the concentration of each antigen calculated as microlitres of the patient's serum per 100 mg dry intima. If all plasma proteins entered the intima and were retained in same proportions, the concentration in terms of $\mu l/100$ mg would be the same for each antigen, but in eight samples of normal intima, the relative concentrations expressed as percentage of the concentration of β-LP were: *albumin*-16.5%; α-*lipoprotein*-18.5%; α_2-*macroglobulin*-45.0%. A plot of relative concentration against molecular weight gave a straight line, and a straight line with a steeper slope was also obtained with five gelatinous lesions in which the mean β-LP concentration was 2.6 times greater than the concentration in normal intima (Smith and Crothers, 1975).

It is unlikely that β-LP with a molecular weight of 2×10^6 crosses the endothelium seven times faster than albumin with a molecular weight of 68,000, and this is not in accord with experimental studies (Stein and Stein, 1973; Bell et al., 1974a, 1974b). If there were specific binding of β-LP, a change in the slope of the line would be expected between α_2-macroglobulin and β-LP, but the relationship remains linear both in normal intima and lesions. This suggests that the steady state concentrations of electrophoretically mobile plasma proteins in

Table 2. The relation between LD-lipoprotein and fibrinogen. Concentration in intima — mg/100 mg dry tissue

	LD-lipoprotein	Residual cholesterol	Soluble fibrinogen	Insoluble 'fibrin'
Normal intima (9)[a]	5.2	3.7	2.2	2.0
Gelatinous thickenings (11)	11.9	3.5	6.5	3.5
Fibrous plaques (9)				
Caps	3.5	11.2	1.5	4.5
Atheroma lipid	3.6	97.8	4.0	10.3

[a]Number of samples.

intima result from non-specific molecular sieving by the extracellular matrix, in which retardation is proportional to molecular weight (Laurent et al., 1963; Iverius, 1973).

The Immobilized LP Fraction

Intimal LP that is electrophoretically and immunologically intact may be able to re-equilibrate with the plasma, but where a large amount of cholesterol is accumulating, it seems probable that lipid is precipitated, either by splitting off the apoprotein or by its irreversible denaturation. The low concentration of LP found in the atheroma lipid fractions of plaques (Table 2) may reflect a rapid rate of destruction rather than decreased ingress or increased egress. While attempting to study this irreversible destruction, we unexpectedly found an 'immobilized' LP fraction. The immobilized LP has been studied by removing and measuring the 'mobile' LP by electrophoresis directly from the intima into an antibody-containing gel, recovering the residual tissue from the agarose plates, incubating it with enzyme solution and measuring, by electrophoresis on fresh immunoassay plates, the amount of LP that has been released.

The concentration of the immobilized LP, and its relation to mobile LP and accumulated residual cholesterol are shown in Table 3. In normal intima, there is only a small amount of immobilized LP, and it is unchanged in fatty streaks and nodules containing numerous fat-filled cells although mobile LP is consistently low in these lesions (Smith and Slater, 1972, 1973). In gelatinous lesions the concentration of immobilized LP doubles although it remains small compared with the mobile LP, but in the amorphous atheroma lipid, it increases ten fold, and its concentration becomes two or three times greater than the concentration of mobile LP. Thus, the total LP concentration in atheroma lipid is as high as in the gelatinous precursor lesions, but most of it is in the immobilized form. For all intimal samples that are free of fat-filled cells, the concentration of immobilized LP is highly correlated with the concentration of the residual cholesterol (not mobile on electrophoresis) that has accumulated in the tissue ($r = 0.702$; $p \ll 0.001$); this suggests that immobilization of the LP may be an intermediate step in the irreversible deposition of extracellular cholesterol in atherosclerotic lesions (Smith et al., 1976b). By contrast, the mobile LP concentration shows a slight negative correlation with residual cholesterol ($r = -0.216$; $p = 0.02$). For all tissue samples, there was no correlation between mobile and immobilized LP concentrations, but in the atheroma lipid fractions, they were highly correlated ($r = 0.745$; $p < 0.001$). Thus, in high-lipid gelatinous plaques, both mobile and immobilized LP concentrations were high, whereas in the atheroma lipid underlying tough, white caps both were low.

The immobilized LP was released most effectively by incubation of the tissue with plasmin (Lysofibrin®, Novo) or a crude collagenase with general protease activity (Sigma Type 1). In Table 4 it can be seen that incubation with pure collagenase released only a third as much LP as incubation with plasmin. Incubation with chondroitinase ABC released only a quarter of the LP released by plasmin, and the difference from incubation with buffer was of borderline significance ($p < 0.02$).

The highest concentrations of immobilized LP were found in samples of amorphous atheroma lipid, and this is the tissue that contains the highest concentration of insoluble fibrin (Smith et al., 1976a). In 24 samples of atheroma lipid, there was a significant correlation between the concentrations of immobilized LP and insoluble fibrin ($r = 0.793$; $p \ll 0.001$). Since plasmin is highly effective in releasing immobilized LP, these observations invite the speculation that LP is immobilized by some form of insoluble fibrin. Fibrin seems to be formed within the intima from plasma fibrinogen that has entered the intima together with LP and other plasma proteins, so this idea has the interesting corollary that there may be a synergism between plasma LP and fibrinogen in the accumulation of lipid in lesions.

Table 3. The concentrations of 'mobile' and 'immobilized' lipoprotein in intima

| Concentration: mg/100 mg dry tissue | Fatty nodule (4)[a] | Adult normal (12) | Gelatinous | | Amorphous lipid (37) |
			Thickening (23)	Edge of plaque (9)	
'Mobile' LP	2.6	4.3	11.0	7.9	3.9
'Immobilized' LP	0.8	0.8	1.6	1.5	8.3
Total	3.4	5.1	12.6	9.4	12.2
Residual cholesterol	33.0	3.2	3.8	5.2	88.1

[a]Number of samples.

Table 4. Comparison of release of lipoprotein by plasmin and other enzymes

	Number of pairs	% of release by plasmin
Saline or buffer	70	17
Chondroitinase ABC	53	27
'Crude' collagenase	17	100
'Pure' collagenase	5	32
Trypsin	4	89

Immobilization of LP Compared With Other Plasma Proteins

The experiments described above do not tell us if LP is immobilized by specific binding or by non-specific trapping in the extracellular matrix. To obtain some information on this, we examined the relative concentrations of LP, α_2-macroglobulin, α_1-antitrypsin and albumin that were present in the fresh tissue (mobile fractions) and that were released from the residual tissue after incubation with plasmin. In order to minimize errors arising from inhomogeneity of the tissue, differences in enzyme effectiveness and errors in dry weight, all samples were run on double antibody plates; the antigens first into an anti-LP gel, and then encountered antiserum specific for one of the other three antigens. Each of the other antigens could then be assessed directly against LP in the same tissue sample. The results obtained from the atheroma lipid centres of six fibro-gelatinous plaques are shown in Table 5. Of the antigens chosen, α_2-macroglobulin and α_1-antitrypsin have about the same concentration in plasma as LP; the former is a large molecule (mol wt 820,000) and the latter a small molecule (mol wt 54,000). Albumin is a small molecule (mol wt 68,000) but its concentration in plasma is 10-20 times greater than the concentration of LP. The amount of LP immobilized is more than 200% of the mobile LP concentration, whereas for the other antigens the immobilized fraction is only 12-20% of the mobile fraction, and there is no difference between the large α_2-macroglobulin and the two low molecular weight proteins. This strongly suggests that LP is immobilized by some form of specific binding, and not by non-specific mechanical trapping in the extracellular matrix.

Table 5. Comparison of the immobilization of different plasma proteins in the amorphous lipid centres of fibro-gelatinous plaques (6 plaque: mean residual cholesterol 83 mg/100 mg dry tissue)

	'Mobile' protein concentration µl patients serum/100 mg	'Immobilized' protein released by plasmin % of mobile protein
L.D.-lipoprotein	815	211
α_2-macroglobulin	540	16
α_1-antitrypsin	126	20
Albumin	160	12

Summary and Conclusions

The steady state concentration of immunologically intact and electrophoretically mobile low-density lipoprotein (LP) in intima is dependent on plasma LP level, blood pressure and intimal morphology. Within the intima, it appears to be enriched relative to other plasma proteins by a process of non-specific molecular sieving. It is not clear if the increased intimal concentrations observed in hypertensive patients result from increased rate of entry due to stretching, increased retention due to changes in intimal structure, or a combination of both these factors.

In tissue samples that have accumulated extracellular atheroma lipid, LP concentration appears to be low. This is because two-thirds of the LP has become 'immobilized', and incubation with proteolytic enzymes is required in order to release it. The concentration of immobilized LP is highly correlated with the accumulation of cholesterol in lesions, suggesting that immobilization may be an intermediate step in the irreversible deposition of cholesterol from LP. Comparison with other plasma proteins suggests that the immobilization represents specific binding of LP rather than non-specific trapping in the extracellular matrix. There is no information on the factors involved in the transfer of LP into the immobilized pool, and the results do not suggest that the two pools are in equilibrium.

Plasmin is highly effective in releasing immobilized LP from intima, and the concentration of immobilized LP is highly correlated with the concentration of insoluble 'fibrin'. This invites the speculation that deposition of fibrin is in some way associated with immobilization of LP. Even if this idea is wrong, the experimental results suggest that increased fibrinolytic activity in plasma and intima might release previously immobilized LP, and thereby reduce the deposition of cholesterol in lesions.

CONNECTIVE TISSUE IN ATHEROSCLEROSIS*

M. Daria Haust**

In introducing the subject of the workshop on "Connective Tissues in Athero-sclerotic Lesions" he chaired in September, 1975, at the International Workshop — Conference on Atherosclerosis at London, Ontario, Canada, Dr. Robert More, paraphrased the importance of connective tissues in atherosclerotic lesions by stating: "No connective tissue, no serious disease." (More, 1976) This remind-er was no doubt necessitated by the circumstance that for several decades the investigators concerned with atherosclerosis were preoccupied with lipids which overshadowed every other aspect of the disease and the underlying lesions. Yet, the connective tissue is the most prominent and clinically important component of the atherosclerotic lesions, particularly those in the medium size arteries, such as the coronary and cerebral vessels; it is this ever-enlarging component of the lesions that is responsible for the encroachment upon the lumen and the ensuing consequences.

Recently, there has been an awakening interest in the connective tissues of atherosclerotic lesions prompted, at least in part, by the sustained fascina-tion with the role of smooth muscle cells in these lesions; that these cells are, indeed, elaborating all connective tissue components in atherosclerotic lesions was suggested first almost 20 years ago (Haust et al., 1957; Haust and More, 1958), and substantiated thereafter by histochemical (Haust et al., 1960) methods, and by electron microscopy (Haust and More, 1963, 1966).

It would be, however, misleading to imply that all the connective tissues of the lesion are produced by the smooth muscle cells (SMC) — a fact often over-looked in the present day era of enthusiasm for these cells. In many lesions that are "progressing" or "growing", mural thrombi contribute to this growth; a portion, or even the bulk of the thrombi may be "converted" to connective tissues by the conventional means of organization. The cell involved in this process is the fibroblast, rather than the SMC. Moreover, the connective tissue elaboration by conventional means takes place in the presence of a vasculariz-ed milieu, since proliferating capillaries are part and parcel of this ortho-dox organization by fibroblasts; the tissue with SMC as the connective tissue (CT) elaborators on the other hand is totally avascular (Haust et al., 1960). The latter difference may be significant.

Notwithstanding the new knowledge acquired with respect to the connective tis-sues in atherosclerotic lesion, many questions remain unanswered. Thus, it is not known, for example, why there is a propensity for CT accumulation in ather-osclerosis; is it because of a stimulus to increased production? If so, what is the stimulus? Until recently it was assumed that hypercholesterolemia per se may represent such a stimulus, but recent experimental evidence does not sup-port this contention in such simplistic terms. Some new data suggest that hy-percholesterolemia may be indirectly involved in stimulating collagen synthe-sis via a hepatic mediator (nonlipid, heat-stable, very small molecular) (Rönne-man et al., 1976). However, in other studies, the collagen level in aortas of

*Supported by grants-in-aid of research T.3-11 from Ontario Heart Foundations, Toronto, Ontario, and MT-1037 from the Medical Research Council of Canada.
**The author wishes to thank Mrs. Mary-Lou Duffy for capable typing of the man-uscript.

rabbits with hypercholesterolemia of 30-, or 60-day duration was not increased (Langner and Modrak, 1976), and in pigeons with experimentally produced hypercholesterolemia there was little increase both in collagen and in proline hydroxylase activity in fatty streaks *or* plaques, whereas collagen was increased in the long-standing spontaneously occurring lesions in these birds (St. Clair et al., 1975). The last quoted studies would indicate that collagen increased by some other means than in direct response to hypercholesterolemia.

It is also not known whether the CT's all increase in the same proportion as they occur in the normal arterial intima (or wall as a whole); are the newly elaborated components in biochemical and structural terms "normal"; are those elaborated by SMC identical to those that are produced in the artery by conventional means (i.e., by thrombus organization in the plaque)?

Recently accelerated work in the field of CT's as these relate to atherosclerosis suggests that answers to many problems may be forthcoming in the foreseeable future.

The purpose of this presentation is to review *briefly* the normal arterial CT components (with special reference to intima), and to summarize the present status of knowledge of each of these components in atherosclerotic arteries. In view of space restrictions, the reader will be referred to other relevant reviews whenever possible.

Defined morphologically, the connective tissue (CT) of the arterial wall consists of:
1. The ground substance
2. The basal laminae
3. The extracellular microfibrils, *not* associated with other CT components
4. Elastic tissue elements (laminae, lamellae, fibers and "units") and
5. Collagen fibrils

In biochemical terms, the intercellular matrix of the arterial wall may be divided into *four* major macromolecular classes:
1. Proteoglycans
2. Structured glycoproteins
3. Elastin and
4. Collagen(s)

The problem of an apparent discrepancy between the two "classifications" has been recently resolved with the identification of four (molecular) classes of collagen (Miller and Matukas, 1974), and the recognition that the structured glycoproteins (Robert and Dische, 1963) are largely the biochemical equivalent of the microfibrils (Haust, 1965); the latter are present in a "free" form in the intercellular space and constitute one of the two components of the elastic tissue (Haust et al., 1965), the other being elastin (Robert et al., 1971; Franzblau and Lent, 1968).

The following presentation will be based on the morphologically defined CT, and whenever necessary, cross reference will be made to the biochemically defined components.

1. The Ground Substance

The concept of an extracellular matrix embedded in which were all formed connective tissue elements originated on the basis of morphologic appearance of a gel-like substance; it not only "harbored", but also was considered to be involved in the formation of the above CT elements. Whereas this concept did change fundamentally, the major organic components of the ground substance, i.e., the acid mucopolysaccharides (AMPS) (= glycosaminoglycans) that confer upon it its properties, still are believed to be of considerable importance in the formation, maintenance and function of the formed CT components (Haust, 1973)

In view of the above, it is perhaps understandable (but not correct) that only the status of the glycosaminoglycans rather than the ground substance as a whole is being considered in discussions. The glycosaminoglycans (this terminology is used interchangeably with: AMPS) are present as protein complexes in the arterial tissue (with the possible exception of the hyaluronic acid) and as such are referred to as proteoglycans (PG). In the accounts to follow these substances will be representing the ground substance of the morphologists.

In the *normal arteries* all three sulphated chondroitins, heparan sulphate and hyaluronic acid are found in man and most of the animals examined. Recently, the presence of heparin in the adventitia (Murata et al., 1975), and a "new" PG molecule consisting of both dermatan sulphate and the chondroitin 4/6-sulphate were reported (Eisenstein and Kuettner, 1976). Apparently, there is a considerable variation in the content and ratios of the various AMPS not only from species to species, but also at a different level of a given artery (Engel, 1971), from intima to adventitia (Murata et al., 1975) and even from season to season (Helin and Lorenzen, 1976).

The glycosaminoglycans are believed, among others, to have an affinity for lipids (Bihari-Varga and Vegh, 1967), and an anticoagulant property (Murata et al., 1975), and to restrict the passage of substances from the blood through the endothelium (Klynstra, 1974). It was reported recently (Eisenstein and Kuettner, 1976) that the PG's are not entirely structureless but rather structured in orders of molecular complexes. As such, they are believed to be associated with collagen, plasma membrane of the SMC, interfibrillar stroma and the surface of elastic fibers in young animals. The "new" PG molecule has reportedly antithrombotic properties and is capable of inhibiting endothelial growth (Eisenstein and Kuettner, 1976).

Much work has been carried out on the role of glycosaminoglycans *in atherosclerosis*, and the reader is referred to a review article for details (Berenson et al., 1971). The affinity for lipids is reported to be consistently increased. Some work indicates that the specific enzymes for the biosynthesis of AMPS in the liver decrease and the levels of enzymes of degradation increase in both the liver and aorta (Vijayakumar and Katup, 1975), implying an overall decreased synthesis and an increased degradation; the problem does not appear to be that simple, however, as is illustrated by the results of other recent studies from the same laboratories. These imply that there are increases in some and decreases in other AMPS, and that these also vary considerably with the stage of the disease (Vijayakumar et al., 1975).

Further work is required for the assessment of the role of AMPS of the artery in atherosclerosis.

2. The Basal Laminae

Until a few years ago the basal lamina (BL) in the arterial wall would not have been included in the discussion on CT. It was documented, however, that the BL consists largely of a special, type IV collagen (Miller and Matukas, 1974). As the width of the BL exceeds in light microscopic PAS preparations that observed by the electron microscope (EM), it is reasonable to assume that in addition to the specific collagen, some (poly)-saccharidic substances are also contained within the BL.

In *normal arteries* wall both the basal (nonluminal) portion of the endothelial cells and the entire SMC's are surrounded by the BL. At times, several SMC's are enclosed within a common BL (Haust and More, 1963, 1966). In suitably prepared specimens, an electron dense, finely fibrillar, inner, and an electron-lucent, ill-defined outer layer may be distinguished.

The intimal BL of both cell types often is associated with the de novo formation of elastic tissue units, particularly with their microfibrillar component (Haust, 1965; Haust et al., 1965).

Very little is known about the BL in *atherosclerotic* arteries. It was observed that in several forms of the lesions there is a considerable proliferation and thickening of the BL, particularly that of SMC's (Haust, M.D., unpublished observations). To the best of the author's knowledge, no data relevant to the possible alterations in chemical composition are available in the literature.

3. Microfibrils (MF)

These represent the smallest structured (or formed) CT elements. It was established in the early part of the last decade that they are consistent components of the extracellular space, both free and associated with the elastic tissue (Haust, 1965; Haust et al., 1965).

The ultrastructural appearance and dimensions of the MF in *normal arteries* may vary from one preparation to another, and the diameter has been reported from approximately 20 Å to 140 Å. In some preparations, the fibrils appear to have a helical configuration. It has been proposed on morphologic grounds that the MF are a common structural component of collagen and elastic tissue (Haust, 1965), but this has not been confirmed to date.

It was possible to isolate MF and analyze their composition. They contain a characteristic protein moiety and are regarded as the so-called structural glycoproteins (SGP) (27). They have the new effect of a negative charge.

In *atherosclerosis* arteries there is quite a striking proliferation of MF in some lesions, particularly in the white fibrous plaques (Haust and More, 1966). There is reportedly an increase of the salt-soluble, stroma-bound SGP (= microfibrils) in the lesion-free parts of the human aorta (Ouzilou et al., 1973), and an increase in atherosclerotic plaques; the ratio of the SGP-MF to elastin is increased (Robert and Robert, 1976). It is of interest that the SGP have been reported to be "immunogenic" and promote sclerosis.

The MF are believed to provide pathways for calcium salt deposition in CT, and there is morphologic evidence to support that contention (Haust and Geer, 1970). Whether this applies also to the mode of calcification in atherosclerotic arteries, has not been explored.

It is not known whether the structure and chemical composition of the MF is altered in lesions.

4. Elastic Tissue

In *normal arteries* the smallest morphologically defined element of elastic tissue, i.e., the "unit" is composed of a central homogeneous core of electron lucent or moderately dense substance surrounded by regularly spaced microfibrils. Fusion of these units gives rise to larger elastic tissue elements (Haust et al., 1965). In developing tissues, and in young animals and man, the microfibrillar component in these larger elements is still prominent, but with advancing age it is not easily discernible.

It is believed at present that the MF, in analogy to those occurring free in the intercellular space, are the equivalent of the negatively charged structured glycoproteins upon which the second component of the elastic tissue visible as the core, aggregates by coulombic forces. This component is the still soluble precursor, tropoelastin, that upon cross-linking catalysed by the specific enzyme lysine oxidase, becomes the insoluble polymer elastin. The elastin has a characteristic protein different in composition from that of MF, and is positively charged. It is rich in the amino acids desmosine, isodesmosine and lysinonorleucine (Kramsch et al., 1974), i.e., amino acids involved in the cross-linking.

Recently, Franzblau and his colleagues obtained a soluble elastin species with high molecular weight of 130-140,000 daltons (Foster et al., 1976). The above large molecular weight substance was readily degraded to several other species including that of 72,000 daltons tropoelastin in the presence of specific proteases. The investigators proposed, therefore, in analogy to the collagenesis, that a soluble precursor of elastin, the proelastin with molecular weight of 130-140,000 daltons is secreted into the extracellular space. Upon the action of specific proteases (in analogy to procollagen peptidase) some segments of the molecule are removed yielding (?several species of?) the soluble tropoelastin. In the presence of specific enzymes, cross-linking of the tropoelastin molecules results in the formation of the insoluble elastin (Mecham et al, 1976).

The half-life of normal mature elastin is believed to approximate the life span of the animal (Slack, 1954). The elastin is a protein-lipid complex with approximately 2% lipids and 98% protein. There is recent evidence (Jordan et al., 1974) that naturally occurring hydrophobic ligands, such as free fatty acids and bile salts, bind to elastin in vitro yielding it approximately five times more susceptible to elastolysis by elastase; the linoleic acid seems to be the most effective fatty acid.

In *atherosclerotic* there are considerable changes in the elastin. There are no data available regarding the turnover rate of elastin in atherosclerosis. In vivo synthesis is increased as indicated by an increased uptake of intravenously injected radioactive lysine into the lysine and desmosine residues. An increased content of free fatty acids in elastin of lesions increases further with advanced atherosclerosis (Kramsch and Franzblau, 1976), and this may play a role in increased degradation.

The most striking changes in elastin of atherosclerotic aortae consist of an increased amount of polar amino acids (aspartic acid, theonine, serine, glutamic acid, lysine, histidine, and arginine), decrease in cross-linking amino acids (desmosine, isodesmosine and lysinonorleucine), and an increase in the lipid content from 2% to as high as 37%; the latter varies with species. Much of the lipid is cholesterol ester (Kramsch et al., 1974). It is believed that the increase in the polar amino acids is the prerequisite for the increased lipid binding. The mechanism of that binding appears to be a transfer largely of cholesterol ester of LDL and VLDL from either serum or artery itself to the altered elastin (Kramsch and Franzblau, 1976). It is still debatable what might be the cause of the altered content in amino acids of the elastic tissue, and whether, indeed, the effect is of extraneous rather than structural (i.e., internal) nature. It has been considered that firm binding of elastin with microfibrillar substance, AMPS, collagen, or even the enzymes elastase or lysyl oxidase may be responsible for the change. Of interest is the observation that at a certain stage the cultured arterial SMC synthesize an alkali-insoluble elastin rich in polar amino acids (Kramsch and Franzblau, 1976). Polar amino acids were also increased in purified elastin derived from calcified plaques (Keeley and Partridge, 1974).

The fatty acids of the elastin-bound lipid change their pattern with increasing severity of atherosclerotic lesions and even in the lesion-free wall; thus, the proportion of the long chain (C >18) fatty acids increases and "odd" chains with known toxicity appear (Robert and Robert, 1976).

As mentioned above, the ratio of the SGP-MF to elastin in diseased atherosclerotic arteries.

5. Collagen Fibrils

Collagen in its conventional, 640 Å banded, fibril form is ubiquitous in the
normal artery; it may be scattered at random or arranged in discrete bundles.
It is often associated with the elastic tissue components and the BL.

Collagen is secreted in its soluble precursor, the parent form procollagen;
this is a triple-coiled substance, the coils consisting of specific α-chains.
There are five different genetically determined α-chains that in various (known)
combinations give rise to four different types of collagen (type I – IV) (Miller and Matukas, 1974). In the artery there are two types: type I collagen (usually known to be associated with fibroblasts) amounts to 30% and type III (also
present in uterine tissues) amounts to 70% (McCullagh and Balian, 1975).

When the procollagen molecules reach the extracellular space, the terminal
(noncoiled) parts are removed by the action of a specific enzyme procollagen
peptidase with the resultant soluble tropocollagen. Oxidation of lysyl and hy-
droxylysyl residues results in the formation of insoluble (fibril) collagen
units which upon cross-linking yield the insoluble 640 Å collagen fibril (Miller and Matukas, 1974; Grant and Prockop, 1972).

The collagen of the normal artery does not have antigenic properties, its affinity to lipids is moderate (Nikkari and Heikkinen, 1968), and turnover rate slow
(Kramsch and Franzblau, 1976); it accounts for approximately 5% of all (arterial) protein synthesis, the rate of which for collagen is approximately 97 ng/g/
4h (McCullagh and Ehrhart, 1974).

In *atherosclerotic* arteries the synthesis of collagen increased to that of 14%
of all proteins. The rate of synthesis increased approximately to 476 ng/g/4h
in moderate lesions, and 1954 ng/g/4h in severe plaques. The turnover rate was
accelerated in lesions and there was an increase in insoluble collagen in the
plaques. The affinity to lipids also increased considerably; the 8%-10% cholesterol was bound to insoluble collagen in the plaques (McCullagh and Ehrhart,
1974). Also remarkable was the reversal in the proportion of the two different
types of collagen: 65% of type I and 35% of type III collagen was found in the
plaques (McCullagh and Balian, 1975). The collagen exhibited antigenic properties and a small amount of collagen-bound IgG appeared to be synthesized locally (Hollander et al., 1974). There was also evidence that 16% of AMPS of the
plaques were firmly bound to the insoluble collagen.

It is significant that collagen content was increased overall in naturally
occurring atherosclerotic lesions of pigeons, whereas no such change could be
observed in the birds on hypercholesterolemic diets (St. Clair et al, 1975).

There is little doubt that much work on connective tissues in atherosclerosis
is under way in numerous laboratories, and that new information may be expected
to be forthcoming continously.

IMMUNOLOGIC MECHANISM OF ATHEROSCLEROSIS*

J. L. Beaumont and V. Beaumont

At the Third International Symposium on Atherosclerosis held in Berlin in 1973, it was possible to collect enough facts to support the hypothesis that immunologic factors could be atherogenic (Beaumont and Beaumont, 1974a).

Since then the knowledge of these factors increased and additional data were acquired. However, in 1976 it remains premature to attempt a description of what would be an "immunologic mechanism" of atherosclerosis.

In this report we will try to give an overview of: (1) the complexity of the natural history of atherosclerosis and its complications with which immune factors may interfere, (2) the facts on which the hypothesis of an immunologic mechanism is based, (3) the molecular interactions by which immune reactions may be harmful for the arterial wall.

The Mechanism of Atherosclerosis

1. The Complexity of Factors Involved in Atherogenesis and Ischemic Diseases

The exact mechanism of atherosclerosis is still largely unknown since the atherosclerotic lesion remains silent for years, before it is revealed by its ischemic consequences (Strong et al., 1972). At that time, which is known as the clinical period of the disease, atherosclerosis is often complicated by thrombosis, and other ischemic factors may be involved (Fig. 1). According to this natural history, the factors of atherosclerosis cannot without caution be equated with the factors of ischemic diseases (the so-called "risk factors"): (a) In the course of the long period of clinical latency, the factors of the original lesion may have disappeared or have become blended with others which may mask them. (b) The thromboses which may inaugurate the clinical period, although they initiate at the site of endothelial lesions on atherosclerotic plaques, may have factors of their own. (c) The ischemia itself may be induced or enhanced by factors associated with the atherosclerotic stenosis and with their thrombotic complications. (d) Lastly, death in ischemic disease is sometimes ascribable to factors of its own, superadded to the ischemic factors, for instance dysrhythmias in ischemic heart disease.

Among the risk factors which prospective studies have shown to be associated with ischemic diseases are thus found simultaneously: atherogenic factors, thrombogenic factors, factors of ischemia distinct of these, and factors of death, where death was included as a criterion of the study (Gordon and Kannel, 1972; Haust and Moore, 1972; Kannel et al., 1971; Stamler et al., 1972). Knowledge and analysis of this complex of factors is necessary if an eventual immunologic mechanism is to be found. This research will have to deal with a set of already known factors which are listed in Figure 1 and keep place for unknown factors. Of course, part of this complexity may be solved by experimentation in animals, but extrapolation of their results to man remains hazardous.

---

*Université de Recherches sur l'Athérosclerose de l'Institut National de la Santé et de la Recherche Médicale (INSERM U 32), Hôpital Henri-Mondor, F-94010 CRETEIL (France).

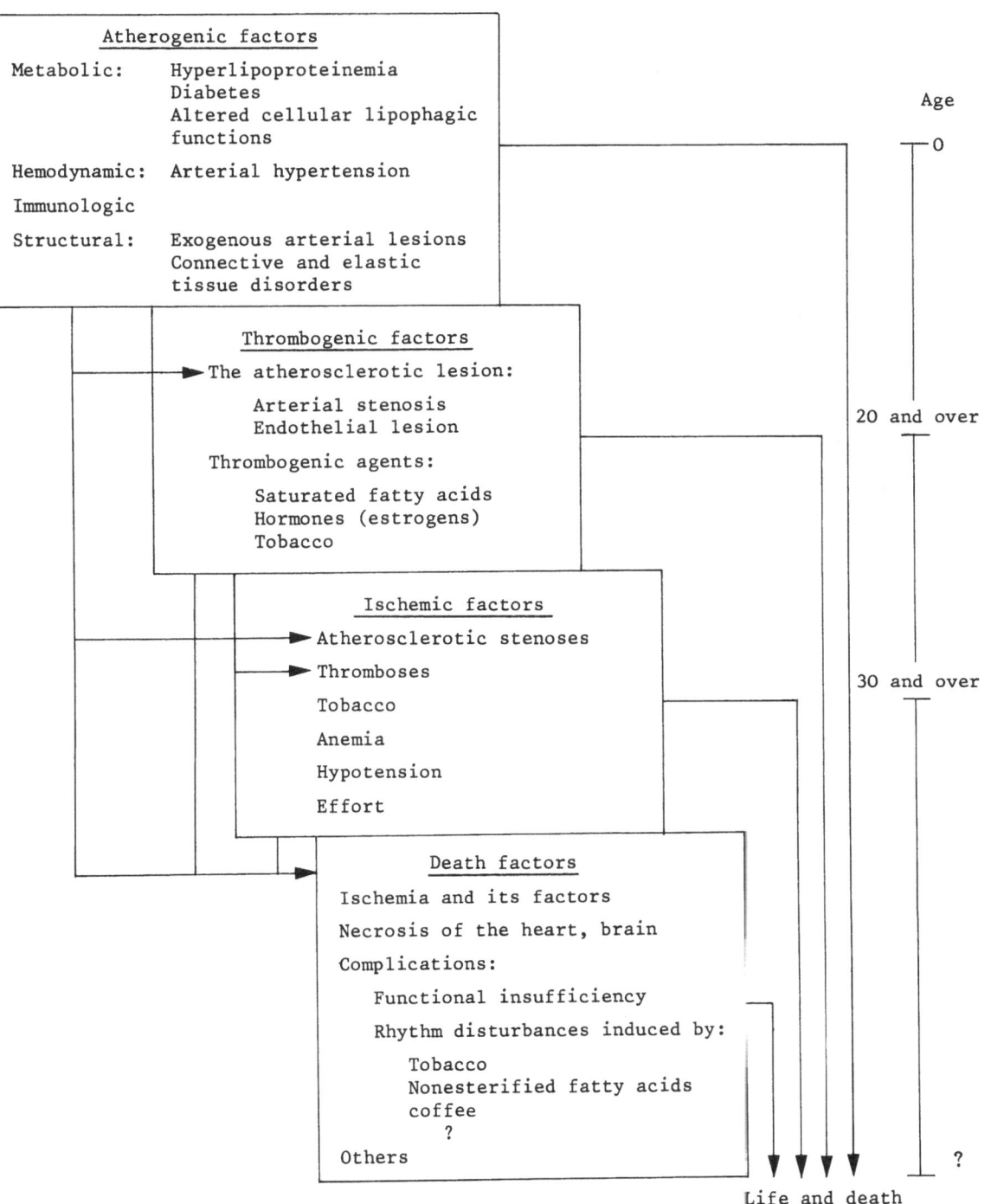

Figure 1. Factors of atherosclerosis and its complications. Their accumulation during life time

37

Finally, it is obvious that if a correlation if found between an immunologic event and one of the steps of atherosclerotic ischemic disease, its exact mechanism will still have to be discussed. For example, a correlation with ischemia may be met through thrombogenesis as well as through atherogenesis. Moreover a correlation with arterial damage may arise through a direct immunologic injury to the vessel wall or through the induction of an atherogenic condition such as hyperlipidemia or arterial hypertension. Indeed, it seems at the present time that there may be several atherogenic immunologic mechanisms and that thrombogenic immunologic mechanisms may also be implicated in ischemic diseases.

2. The Pathogenesis of Atherosclerosis

Since the last century, there have been two opposite theories. In one, the cholesterol-rich atherosclerotic lesion is due to infiltration of the arterial wall by molecules coming from the circulation blood. In the other, the arterial lesion is primary, affecting the connective and elastic tissue structures and the cells which produce them, and the lipid infiltration is secondary. To the first of these theories must be added the thrombogenic theory, according to which the infiltration of the wall is subsequent to the formation of multiple mural thrombi.

At present, it seems necessary to conciliate these theories because it is obvious that atherosclerosis may result either from an abnormality in the circulating blood or primary arterial damage. Such a conciliation is possible if attention is focused on the circulation of cholesterol-rich macromolecules in the normal arterial wall and if it is considered that atherosclerosis may be the result of an abnormal circulation of these macromolecules (Beaumont, 1964, 1975). This theory is based on the following facts:

a) There are no capillaries in the intima or in the inner layer of the media of the large and medium arteries. This conformation makes exchanges with the circulating blood rather slow.

b) The cholesterol molecule is not catabolized by mammalian cells and is not synthesized in appreciable amounts by the arterial wall.

c) The cholesterol molicule is almost insoluble in water, except when it is combined with the circulating lipoproteins.

d) A constant flow of macromolecules, especially of serum lipoproteins, goes acriss tge arteruak ubtuna abd nedua (Smith and Slater, 1973; Stein and Stein, 1972; Wlaton, 1973; Zolversmit and Mewman, 1966). Lipis including cholesterol are transported by the lipoproteins and thus circulate easily in this form.

e) Most of the molecules which cross the arterial intima are easily metabolized, even when the carrier molecule is broken down, since the chemical elements of which they are made are soluble or degradable in soluble fractions. This is not the case for the cholesterol molecule which, if its carrier lipoprotein is destroyed, has to be excreted by the artery after its incorporation in another soluble macromolecule.

According to this theory, the amount of cholesterol excreted by the artery during a given period under normal conditions is equal to the amount of cholesterol entering it from the blood and no deposit is formed. Cholesterol deposits and atheroma form when the amount of blood cholesterol entering the arterial wall is increased and thereby exceeds the excretion capacity; or when the maximal excretion capacity of a diseased artery is abnormally decreased and thus falls below the value of a normal entry of cholesterol. It is thus possible to distinguish between atherosclerosis due to an increased penetration of the artery by lipid-rich blood macromolecules, atherosclerosis due to a decrease in the exit rate of lipid carrying macromolecules, and finally atherosclerosis of mixed origin, due to a combination of these two mechanisms.

This theory enables all known factors to be taken into account (Beaumont, 1964, 1975). It would admit several different immunologic mechanisms inducing either increased penetration or decreased excretion of lipid-loaded macromolecules or a combination of both mechanisms. It admits also many other nonimmunologic mechanisms.

The Immunologic Factors of Atherosclerosis and Its Complications

1. *Ischemic Disease and Genetic Markers Related to the Immune Response*

Recently it was claimed (Mathews, 1975) that national death rates from ischemic heart disease are significantly correlated with the frequency of antigen HLA 8 and haplotype HLA 1-8 in the population. These histocompatibility genes are known to determine patterns of immune response in animals and man. HLA 8 was also found to be linked to genes which predispose to several autoimmune diseases such as myasthenia gravis and chronic active hepatitis, and also Addison's disease, juvenile onset diabetes mellitus and Grave's disease. The validity of this correlation needs confirmation and more work will be necessary to elucidate the underlying mechanisms. However, it was added (Mathews, 1975) that serum cholesterol levels in a population seem to be correlated with the HLA 8 frequency and also that high death rates from ischemic heart disease and high levels of serum cholesterol in Finland may be related to the combined effects of HLA 8 and W 15 antigens.

2. *Immunopathology and Atherosclerosis*

a) Immunization Induced Arteriopathies

It is well-known that injury to the arterial tissue results from repeated injections of antigens in the appropriate experimental conditions of serum sickness and it was demonstrated that the fresh histologic lesions were due to the trapping of soluble circulating antigen-antibody complexes in the arterial wall (Saphir et al., 1958; Germuth et al., 1967; Cochrane, 1968). The subsequent arteritis is wide spread and involves mainly small arteries and capillaries. However deposits of immune complexes were also seen in the aorta and the coronary arteries at sites where hydrodynamic conditions were favorable (Kniker and Cochrane, 1965). Moreover, it was demonstrated that major lesions of large and medium arteries can also be induced by immunization (Minick and Murphy, 1973; Scebat et al., 1966; Levy, 1967).

Under these conditions, the early lesions are not characteristic of atherosclerosis. They are much more destructive with early and severe alterations of the elastic structure of the vessel and contain little or no lipid. However, it was possible to induce typically atherosclerotic plaques in rabbits by a combination of immunization course and a long-term cholesterol enriched diet (Minick and Murphy, 1973; Scebat et al., 1966). In these experiments atherosclerosis can be induced even when the enriched diet is given after ending the immunization process (Minick and Murphy, 1973). This observation suggests that the immunization process induces an arterial injury and that atherosclerosis is secondary to the abnormal metabolism in the injured artery (Minick and Murphy, 1973; Levy, 1967). This hypothesis would fit the already known nonspecificity of antigens which may induce arterial lesions (Beaumont and Beaumont, 1968) and also with the general concept that any kind of injury may be responsible for secondary atherosclerosis (Rossle, 1944; Haust, 1971; Hardin et al., 1973), if secondary conditions are appropriate such as hyperlipidemia (Minick and Murphy,

1973) or arterial hypertension (Wilens, 1965). However, the mechanism of the early immunologic lesion remains open to question. Obviously, in many experiments it is the result of immune complex filtration through the arterial wall. However, it was claimed that antiartery and antielastin antibodies were involved in other experiments (Scebat et al., 1967; Dallochio et al., 1968; Szigetti et al., 1960; Robert et al, 1967; Robert et al., 1970; Stein et al., 1965). On the other hand, it may be recalled that immunization procedures may induce hyperlipidemia and sometimes autoimmune hyperlipidemia (Beaumont and Beaumont, 1968; Beaumont et al., 1969) which may be atherogenic by themselves. The role of complement in the production of atherosclerosis may be important since complement is an important factor in arterial wall lesions induced by vitamin D poisoning (Geertinger and Sorensen, 1970).

b) Human Diseases Related to Experimental Immunization Arteriopathies

Before all it may be stated that atherosclerosis is rather unusual in human autoimmune diseases in which damage to the vascular wall may be encountered. Atherosclerosis was not reported to occur in Horton's disease, Takayasu's disease or panarteritis. In these diseases, the arterial lesions are very different and do not include atheroma. On the other hand, they resemble closely immune lesions and usually associate a granulomatous tissue and a fibrosis with more or less giant cells. These arteritis may affect large vessels and induce thrombosis. For example, examples of coronary arteritis were reported in these diseases including Takayasu's (Rosen and Gaton, 1972).

However, typical coronary and aortic atherosclerosis with subsequent ischemia may be encountered in systemic lupus erythematosus (Rich and Gregory, 1947; Meller et al., 1975; Kong et al., 1962; Tskralides et al., 1974) and perhaps in rheumatic cardiac disease and rheumatoid arthritis (Minick and Murphy, 1973). In SLE when autopsies are made after death following myocardial infarction, widespread coronary arteritis with necrotizing lesions and occlusion in the small vessels may be found (Brigden et al., 1960) and also, in other cases, typical occlusive atherosclerotic plaques, which may be complicated by thrombosis (Meller et al., 1975; Kong et al., 1962; Tskralides et al., 1974). There is little doubt that this atherosclerosis is due to the SLE because it happens before 30 years of age, often in women, and in the absence of other risk factors. However, although it is very likely, the immune mechanism of the atheroma was not proved and deposition of immune complexes were not yet found in the arterial wall as they were in the glomeruli (Meller et al., 1975). Arteritis and sclerotic lesions of the aorta were seen in rheumatoid arthritis (Bauer et al., 1951; Bywaters, 1957) and also in rheumatic heart disease (Minick and Murphy, 1973). However it is difficult to make sure that these diseases can induce typical atherosclerosis since (1) in almost all cases, reports deal with sclerosis and not with atheroma, and (2°) atherosclerosis is found in patients over 40, an age after 40, an age after which this lesion is common.

Another example of possible immune atherosclerosis in man is given by the arterial disease which may develop in heart or kidney homotransplants (Hadjiisky et al., 1971) and which was called occlusive disease of the transplant (Dempster, 1969) or graft atherosclerosis (Kosek and Biebler, 1970). Indeed, many years before, Yamanouchi (1911) demonstrated that in arterial homografts but not in autografts there was a proliferative intimal thickening accompanied by medial thinning and fragmentation of the elastic lamellae. These findings were confirmed and it was also shown that the lesions may lead to typical atherosclerosis in hypercholesterolemic (Fisher and Fisher, 1956) and also in normocholesterolemic rabbits in long-term experiments (Bowyer et al., 1974). This occlusive arterial disease is one of the main problems for the survival of heart (Lower and Shumway, 1970) and kidney (Lower and Shumway, 1970) transplants in man. They sometimes (Hadjiisky et al., 1971; Dempster, 1969; Kosek and Biebler, 1970; Hamburger and Dormont, 1968; Thomson, 1969) but not always resemble atherosclerosis: fibrous thickening of the intima and injury to the elastic fibers are almost constant findings, atheroma and thrombi are not. The arterial wall is usually more or less infiltrated by lymphocytes (Hadjiisky et al., 1971). On the other hand, if there is no doubt that an immune process is responsible for the early lesions, associated risk factors may favor their evolution towards atherosclerosis. However, they may occur even in the absence of hypercholesterolemia (Thomson, 1969).

c) Autoimmune Hyperlipidemia (AIH)

AIH was described in 1964-65 (Beaumont, 1965). It is the result of an inhibition by autoantibodies of the lipolysis of circulating lipiproteins which leads to their accumulation in the blood (Beaumont, 1970, 1969). In myeloma cases in which a sufficient amount of molecules were provided, the activity of the purified antibodies was located to their antibody sites on the Fab fragment of the molecules (Beaumont, 1969; Beaumont et al., 1970). Different AIH types which were induced by different antibodies reacting specifically with different sites were reported (Beaumont and Beaumont, 1974a; Beaumont, 1970, 1969; Beaumont et al., 1974). In these different types, different steps of the complex lipolytic process are inhibited so that the hyperlipoproteinemia pattern may be different from one case to another (Beaumont and Beaumont, 1974a).

In the antilipoprotein type, inhibition of lipolysis is due to antibodies which react with the surface of the lipoproteins at sites which are necessary for a correct enzyme attack. Several subtypes were described including IgA anti-Pg, and IgG anti-AS (Beaumont, 1969) myelomas; other subtypes do exist. Hyperlipidemia may be of type II b, III or V. Spontaneous agglutination of lipid particles may be seen in the circulating blood (Beaumont and Lorenzelli, 1972). Fat tolerance and vitamin A tolerance tests give abnormally high and prolonged blood levels. Production of post heparin lipoprotein lipase activity in vivo is normal, but lipoprotein lipase activity may be inhibited in vitro in appropriate conditions (Beaumont et al., 1976).

In the antienzyme type, inhibition of lipolysis may be due to antibodies which interfere either with the activated lipase molecules or with their production. At the present time, only antiheparin antibodies were described (Glueck et al., 1969; Beaumont and Lemort, 1970; Glueck et al., 1972). Likely there are subtypes. Hyperlipidemia may be of type I, IV or V. There is no agglutination of circulating lipid particles and the fat tolerance and vitamin A tolerance tests are abnormal. The post heparin lipase activities are diminished. In some instances, it was found that production of circulating lipase activity may be restored by increasing the amount of heparin injected (Glueck et al., 1969).

AIH is the result of a disturbed immunoglobulin production which in most of the cases remains still unknown. It may be associated to myeloma when the immunoglobulin produced has the appropriate activity. It may also occur in association with lymphoma, S.L.E. and rheumatoid arthritis. Recently it was found in two nephrotic syndromes (Beaumont et al., 1974). However, more often it seems primary and additional research will be necessary to understand its exact mechanism. In animals, AIH could be produced by immunization procedures (Szigetti et al., 1960; Beaumont et al., 1969) and it may be associated with the development of tumors like the Walker carcinoma in rats (Posner, 1960) and the Greene lymphoma in hamsters (Albrink and Albrink, 1971; Beaumont and Beaumont, 1974b).

The frequency of AIH is not known since there is not yet any simple diagnostic test suitable for epidemiologic studies. However, it is felt that it may be rather frequent since, in the nonmyeloma cases, the blood lipoprotein pattern faces one or the other of the common types of primary hyperlipoproteinemia. Presumptive signs and diagnostic tests were reviewed before (Beaumont and Beaumont, 1974a). According to systematic research of spontaneous agglutination of lipid particles in the serum which is in progress, a figure of 20% of antilipoprotein AIH may be an approximate of the frequency of this type of AIH among hyperlipoproteinemia with milky serum.

Atherosclerosis is one of the possible tissue complications of AIH. Clinically defined ischemic diseases are frequently associated with myeloma AIH, although they are rather unfrequent in myeloma without AIH (Beaumont et al., 1970). In one very well-documented case of AIH associated with a benign monoclonal IgA followed for 22 years, Lewis et al. (1975) observed the development of severe peripheral atherosclerosis with typical atheroma, fibrosis, thrombosis, and also a "diffuse aneurysmal disease". The lesions were seen on angiograms and on histologic examination of arterial samples which were taken when a by-pass graft was performed. A deposition of IgA-lipoprotein complexes was found in the arterial wall (Lewis and Lazzarini-Robertson, 1974). They were in greater amount in the atherosclerotic areas than in the less involved areas (Lewis et al., 1975). In nonmyeloma AIH, ischemic diseases were also found associated in a possibly significant way according to the age of the patients and to the absence of other arterial risk factors (Beaumont et al., 1967). However, it may be that some types of AIH are atherogenic while others are not. Moreover, the mechanism by which AIH induces atherosclerosis may be different for antilipoprotein and antienzyme (anti-heparin) types. In both, there is a hyperlipidemia which is by itself a factor of atherosclerosis. Additionally, in the antilipoprotein type, the circulating Ig-Lp soluble complexes may be harmful by themselves. Some of them may move through the arterial wall like other circulating macromolecules and, as they are rather unstable, they may precipitate in the intima and induce accumulation of lipids and cholesterol. It is noteworthy that the Ig-Lp complexes which were studied until now do not fix complement. This may explain why they do no immediate and dramatic damage to the wall and do not induce arteritis as in the postimmunization immune complex disease. According to this, atherosclerosis in antilipoprotein AIH would be an "autoimmune cholesterol-rich complex disease (Beaumont and Beaumont, 1974a). In antiheparin AIH, there are no circulating complexes but a thrombotic tendency may be associated to the hyperlipidemia and may contribute to the atherosclerotic lesion.

AIH associated with monoclonal gammapathia is influenced by immunosuppressive treatment which was found to reduce both the gamma globulin and the lipoprotein levels (Sobel et al., 1976; Lewis et al., 1973). However, this treatment is not indicated in nonmyeloma cases.

3. Immunopathology and Thrombosis

It is well-known that antigen-antibody interactions can interfere in vivo with the coagulation system through the complement system. This may produce or favor thrombosis. However, it is not known if obstruction of large or medium arteries may result from this mechanism. Moreover, it is likely that when ischemia results of antigen-antibody reactions in vivo, it is due to thrombosis secondary to arterial wall damage. Among the arterial disease which may be secondary to immune reactions leading to arterial damage and thrombosis, the vascular risk of oral contraceptives may take place (Beaumont and Lemort, 1976). A case of pulmonary artery thrombosis associated with an ethinyl estradiol oral contraceptive was described, in which a circulating monoclonal IgG λ was found to react specifically with ethinyl estradiol. This reaction was antibody-like since two sites having the same affinity (K_a: 2.7 x 10^7 M^{-1}) were found on each IgG λ molecule (Beaumont and Lemort, 1976). About this observation, it may be remembered that at least in one case of death secondary to a Budd-Chiari syndrome induced by oral contraceptives, the intima of the vessels were found to be diffusely damaged (Rothwell-Jackson, 1968).

The Immunologic Mechanism of Atherosclerosis

1. The Antigen-Antibody Molecular Interactions

The secondary effects of any immune reaction are the results of very specific molecular interactions of high affinity. In these interactions, the reactive sites of an immunoglobulin (Ig) which are its antibody (Ab) sites react with a complementary structure which is called the antigen determinant of the antigen (Ag). The reacting Ab may be soluble and induce serum reactions or remain attached to a lymphoid cell, which are the carriers of cellular immunity. The reacting Ag may also be soluble or attached to a membrane. The Ab-Ag interaction may involve other molecules and cells such as complement, histamine and kinins, macrophages, and polymorphonuclear leukocytes.

The secondary effects of an Ab-Ag reaction in vivo depend on the nature of the nature of the reacting Ag and Ab.

If the Ag circulates in a soluble form, the Ag-Ab complexes may be insoluble and precipiting and then they are readily taken up by macrophages. On the other hand, the Ag-Ab complexes may be soluble and then they can infiltrate the tissues and produce an immune complex disease.

If the Ag has a physiologic function, this can be blocked by the Ab and a metabolic trouble will result. This is the case when the Ag is an enzyme or any structure involved in the activity of an enzyme. AIH is an example of such an immune metabolic disease.

If the Ag-Ab complexes react with complement (this depends firstly on the structure of the Ig Ab), cytolysis and inflammation will result in the tissues. If they do not react with complement, the Ag-Ab reaction may cause no immediate damage to the tissues.

If the Ag is attached to a cell or part of the structural constituents of a tissue, the damage induced by an Ag-Ab reaction will depend similarly on the physiologic function of the Ag and on the involvement of the complement and kinin systems.

2. The Atherogenic Ag-Ab Reactions

It is not possible to say at present that one particular sequence of molecular reactions can bring an Ag-Ab reaction to be atherogenic. On the contrary, it seems that several sequences can induce an arterial wall disease. For example, in AIH the arterial lesions may be secondary to the increase in the amount of circulating lipoproteins which is induced by the antienzyme type of AIH. In this case, atherosclerosis is the result of hyperlipidemia and there is no immune reaction in the arterial wall. On the other hand, in AIH too, the arterial lesions may be secondary to the infiltration of the wall by cholesterol-rich Ag-Ab complexes. In this case, atherosclerosis is the result of a variety of autoimmune complex disease.

In the immunization model of arteriosclerosis, the lesions may be due to Ag-Ab complexes of different composition or, more hypothetically to antiartery, including antielastin, antibodies. In these models, it is likely (Minick and Morphy, 1973) that the Ag-Ab reaction induces first an arteritis which is the result of the immunologic injury to the arterial wall. This injury, like any other type of injury (Haust, 1971) may lead to secondary atherosclerosis.

3. Immunologic Factors in the Pathogenesis of Atherosclerosis and Its Complications

The different immunologic factors which are already known or may be expected fit easily into the theory of atherogenesis described above. In this theory, atherosclerosis is the result of a disturbed flow of molecules and especially of cholesterol through the arterial wall. a) Ag-Ab reactions may alter primarily the entry of these molecules into the artery when they alter the amount and the pattern of circulating lipoproteins. b) Ag-Ab reactions may alter primarily the ex-

cretion capacity of cholesterol by the artery when they damage the arterial wall.
It may be kept in mind that Ag—Ab reactions may also be thrombogenic in different
ways.

4. Origin of the Immunologic Atherogenic Factors

It must be pointed out first that, although several different hypothesis were
formulated, none would explain all the observed facts. One of the most attractive
of these theories states that the antigenicity of degraded elastin is the root of
an immunologic injury to the arteries and is related to the general mechanism of
aging. But there is yet no confirmation of such a process in human beings and it
does not include the risk factors of the human disease.

It is felt that it would be better to look for theories which would be coherent
with all known facts. Along these lines, the immunologic mechanism of atherosclerosis appears still multifactorial and not unique like the mechanism of atherosclerosis itself.

However, this does not diminish the interest of studying these mechanisms at a
cellular and molecular level. We feel that important advances in knowledge of
the disease and of its treatment would be the result of these efforts.

WORKSHOP 1. Dynamics of Lipoproteins and Lipids in the Arterial Wall

Chairmen: A.J. Day, Australia
          K. Wada, Japan

Participants: T. Yasugi, Japan
              J. Patelski, Poland
              R. Mahley, USA
              A.J. Day, Australia

INTRODUCTION

A.J. Day

Atherosclerosis is characterised by lipid accumulation in the arterial intima and the composition of the various lesions have now been well-documented. The two components which accumulate to the greatest extent are cholesterol ester and phospholipid. The mechanisms of their accumulation, however, is still not clear. There are at least three processes which contribute.

1. Lipoprotein entry from the plasma.
2. Arterial wall synthesis and metabolism.
3. Differential removel of lipid components from the arterial lesion.

1. Lipoprotein Entry From the Plasma

The normal endothelium appears to be practically impermeable to low-density lipoprotein. Cholesterol ester which is present in low-density lipoprotein can only be detected in low concentration in the early intima in infants and in animal arteries free of atherosclerotic disease. When the lesion develops, low-density lipoprotein can be identified by immunohistochemistry and immunochemistry and its entry is facilitated by hypertension, by platelet adhesion or by the lipid accumulation itself.

There are several questions which remain unanswered relating to the transport of lipoprotein into the atherosclerotic lesion and might appropriately claim the attention of this workshop. Information is accumulating about the transport of large molecular weight particles across the endothelium, but virtually no information is available regarding the mechanism of transport of lipoprotein across endothelium. The question of vesicular transport and whether this is energy-dependant remains open. Where lipoprotein entry is increased as it is in the atherosclerotic lesion, it is still not clear whether this represents some breakdown of a barrier or the speeding up of the normal slow transport of lipoprotein. Further information is therefore necessary regarding the penetration of lipoprotein in the arterial intima and on the mechanism of hypertension and platelet aggregation in facilitating lipoprotein entry into the atherosclerotic lesion.

2. Arterial Wall Synthesis and Metabolism

The accumulation of phospholipid and of cholesterol ester in the atherosclerotic lesion results from the dynamic balance of their entry, formation and degradation and enzymes associated both with phospholipid synthesis and degradation and of cholesterol ester synthesis and hydrolysis have been studied fairly extensively in the arterial wall. There are, however, a number of unanswered questions. The relative contribution of the serum and of arterial wall synthesis *in situ* to cholesterol ester accumulation is still undecided and while extensive work has been carried out recently on cholesterol esterifying and hydrolyzing activity, it is still not clear whether increased synthesis or decreased hydrolysis of cholesterol ester is associated with atherogenesis. Little work has been done on the modification of enzymes associated with either phospholipid or cholesterol ester formation in the arterial wall and some of these questions might legitimately be asked in the context of this workshop.

The characteristic cell of the atherosclerotic lesion is the foam cell and considerable work is being carried out in a number of laboratories on the role of smooth muscle cells in atherogenesis. It is believed that these cells develop into established foam cells and work done in tissue culture has established that low-density lipoprotein introduced to the smooth muscle cell leads to its proliferation, to cholesterol ester formation and to inhibition of cholesterol synthesis in these cells.

The mechanism of foam cell formation, however, is still unclear. It has not been possible to produce established foam cells in culture. Although smooth muscle cells accumulate lipid, the quantity which accumulates is less than that shown to be present in established foam cells. The role of other cells in the production of foam cells is still unclear and recent interest in the development of macrophages into foam cells has been reactivated by the identification of catalase B-positive cells in established atherosclerotic lesions. Whether the lipid in foam cells arises primarily from phagocytosed lipoprotein or as lipid synthesized in the cell is still unknown. The question of foam cell breakdown and of collagen formation is also relevant to atherogenesis and more information in this area is necessary.

3. Differential Removal of Lipid From the Atherosclerotic Lesion

The arterial wall is in a dynamic state with regard to its lipid content. Lipid is being synthesized and degraded, lipid is entering and being removed. The processes indicated above all relate to the dynamic changes associated with lipid accumulation during atherogenesis. Considerable interest has arisen recently in the possibility of regression of atherosclerotic lesions and a number of questions with regard to arterial wall models in this respect remain open. It is of importance to determine whether lipid can be removed from cell or arterial wall systems in vitro and, if such removal can be effected, what significance this has with respect to regression of the atherosclerotic lesion. The following papers relate to some of the above questions and we will address ourselves to answering some of these questions in the context of the four papers to be presented.

UPTAKE OF SERUM LIPOPROTEINS INTO THE ARTERIAL WALL

T. Yasugi

It is well-known that serum low-density lipoproteins (LDL) and very low-density lipoproteins (VLDL) play an important role in the development of atherosclerosis. High-density lipoproteins (HDL) are considered antiatherogenic. Fluorescent antibody techniques indicate that in thoracic aorta from normal rabbits LDL cannot be identified. In rabbits receiving a diet containing 1% cholesterol, LDL can be clearly identified in the intima. This evidence suggests that serum LDL enters the arterial wall of the hyperlipidemic rabbit.

In the present paper, data is presented relating to the entry of serum lipoproteins into the arterial wall and the mechanism of lipoprotein entry and the factors which effect it are considered.

Two procedures have been employed. Isolated arterial wall obtained from male rabbits was incubated for 2 hours in vitro in a Warburg apparatus in order to measure the uptake of ^{14}C-cholesterol labeled lipoproteins. During the incubation period, 100% oxygen was administered and various humoral factors were added to the incubation medium in order to investigate the effect of these substances on lipoprotein entry. Radioactivity was counted by liquid scintillation counting. The second procedure was an in vivo approach using immunofluorescent techniques to identify the antigens of lipoproteins in the arterial wall.

The entry of LDL and HDL into the arterial wall in vitro was appreciably less when dead tissues without oxygen consumption and tissues which were boiled were studied in comparison with viable tissue with an adequate oxygen supply. This suggested that the mechanism of lipoprotein entry in viable tissue was due to active transport.

In the tissues without oxygen consumption, the uptake of lipoprotein was linearly related to concentration. This is possibly due to entry of lipoprotein into the dead tissue by physicochemical diffusion. In the viable tissues, a high uptake of LDL was observed with a low concentration of lipoprotein in the incubation media with a plateau of lipoprotein entry at higher concentrations. This may be due to lipoprotein entry as an active transport.

In order to investigate the role of endothelial cells in lipoprotein uptake, the endothelial side of the arterial wall was coated by a cyanoacrylate monomer. The isolated arterial tissues were then incubated with labeled lipoproteins as described above. The lipoprotein uptake of coated tissues was only 15% with respect to LDL and 25% with respect to HDL, that of corresponding noncoated tissues. These results indicate that the intimal side of the arterial wall is important in lipoprotein entry.

When endothelium was injured by a sharp knife, the entry of both LDL and HDL into the arterial wall was increased. This evidence is consistent with other papers reporting acceleration of experimental atherosclerosis in the rabbit when the intima was injured by catheters.

The arterial wall was exposed to LDL for 6 hours in the in vivo study. In order to make the LDL clearly visible, the incubated LDL was concentrated up to ten times the normal serum concentration. Immunofluorescence for LDL was clearly visible in the tissue, especially on the intimal side. This suggests the importance of endothelial cells to lipoprotein uptake into the arterial wall.

In human middle cerebral arteries (56-year-old male patient with hypertension), large vesicles with a diameter of around 6000–9700 Å are visible. In the inside of the large vesicles, smaller vesicles with diameters around 270 Å are seen. This may be interpreted as the entry of LDL into the endothelial cell by pinocytosis.

From the above results, the following conclusions might be drawn. The entry of serum lipoproteins into the arterial wall occur by active transport, namely pinocytosis by the endothelial cell. It is difficult to consider entry as simple physico-chemical diffusion of serum lipoproteins into the arterial wall or as passive transport through the intercellular junction.

The effects of several humoral factors on lipoprotein entry into the arterial wall were also considered. Additions of hog renin, in various concentrations, to the incubation medium did not show any significant effect on the uptake of LDL or HDL into the arterial wall. Renin injected into the rabbit vein with a continuous infusion pump for 6 hours in a concentration of 0.15 Goldblatt U/kg/min showed no effect on the immunofluorescence to LDL in the arterial tissue.

Epinephrine did not influence lipoprotein entry. Following its infusion, continuously for 6 hours in a concentration of 0.3 µg/kg/min, no immunofluorescence to LDL was observed in the arterial wall. Addition of norepinephrine into the medium did not significantly influence the uptake of either LDL or HDL. Infusion with norepinephrine continuously for 6 hours in a concentration of 3.0 μg/kg/min did not result in any immunofluorescence to LDL.

The effect of angiotensin II was also studied. The action time of angiotensin II may be too short to be evidences during the 2 hours duration of the incubation study, so that studies both with one shot and intermittent additions of angiotensin II into the medium at intervals of 15 min were performed. While no influence was observed in the one shot study, significant effects were observed in the intermittent administration study. Angiotensin II significantly increased the uptake of both LDL and HDL into the arterial wall. Angiotensin II infused continuously for 6 hours in a concentration of 0.1 μg/kg/min produced immunofluorescence to LDL on the intimal side of arterial wall.

It is difficult to explain why only angiotensin II increased lipoprotein uptake. It is suggested that the constriction of the artery may not relate to this phenomenon, because both angiotensin II and catecholamines constrict the artery. Angiotensin II may be considered to increase the permeability of the artery.

Following the study of the action of angiotensin II on lipoprotein uptake, the effect on insulin was studied. Addition of insulin into the incubation medium increased significantly the LDL entry. No significant effect on HDL entry was observed, however. Continuous infusion of insulin in a concentration of 1 U/kg/h showed an increase of immunofluorescent LDL on the intimal side of the arterial wall.

The precise mechanism of the humoral factors described above are still being studied.

ENZYMES CATALYZING PHOSPHOLIPID-DEPENDENT TRANSACYLATIONS IN THE ARTERIAL WALL

J. Patelski, M. Piorunska-Stolzmann, and A.Waliszewska*

Relationship Between the Metabolism and Accumulation of Lipids in the Arterial Wall

The known different accumulation of cholesterol esters, phospholipids, and glycerides in the arterial wall is closely related to complex interactions of the compounds and enzymes catalyzing their synthesis and decomposition.

The relationship between the metabolism and accumulation of cholesterol esters and triglycerides may be summarized as follows: in different types of hyperlipemia, a relatively high increase in hydrolysis of triglycerides can prevent their retention but favor the accumulation of cholesterol esters by increased ATP-dependent synthesis and decreased hydrolysis of these esters (Patelski et al., 1968, 1970; Patelski, J., Plotast, B., Majewski, W., Zapalski, S., unpublished observations). On the other hand, a relatively low increase in hydrolysis of triglycerides can favor the retention of triglycerides rather than synthesis of cholesterol esters.

Possible interactions of cholesterol ester and phospholipid metabolism in the arterial wall result from the presence of lecithin-cholesterol acyltransferase

_____

*The authors wish to thank Nattermann and Cp., Cologne, for their support.

48

(Abdulla et al., 1968; Patelski and Piorunska, 1975) and the cholesterol ester-lysolecithin acyltransferase activity (Patelski and Piorunska, 1975). However, not much is known about the enzyme-substrate-product interactions.

The present work deals with the LCAT* -catalyzed synthesis and deacylation of cholesterol esters and the activity of lysolecithin-lysolecithin acyltransferase (LLAT) in the aorta.

Enzyme-Catalyzed ATP-Independent Transacylations Involving Lecithin, Cholesterol, Cholesterol Ester and Lysolecithin

The enzyme activities were assayed by measuring products formed in the reaction mixtures at optimum experimental conditions. The reaction mixtures in 4 ml total volume contained EDTA (10^{-3} mol/l), reduced glutathione (10^{-4} mol/l), substrate (Sigma, U.S.A.) hydrolysis (Patelski et al., 1970), buffers, and water extracts of proteins from acetone-butanol powders from pig aortas (Patelski et al., 1967) as follows: (1) egg yolk lecithin (3×10^{-3} mol/l) and cholesterol (10^{-3} mol/l), (2) cholesteryl oleate (10^{-3} mol/l) and lysolecithin (3×10^{-3} mol/l), (1, 2) tris/hydroxymethyl/aminomethane (2.5×10^{-2} mol/l), at pH 8.0, and 1.1 ± 0.1 mg of protein/ml of the enzyme extract, (3) lysolecithin (6×10^{-3} mol/l), phosphate buffer (3×10^{-2} mol/l), at pH 7.0, and 0.5 mg of protein of the enzyme extract. Incubation followed in glass-stoppered test tubes placed in a Dacie electric cell suspension mixer at 30°C for 30 (3) and 60 min (1, 2). Control reaction mixtures (1, 3) without enzyme, (2) without lysolecithin (for cholesteryl) oleate hydrolase activity), and (2) without cholesteryl oleate (for lysolecithin-lysolecithin acyltransferase activity) were used. Total lipids were extracted with chloroform-methanol (2:1, v/v), and the reaction products were separated by thin-layer chromatography and determined chemically (Patelski et al., 1970). Results are expressed in nEq. of esterified (1) and released cholesterol (2) and lecithin formed (3) per min per mg of protein of the enzyme extract (mU/mg). Protein was determined as previously (Patelski et al., 1970), and ATP was carefully proved absent by the Boehringer UV test for ATP.

The concentration of lecithin formed is approximately 30% lower as compared to that of cholesterol released in the reaction mixtures with lysolecithin and cholesteryl oleate. This results from subsequent hydrolysis of lecithin by the thermoresistant phospholipase A which acts at the same optimum pH 8.0, as was found at optimum experimental conditions for the LCAT-catalyzed decomposition of cholesteryl oleate.

The rates of synthesis and decomposition of cholesterol esters by LCAT are not significantly different from each other (Table 1). However, both pH 7.0 and 8.0 are optimal for the former reaction to proceed, whereas the latter is negligible at neutral pH and reaches its maximum rate only at the alkaline pH. Optimum pH for LLAT also is 7.0 (Fig. 1) and the enzyme specific activity is over three and one half times higher as compared with LCAT.

The optimum phospholipid and cholesterol or cholesterol ester concentration for LCAT amounts to 3 and 1 mmol/l respectively. The enzyme is inhibited by higher concentrations of the substrates. Substrate saturation of LLAT is only reached at 6 mmol concentration of lysolecithin (Fig. 2).

---

*LCAT = lecithin:cholesterol acyltransferase (EC 2.3.1.43), LLAT = lysolecithin:lysolecithin acyltransferase (EC 2.3.1), phospholipase A = phosphatide acyl-hydrolase (EC 3.1.1.4), cholesterol-ester hydrolase = sterol-ester hydrolase (EC 3.1.1.13).

Table 1. Enzyme activities of pig aorta

Enzyme	pH Optimum	Acitivity (mU/mg)
Lecithin – cholesterol	7.0	2.7 ± 0.69^{a} (ce)
⇌	8.0	2.0 ± 0.51^{b}
Cholesteryl oleate – lysolecithin acyltransferase	8.0	2.5 ± 0.56^{b} (c)
Lysolecithin – lysolecithin acyltransferase	7.0	9.7 ± 0.48^{c} (1)

[a] $\bar{x} \pm$ SEM from series of estimates, N = 4.
[b] $\bar{x} \pm$ SEM from series of estimates, N = 6.
[c] $\bar{x} \pm$ SEM from series of estimates, N = 5.

(ce) = cholesterol esters, (c) = cholesterol, (1) = lecithin.

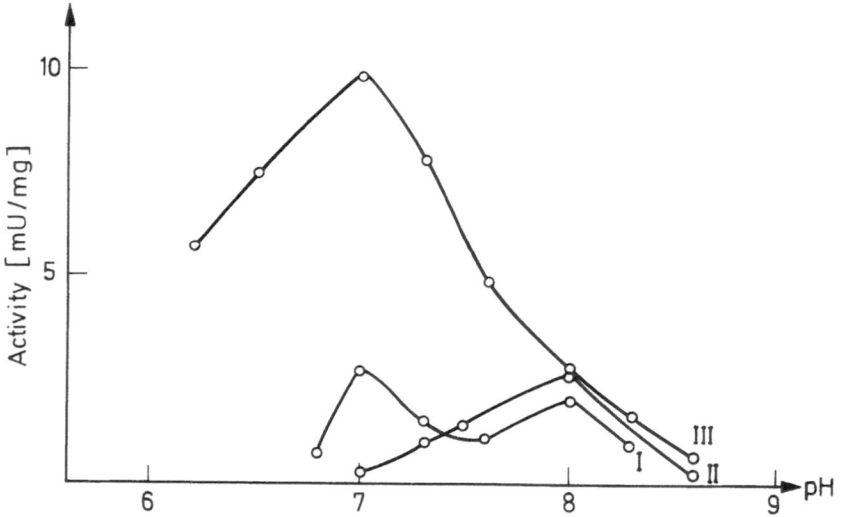

Figure 1. Effect of pH on lecithin – cholesterol (1), cholesteryl oleate – lyso-lecithin (2), and lysolecithin – lysolecithin (3) acyltransferase activities

Interactions of Arterial Enzymes and the Phospholipid and Cholesterol Substrates Products

As shown by the results, enzymes catalyzing the ATP-independent transacylations in the arterial wall can utilize both lecithin and cholesterol esters as donors, cholesterol as acceptor, and lysolecithin as both acceptor and donor of fatty acyls (Fig. 3) depending on pH, substrate product concentrations, and other conditions.

The fatty acyl exchange between lecithin and cholesterol esters has been hypothesized (Patelski, 1976) to render the cholesterol esters more susceptible

(Patelski et al., 1975) to hydrolysis. The double function of lysolecithin acting both as fatty acyl acceptor and donor can favor synthesis rather than deacylation of lecithin. This is consistent with the accumulation of lecithin rather than lysolecithin at increased phospholipase A activity (Patelski et al., 1970; Eisenberg et al., 1968). The relative importance of the ATP-independent transacylations and other enzyme activities involved in the metabolism of phospholipids and cholesterol esters in the arterial wall is not known.

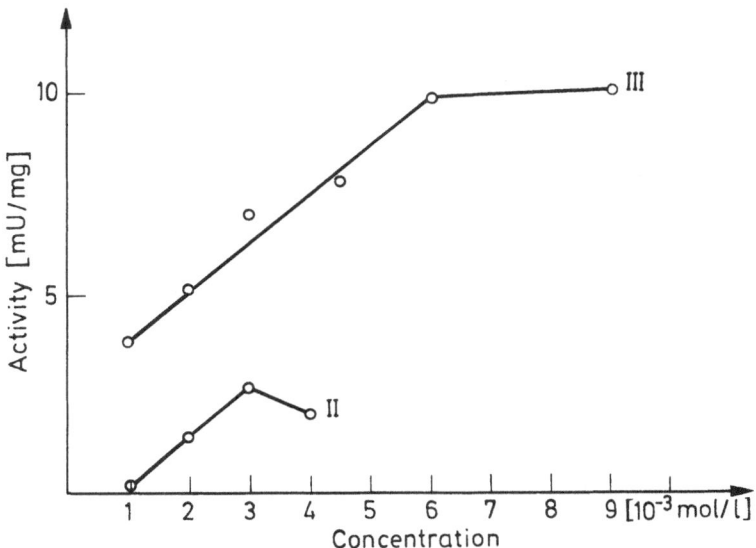

Figure 2. Effect of substrate concentrations on cholesteryl oleate – lysolecithin (2) and lysolecithin – lysolecithin acyltransferase (3) activities

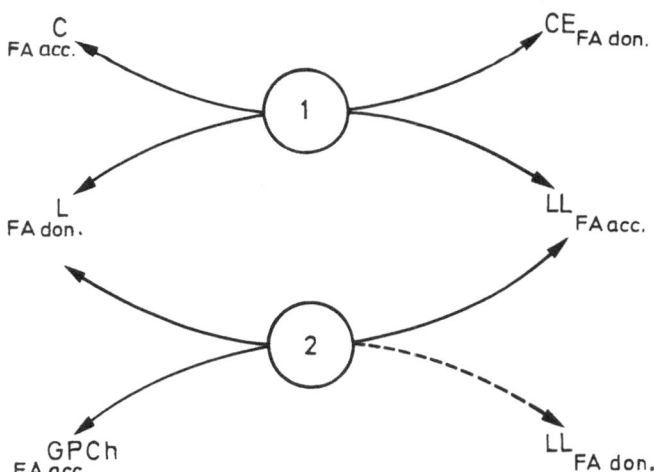

Figure 3. Fatty acyl (FA) acceptors (acc) and donors (don): C = cholesterol, CE = cholesterol esters, L = lecithin, LL = lysolecithin, GPCh = glycerylphosphoryl choline in enzyme – catalyzed transacylations: 1 = lecithin – cholesterol acyl-transferase, 2 = lysolecithin – lysolecithin acyltransferase

HEPARIN-MANGANESE PRECIPITABILITY OF CANINE LIPOPROTEINS AS CORRELATED WITH BINDING TO THE CELL SURFACE RECEPTORS ON FIBROBLASTS

Robert W. Mahley and Thomas L. Innerarity

Introduction

The binding of specific lipoproteins to cell surface receptors on fibroblasts and smooth muscle cells initiates a series of events which result in uptake and degradation of the lipoproteins, the accumulation of cholesteryl esters, and the regulation of cholesterol synthesis. The specificity for binding certain lipoproteins and not others may reside with the apoprotein content of the lipoproteins. The two classes of lipoproteins demonstrated to bind to the same cell surface receptor include those which contain the B-apoprotein (LDL) (Goldstein and Brown, 1974) and those which contain the arginine-rich apoprotein (e.g., the HDL_c of the cholesterol-fed swine) (Bersot et al., 1976). Previously, we also demonstrated that an HDL_c fraction from coconut oil-cholesterol-fed dogs had only the arginine-rich apoprotein and was as effective in delivering cholesterol to canine smooth muscle cells as were the LDL (Mahley, 1976). These findings suggested that if the protein were the important determinant for binding, then the receptor recognized both the B- and the arginine-rich apoproteins. The B and ARP may have in common a structural sequence or a similarly charged region which might be responsible for the binding of lipoproteins to the same cell surface receptor. That surface charge is important has been suggested by the studies of Goldstein et al. (1976) in which glycosaminoglycans, in particular heparin, competed with the receptor on fibroblasts for binding with human LDL. The negatively charged heparin is thought to bind to LDL at regions of positive charge (Iverius, 1972), which may also be the portion of the molecule that binds to the receptor.

To investigate further the properties of lipoproteins responsible for specific binding to the cell receptor, various lipoproteins from normal and tallow-cholesterol-fed dogs have been studied with respect to binding, uptake, and degradation by human fibroblasts in tissue culture. Dogs on control chow have lipoproteins similar to human VLDL, LDL, and HDL. In addition, there are α_2-migrating lipoproteins of density between 1.03 and 1.08 (referred to as HDL_1) which lack the B-apoprotein and contain primarily the A-I and the arginine-rich apoproteins (Mahley and Weisgraber, 1974a). After cholesterol feeding, the HDL_1 become major cholsterol-transporting lipoproteins (referred to as HDL_c) (Mahley and Weisgraber, 1974b). Depending upon the metabolic and dietary conditions, the HDL_c, which always lack the B-apoprotein, contain the A-I apoprotein and a variable amount of the arginine-rich apoprotein, which ranges from virtually the only protein to a minor apoprotein constituent. It was found that the HDL_1 and HDL_c were variably precipitated by heparin and manganese and that the most readily precipitable HDL_1 and HDL_c were those in which the concentration of the arginine-rich apoprotein were greatest. Thus, by use of the heparin-Mn precipitation, subfractions of HDL_1 or HDL_c, which had different apoprotein contents, could be obtained. Comparison of the precipitable vs. nonprecipitable HDL_1 and HDL_c with respect to binding and degradation by fibroblasts was studied in an attempt to define more clearly the properties of lipoproteins responsible for binding to cell surface receptors.

Results

1. Heparin-Manganese Precipitation of Canine Lipoproteins

Using standard procedures for lipoprotein precipitation with heparin-Mn (Cornwell and Kruger, 1961), it was possible to precipitate 95 - 99% of the dog LDL. The HDL_1 and HDL_c isolated from d = 1.02 - 1.063 were 50 - 80% precipitable with a single precipitation when 1 mg heparin and 4.8 mg $MnCl_2$ were added to 1.5 mg lipoprotein protein. The typical dog HDL (d = 1.087 - 1.21) were less than 10% precipitable. When the heparin and manganese concentrations were increased by multiple additions of the reagents, progressively more of the HDL_1 or HDL_c could be precipitated. With the stepwise addition of heparin-Mn, it was possible to obtain several different precipitated HDL_1 or HDL_c fractions, which could be resolubilized in $NaHCO_3$, and a final supernatant fraction. Dialysis of the lipoprotein fractions against $BaCl_2$ resulted in the complete precipitation of the heparin from the fractions. The various subfractions of HDL_1 and HDL_c were characterized with respect to chemical composition, size by negative staining electron microscopy, and apoprotein content by polyacrylamide gel electrophoresis. The precipitated HDL_1 or HDL_c could be totally resolubilized and retained their α_2-mobility by electrophoresis as well as other characteristics shown later. These lipoprotein fractions were then used in tissue culture experiments.

2. *Binding and Degradation of Heparin-Precipitable and -Nonprecipitable Lipoproteins*

When iodinated canine LDL were incubated with human fibroblasts, the LDL were bound to the cell surface receptors, internalized, and the protein degraded. Competitive binding studies using two different preparations of HDL_1 from control dogs at a concentration of 20 µg protein/ml resulted in a displacement of 55 and 75% of the ^{125}I canine LDL. Since similar variability had been observed with the degree of heparin-Mn precipitability, a comparison of heparin-precipitable and -nonprecipitable HDL_1 with respect to differences in competitive binding and degradation by fibroblasts was undertaken. As shown in Figure 1, the heparin-precipitable HDL_1 were much more effective in displacing the ^{125}I LDL from the cell surface receptors than the HDL_1 which remained in the supernatant after heparin-Mn treatment. Likewise, the precipitable HDL_1 competed more effectively with ^{125}I LDL for degradation than did the nonprecipitable HDL_1.

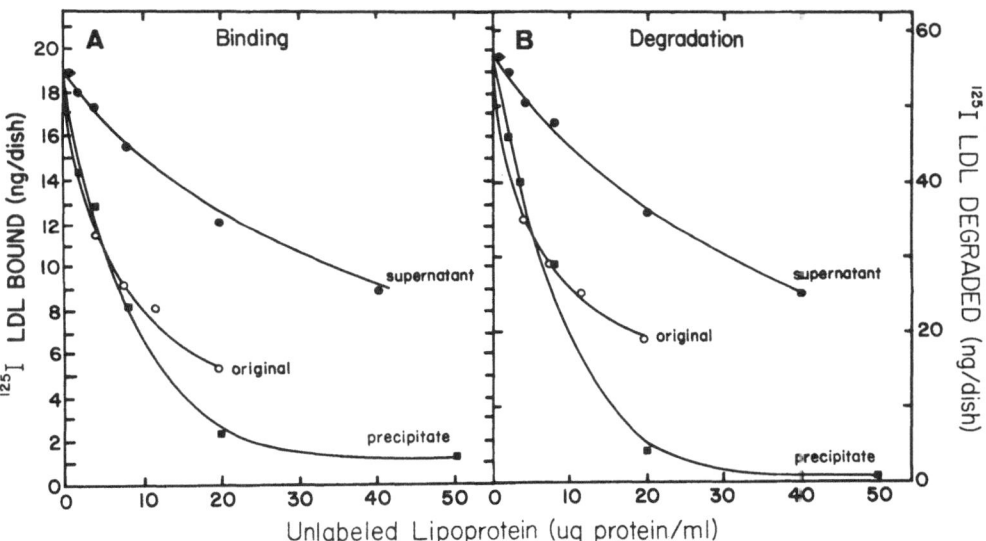

Figure 1. Ability of the original HDL_1, heparin-Mn precipitable HDL_1, and the HDL_1 which remained in the supernatant to compete with canine ^{125}I LDL for binding and degradation in human fibroblasts. Procedures for maintenance of the cells in culture and for performance of the assays were described elsewhere (Goldstein and Brown, 1974; Bersot et al., 1976). On day 7 the media was replaced by 10% canine lipoprotein-deficient plasma, 2.5 µg/ml canine ^{125}I LDL (287 cpm/ng protein), and the unlabeled lipoproteins at the concentrations indicated. HDL_1 were precipitated using 2.5:1:4.8 lipoprotein protein:heparin:$MnCl_2$ (w/w). 63% of the HDL_1 was precipitated and 96% of the starting HDL_1 was recovered in the precipitate and supernatant

To document further the association between heparin precipitability and binding to cell surface receptors, heparin-Mn was added to HDL₁ in progressively higher concentrations to obtain HDL₁ with various degrees of susceptibility to precipitation. Four precipitates and the final supernatant were compared. As shown in Figure 2, the most readily precipitable HDL₁ (labeled 1st precipitate) were the most effective in competing with the iodinated LDL for binding and degradation. Displacement of ^{125}I LDL was progressively less with each successive precipitation and least with the HDL₁ which remained in the supernatant of the last precipitate.

The original HDL₁ and its subfractions were characterized with respect to physical and chemical properties (Table 1). The HDL₁ subfraction which precipitated at the lowest concentration of heparin-Mn and which competed most effectively for binding and degradation (labeled ppt. I) contained qualitatively more of the arginine-rich apoprotein than the original HDL₁. Progressively less arginine-rich apoprotein was present in each of the successive precipitates (II through IV) and none was seen in the supernatant HDL₁ by polyacrylamide gel electrophoresis. The chemical composition of the subfractions revealed that the first precipitate contained more cholesterol and less protein than the other precipitates or the supernatant. The total cholesterol to protein ratio, which reflected the changes in composition, decreased from 3.7 in the first precipitate to 1.1 in the supernatant HDL₁. The mean particle size decreased from the first through the fourth precipitates, with the supernatant having the smallest particle size. However, the change in mean particle size was only 40 Å. The supernatant HDL₁, which were very ineffective in displacing ^{125}I LDL from the binding sites, were

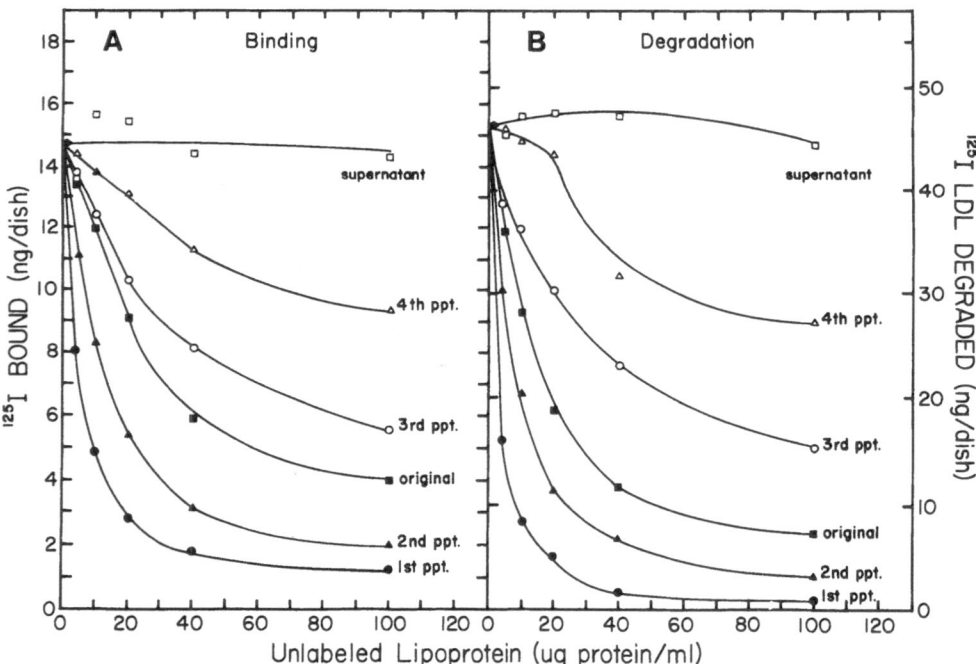

Figure 2. Ability of canine HDL₁, the four precipitated HDL₁ fractions, and supernatant HDL₁ to compete with canine ^{125}I LDL for binding and degradation. Studies were performed as indicated in Figure 1 except that 2 μg/ml ^{125}I LDL (625 cpm/ng protein) was added to the incubation media. Heparin and MnCl₂ were added stepwise. The portions of the total starting HDL₁ protein which were recovered in each fraction (ppt. I - ppt. IV, and the supernatant) were 15, 25, 24, 24, and 15% respectively

218 Å in diameter (approximately the size of LDL), indicating that particle size may not have been an important determinant of the cell surface receptor specificity under these conditions.

HDL_C from cholesterol-fed dogs were also variably precipitated by the heparin-Mn procedure. When tested for their effects on competitive binding and degradation, the precipitated HDL_C were much more effective in displacing the iodinated LDL from the cell surface receptors than the HDL_C in the supernatant (Fig. 3). The HDL_C which precipitated were enriched in the arginine-rech apoprotein as compared to the HDL_C in the supernatant.

To demonstrate that the precipitation, resolubilization, and dialysis procedures did not alter the binding and degradation properties of the lipoproteins, canine LDL and LDL which had been precipitated by heparin-Mn and resolubilized were compared in the tissue culture procedure. The original LDL and the totally precipitated LDL gave identical results with respect to competitive binding and degradation. HDL (d= 1.087-1.21) were also subjected to the heparin-Mn procedure. The HDL which remained in the supernatant (>99% of the total) and the original HDL gave identical results and did not compete with ^{125}I LDL for binding or degradation.

Table 1. Characterization of HDL_1, precipitated HDL_1, and supernatant HDL_1

Apoproteins[a]	Ppt. I[b]	Ppt. II	Ppt. III	Ppt. IV	Super-natant	Original
B	0	0	0	0	0	0
ARP	++++	+++	++	+	0	++
A-I	+	++	++	+++	++++	++
C's	++	++	++	+	+	++
% Composition						
T. cholesterol[c]	43.8	38.8	38.1	34.9	28.5	37.4
Phospholipid	44.4	47.1	45.4	45.5	44.5	45.6
Protein	11.8	14.1	16.5	19.6	27.0	17.1
TC/PL	1.0	0.82	0.84	0.77	0.64	0.82
TC/protein	3.7	2.8	2.3	1.8	1.1	2.2
Diameter, Å[d]						
Mean	256	259	223	221	218	252
Range	180-360	160-340	180-300	160-320	180-300	160-380

[a]Qualitative assessment of the prominence of the apoproteins in the lipoprotein fractions as determined by polyacrylamide gel electrophoresis.

[b]Ppt. I was the HDL_1 fraction which precipitated at the lowest concentration of heparin-Mn (4:1:4.5). Ppt. IV precipitated at the highest concentration of heparin and the supernatant HDL_1 remained nonprecipitable at this concentration.

[c]The % esterified cholesterol was not different among the fractions (ranged: 65-68% of total).

[d]200 particles measured.

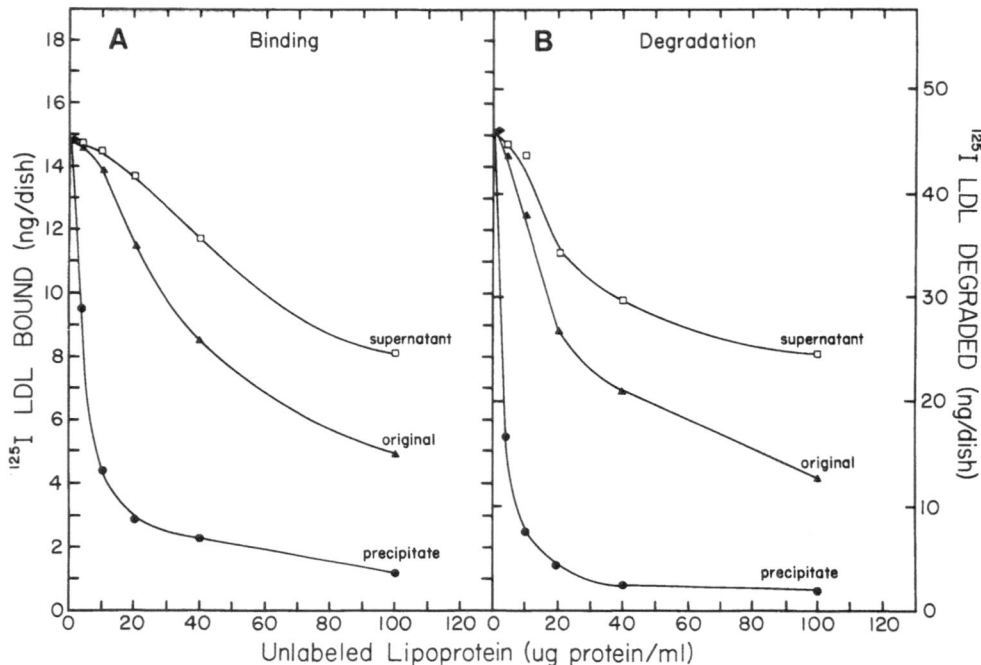

Figure 3. Ability of the cholesterol-induced HDL_c, the heparin-Mn precipitable HDL_c, and the nonprecipitable HDL_c (supernatant) to compete with the canine ^{125}I LDL for binding and degradation. The conditions were as described in Figure 2, and 1.5:1:4.8 lipoprotein protein:heparin:$MnCl_2$ was used. 70% of the HDL_c was precipitable

Summary

To determine the nature of the specificity of the cell surface receptors on fibro-blasts, HDL_1 from control dogs and HDL_c from cholesterol-fed dogs were subfrac-tionated by the heparin-Mn precipitation method. The subfractions of HDL_1 and HDL_c were compared with respect to their ability to be bound and degraded by human fibroblasts. The subfractions which were most readily precipitated by hep-arin were the most efficient in competing with LDL for binding and degradation. The most striking characteristic of the precipitated HDL_1 and HDL_c which were most efficiently bound and degraded was the occurrence of the arginine-rich apoprotein as a major apoprotein constituent.

It is reasonable to speculate that a single lipoprotein property may be respon-sible for binding both to heparin and to the cell surface receptor; moreover, this may represent a positively charged region on the lipoprotein surface. That this property of the lipoproteins resides with the protein moiety is suggested by studies of glycosaminoglycan interaction with lipoproteins (Iverius, 1972; Nishida and Cogan, 1970; Day and Levy, 1975) and of cell surface receptor binding (Goldstein et al., 1976) which demonstrate that alterations in the protein by acetylation, succinylation, and maleation interfere with both binding properties. In conclusion, there may be similar positively charged regions on the surface of all lipoproteins which interact with the cell surface receptor; furthermore, the ability to bind to the receptor may be a property of either the B-apoprotein or the arginine-rich apoprotein.

SYNTHESIS AND REMOVAL OF FREE CHOLESTEROL AND OF CHOLESTEROL ESTER BY SMOOTH MUSCLE CELLS IN TISSUE CULTURE

A.J. Day, M. Sheers and S. Kar

Introduction

The key cellular event in early atherogenesis is the proliferation of smooth muscle cells from the intima-medial region of the artery and their conversion to lipid containing foam cells. It has been shown that these cells will multiply when exposed to low-density lipoprotein (Dzoga et al., 1971) and the entry of this fraction into the intima presumably triggers off both the cellular and metabolic events of early atherogenesis.

Smooth muscle cells from normal arteries can be grown in tissue culture and a number of studies have been carried out on their metabolism of lipid. The smooth muscle cell in culture forms a convenient model, therefore, to study the formation of cholesterol ester and the removal of both cholesterol and cholesterol ester from these cells.

It has been reported that the incorporation of acetate into cholesterol by these cells is inhibited by low-density lipoprotein (Weinstein et al., 1976).

It has also been reported that cholesterol esterification is stimulated when smooth muscle cells in culture are exposed to low-density lipoprotein (St. Clair, 1976).

The removal of cholesterol from aortic smooth muscle cells has also been shown to be accelaterated by the addition of high-density lipoprotein to the incubation medium (Stein et al., 1975).
In the present study, the synthesis and removal of both cholesterol and of cholesterol ester from smooth muscle cells in culture has been studied using ^{14}C-labeled acetate or ^{3}H-labeled cholesterol in lipoprotein as precursors for cholesterol and cholesterol esters in the cell.

Methods

Aortas were obtained from 2-4 week-old normal rabbits. The adventitia was removed and explants set out in Falcon flasks for tissue culture. Growth occurred under such circumstances in 5-6 days and by 10-14 days growth had extended into the surrounding area. At approximately 14 days from primary planting, the explants and their outgrowing cells were trypsinized and aliquots placed into Leighton tubes for metabolic study. They were allowed to grow to confluence and when growth was stationary, ^{14}C-labeled acetate and ^{3}H-cholesterol labeled lipoprotein were added and their incorporation into lipid fractions and the subsequent removal of these lipid fractions investigated.

Results and Discussion

Two series of experiments are reported. In the first, smooth muscle cells were incubated in a medium containing 9/% basal eagles medium with 5% foetal calf serum added, together with a supplement of either 5% normal rabbit serum or of 5% hyperlipemic rabbit serum. ^{14}C-labeled acetate or ^{3}H-cholesterol labeled lipoprotein were added in order to study the uptake of these precursors and their incorporation into the cell cholesterol and cholesterol ester pool. After 24 hours of incubation, the medium was removed and the cells washed with saline. The labeled lipid was then extracted with chlorofrom-methanol (2:1) and the lipid extracts separated by thin layer chromatography. Lipid analysis was carried out either by densitometry (for cholesterol and cholesterol ester) or by the microassay of Bartlett (1959) for lipid phosphorus.

Table 1. Uptake and incorporation of [1-^{14}C-] acetate into lipid fractions by smooth muscle cells in culture

| | Experiment I[a] | | Experiment II[b] | | Experiment III[b] | |
	Normal	Hyper-lipemic	Normal	Hyper-lipemic	Normal	Hyper-lipemic
Phospholipid	68458	70958	2604	3926	4541	4430
Triglyceride	3038	4318	163	509	181	389
Cholesterol (free)	35539	8681	923	502	1180	375
Cholesterol (ester)[c]	3235	3990	48	101	34	39
% Cholesterol ester[c]	8.4%	31.7%	4.91%	16.8%	2.80%	9.35%
Cholesterol ester — fatty acid	1838	6083	72	314	53	167

[a]Dpm/25 ml. [b]Dpm/10^6 dpm I.M./μg lipid Pi. [c]Digitonin precipitable sterol.

Table 1 gives the data for the uptake and incorporation of ^{14}C-labelled acetate into various lipid fractions by the smooth muscle cells in culture. The presence of hyperlipemic serum in the incubation medium is associated with suppression of cholesterol synthesis. The incorporation of ^{14}C-labelled acetate into cholesterol ester-cholesterol, however, is increased in the cells exposed to hyperlipemic serum.

The increased formation of cholesterol ester is more apparent when the incorporation of ^{14}C-labelled acetate into cholesterol ester fatty acid is observed. In each experiment, there is a diversion of synthesized fatty acid to cholesterol ester in the presence of hyperlipemic serum.

The ^{3}H-cholesterol labelled lipoprotein was taken up more readily from the normal serum than from the hyperlipemic serum, but more marked esterification of the exogenously introduced cholesterol was apparent when hyperlipemic serum was added to the incubation medium. The stimulation of cholesterol ester synthesis from exogenously introduced cholesterol was similar in magnitude to that from the cholesterol synthesized from acetate.

In the second series of experiments, the removal of endogenously synthesized cholesterol was compared with that of cholesterol introduced as lipoprotein from the incubation medium. The removal rate of cholesterol ester from the cells was also compared with that of free cholesterol. Cells were pulse labelled for one day with ^{14}C-labelled acetate and ^{3}H-labelled cholesterol in lipoprotein, in an incubation medium containing 5% normal serum. After the 1-day pulse, on-labelled incubation medium was added, either normal or hyperlipemic. Duplicate or in some cases, triplicate samples were taken for analysis at daily intervals for 4 days.

Figure 1 shows the free cholesterol ester, cholesterol and liquid P content of the cells at the various time intervals. There were no appreciable changes in the phospholipid or free cholesterol content of the cells with time, or between the groups incubated with normal or hyperlipemic serum. In the cells incubated with normal serum, the cholesterol ester concentration remained constant. Where hyperlipemic serum was added, however, the cholesterol ester content increased markedly so that by 4 days it was approximately five times that of the cells grown in normal serum.

The removal of phospholipid, cholesterol and cholesterol ester synthesized from ^{14}C-labelled acetate in relation to time is plotted on a semilog basis in Figure 2.

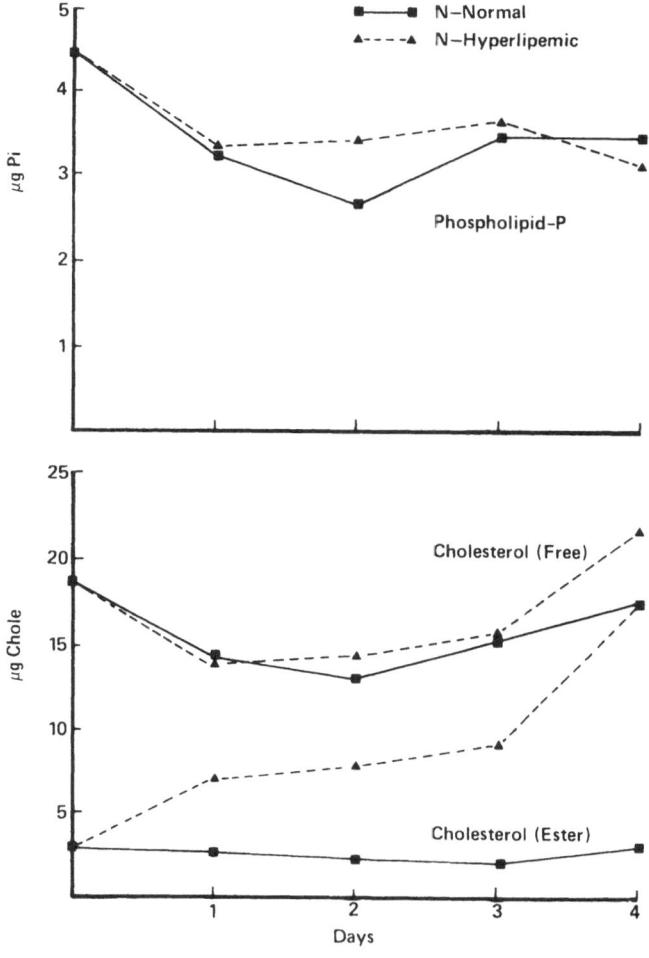

Figure 1. Chemical composition of smooth muscle cells in culture grown in the presence of normal and hyperlipemic serum

The curves are calculated from specific activity data for each fraction. The removal rate for the synthesized phospholipid is similar in the presence of normal or hyperlipemic serum. The removal of free cholesterol synthesized from ^{14}C-labelled acetate is accelerated in the presence of hyperlipemic serum presumably by exchange with the lipoprotein in the incubation medium. The removal rate for cholesterol ester is slower than that for free cholesterol but it is still removed at a significant rate over the 5-day period studied. Corresponding removal rate and calculated turnover half-times for the exogenously introduced cholesterol ester formed from it were observed.

The efflux of free cholesterol into the incubation medium (endogenous ^{14}C or exogenous ^{3}H-lipoprotein) is shown in Figure 3. It is apparent that for both hyperlipemic and normal serum the disappearance of labelled cholesterol from the cells can be accounted for by its appearance in the incubation medium. The corresponding data for cholesterol ester and phospholipid synthesized from acetate is shown in Figure 4. It is apparent that only a small proportion of the loss of these components from the cells can be accounted for by their appearance in the incubation medium. It is concluded, therefore, that cholesterol ester removal from the cells is dependant on hydrolysis and is facilitated by increasing the exchange of free cholesterol into the incubation medium.

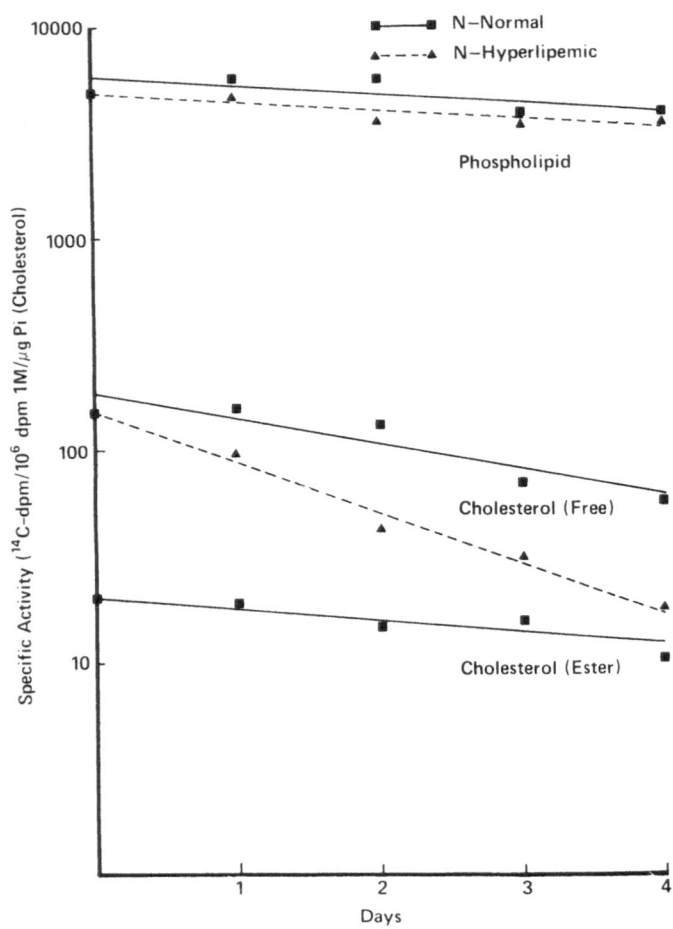

Figure 2. Removal of labelled phospholipid, cholesterol and cholesterol ester from smooth muscle cells in culture grown in the presence of normal and hyper-lipemic serum

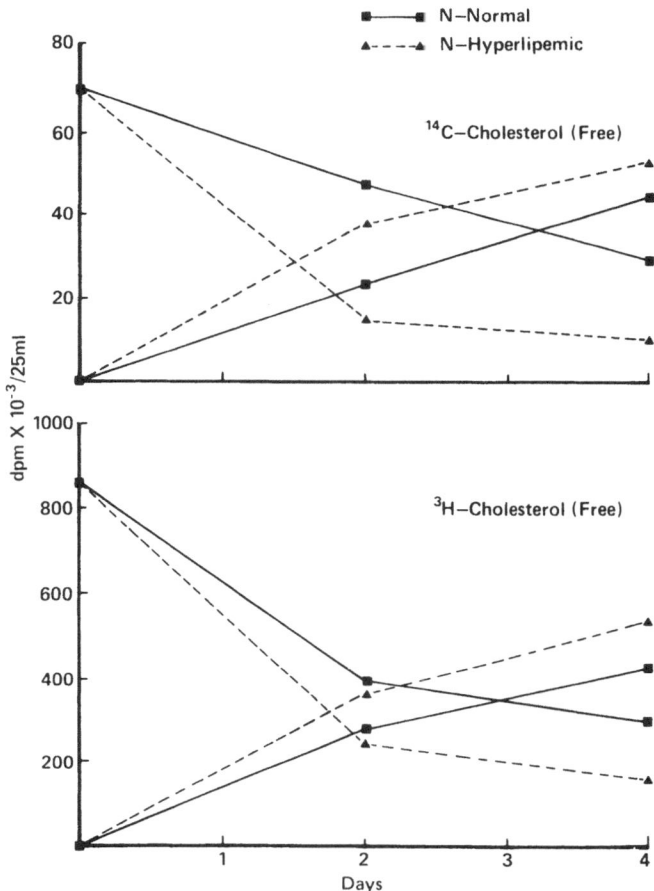

Figure 3. Efflux of endogenously (^{14}C) and exogenously synthesized cholesterol (^{3}H) from smooth muscle cells in culture grown in the presence of normal and hyperlipemic plasma. Falling curves represent cpm present in the cells while the rising curves represent the appearance of the respective fraction in the incubation medium

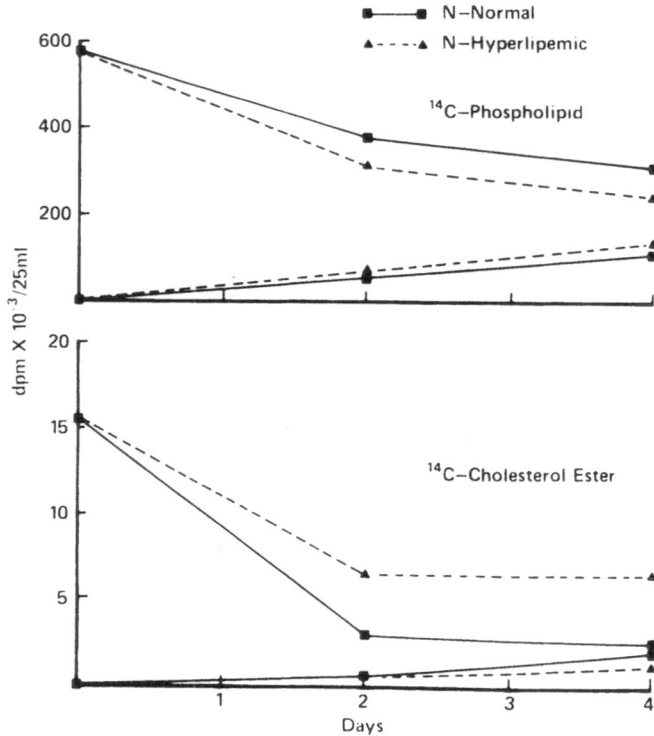

Figure 4. Efflux of endogenously synthesized phospholipid and cholesterol ester from smooth muscle cells in culture grown in the presence of normal and hyperlipemic serum. Falling curves represent dpm present in the cells while the rising curves represent the appearance of the respective fraction in the incubation medium

Summary

1. Smooth muscle cells in tissue culture show both an inhibition of cholesterol synthesis and a reciprocal accentuation of cholesterol ester formation when exposed to hyperlipemic serum.
2. Both endogenously synthesized cholesterol and exogenously introduced cholesterol penetrate to sites of cholesterol esterification in the cell and formation of cholesterol ester from both sources is stimulated.
3. Removal of free cholesterol (presumably by isotopic exchange) is accelerated in the presence of hyperlipemic serum.
4. Cholesterol ester removal from smooth muscle cells in culture is accelerated via its hydrolysis to free cholesterol and the subsequent removal of the formed free cholesterol from the cells.

PHYSICAL THEORY OF THE PERMEABILITY OF VASCULAR WALLS TO CHOLESTEROL AND ALBUMIN IN RELATION TO HEMODYNAMIC FACTORS

Syoten Oka
Department of Physiology, Kyorin University, School of Medicine, Mitaka, Tokyo/Japan

With regard to the role of hemodynamic factors in the development of atherosclerosis, the permeability of vascular walls to cholesterol and albumin is studied theoretically. Our theory is based on polymer physics and the theory of rate processes, the results being in good agreement with the experiment findings: i) the permeability P increases with the square of wall shear stress, ii) P increases with stretch ratio $\lambda^2-1)^2$, iii) P is enhanced by pulsatile strains, iv) P is significantly enhanced in the presence of vibration, v) P increases by increased circumferential tension due to hypertension, vi) positive circumferential tension is in general closely related with atherosclerosis, while it is not the case with negative circumferential tension, and vii) systolic pressure is more significant than diastolic pressure in the development of atherosclerosis due to hypertension.

STUDIES ON THE PERMEABILITY FACTOR IN ATHEROSCLEROSIS
1. PURIFICATION OF THE PERMEABILITY FACTOR OF RENAL ORIGIN

Toshiro Ooyama, Hajime Orimo, Kyoko Kawamura, and Mototake Murakami
Department of Internal Medicine, Municipal Geriatric Hospital, Tokyo/Japan

It has been recently reported that the permeability factor (PF) of renal origin is involved in the development of angionecrosis. The purpose of this report is to describe the preparation and purification method of non-renin PFs. The first step of the preparation procedure was the homogenization and the extraction of kidney tissue. Extract was separated to 4 PF fractions, namely 1,2,3 and 4, by Sephadex G-50 chromatography. Since PF3 and 4 which eluted in retarded fraction showed no renin activity, further purification of PF3 and 4 was performed. After concentrating PF 3 and 4, chromatography on Hydroxyl apatite was done. Throughout this step, PF3 and 4 were purified at 3 and 3.6 times respectively. Finally PF4 purified by Hydroxyl apatite was applied to DEAE-Sephadex A-50 and was fractionated. Throughout this step, PF4 was purified at 36 times of that of starting material. Physicochemical properties of these substances will be discussed.

STUDIES ON THE PERMEABILITY FACTOR IN ATHEROSCLEROSIS
2. PHARMACOLOGICAL PROPERTIES AND THE BIOLOGICAL SIGNIFICANCE OF THE PERMEABILITY FACTOR OF RENAL ORIGIN

Hajime Orimo, Toshiro Ooyama, Kyoko Kawamura, and Mototaka Murakami
Department of Internal Medicine, Municipal Geriatric Hospital, Tokyo/Japan

It has been recently reported that the permeability factor (PF) of renal origin other than renin is involved in atherogenesis. PF3 and 4 have been highly purified from renal extract of normal Wistar rats using chromatography on Sephadex G-50, Hydroxyl apatite and DEAE-Sephadex A-50 in this order. These substances did not contain any renin activity and protease activity. Its molecular weight was approximately 10000 and 5000 respectively. Permeability activity of PF3 and 4 lasted for 15-60 minutes and was partially inhibited by antihistamin. Such effect of PF4 was completely abolished by the heat treatment (56ºC) for 30 minutes, whereas that of PF3 was not affected. Intravenous administration of PF3 to normal rat resulted in a rise of hematocrit and a fall in plasma volume. Thus, we have confirmed the presence of renal PF other than renin in the kidney extract of normal rat. Effects of PFs on small artery and arteriole will be discussed.

ELECTRON MICROSCOPIC STUDY ON ATHEROGENESIS OF CEREBRAL AND CORONARY ARTERIES OF RABBITS

Takeshi Kurozumi and Kenzo Tanaka
Department of Pathology, Faculty of Medicine, Kyushu University, Fukuoka/Japan

There might be some differences in the atherogenesis among various arteries, and, in particular, cerebral artery shows resistance to the cholesterol induced atherosclerosis. In this study, cerebral and coronary arteries of cholesterol-fed rabbits with renovascular hypertension were examined at the ultrastructural level with reference to the changes of the vascular permeability. Foam cell accumulation was observed in the intima of coronary artery corresponding to the increased vascular permeability. Cerebral artery showed neither foam cell accumulation nor increased vascular permeability, but endothelial cells were detached from the basal lamina causing widening of the subendothelial space where electron dense materials were deposited. These findings might suggest the initial phase of atherosclerosis of cerebral artery. Evolution and progression of atherosclerosis of cerebral artery will be discussed, in comparison with those of coronary artery.

STUDIES ON THE PERMEABILITY TO LIPIDS AND LIPOPROTEINS OF INFLAMED SKIN CAPILLARIES (CANTHARIDINE-BLISTER-FLUID) IN HYPERLIPOPROTEINEMIAS (TYPE II a/b; IV)

W. Schwartzkopff and K. Peslin
Medical Clinic, Free University, Berlin-West/BRD

One factor in the pathogenesis of atherosclerosis is an alteration in permeability to lipids and lipoproteins in the wall of the greater vessels, of the arterioles and of the capillaries. A model to study the permeability of capillaries is the cantharidine blister fluid (CBF) and the filtrate which is passing through the membrane of the cantharidine-blister-base after applying negative pressure from 40 to 100 torr.
The concentration of lipids etc. is lower in the blister fluid than in the serum. There is no relation between the sieving quotient C2/C1 of proteins (0.65) and of lipids in type IIa (0.49), in type IIb (0.41), and in type IV (0.38). The concentration of lipids and lipoproteins in the CBF was not strictly correlated to those of the serum. In type IV the diffusion of the TG was more restricted (0.39) than in type II b/a (0.40). The three fractions of lipoproteins (LDL, VLDL, HDL) had nearly the same relative distribution in the CBF an in the serum. The percentage of LDL and VLDL was in the CBF lower than in the serum. There is no difference of concentration for the HDL between both fluids. The sieving quotient C2/C1 for the lipoproteins etc. was different in the three HLP-types. TG, VLDL, CH and LDL were mostly restricted in type IV (C2/C1: TG = 0.39; VLDL = 0.38; CH = 0.36; LDL = 0.35). But the concentration of CH and LDL in the CBF was greater in type IIa/b than in type IV. The volume of capillary filtrate (ml/cm^2/min/mm HG) was proportional to the negative pressure. With increasing filtrate volume the concentrations of lipids etc. decreased especially those of cholesterol and LDL. High blood pressure restricts the diffusion of cholesterol and LDL and promotes the deposition of these lipids in the vascular wall.

MOTILITY OF ARTERIAL SMOOTH MUSCLE CELL AND ATHEROSCLEROSIS

Nobuhiko Shibata, Akira Wada, Toru Yamagami, und Seiichi Toyama
The Center for Adult Diseases, Osaka, Osaka/Japan

Histological and biochemical investigation of aortic wall in experimental and
clinical atherosclerosis are presented in this study. At the initial stage (within a week) of cholesterol feeding to rabbits, lipid were observed histologically
in the intima of aorta, suggesting infiltration of lipid to the area directly
bathing with plasma. In the following early stage, smooth muscle cells in the
media located adjacent to the intima, which were originally arranged parallel
each other to the endothelial surface, were found to be arranged perpendicularly
to the surface and to be going to imigrate through intimal elastic lamina to the
intima. After two to three weeks, smooth muscle cells were accumulated in the
intima and they changed to so called "foam cell" probably due to phagocytosis of
lipid. The lipid containing cells which are thought to be derived from the foam
cells concerning with the first cellular response in atherosclerosis were further
studied in clinical atherosclerosis, demonstrating the intracellular localization
of the contractile protein and finding that myosin and actin content measured as
extracted contractile protein and the calcium sensitivity of the protein decreased as the disease advanced.

PREVENTION OF EXPERIMENTAL ATHEROSCLEROSIS IN RABBITS ON THE BASIS OF AUTOIMMUNE THEORY OF PATHOGENESIS

Anatoli Klimov, Yuri Zubzitsky, Vladimir Nagornev, Tatiana Loviagina, and Larisa
Petrova-Maslakova
Institute for Experimental Medicine, Leningrad/ USSR

It has been shown on the autopsy materials and in experiments on rabbits that
autoimmune complex consisting of the altered pre-β-lipoprotein (antigen) and
IgG (antibody) appears in the blood plasma and the arterial wall during the development of atherosclerosis. C_1^3 complement is fixed to this complex.
Tolerance to experimental atherosclerosis has been achieved through immunization
of newborn rabbits with a fraction of pre-β-lipoprotein (VLDL) isolated from
the serum of adult rabbits with experimental atherosclerosis.
In the plasma of immunized (in contrast to nonimmunized) rabbits there were no
circulating autoimmune complexes and the content of arginine-rich apolipoprotein
was very low when the animals has been kept on atherogenic diet 4 months after
immunization.

THE PERMEABILITY TO PLASMA MACROMOLECULES OF AORTIC ENDOTHELIUM IN COCKERELS

Søren Christensen and Henning Nielsen
Departments of Physiology and Medical Biochemistry, University of Aarhus,
Aarhus/Denmark

Estrogen-treated, hyperlipidemic, donor cockerels were injected with 2.5 mCi
32-P-phosphate per kg b.w. and exsanguinated after 24 hours. The phosphoprotein-
32-P of the donor plasma showed one concentration max. during elution from
Sepharose 6B columns corresponding to a MW of 0.8×10^6. The major part of the
phospholipid-32-P eluted corresponding to a MW about 3.4×10^6.
Normolipidemic birds were transfused with the labelled plasma and sacrificed at
7, 60, 300 and 600 minutes. Aortic intima-media was studied for uptake of 32-P-
labelled phosphoproteins, phosphatidylethanolamine, phosphatidylcholine, sphin-
goyeline and the acidic phospholipids plus lysolecithin. Further, the average
plasma conc.'s of labelled substances were determined. Intimal clearances (μl
$cm^{-2}h^{-1}$) were calculated for the five substance groups. Significant positive cor-

relations were present between phosphoprotein intimal clearances and the intimal clearances of any of the four P-lipid groups. The term $\mu l\ cm^{-2} hour^{-1}$ is equal to $2.78 \times 10^{-7}\ cm\ sec^{-1}$, and the results may possibly be taken as permeability coefficients for the endothelium. We obtained for phosphoprotein a value of $3.8 \times 10^{-8}\ cm\ sec^{-1}$, and for phosphatidylethanolamine and phosphatidylcholine, 2.4 and $2.3 \times 10^{-8}\ cm\ sec^{-1}$, respectively. The phospholipids were probably taken up as components of plasma lipoproteins, functioning as tracers for these.

ULTRASTRUCTURE OF THE AORTIC SURFACE IN FOCAL AREAS OF IN VIVO EVANS BLUE UPTAKE IN THE RABBIT

Knud Kjeldsen and Henrik Klem Thomsen
Department of Clinical Chemistry CL, Rikshospitalet, Copenhagen/Denmark

The aortic endothelial cell morphology was investigated in areas showing Evans Blue dye uptake and compared to areas not showing Evans Blue dye uptake. In 'white' areas the endothelial cells measured 50-80 x 10-15 μm and were oriented with their longitudinal axis parallel to the direction of the blood flow. The intercellular junctions were covered by a number of interdigitating endothelial flaps. In 'blue' areas the endothelial cells showed a more irregular pattern, had more protruding nuclei and were shorter, measuring 40-60 x 10-15 μm. The endothelial flap arrangement was identical. No 'stomata' or 'stigmata' were observed.
In the 'blue' areas a number of dilated, insufficient junctions were seen, possibly due to contraction of the endothelial cells. The hypothesis is put forward, that the intercellular junctions and the endothelial flaps together form a selective and dynamic structure regulating intimal transport of macromolecules. It is also suggested that the characteristic ultrastructure of the 'blue' areas contribute to the understanding of the increased permeability and accelerated atherogenesis in areas of dye uptake.

HYPOTHESIS ON THE CIRCULATION OF LIPIDS WITHIN FIBROUS PLAQUES

Clarke Stout
Department of Pathology, University of Texas, Medical Branch, Galveston, TX/USA

The present report is an attempt to determine the nature of the circulation of plasma components within fibrous plaques by studying the pattern of lipid distribution and gelatinous lesions within the plaques. The material was obtained from aortas from 405 mammals and birds dying in the Oklahoma City Zoo. Analysis of the pattern of lipid distribution in 187 lipid containing aortic fibrous plaques suggested that most of the lipids entered the plaques at the shoulders and circulated from there toward the centers, usually in the outermost layers (the layer adjacent to the media) of the plaques. Analysis of step serial sections from 3 aortic fibrous plaques from an ostrich showed that gelatinous lesions appeared to originate at plaque shoulders and occasionally to penetrate toward the plaque centers, again in the outermost layer of the plaque. These morphologic findings suggest a lateral circulation of plasma components through fibrous plaques, and provide a mechanism for the accumulation of lipids within the deeper layers of fibrous plaques. Alterations in this circulation could play a role in the conversion of fibrous plaques to atheromatous plaques.
(Supported in part by HE 08725, USPHS.)

HOW DO BLOOD PLASMA PROTEIN AND LIPID ENTER THE ARTERIAL WALL? LIGHT AND ELECTRON MICROSCOPIC STUDIES ON THE HUMAN CEREBRAL ARTERIES

Yoji Yoshida, Hiroko Shinkai, Noriyuki Sakata, and Genju Ooneda
Department of Pathology, School of Medicine, Gunma University, Maebashi/Japan

One of the key points of atherosclerosis research is to clarify how blood plasma constituents enter the arterial wall. We have had limited information concerned with this problem in human arteries. Light microscopic study on the human cerebral arteries often revealed that foam cells and extracellular lipid insudated into both periphery of the thickened intima and at junctions between each layer of the laminatedly thickened intima. Furthermore, electron microscopy frequently showed degeneration and necrosis with resultant desquamation of endothelial cells covering these predilection sites of lipid entry. These endothelial injuries might result from a tearing force which was produced at the junctions of each layer of the arterial wall, since smooth muscle cells existing in each layer contracted in different directions due to their specific arrangement. Localized medial hypertrophy and injured internal elastic lamina were almost always observed at the sites where inner layer of the thickened intima containing a lot of smooth muscle cells attached to the media. These changes would suggest that the above mentioned force might occur there.

CHOLESTERYL ESTER AND TRIGLYCERIDE HYDROLYSIS BY A LYSOSOMAL ENZYME FROM RABBIT AORTIC TISSUE

Peter Brecher, Hae Yung Pyun, and Aram V. Chobanian
Cardiovascular Institute, Boston University School of Medicine, Boston, MA/USA

A sensitive and reproducible method for assaying aortic cholesterol esterase was developed using phospholipid vesicles as a vehicle for introducing cholesteryl oleate into aqueous systems. We demonstrated the presence of cholesterol esterase with an acid pH optimum in subcellular fractions of rabbit aortic homogenates. Cofactors were not required for enzymatic activity and specificity studies indicated that both cholesteryl esters and triglycerides were hydrolyzed whereas the phospholipid contained in the vesicles was not affected. Subcellular fractionation studies supported a lysosomal origin for the lipolytic activity. In comparative studies, atherosclerotic lesions contained several-fold more activity than non-involved aortic segments with respect to both cholesteryl ester and triglyceride hydrolysis. Increases in activity of several other lysosomal enzymes were also observed in the atherosclerotic segments. These studies indicate that in contrast to the previously reported observations with non-lysosomal cholesterol esterase, the activity of a lysosomal esterase is increased in atherosclerotic tissue along with that of other lysosomal enzymes. The proportionate increases in hydrolysis of both cholesteryl ester and triglyceride suggest that a single lipolytic enzyme may be involved in this process.

IDENTIFICATION OF FIVE EXISTENCE FORMS OF LIPIDS ACCUMULATING IN ATHEROSCLEROSIS

Yoshiya Hata and Toshiharu Ishii
Department of Medicine and Pathology, Keio University, School of Medicine, Tokyo/Japan

One of the major biochemical changes in human and experimental atherosclerosis is the accumulation of lipids, particularly cholesteryl esters and phospholipids, in the arterial tissues. However, the physico-chemical state of lipids and their localization within the lesion have not been clearly identified in the environment of arterial tissues.

By using ordinary and polarizing light microscopy, together with silver nitrate staining and immunofluorescent method, we have identified 5 forms of existence in lipids accumulating in atherosclerotic lesions: (i) lipids bound to cell membranes and interstitial substances, (ii) lipids in the soluble form of lipoproteins incorporated into the cytosol and insudated into the intercellular space of intima and medial cells, (iii) lipids as anisotropic inclusions mostly present in the cytosol of modified smooth muscle cells, (iv) lipids as isotropic inclusions present mainly in the extracellular space, and (v) lipids in the form of solid crystals separated out in the lesion tissues.

Identification of these 5 forms of lipids makes us enable to investigate the role of lipids in atherogenesis with a more comprehensive view.

INFLUENCE OF ATHEROSCLEROSIS, HIGH-FAT DIET AND DIABETES ON AORTIC ACYL-CoA HYDROLASE ACTIVITY

Sam Hashimoto and Seymour Dayton
VA Wadsworth Hospital Center, and UCLA School of Medicine, Los Angeles, CA/USA

During atherogenesis, cholesteryl ester synthesis in aortic microsomes is augmented. Since the rate of cholesteryl ester synthesis is dependent in part on the acyl-CoA concentration, slowed degradation of acyl-CoA would favor increased cholesteryl ester synthesis. We have tested the possibility that imparied hydrolysis of acyl-CoA may contribute to atherogenesis. Acyl-CoA hydrolase activity was reduced in atherosclerotic microsomes (rabbit) to approximately 40% of the normal activity, supporting the hypothesis. The influence of nutritional status and diabetes on the activity of this enzyme was investigated. Fasting rabbits for 16 hr diminished the acyl-CoA hydrolase activity about 30%. The type of fat in the diet influences the acyl-CoA hydrolase activity: oils containing 75% oleic acid (high-oleic safflower oil) and containing 80% linoleic acid (conventional safflower oil) lowered the acyl-CoA hydrolase activity in comparison to a more saturated fat (cocoa butter). Aortic microsomes from rats made diabetic by streptozotocin exhibited higher acyl-CoA hydrolase activity than normal. The results show that conditions associated with human atherogenesis (diabetes and saturated fat diet) increase rather than suppress the activity of this enzyme. Possible inferences: other, more potent mechanisms are dominant in these situation; or high acyl-CoA hydrolase activity does not mitigate atherogenesis. (Supported in part by Arthur Dodd Fuller Foundation and by NIH Grant HE-03734.)

FATTY ACID SYNTHESIS IN DOG AORTAS AND IN CORONARY ARTERIES

Ingeborg R. Kupke
Huntington Memorial Hospital, Pasadena, University of Southern California, Los Angeles, CA/USA
Pediatric Clinic, University of Düsseldorf, Düsseldorf/BRD

The incorporation of ^{14}C-acetate into the acylglycerol-fatty acids synthesized by chain elongation (FA >C 16) was studied in perfused dog aortas and in coron. arteries. The FA were separated by TLC and by radio-GLC. (Data as percent ^{14}C-activity of total FA in acylglycerols.)

Diacylglycerols (DG)	Adventitia	Media	Intima	Coron. artery
control	51.4 ± 6.4	77.7 ± 3.1	47.0 ± 4.0	53.9
atherogenic diet	66.3 ± 8.6	90.4 ± 0.9	63.8 ± 6.7	78.5 ± 1.8
Triacylglycerols (TG)				
control	49.8 ± 5.6	61.1 ± 6.0	58.9 ± 8.9	46.6 ± 0.6
atherogenic diet	-	76.5 ± 4.3	76.6 ± 7.1	82.4 ± 2.9

As compared to the other aortic layers of the controls, the DG of the media are the predominant acceptors for FA >C16 (P <0.0025). Apparently, chain elongation

as an ATP saving process is favored in the media suggesting artificial or physiological hypoxia in this layer. This hypoxic effect is pronounced by the diet.
Under the influence of the diet, the TG of the media (P <0.05) and of the coron.
arteries (P <0.0005) incorporate higher amounts of FA >C16. However, the coron.
arteries are more severely affected, as compared to the aortas (Kupke, 1972).

CHOLESTEROL CONTENT IN ARTERIAL TISSUE AND IN SERUM LIPOPROTEINS IN MAN

Göran Bondjers, Anders Gustafson, John Kral, Tore Scherstén, and Lars Sjöström
Department of Internal Medicine I, Göteborg University, Göteborg/Sweden

A decreased level of cholesterol in serum high density lipoproteins (HDL) is
suggested to be related to the development of atherosclerosis in man. - In thirteen individuals (11 females and 2 males) operated on for obesity by an intestinal shunt, the cholesterol content of mesenteric arterial tissue was related to
the cholesterol content of serum lipoprotein fractions. - There was a positive
correlation (r_s = 0.545) between LDL- and arterial tissue cholesterol while
there was a negative relationship between the cholesterol concentrations in HDL
and arterial tissue (r_s = -0.804). In this small group of subjects there were
no interrelationships among cholesterol content in various lipoprotein fractions
or with serum lipid values. - With the background of recent experience in studies
of cholesterol transfer in vitro in experimental animals and in man, it is suggested that HDL may participate in the elimination of cholesterol in arterial
tissue. Therefore, decreased HDL-cholesterol may precede the development of atherosclerotic arterial disease, rather than being a secondary effect of it. Thus,
low HDL-cholesterol should be regarded as an additional risk factor for the
development of atherosclerotic arterial disease.

INHIBITION OF CHOLESTEROL UPTAKE INTO THE ARTERIAL WALL BY 7-KETOCHOLESTEROL

R.J. Bing, J.S.M. Sarma, R. Fischer, and Y. Maruyama
Huntington Institute of Applied Medical Research and Huntington Memorial Hospital,
Pasadena and the University of Southern California, Los Angeles, CA/USA

The effect of an inhibitory steroid, 7-ketocholesterol on cholesterol uptake by
the arterial wall of human and animal coronary arteries was studied in vitro and
in vivo. In vitro: prior to adding to perfusate 7-ketocholesterol and ^{3}H-choles-
terol were bound to plasma lipoproteins by sonication. In vivo: i.v. injection
of 7-ketocholesterol was solubilized with bile salts. When 7-ketocholesterol was
fed it was suspended in a mixture of bile salts and lecithin. ^{14}C-7-ketocholes-
terol was used for turnover studies in vivo. In in vitro perfusion, 7-ketocholes-
terol inhibited uptake of cholesterol by the arterial wall by 90%. I.V. injection
of solubilized 7-ketocholesterol into rabbits inhibited cholesterol uptake by the
arterial wall by 30%. No inhibiton was noticed after gastric feeding. ^{14}C-7-keto-
cholesterol is chiefly excretet in the bile with little deposition in the arterial
wall.

PHOSPHOLIPID METABOLISM IN ARTERIAL WALL

Akio Kikuchi, Hiroshi Shigematsu, Kazuo Aihara, Yoshiya Hata, and Yuichiro Goto
Department of Medicine, Keio University, School of Medicine, Tokyo/Japan

To elucidate the role of phospholipids (PL) in progression and regression of atherosclerosis, 50 μCi of emulcified ^{14}C-dilinoleyol lecithin was injected into 25

fasting rabbits fed normal pellets (body wt. 3120±350 g). ^{14}C-Lecithin was rapidly incorporated into lipoprotein PL and transfered to lipoprotein cholesteryl esters (CE) in VLDL+LDL and HDL fractions. The half life time gained from the specific activity (SE) curves were 15 hours for VLDL+LDL-PL and 20 hours for HDL-PL. The ratios of DPM of CE/PL were e.g. 0.43 in VLDL+LDL and 0.30 in HDL at 24 hours. Labelled lipoprotein lipids were also incorporated into aortic tissue, whose uptake curve consisted of three phases: the first steep rise in 1 hour, the second rapid decrease in 6 hours, and the third almost stationary phase in 48 hours. From CE fraction of aortic tissue, no significant counts were gained, thus the DPM ratios of CE/PL in serum lipoproteins were not maintained in the arterial tissue. These results indicated that the uptake of lipids in normal arteries with an integrated endothelium occurred predominantly in the form of molecular flux, rather than a penetration of lipoproteins in a particulate form across the cell wall.

RELATIONSHIP BETWEEN LOW DENSITY LIPOPROTEIN STRUCTURE AND ITS INTERACTION WITH ARTERIAL WALL COMPONENTS: A PROCESS PROBABLY CONTRIBUTING TO HUMAN ATHEROGENESIS

Germán Camejo, Harry Acquatella, Salvador Waich, and Fernando Lalaguna
Instituto Venezolano de Investigaciones Ceintíficas (IVIC), Apdo. 1827, Hospital Universitario and Hospital Carlos Arvelo, Caracas/Venezuela

A particle made of proteoglycan and lipids has been isolated from human arterial intima media (Camejo et al., Atherosclerosis, 21:77, 1975), and it specifically forms insoluble complexes with serum LDL. Serum LDL from 55 acute ischemic heart-disease patients form almost twice the amount of insoluble complex with the arterial lipoprotein complexing factor (LCF), than 50 apparently healthy controls (P <0.005). Also, 56 chronic ischemic patients have LDL with a higher affinity for the arterial factor than 103 controls (P <0.02). The LDL of high reactivity towards the arterial factor (LCF) has differences of surface charge measured by isoelectric focusing, lipid composition and apoprotein pattern, established by SDS-pore gradient acrylamide gel electrohporesis, when compared with LDL of low reactivity towards the arterial factor. It is proposed that this structural change leading to a higher reactivity towards arterial components could be another factor controlling the extent of LDL trapping in the arterial wall and the development of the atherosclerotic lesion.

HIGH DENSITY LIPOPROTEIN (HDL) DEPENDENT ELIMINATION OF CHOLESTEROL FROM NORMAL ARTERIAL TISSUE IN MAN

Göran Bondjers, Gun Olsson, Lise-Lotte Nyman, and Sören Björkerud
Department of Internal Medicine I, University of Göteborg, Göteborg/Sweden

HDL-cholesterol is low in patients with clinical complications to atherosclerosis. However, it may be disputed whether this represents a primary or secondary event in the pathophysiology of the disease. In the present study cholesterol transfer in vitro between HDL and arterial tissue from young human subjects without known complications of atherosclerosis was investigated. - Arterial biopsies were obtained in mesenteric tissue from patients operated on for obesity by intestinal shunt. The arteries were incubated with HDL from the same subjects. - The cholesterol concentration of the incubation medium increased during a 4 hr incubation. Simultaneously, the cholesterol concentration of the tissue decreased, suggesting actual elimination from the tissue. For each individual, cholesterol transfer was not affected when the lipoprotein concentration in the medium changed from 12.5 to 100% of that in serum. On the other hand, elimination decreased with increasing total serum cholesterol of the patients. - The results suggest that HDL promotes cholesterol elimination from normal arterial tissue in man. Therefore, sufficient levels of HDL may be necessary for the maintenance of normal tissue cholesterol concentrations. Consequently, changes in HDL may precede the development of atherosclerosis, rather than being a secondary effect of it. Obviously, the decreased HDL-dependent cholesterol elimination in hypercholesterolemia may prove to have important pathophysiological implications.

COMPARATIVE STUDY OF LIPOPROTEINS OF THE HUMAN PLASMA AND AORTIC WALL: APOLIPOPROTEIN AND FATTY ACID COMPOSITION

Anatoli Klimov and Alexander Denisenko
Institute for Experimental Medicine, Leningrad/USSR

Immunological identity of apo-ala, apo-glu, apo-ser, apo-gln I and apo-gln 2 of serum lipoproteins and lipoproteins of the aortic tissue fluid prepared according to earlier described method (A.N. Klimov et al., Atherosclerosis, 1974, 19, 243) was shown by immunodiffusion technique.
Fatty acid composition of cholesteryl esters, triglycerides, and phospholipids extracted from the serum VLDL, LDL, and HDL was very similar to those extracted from the aortic tissue fluid lipoproteins.
The data obtained indicate that aortic lipoproteins are likely to be derived from the circulation.

IMMUNOHISTOLOGICAL STUDIES OF ARTERIAL LIPOPROTEIN ACCUMULATION

M. Harada, T. Yasugi, T. Shimizu, I. Kobayashi, H. Matsumoto, K. Hoshino, and M. Hatano
Department of Medicine, Nihon University, School of Medicine, Tokyo/Japan

Fluorescent antibody technique has been employed to identify native tissue antigens in study of rabbit aortic LP. Specific antibody to serum LDL has been used as a histochemical stain to demonstrate the presence of LP in the wall. Histological materials from aorta have been obtained from normal, 1%-cholesterol fed, renovascular hypertension lorded and immunological treated (BSA) rabbits. Result: 1) Immunofluorescin (IF) in the aortic wall was not observed in the normal group. 2) In the chol. fed group, IF was observed 1 week after the administration. And, the degree of the LP accumulation of the aorta appeared in proportion to extent and duration of lipidemia. 3) In the hypertensive group, LP was found inside the intima without lipidemia and increased with time course. 4) In the BSA group, LP invaded the intima within 1 week after the administration, then, decreased gradually 2-3 week later. Conclusion: Lipidemia affected the LP accumulation in the arterial wall. Hypertension and immunological reaction also may accerelate the uptake of serum LP into the arterial wall. However, influence of immunological reaction seems to be temporary.

UPTAKE OF LOW DENSITY LIPOPROTEIN AND ALBUMIN BY RABBIT AORTIC INTIMA-MEDIA IN VIVO AND IN VITRO

Santibrata Ghosh, Jacob N. Finkelstein, and John S. Schweppe
Department of Biochemistry, Northwestern University Medical School, Chicago, IL/USA

A knowledge of the mechanism of lipoprotein uptake by arterial wall is critical to our understanding of the atherosclerotic process. We have measured the uptake of ^{125}I labeled low density lipoprotein (LDL) and albumin (SA) in vivo in rabbit thoracic aorta. From a kinetic analysis of the uptake at different times, we have calculated the rates of arterial influx and efflux for these molecules. LDL showed an increased influx over albumin indicating an enrichment of LDL in aorta, compared to SA. A similar higher uptake of LDL compared to albumin by the intima-media of thoracic aorta was found in *in vitro* incubations (lactated Ringer's buffer, 37°C). Using this model system the effect of various factors on the uptake was determined with a view to elucidating the mechanism of the uptake process. The concentration dependence of uptake showed that it was non-saturable for SA, whereas for LDL there was a saturable as well as a non-saturable aspect. The saturable uptake of LDL was inhibited by VLDL but not by HDL. Inhibitors like cyanide, and low temperature (4°C) inhibited the saturable uptake of LDL but not the uptake of albumin or inulin. The above results are consistent with the saturable uptake of LDL being a receptor mediated endocytotic process.

WORKSHOP 2. Hypertension, Arteriolar Disease and Atherosclerosis

Chairmen: H. Jellinek, Hungary
           G. Ooneda, Japan

Participants: I.K. Shkhvatsabaya, UdSSR
              R.F. Scott, USA
              H. Jellinek, Hungary
              Y. Yamori, Japan
              Y. Yoshida, Japan

POSSIBILITIES OF HYALINE FORMATION IN THE VESSEL WALL, LIGHT- AND ELECTRON MICROSCOPIC STRUCTURE: PROBLEMS OF NOMENCLATURE

H. Jellinek

With the collaboration of I. Hüttner

"Hyaline" is a collective term which was generally employed in vascular pathology to denote the substance taking on a homogenous blue trichrom stain. Lendrum (1963, 1967) was the first to attempt identification of various forms of hyaline by staining techniques developed specially for this purpose. However, nomenclatural confusion still prevails with respect to the definition of hyaline and fibrinoid and the transistory stage between the two.

Two main forms of hyaline are encountered in vascular changes, viz:
1. Primary hyaline
2. Secondary hyaline

1. Increase of vascular permeability disorder plays an important role in the formation of the primary hyaline (Bálint et al., 1974; Elemér et al., 1975; Hüttner et al., 1968, 1969a, 1969b, 1969c, 1970; Jellinek, 1974; Jellinek et al., 1966, 1967, 1969, 1970; Kerényi and Jellinek, 1972; Kerényi et al., 1966, 1975; Veress et al., 1970.) Increased permeability disorder results either in plasmatic vasculosis or intimal edema which initially contains proteins of small molecular size; these accumulate in the subendothelial space, causing distension thereof (Constantinides and Robinson, 1969; Dustin, 1962; Eto et al., 1975; French, 1966; Frost, 1972; Gardner and Matthews, 1969; Giese, 1961; Haust, 1971; Nelson et al., 1975; Ooneda et al., 1965; Shainoff et al., 1972; Shimamoto and Numano, 1969; Shimamoto et al., 1969, 1973; Shimamoto and Sunaga, 1972; Still, 1967; Trillo et al., 1970; Weber et al., 1973; Wiener et al., 1965). At this stage, the lesion is stained blue by azan stain and yellowish by Mallory's phosphotungstic acid stain (hereafter referred to as Mallory's stain).

The plasma substances taking on blue azan and yellow Mallory's stain show a granular structure on electron microscopic examination. As the initial signs of permeability increase, the endothelial cells become rich in organelles, and a basement membranelike granular substance appears in the subendothelial space. These two types form the electron microscopic substrate of primary hyaline (Fig. 1).

The above types of change are found in rapidly developing disorders of permeability, the most striking example of which are the vascular lesions associated with allergic mechanisms. In such cases, accumulation of plasma proteins of small molecular weight causes widening of the vessel wall which takes on blue azan and yellow Mallory's stain.

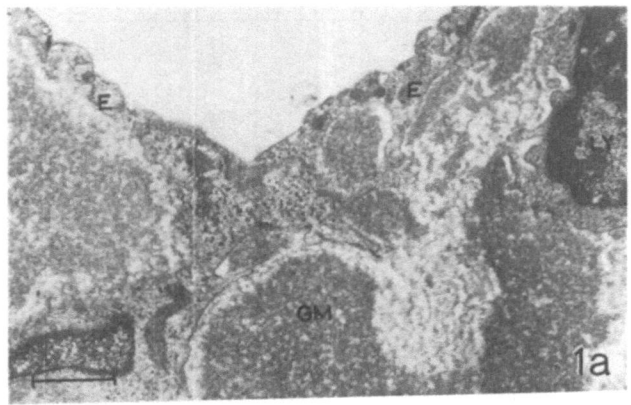

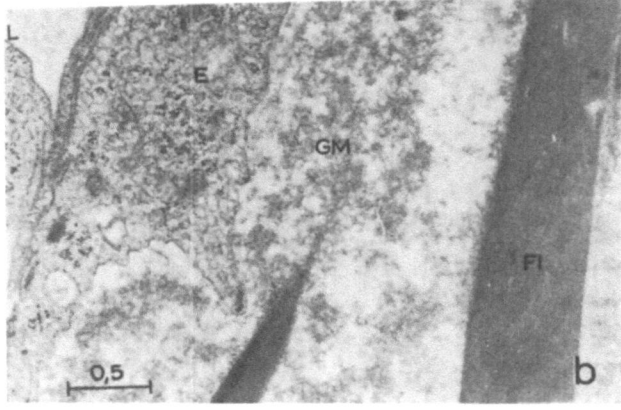

Figure 1. (a) A granular matter (GM) accumulates beneath the endothelial cells
in the initial stage of plasma influx. LY: lymphocyte. (b) On severe vascular
injury, apart from the granular matter (GM), fibrin (FI), showing a well-defined
periodicity, is also deposited beneath the endothelial cells (E). L: vascular
lumen

Such lesions are found for example in small arteries of the spleen, as accompanying phenomena of various kinds of inflammatory (infectious) conditions. A
similar change could be produced experimentally by inducing lymph stasis which
resulted in mural retention of plasma owing to interference with transport across
the vessel wall. Initially, the intramural plasma deposition stains blue with
azan. Similar phenomena were also encountered in the initial stage of plasma accumulation in slowly progressive hypertension.

The above change represents the primary hyaline. Its development is due to moderate injury of the vessel wall by various factors. The process of primary hyaline
formation is reversible, because if plasma flow across the vessel wall ceases,
the intramural plasma deposition becomes absorbed and the lesions heal completely.

2. Chiefly the same factors are also responsible for the development of the
secondary hyaline, but in this type of change apart from plasma substances, fibrinogen and fibrin also become deposited inside the vessel wall, and the final
stage is their transformation, viz. the production of a basement membrane-like
substance. The process of secondary hyaline formation has several stages:

a) The development of secondary hyaline is usually introduced by acute vascular
changes. The primary hyaline progresses to a characteristic fibrinoid lesion as
vascular injury increases. In light micrographs, the vascular fibrinoid takes on

red azan and black Mallory's stain. Appearance of fibrinogen, viz. fibrin in the subendothelial space, can be held responsible for these colors. The presence of fibrinogen or fibrin is shown by increased birefringence under the polarization microscope, and the characteristic structure of fibrin is demonstrable by phase contrast microscopy.

b) The azan-positive and Mallory-positive subendothelial fibrinoid shows characteristic structural details on electron microscopic examination. At the beginning of plasma flow across the vessel wall, only the accumulation of a basement membrane-like substance is seen. This also corresponds with the electron microscopic appearance of the primary hyaline. Later, apart from the accumulation of plasma substances, precipitation of fibrin showing a regular periodic structure (periodicity: 220) takes place. The amount of granular plasma substances and of fibrin tends to increase, depending on the degree of injury, until they become agglomerated, resulting in the formation of crystalline bodies (Ooneda et al., 1965; Figs. 1-3). The crystalline bodies usually exhibit a striation of 1600-2200 Å periodicity, the structure of which has been studied by us in greater detail.

Kerényi's (Kerényi et al., 1966) examinations have disproved the tendency of regarding the striation as an artifact. The latter judgement was based on the observation that fewer striated crystalline bodies are encountered on processing

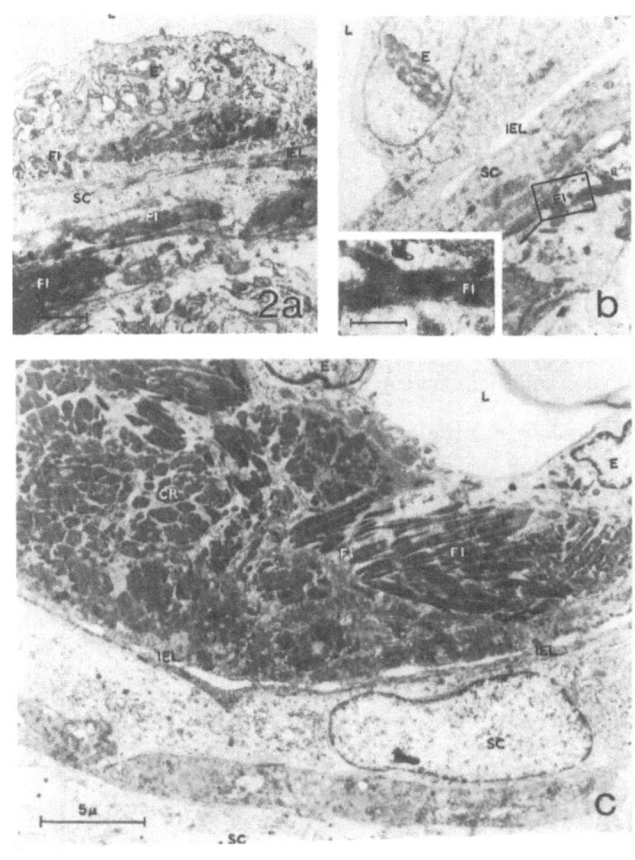

Figure 2. (a) Note deposition of fibrin (FI) in the broadened subendothelial space. The same can be seen in Figure 2 (b) *Insets*: elementary structure of fibrin with fibrillar elements spaced at 60 Å. (c) Apart from fibrin structures, developing crystalline bodies are also seen in the broadened subendothelial space L = lumen, E = endothelial cell, IEL = internal elastic lamina, SC = smooth muscle cell

with a diamond knife than with a glass knife. However, the opposite tendencies of the striation pattern weighed against its being an artifact.

Kerényi et al. (1966) established on tilting the preparations that the distance of periodicity did not change.

On tilting preparations containing crystalline bodies of broad periodocity at $\pm 15^\circ$ angle to the striation as an axis, no alteration of the periodicity occurred, and changes in dimension at 0° angle were only those related to projection. It follows that the broad periodicity is clearly not a summation phenomenon.

According to certain data in the literature and our own experience, the broad periodicity can be regarded as the morphologic manifestation of biochemical heterogeneity. On digestion of ultrathin preparations with 1.25% trypsin, the broad-periodicity crystalline bodies became almost homogeneous, only the 90-110 Å striation, generally characteristic of fibrin, having persisted in them.

c) The crystalline bodies aggregate more and more densely as time progresses. The granular substances originally filling the interspaces between them disappear gradually until they cling together and finally, a greyish mass, still showing periodicity in places, fills the entire subendothelial space (Figs. 3a and 3b). At this stage, reactions to azan and Mallory's stains gradually display bluish and yellowish hues, respectively, in light micrographs, red and black colors being seen only sporadically in those places in which the fibrin structures are still preserved. This transitory stage is referred to as the fibrinoid, viz. hyaline change (Figs. 3a and 3b).

d) The substance localizing subendothelially between endothelial cells and internal elastic membrane tends to become more and more homogeneous in a later stage. The last indications of striated pattern disappear and at this stage, the subendothelial lesion takes on blue azan and yellow Mallory's stain. Electron microscopically myeline figures and lipid-like substances are demonstrable at this stage, which ensues as a rule after 6-8 weeks. The electron microscopic substrate seen in the hyaline change accounts for the characteristic sudanophilia of hyalinosclerosis, which had previously been attributed to the lipids. The appearance of lipids is a secondary phenomenon, due in all probability to the permeability-decreasing, filtrating effect of the broadened subendothelial hyaline substance.

e) Depolarization of fibrin is an important element in the process of hyalinization. The fibrin structures and crystalline structures described above may also show the phenomena of degradation without previous merging and homogenization (Fig. 4). Light granular details appear in the depolymerized fibrin at the central parts of the crystalline bodies, and these result in the disappearance of fibrin, often showing a very variated appearance as they grow larger. The fibrinolytic activity of the cells plays an important role in fibrin depolymerization, to judge from in vitro experimental and practical observations (Clark and Collins, 1969; Krakow et al., 1972; Pauit et al., 1972; Shainoff et al., 1972; Todd, 1959; Warren and Khan, 1974).

f) In places, active cellular phagocytosis is responsible for fibrinolysis. In such cases, fibrin, still showing a regular periodicity, can be identified inside the cytoplasm (Fig. 5), whereas in other places, depolymerization of fibrin gives rise to the formation of membrane-coated fibrin residues showing a lysosomal structure.

g) Injury of the vascular wall causes destruction of the muscle cells also in the media (Kerényi et al., 1966, 1975; Kerényi and Jellinek, 1972), and cell deterioration is due to the influx of plasma. Inflowing plasma and the deteriorating muscle cells join to form the medial part of the vascular fibrinoid, in which the subendothelial fibrin is substituted by the necrotic degradation products of muscle cells. Fibrin is also demonstrable in the media, but crystalline bodies

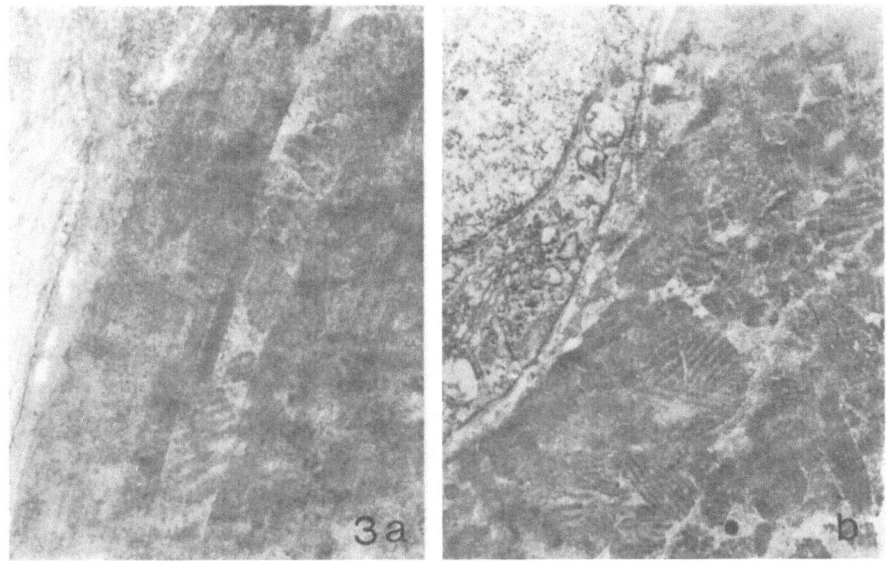

Figure 3. (a) Apart from structures showing the regular periodicity of fibrin, bodies exhibiting a broad striped pattern are also seen in the subendothelial space. The latter bodies represent the transitory stage. (b) Only bodies showing the broad striation are now seen in the subendothelial space

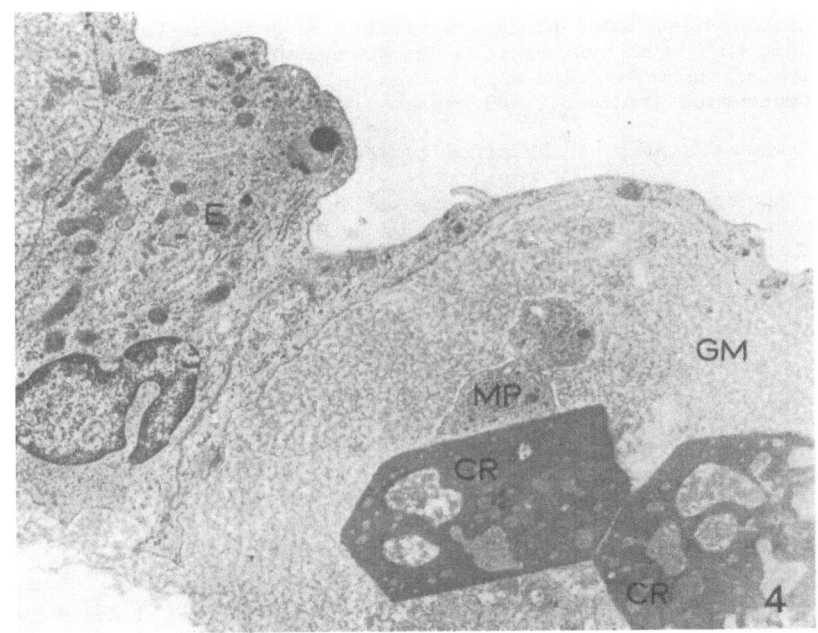

Figure 4. Crystalline bodies (CB) showing depolymerization appear between the granular matter (GM) beneath the endothelial cells (E). Transformation begins at the central parts. MP: cell process

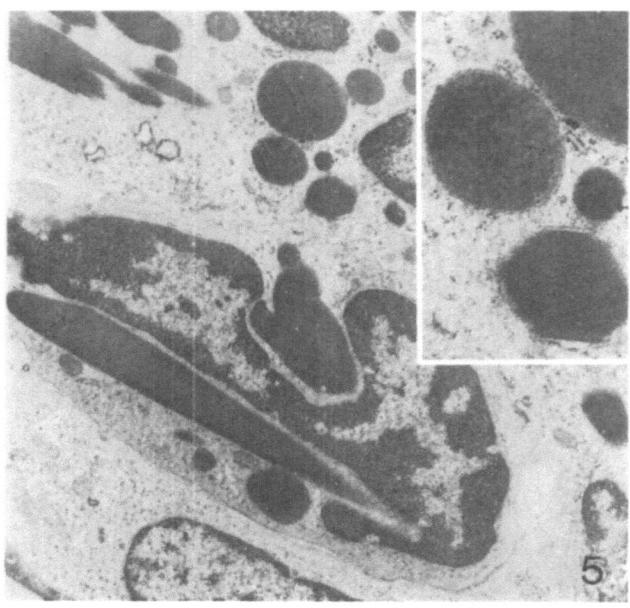

Figure 5. Details of fibrin are enclosed by a phagocyte. Inset: in places fibrin residues are surrounded by lysosome-like details of membrane

never develop in this region (Figs. 2a and b). This indicates that the milieu in the subendothelial space favors the formation of crystalline bodies from fibrin.

The deteriorating medial muscle tissue is gradually replaced by regenerating muscle cells. These produce a stratified basement membrane (Fig. 6) which, in addition to the hyaline from the subendothelial fibrinoid, account for hyalinization of the media. The medial hyaline shows in places a granular, in places a homogeneous structure, and may also retain the basement membrane character.

Various examples can be cited to affirm the correctness of the above statements.

If the vascular injury is either durable or severe, the form of primary hyaline described in the spleen transforms to a characteristic vascular fibrinoid, exhibiting muscle cell necrosis and positive reaction to azan and Mallory's stains. In hypertensive vascular injury and experimental hypertension of short duration, only the initial influx of plasma takes place. However, the elastic membrane plays an important role in plasma flow across the vessel wall. The elastic fiber acts as a barrier but changes itself as a consequence of the increased influx of proteins, to judge from the increase in its digestibility by elastase (Jellinek, 1974).

In view of the foregoing considerations, the development of the vascular fibrinod can be easily followed up on the light microscopic level by polarization and phase contrast microscopy but especially by electron microscopy. Primary and secondary forms of the vascular hyaline can be distinguished. The development of the secondary hyaline was studied and clarified in this laboratory. The main factors in this process are the transformation of fibrin and accumulation of a basement membrane-like substance produced by muscle cells and endothelial cells. Appearance of lipids in these lesions is only a secondary phenomenon.

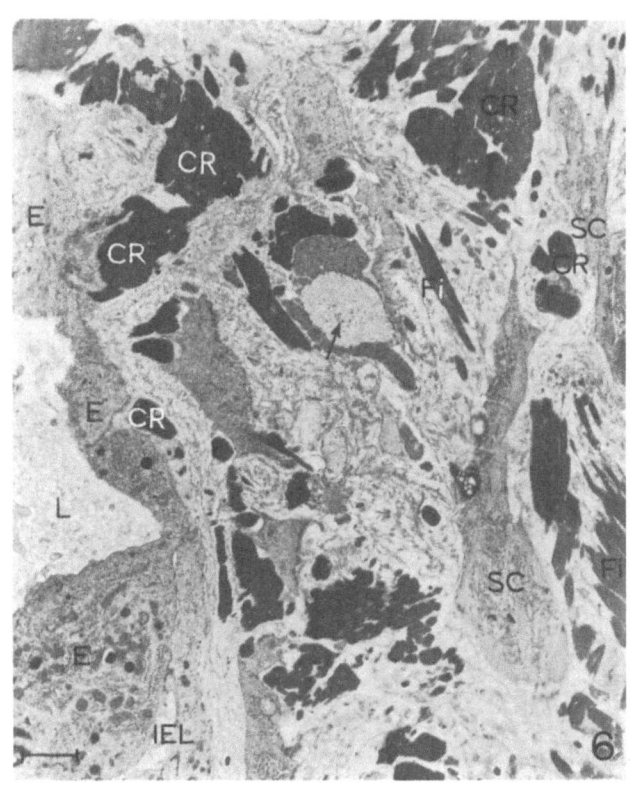

Figure 6. After the gradual degradation of fibrin (FI) and crystalline bodies (CB), transformation of these substances causes hyalinization along with increasing amounts of the basement membrane-like substance produced by smooth muscle cells (SC) and endothelium (E). Arrow: depolymerized fibrin. L: lumen, IEL: internal elastic lamina

HYPERTENSION, STROKE AND ATHEROGENESIS IN EXPERIMENTAL MODELS

Yukio Yamori, Ryohichi Horie, Michiya Ohtaka, Yasuo Nara, and Masaichi Fukase

By the establishment of proper animal models for hypertension, stroke, and atherogenesis, it has been possible to greatly accelerate studies on not only the pathogenesis but also the interrelation of these pathologic states.

Establishment of Animal Models for Hypertension, Stroke and Atherogenesis

Spontaneously hypertensive rats were established by selective breeding from a couple of Wistar-Kyoto rats with mild or borderline hypertension (Okamoto and Aoki, 1963). These rats are now in the F_{42} generation and maintained at our laboratory, genealogically classified into ten substrains with different characteristics. The common feature in SHR is primary hypertension which develops spontaneously with the aging process without any apparent organic lesions; this hypertension is determined by gene-environment interactions and is caused by increased peripheral vascular resistance. Because pathophysiologic features are similar to essential hypertension in man, SHR are regarded as the best animal model for essential hypertension in man (Yamori and Okamoto, 1974; Institute of Laboratory Animal Resources, 1976).

Stroke-prone SHR (SHRSP) (Okamoto et al., 1974; Yamori et al., 1974) — the offspring selectively bred from among SHR which had cerebravascular lesions at autopsy — develop cerebral hemorrhage and/or infarction (so-called stroke) in more than 80% of the population (Figs. 1 and 2). The basic pathologic lesions are arterionecrosis and thrombosis, so that such can be called arterionecro-thrombogenic stroke (Yamori, 1976a; Yamori et al., 1977). Because of their pathologic and pathogenetic similarities (Yamori et al., 1976e), these SHRSP are regarded as the best animal models so far for stroke in people with hypertension.

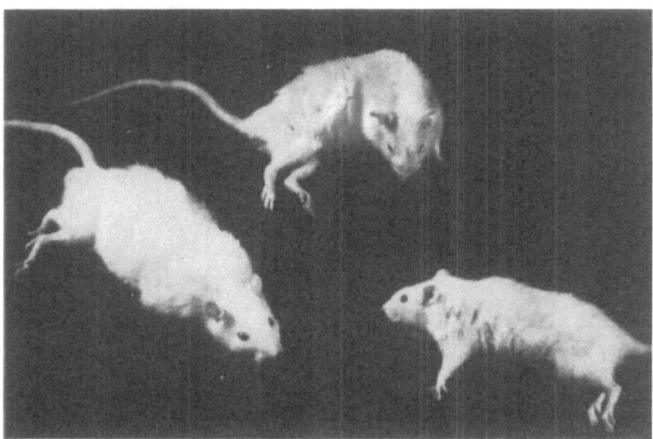

Figure 1. SHRSP with late symptoms of stroke such as paralysis, paresis, hypokinesia, lethargia, urinary incontinence, etc.

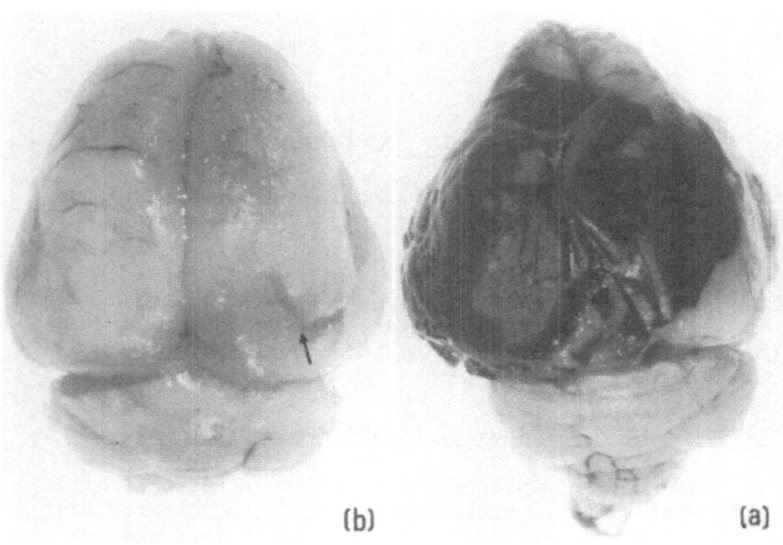

Figure 2. Macroscopical findings of massive hemorrhage(a) and infarction(b) (indicated with an arrow)

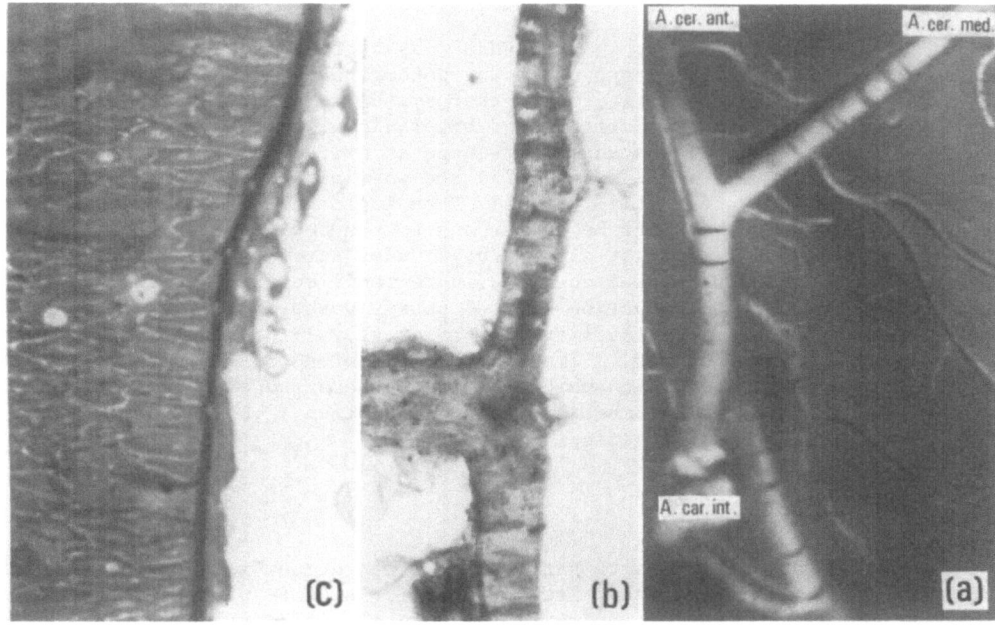

Figure 3. Acute arterial fat deposits in ALR: (a) Ring-like fat deposits in the circle of Willis demonstrated by barium-contrasted Sudan-staining method, (b) Sudanophilic ring-like fat deposits detected in extirpated superior cerebellar arteries, (c) Foam cells noted in intima and media of basilar artery with fat deposits

SHR (Yamori et al., 1975a, 1976c) and *arteriolipidosis-prone rats* (ALR) (Yamori, 1976a, 1977; Yamori et al., 1977) — which have been established by selective breeding for greater reactive hypercholesterolemia from among SHR — develop not only hypercholesterolemia but also ring-like arterial fat deposits within a few weeks when fed on a hypercholesterolemic diet (Fig. 3). These deposits are noted in mesenteric, cerebral, and other arteries; such lesions in the cerebral arteries are especially good models for cerebral arteriosclerosis, as they cannot be easily obtained within such a short period in other animals.

Mechanism of Hypertension in SHR

To a large extent, hypertension in SHR is genetically determined by the additive made of inheritance of a small number of major genes (Tanase et al., 1970). Environmental factors such as stress and salt loading accelerate or augment the hypertension (Yamori et al., 1969). Various experimental findings directly or indirectly indicate that neurogenic factors are important in the initiation mechanism of labile hypertension (Yamori, 1976b, 1976c). Functional and metabolic alterations of vasculatures are involved primarily or secondarily (Yamori, 1976b, 1976c, 1974, 1976d). Structural vascular alteration, caused through enhanced vascular protein metabolism, increases peripheral vascular resistance and finally stabilizes hypertension (Yamori, 1976, 1976c). Although biochemical lesions induced by major genes are not yet pinpointed, the insufficiency of central inhibitory mechanisms of blood pressure regulation seems to be involved at least in the initiation of neurogenic hypertension (Yamori, 1976b, 1976c).

Mechanism of Stroke in SHRSP

Statistical analysis on more than 1200 SHRSP has clarified that rapidly developing severe hypertension is important in the pathogenesis of stroke (Okamoto et al., 1974). It has also clarified that other systemic factors are an alteration of the physicochemical characteristics of arterial walls (Yamori and Sasagawa, 1975), and that a humoral substance (Matsunaga et al., 1975) or changes of platelet function (Okuma and Yamori, 1975) are possibly involved in causing vascular lesions (Matsuhaga et al., 1975). Pathologic investigation has proven that predilection sites for stroke correspond to the boundary zone, mainly fed by recurrent branches (Yamori et al., 1976e). Under severe hypertensive state, these local factors cause marked decrease in regional cerebral blood flow (Yamori et al., 1976f). Prolonged reduction of rCBF causes vascular damage due to hypoxia, which increases vascular permeability (Yamori et al., 1975b) and finally induces arterionecrosis (Yamori et al., 1976a, 1976b). Arterionecrosis is the basic lesion for microaneurysm formation which results in hemorrhage when ruptured and also the basic lesion for thrombosis causing infarction, i.e., stroke in this model is arterionecro-thrombogenic stroke.

Mechanisms of Atherogenesis

For hypertensive and normotensive rats, three preparations for atherogenesis have been established (Table 1). These are now used for studies on the pathogenetic mechanism, regression, and prophylaxis of atherosclerotic lesions (Yamori, 1976a; Yamori et al., 1977, 1976a). *Preparation I* is the hypertensive model (SHR or experimental hypertensive rats) fed on a hypercholesterolemic diet. Especially ALR quickly develop hypercholesterolemia as well as ring-like arterial fat deposits within a few weeks in systemic and cerebral arteries (Yamori, 1976a, 1977; Yamori et al., 1977). *Preparations II and III* are normotensive models fed on a hypercholesterolemic diet; the former are rats with bilateral carotid arteries ligated (Yamori et al., 1976d), and the latter are prehypertensive or antihypertensive agent-treated SHR. Within several weeks, ring-like fat deposits in the cerebral arteries develop in the former; and the latter, such deposits develop mainly in other arteries. Analytic studies in these three preparations indicated that hypertension, hemodynamic derangement, genetic disposition, and vascular permeability related to vasospasms had dilatation and are all important in the development of acute arterial fat deposition (Yamori et al., 1976a, 1976b).

Table 1. Models for atherogenesis in rats

Classification	Arterial lesion	
	Cerebral	Systemic
Hypertensive Models		
Yamori's preparation I SHR; "Arteriolipidosis-prone rat (ALR)" Experimental hypertensive rats	++	++
Normotensive Models		
Yamori's preparation II Rats with carotid artery ligation	+	-
Yamori's preparation III Antihypertensive agent-treated SHR or ALR Prehypertensive SHR or ALR	-	+

Interaction Between Hypertension, Stroke, and Atherogenesis

Studies in these models have clarified that hypertension is a direct cause of arterionecro-thrombogenic stroke and that it accelerates artherogenesis when accompanied with lipidemia. Lipidemia causes atherogenesis, but it attenuates severe hypertension partly through the reduction of vascular reactivity; it rather decreases arterionecro-thrombogenic stroke (Yamori et al., 1976a, 1976b). Control of hypertension was confirmed to be one of the most effective prophylaxes for both stroke and atherogenesis (Yamori et al., 1976a, 1976b).

HYPERTENSION AND CEREBRAL ATHEROSCLEROSIS

Y. Yoshida, H. Shinkai, T. Sekiguchi, and G. Ooneda

The object of this study is to determine whether atherosclerosis associated with hypertension more severely affects cerebral arteries than other visceral arteries to define the microscopic features of intracerebral atherosclerosis.

Materials and Methods

The grade of atherosclerosis in the large cerebral arteries at the base of the brain was determined in 114 randomly obtained autopsy cases at Gunma University. After fixation with 10% formalin, cross sections of the arteries were made at 22 defined sites in each case (Fig. 1). Narrowing of the lumen was graded as follows: grade 0, no narrowing; grade 1, intimal thickening producing less than 25% lumen narrowing; grade 2, 25–50%; grade 3, 50–75%; and grade 4, over 75%. The sum of the grades at the 22 sites was designated the cerebral atherosclerotic index in each case.

A similar analysis was made on the intracerebral small arteries. In carrying out this study, microscopic specimens were prepared from the basal ganglia of 26 age-matched normotensive (blood pressure, less than 140/90 mm Hg) and hypertensive (200/110 mm Hg or more) cases aged 30–79 years. Grades of intracerebral atherosclerosis (I/R x 100), evaluated from the ratio of the thickness of the intima (I) to the original radius (R) of arteries, were designated as follows: grade 1, ~25; grade 2, 26 or 50; grade 3, 51–75; grade 4, 76–100. I und R were calculated from the length (l) of the internal elastic lamella and the length (l') of the endothelial lining which were measured on histologic cross sections stained for elastin, according to the following formulas: $I = R-r$, $2R = \frac{l}{X\pi}$, and $2r = \frac{l'}{X\pi}$ (r designates diameter of the narrowed lumen and X designates magnifiying power).

Histologic features of intracerebral atherosclerosis were studied in 24 cases of basal ganglionic infarction with hypertension. After injection of contrast medium into the cerebral arteries, the brain tissue was cleared with tetrahydronaphthalene and examined using routine histologic techniques. On cases autopsied within 3 hours of death, immunoperioxidase techniques against fibrinogen and β-lipoprotein were performed.

In order to determine whether hypertension has a greater enhancing effect on the development of atherosclerosis in cerebral arteries than on arteries elsewhere, 96 coronary arteries were examined from a total of 114 cases studied. The coronary arteries were cut transversely at eight defined sites and the luminal narrowing graded in the same way as in the cerebral arteries (Fig. 1). The sum of the grades at the eight sites was taken as the coronary sclerotic index in each case.

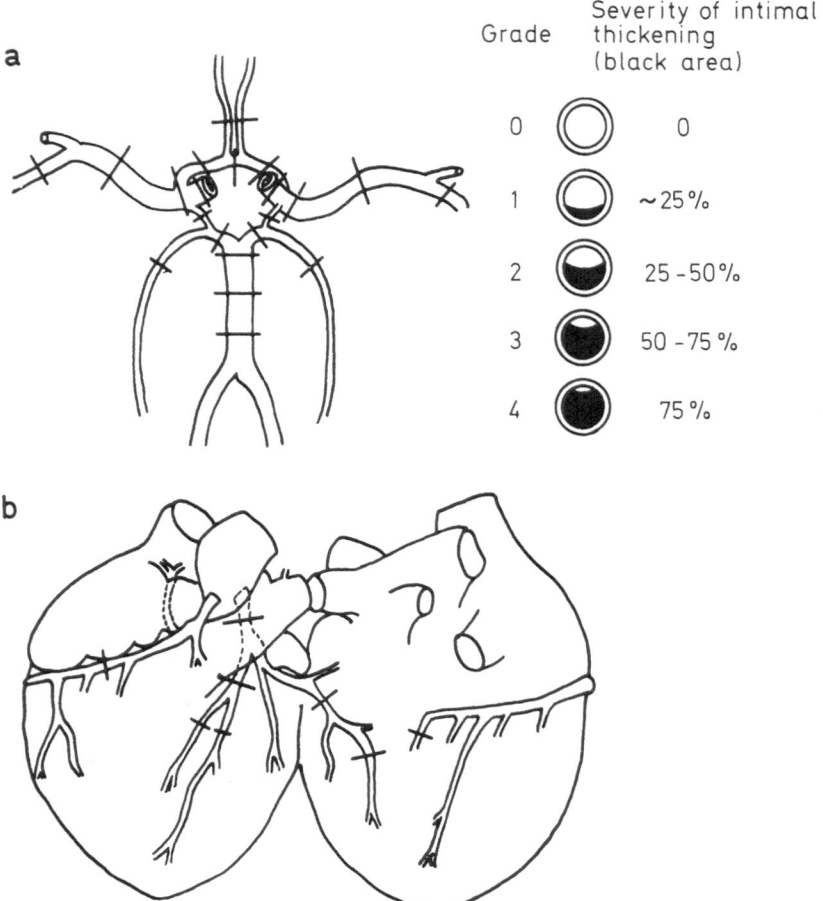

Figure 1. The cerebral (A) and coronary arteries (B) were cut transversely at the points marked by the lines. The most severe grade among several sections in each portion represented the atherosclerotic grade of the portion

Hypertension was generally defined as blood pressure higher than 160 mm Hg systolic and 95 mm Hg diastolic.

Results and Discussion

Cases with cerebral atherosclerosis indices higher than 20 were designated as severe cerebral atherosclerosis. Cases of cerebral infarction, excluding those due to known cerebral embolism, always had indices higher than 18. Those with grades under ten were taken as normal since such was the range observed in all the normotensives under 40 years of age.

All the hypertensive cases aged more than 40 years showed atherosclerotic grades greater than ten. Thirty-six of 42 cases of severe sclerosis (85.7%) were hypertensives (Fig. 2).

Coronary sclerosis was also increased among hypertensives, but less markedly than cerebral sclerosis. A grade of ten or higher was designated as severe coronary sclerosis.

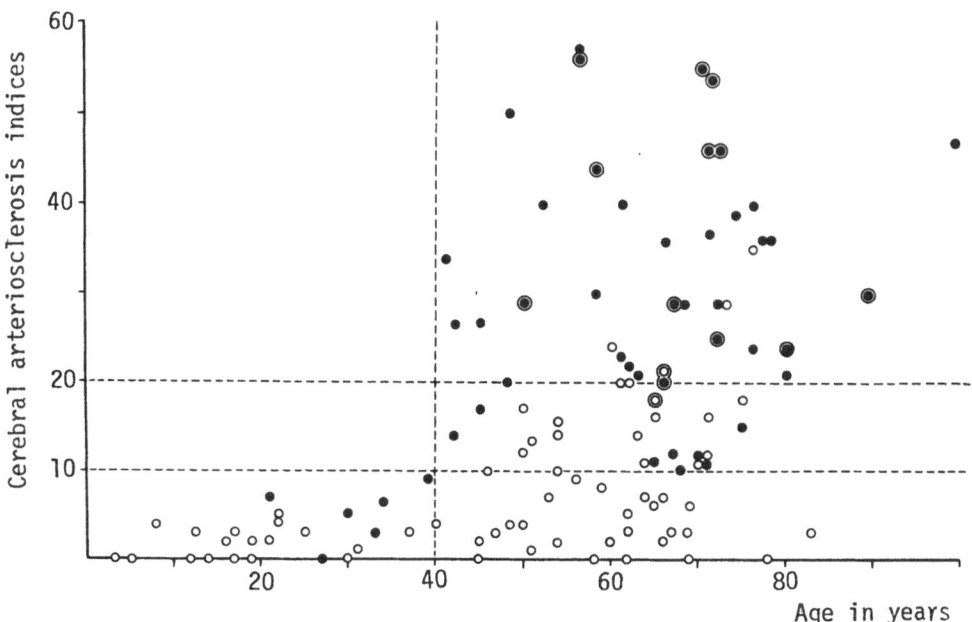

Figure 2. Cerebral atherosclerosis indices of 114 cases. • hypertensives, ○ normotensives, ◎ cases with cerebral infarction

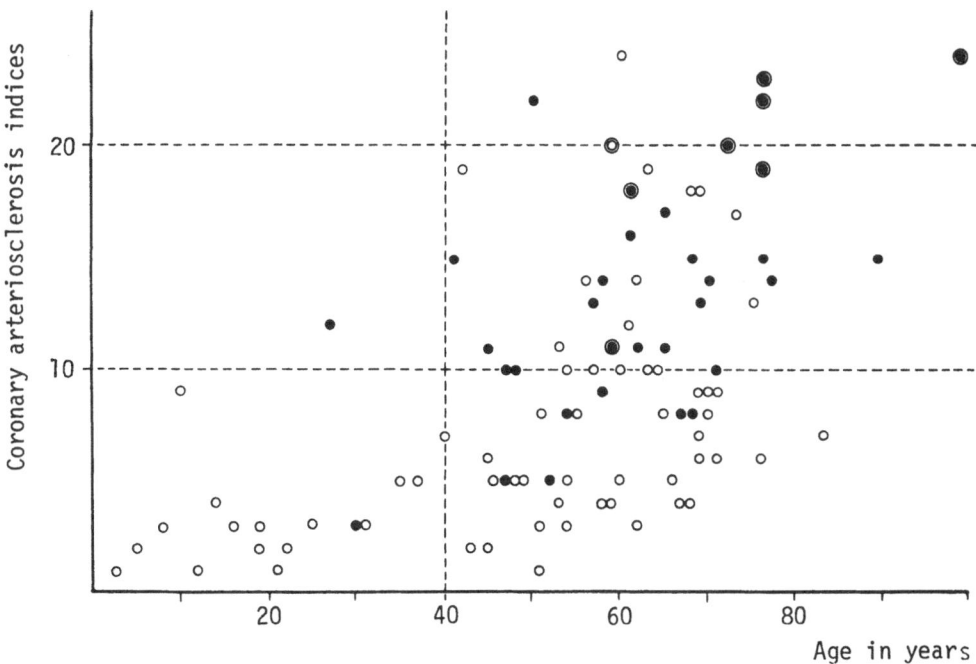

Figure 3. Coronary atherosclerosis indices of 96 cases. • hypertensives, ○ normotensives, ◎ cases with myocardial infarction

Cases with myocardial infarction had grades above 11. Twenty-six out of 42 severe coronary sclerotic cases (61.9%) were hypertensive (Fig. 3). Thus, the incidence of hypertension among cases with severe coronary sclerosis was significantly lower than among those with severe cerebral sclerosis (P <0.02).

Out of the 372 intracerebral arterial segments examined histologically from hypertensive subjects, 80, or 21.5%, showed atherosclerotic involvement of a grade greater than two. In normotensives, however, only six out of 379 or 1.6% of arterial segments examined showed such involvement (Fig. 4). There was thus a significant difference between the two groups (P <0.01).

In the cases with basal ganglionic infarction, out of 129 arteries graded two or higher, 48.1% showed atherosclerosis or intimal lipoidosis (foam cell and/or ceroid accumulation in the intima without fibrosis), 27.1% fibrocellular intimal thickening, 17% intimal edema, and 7.8% pseudocalcification with atherosclerosis of intimal edema. Of the 33 arteries having the highest sclerotic grade, 57.6% were involved by atherosclerosis or intimal lipoidosis and 24.2% showed intimal edema.

Among lesions of proximal intracerebral arteries more than 300 μ in diameter, fibrocellular intimal thickening and atherosclerosis were predominant. The ath-

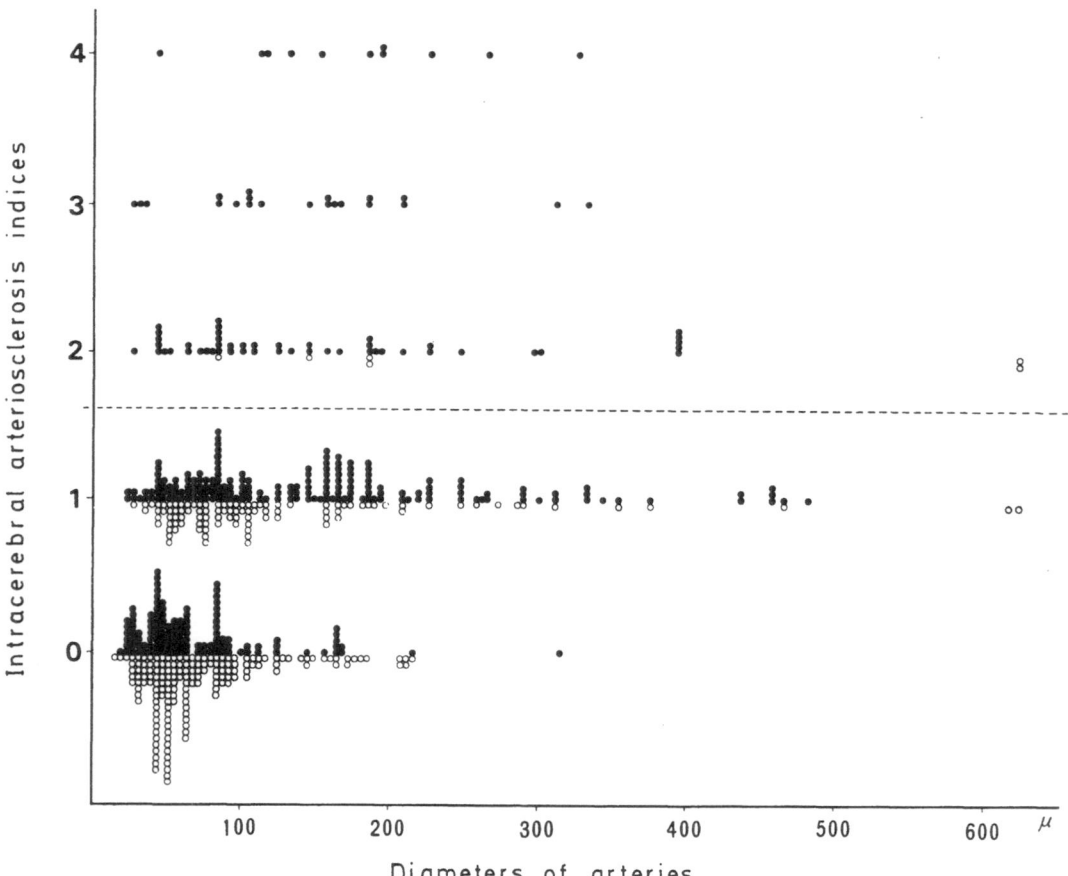

Figure 4. The number of intracerebral arteries with sclerotic indices of grade two or more is significantly larger in hypertensives (•) than in normotensives (o)

eromata in the latter were formed by disintegration of collagen fibers swollen with lipid-rich plasma infiltration (fiber disintegration type; Ooneda et al., 1973a).

In arterioles less than 200 μ in diameter, various lesions (for example, intimal lipoidosis, atheroma, foam cell disintegration type; Ooneda et al., 1973b; intimal edema) were produced without a preceding fibrocellular intimal thickening, that is, plasma infiltration occurred without the intimal thickening. As a matter of fact, immunoperoxidase techniques revealed that the arterioles showed foam cell lesions with β-lipoprotein and fibrin stagnation in the intima without the fibrocellular intimal thickening.

Intracerebral arteries in the hypertensives were involved not only by atherosclerosis but plasmatic arterionecrosis (Ooneda et al., 1973a, 1973b; Shinkai et al., 1976) as well. The arterionecrosis was observed most frequently in arteries with diameters ranging from 100 to 300 μ. In order to determine the reason for this predilection, the medial thickness and diameter were examined in variously sized intracerebral arteries. The ratio of the medial thickness to the diameter was smaller in the arteries ranging from 100 to 300 μ in diameter than in other sized arteries. It can be surmised that the thinner the wall, the more easily the wall can be damaged, as the tension applied to the wall will increase according to Laplace's formula.

Furthermore, blood flow disturbances or hypoxia in the intracerebral arteries could be considered an additional factor in the development of hypertensive vascular disease. Occasionally, plasmatic arterionecrosis was seen in the distal segments of the intracerebral arteries in which bifurcations of the proximal segments of these arteries were stenosed by atherosclerosis.

Summary

Hypertension accelerated cerebral atherosclerosis more markedly than coronary sclerosis. Intracerebral atherosclerosis was found out to the distal segments less than 100 μ in diameter (with significantly higher incidence in hypertensives).

Fibrocellular intimal thickening and atherosclerosis, which always was preceded by the former, were prevalent in the proximal parts of intracerebral arteries more than 300 μ in diameter. Arterial lesions which occurred in the distal segment less than 200 μ in diameter were formed without being preceded by fibrocellular intimal thickening. Cerebral arteries from 22 out of 24 hypertensive cases with basal ganglionic infraction showed arterionecrosis. Most of it was found in arteries ranging from 100 μ to 300 μ in diameter, presumably due to the thinner medial layer of these arteries. In addition to hypertension, blood flow disturbances of hypoxia may be a causative factor in the development of the arterionecrosis.

EFFECT OF HYPERTENSION ON THE ENTRY OF ^{125}I-LABELED LDL INTO ARTERIAL INTIMA IN CHOLESTEROL FED RABBITS

Kenneth N. Bretherton, Allan J. Day, and Sandford L. Skinner
Department of Physiology, University of Melbourne, Melbourne/Australia

Entry of ^{125}I-labeled low density lipoprotein (LDL) into the arterial intima was studied during 6 hours in normotensive (NT) and hypertensive (HT) rabbits fed cholesterol for 9 and 4 weeks respectively. Studies were also made in HT and NT cholesterol fed rabbits in which blood pressure was reduced acutely with hydralazine.
In all groups influx was greatest in the aortic arch and least in the abdominal aorta. LDL influx was proportional to intimal cholesterol concentration, such that when corrected for differences in cholesterol concentration, no effect of hypertension or hydralazine on influx was detected. Comparison between the rate of LDL influx and rate of intimal cholesterol accumulation indicated that the two were not necessarily related.
The findings are consistent with the hypothesis that elevated serum lipoproteins promote both increased lipoprotein entry and increased retention of lipoprotein cholesterol within the arterial wall. Hypertension accelerates the development of atherosclerosis by further augmenting the degree of lipid retention.

INFLUENCE OF MUSCULAR TRAINING ON ARTERIAL WALL CELLS REACTION

W.H. Hauss, G. Schmitt, K.P. Backwinkel, and R. Lehmann
"Institut für Arterioskleroseforschung" and "Medizinische Klinik und Poliklinik der Universität Münster, Abt. Innere Medizin B", Münster/BRD

In former studies we have shown that arterial hypertension, muscular exercise, infectious diseases and bacterial toxins induce cell proliferation in the intima, media and adventitia of rats aortas (demonstrated by measuring the incorporation rate of 35S-sulphate(1,2)*. Muscular exercise is considered to prevent diseases esp. arteriosclerosis, but convincing evidence is lacking. We studied this problem by three groups of 7-14 wistar male rats of equal age with a bodyweight of 140-160 grams, kept on constant conditions: one control group, one damaged by muscular stress and by i.p. staphylotoxin injection and one group damaged in the same way after being trained in the manner Fig. 1 shows. While running stress and toxin injection induced a big reaction in the arterial wall cells of untrained animals (group 2), raising the uptake of 35S-sulphate into the SMPS to the three-fold, the same damage in trained animals (group 3) did not alter the metabolism significantly (see Fig. 2). The preceding muscular training has obviously protacted or adapted the arterial wall cells against resp. to both stressors. We suggest that these animal experiences can give an information about the preventing quality of human sport. It must be unspecifically working, eliminating the effect of muscular stress and toxin injection. I thank the Landesversicherungsanstalt Westfalen in Münster, who sponsored these experiences.

---

* 1. W.H. Hauss, G. Junge-Hulsing, U. Gerlach: Die unspezifische Mesenchymreaktion. Stuttgart: Thieme, 1968. 2. W.H. Hauss: The Role of the Mesenchymal Cells in Arteriosclerosis. Front. Martix Biol., Vol. 2, pp. 89-124. Basel: Karger 1976.

Animal group		1. Week till to 5. Week	6. Week			
			1. day	2. day	3. day	4. day
I	Control animals untrained without toxin without running stress				^{35}S-sulphate injection	+
II	Control animals untrained with toxin with running stress		6 h running stress	6 h running stress	1 x toxin injection then ^{35}S-sulphate injection	+
III	Experimental animals trained* with toxin with running stress	3 x ½ h till to 3 x 5 h running a day	6 h running stress	6 h running stress	1 x toxin injection then ^{35}S-sulphate injection	+

*Training in activity weels (5 turns/min.) on 3 days per week with one day inter-mission.

Figure 1. Experimental arrangement of the training program

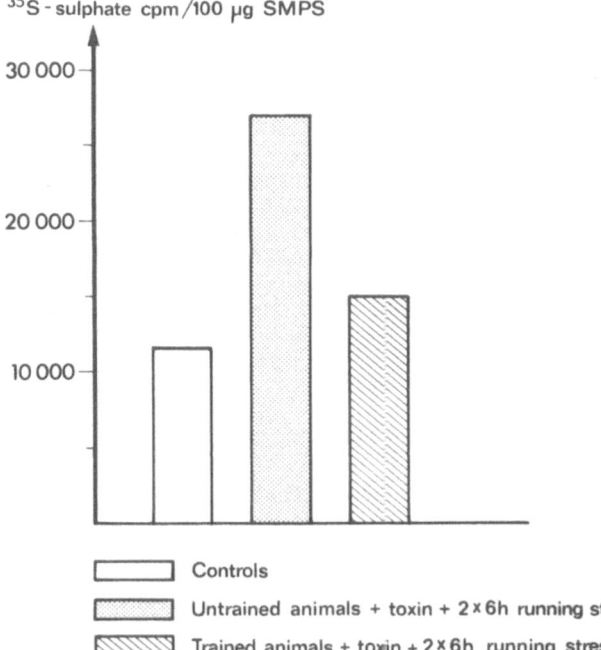

^{35}S - sulphate cpm/100 µg SMPS

☐ Controls

▨ Untrained animals + toxin + 2 x 6h running stress

▧ Trained animals + toxin + 2 x 6h running stress

Figure 2. Changes in mesenchymal metabolism in aortas of rats in untrained animals and in trained animals after damaging by combination of running stress and toxin injection.
(^{35}S-sulphate incorporation into the SMPS of aorta)

HYPERTENSIVE ARTERIOPATHY AND ATHEROSCLEROSIS: HISTOMETABOLIC AND ULTRASTRUCTURAL AORTIC CHANGES DURING THE SHR ONTOGENESIS

P. Hadjiisky, J. Renais, and L. Scebat
Centre de Recherches Cardiologiques, Hôpital Boucicaut, Paris/France

Aortic ultrastructure, 27 enzyme activities and some macromolecular substances were comparatively studied in spontaneous hypertensive rats (SHR) (Okamoto-Aoki) and normotensive (NT) Wistar rats, 3, 5, 11 and 16 months old.
The earliest aortic changes (*3rd month*) were only histoenzymatic: 5-Nase and LDH increase in the entire wall; some oxydo-reductases increase in the intima. *In 5 to 11 month old SHR* (stable hypertension) the smooth muscle cells (s.m.c.) are metabolically and morphogenetically activated: increase of histoenzymatic activities linked with lipolysis, GAG anabolism, glycolysis cell respiration, energizing metabolism and nucleotid esterolysis; hyperplasia of cells and cell organelles including myofilaments, cell hypertrophy. This s.m.c. reaction has led to the diffuse medial thickening and the interstitial fibrosis. In the *16 month old SHR*, irreversible lesions appeared: medial necrosis, cicatricial fibrosis, decrease of oxydo-reductases, and increase of lysosomial E A in some cellular foci, decrease of lipolysis-linked E A. It is suggested that three of these changes are susceptible to favour the atherogenesis: (1) diffuse medial thickening, (2) medial fibrosis, (3) decrease of aortic wall lipolysis.

HYPERTENSION AND ATHEROSCLEROSIS IN DIFFERENT ARTERIAL SEGMENTS

Lars Aage Solberg
Department of Pathology Ullevål Hospital, Oslo/Norway

Five arterial segments (aorta, coronary, carotid, vertebral and intracranial arteries) from 543 autopsied cases were graded for the degree of atherosclerosis. Multivariate statistical methods were used to study the relationship between hypertension and eight variables (age, sex, heart weight, and raised atherosclerotic lesions in the five arterial segments). The findings indicate a very strong independent relationship between hypertension and the degree of atherosclerosis in the intracranial arteries compared with the degree of atherosclerosis in the other arterial segments. Hypertension was also relatively strongly related to vertebral atherosclerosis and some weaker related to coronary atheroclerosis. The relationship to aortic and carotid atherosclerosis was weak. The findings indicate that hypertension is a stronger atherogenic factor in the intracranial arteries than in the other arterial segments examined.

THE USE OF CROCETIN FOR HYPERTENSION

John L. Gainer, Joseph D. Pool, and John W. Dailey
University of Virginia, Charlottesville, VA/USA

There appears to be a link between atherosclerosis and hypertension, although such has not been established definitely at the present time. However, it would seem reasonable to test the effect of antiatherosclerotic drugs for their use for hypertension. Crocetin, a carotenoid compound, has been shown previously to reduce serum cholesterol and triglycerides levels as well as lessening vascular damage in cholesterol-fed rabbits. This study was to test the effect of crocetin on hypertension.
Spontaneous hypertensive rats were treated with crocetin for 7 months. Blood pressures were measured weekly using the tail-cuff method. The use of crocetin resulted in a statistically significant reduction (p <0.005) in the blood pressure. When the crocetin treatment was stopped, the blood pressures in the treated rats returned to that of the controls in six weeks. Since the SHR has been shown

to be a good model for human hypertension, crocetin may be useful in treating
hypertension.

CEREBRAL INFARCTION, HEMORRHAGE AND ATHEROSCLEROSIS

Lars Aage Solberg
Department of Pathology, Ullevål Hospital, Oslo/Norway

Five arterial segments (aorta, coronary, carotid, vertebral and intracranial
arteries) from 543 autopsied cases, were graded for the degree of atherosclerosis.
Multivariate statistical method were used to study the relationship between cerebral infarction, hemorrhage and atherosclerosis. Eight variables were used (age,
sex, heart weight, hypertension and raised atherosclerotic lesions in the five
arterial segments). The findings indicate a strong independent relationship between cerebral infarction and intracranial atheroscleoris, and some weaker relationship between cerebral infarction and vertebral and coronary atherosclerosis.
The relationship to the other factors including hypertension was weak. There was
a strong independent relationship between cerebral hemorrhage and hypertension,
and some weaker relationship between cerebral hemorrhage and intracranial atherosclerosis. The relationship to the other factors was weak. The study demonstrate the importance of hypertension compared with atherosclerosis in the pathogenesis of cerebral hemorrhage. The study also demonstrate the importance of
cerebral atherosclerosis compared with hypertension in the pathogenesis of cerebral infarction.

WORKSHOP 3. Epidemiology of Atherosclerosis and Geographic Differences in Risk Factors

Chairmen: J.P. Strong, USA
T. Omae, Japan

Participants: L.A. Solberg, Norway
H.H. Sternby, Sweden
M. Hanefeld, DDR
M.R. Garcia-Palmieri, PR
G. Stemmerman, USA
S. Hatano, Japan
G. Crepaldi, Italy
J.P. Strong, USA
T. Omae, Japan

AN INTRODUCTION TO THE EPIDEMIOLOGY OF ATHEROSCLEROSIS

Jack. P. Strong

With the collaboration of M.L. Richards†, Margaret C. Moore, Margaret C. Oalmann, and Richard E. Tracy

My main point will be to discuss the relationship of epidemiological variables or risk factors to the prevalence and extent of atherosclerotic lesions in the wall of the coronary arteries and the aorta. Figure 1 illustrates the relationship of the risk factors to atherosclerotic lesions and coronary heart disease. I will emphasize the epidemiology of the underlying arterial lesions rather than the epidemiology of coronary heart disease per se.

Risk factors for CHD	Sequence of events in CHD
Age	
Sex	
Race	
Geographic location	Atherosclerotic lesions
Elevated serum lipids	┼
Hypertension	
Cigarette smoking	Occlusive episode
Diabetes	↓
Physical inactivity	
Obesity	Coronary heart disease
Mineral content of water	
Other factors	
	LSU PATH '74

Figure 1. Risk factors for coronary heart disease and atherosclerotic lesions

As workshop chairman, I reflected on knowledge about risk factors and atherosclerotic lesions, as evinced at the Second International Symposium in Chicago
in 1970. The summary of a paper titled "Risk Factors and Atherosclerotic Lesions"
(Strong and Eggen, 1970) from that symposium reads:

"Date from the International Atherosclerosis Project (IAP) and other recent
autopsy surveys are used to illustrate the association of risk factors for coronary heart disease to coronary atherosclerotic lesions. Coronary atherosclerosis
is found to vary with age, sex, geographic location, and race. Lesions seem to be
related to serum cholesterol and dietary fat when comparing populations, but insufficient data are available to confirm such associations on an individual basis
within a population. Lesions are greater in hypertensive and diabetic individuals
than in those without these conditions. Lesions are also greater in heavy cigarette smokers than in nonsmokers. No consistent association of atherosclerotic
lesions is observed with physical activity or obesity. There is much variability
in extent of coronary atherosclerosis among individuals of similar race, sex,
age, geographic location, disease, and smoking habits. Thus, there are other important factors involved in development of atherosclerosis that have yet to be
determined."

How much have we learned since that symposium? Much of that paper's information
derived from the International Atherosclerosis Project, from incomplete studies
of deceased New Orleans men on the relationship of atherosclerotic lesions to
smoking habits, and from Sternby's (1968) autopsy studies. Carefully collected
antecedent information on risk factors was not usually available in these autopsy
studies, and sometimes such information was gathered from routine autopsy proto-
cols. In other instances, standardized schedules that had been carefully tested
on pairs of living subjects were used to gather information from decedents' surviving relatives.

Perspective on Objectives

The current workshop assignment challenged me to assemble new information from
our own studies and to suggest participants for the workshop who might have new
and exciting information gathered since the Second International Symposium.

Cigarette Smoking and Atherosclerosis

We completed our study of the association of cigarette smoking and atherosclerosis in 1320 New Orleans men aged 25-64 years who underwent autopsy (Strong and
Richards, 1976). Aortic and coronary lesions were evaluated visually in coded
specimens and objectively by analysis of radiographs. Interviewers, using schedules previously tested on pairs of living persons, obtained from relatives estimates of cigarette smoking habits of the deceased subjects. Data were analyzed
for black and white men in the total sample of cases and also in groups according
to the presence (selected disease group) or absence (basal group) of diseases
thought to be associated with smoking (e.g., emphysema, lung cancer) or with
coronary heart disease (e.g., myocardial infarction, hypertension, diabetes,
stroke). Figures 2 and 3 show for the total sample the extent of coronary and
aortic atherosclerosis by smoking category and race. Atherosclerotic involvement
of aorta und coronary arteries was greatest in heavy smokers and least in nonsmokers of both races in the total sample of cases, the basal group, and the
selected disease group. Thus, our findings seem to indicate that the relationship
of cigarette smoking to ahterosclerosis and CHD is not limited to events at the
terminal occlusive episode.

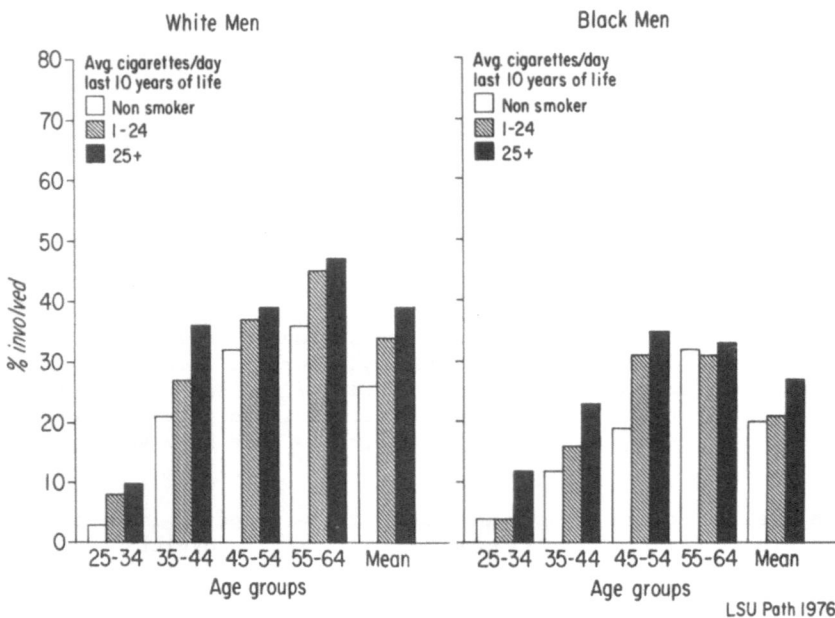

Figure 2. Mean percent of coronary intimal surface involved by raised lesions for total sample of cases

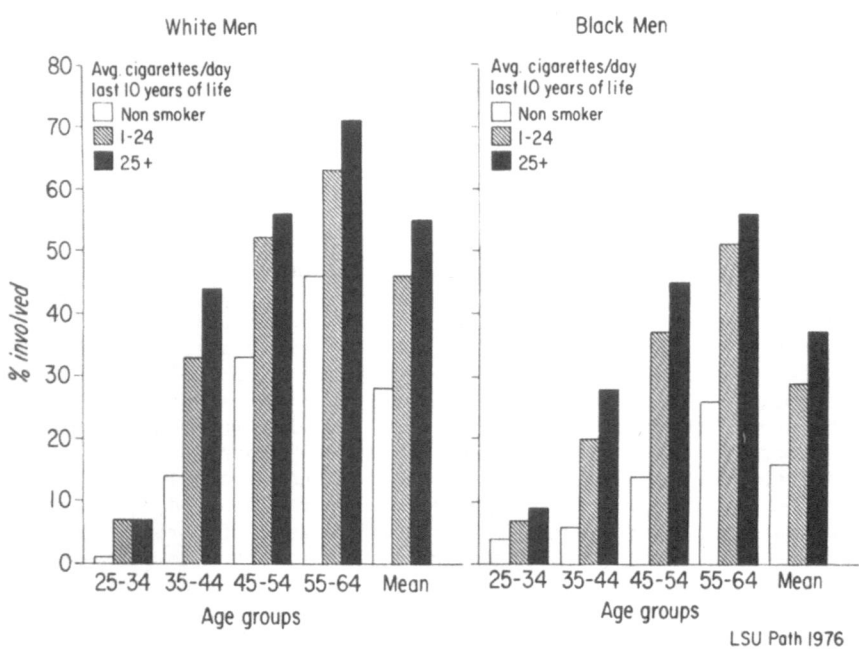

Figure 3. Mean percent of abdominal aorta intimal surface involved by raised lesions for total sample of cases

Diet and Atherosclerosis

Research nutritionists, using procedures previously tested and validated (Moore et al., 1967, 1970), obtained individual dietary histories for a subsample of 253 cases of the deceased men included in the smoking study. Data derived from the dietary histories were analyzed to study possible association of nutrient intakes during the subject's last year of life with the extent of raised lesion involvement in the three main coronary arteries, as measured at autopsy (Moore et al., 1976). We are aware of the limitations inherent in our study (e.g., highly selective autopsy sample, retrospective dietary data on deceased persons); nevertheless, we are intrigued by the findings and present them as hypotheses to be tested by other investigators.

The diet-lesion relationships examined on the basis of groupings of the nutrient-to-calorie ratio distribution are shown in Table 1 for different dietary components. The results suggest that, in general, the increased consumption of vegetables may relate to a decreased atherosclerotic involvement.

Table 1. Mean of nutrient-to-calorie ratios by tertile of nutrient to calorie ratios[a] and mean percent raised coronary lesion involvement in each tertile for 253 men who underwent autopsy (New Orleans/LA)

Dietary component	Mean daily nutrient:calorie ratio by tertile			Mean percent raised coronary lesion by tertile for nutrient:calorie ratio		
	Low (N=84)	Middle (N=85)	High (N=84	Low (N=84)	Middle (N=85)	High (N=84)
Protein, total	12	15	19	31	27	36
Animal	7	11	15	26	29	39[d]
Vegetal	3	4	6	39	30	25[d]
Fat, total	29	37	43	25	35	35[c]
Animal	19	26	33	27	34	33
Vegetal	5	8	13	29	30	36
Fatty acids, saturated	11	15	18	26	31	37
Fatty acids, unsaturated	16	19	23	28	30	36
Fatty acids, polyunsaturated	4	5	6	30	29	35
Cholesterol	139	181	265	31	29	35
Carbohydrates, total	39	46	54	36	32	26
Sugars	10	21	33	26	32	34
Starch	13	18	25	42	29	23[e]
Fiber	87	131	200	35	30	29

[a] Percent calories contributed, excepting cholesterol and fiber, which are expressed as mg per 1000 kcal.

[b] Exluding fish fat.

[c] Significant difference and linear trend. P <.05.

[d] Significant difference and linear trend. P <.01.

[e] Significant difference and linear trend. P <.001.

We found significantly greater atherosclerotic involvement with higher levels of animal protein and total fat (including animal and vegetable fat consumption). The higher the level of animal fat, saturated fatty acids, and cholesterol consumption, the greater the *trend* toward forming more lesions, in keeping with current hypotheses. Surprisingly, contrary to current hypotheses, use of vegetable fat, all unsaturated fat, and polyunsaturated fat showed the same *trend* to form more lesions with higher levels. Although these trends did not satisfy tests of significance at the $P < .05$ level, they indicate that almost all means of estimating dietary fat intake by our methods showed at least a trend toward finding more lesions among those who consumed more fat (or more of a specific type of fat).

A negative association was significant between the extent of atherosclerotic lesions and the amount of vegetable protein and starch consumed. Fewer lesions were found where more calories from vegetable protein and starch had been eaten. The significance of the negative association of starch and lesions was much stronger ($P < .001$) than that of any other positive or negative associations. This finding, taken at face value (noting the above limitations), suggests that dietary starch may be protective against atherosclerosis. Or are the data, taken as a whole, only indicating that persons who consume more vegetables (vegetable protein, starch, fiber findings in the right direction, but not significant) eat less of the rich foods that contain the commonly implicated atherogenic substances?

We believe that our study provides — for the first time on a case-related basis in humans — evidence of significant relationships between nutrient intake and extent of atherosclerotic lesions, and, furthermore, that the hypotheses generated merit further investigation. Will the longitudinal epidemiological studies of cardiovascular diseases with autopsy follow-up and carefully collected antecedent data confirm these findings?

Epidemiological Studies With Autopsy Follow-Up

Although earlier studies lacked pathologic follow-up for evaluating autopsy findings, several recent long-term epidemiological investigations have incorporated such follow-up with standardized methods for evaluating atherosclerotic lesions in patients undergoing autopsy. The recent studies have limitations, however, because not all study subjects who died could be identified nor could every autopsy be done by the standardized method for evaluating atherosclerotic lesions. Nevertheless, these studies probably provide the best way of studying the relationship of antecedent risk factors measured during life to atherosclerotic lesions — to the first stage of the process that ends in coronary heart disease (Fig. 1). All of the studies that meet these criteria and of which I am aware will be included in the various reports of this workshop. Those reports confirm many of the findings from previous studies reported above and also provide new information on the association of atherosclerotic lesions and risk factors. Some of these statistically significant relationships (some highly significant) have been demonstrated with only a handful of cases, a fact that, rather than detracting from the value of the studies, indicates how strong a relationship must be for it to be found significant with the small numbers present to date. More subtle significant relationships are expected from these same studies as surveillance and follow-up continue and the number of cases for analysis increases.

Community-Wide Studies of Atherosclerosis

Community-wide studies of deceased persons in settings where a high percentage of autopsies are performed may help complete both the clinical and epidemiological picture. We are now conducting such a study in New Orleans, an intensive investigation of 25 - 44-year-old black and white men who underwent autopsy (Oalmann et al., 1973). Our preliminary findings on the relationship of serum cholesterol levels (determined only once — at post mortem) and the extent of lesions differed between black and white men, with only the white men having a significant correlation. On the other hand, preliminary findings from the same study suggest that morphologic lesions reflecting hypertension are significantly related to the extent of lesions in the blacks, but not in the whites. Furthermore, the differences in the extent of lesions between white and black men in New Orleans may not now be as great as they were when reported several times in the past. This finding suggests that environmental changes may be decreasing the racial differential in the extent of coronary and aortic atherosclerosis. More cases and more refinement of analyses are needed before the tentative findings of this study can be confirmed.

New Data from this Workshop Concerning Known CHD Risk Factors

Papers in this workshop clearly show — for the first time — a significant positive association between serum cholesterol levels (even if measured only once during life or at post mortem) and the extent of atherosclerotic lesions measured carefully at autopsy. The relationship of blood pressure levels carefully measured by standardized techniques at one or more times during life and the extent of atherosclerosis measured at autopsy is clearly confirmed in practically every study that is reported in this symposium. Tentative findings from the New Orleans studies suggest the strength of the associations between serum lipids and blood pressure to arterial lesions may differ between two racial groups in that city.

Some of the studies in this symposium show a clear-cut and significant association between cigarette smoking habits and the lesions of atherosclerosis in both coronary arteries and the aorta. In other studies, a significant relationship was shown for only one arterial segment; in one study no significant relationship was shown, although the correlation was positive. With the large variability in extent of atherosclerosis that exists in the most homogeneous populations, large numbers of study subjects may be needed to show significant relationships. Another explanation for failure to show consistent significant relationships among the various studies could be that cigarette smoking as a lesion-related risk factor may require (1) greater usage than is present in those populations not showing the effect, or (2) a greater "baseline" foundation of atherosclerosis before this risk factor has any effect. Furthermore, biases due to selection or methodology could cause discrepancies in findings from the different studies.

So What Else is New?

From the findings and the reports of this workshop, some new hypotheses that need further testing are proposed as questions:
1. Is the blood glucose level truly related to the extent of atherosclerotic lesions?
2. Does complex carbohydrate in the diet "protect" the body against the lesions of atheroclerosis?
3. Is obesity an independent risk factor for the arterial lesions of atherosclerosis?
4. Does nutrition in early life influence extent of atherosclerosis in adult life?
5. What about other suspected risk factors, such as the physical activity of work and leisure, stress, and the chemical composition of drinking water?

What are Some Future Frontiers?

Levels of serum cholesterol measured during life have now clearly been shown to be associated with the extent of atherosclerosis at autopsy. Would a more careful characterization of lipoprotein levels and components give stronger associations with the extent of lesions? Would lifetime data on levels of lipoproteins, blood pressure, and smoking habits (and measurement of their cumulative effects) result in higher correlations and explain a greater portion of the variability of atherosclerotic lesion involvement than we find within homogeneous groups (Strong, 1976). I suspect that with better evaluation of the cumulative effect of risk factors more and more of the variability in lesions will be explained by the known risk factors. Nevertheless, arterial "susceptibility" remains to be investigated, and the true mechanism of action of the risk factors remains to be defined with certainty.

ASSOCIATION BETWEEN RISK FACTORS AND ATHEROSCLEROTIC LESIONS BASED ON AUTOPSY FINDINGS IN THE OSLO STUDY: A PRELIMINARY REPORT*

Lars A. Solberg, Ingvar Hjermann, Anders Helgeland, Ingar Holme, Paul A. Leren, and Jack P. Strong

Atherosclerosis results from many interacting factors working during a long period. The geographic differences in the extent of atherosclerotic lesions (McGill, 1968) indicate the importance of the environment. Within one population the extent of atherosclerotic lesions differs among persons (Tejada et al., 1968) because of individual differences in susceptibility to atherosclerosis and in differences in exposure to risk factors. We probably know only a few of the risk factors. Some risk factors lead to atherosclerotic lesions, to complications of the lesions, and thereby to the occlusion of vessels. Risk factors for coronary heart disease may also act directly on the myocardium and its conductive system. These risk factors and clinical atherosclerotic disease, particularly coronary heart disease (Westlund and Nicolaysen, 1972). Less information is available about risk factors and the extent of atherosclerotic lesions. Some of the factors known to be associated with clinical coronary heart disease have been studied retrospectively for their association with atherosclerosis (Robertson and Strong, 1968; Strong and Richards, 1976). Before our present report, no prospective studies had examined risk factors and coronary atherosclerotic lesions in the same persons, mainly because reliable measurements of atherosclerotic lesions can only be obtained after death.

In this report from the prospective Oslo study (Leren et al., 1975), we compared recorded risk factors before death with quantitated coronary raised atherosclerotic lesions at autopsy in the same persons.

Materials and Methods

The Oslo study (Leren et al., 1975) is an epidemiological investigation of coronary heart disease risk factors in Oslo men. All men, aged 40-49 years, were invited to a health examination that included a blood sample for lipid examination, measurement of blood pressure, and questions about smoking habits. The screening procedure and laboratory methods are described elsewhere (Leren et al., 1975).

At autopsy, coronary arteries were collected from 49 men, aged 40-53 years at the time of death. No clinical evidence of coronary heart disease existed in these men at the time of screening. Details of dissection and preparation of arteries are given in the report from the International Atherosclerosis Project (Guzmán

*The study is supported by the city of Oslo. Norwegian Council on Cardiovascular Diseases in part by Grants HL-08974 and HL-14496 from the National Heart, Lung, and Blood Institute, National Institutes of Health, U.S. Public Health Service, Bethesda, MD/USA.

et al., 1968). In brief, coronary arteries were removed at autopsy, opened longitudinally, fixed in formalin, stained with Sudan IV by standardized techniques,
and graded for the percent intimal surface involved with atherosclerotic lesions.
The grading results of raised atherosclerotic lesions (RL) were compared with
previously recorded risk factors: serum cholesterol, triglycerides, systolic and
diastolic blood pressures, and daily number of cigarettes smoked. Simple correlation coefficients were computed, and multivariate linear regression analysis was
performed, using serum cholesterol, systolic blood pressure, and number of cigarettes smoked daily as explanatory variables.

Results

Table 1 shows the simple correlation coefficients between RL and the different
risk factors. The coefficients are statistically significant for serum cholesterol and systolic and diastolic blood pressures. The coefficients for triglycerides
and number of cigarettes smoked daily were not statistically significant. Correction for age decreased the coefficients for RL and serum cholesterol only. The
multivariate linear regression analysis included serum cholesterol, systolic blood
pressure, and number of cigarettes smoked daily as explanatory variables. The partial correlation coefficient was higher compared with the simple correlation
coefficient for serum cholesterol only, .32 before and .34 after correction for
age. For the other risk factors, the simple and partial correlation coefficients
were identical. The multivariate analysis revealed that about 20% of the variation of RL can be explained from the three variables, serum cholesterol, systolic
blood pressure, and number of daily cigarettes; 80% of the variation remains unexplained.

Figure 1 shows RL and serum cholesterol in the individual cases. The individual
variation in RL is large, but the mean and the median of RL increase with increasing value of serum cholesterol. Figure 2 shows the same for RL and systolic
blood pressure. The trend is the same for diastolic blood pressure. The individual variation of RL for different values of triglycerides and number of daily
cigarettes smoked is large. However, little or no increase occurs in mean and
median of RL by increasing values of triglycerides and number of cigarettes
smoked.

Table 2 shows the mean values for RL and the risk factors in patients with and
without coronary heart disease. The average age was the same. Persons having coronary heart disease had significantly more RL than those having no coronary heart
disease (P <0.05). The CHD cases also have higher values for risk factors than
the non-CHD cases. The differences, however, are not statistically significant.

Table 1. Correlation coefficients between risk factors and coronary raised
atherosclerotic lesions in Oslo men who underwent autopsy

	Not corrected for age	Corrected for age
Cholesterol	0.29[a]	0.31[a]
Systolic BP	0.34[a]	0.34[a]
Diastolic BP	0.34[a]	0.34[a]
Triglycerides	0.15	0.17
Cigarettes	0.12	0.14

[a] $P < 0.05$.

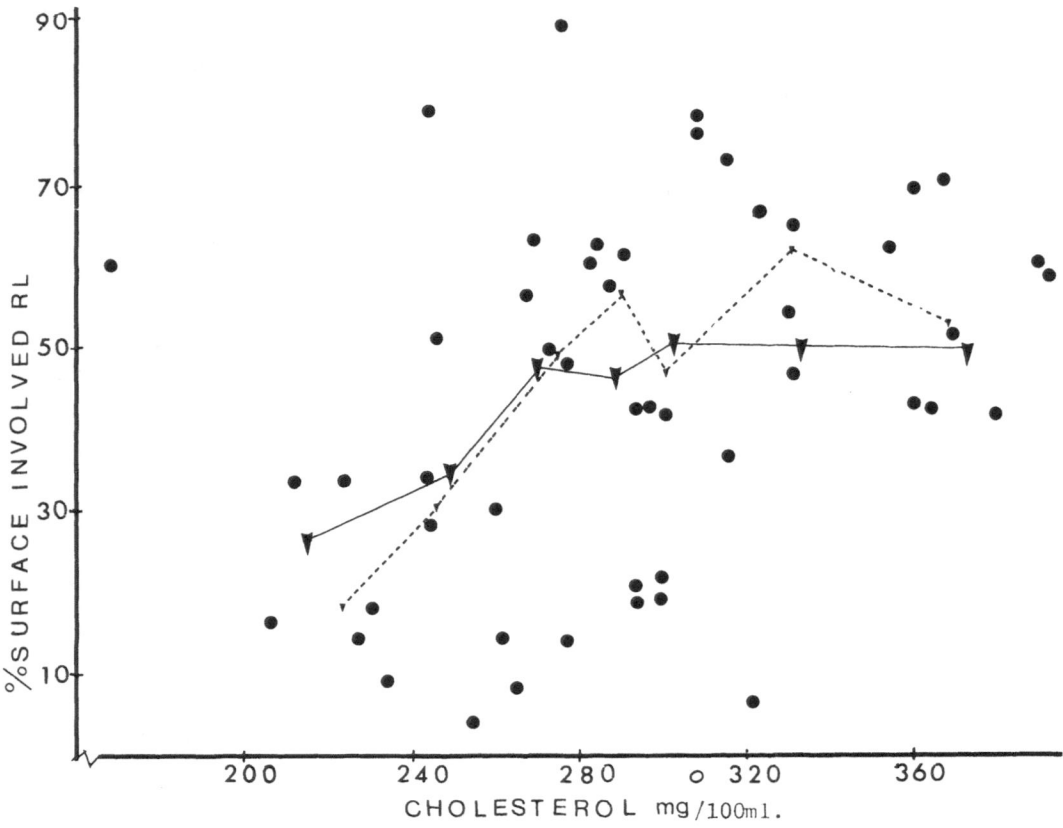

Figure 1. Raised atherosclerotic coronary lesions in individual cases, mean and median, by increasing values of serum cholesterol. —— mean; ----- median (Oslo study)

Table 2. Mean values of risk factors and coronary raised atherosclerotic lesions (RL) in Oslo men with and without coronary heart disease (CHD) who underwent autopsy

Case category	RL[a]	Age	Choles-terol	Tri-glycerides	Ciga-rettes	Systolic BP	Diastolic BP
CHD, 24 cases	55	48	301	2.95	14.9	152	94
Non-CHD, 25 cases	31	48	285	2.40	12.4	142	91

[a]P <.05.

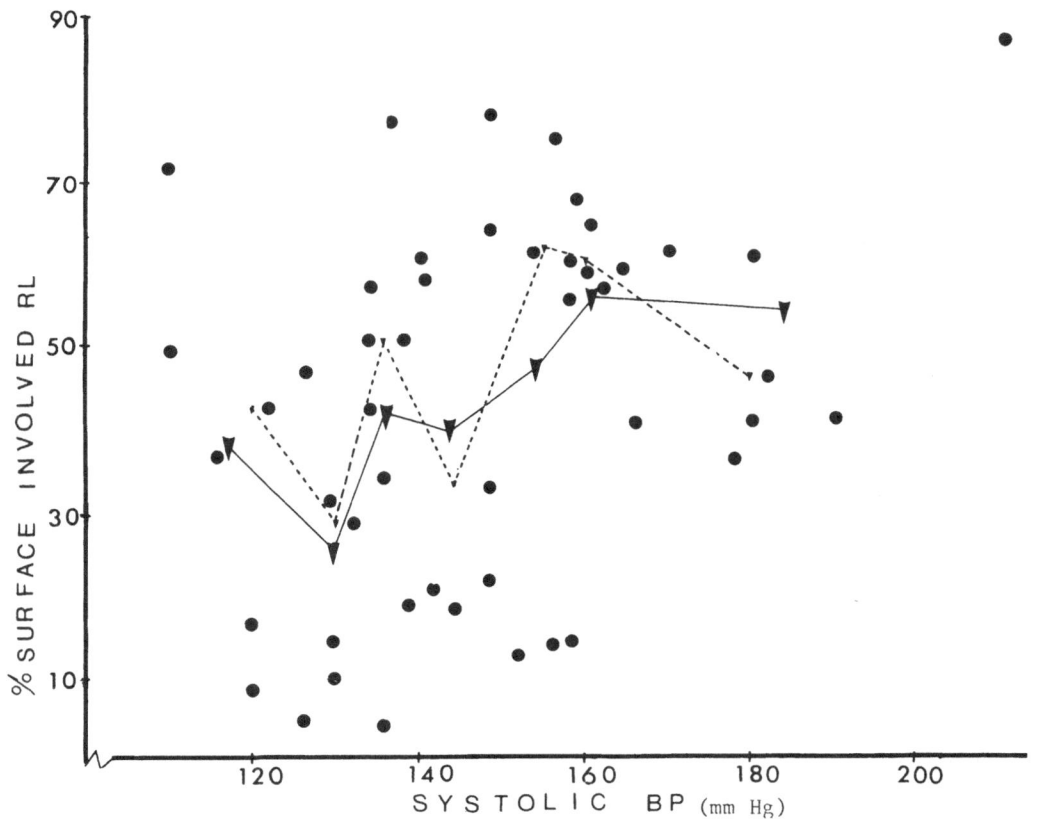

Figure 2. Raised atherosclerotic coronary lesions in individual cases, mean and median, by increasing values of systolic blood pressure. ——— mean; ----- median (Oslo study)

Discussion

We probably know only a few of the pathogenetic factors in atherosclerosis. Among them, serum cholesterol, blood pressure, and smoking habits seem to be the most accepted. Everyone is exposed to risk factors, but the degree of atherosclerotic lesions varies by age (Eggen and Solberg, 1968). Measurement of atherosclerotic lesions in one age group showed a large variation in RL because of individual differences in susceptibility to atheroclerosis and in exposure to risk factors. We anticipate a large variation in RL when we compare a single risk factor with the extent of RL because that is not the only factor. One factor alone explains only a part of the individual variation in RL. The multivariate analysis in this study using serum cholesterol, systolic blood pressure, and number of daily cigarettes smoked as explanatory variables, indicates that these three factors explain only 20% of the variation in RL: about 80% remains unexplained. The study has, however, limitations that may reduce the correlation. One limitation is the small number of cases considering the large individual variation in RL. Another limitation is that the study is based on *one* measurement of risk factors. Those risk factors are recorded in different periods before death, from a few weeks up to 4 years. We have no information about the level of risk factors in the decades before. Therefore, we cannot measure the influence of the risk factors previously. The results in this study indicate only crude estimates between risk factors and RL. Despite these limiations, our study shows a statistically significant correlation between RL and serum cholesterol and between RL and level of blood pressure. The findings indicate strongly that serum cholesterol and blood pressure are of importance for development of atherosclerotic lesions. The relative importance of these factors cannot be determined from our study. The lack of significant correlation between RL and triglycerides and between RL and smoking habits does not exclude those as risk factors for atherosclerotic lesions. Triglycerides and smoking may be weaker atherogenic factors compared with serum cholesterol and blood pressure. A larger study might well show significant correlation.

Summary

In the prospective Oslo study, coronary arteries from 49 men who underwent autopsy, aged 41 - 53 years, were graded for the extent of intimal raised atherosclerotic lesions. The grading results were compared with risk factors recorded before death. The results showed statistically significant correlation coefficients for serum cholesterol and systolic and diastolic blood pressures. The coefficients for triglycerides and number of daily cigarettes were not statistically significant.

ATHEROSCLEROSIS AND RISK FACTORS

Nisl H. Sternby

In 1969 (Fig. 1), a population-related clinical study of cardiovascular diseases was performed in Malmö, Sweden, on men born in even months during 1914. The main purpose was to evaluate the role of smoking, especially in the development of peripheral arterial disease. During the next 5 years, 41 men died and 33 of those were subject to detailed autopsies, including collection of various arteries. Overall mortality was 5.8%, but only 2.3% of the non-smokers and ex-smokers died, whereas 8.0% of the smokers died. Smoking was especially associated with death from neoplasia: only 0.4% of the non-smokers and ex-smokers, but 3.4% of the smokers died of cancer. Corresponding figures for cardiovascular diseases were 1.1% and 2.3%, respectively. Hypertension was associated with increased frequency

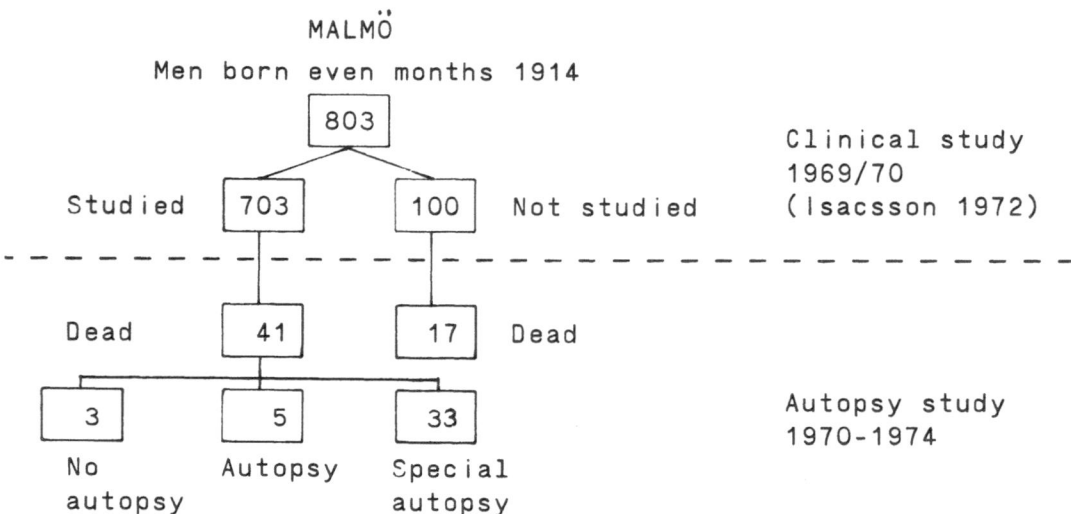

Figure 1. Number of cases studied clinically and at autopsy

of cardiovascular death, whereas hyperlipidemia was as common among subjects dying of neoplasia as among those dying of cardiovascular diseases.

Atherosclerosis was studied on stained arteries sealed in plastic bags. Specimens were available from five non-smokers and ex-smokers and 28 smokers. Table 1 compares atherosclerosis in various arteries in relation to smoking habits. Smokers had more aortic and peripheral atherosclerosis but not more coronary and cerebral atherosclerosis.

The influence of other risk factors was studied in 28 smokers (Table 2). Hypertension was strongly related to severe atherosclerosis in all arteries, whereas the effect of hyperlipidemia was uncertain but possible in the coronary arteries.

Table 1. Extent of atherosclerosis (percent of intimal surface area) in various arteries in men aged 56 – 60 and in relation to smoking habits

		Aorta	Coronary arteries	Cerebral arteries	Peripheral arteries
Total amount	Non Ex- smokers	50	59	28	35
	Smokers	64	51	20	44
Raised lesions	Non Ex- smokers	38	56	21	28
	Smokers	52	45	9	40

Table 2. Extent of atherosclerosis (percent of intimal surface area) in various arteries in men aged 56 – 60 and in relation to smoking, hyperlipidemia, and hypertension

		Smoking	Smoking and hyperlipidemia	Smoking and hypertension ($\pm$ hyperlipidemia)
Aorta	Total amount	60	56	77
	Raised lesions	46	44	72
Coronary arteries	Total amount	44	53	70
	Raised lesions	38	46	67
Cerebral arteries	Total amount	18	13	35
	Raised lesions	7	3	26
Peripheral arteries	Total amount	46	32	74
	Raised lesions	38	26	69

Some results from a WHO-organized epidemiological study of atherosclerosis in Europe (Kagan et al., in press) were reported. Lifsic, Yalta, USSR, studied the influence of smoking and of alcohol consumption on the development of atherosclerosis. Cigarette smoking was associated with an increased extent of raised aortic lesions but not with coronary atherosclerosis or stenosis or with myocardial infarction. Alcohol consumption was positively associated with extent of raised aortic lesions and especially of aortic calcification; in the coronary arteries the association was only with extent of calcified lesions. But myocardial and cerebral infarction was negatively associated with alcohol consumption.

In this European study, obese persons were found to have more atherosclerosis than thin persons had. The difference was greatly reduced when subjects with hypertension and diabetes were excluded. Obese persons did not have, however, significantly more atherosclerosis than subjects belonging to a standardized average atherosclerosis group; and if obesity has any effect on atherosclerosis, it accounts for only a small fraction of the total variation between subjects. On the other hand, the association between obesity and fresh myocardial infarction was significant, especially in men.

In men aged 40 – 59, incidence of sudden heart death and coronary heart disease was greater in those with sedentary than in those with strenuous occupations. An association of extent of raised coronary lesions with inactivity was evident.

The association between water hardness and atherosclerosis and frequently of myocardial infarction in the European study was not clear. Atherosclerosis was less extensive and myocardial disease was generally less frequent in the town with highest water hardness (Yalta, USSR), and they were greater (more extensive or more frequent) in the town with lowest water hardness (Prague, CSSR). In cities with intermediate values of water hardness, however, measures of atheroclerosis and myocardial infarction varied considerably. The influence of water hardness, if any, seemed to be much less than other factors.

CORONARY RISK FACTORS IN ADULTS: THE INFLUENCE OF NUTRITION IN EARLY LIFE

M. Hanefeld, W. Leonhardt, and H. Haller

The Dresden Study (Hanefeld et al., 1973), which was started by our group in 1971 and 1972, originally was designed to analyze:
1. The prevalence of coronary risk factors in a representative population group aged between 15 and 70 years, 2. the implications of these factors, and 3. dependence of specific variables on sex and age.

Therefore, the following program was carried out with 1216 persons (639 females and 577 males) selected at random who were working in factories and colleges within a limited area around Dresden (Fig. 1).

The variables shown at the top were recorded and correlations, percentiles, and prevalence of the disorders were calculated. About 90% of the persons asked volunteered to take part in the test. Persons with acute diseases and pregnant women were excluded.

As in other highly developed industrialized countries whose societies have a problem of overnutrition and low physical activity, we found a tremendously high percentage of metabolic diseases and hypertension (Table 1).

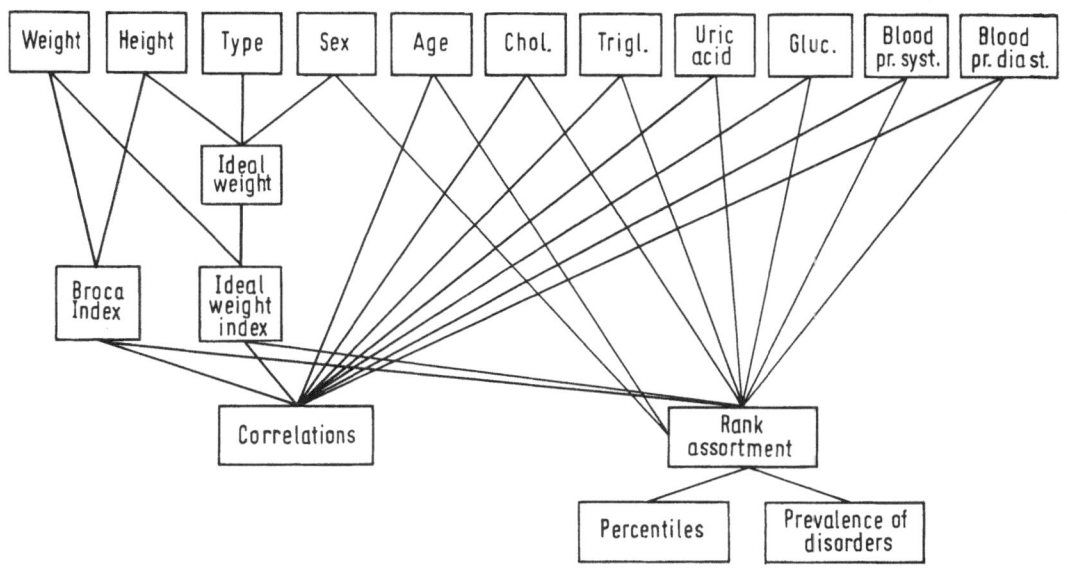

Figure 1. Program of the Dresden study

Table 1. Prevalence of risk factors in the Dresden study (n = 1216)

	Limits	Prevalence (%)
Diabetes mellitus	Fasting blood sugar >130/dl and/or known diabetes	2.0
Hyperuricemia	Uric acid ⩾6 mg/dl (F) ⩾7 mg/dl (M)	3.8
Hyperlipoproteinemia	Triglycerides ⩾250 mg/dl and/or cholesterol ⩾300 mg/dl	7.4
Obesity	Ideal weight index >1.3 (F) >1.2 (M)	8.2
Hypertension	≥160/95 mm Hg	17.2
Smoking	⩾1 g tobacco/d	30.3

By analyzing the total material, a close implication between these factors was found to exist. As is known from numerous other epidemiological studies, all factors correlated significantly with age. The correlation coefficients to age increased in this order: uric acid, glucose, triglycerides, cholesterol, blood pressure, and weight.

However, a detailed analysis of the age-dependent curves of the measurements resultet in distinct discontinuities of the curves. Thus, men aged 31 – 36 years showed a maximum for the mean triglyceride and cholesterol levels followed by a minimum at an age 36 – 41 years. In comparison, the curves given by Keys et al. (1972) for cholesterol showed a continuous increase until age 60 years.

In animal experiments, Hirsch et al. (1966) and Oscai et al. (1974) showed that variations in nutrition and physical activity in critical phases of early postnatal and prepubertal life permanently influence adipose tissue cellularity. Dörner and Mohnike (1973) demonstrated a significantly lower frequency of diabetes in adult men born in periods of food shortage. So the question arose for us whether the extremely different nutritional conditions resulting from years of peace and war in the childhoods of the tested population could influence the outcome and level of risk factors.

Materials and Methods

Therefore, the age-dependence curves of the measurements were computed as sliding 5-year average values for both sexes. For example, to compute the average cholesterol value for those aged 30, we used all values from persons aged 28 – 32 years. In that way, about 60 dates were pooled for every average value between ages 19 and 67 years. The average values for the categories below 19 and 67 years could only be computed as 3-year means with pools of 10 – 20 persons.

The data for food supply were based on statements made by v. Tyszka (1934), Woerrmann (1944), Ziegelmayer (1947), Holtmeyer, and others, as well as on the materials of Saxonian archives and on food ration cards.

Results

The curves for triglycerides, cholesterol, and glucose levels and weights clearly displayed maxima at the age group of 31 – 36 years followed by minima at the age group fo 36 – 41 years. The uric acid minimum occurred about 3 years later. A second minimum seemed to occur at the group age of 50 – 56 years (Fig. 2).

The probands between 31 and 35 years of age were born in years in which the supply of calories was normal. Minima of risk factors showed probands aged 36 – 41 years, born at the time of the world depression, had very low caloric intakes between ages 7 and 12 years.

In women, the minima were less clearly pronounced and concern mainly cholesterol, glucose, and uric acid levels.

Using the Student t test, we then tried to find out whether the differences between the minima and maxima were statistically significant. For that reason we selected for each measurement the age group in which a maximum was followed by a minimum (Table 2).

Discussion

In accordance with numerous epidemiological studies, our results showed the great differences of average values for various risk factors in different age groups. In comparison with epidemiological studies in Scandinavia, Switzerland, and the United States (Carlson and Ericson, 1975; Hartmann, 1974; Keys, 1969) the average values of blood lipids in our population were generally lower, but they corresponded in their maxima with those of the above-mentioned countries. The most interesting aspects of our curves were their minima of risk factors. Thus, the question arises whether the minima for persons between 36 and 41 years of age can be correlated with low food supply in critical developmental phases of ontogenetic differentiations, i.e., perinatal and prepubertal periods. Men aged 36 – 41 born during the world depression showed minimal values of triglycerides, cholesterol, and glucose. They were 7 – 12 years old at the beginning of a tremendous food shortage and 13 – 18 when nutrition became normal. Women of these age groups showed the same tendency, but less pronounced. In those critical periods, environmental signals like food supply may determine the level of neuronal behavioral systems and of metabolite- and hormone-regulating systems (Dörner, 1974). Further arguments in support of this hypothesis — additional to the above-mentioned results of animal experiments — provide data recently published by Dörner (1974) and Okamoto (1965).

1. Children of diabetic mothers become diabetic significantly less frequently than do children of diabetic fathers.
2. A significant relationship exists between weight put on in the first postnatal trimester and the weight index in maturity.
3. In the F_4-F_5 generations of alloxan diabetic rats, rabbits, and guinea pigs spontaneous diabetes occurred.

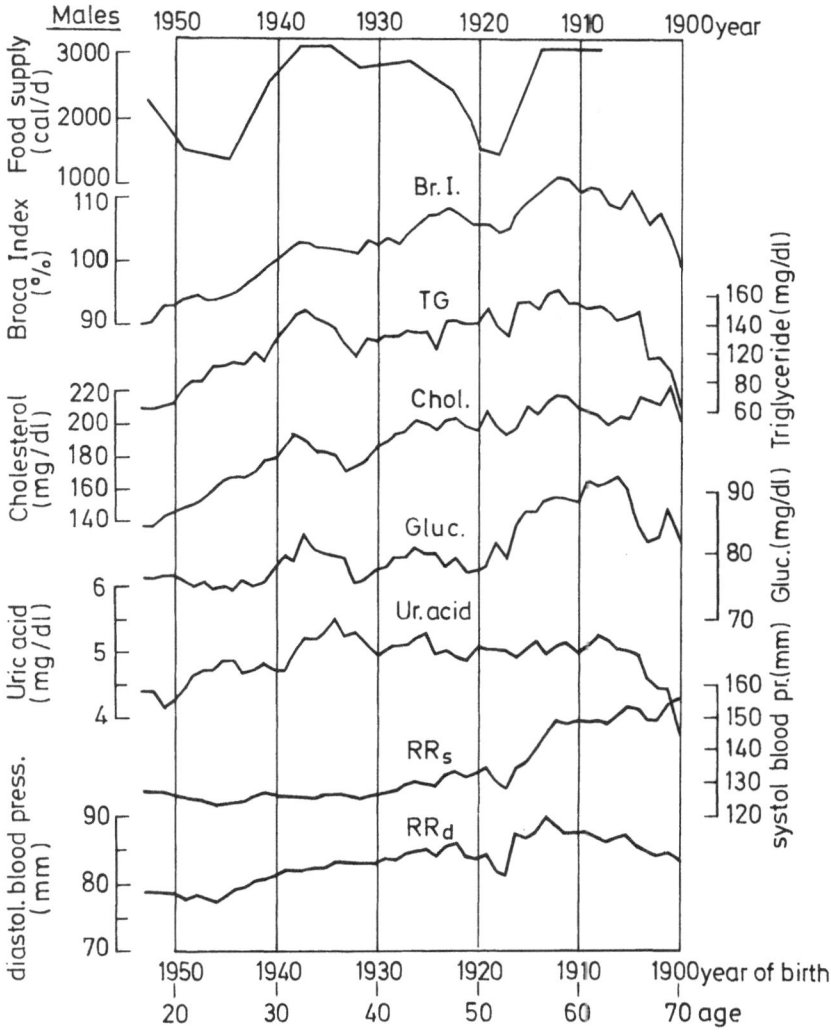

Figure 2. Relations between coronary risk factors, age, year of birth, and food supply

Table 2. Significance of maxima - minima configurations

Variable	Sex	mg/dl		Age	Maximum yr. of birth	mg/dl		Age	Minimum yr. of birth	P
TG	M	147	±85	32-36	1935-1939	116	±52	37-41	1930-1934	<0,05
Chol.	M	194	±50	31-35	1936-1939	172	±48	36-40	1931-1935	<0,025
	F	178	±50	28-31	1940-1943	155	±61	35-38	1933-1936	<0,025
Gluc.	M	83,9±24,4		32-36	1935-1939	75,2± 9,2		37-41	1930-1934	<0,05
	F	75,7± 9,3		24-27	1944-1947	70,8±10,5		35-38	1933-1936	<0,02
Ur.ac.	M	5,5± 1,6		35-39	1932-1936	4,9± 1,3		40-43	1928-1931	<0,05
	F	3,7± 0,9		16-29	1942-1955	3,5± 1,0		30-43	1928-1941	<0,05
Ur.ac.	F	4,1± 0,9		50-53	1918-1921	3,4± 1,1		56-59	1912-1915	<0,005
RR diast. (mmHg)	M	86,0± 9,8		46-51	1920-1925	79,0±11,1		52-55	1916-1919	<0,01

In summary, our data suggest that a low caloric intake during the perinatal and prepubertal growth might lead to lower levels of blood lipids, glucose, and uric acid in adults. Apart from the caloric intake, one must of course take into account other factors, such as protein and fat content of the food during the war and postwar years. We are aware of the speculative character of the interpretation of our data, but we believe that the interpretation should be reported and the problems further investigated.

THE RELATION OF ANTE MORTEM FACTORS TO ATHEROSCLEROSIS AT NECROPSY*

Mario R. Garcia-Palmieri, Maria I. Castillo, Margaret C. Oalmann, Paul D. Sorlie, and Raúl Costas, Jr.

Results from the International Atherosclerosis Project showed that coronary atherosclerotic lesions were less extensive and less severe among Puerto Ricans than among United States mainland decedents (Tejada et al., 1968).

An epidemiological prospective study has been in progress in Puerto Rico since 1965 in an effort to explain the low coronary heart disease (CHD) mortality by studying the influence of so-called risk factors on the development of the disease. Since 1965, the study has followed up 6843 urban and 2981 rural men aged 37 - 79 at entry. All were characterized for CHD risk factors at entry. Sizeable urban-rural differences in the level of traditional CHD risk factors and in myocardial infarction prevalence were noted (Garcia-Palmieri et al., 1970).

The study has also shown that CHD incidence in Puerto Rico is half that found in Framingham, Massachusetts, and is almost the same as that of Honolulu Japanese (Gordon et al., 1974).

*
This investigation was supported in part by Contracts PH 43-63-620 and NO1 HV 42902 from the National Heart, Lung and Blood Institute, National Institutes of Health, U.S. Public Health Service, Bethesda, Maryland, the University of Puerto Rico, and by grants HL-08974 and HL-14496 from the National Heart, Lung and Blood Institute to the Louisiana State University Medical Center.

As part of the protocol, all later deaths were documented. Because half of the decedents underwent autopsy, special procedures were introduced to determine aortic and coronary atherosclerosis in a subgroup of those autopsy subjects; the intent was to relate atherosclerotic findings in the urban and rural populations to antecedent risk factors routinely measured.

Methods

During the routine examinations, participants were interviewed to ascertain socioeconomic, dietary, and medical data. A physical examination oriented to detection of cardiovascular disease was done. The total vital capacity was measured and an electrocardiogram taken. Urine was examined for glucose and albumin, and blood for hematocrit, glucose, cholesterol, and glyceride levels. Details of the study design and laboratory methods are presented elsewhere (Colón et al., 1969).

Subjects were reexamined every 2 1/2 – 3 years. On the death of a participant, medical information was sought from the hospital, physician, or next of kin. Results of all autopsies were obtained. Pathologists and morgue attendants at two locations performing most of the autopsies in the area were altered to identify cases that might belong to the study population, and to save the coronary arteries and aortas for special studies. For a variety of reasons related to work conditions, fewer than half the possible specimens were collected.

The research autopsies used a protocol similar to the one designed by the International Atherosclerosis Project (Guzmán et al., 1968) to determine the extent of atherosclerosis. The specimens were stained with Sudan IV and were evaluated by the visual grading system to assess the percentage of intimal area of coronary artery or aorta showing fatty streaks, fibrous plaques, complicated lesions, or calcification. The sum of percentage intimal involvement with fibrous plaques, complicated lesions, and calcification (i.e., all *raised lesions*) constituted the measure of atherosclerosis used in this report. For each case, the aorta and the three coronary arteries were graded separately and independently by five pathologists. The value for a subject's degree of coronary atherosclerosis was the mean of the 15 gradings (three arteries by five pathologists). For some persons, fewer than 15 gradings were done. The value for aortic atherosclerosis was the mean of five gradings.

We used linear regression analysis and simple correlation coefficients to analyze the relationship of atherosclerosis at autopsy to baseline characteristics. Linear regression coefficients and their standard errors were determined. A t test of the difference between the ural and urban coefficients was done; the footnotes in Tables 1 and 2 show when the difference was statistically significant under the null hypothesis. The normal test statistic for the difference in correlation coefficients was done, testing whether the correlations were different in the cardiovascular and noncardiovascular death groups. Scatterplots of atherosclerosis on selected factors were drawn, showing that the significant coefficients were not due to extreme atherosclerosis in persons with high values of the independent variables.

Results

Ninety-two of the subjects who took the initial examination and whose death was known by February, 1974 underwent this special pathology study. Although the total autopsy rate was about 50%, only subjects undergoing autopsy at the Medical Center and Institute of Legal Medicine were accessible for the special autopsy protocol. Death occurred an average of 5 years after the initial examination, with the range being from less than 1 year to 9 years. All 92 subjects had a satisfactory aorta specimen for evaluation. For a limited time, some coronary material was taken seriatim for special biochemical studies. In those cases, the remaining coronary material was used for grading. In three subjects, the coronary arteries could not be properly evaluated.

The urban population had more atherosclerosis in the coronary arteries than did the rural, though this difference was not significant (Fig. 1). High involvement with coronary atherosclerosis (above 60%) was only found in the urban population. On the other hand, the severity of aortic atherosclerosis was similar for both rural and urban populations (Fig. 2). The correlation between atherosclerosis in the coronary arteries and aorta was only .38. A high degree of aortic involvement can exist with almost no coronary atherosclerosis.

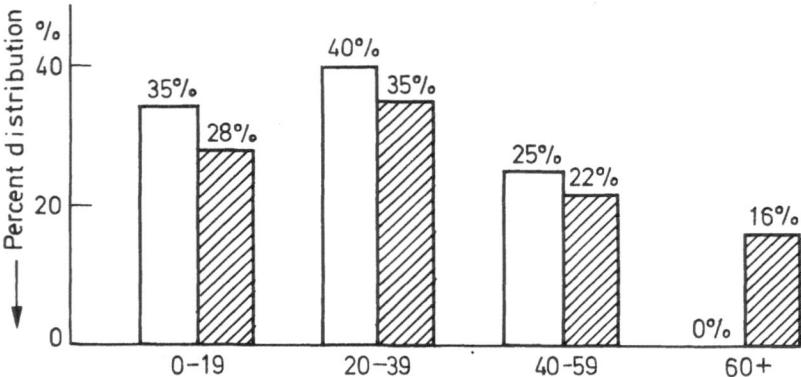

Figure 1. Distribution of atherosclerosis in the coronary arteries
☐ rural: N = 20, mean % involvement with raised lesions = 27.6
▨ urban: N = 69, mean % involvement with raised lesions = 33.7

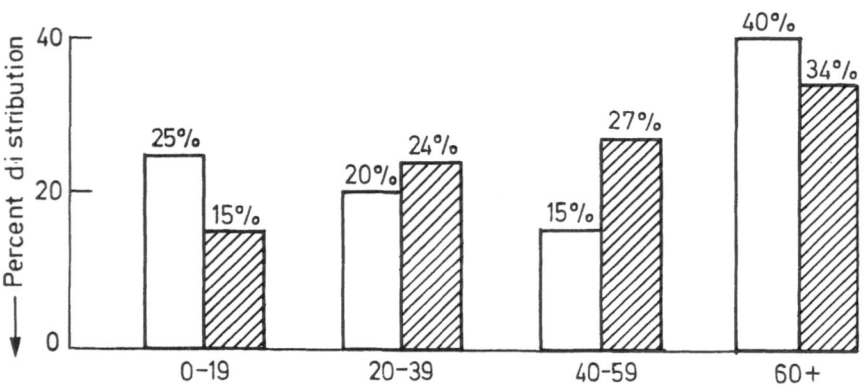

Figure 2. Distribution of atherosclerosis in the aorta
☐ rural: N = 20, mean % involvement with raised lesions = 44.1
▨ urban: N = 72, mean % involvement with raised lesions = 45.3

Table 1. Association of atherosclerosis in the coronary arteries with ante mortem characterisitcs; linear regression model coefficients

Characteristic		Regression coefficients			T test of coefficients H_o:rural-urban
		Total	Rural	Urban	
	N	89	20	69	
Age at death		0.000	0.505	-.178	NS
Relative weight		.023	-.173	.043	NS
Cigarettes/day		1.662	9.441	.485	NS
Serum cholesterol		.151[a]	.505[b]	.124[b]	b
Serum triglycerides[c]		.077[b]	.323[b]	.064[b]	NS
Blood glucose		.163[b]	.138	.160[b]	NS
Hematocrit		.194	1.925	-.043	NS
Systolic blood pressure		.107	-.138	.243[a]	a
Diastolic blood pressure		.295[b]	-.137	.389[b]	NS
Caloric intake		-.002	-.002	-.002	NS
Starch intake		-.027	-.001	-.029	NS
Physical acitvity index		-.518	.302	-1.082[b]	b
Income		.018	.000	.017	NS
Education		3.237	-5.256	4.836[b]	b
Calories/relative weight		-.228	.174	-.297	NS

[a] $P < .01$; $NS_p > .05$. [b] $P < .05$. [c] Fasting (n-57, 12, 45 respectively).

In the coronary arteries, the severity of atherosclerosis was significantly related to serum cholesterol, serum triglycerides, blood glucose levels, and diastolic blood pressure (Table 1). Lipid variables and blood pressure seemed to differ between the urban and rural populations. The regression of atherosclerosis on serum cholesterol was significantly larger in the rural than in the urban population. The regression on triglyceride showed a similar urban-rural contrast, but that contrast does not reach statistical significance. The relationship between blood pressure and coronary atherosclerosis could only be demonstrated in the urban population. Lower physical activity was associated with greater atherosclerosis in the urban but not the rural group. A greater amount of schooling was also related to more severe coronary atherosclerosis in the urban group, whereas in the rural population the opposite if anything applies. In the aorta, atherosclerosis was significantly associated with age at death, amount of cigarette smoking, levels of serum cholesterol, blood glucose, and hematocrit and caloric intake (Table 2). Although there appear to be some differences in the strength of the associations for the urban and rural populations, the only urban-rural contrast that was statistically significant was that for cigarette smoking with the rural group showing the stronger association.

In both the coronary arteries and the aorta, serum cholesterol was a significant factor in atherosclerosis with almost identical regression coefficients. Scatter-plots showed that the significant association was not the result of very high cholesterol levels.

Cause of death was apparently associated with atherosclerosis, because the average extent of atherosclerosis was significantly greater in those dying of cardiovascular causes.

Table 2. Association of atherosclerosis in the aorta with ante mortem characteristics; linear regression coefficients

| Characteristic | | Regression coefficients | | | T test of coefficients |
		Total	Rural	Urban	H_o:rural-urban
	N	92	20	72	
Age at death		1.144[a]	1.216	1.147[b]	NS
Relative weight		-.217	-.412	-.186	NS
Cigarettes/day		8.857[a]	24.078[a]	7.189[a]	[b]
Serum cholesterol		0.137[b]	0.506	0.116[b]	NS
Serum triglycerides[1]		.018	.412[b]	.001	NS
Blood glucose		.114[b]	.468	.103[b]	NS
Hematocrit		1.094[b]	2.525	.859	NS
Systolic blood pressure		.119	.078	.141	NS
Diastolic blood pressure		.154	.480	.092	NS
Chloric intake		-.007[b]	-.019	-.005	NS
Starch intake		-.051	-.098	-.039	NS
Physical activity index		-.335	-.995	.139	NS
Income		-.005	.027	-.012	NS
Education		-2.209	-5.387	-1.771	NS
Calories/relative weight		-.489	-1.888	-.319	NS

[a] $P <.01$; NS $P >.05$. [b] $P <.05$. [c] Fasting (n-59, 12, 47 respectively).

Discussion

The data presented here are considered as a preliminary report because ours is an
ongoing project. Clearly, it is not reasonably to make direct inferences from
this highly selected autopsy subsample to the general population because of the
well-known selective influences related to death and autopsy (McMahan, 1968).
Nevertheless, an unusual and important feature of this study is that baseline
characteristics were obtained an average of 5 years before death and in general
before the appearance of the terminal illness. This type of study is urgently
needed to clarify many unsolved questions concerning the true influence of risk
factors on atherogenesis in humans. A perusal of the literature fails to provide
such information.

The findings in this study revealed that aortic atherosclerosis was of similar
severity in the urban and rural groups. Coronary atherosclerosis, on the other
hand, was more severe in the urban than the rural decedents. The latter observation is consistent with the confirmed findings of a higher incidence of clinical
coronary heart disease in the urban population and might be more meaningful when
a larger number of special autopsie is available.

The degree of atherosclerosis in the coronary arteries of the 92 subjects was
related to their baseline levels of serum cholesterol, blood glucose, serum
triglycerides, and diastolic blood pressure ($P <0.05$). Although the urban and
rural populations seem to differ in the factors associated with coronary atherosclerosis, serum cholesterol was a significant factor in both groups.

The significant factors encountered in aortic atherosclerosis included serum
cholesterol, cigarette smoking, and blood glucose. The only two variables significantly associated with atherosclerosis in both the coronary arteries and aorta
were serum cholesterol and blood glucose levels.

A strong and consistent association of cigarette smoking with the extent of aortic atherosclerosis was noted in both urban and rural groups. This observation is consistent with the findings reported in similar studies (Sackett et al., 1968; Strong and Richards, 1976).

We are processing and analyzing more than 50 additional special autopsies and looking forward to any further light that might be obtained on this subject. Monitoring of all deaths continues.

The importance of performing special autopsy studies by a systemic and reproducible method in subjects that die while participating in prospective epidemiological studies in which systematic ante mortem information has been obtained cannot be overemphasized.

ATHEROSCLEROSIS AND ITS RISK FACTORS IN THE HAWAIIAN JAPANESE*

G.N. Stemmermann, G.G. Rhoads, and W.C. Blackwelder

The mortality for coronary heart disease (CHD) among the Japanese of Hawaii is intermediate between the rates for indigenous Japanese and U.S. whites, and indications are that the gap between the Hawaiian Japanese and the Hawaiian Caucasian rates has narrowed (Gordon, 1957; Worth et al., 1975). A tripartite study of Japanese men in Hiroshima, Japan, in Honolulu, Hawaii, and in Northern California (the Ni-Hon-San Study) was undertaken to discover the reason for the upward trend of CHD among the migrant Japanese. Dietary analyses indicate that, in contrast to that of the indigenous Japanese, a larger proportion of the Hawaiian Japanese diet is composed of animal fat and animal protein and a smaller proportion is composed of carbohydrate (CHO). A larger proportion of the Hawaiian CHO load is composed of simple CHO (e.g., sugar), as compared to complex CHO (e.g., rice). The Hawaiian Japanese are heavier, have thicker skinfolds (but are only slightly taller), have higher blood hematocrit levels, have higher levels of serum cholesterol and uric acid, and have more frequent glucose intolerance than the indigenous Japanese (Kagan et al., 1974).

If a study subject dies in either Hiroshima or Honolulu, permission for autopsy is requested. If the autopsy is performed at the Kuakini Medical Center in Honolulu or the RERF Laboratory in Hiroshima, the great vessels are dissected according to a detailed protocol. The degree of coronary and aortic atherosclerosis is estimated by a panel method (Gould et al., 1972). The vessels are matched to photographs, and the most appropriate of seven intervals is selected as the grade of severity. A grossly occluded vessel that cannot be opened longitudinally is automatically coded grade 7. Comparison between autopsy findings of Hiroshima and Honolulu indicate that Hawaiian Japanese have larger hearts, more numerous fatal infarcts, and more severe degrees of both aortic and coronary atherosclerosis (Stemmermann et al., 1976). Both severe coronary atherosclerosis and myocardial infracts were encountered at a younger age in Hawaii than in Japan. The degree of aortic atherosclerosis was positively associated with heart weight in both countries, but for coronary arteries a positive correlation with heart weight was found only in Hawaii.

To determine whether the patterns of vascular disease in the Hawaiian Japanese were related to one or more epidemiological variables, we correlated examination data with the Honolulu autopsy findings. Because several of the variables are

_____
*
These studies are funded by Contract #PH-43-NHLI-65-1003C-NO1-HL5-1003 to Kuakini Medical Center from the National Heart and Lung Institute, National Institutes of Health.

Table 1. Correlation coefficients among selected autopsy and examination variables

| Variables | Atherosclerosis grade | | Heart weight (grams) |
	Aorta (124 specimens	Mean coronary (109 specimens)	(223 specimens)
Age at death	.30[a]	.11	-.07
Exam variables:			
Height	-.12	.09	.14[b]
Relative weight (%)	-.10	.27[a]	.34[a]
Cigarettes/day	.14	.21[b]	-.07
Cholesterol (mg/dl)	.24[a]	.35[a]	.18[a]
Triglycerides (mg/dl)	.14	.23[b]	.13[b]
Uric acid (mg/dl)	-.05	.10	.17[b]
Glucose (mg/dl)	.15	.20[b]	.08
Hematocrit (%)	-.03	.19[b]	.04
Blood pressure:			
Systolic (mm Hg)	.29[a]	.14	.31[a]
Diastolic (mm Hg)	.05	.11	.26[a]
Pulse (mm Hg)	.35[a]	.11	.21[a]
Vital capacity (L)	-.23[a]	-.10	-.05
24-h dietary recall:			
Calories	-.10	-.23[b]	-.04
Starch (gm)	-.05	-.23[b]	.04
Saturated fatty acids (gm)	-.09	-.11	-.06
Alcohol (gm)	-.08	-.11	-.11
Mean coronary grade	.50[a] (96)	-	.46[a]
Aorta grade	-	.50[a] (96)	.16

[a]Significant at .01 level. [b]Significant at .05 level.

When a correlation coefficient is based on less than 95% of the specimens available (because of missing data), the number of observations is indicated in parentheses.

interrelated (e.g., age and systolic blood pressure), they were also analyzed in relation to the atherosclerotic process after other variables were taken into account. Table 1 indicates that, in univariate analysis, the serum cholesterol was the only variable significantly related to atherosclerosis in both the aorta and the coronary arteries. Aortic atherosclerosis was also related to age at death and blood pressure, and was inversely related to vital capacity. The coronary grade was positively associated with relative body weight, heart weight, cholesterol levels, the number of cigarettes smoked per day, 1-hour postprandial glucose level, and serum triglycerides and hematocrit levels; it was inversely related to the daily caloric intake and starch consumption. After multivariate analysis, the association of aortic atherosclerosis with cigarette smoking was strengthened. Triglycerides, glucose, and hematocrit levels were not significantly related to coronary atherosclerosis after other variables were considered in this multivariate analysis. The independent significant relationship between cholesterol level and aortic and coronary atherosclerosis is consistent with what one would expect from other published results. The clear relation of systolic blood pressure to aortic atherosclerosis in Hawaiian Japanese was not unexpected; although the correlation with coronary atherosclerosis was positive, it was not statistically significant. Notably, cohort men who died without myocardial infarction had higher mean blood pressures than the cohort as a whole.

Prospective studies in the United States have consistently identified cigarette smoking as a major CHD risk factor (Doyle et al., 1964), but this has not been reported in Japan (Johnson et al., 1968). It is an important risk factor for clinical CHD in Hawaiian Japanese, and the present study shows a positive association with coronary atherosclerosis in both univariate and multivariate analyses. Cigarette smokers tend to be thinner and younger than other persons, and, when that is accounted for, the strength of the association with both aortic and coronary atherosclerosis is enhanced.

In Hawaiian Japanese obesity is a strong clinical risk factor for CHD, and in our study body weight was significantly related to coronary, but not aortic, atherosclerosis. That finding is not consistent with an international study, the results of which could not relate the degree of atherosclerosis to the thickness of the abdominal panniculus.

Table 1 shows the correlation of heart weight with selected variables. The strongest associations are with blood pressure, relative weight, and mean coronary grade. Weaker associations were found with cholesterol and uric acid levels. Multiple regression analyses indicated significant independent associations with heart weight for old infarct, valvular disease, myocardial infarction, cancer death (negative), blood pressure, and relative body weight and height, whereas those for cholesterol, triglycerides, and uric acid levels were lost (Table 2).

Table 2. Associations of heart weight with selected variables

Variables	Regression coefficients	
	Simple	Multiple[a]
Mean coronary grade	28.8[b]	NS
Aorta grade	11.9	NS
Exam variables:		
Height (cm)	6.25[c]	6.23[c]
Relative weight (%)	2.34[b]	1.61[b]
Cholesterol (mg/dl)	.415[b]	NS
Triglycerides (mg/dl)	.097[c]	NS
Uric acid (mg/dl)	1.04[c]	NS
Systolic blood pressure (mm Hg)	1.39[b]	.710[b]
Diastolic blood pressure (mm Hg)	2.08[b]	NS
Total vital capacity (dl)	−.912	NS
Alcohol (gm)	−.302	NS
Old myocardial infract[d]	76.0[b]	43.0[b]
Valvular heart disease[d]	119[b]	67.7[b]
Cancer death[d]	−92.8[b]	−65.4[b]

[a] Multiple regression was done via a step-down procedure beginning with the set of variables shown; coefficients are for the final step. Multiple correlation (final step) = .61 (n = 196).

[b] Significant at .01 level. [c] Significant at .05 level.

[d] Entered as binary (0,1) variables.

NS: Variable included in first step, deleted as not significant at .05 level.

The substantial association of heart weight with coronary atherosclerosis seems largely explainable by this strong relation between coronary grade and previous myocardial infarction. Coronary grade averaged 5.3 for 28 men with old infarct and 2.8 for 81 men without infarct.

ATHEROSCLEROSIS IN RELATION TO PERSONAL ATTRIBUTES OF A JAPANESE POPULATION IN HOMES FOR THE AGED

Shuichi Hatano and Toshihisa Matsuzaki*

A group of residents in Tokyo metropolitan homes for the aged, comprising 731 men and 1241 women aged 60-94 underwent annual health examinations in 1972. They had mean lower serum cholesterol levels but similar body builds, skinfold thicknesses, and diastolic blood pressures when compared with a general Japanese group of the same age in Koganei City, Tokyo.

The majority of such patients are admitted to the affiliated hospital when they become severely ill, and the autopsy rate in our hospital has been over 80%. Because of the group's representativeness, and the high autopsy rate, the investigation of persons undergoing autopsy would permit estimating atherosclerosis among the aged Japanese, by and large.

A study of atherosclerosis among 100 men and 86 women, residents of the homes who underwent autopsy, was done to study: (1) the extent of atherosclerosis in the elderly Japanese who lived a traditional Japanese life, which is supposed to be less atherogenic, over a long period, (2) the relevance of atherosclerosis to cardiovascular diseases in the aged, and (3) to what extent personal attributes and behavior observed in the aged are related to atherosclerosis.

Methods

The degree of atherosclerosis was macroscopically graded into five classes. The extramural coronary arteries were sectioned at intervals of a few millimeters, and the degree of narrowing was graded by macroscopic observations at each section with cutoff points at narrowing of 25%, 50%, 75% and 90% of the lumen. The intracranial arteries were graded in a similar manner (Kameyama, 1974).

Altogether during 4 years since the health exam in July, 1972, 186 patients were hospitalized, died, and subsequently underwent autopsy (Table 1). More than half belonged to the age brachet 75-84 for both men and women. The mean age at death was 78 in men and 80 in women.

We compared selected personal attributes and behavior characteristics that were examined when the subjects were healthy with atherosclerotic indices, namely, either a macroscopically graded degree of atherosclerosis (in larger arteries), or a degree of narrowing of the arterial lumen (the intracranial arteries and the coronary arteries).

We compared the frequency of ischemic lesions in the brain and the myocardium between the groups having different atherosclerotic indices of the perfusing arteries.

----

* The authors thank the staffs in the Department of Clinical Pathology, Tokyo Metropolitan Geriatric Hospital: Drs. Shohichi Ohtsu, Hroyuki Shimada, and colleagues who carried out general autopsy, and Drs. Masakuni Kameyama, Masanori Tomonaga, and colleagues for neuropathology.

Table 1. Number of subjects who underwent annual health examination and autopsy (Tokyo metropolitan homes for the aged 1972-1976)

Age (year)	Men	Women	Mean and women
60 - 64	5	1	6
65 - 74	27	17	44
75 - 84	53	47	100
85 - 94	15	21	36
All ages	100	86	186
Mean age	77.8	79.8	78.9

Results

1. Atherosclerosis by Age and Sex

The degree of atherosclerosis in the arteries generally did not differ much after age 65. A slightly severer degree of atherosclerosis and more frequent secondary lesions, such as calcification or ulcers, were observed in the aorta in a group aged 80 and more than in a younger group.

In an old-age population, sex differences in biological variables usually diminish. Stenosis of the coronary arteries, however, was more extensive in men than in women. The frequency of cases with stenosis (luminal narrowing of more than a half section) in any coronary artery was 84% in men and 69% in women, and that with stenosis in more than one artery was 58% in men and 44% in women.

2. Personal Factors. Behavior and Atherosclerosis

Table 2 shows the weak but statistically significant correlations. Blood pressure correlated with the degree of atherosclerosis of the intracranial arteries. Serum cholesterol level correlated with atherosclerosis in the main trunks of the aorta. Atherosclerosis of the aorta itself was not correlated with any of the listed factors. Coronary artery stenosis correlated with diastolic blood pressure, skinfold thickness, and serum cholesterol and hematocrit levels but only in women. Those data coincided, in part, with a preceeding report on another Japanese population in a home for the aged in Tokyo.

The hypertensives, once detected at the annual health examination, were invited to the clinic for control. The blood pressure distribution of treated hypertensive patients was thus available. Despite medication, the hypertensives showed higher mean pressure and higher frequency of hypertension. The blood pressure gradient, however, must have narrowed and the power of association with atherosclerosis would have been underestimated in this series of treated patients.

We studied the relation of smoking and drinking habits to degree of atherosclerosis among men (Table 3). Daily smoking was associated with a higher frequency of coronary stenosis, but the dose-response relationship was not clear. Drinking alcoholic beverages was associated with a higher frequency of calcified lesion or ulcer in the aorta.

Table 2. Correlation coefficient between personal attributes and atherosclerotic indices (Tokyo metropolitan homes for the aged 1972-1976)

Attributes	Atherosclerosis in						
	A.cerebri media	A.basilaris	A.carotis	A.subclavia	A. iliaca	Aa. coronariae No. of arteries with stenosis	No. of stenoses
Blood pressures							
Systolic		0.25^a(M)			0.28^a(M)		
Diastolic	0.24^a(F)	0.25^a(M) 0.24^a(F)					0.23^a(F)
Skinfold thickness						0.24^a(F)	0.36^b(F)
Serum cholesterol			0.30^b(M) 0.33^b(F)	0.40^b(F)	0.32^b(F)		0.25^a(F)
A/G ratio of serum protein		0.25^a(M)					
Hematocrit							0.26^a(F)

^{a}P <0.05. ^{b}P <0.01. M = men; F = women.

Table 3. Smoking and drinking habits and atherosclerosis in men (Tokyo metropolitan homes for the aged)

Smoking and coronary artery stenosis

Smoking	Stenosis		
	No	Yes	Total
No	6	8	14
Yes, daily	8	67	75
Total	14	75	89

P <0.05.

Drinking and aorta calcification

Drinking	Complicated or calcified lesions		
	No	Yes	Total
No and occasionally	48	20	68
Yes, daily	6	12	18
Total	54	32	86

P <0.05.

3. Atherosclerosis and Ischemic Lesions

Among patients having coronary arterial occlusion, more than half had fresh myocardial necrosis, and when scars are included, more than 80% had myocardial damage.

Two of 24 patients having fresh myocardial infarction had no occlusion. Disseminated intravascular coagulopathy was often seen in such conditions.

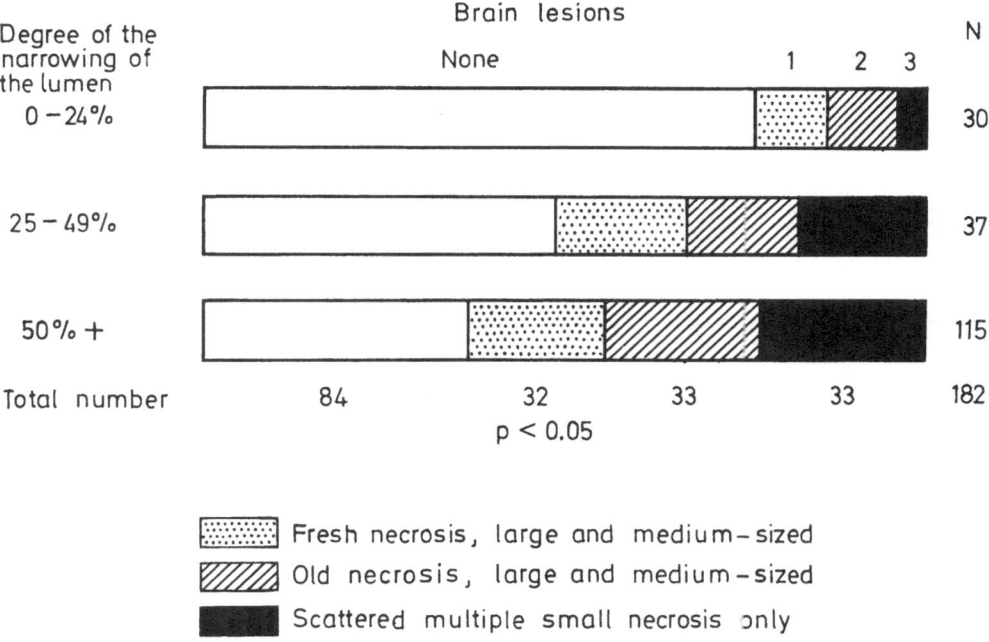

Figure 1. Relative frequency of ischemic brain lesions by degree of stenosis of the middle cerebral arteries (Tokyo Metropolitan Geriatric Hospital 1972-1976)

The frequency of fresh necrosis and scattered multiple small necroses of the brain increased with the increase in the degree of narrowing of the middle cerebral artery (Fig. 1). We found similar results for the degree of narrowing of the basilar artery and for the degree of atherosclerosis in the carotid artery.

Summary and Conclusions

Of 1972 residents in Tokyo metropolitan homes for the aged, 186 subjects died in Tokyo Metropolitan Geriatric Hospital and underwent autopsy during 0-4 years of follow-up since the annual health exam in July, 1972.

Coronary arterial stenosis or occlusion was not rare among the aged Japanese. The rather high frequency, however, was not directly comparable with the IAP results or other studies because methods differed.

In the old persons, the degree of atherosclerosis did not change much with age; however, sex differences were still observed in the extent of coronary stenosis.

Atherosclerosis of perfusing arteries was associated with cerebral or myocardial infarction in old patients, too.

A small fraction of brain and myocardial damage was caused by other than the atherosclerosis, but its frequency was much lower than that of the atherosclerosis.

Various personal factors and behavior characteristics seemed to correlate with the degree of atherosclerosis or stenosis. The extent of relationship for each factor to atherosclerosis of arteries varied among different sites: blood pressure correlated with atherosclerosis in the intracranial arteries, iliac artery, and coronary arteries; serum cholesterol level correlated with atherosclerosis of the coronary arteries and major trunks of the aorta, but not to the same extent as that of the intracranial arteries; skinfold thickness correlated with atherosclerosis of the coronary arteries. Smoking correlated with atherosclerosis of the coronary arteries, and alcohol drinking with secondary lesions of the aorta. The association of personal factors with atherosclerosis of the coronary arteries appeared to be significant in women, but not in men.

FREQUENCY OF CORONARY AND PERIPHERAL ARTERY DISEASE IN HYPERLIPO-PROTEINEMIA
A Cooperative Study Among Italian Lipid Clinics*

G. Crepaldi

Recent reports show that during the past 20 years mortality resulting from cardio-vascular disease (CVD) has been increasing steadily in Italy as in the rest of the industrialized world (Crepaldi et al., 1976).

The statistics on general mortality in Italy show that the number of deaths from CVD rose from 36/10,000/year in 1951 to 45/10,000/year in 1972. For coronary artery disease (CAD), the data show mortality rising from 4/10,000/year in 1952 to 16/10,000/year in 1971.
According to national statistics, the frequency of CVD in the Italian hospital population was 7/1000 in 1961 as compared with 14/1000 in 1971.

More reliable data concerning CAD incidence has been provided recently by Menotti's epidemiological study (Italy) as part of the "Seven Country Study" (Keys, 1970). In the two small towns studied by Menotti et al. (unpublished observations, 1976), CAD incidence was about 10/100/year among men, practically the same as the incidence reported for men in the United States.

The Framingham (Kannel et al., 1971) and "Seven Country" (Keys, 1970) studies concluded that the differences in CAD incidence relate to differences in serum cholesterol levels. Dietary surveys (Stamler, 1967) indicate that differences in cholesterol concentrations may relate to diet — and more specifically to percent intake of saturated fat.

Mean cholesterol levels were studied in three population samples (age range 20 – 60 years) by three lipid clinics in Italy (Bologna, Rome, and Naples). The highest levels, for both cholesterol and triglycerides, were observed by the northern clinic (Bologna), whereas the lowest levels were reported by the southern clinic (Naples). Dietary surveys of the populations of those areas revealed a strict relationship between the degree of hyperlipidemia and total calorie and saturated fat intake.

---

*Italian Lipid Clinics:
 - Bologna: S. Lenzi, G.C. Descovich, C. Ceredi, P. Meliota, U. Montaguti
 - Milan: R. Paoletti, L. Sirtori, G. Conti
 - Naples: M. Mancini, P. Oriente
 - Padua: R. Fellin, G. Briani, E. Manzato
 - Palermo: S. Strano, G. Avellone, A. D'Eredità
 - Perugia: S. Ventura, U. Senin
 - Rome: G. Ricci, A. Menotti
 - Siena: G. Weber, B. Bertelli
 - Venice: P. Avogaro, G. Cazzolato
 - Verona: C. Dal Palù, A. Pagnan.

With the collaboration of the Institute of Genetics (Bologna), S. Cavicchi, D. Conti, and the Institute of Mathematics (Modena), G. Mannino.

Prevalence of Hyperlipidemias

The risk of premature CAD — at least among men — rises directly as serum cholesterol levels rise. This relationship is particularly evident in patients in whom
the serum cholesterol level is high because of familial hyperbetalipoproteinemia
(type II), although studies of such subjects reveal considerable variation in the
incidence of CAD (Jensen et al., 1967; Patrassi and Crepaldi, 1971; Slack, 1969;
Stone et al., 1974). An increased risk of CAD and peripheral artery disease (PAD)
has been observed in patients with Fredrickson's type III and IV hyperlipidemias
(Patrassi and Crepaldi, 1971).

A series of patients affected with different types of hyperlipoproteinemia have
been studied by ten lipid clinics in Italy (Table 1). A total of 3359 subjects —
2010 men and 1349 women — were examined. Of those patients 43.7% were affected
with type IIa, 22.9% with type IIb, 30.4% with type IV, 2.4% with type V, and
fewer than 1% with type III. Only three patients (observed at the Padua Clinic)
were affected with type I. All of the lipid clinics used the World Health Organization's "classification of hyperlipidemias and hyperlipoproteinemias" (WHO,
1972) as the basis for lipid typing.

Despite the homogeneous distribution of the patients observed by the ten lipid
clinics, the incidence of specific types of hyperlipoproteinemias varied greatly;
for example, in the Milan, Palermo, and Siena populations type IV exceeded 40%
(Table 2). At the same time, the lowest percentage of type IV and the highest of
type IIa were noted in the Roman population.

More men than women and more northerners than southerners were examined in this
country-wide survey. Although type IIa was more prevalent among women, type IV
was more frequently observed among men (Table 3). This finding was true for both
northern and southern Italy.

Our results were confirmed by the retrospective study carried out in Brisighella
(Italy) (Lenzi, S., Descovich, G., unpublished data, 1976). That study showed
that the women of that small Italian town were prevalently hypercholesterolemic,
whereas the males were prevalently hypertriglyceridemic, when 260 mg/dl was used
as the cut-off point for the normal cholesterol level and 190 mg/dl that for the
normal triglyceride level.

For men, age was significantly correlated with the type of hyperlipoproteinemia. This
finding was confirmed by the fact that the greatest number of men classified as having
type IIa and type IIb hyperlipoproteinemias were in the age range between 50 and
54 years, whereas those having type IV and V were mostly between 45 and 49 years.

Moreover, for each type of hyperlipoproteinemia, the number of men was greater
for the early decades of life, but the number of women was greater for the latter
decades.

Table 1. Primary hyperlipoproteinemias total No. 3359 (M = 2010; F = 1349)
(Lipid clinic cooperative study, Italy)

Type	Males	Females	All	Prevalence
I	1	1	2	0.06%
IIa	645	823	1468	43.70%
IIb	484	284	768	22.90%
III	11	9	20	0.60%
IV	800	221	1021	30.40%
V	69	11	80	2.40%

Table 2. Percent excess values (Lipid clinic cooperative study, Italy)

	BMI ($>\bar{x}$ + 1 SD)				FBS (>120 mg/dl)				SUA (>6,0 mg/dl)		
	IIa	IIb	IV		IIa	IIb	IV		IIa	IIb	IV
Northern	23.5	40.8	42.5	Northern	3.8	8.6	10.4	Northern	15.3	60.2	71.1
Southern	28.7	33.0	41.7	Southern	2.8	5.4	5.6	Southern	27.9	38.5	53.7
All	24.9	38.8	42.2	All	3.6	7.9	9.1	All	18.3	55.6	66.5

Table 3. CAD and PAD percent frequency in hyperlipoproteinemias (Lipid clinic cooperative study, Italy)

		IIa	IIb	IV	Northern Italy	Southern Italy
CAD	Males	35.2	30.9	28.2	31.7	27.6
	Females	38.1	38.0	41.9	41.4	29.9
	All	36.8	33.6	31.1	35.5	28.4
PAD	Males	21.0	23.9	20.4	22.9	16.7
	Females	20.3	27.9	23.7	25.3	12.3
	All	20.5	25.3	21.2	23.9	15.3

Although the incidence of diabetes in type IIa subjects is equivalent to that found in the normal population, it is greater among persons having types IIb and IV hyperlipoproteinemias, with the highest incidence occurring with the latter. The percentage of hyperglycemia in the subjects having type IIa, IIb, and IV was much lower in southern Italy.

Mean serum uric acid levels were higher among persons having type IV and IIb hyperlipoproteinemias. The percentage of type IV subjects having hyperuricemia was about 75%. Similar to the findings for diabetes, the frequency for hyperuricemia among subjects having type IV and IIb was greater in northern Italy.

Although the body mass index is normal among persons having type IIa conditions, it is increased among those having type IIb and IV. Percent excess values were 42% for type IV and 38.8% for type IIb (Table 2).

Mean values of both systolic and diastolic blood pressure were similar in all three types. The percentage of hypertensive patients was not significantly different among the three types. The percentage of hypertensive subjects in our hyperlipemic group was about the same as that in the Brisighella population, when the same cut-off points were used.

Frequency of CAD and PAD

The highest percent frequency of CAD was observed with type IIa (36.8%), whereas the highest prevalence of PAD was noted with type IIb (25.3%) (Table 3). CAD prevalence was 33.8% and incidence of myocardial infarction 7.44% in the group of hyperlipemics taken as a whole. Among men, the highest incidence of CAD was noted with type IIa, whereas among women it occurred with type IV.

The percent frequency of CAD was higher for women (41.4%) and men (31.7%) from northern Italy than for their southern counterparts. CAD percent frequency was always higher in the northern population for both men and women.

The percent frequency of PAD was higher among women affected with type IIb and IV hyperlipoproteinemias than among the men having these types. The geographic distribution shows PAD was more frequently observed in the north than in the south for both men and women. The higher frequency of CAD and PAD in the northern population can be correlated with other risk factors, such as diabetes, hyperuricemia, and excess body weight, which are more frequently observed in those patients.

When the prevalence of certain risk factors is evaluated (Table 4) in association with hyperlipidemia, smokers having hyperlipidemia have a greater risk than smokers not having hyperlipidemia. When all risk factors are considered, CAD prevalence is about the same as that of hyperlipidemia plus hypertension (Crepaldi et al., 1976). This finding is true for both men and women.

In the same way, for persons having type IIb hyperlipidemia, the risk is greater if they smoke than if they do not, but those having hyperlipidemia and hypertension have an even greater risk. The percent decrease in PAD prevalence noted for women was statistically significant, but that for men was not.

In type IV, smoking did not affect CAD prevalence, whereas hypertension induced a statistically significant increase for both women and men. That hypertension is an important adjunctive risk factor that increases CAD incidence in hyperlipoproteinemias should be emphasized.

Table 4. Risk factors and CAD prevalence in primary hyperlipoproteinemias (Lipid clinic cooperative study, Italy)

	CAD% – Type IIa		CAD% – Type IIb		CAD% – Type IV	
	Males	Females	Males	Females	Males	Females
Hyperlipemia	18.2	28.6	28.1	23.1	28.7	36.4
Hyperlipemia + smoking	35.0	39.1	25.0	34.1	22.8	13.8
Hyperlipemia + hypertension	39.2	48.2	27.2	52.9	35.4	59.1
All factors	48.2	48.8	42.8	35.3	36.1	41.2
	$X^2=33.09$	$X^2=40.55$	$X^2=16.41$	$X^2=27.01$	$X^2=19.02$	$X^2=23.90$
	P <0.005	P <0.005	N.S.	P <0.005	P <0.02	P <0.005

CONCLUDING REMARKS ON THE EPIDEMIOLOGY OF ATHEROSCLEROSIS

T. Omae

As some speakers have described, risk factors of coronary atherosclerosis may not be exactly the same as those of aortic atherosclerosis. Several years ago a collaborative study by two study groups, Kyushu University and University of Minnesota, on stroke and cerebral atherosclerosis in the Japanese and Caucasian populations, showed that atherosclerosis of the circle of Willis was of the same degree — or even more advanced — in the Japanese compared with that in the Minnesota subjects. Cerebral angiograms of the stroke patients showed that the Caucasians had more frequent occlusive lesions in the extracranial arteries than the Japanese, and the situation was reversed for the frequency of severe occlusions in the intracranial arteries. Racial differences may explain these disparities.

Among our patients, hypertension was by far more important than hypercholesterolemia as a risk factor of cerebral atherosclerosis and cerebral infarction. Hypertension may also accelerate coronary atherosclerosis, but the correlation of hypertension with coronary atherosclerosis was not as strong as that with cerebral atherosclerosis. In our experience, elevation of systolic blood pressure correlated more with coronary atherosclerosis than did elevation of diastolic blood pressure. Furthermore, the correlation of blood pressure with coronary atherosclerosis was not as consistent. Sometimes the correlation was absent, depending on the selection of ante mortem blood pressure recordings.

When risk factors of atheorsclerosis are discussed, correlation of one factor with another should be considered carefully. For example, obesity may be associated more frequently with such factors as hypertension, abnormal GTT, hyperuricemia, lack of physical activity, and increase in caloric intake. Therefore, when only one factor is taken and the factors associated with it are ignored, the most appropriate conclusion may not be reached.

There is one other point I would like to make. The risk factors that we have discussed in this workshop were based on the data at cross-sectional examinations. Body weight, blood pressure, some of the blood chemistries, and other factors can change considerably with time. The time-course of those variables should also be considered in preparing the second step of such an epidemiological study.

ABSTRACTS

SOCIO-ECONOMIC FACTORS IN CHD EPIDEMIOLOGY IN MIGRATING POPULATIONS

Daniel Brunner
Donolo Institute of Physiological Hygiene, Tel Aviv University, Tel Aviv/Israel

The effect of changing life pattern on CHD-epidemiology and coronary risk factors is demonstrated in Oriental Jews who immigrated from underdeveloped countries to Israel 25 years ago. CHD mortality rates increased from 1950 to 1973 in Oriental-born males 45-59 years old from 110 to 240, and in 60-74 years old from 220 to 1100 per 100,000. The CHD mortality rates of European-born males were significantly higher, of females not different from that of Oriental Jews.
Recently performed post-mortem studies of 115 European-born, and 72 Oriental-born fatal victims of road accidents showed significant differences in the degree coronary atherosclerosis.
Even 20 years after their immigration to Israel, Oriental Jews had significantly lower serum cholesterol levels than European-born subjects. In 1955, Yemen-born diabetics, when compared with matched European-born diabetics, showed a very low incidence or absence of vascular complications. 20 years later, no difference in the prevalence of atherosclerotic complications in diabetics of different ethnic origin exists.
Higher body weight and height, blood pressure and cholesterol were measured in Yemenites living more than 35 years in Israel when compared with more recently arrived Yemenite Jews.

CORONARY RISK FACTORS IN AUSTRALIAN MEN

Jean Palmer, Boonseng Leelarthaepin, Clyde McGilchrist, and Ralph Blacket
Department of Medicine, University of New South Wales, Prince Henry Hospital, Sydney/Australia

Four hundred fifty eight men, age thirty to sixty with coronary disease were compared with seven hundred forty healthy men of the same age. Univariate analysis showed the coronary men to be shorter, heavier, to have higher serum lipids, serum urate and blood pressure and to be heavier smokers than the normal controls. Stepwise discriminant analysis showed that over the whole age range height, serum urate, serum cholesterol, age and systolic blood pressure were the most significant discriminants of coronary men. In men under forty nine the order of importance was serum cholesterol, height, serum urate and systolic blood pressure. In men over forty nine the order was serum urate, height and serum cholesterol. The findings emphasize the greater concentration of risk factors in younger men with coronary heart disease. The significance of body weight and cigarette smoking was clear in the univariate analysis. The stepwise discriminant analysis did not take into account changes in body weight and smoking habits between infarction and examination. Further data taking these factors into account will be presented.

EPIDEMIOLOGICAL STUDY OF CORONARY ARTERY DISEASE AND CEREBRO-VASCULAR DISEASE IN TAIWAN. RISK FACTORS

Cheng-Jen Hsu, Jui-San Chen, Ching-Min Chen, and Wen-Ping Tseng
Department of Medicine, National Taiwan University Hospital, Taipei, Taiwan/Republic of China

In our prospective epidemiological study of coronary artery disease (CAD) and cerebrovascular disease (CVD) in Chinese over 40 years of age in Taiwan, 1058 urban (Taipei) and 670 rural (Sanchih) inhabitants were studied with epidemiological random sampling method. Prevalence rate of CAD was 2.647 (male 3.015, female 2.109) for urban, and 0.597 (male 0.794, female 0.342) for rural population. There is a significant difference between urban and rural population. Prevalence rate of CVD was 1.229 (male 1.843, female 0.434) for urban, and 1.194 (male 1.058, female 1.37) for rural population. There is some difference between male and female urban inhabitants, but no difference between urban and rural population. CAD is related significantly with activity, body weight, systolic and diastolic pressure, blood sugar, abnormal lipoprotein typing, serum cholesterol, triglyceride and uric acid. CVD is related significantly with the same factors as in CAD except serum cholesterol and abnormal lipoprotein typing. Lower activity, more obesity, more abnormal lipoprotein typing, higher serum triglyceride and uric acid were found in urban population and these would be responsible for higher prevalence rate of CAD among urban population.

EPIDEMIOLOGY OF RISK FACTORS FOR CORONARY HEART DISEASE (CHD) IN A FREE LIVING POPULATION

José Neuman, María P. Neuman, Elina Valero, and Daniel Lindental
Instituto de Obra Social del Bjército, Buenos Aires/Argentina

A project of detection and treatment of multiple risk factors (RF) toward CHD has been started. Up to now, 780 subjects have been screened and 462 are apparently normal. Medical history, physical examination, ECG, chest-X ray plate, routine laboratory, cholesterol, triglycerides and agarose gel electrophoresis were performed. The frequency (%) of RF in "normal" population is: hyperlipoproteinemia (HLP) 44, hypertension ($\geq$160-95) 17, smoking habits (>10 cigarettes daily) 39, stress 49, overweight (weight/height >1.1) 41, sedentariness 45, family history of CHD 8, diabetes 6, ECG abnormalities 5. Of this population, 5% have no RF. Type IV HLP ist significantly more prevalent (P <0.001) in males than females: 30.4 (70/230) vs 13.4% (31/232). No sex differences were found for types IIa (11.5%) and IIb (10.6%). Males in the 5th and females in the 6th decade showed the highest frequency of HLP. An extra pre-B lipoprotein band was detected in 25% of the subjects.

ATHEROSCLEROSIS OBLITERANS OF THE LOWER EXTREMITY IN JAPANESE

Kiyoshi Inada
Department of Surgery, Gifu University, School of Medicine, Gifu/Japan

Atherosclerosis obliterans is recently increasing in Japan, though not common in Western countries. Clinical features of these patients were analysed to compare with those of reported series in English literatures. Average age of the series, sex distribution, symptomatology, method of treatment and prognosis were similar in both, though incidence of diabetes is low and aortic occlusion is not common in Japanese.
Blood cholesterol, triglyceride and β-lipoprotein determination were performed in patients with atherosclerosis obliterans and with Buerger's disease as control. The mean levels of these lipid were very much the same in both groups. Hypercoagulability was found in most of these patients, though there were no significant differences between both groups, too.

ROLE OF HYPERLIPOPROTEINEMIA IN THE NATURAL HISTORY OF PERIPHERAL ARTERIAL DISEASE

R.M. Greenhalgh, G.W. Taylor, M.J.P. Higgins, and Gillian Harcourt
Professorial Surgical Unit, St. Bartholomew's Hospital, London/Great Britain

Resting ultrasonic systolic ankle/brachial pressure index has been used to follow 200 patients with angiographic evidence of stenosing peripheral arterial disease in the arteries supplying their lower limbs. 54% of patients had a raised serum lipoprotein level. Results are available on 67 limbs after 2.5 years and 260 limbs after 6 months. From age and sex matched control studies the upper limit for triglyceride was taken as 160 mg per 100 ml and for cholesterol as 270 mg per 100 ml. A change of 5% in the pressure index was regarded as significant. After 2.5 years with normal lipid levels, 16 limbs were improving, 6 worsening and 10 were the same. With raised lipid levels 7 limbs were improving, 16 worsening and 12 were unchanged (X^2 = 8.13 P <0.02). A controlled serum lipoprotein level is associated with an improving pressure index and better prognosis.

FASTING SERUM LIPOPROTEIN DIFFERENCES ACCORDING TO TYPE AND SITUATION OF PERIPHERAL ARTERIAL DISEASE

R.M. Greenhalgh, G.W. Taylor, and J. Kaye
Professorial Surgical Unit, St. Bartholomew's Hospital, London/Great Britain

The fasting serum lipoprotein types of 306 patient with various arteriographic types of peripheral arterial disease have been compared with 150 age and sex matched control patients without arterial disease. In all groups except 22 patients with intracranial aneurysms, the serum lipoprotein types are raised. However, there are striking differences between the sera of 145 patients with stenosing arterial disease (IIa 4, II6 9, II 1, IV 4 7, V 0) and 69 patients with dilating (aneurysmal) disease. (IIa 9, IIb 1, III 6, IV 8, V 1) and 43 patients with carotid artery stenosis (IIa 8, IIb 9, III 0, IV 6, V 0). The male to female ratio is 13 to 1 in all groups. 27 short stature women with stenoses only at the lower end of the aorta were different again (IIa 14, IIb 4, III 1, IV 2). Lipoprotein types are different according to site and nature of peripheral arterial disease. F test P <0.001.

LONG TERM FOLLOW UP STUDY AND PROGNOSTIC FACTORS IN INTERMITTENT CLAUDICATION

R. Cristol, B. Graisely, and A. Audebert
Service Pr. Debray, Hôpital Saint Antoine, Paris/France

Ninety patients (72 men, 18 women) with intermittent claudication and angiographically documented atherosclerosis were followed up 5-14 years to determine the possible role of prognostic factors on the occurrence of cerebrovascular or coronary events and the evolution of treadmill walking performance. No significant difference could be found between patients with (50 cases) and without (40 cases) such events, cerebrovascular and/or coronary concerning the age of onset of claudication (58 ± 9 years, 53 ± 8 years) the duration of survey (8.6 years/8.4 years) the incidence of relapsing smokers (56%/46%) of glucose intolerance (42%/46%) and of serum lipid anomalies (68%/66%) the systolic (17 ± 3/16 ± 2.6) or diastolic (9.3 ± 1, 8.9 ± 1) blood pressure. A significant difference appeared between the patients with improved or stabilized walking performance (16 and 48 cases) versus those who impaired it (26 cases) as for relapsing smoking (24%, 54% versus 94%) and systolic (14.7 ± 1, 16.8 ± 2.5 versus 17.6 ± 3.6) or diastolic (8.4 ± 0.7, 9.2 ± 0.9 versus 9.6 ± 1.3) but not for lipid or glucose anomalies.

HYPERLIPOPROTEINEMIA (HLP) AND DIABETES MELLITUS (D.m.) AS RISK FACTORS IN PERIPHERAL VASCULAR DISEASE (PVD). THE INFLUENCE OF AGE

Karl Heinrich Vogelberg, Peter Berchtold, Hinz Berger, F. Arnold Gries, and Theodor Stolze
Diabetes Research Institute and 2nd med. Department, University of Düsseldorf/ BRD

The severity of PVD was assessed angiographically with a sclerosis index (S.I.) in patients with clinical signs of PVD. 75 patients displayed HLP, 15 D.m. and 31 were without metabolic risk factors. The influence of age as a risk factor was studied. Patients with type III HLP showed the highest S.I. The number of risk factors was correlated to overweight and to the S.I. Only in type IIa an age in-dependent correlation between serum cholesterol and the S.I. was demonstrable. In patients with both hypertriglyceridemia and hypercholesterinemia or hypertri-glyceridemia alone the S.I. was age dependent. The S.I. was not different in chemical and clinical D.m. A correlation between age and the S.I. was shown in diabetics.
Conclusion: The most important age independent metabolic risk factor in PVD is hypercholesterolemia. In hypertriglyceridemia and D.m. age plays a predisposing role for the development of PVD. The degree of glucose intolerance appears not to be important as risk factor. Obesity was not associated with PVD.

PRELIMINARY REPORT: PREVALENCE OF GALLSTONES IN MEN WITH TYPE II HYPERLIPOPROTEINEMIA (HLP) IN THE CORONARY PRIMARY PREVENTION TRIAL

Alick Little, Helmut Schrott, Bruce Bird, William Connor, William Cohen, Harold Stolberg, Douglas Sanders, George Steiner, Maurice Mishkel, and Glen Jones
Department of Medicine, University of Toronto, Toronto, Ontario/Canada

Previous reports suggest a possible association of gallstones with HLP or its treatment. 730 men, ages 35-59, with type II HLP were selected at the Un of Iowa, McMaster & Toronto: cholesterol (C) >265, β-C>190, triglyceride (TG) <300 mg%, no abdominal pain, gross obesity, ischemic vascular disease, diabetes, hypertension, thyroid or other serious disease. 14 hr after ingesting 3 g of telepaque, multiple x-rays were made of the gall bladder, free of overlying gas. If the gall bladder was poorly visualized these were repeated after 3 g of telepaque on 2 successive evenings. Of the 730 men, 15 were not x-rayed because of previous cholecystectomy, 30 had gallstones visualized, 3 had non-function and 3 had poor function and 679 had normal cholecystograms. Equating non and poor function with stones the total prevalence of gallstones in primary type II HLP is 7% (51/730). Prevalence is different (P <.0002) in Iowa, 4.1% (16/393) and Toronto-Hamilton, 10.4% (35/337). Mean plasma HDL-C, total TG and age (but not total C or LDL-C) were significantly higher in subjects with gallstones. Discriminant function analysis separated sub-jects best into groups with and without gallstones using plasma HDL-C, total TG and age (P = .005, .01 and .06 respectively).
Supported by Contract No. NIH-NHLI No1-NV-2-2917-L, under the Lipid Research Clinic Program, Dept HEW and by an Ontario Heart Foundation Grant.

WORKSHOP 4. Measurement of Triglyceride Turnover

Chairmen: E. Nikkilä, Finland
          I. Fukui, Japan

Participants: G. Steiner, Canada
             J.D. Brunzell, USA
             S. Rössner, Sweden
             H. Nakamura, Japan

KINETICS OF VLDL SUBFRACTIONS

Georg Steiner and Dan Streja

Of the methods to measure VLDL triglyceride (TG) turnover in humans, the simplest is that utilizing ^{3}H-glycerol. We showed that when simultaneous measurements were made with the radioglycerol method and the lipolytic rate method, a method which depends on different assumptions, similar turnover rates were obtained (Steiner and Murase, 1975). This paper will describe how the radioglycerol procedure has been used in humans in order to determine 1) whether VLDL behaves as a single homogeneous pool, 2) whether large VLDL is the only precursor for small VLDL, 3) whether LDL-TG is derived only via the smallest VLDL particles, and 4) the proportion of VLDL-Tg glycerol derived from plasma glycerol.

For the studies, VLDL was separated by density gradient ultracentrifugation (Lossow et al., 1969) into VLDL I (Sf 100-400, 400-750 Å), VLDL II (Sf 60-100, 340-400 Å), and VLDL III (Sf 20-60, 240-340 Å). LDL was obtained by Mn-heparin precipitation (Fredrickson et al., 1967) of the VLDL infranatant. When the plasma VLDL-TG concentration was 50 mg/dl, equal amounts of VLDL-TG were present in all three fractions. The proportion of VLDL-TG in the VLDL I fraction increased to 60%, and fell in the VLDL III fraction to 10% at plasma VLDL-TG concentration of 1000 mg/dl.

When $2-^3$H-glycerol was constantly infused, its specific activity plateaued within a few minutes. By 8 hours, VLDL-TG glycerol's specific activity was also constant. The ratio of the specific activity of the latter to that of the former indicated the proportion of VLDL-TG glycerol which was derived from plasma glycerol (Fig.1). The specific activity, and hence the proportion of TG glycerol derived from plasma glycerol was highest in the smallest VLDL (VLDL III) and lowest in the largest VLDL. The disparity between the two increased as the plasma VLDL-TG levels rose.

A single injection of $2-^3$H-glycerol was also given, and the specific activities of the TG in the VLDL subfractions were followed (Fig. 2). In 11 of 13 studied in this way, the peak specific activity of VLDL III exceeded that of VLDL I. Again the disparity increased as the plasma VLDL-TG level rose. As Zilversmit (1960) clearly indicated, one compound (e.g., large VLDL in the present studies) cannot be the sole precursor of another (e.g., small VLDL) if the specific activity of the product exceeds that of the putative sole precursor. The specific activity curves also showed that the slope of the decline of VLDL III specific activity was flatter than that of VLDL I. In all 13 studied, the slope of the VLDL III curve was 55 ± 4% of that of the VLDL I curve. This could have been because the larger VLDL had a faster fractional turnover, in a manner analogous to that which has been shown for larger chylomicrons (Quarfordt and Goodman, 1966). The VLDL III curve could also have been flatter than that for VLDL I if $2-^3$H-glycerol incorporation into VLDL III continued for longer than that into VLDL I.

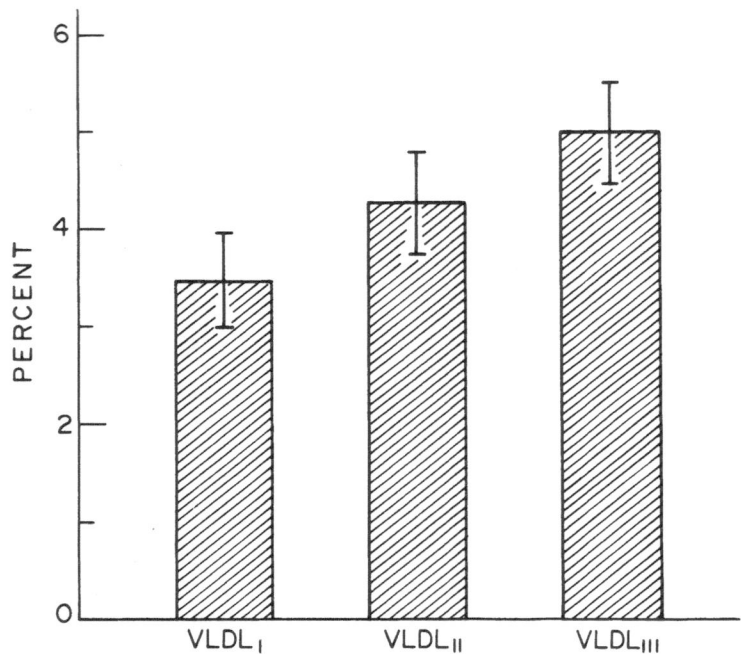

Figure 1. The percentage of TG glycerol in VLDL subfractions derived from plasma glycerol. Glycerol-2-^{3}H was infused constantly for 10 h. The VLDL-TG glycerol specific activities plateaued by 8 h. The percentage of TG glycerol derived from plasma glycerol was obtained by dividing the VLDL-TG glycerol plateau specific activity by the plasma glycerol plateau specific activity. Data given as the mean of this ratio x 100 ± SE (n = 6)

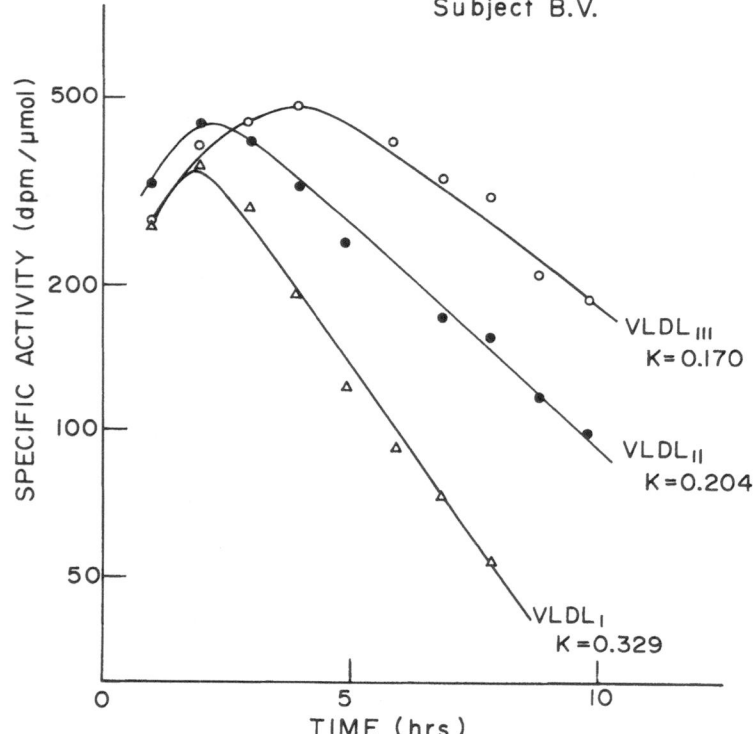

Figure 2. Specific activity of TG glycerol in subfractions of VLDL after a single injection of glycerol-2-^{3}H

The TG specific activity in LDL was also examined (Fig. 3). The same data were obtained whether the fraction was isolated by Mn-heparin precipitation of the VLDL intranatant or by spinning and washing the VLDL infranatant at d=1.063. This fraction was largely composed of LDL, but probably also had some remnants of VLDL. In the lower right panel of Figure 3, it may be noted that the LDL and total VLDL-TG curves cross in a way which would be consistent with all LDL-TG coming via VLDL. This was also the case with the LDL curve and that for VLDL I or VLDL II, but not with the LDL and VLDL III curves. Althoug the peak specific activity of TG of LDL was less than that of VLDL III, the peak occurred before the LDL curve crossed the curve of VLDL III. Zilversmit (1960) has shown that, if a precursor is to be the only precursor of a particular compound, the peak specific activity of the product cannot be reached before the product curve crosses that of the putative sole precursor. Hence, VLDL-TG could not have been the sole precursor for the LDL-TG.

Conclusions

The curve describing the decline of VLDL-TG specific activity after a single dose of radioactive glycerol has occasionally deviated from a monoexponential pattern (Kekki and Nikkila, 1975). One possible explanation offered to account for such a bend has been a possible recycling of radioactive glycerol released after hydrolysis of the labeled VLDL-TG.

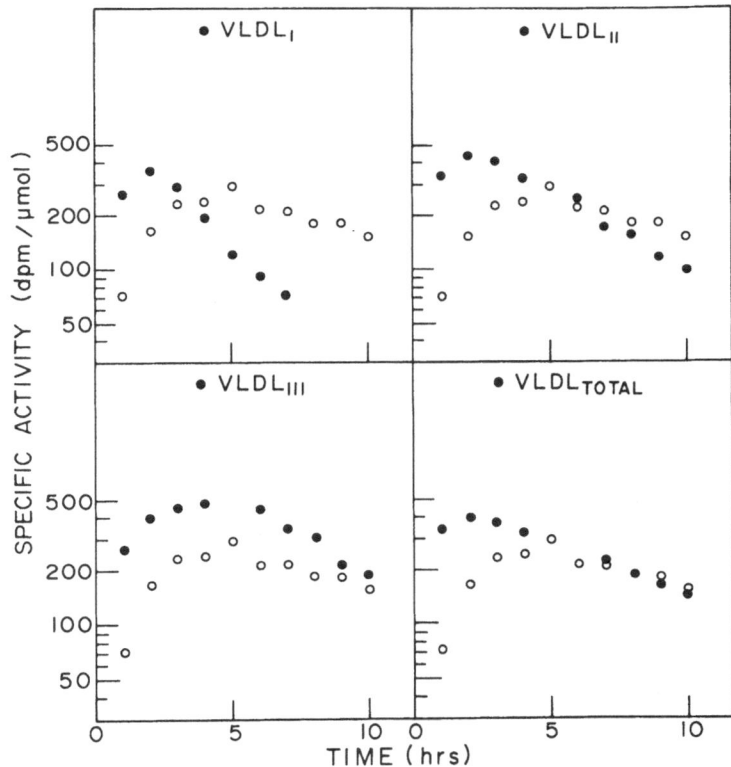

Relationship between specific activity in VLDL $_{I, II, III}$ and VLDL$_{TOTAL}$ and LDL (o) in subject B.V.

Figure 3. The specific activity of TG glycerol in LDL compared to that of total VLDL and that of each of three subfractions of VLDL following a single injection of glycerol-2-^{3}H

However, we found the proportion of VLDL-TG glycerol derived from plasma glycerol was too small (Fig. 1) to explain any bend in this way. Another possible explanation was suggested by the observation that VLDL did not behave as a single homogeneous pool. A noticeable bend, therefore, could occur if there were a large enough discrepancy between the contribution of the steep slope of the large VLDL to the early portion and of the flat slope of the small VLDL to the late portion of the whole VLDL curve (Fig. 2).

We observed that, during a glycerol infusion, the plateau TG specific activity of small VLDL exceeded that of large VLDL (Fig. 1) and that, after a bolus injection of glycerol, the peak specific activity of small VLDL also exceeded that of large VLDL (Fig. 2). This indicated that large VLDL was not the sole precursor of TG in small VLDL but that the entire spectrum of VLDL particles could be produced directly. Barter and Nestel's (1972) demonstration that palmitate in the TG of small VLDL was produced via large VLDL suggested that palmitic acid, in contrast to glycerol, was primarily incorporated into the TG of large VLDL. Thus, small VLDL-TG may have been produced both directly and via large VLDL.

Two possibilities could have accounted for the demonstration (Fig. 1) that the proportion of TG glycerol derived from plasma glycerol differed in large and small particles. The first was that the cell had multiple pools of immediate precursor for VLDL-TG glycerol, each receiving a different contribution of glycerol from the plasma. The second was that there were two sites of VLDL synthesis, one producing predominantly larger particles and receiving less glycerol from the plasma than the other. The second possibility was considered more likely for the following reasons. Both the intestine and the liver have been shown to produce VLDL (Ockner et al., 1969; Steiner et al., 1975). The intestine (Kayden et al., 1967), but not the liver (Senior and Isselbacher, 1962), readily esterified fatty acids to 2-monoglyceride. Hence, the proportion of TG glycerol derived from plasma glycerol could have been smaller in intestinal VLDL than in hepatic VLDL.

The degradation of VLDL did not necessarily require an orderly cascade from larger to smaller particles before remnants and LDL were produced. The curves in Figure 3 showed that small VLDL (VLDL III) was not the only precursor for LDL-TG. Rather, they indicated that LDL and/or remnants were produced directly from cell parts of the VLDL spectrum.

These studies, therefore, suggested the following model. All parts of the VLDL spectrum could be produced directly. Large VLDL could, but need not necessarily be degraded so small VLDL. LDL and/or remnants may have been made directly from the entire VLDL spectrum.

COMPARISON OF METHODS OF PLASMA TRIGLYCERIDE TURNOVER

Alan Chait, John J. Albers, and John D. Brunzell

Introduction

Over the past several years, a kinetic approach has been widely used in an attempt to determine whether either overproduction or impaired removal of very low-density lipoproteins (VLDL) is the fundamental mechanism underlying the elevated triglyceride (TG) levels seen in many primary and secondary hyperlipidemic states. No method of measuring TG or VLDL turnover has gained universal acceptance since none has been adequately validated. Therefore, a comparison of data between studies is often difficult, and conflicting conclusions have been claimed as to the prime mechanism of the TG elevation in endogenous hypertriglyceridemia (Farguhar et al., 1965; Bierman et al., 1970; Boberg et al., 1972; Havel et al., 1970). In addition to methodologic considerations, differences in results and conclusions may partly be accounted for by marked differences in patient selection and heterogeneity of subjects studied.

The main methods used in the determination of TG and VLDL turnover are:
1. TG splanchnic secretion: chemical measurement Boberg et al., 1972
2. Radiopalmitate incorporation into TG Boberg et al., 1972; Havel et al., 1970
3. Radioglycerol TG disappearance Farguhar et al., 1965; Nikkilä and Kekki, 1971
4. Radioiodine B-apoprotein disappearance Bilheimer et al., 1972; Sigurdsson et al., 1975
5. Lipoprotein lipase related TG removal Bierman et al., 1970; Porte and Bierman, 1969
6. Particulate TG disappearance: Intralipid Boberg et al., 1969

The purpose of this study is to compare TG turnover as measured by three different techniques, each of which depends on different assumptions. The similarity of results obtained by all three methods suggests that the assumptions on which they are based are correct, or if incorrect, the effects of these assumptions play an insignificant role. It also suggests that these methods may be valid indices of TG turnover.

Methods

1. Radioglycerol Method

The method used is essentially that described by Farquhar et al. (1975), which measured the disappearance rate of endogenously labeled TG following a bolus injection of H^3-glycerol. An injection of 150 µCi H^3-2-glycerol was given intravenously after an overnight fast. Blood samples are obtained for the next 8 hours during which time the patient is fasting. Lipids are extracted by the Folch procedure (Folch et al., 1957), and phospholipids removed by adsorption to silicic acid. No prior separation of VLDL is performed as it has been shown that the turnover measured by this technique is essentially the same whether determined on whole plasma or on VLDL (Kekki and Nikkilä, 1975; Steiner and Murase, 1975). The log linear portion of the disappearance curve is used to calculate the TG fractional catabolic rate; when multiplied by TG pool size (plasma TG concentration x plasma volume), a measure of TG turnover rate is obtained.

2. Endogenous Lipolytic Rate During Maximal Heparin Infusion (Lipoprotein Lipase Related TG Removal)

This method of Porte and Bierman (Porte and Bierman, 1969; Brunzell et al., 1973) depends on the assessment of the in vivo lipolytic rate as measured in vitro by the interaction of the subjects lipoprotein lipase released into plasma by heparin against their own endogenous TG. A pulse injection of heparin (2280 U/m^2) followed by a constant infusion of 1980 U/m^2 has been shown to result in a maximal release of lipolytic activity in plasma. This test is performed in the fasting state after 10-14 days on a fat-free formula diet at which time the subject has reached a steady andogenous TG concentration. During the heparin infusion, plasma TG concentration falls and plasma free fatty acids rise, each to new steady state levels. At these new steady state conditions, blood is drawn and immediately incubated in vitro for determination of the rate of free fatty acid release from the subject's own endogenous lipoprotein TG by lipoprotein lipase. As TG levels are constant, the rate of lipolysis is assumed to equal the rate of TG input into plasma. This turnover rate is calculated as follows:

Turnover rate (mg/kg/h)=

$$\frac{\text{lipolytic rate (µmol/l/min) x 60 x plasma volume (l) x 850/3}}{\text{weight (kg)}}.$$

Fractional catabolic rate (h^{-1}) was assessed as $\dfrac{\text{turnover rate (mg/h)}}{\text{pool size (mg)}}$.

3. *Radioiodinated B-Apoprotein Disappearance*

Blood is taken from the subject following an overnight fast. After ultracentrifugation at 10^8 g·min (Havel et al., 1955), the VLDL obtained is washed once at
d = 1.006 and iodinated by the iodine monochloride method (McFarlane, 1958), as
modified for lipoproteins (Langer et al., 1972). Following one further recentrifugation at d = 1.006 for 10^8 g·min, the iodinated lipoprotein is passed through
a millipore filter before reinjection into the subject from whom it was obtained.
Preparation of the iodinated lipoprotein takes no longer than 72 hours. Blood is
sampled over a 24-hour period after injection, during which time the subjects
consume their normal daily caloric requirements as fat-free formula feedings.
VLDL is separated from the samples by ultracentrifugation and counted for radioactivity. The radioactivity in lipids is determined by the Folch technique
(Folch et al., 1957); counts in apoB and apoC are separated by the tetramethylurea method of Kane et al. (1975). ApoB concentration in plasma and VLDL is measured by radioimmunoassay (Albers et al., 1975). The fractional catabolic rate
is determined from the slope of the apoB specific activity time curve and VLDL-
apoB pool size from the VLDL-apoB concentration and the plasma volume. By a
knowledge of the ratio of plasma VLDL-TG-apoB, which remains constant during the
study, TG turnover can then be extrapolated from the apoB turnover rate.

4. *Study Protocol*

Turnover as measured by the apoB and glycerol techniques was compared while on a
formula diet, 40% of the calories were supplied as fat. As the heparin infusion
technique can only be used during the consumption of a fat-free diet, it was
necessary for TG turnover measurements by this method to be compared with that
measured by the radioglycerol method while on the same diet.

Therefore, each patient underwent two periods of formula feeding each of 2-weeks
duration. Toward the end of the initial fat-containing period, TG turnover was
measured by the glycerol technique, and blood was obtained for iodine labeling
of VLDL in vitro. On the day of reinjection of iodinated VLDL, the diet was
switched to a high-carbohydrate (85% of calories), essentially fat-free diet.
The glycerol technique was repeated at the end of 2 weeks on this diet, followed by the heparin infusion technique 2 days later.

Results and Discussion

A close relation existed among kinetic measurements made in 13 subjects with
plasma TG levels ranging 117 - 1750 mg/dl (Table 1). On the fat-containing diet,
TG turnover (mg/kg/h), as measured by the glycerol technique, and apoB turnover
were significantly correlated (n = 10, r = 0.67, p <0.05), as were the fractional catabolic rates (r = 0.76, p <0.01) (Table 2). Mean values for TG turnover
as measured by these two techniques were 19.2 ± 6.0 (mean ± SD) mg/kg/h and 15.6
± 7.8 for the H^3-glycerol and iodinated apoB methods, respectively (Table 3).

Measurements made by the two techniques used during the fat-free feeding period
were also similar. Turnover rates measured by glycerol and during heparin infusion were significantly correlated (n = 12, r = 0.69, p <0.02), as were the
fractional catabolic rates (r = 0.71, p <0.01) (Table 2). The mean TG turnover by
these two techniques were in close agreement, being 21.0 ± 8.4 mg/kg/h and 22.2
± 7.8 for the glycerol and heparin infusion techniques, respectively (Table 3).
Mean TG turnover measured by the glycerol method did not increase significantly
on the fat-free, high-carbohydrate diet; marked individual variation was, however, observed. Moreover, measures of TG turnover on the fat-containing diet

Table 1

		40% Fat-containing diet					Fat-free diet (85% CHO)				
		TR			k_1 (h⁻¹)			TR (mg/kg/h)		k_1 (h⁻¹)	
Subject	TG (mg/dl)	Glycerol (mg TG/kg/h)	ApoB (mg apoB/kg/h)	Glycerol	ApoB	TG (mg/dl)	Glycerol	Heparin	Glycerol	Heparin
WC	117	15.24	.498	.274	.299	125	16.26	9.30	.265	.170
DT	272	14.10	.528	.137	.152	384	15.78	13.26	.100	.086
DM	288	14.58	.433	.114	.182	---	---	---	---	---
AR	311	18.54	.438	.147	.108	723	16.32	24.24	.054	.102
AH	362	22.14	.410	.126	.047	539	10.08	21.48	.038	.089
CT	415	12.00	.458	.085	.125	916	14.16	22.74	.044	.085
SE	436	18.42	.563	.139	.125	864	27.18	20.52	.102	.111
RM	462	21.84	.310	.132	.071	1230	25.08	29.16	.054	.074
JH	---	---	---	---	---	513	30.06	24.72	.149	.120
LS	604	19.14	.301	.104	.039	1750	38.88	39.30	.071	.085
BR	---	---	---	---	---	613	14.88	15.84	.073	.083
RB	---	---	---	---	---	633	21.84	29.46	.090	.137
CG	818	33.06	1.120	.128	.110	907	19.92	21.60	.064	.086

TR = Turnover rate. k = Fractional catabolic rate

Table 2. y = bx + a

	n	a	b	r	p
40% fat-containing diet					
Turnover (mg/kg/h) ApoB vs. glycerol	10	10.18	17.25	0.67	<0.05
Fractional catabolic rate (h⁻¹) ApoB vs. glycerol	10	.074	.517	0.76	<0.01
Fat-free diet (85% carbohydrate)					
Turnover (mg/kg/h) Heparin vs. glycerol	12	4.68	.715	0.71	<0.02
Fractional catabolic rate (h⁻¹) Heparin vs. glycerol	12	.102	1.898	0.85	<0.01

Table 3. Comparison of TG turnover methods (mg TG/kg/h)

	H^3-glycerol	I^{125} apoB	LPL removal
Fat-containing diet	19.2 ± 6.0	15.6 ± 7.8	
Fat-free diet	21.0 ± 8.4		22.2 ± 7.8

showed no significant correlation with those on the fat-free diet. [Glycerol (fat-free diet) vs. apoB r = 0.18, p >0.1; heparin vs. glycerol (fat-containing diet) r = 0.22, p >0.1; heparin vs. apoB r = 0.30, p >0.1].

The H^3-glycerol method has the advantage of technical case: it, however, assumes insignificant recycling of the label during the initial decay curve. A slow component of the decay curve may be seen if observations are continued for an extended period of time. This may represent recycling or a slow TG pool turnover, which may in fact be a subspecies of VLDL or some form of remnant particle. It has been suggested (Grundy et al., 1975) that in view of this "tailing" effect, multicompartmental analysis should be used in the calculation of TG turnover by this technique. However, the similarity of results obtained by this and the other two methods suggests that for practical purposes multicompartmental analysis may in fact not be necessary.

The major disadvantage with the iodinated apoB method is that it is too laborious and time-consuming to undertake on a large scale. In common with the other methods of turnover measurement, it is difficult to validate adequately. A shortcoming may relate to the heterogeneity of VLDL, subclasses of which may have different turnover rates. The method used in the present study would measure the net effect of these. As with all tracer experiments in which the radioactive material is prepared in vitro, one has to assume that the tracer has the same metabolic and kinetic properties as does the native particle. The lack of a rapid disappearance phase of tracer soon after its injection, as well as the similar fractional catabolic rates between iodinated apoB and endogenously labeled plasma TG, suggests that this is in fact so. Tailing may also be observed at a late stage using this method, but as the decay is strictly a single exponential for at least three to four half-lives, it would seem valid to use this initial decay rate in the determination of apoB turnover rates.

The heparin infusion technique avoids the use of radioisotopes but is limited by the inability to adequately determine TG turnover rates during the consumption of fat-containing diets because the released enzyme will presumably affect lipoproteins of exogenous and endogenous origin at different rates. In order to measure endogenous TG production rates, exogenous TG must be eliminated from the blood by maintaining subjects on fat-free, high-carbohydrate diets. This method assumes that all TG removal is lipoprotein lipase-related and that all functional lipoprotein lipase is released into plasma during the heparin infusion. A further assumption is that the 10% increase in free fatty acid levels resulting from lipolysis in the circulation does not result in increased TG production. While none of these assumptions has been adequately validated, indirect support for their validity is obtained by the similarity of results between this method and the radioglycerol method. Steiner and Murase (1975) have also shown a significant correlation between production rates determined by the same two methods. However, in contrast to the present findings, mean values using the heparin procedure were one-third higher than those obtained with H^3-glycerol (Steiner and Murase, 1975). The reason for the difference between their findings and those of the present study are not clear, but may relate to the long period of starvation prior to the heparin infusion used by Steiner and Murase. It is conceivable that starvation-induced elevation of free fatty acids, in conjunction with the increase consequent on heparin induced in vivo lipolysis, may have resulted in enhanced hepatic TG production.

The correlations among the three methods for assessment of TG turnover demonstrated in this study thus suggest that, despite very different assumptions, each is valid as an index of plasma TG turnover over a wide range of plasma TG levels. The lack of correlation between values compared on the fat-containing diet with those on the fat-free diet emphasizes the importance of using comparable diets when comparing TG turnover among individuals.

THE INTRAVENOUS FAT TOLERANCE TEST WITH INTRALIPID — VALIDITY, APPLICATIONS, AND LIMITATIONS

Stephan Rössner

Determinations of plasma concentrations of serum lipids or lipoproteins will give an estimate of the pool size of these plasma constituents but will not give information about the amount secreted into the circulation per unit time or the amount eliminated from plasma per unit time. Such dynamic measurements have awakened increasing interest because they give considerably more information about the lipoprotein turnover and add to our knowledge of the pathophysiologic mechanisms causing hyperlipoproteinemia. Various methods have, therefore, been developed to study these parameters. However, no ideal tracers for endogenous TG have been found as yet. Several methods using precursors and labeled substances have been developed, but such procedures have generally been laborious and criticized for being imprecise. Doubt has also been cast on the reliability of the outcome of these methods because of the underlying assumptions for each technique.

When it was demonstrated that Intralipid® closely resembled chylomicra in vivo and in vitro, the intravenous fat tolerance test (IVFTT) was developed as a simple tool to assess the fractional removal rate of exogenous TG from the circulation (Boberg et al., 1969). Evidence for a common metabolic pathway for exogenous and endogenous plasma TG favored the hypothesis that the IVFTT fractional removal rate might reflect the fractional catabolism of VLDL (Brunzell et al., 1973).

Methodology

The IVFTT is performed in the following way (Rössner, 1974). After an overnight fast, venous blood for analysis of serum lipids and a nephelometric determination of the plasma blank value is taken. A single dose injection of 1 ml/kg body weight of 10% Intralipid® is given intravenously and venous blood is sampled at timed intervals for 40 min. The light scattering index of plasma diluted 1:100 with saline is determined by nephelometry as a measure of the amount of Intralipid® triglycerides. The elimination of the emulsion from the blood stream is a first order reaction which can be calculated in a semilogarithmic plot by the method of least squares and expressed as k_2%/min.

Both short- and long-term reproducibility of the test is very high. Comparisons of the long-term reproducibility of the k_2 value and fasting plasma TG concentrations from the same day demonstrate that for the plasma TG concentration the coefficient of variation was 33%, whereas the corresponding IVFTT k_2 value was 14% in subjects in steady state with regard to diet, drugs, and diseases known to affect lipid metabolism. These data may reflect the fact that the plasma TG concentration is determined both by secretion and removal and that variations in removal explain one part of the plasma TG concentration changes.

Removal Sites for Intralipid®

The arteriovenous concentration differences of Intralipid® during a constant infusion have been studied in man in several tissues (Rössner, 1974), and the following results were obtained. Intralipid® was significantly removed in the myocardium, the splanchnic region, the forearm skeletal muscle, and subcutaneous tissue. No net removal was observed in the liver. The results are summarized in Table 1.

The results from studies on human forearm with catheters in deep veins, mainly draining skeletal muscle, and in superficial veins, mainly draining subcutaneous tissue, suggest that skeletal muscle may play a major role in the initial removal of Intralipid® TG from the circulation compared to adipose tissue. This view is supported by the recent findings of Heaf et al., who injected heparin intra-arterially and then determined the immediate release of lipoprotein lipase activity after the first heparin passage through these tissues. Considerably more lipoprotein lipase activity was found in blood from deep veins than in superficial veins, suggesting that lipolysis can take place in skeletal muscle.

IVFTT k_2 Versus Plasma TG

There is a negative correlation between the IVFTT k_2 value and the total plasma as well as the VLDL-TG concentration. This relationship corresponds to a straight line in a double logarithmic system. Much discussion has focused on the question whether the k_2 value is dependent on the plasma TG pool size or whether it is a process independently reflecting the TG fractional removal rate. In some situations, an increased k_2 is found concomitant with a plasma VLDL-TG reduction which would indicate that the amount of TG removed from the circulation per unit time is unchanged. (Fig. 1). However, there are several situations where the TG concentration and k_2 value may change independently. A schematic representation summarizing results from several studies is shown in Figure 1. In summary, this Figure demonstrates that several drugs, diseases, and diets may lead to various changes in the relationship between k_2 and the plasma TG pool size. These studies support the concept that the IVFTT may be used to give an index of the plasma TG removal rate and thus indicate whether serum TG changes are mainly the results of increased secretion or impaired removal.

Table 1. Fractional removal rate and removal of infused Intralipid® in human tissues. The data were obtained from four different studies and each study was calculated separately

	Fractional removal rate, % of arterial concentration	Removal of infused Intralipid® %
Myocardium	6	14
Splanchnic viscera	5	25
Liver	0	0
Skeletal muscle	10	47
Subcutaneous tissue	6	13

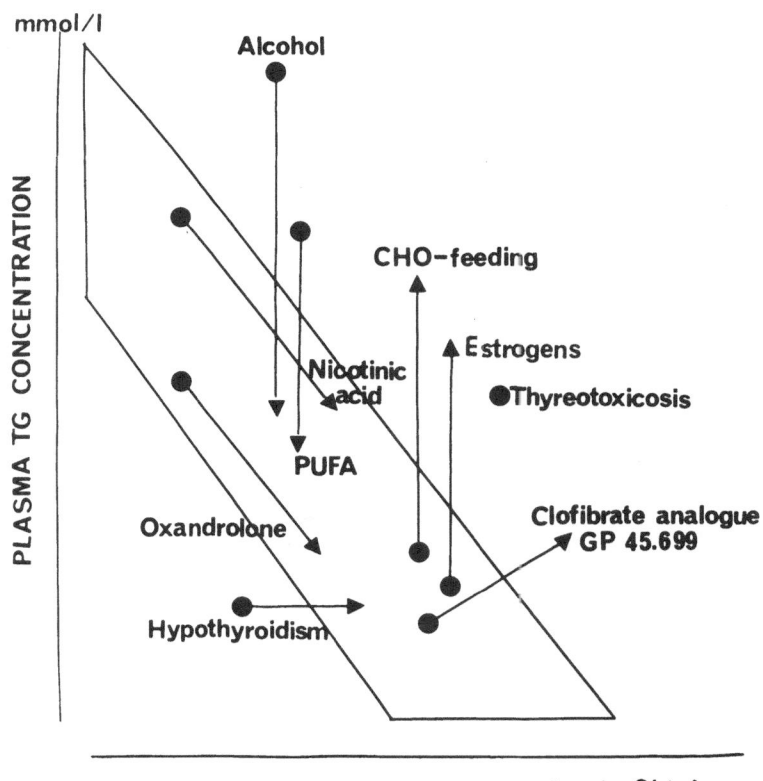

Figure 1. Relationship between the IVFTT k_2 value and the plasma TG concentration. Schematic representation of the effects of some drugs, diets, and diseases. "Normal" range of TG turnover indicated, logarithmic scales

IVFTT k_2 *Correlation to Lipase Activity and the FIAT Process*

Although no correlation between the total postheparin lipolytic activity in k_2 has been found in previous studies, Huttunen and co-workers recently demonstrated that the k_2 value was positively correlated to the early lipoprotein lipase activity, when the hepatic lipase TG was inhibited (Huttunen et al., 1975). During starvation of the obese subjects investigated in these studies the correlation disappeared. A possible explanation for this finding, put toward by these authors, may be the fact that starvation increases the lipase activity in heart and skeletal muscle and that Intralipid® removal might, therefore, be shifted more toward the active tissues. A further critical step for the removal of TG from the circulation is the fatty acid incorporation into adipose tissue (FIAT) that takes place after hydrolysis (Walldius, 1976). The FIAT value has been shown to be an important factor in the determination of the serum TG concentration and has been found low in hypertriglyceridemia. Figure 2 shows that there is a significant positive correlation between the k_2 and the FIAT values.

IVFTT k_2 *and Endogenous VLDL-TG Catabolism*

Direct comparison between the IVFTT k_2 and the fractional removal rate of endogenous VLDL-TG has been carried out. Using the so-called "splanchnic secretion method" a highly significant positive correlation was obtained (r = +0.71) (Rössner et al., 1974). Furthermore, Nicoll and co-workers recently demonstrated that

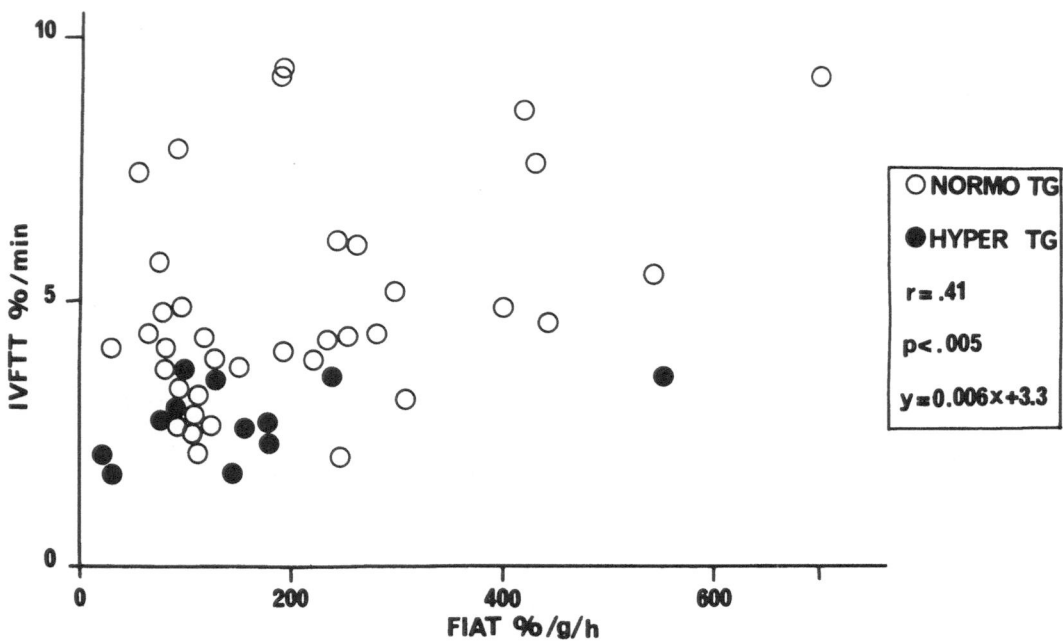

Figure 2. Relationship between the fatty acid incorporation into adipose tissue (FIAT) process and the IVFTT k_2 in subjects with a wide range of serum TG concentrations

there is a strong positive correlation between IVFTT k_2 and the fractional catabolic rate of VLDL $\frac{1}{m}$ = B apoprotein (r = +0.87) (Nicoll et al., 1976). This correlation was obtained in subjects with a wide range of k_2 and VLDL-TG values. This is of importance since it has been argued that IVFTT can be applied only provided the endogenous TG pool size is not too large. In these studies, the k_2 values were considerably higher than the corresponding values obtained for endogenous VLDL fractional turnover rate. This could be due to the difference in particle size, since it has been demonstrated that larger lipoprotein particles are removed more rapidly than smaller ones (Quarfordt and Goodman, 1966).

IVFTT in Epidemiological Studies

In a large sample of several hundred asymptomatic hyperlipidemic subjects and control groups, a continuous negative relationship between k_2 and plasma TG concentration is found (Rössner, 1974; Lewis et al., 1976). Female subjects were found to have faster k_2 values than males. A considerable overlap between k_2 values in subjects with and without cardiovascular disease was found (Fig. 3). The IVFTT, therefore, in general does not seem to be a more sensitive discriminator between subjects with vascular disease and control than the VLDL-TG concentration. However, in some patients hypertriglyceridemia seems to occur without indication of a TG removal defect. The IVFTT might help to distinguish subjects with impaired TG clearance from plasma which may have implications for the choice of lipid-lowering therapy.

Summary

The fractional removal rate of the TG emulsion Intralipid® reflects the turnover rate of endogenous plasma TG, although the fractional turnover rate for these exogenous TG particles is higher. The reproducibility of the test is high, the test can be performed repeatedly and is very easy to apply in large-sclale studies

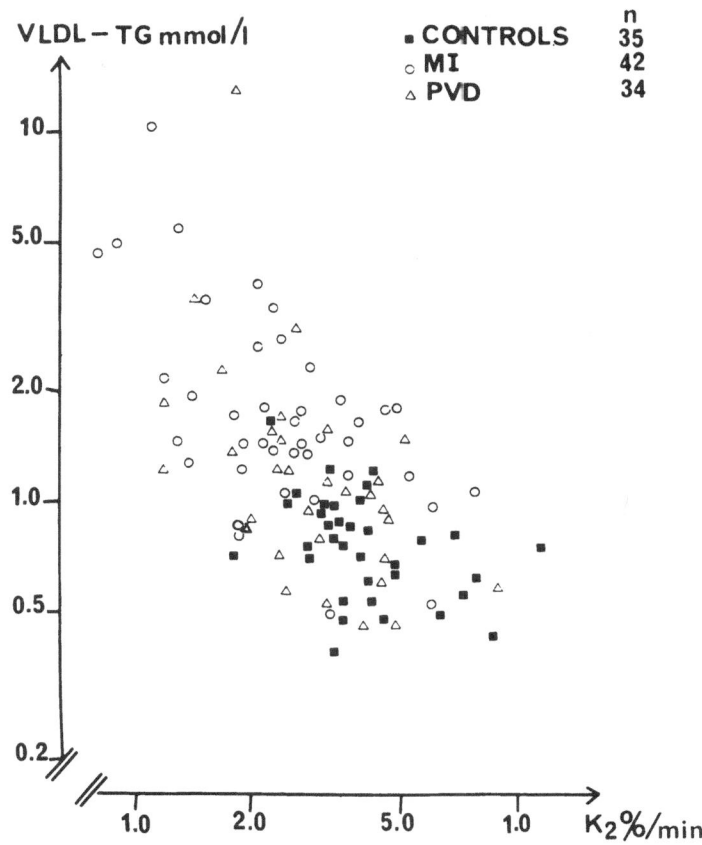

Figure 3. Relationship between k_2 value and VLDL-TG concentration in controls, subjects with myocardial infarction (MI) and peripheral vascular disease (PVD). Logarithmic scales

on TG turnover. The IVFTT k_2 value is not a passive reflection of the plasma TG pool size, but rather an indicator of TG-removing processes. Studies on Intralipid® removing sites have demonstrated that skeletal muscle in particular may play an important role in the removal of thse exogenous TG particles.

The use of the IVFTT in epidemiological studies has shown a k_2 overlap between normal and hyperlipidemic subjects, and in such large subjects, the IVFTT did not discriminate better than the VLDL-TG concentration between subjects with or without vascular disease. However, in individual subjects, the IVFTT may help to elucidate the mechanisms leading to hyperlipidemia and thus be of importance for the choice of therapy.

TRIGLYCERIDE TURNOVER IN DIABETIC STATES OF DOGS

Haruo Nakamura

The level of triglyceride in the plasma has received the growing attention as a possible risk factor to the pathogenesis of vascular disease. However, regulatory mechanism of plasma triglyceride level appeares to involve various determining factors. In simple terms, plasma triglyceride levels are linked directly to the influx of triglyceride into the plasma and to the clearance (outflux) of triglyceride out of the plasma.

The plasma level of triglycerides in human and animal is highly variable and depends on the type of disease, degree of control, age of the subjects, previous diet, obesity, kinds of diabetogenic agents and the presence or abscence of complications.

Present study is conducted to assess these regulatory mechanisms in determining the plasma triglyceride level in control and alloxan-diabetic dogs, and to observe whether there is any different behavior to these regulartory processes depending upon the specific fatty acid as a precursor.

1. Plasma triglyceride turnover by using radioactive fatty acid 10 alloxan-diabetic dogs with fasting blood sugar over 200 mg% were used for this study. 75 mg/kg of alloxan was injected 3 days prior to the study. Dogs anesthetized with pentobarbital were catheterized in portal and hepatic vein and femoral artery. Radioactive fatty acids in 2% bovine serum albumin was continuously and constantly infused and blood samples for chemical analysis were started to be obtained 1 hour after the initiation of the infusion.

For the calculation of the triglyceride kinetics, FFA is generally considered to be major precursor of triglyceride and thus the equations of the kinetics were developed by Ryan and Schwartz in 1965. However, this is undoubtedly oversimplified.

The rate of appearance of labeled triglyceride (dpm/min) was determined by taking the difference between labeled triglyceride dpm/min at a certain time difference, multiplying by the plasma volume.

The rate of appearance (dpm/min) devided by the rate of infusion of FFA gives the proportion of labeled FFA converted to labeled TG. Using the reasonable assumption that the infused labeled FFA are incorporated into TG in the same proportion as the endogenous FFA, this proportion is then multiplied by the average total influx rate of FFA during this time and devided by 3 to determine the average TG influx rate.

Since the blood samples were taken in the portal and hepatic vein, this can ignore the removal of labeled TG from the plasma compartment by peripheral tissues. The clearance of plasma TG was calculated by dividing the plasma TG influx by the plasma TG concentration. Turnover time in minutes is determined by dividing the plasma volume by the clearance.

Table 1 shows the results of this FFA uptake in the liver and non-hepatic splanchnic area by using $1-{}^{14}C$-palmitate.

FFA in the arterial blood in diabetic dogs were markedly elevated and thus hepatic uptake was also high.
FFA uptake in liver and non-hepatic splanchnic area was found to have a significant correlation with arterial FFA concentration.

Livers in diabetic dogs removed a much large amount of FFA per unit time and released more triglyceride.

However, non-hepatic splanchnic area removed FFA less than liver and net release of triglyceride from this area was not found.

Therefore, it is considered that influx of triglyceride is mostly responsible for the its secretion from the liver in this present experimental condition, which is consistent with the results of Spitzer et al.

Table 1. FFA extraction by liver and nonhepatic splanchnic area

	Control	Diabetic
Arterial FFA (μM/1)	456 ±58	1652 ±194
Arterial TG (mg%)	98 ±13	216 ± 35
Hepatic extraction of 1-^{14}C-palmitate (%)	33.5±3.1	29.6±3.2
Hepatic FFA uptake (μM/min.)	71 ±15	236 ± 56
Hepatic $\frac{^{14}C \ TG \ output}{^{14}C \ FFA \ uptake}$ (%)	14.1±4.2	21.1±7.5
Splanchnic FFA uptake (μM/1)	26 ± 5	98 ± 4
Splanchnic extraction of 1-^{14}C-palmitate (%)	20.5±1.4	17.2±3.4
Splanchnic $\frac{^{14}C \ TG \ output}{^{14}C \ FFA \ uptake}$ (%)	-0.3±3.5	-3.1±4.5

Table 2 shows the triglyceride kinetics by using palmitate. Influx of triglyceride into hepatic vein in diabetic dogs was about 4 times greater than that of the control dogs. Clearance of triglyceride in diabetic dogs in this experiment was also about twice greater than that of the control dogs. Therefore turnover time of triglyceride was shorter in diabetic dogs than in control dogs. Triglyceride concentration in diabetic dogs was doubled.

Table 3 shows the triglyceride kinetics obtained by using oleate. The influx of triglyceride in diabetic dogs was again increased significantly. Clearance was also increased in the diabetic dogs. Turnover time was also shortened in diabetic dogs.

It is interesting to observe the difference of influx by using either palmitate or oleate. Influx of oleate is a little greater than palmitate, though this is not statistically significant.

As stated earlier, there was a significant positive correlation between arterial FFA concentration and the hepatic uptake. And in FFA composition in diabetic, percentage of oleic acid was the greatest, occupying almost 4C% in FFA. This could lead to accelerated esterification of oleic acid into triglyceride in the liver. There might be heterogenous in kinetic behaviors which are operative in vivo depending upon the kinds or the concentration of fatty acids.

Increased concentration of triglyceride in diabetic dogs appeared to be responsible for the marked increase of the triglyceride influx from the liver. However, there was no correlation found between the magnitude of the triglyceride influx and the triglyceride concentration in the plasma. Also, the extent of clearance could not either explain the triglyceride concentration.

But the most pronounced change in triglyceride kinetics of the diabetic dogs was the increased influx.

This finding was supported by the following experiment.

2. Triglyceride secretion rate by using Triton WR 1339. 9 control and 9 alloxan-diabetic dogs were anesthetized and catheters were placed in femoral artery and vein. After certain period of observation, Triton WR 1339 was injected in the dose of 150 mg/kg, of body weight.

Table 2. TG kinetics (1)

Palmitate	Influx (μm/min.)	Clearance (plasma/min.)	Turnover (min.)
Control (n=10)	0.43 ± 0.23	0.351 ± 0.178	3969 ± 470
Diabetic (n=10)	1.654 ± 0.236	0.724 ± 0.263	2325 ± 611
	P<0.01	P<0.01	P<0.01

(Mean ± S.D.)

Table 3. TG kinetics (2)

Oleate	Influx (μm/min.)	Clearance (plasma/min.)	Turnover (min.)
Control (n=10)	0.394 ± 0.214	0.335 ± 0.196	4215 ± 575
Diabetic (n=10)	1.719 ± 0.454	0.779 ± 0.326	2215 ± 785
	P<0.01	P<0.01	P<0.01

(Mean ± S.D.)

After the start of the injection, triglyceride increases up to 2 hours lineally. In this situation, FFA also shows the sharp rise in the early phase and cholesterol also shows gradual increase with triglyceride.

Triglyceride secretion rate could be measured until 2 hours in this equation, which might have a possibility to overestimate the secretion rate, because of the sharp rise of FFA in the initial part of the experiment.

The plasma which has Triton shows the decrement in electrophoretic mobility and thus, α moves with β-lipoprotein. After the injection of heparin, lipoprotein lipase activity measured by Ediol showed the increased activity but it did not induce the increase of FFA or did not affect any lipoprotein electrophoretic pattern. Intravenous fat tolerance test also showed the complete block of clearance.

Table 4 shows the body weight, blood sugar and secretion rate in alloxan-diabetic dogs. The secretion rate in diabetic dogs in this experiment also showed the acceleration. Compared with that of control, it showed 2-3 times greater in diabetic dogs. The results were far greater than the data obtained by using radioactive fatty acids.

The application of radioactive fatty acids to kinetic study of triglyceride has possibilities to underestimate the results, as was pointed out previously by many papers.

Recycling of the fatty acids, uptake of triglyceride in the liver were the most important technical problems since it is based on the assumption that all plasma triglyceride fatty acids is derived directly from plasma FFA and none is coming from hepatic fatty acid synthesis or storage fat pool. Dietary characteristics

Table 4. Body weight, glucose, and secretion rate in normal and alloxan-diabetic dogs

	B.W. (kg)	B.S. (mg%)	S.R. (mg/kg/h)
Diabetic (n=9)	11.9 ± 0.6	453.3[a] ± 81.5	25.2[a] ± 4.8
Normal (n=9)	15.4 ± 1.7	103.0[a] ± 3.0	8.8[a] ± 2.5

[a] $p < 0.001$. (Mean ± SE)

and the level of plasma triglyceride should be also considered when this method was applied.

Concerning the procedure of Triton, this method has a possibility to overestimate the influx rate in the experimental animal. This method is able to block the removal process of the triglyceride in the peripheral tissues, but it promotes the mobilization of fatty acids and it may stimulate the secretion of triglyceride either by direct effect or indirect process.

Both methods, however, can support the increase of triglyceride influx in alloxan-diabetic dogs in this experiment. Metabolic states in alloxan-induced diabetes may vary depending upon the days after the injection and dosage of alloxan. Present experiment was performed in rather acute stage after the alloxan-injection. Therefore, hypertriglyceridemia in this acute stage may change according to the time passing. Since insulin deprivation may exert the retardation of lipoprotein lipase activity, impairment or removal process would be the major role on the development of hypertriglyceridemia in later phase of the alloxan-diabetes.

Further experiment will be required to observe whether these regulatory mechanisms will be shifted toward to impaired removal from the overproduction.

A part of this study was supported by the grant of adult disease foundation.

ABSTRACTS

TRIGLYCERIDE TURNOVER AND BILE ACID KINETICS IN VARIOUS TYPES OF HYPERLIPOPROTEINEMIA

Bo Angelin, Kurt Einarsson, Kjell Hellström, and Barbro Leijd
Department of Medicine, Karolinska Institutet at Serafimerlasarettet, Stockholm/ Sweden

Earlier reports have shown a normal cholesterol balance in hyperlipoproteinemia type IIa and IIb, while type IV pattern is usually associated with an increased steroid excretion, mainly as bile acids. To investigate the possible relationship between cholesterol/bile acid and triglyceride metabolism, the kinetics of ^{14}C-cholic acid and ^{14}C-chenodeoxycholic acid were studied in 20 patients with type IIa, 6 with type IIb and 14 with type IV hyperlipoproteinemia. They were also characterized with regard to endogenous triglyceride turnover by means of plasma radioactivity determinations after the intravenous administration of ^{3}H-glycerol. In type IIa and type IV subjects and in the total material there was a correlation between bile acid turnover and triglyceride synthesis. However, the latter parameter was better correlated to cholic acid formation than the total bile acid production. The present findings suggest a close relationship between cholesterol/bile acid and triglyceride synthesis.

PLASMA TRIGLYCERIDE TURNOVER IN FASTING OBESE HUMANS

G. Steiner, D. Straja, and E.B. Marliss
Department of Medicine, University of Toronto, Toronto/Canada

Free fatty acids (FFA) may be oxidized to ketones or esterified to triglycerides (TG). Animal studies suggest that the proportion of FFA metabolized in either direction is determined by the relative concentration of insulin and glucagon. To examine this in man, we studied a group of obese (155-237% ideal weight, otherwise normal) subjects in two states; postabsorptive and prolonged fasted (3-5 weeks), and compared them to lean postabsorptive subjects. After prolonged fasting the obese lost 10% of their initial weight; mean plasma, insulins fell by 50%; glucagon was unchanged; and the insulin/glucagon molar ratio fell from 3.4 to 2.2 (P <0.05). Concurrently, plasma FFA rose (from 511 ± 74 to 854 ± 140 μM); blood ketones rose (βOH-butyrate from 0.12 ± 0.04 to 4.7 ± 0.5 mM, acetoacetate from 0.02 ± 0.01 to 0.8 ± 0.1 mM); and plasma TG fell (from 114 ± 17 to 82 ± 9 mg/dl). The hyperketonemia results mainly from increased ketone production. In the obese the postabsorptive TG turnover rate (5.4 ± 0.7 mg/kg-hr) was indistinguishable from that in lean subjects with comparable TG levels. After prolonged fasting, the TG turnover in the obese fell to 2.6 ± 0.4 and the relationship between TG concentration and turnover was consistent with TG removal being impaired. The data suggest that: (1) in man TG turnover in the postabsorptive obese is comparable to that in the lean; (2) TG removal is impaired in obese during fasting; and (3) in man, as in animals, coincident with a fall in the insuling/glucagon molar ratio ketone production increases and, despite an increase in FFA availability, TG turnover falls.

REGULATION OF TRIGLYCERIDE METABOLISM BY ESTROGEN: INHIBITION OF TURKEY POST-HEPARIN PLASMA AND ADIPOSE TISSUE LIPOPROTEIN LIPASES BY AN ESTROGEN-INDUCED PROTEIN

Jim Kelley, Devaki Ganesan, Rollin Thayer, and Petar Alaupovic
Lipoprotein Laboratory, Oklahoma Medical Research Foundation, Oklahoma City, OK/USA

At the onset of egg production in female turkeys or upon administration of estrogen to male turkeys, the post-heparin plasma lipolytic activity (PHLA) is greatly decreased and the plasma triglyceride (TG) levels increase to >2000 mg/100 ml. Three post-heparin lipases were purified: the C-I activated lipoprotein lipase; the C-II activated lipoprotein lipase; and the protamine insensitive triglyceride lipase (TGL). The activity of all three lipases were decreased in laying birds and in estrogen treated birds.
Incubation of increasing volumes of laying turkey plasma with the purified lipoprotein lipases (LPLs) caused a marked decrease in lipolytic activity. Phosvitin, an estrogen-induced protein, which appears in plasma of estrogen-treated or laying birds was tested for its effect on the purified LPLs and TGL. At levels of 3 µg, phosvitin caused marked inhibition of the LPLs (>80% of control values) but had no effect on the TGL. Adipose tissue lipoprotein lipase was more strongly inhibited by phosvitin than the plasma LPLs. Our results when combined with observations of others suggest that estrogens cause an increase in plasma TG levels by two mechanisms: 1) increased synthesis of TG by the liver and 2) inhibition of plasma and adipose tissue LPLs by phosvitin.

FATTY ACID INCORPORATION INTO HUMAN ADIPOSE TISSUE AND OTHER ADIPOSE TISSUE CHARACTERISTICS RELATED TO SERUM TRIGLYCERIDE CONCENTRATION

Göran Walldius
King Gustaf V Research Institute, Karolinska Hospital, Stockholm/Sweden

Fatty acid incorporation into adipose tissue, FIAT, the process involved in removal of plasma triglyceride (TG)-fatty acids liberated by lipoprotein lipase, is often low in hypertriglyceridemia (HTG) and low FIAT may contribute to the development of HTG. In this study the negative correlation between FIAT and TG was analyzed by measuring other variables that might be related to FIAT and/or TG. FIAT determined by an isotopic technique, and glycerol release from needle biopsy specimens from subcutaneous fat, fat cell size and number, the fatty acid spectrum in fat glycerides and the k-value of the intravenous glucose tolerance test were measured in 109 males with different types of HTG.
FIAT per cell was positively correlated with fat cell size and lower in hyper- then in normotriglyceridaemic subjects. Stearic acid correlated positively with FIAT and linolenic acid negatively with the k-value. The k-value and glycerol release were not related to FIAT. The negative correlation between TG and FIAT remained significant when all measured variables were kept constant in partial correlation analysis. In stepwise regression analysis with TG as the dependent variable the highest multiple correlation was obtained by combining FIAT/gram with the content of stearic and linolenic acid, R = 0.79, P <.001. The results suggest that these three variables to a large extent determine TG levels probably by mechanisms related to removal characteristics of individual fatty acid.

MECHANISM OF ACTION OF INTRAVENOUS PHOSPHATIDYL CHOLINE ON LIPOLYSIS: A COMPARISON WITH HEPARIN

A.N. Howard, B. Brown, and J. Patelski

Department of Medicine, University of Cambridge, Cambridge/England and
Department of Biochemistry, Medical Academy, Poznan/Poland

Intravenous polyunsaturated phosphatidyl choline (EPL solution, 10% w/v in 4% sodium deoxycholate) has a clearing effect on lipaemic serum in subjects given a fatty meal, the effect being similar to heparin (HEP). A single injection of EPL soln. (100 mg/kg) in the normal rabbit gave a 50% increase in serum lipase and a 100% increase in lipase content of the liver. HEP (150 i.u./kg) gave a larger increase in serum and small increase in liver. EPL soln. stimulated chiefly liver lipase, since increased activity was seen with M NaCl incubation. HEP stimulated phospholipase in serum and tissues but EPL solution decreased phospholipase in serum and stimulated tissue phospholipase, especially in the liver. Since liver lipase has phospholipase activity, the increase in lipase activity is seen as a direct consequence of substrate stimulation. Groups of rabbits were injected with EPL or egg yolk lecithin (100 mg/kg) as hydrosol or a preparation in 4% sodium deoxycholate (NaDOC), and the effects on liver lipase determined. NaDOC had no effect itself but enhanced the activity of both EPL and egg yolk lecithin. EPL either as a hydrosol or soln. had a greater activity than respective egg lecithin preparations. Thus, the action of EPL on liver lipase is a property of pure EPL but can be further enhanced by its soln. in NaDOC.

WORKSHOP 5. Smoking and Atherosclerosis

Chairmen: H.C. McGill, USA
          N. Kimura, Japan

Participants: Y. Nakayama, Japan
              P. Astrup, Denmark
              H.C. McGill, USA
              J.L. Gainer, USA
              H. Schievelbein, West Germany

EPIDEMIOLOGICAL RESEARCH IN JAPAN ON SMOKING AND CARDIOVASCULAR DISEASES

Yuhki Nakayama

In 1904, the manufacturing and monopoly system of tabacco started in Japan.

Recently, 13% of females and 80% of males smoke cigarettes according to information from the Japanese monopoly. Now, I wish to introduce to you the relationship between cigarette smoking and ischemic heart disease and stroke based on prospective epidemiological research in Japan.

Hirayama's Study

Figure 1 shows Dr. Hirayama's study on 265, 118 adults, aged over 40, living in the area of 29 public health centers, in five selected prefectures. These cohorts were checked for decedents every year since 1965.
Figure 2 shows that the ratio of observed deaths of smokers compared with expected deaths due to cardiovascular diseases is 1.16 in males. For cerebral hemorrhage and cerebral infarction, the effect of smoking is not significant in males.
Figure 3 shows dose response. The risk is increased with the dose.
Figure 4 shows that those who started as teen-agers are high risk cases.

Sasaki's Study

This study (Fig. 5) was made in the Akita prefecture where the incidence of strokes is very high in Japan. All resident 529 men aged 40 - 59 were studied. Response rate was 82%, and follow-ups were made for 15 years.

As seen at the left side of Figure 6, smokers of more than ten cigarettes a day had lower death rates. Stroke, shown on the right side of Figure 6, showed a similar result.

Hisayama Study

Figure 7 shows the Hisayama study. Subjects were 1841 persons aged 40 or more. As can be noted in the middle of Figure 7, out of 579 smokers, 74 persons (12.8%) developed cerebral infarction and 15 persons (2.6%) developed myocardial infarction. However, in this study, cerebral hemorrhage had no definite relation to cigarette smoking.

For the epidemiological study, taking
advantage of the population census of
1965, 29 public health centers in 5
prefectures were indiscriminatly
chosen.
265,118 residents, aged above 40,
were investigated as to their
physical condition and living
habits.

     Rate: 91 - 99%

☐: No. of public health centers

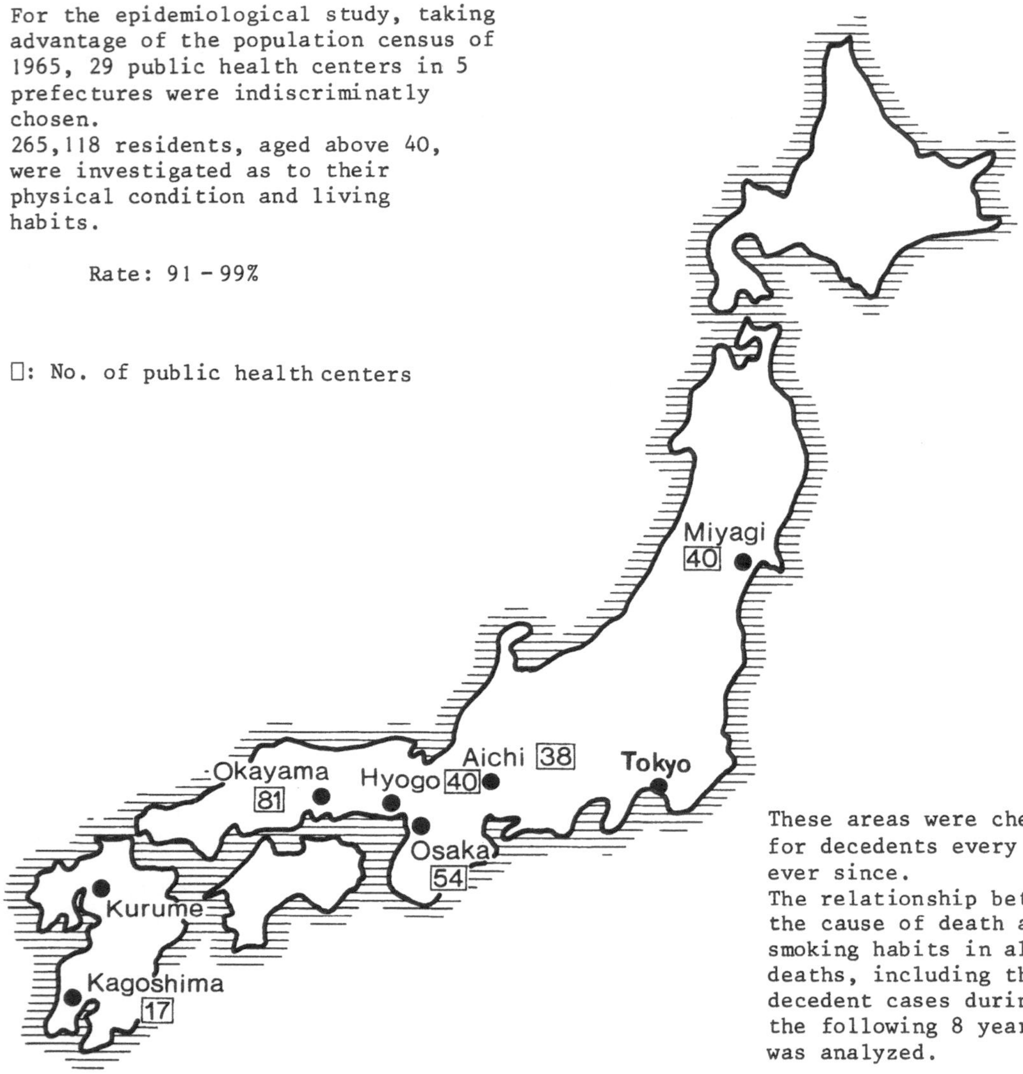

Miyagi
40 ●

Okayama   Aichi 38   Tokyo
81   Hyogo 40 ●

Osaka
54

Kurume

Kagoshima
17

These areas were checked
for decedents every year
ever since.
The relationship between
the cause of death and
smoking habits in all
deaths, including the
decedent cases during
the following 8 years,
was analyzed.

Figure 1. 8-year follow-up Hirayama's study

	Male			Female		
	Smoker observed deaths	Age standardized expected deaths	Ratio	Smoker observed deaths	Age standardized expected deaths	Ratio
All causes of deaths	9,311	7,623.1	1.22[a]	1,327	1,018.9	1.30[a]
Subarachnoid hemorrhage	71	31.7	2.23[a]	22	10.5	2.10[a]
Cerebral hemorrhage	1,373	1,363.5	1.00	208	164.4	1.26[a]
Cerebral thrombosis	680	713.1	0.95	80	90.0	1.11
Other forms of cerebrovascular disease	412	309.9	1.32[a]	56	41.7	1.34[b]
Total	2,536	2,418.2	1.05[b]	366	306.6	1.19[a]
Chronic rheumatic heart disease	29	21.6	1.34	14	9.8	1.43
Ischemic heart disease	611	372.0	1.64[a]	75	47.5	1.57[a]
Other forms of heart disease	477	434.0	1.09[b]	89	71.8	1.23[b]
Hypertensive heart disease	143	62.3	2.29[a]	28	21.0	1.33
Other forms of hypertension	74	56.6	1.30[b]	8	7.5	1.06
Total	1,334	946.5	1.41[a]	214	157.6	1.36[a]
Grand Total	3,870	3,364.7	1.16[a]	580	464.2	1.25[a]

Cerebrovascular disease

Heart disease

[a] $p < 0.001$. [b] $p < 0.05$.

Figure 2. Age standardized 8-year death rate (Hirayama's study)

151

(Standardized Death Ratio)

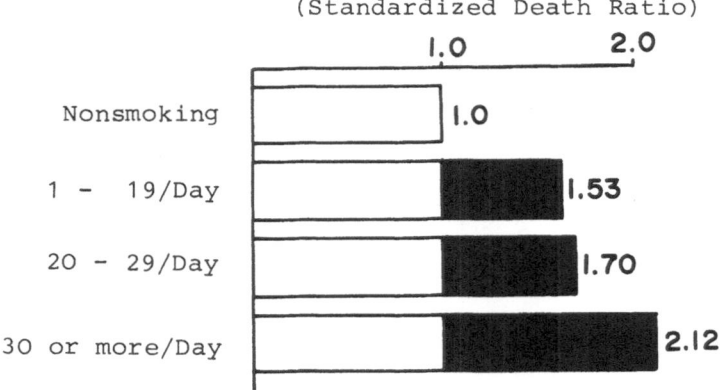

Figure 3. Smoking habits vs. ischemic heart disease (1966-1973 Japan; Hirayama et al.)

(Standardized Death Ratio)

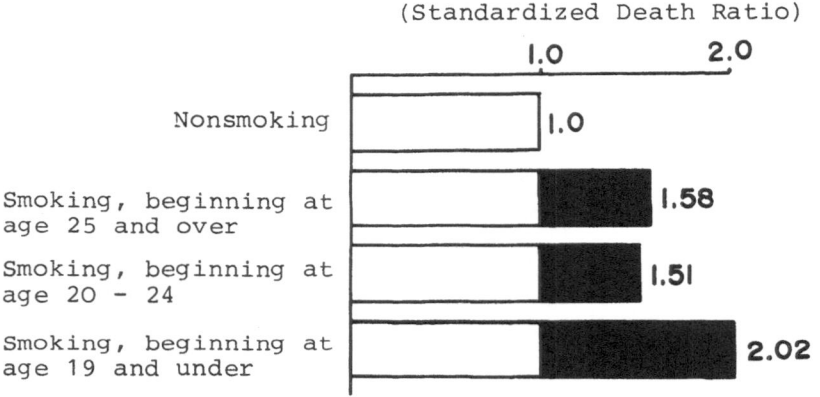

Figure 4. Smoking (beginning age) vs. ischemic heart disease (1966-1973 Japan; Hirayama et al.)

Area: Nishime Village, Akita, Japan
Roster:
Through a questionnaire data on living habits, including cigarette smoking habits, were obtained from all 529 male residents, aged 40 – 69.

Start: 1957

Lost to follow-up: rate 3,6%

Figure 5. 15-year follow-up of nishime village, Akita, Japan

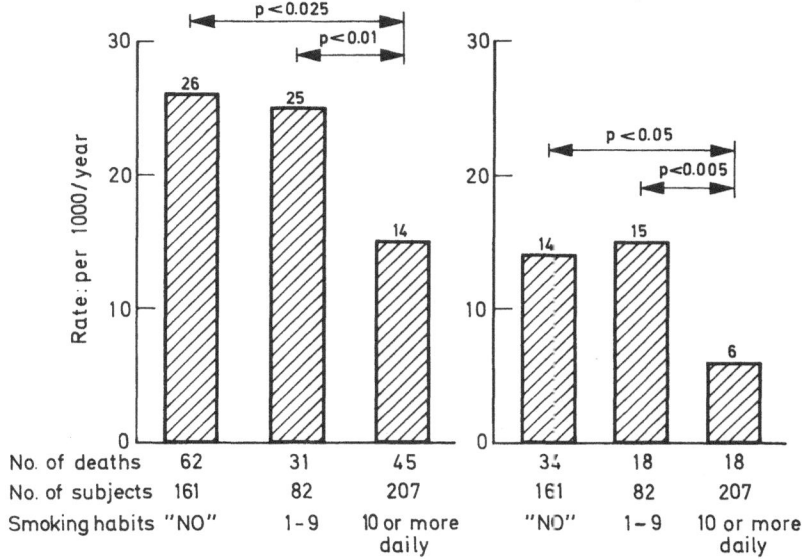

All causes of deaths   Cerebrovascular disease
Sasaki N.

Figure 6. Smoking habits vs. deaths

Risk factors	No. of subjects	Cerebral infarction 109 (cases)	6.7(%)	Myocardial 26 (cases)	Infarction 1.6(%)
Age (60 years of more)	591	87	14.7[a]	16	2.7[a]
Occupation	654	64	9.8[a]	7	1.1
Family history (stroke, hypertension)	493	65	13.2[a]	9	1.8
Heavy drining habits	56	50	89.3[a]	7	12.5[a]
Smoking habits	579	74	12.8[a]	15	2.6[b]
Overweight (+10% or more)	175	29	16.6[a]	8	4.6[a]
Hypertension (WHO)	410	68	16.6[a]	11	2.7[b]
ECG abnormalities (Minnesota code 3-1, 4-1, 2,3)	286	60	21.0[a]	12	4.2[a]
Fundus abnormalities (kw II-IV)	344	56	16.3[a]	12	3.5[b]
Serum cholesterol (200 mg/dl or more)	182	16	8.8	3	1.6

[a] p <0.05. [b] p <0.01.

Figure 7. 10-year follow-up of Hisayama study
Roster: 1841 persons, examined: 1658, rate: 90.1%
Cerebrovascular disease free area: 1621
Lost to ten-year follow-up: rate 0.3%
Start: 1961, age: 40 years or more

Risk factors of cerebral infarction, myocardial infarction (studies on incidence cases)

Cerebrovascular disease free area 1621. Follow-up period Nov. 1961 – Oct. 1971. Statistical analysis between cases with and without risk factors were determined by student t-test

Our 15-year Follow-up Study

This study (Fig. 8) is part of the "Seven Country Studies" conducted by Prof. Ancel Keys. In that study, middle-aged men ranging 40 – 59 were already reported. But, here, I wish to present data on men 40 – 64 years old in our study.

Figure 9 shows the relationship between cigarette smoking and incidence of myocardial infarction. The incidence of myocardial infarction increased with an increas in cigarettes smoked. The risk of the smoker is over three times higher than that of the nonsmoker.

In contrast with Figure 9, the incidence (Fig. 10) of stroke had no definite relation to cigarette smoking.

Figure 11 illustrates the relationship between smoking habits, blood pressure, and stroke. Stroke occurred more frequently among persons who had never smoked cigarettes or had quit smoking cigarettes and had hypertension than among cigarette smokers with hypertension.

Accordingly, the risk of stroke in hypertensives, taken as a whole, decreased with the increas of cigarettes smoked.

Area: Tanushimaru (farmers), Ushibuka (fishermen)

Examination coverage:

General population age 40 – 64, male

Roster:

	No. of men	Examined	Rate
Tanushimaru	639	639	100.0%
Ushibuka	614	612	99.7%

Start:

Tanushimaru	1958
Ushibuka	1960

Lost to follow-up:

Tanushimaru	0.2%
Ushibuka	0.3%

(W.B.)

48 men were found to have smoked kiseru at entry. Data of 8 men were not available because of lack of information.

These 56 men were excluded from this study.

Figure 8

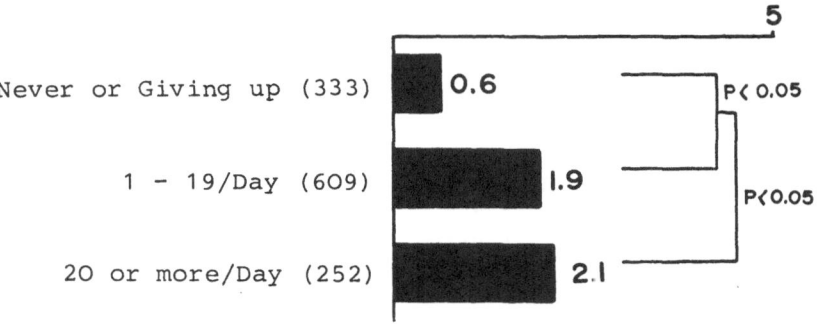

Figure 9. Smoking habits vs. myocardial infarction. 15-year follow-up of rural Kyushu, Japan (Kimura et al.)

Figure 10. Smoking habits vs. stroke. 15-year follow-up of rural Kyushu, Japan (Kimura et al.)

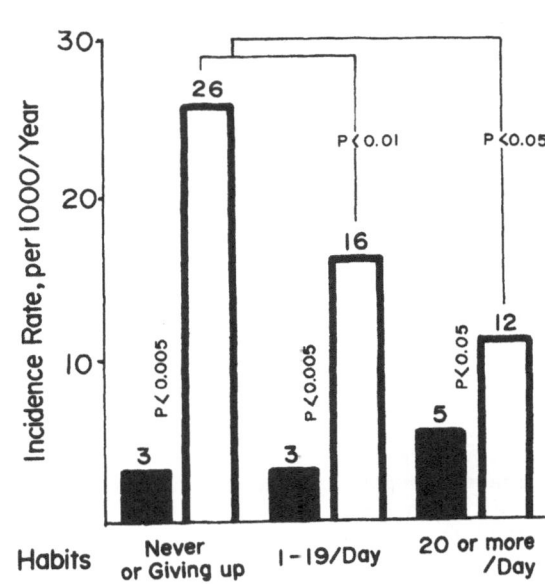

Figure 11. Smoking and blood pressure vs. stroke. 15-year follow-up of rural Kyushu, Japan (Kimura et al.)

☐ hypertensive: 160-90 mm HG or more:

■ nonhypertensive

Conclusion

In addition to our 15-year follow-up experience, I have reviewed three prospective studies in Japan.

We are inclined to think that there might exist a significant correlation between ischemic heart disease and cigarette smoking.

The observed inverse relationship between stroke and cigarette smoking is not explainable. However, our 15-year follow-up experience leads us to surmise that cigarette smoking might inhibit the development of stroke in hypertensive men.

ATHEROGENIC COMPOUNDS OF TOBACCO SMOKE

Poul Astrup

The components of tobacco smoke having a potential atherogenic effect are nicotine, carbon monoxide, cyanide, and nitrogen oxides.

The physiologic and pharmacologic effects of nicotine on the cardiovascular system are well-known and described several times and will not be dealt with in this paper, while investigations concerning the possible atherogenic effects will be discussed briefly.
The main results of the investigations are that nicotine, when administered alone, has no injuring effects on intima, but might lead to the occurrence of moderate fibrosis and of calcifications in the media of aorta (U.S. Public Health Service, 1971; Schievelbein et al., 1970). When nicotine has been administered to hypercholesterolemic or hypertensive animals, no or only very limited additive effects of nicotine on the arterial wall injuries have been observed (Fisher et al., 1973; Grogogeat et al., 1965). It is remarkable, however, that the daily dose of nicotine in the animal studies in general has been several times higher per kg of body weight than the daily amount of nicotine absorbed by heavy smokers. This is demonstrated in Table 1. By assuming that 1 mg of nicotine is absorbed in humans for each cigarette smoked, up to 1200 cigarettes should be smoked and inhaled per day by an individual to absorb similar amounts of nicotine as administered to the animals in the experiments mentioned, where no arterial wall injuring effects of nicotine were observed. Therefore, since such doses of nicotine are unable to produce atheromatosis in rabbits, it is very unlikely that nicotine is the responsible component in tobacco smoke for the increased incidence of atherosclerosis in smokers. So one has to look for other components.
We have focused our interest on carbon monoxide and other compounds which might compete with oxygen in the arterial walls, and our results found so far are reviewed in this paper. First, however, it would be appropriate to mention the results of our hypoxia exposure studies since they are quite similar to our carbon monoxide studies.

For many years, some kind of oxygen deprivation has been considered as an essential part of the various ways of injuring tissues and also of injuring vascular walls, leading to atherosclerosis. To study this process, the most basic experiments of perform would be to study the vascular wall effects of lowering the oxygen content of the breathing air. This has actually also been done in various laboratories, starting in the 1930's in Germany by exposing animals to hypobaric hypoxia. More elaborate studies were performed in 1951 by Grundman who found severe subendothelial edema and medial necrosis in arteries of cats exposed to hypoxia from 1 - 24 hours in low pressure chambers, where the oxygen tension was lowered to near the critical level for death by reducing the barometric pressure.

Table 1. Amounts of nicotine used in experimental studies in rabbits
1. Fisher et al., 1962; 2. Schievelbein, et al., 1965;
3. Grosgogeat et al., 1965; 4. Scott et al., 1973

	Nicotine per kg/day	Corresp. to cigarettes per day in a smoker	Atherogenic effect
Authors:			
1.	0.3	35	none
2.	2.3	160	none
3.	10 mg	700	none
4.	6-18	400-1200	none

In my laboratory, vascular wall injuries were observed in rabbits exposed to
normobaric hypoxia by lowering the oxygen content of atmospheric air to 15% by
adding nitrogen at a normal barometric pressure (Kjeldsen and Klem Thomsen,
1975). The injuries were characterized first of all by a pronounced subendothelial edema, blister formation, and fragmentation of the internal elastic membrane.
Figure 1 is a micrograph of aorta from a control rabbit showing flat continuous
endothelium almost directly attached to the internal elastic membrane. Figure 2
is from aorta of a rabbit exposed for 2 weeks to 15% oxygen. There is a pronounced subendothelial blister formation and fragmentation of the internal elastic membrane. The cells are pushed toward the lumen of the artery, and they are

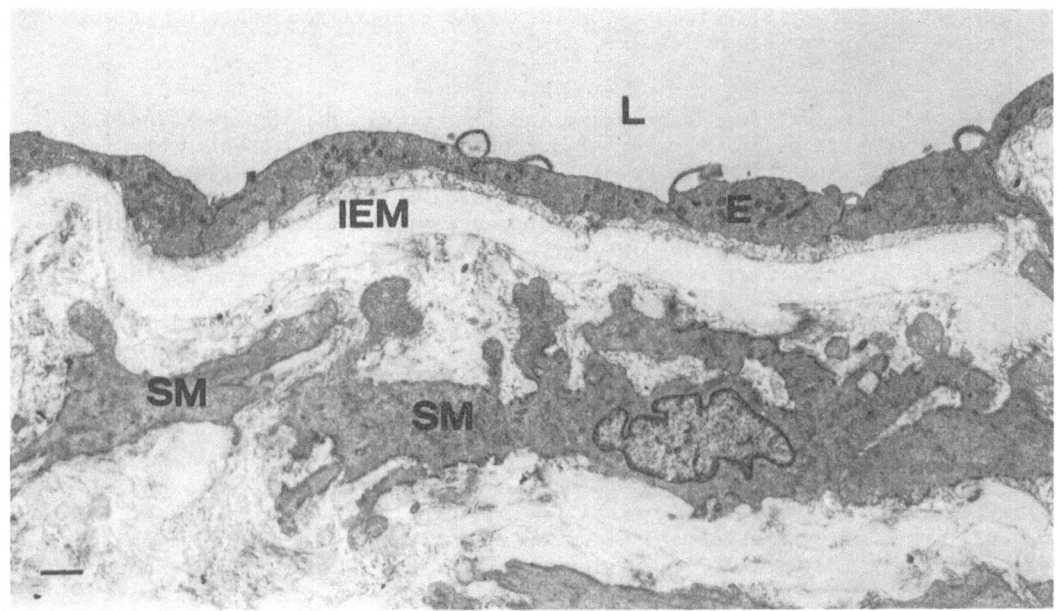

Figure 1. Micrograph of aorta from control rabbit showing flat continuous endothelium connected by tight junctions and almost directly attached to the internal
elastic membrane. E, endothelial cell; IEM, internal elastic membrane; SM, smooth
muscle cell; L, lumen. Bar represents 1 μm

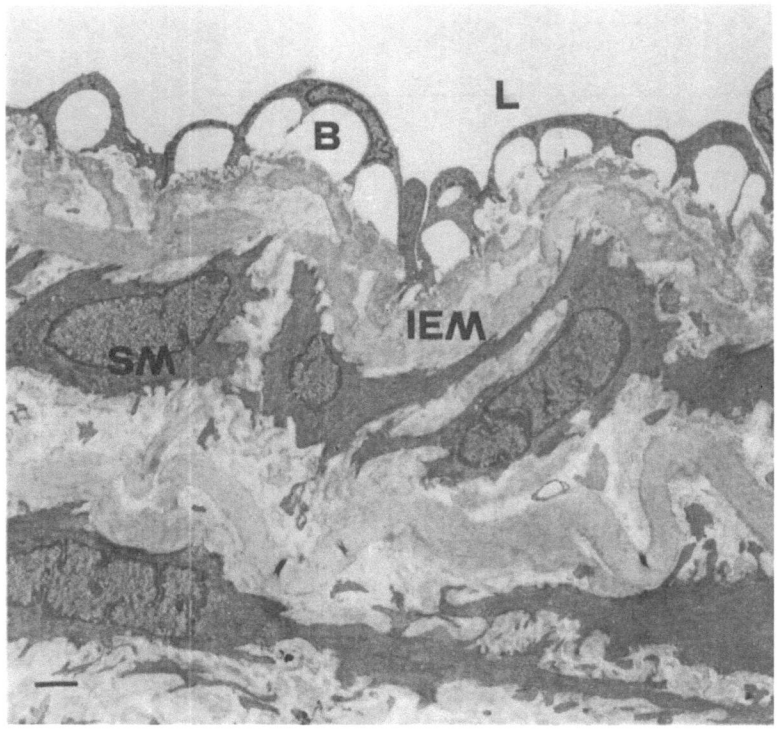

Figure 2. Micrograph from aorta of rabbit exposed for 2 weeks to approximately 15% oxygen. L, lumen; B, blister; IEM, internal elastic membrane; SM, smooth muscle cell. Bar represents 1 μm

attached to the underlying membrane by the remains of thin and occasionally thicker sections of cellular material surrounding the liquid, which has intruded between the cell and the membrane. An edema was dominating the picture also beneath the internal elastic membrane. The scanning pictures showed that the regular pattern disappeared with the occurrence of the blisters beneath the cells, leading to a characteristic cobblestone appearance of the cells. In some areas, the endothelial cells were separated completely from the membrane by the intruding fluid, and a plaque was formed where the folds had disappeared completely. When using cholesterol-fed rabbits, we further observed that normobaric hypoxia enhanced the aortic accumulation of cholesterol more than three times in comparison to a normoxic control group (Kjeldsen et al., 1968). Other investigators have made similar observations. It should, therefore, be considered as an established fact that arterial blood hypoxia is atherogenic.

The mechanism involved is partly an increased permeability of the vascular system as indicated by the microscopic findings, but hypoxia also enhances the accumulation of lipids of myocardium and of arterial walls according to findings by various authors (Harris, 1971; Fillios et al., 1961). Furthermore, exposure to hypoxia increases serum cholesterol for a certain period whether the animals are fed cholesterol or not. In our own experiments with cholesterol-fed animals the hypoxic animals has about 20% higher serum cholesterol values than the control animals, which has to be related to the about 300% higher aortic cholesterol values in the hypoxic animals in comparison to the control animals. This increase in serum cholesterol has probably added to the observed aortic cholesterol accumulation in the various experiments performed.

When talking about arterial blood hypoxia and atherogenesis it is also of interest to discuss the influence of *hyperoxia*. The very few experiments performed for studying this influence indicate a reversal effect by hyperoxia on atherosclerosis (Kjeldsen et al., 1969). The effect seems to be in the regressive phase according to some recent results obtained in our laboratory (Stender et al., 1976).

What is now the significance for atherosclerosis in humans of these experimental findings in animals? If continuous exposure to hypoxia enhances atherosclerosis in man as it does in animals, we should expect to find more atherosclerosis in people living at high altitude than in people living at sea level. This is, however, not the case. This probably cannot be explained exclusively by a less frequent occurrence of risk factors in people living at high altitude. To me it seems more likely that adaptation phenomena occur by long exposure to high altitude, something we do not know much about from either human or animal investigations. But the existence of adaptation concerning endothelial permeability is indicated by the fact that people living at high altitude easily develop lung edema when returning by air from traveling to sea level. It might, therefore, well be that adaptation of some kind protects high altitude dwellers from developing atherosclerosis. The fact, however, that atherosclerosis is very uncommon in high altitude dwellers makes it seem very unlikely that continuously reduced arterial oxygen tensions are of any significance in the pathogenesis of atherosclerosis in human beings.

So, if hypoxia in general should be of importance, we have to continue our discussion about the types of hypoxia caused by compounds competing with oxygen concerning either transport in blood and delivery to the tissues or concerning the cellular oxidative metabolism. Carbon monoxide is of particular interest in this relation, since heavy smokers have up to 20% COHb in their blood.

In my laboratory we have for about 10 years been interested in studying atherogenic effects of carbon monoxide. After *continuous exposure* of rabbits for a few weeks to carbon monoxide, leading to carboxyhemoglobin levels of 16-18%, arterial wall injuries occur, indistinguishable from the lesions found in rabbits exposed to hypoxia (Astrup and Kjeldsen, 1974).

If cholesterol is added in moderate amounts to the food of animals exposed to carbon monoxide, an enhancement occurs of the cholesterol accumulation in the arterial walls. So, when exposing cholesterol-fed rabbits to carbon monoxide continuously for 6-8 weeks, the arterial wall accumulation of cholesterol increases two to three times (Astrup et al., 1967).

Enhancement of cholesterol accumulation by moderate continuous carbon monoxide exposure also occurs in coronary arteries of primates (Webster et al., 1970), and in 4-hour perfusion studies of human coronary arteries, it has been found that a concentration of 15% COHb in the perfused blood increases the cholesterol uptake, while the lipid synthesis in the arterial walls does not change (Sarma et al., 1975).

Concerning the effects of *intermittent* exposure, which means exposure for a certain amount of hours a day for some time, there are conflicting results. By intermittent exposure of rabbits to 180 ppm carbon monoxide 12 hours daily for some weeks, we found in our first experiment a very pronounced atherogenic effect (Astrup, 1972). We have, however, not been able to confirm this result in two new experiments carried out recently, where the serum cholesterol concentration was kept uniform in the nonexposed group by individual cholesterol feeding. Further, Malinow et al. (1976) recently found that 6 hours exposure (30 min of each hour leading to about 20% COHb, for 12 consecutive hours of each day) during 14 months did not lead to enhanced accumulation of cholesterol in the arterial walls of primates. However, the animals were hypertensive, and a heavy cholesterol loading was used as well, which may have masked any possible added atherogenic effect of carbon monoxide. Therefore, the conclusion to be drawn concerning intermittent exposure is that the results are inconsistent and that a wall injuring effect is unproven at present.

The mode of action of carbon monoxide seems to be similar to the mode of action of hypoxia, which also involves an increased permeability of endothelium membranes as a direct influence on lipid accumulation.

Parving in our group has shown that carbon monoxide exposure (20-25% COHb) of men for 3 hours leads to a 50% increase in disappearance rate from the blood of injected serum ^{131}I albumin (Parving, 1972; Parving et al., 1972. The occurrence of increased permeability during exposure to carbon monoxide could also be shown in dogs, where the lymph flow and the protein flux in the thoracic duct increased considerably. It was of interest that the increase in protein flux was more pronounced for the high molecular proteins than for the low molecular ones (Parving et al., 1972). Besides the effect of carbon monoxide on endothelial permeability, there might also be a direct effect on lipid metabolism. So, carbon monoxide exposure increased the serum cholesterol values in our cholesterol fed animals. The increases are moderate, usually about 15% in animals exposed to 200 pp, carbon monoxide, but this increase will of course add to cholesterol accumulation in the carbon monoxide exposed animals. It remains to be clarified to what degree this serum cholesterol increase can explain the enhancement of aortic accumulation in carbon monoxide exposed animals.

We have recently performed an exposure experiment with carbon monoxide and cholesterol-fed rabbits, where we kept the serum cholesterol concentration at the same level in all animals by individual cholesterol feeding. Here, we were unable to demonstrate a difference between the aortic cholesterol content in the exposed group in comparison to the control group.

When, however, we exposed normocholesterolemic rabbits to carbon monoxide, it was possible to demonstrate an increased accumulation of cholesterol in the aortas of the rabbits despite the fact that their serum cholesterol concentrations were lower than in the control group.

The explanation of the apparent difference between the normocholesterolemic and the hypercholesterolemic exposure experiment seems to be that severe hypercholesterolemia is a much more potent atherogenic factor than moderate carbon monoxide exposure, being able to demask the atherogenic effect of the latter.

Other toxic effects of moderate carbon monoxide exposure concern the myocardium, where subendothelial edema, interstitial edema, and injuries of mitochondria can be observed already after 4 hours exposure of rabbits to 100 ppm carbon monoxide (Thomsen and Kjeldsen, 1974). Further, decreased birth weight and heavily increased rate of stillborns are observed, when rabbits are exposed to carbon monoxide (9-10% or 16-18% COHb) during pregnancy (Astrup et al., 1972).

Another compound of tobacco smoke, cyanide, also competes with oxygen. No inhalation experiments with cyanide has to my knowledge been performed in animals, but it is not unlikely that cyanide in the concentrations occurring in tobacco smoke, about 100-300 μg from a cigarette, might influence particularly the endothelium of arteries, which, when disregarding the respiratory tract, will be exposed to higher cyanide concentration than all other cells.

Also, nitrogen oxide may have atherogenic effects, but exposure studies have so far not been published. We have found that exposure of rabbits to 5 ppm nitrogen oxide for 2 weeks leads to the development in the pulmonary arterioles of fluid containing vacuoles inside the arteriolar endothelial cells and/or in the intercellular junctions, and to thickening of the alveolocapillary membrane due to fluid accumulation in the interstitial space.

In conclusion, it should be emphasized that it is of the greatest importance to have all the components in tobacco smoke with pathogenic pulmonary and cardiovascular effects identified with certainty. So far, the interest has been focused mainly on tar and nicotine. The carcinogenic and pharmacologic effects respectively of those two components are well-known. To what extent, however, they are responsible for the pathologic effects of tobacco smoking is unknown. Other compounds such as carbon monoxide, cyanide, and nitrogen oxides may be blamed as well. It is very likely that carbon monoxide in tobacco smoke is at least partly responsible for the harmful effects of smoking on the myocardium, the arterial walls, and the fetus. Cyanide and nitrogen oxides probably harmful effects too. The clarification of the role of the components mentioned are of the greatest importance for our understanding of the involved pathogenetic mechanisms and for a successful prevention of the tobacco smoking diseases.

ABNORMALITIES POTENTIALLY MEDIATING THE EFFECT OF CIGARETTE SMOKING ON ATHEROSCLEROSIS

Henry C. McGill, Jr.

Introduction

It seems unnecessary to document further the strong association of cigarette smoking with the atherosclerotic diseases, particularly coronary heart disease and its sequelae. This association has been observed in almost every clinical and epidemiological study conducted in the past 30 years, and the consistency and strength of the association strongly suggest that there is a causal relationship. It now seems prudent to direct attention to elucidating the mechanisms of this relationship in biochemical and physiologic terms.

Other presentations in this workshop have been concerned with the components of cigarette smoke that are inhaled and absorbed, and with evidence regarding which of these components are responsible for augmenting the incidence of coronary heart disease in cigarette smokers. As can be seen from the other papers, we are not yet certain which component is the culprit. This discussion is concerned with biochemical or physiologic variables that are altered in human cigarette smokers and that may serve as intervening variables in the cigarette smoking effect on atherosclerotic disease. These alterations may yield clues to the mechanism of the cigarette smoking effect.

Clinical Disease or Atherosclerosis

The first major problem in examining the mechanism of the cigarette smoking effect on atherosclerotic disease is to determine whether the effect is on the terminal occlusive episode, on the process of atherogenesis, or on both stages. Most data have been concerned with the association of cigarette smoking with increased incidence of clinical disease and a decrease in incidence after cessation of smoking. Risk of coronary heart disease drops to near normal levels within a year after cessation of smoking, and falls slowly thereafter so that the ex-smoker has normal or below normal risk of coronary heart disease within 10 - 15 years after cessation of smoking (Hammong and Garfinkel, 1969; Rogot, 1974). Since it seems unlikely that advanced fibrous plaques can undergo regression in less than a year, this observation suggests that the cigarette smoking effect is predominantly on the terminal occlusive episode rather than on atherogenesis.

To determine whether cigarette smokers have more atherosclerosis than nonsmokers requires the evaluation of atherosclerosis in the arteries of autopsied persons, and then evaluating the lifetime cigarette smoking habits of these persons. Several reports have agreed that advanced atherosclerotic lesions (principally fibrous plaques and related lesions) are more extensive in cigarette smokers than in nonsmokers. The most thorough of these studies (Strong and Richards, 1976) described the findings in 1320 autopsied men 25 - 64 years of age. Cigarette smoking histories of the subjects were estimated by interviewing surviving relatives and associates using a pretested schedule (McMahan et al., 1976). The coronary arteries of the heavy smokers had about 50% more of the intimal surface involved with fibrous plaques and other advanced lesions than did those of nonsmokers. The abdominal aortas of smokers had twice as much intimal surface involved as did those of nonsmokers. This difference was present in the 25 - 34 year group, but was not present in the few cases under 25 years of age. These data, which are similar to the results of other studies on the association of cigarette smoking and atherosclerosis (Wilens and Plair, 1962; Auerbach et al., 1965; Sackett and Winkelstein, 1967; Sackett et al., 1968; Strong et al., 1969), indicate that cigarette smoking is a strong stimulus to the production of fibrous plaques in the coronary arteries and the abdominal aorta.

No effects have been observed on fatty streaks, which are the predominant lesions in young persons under the age of 25. Such persons have relatively short histories of cigarette smoking exposure and low death rates, making it difficult to obtain significant numbers of cases.

Thus, it appears that at least one effect of cigarette smoking on atherogenesis is to accelerate the formation of fibrous plaques. Recent information regarding characteristics of fibrous plaques suggests potential mechanisms of this effect. For example, Benditt (1974), reviewing the implications of the mutagenic hypothesis of atherogenesis, suggests that carcinogenic substances in cigarette smoke may be responsible for the transformation of selected smooth muscle cells in the arterial intima and the excessive proliferation of some of these transformed cells to form monoclonal fibrous plaques.

Blood Pressure

The effects of cigarette smoking on the major risk factors for atherosclerosis and related diseases also is informative in searching for possible causal mechanisms. Despite the transient elevation of blood pressure induced by nicotine, no epidemiological study of cigarette smokers has demonstrated increased risk of hypertension among cigarette smokers (for example, Epstein et al., 1965); and at least one has shown that smokers have lower diastolic blood pressure (Higgins and Kjelsberg, 1967). It is not possible to assess the possibility that many transient elevations in blood pressure induced by repeated doses of nicotine over many years could affect atherosclerosis.

Diabetes and Glucose Tolerance

Glucose tolerance is slightly impaired in cigarette smokers, but cigarette smoking is not associated with increased prevalence of diabetes (Higgins and Kjelsberg, 1967). Clinical diabetes mellitus is unquestionably a strong risk factor for the atherosclerotic diseases, but the significance of impaired glucose tolerance without clinical diabetes is less well-established (Epstein et al., 1965). The problem of lack of reproducibility of the glucose tolerance test in clinically healthly adults complicates evaluation of this physiologic variable as a mechanism of the cigarette smoking effect. It is especially remarkable that glucose intolerance might be increased in cigarette smokers, since they also are reported to be thinner and less likely to be obese than nonsmokers, and since obesity is a strong risk factor for the development of diabetes mellitus (Medalie et al., 1975).

Szanto (1967) reported increased blood glucose and increased insulinemia in the serum of cigarette smokers. Hyperinsulinemia has been linked to accelareted atherosclerosis in experimental animals and this offers another potential mechanism for the cigarette smoking effect.

Serum Lipid Concentrations

Many epidemiological studies have examined the relationship of cigarette smoking to serum cholesterol and triglyceride concentrations (Acheson and Jessop, 1961; Konttinen, 1962; Konttinen and Rajasalmi, 1963; Higgins and Kjelsberg, 1967; Howell, 1970; Dales et al., 1974; Billimoria et al., 1975). In summary, some studies find higher serum cholesterol concentrations in smokers than in non-smokers, and a nearly equal number find no difference. Differences, when present, are not great, and even if the differences are real, they do not account for the increased incidence of clinical disease and the increased severity of athero-sclerotic lesions in heavy cigarette smokers. Furthermore, in multivariate anal-yses in which cigarette smoking is analyzed as a risk factor independently of other variables, cigarette smoking emerges as a strong independent variable and its effect does not depend on elevated serum lipids.

Coagulation and Thrombosis

Cigarette smokers tend to have a higher incidence of thromboembolic disease (Murphy and Mustard, 1966). Cigarette smoking has not yet been demonstrated to produce a consistent effect on the procoagulants, but many investigators have shown effects on platelet functions. Ashby (1965) showed that platelet stickiness was increased in smokers. Mustard and Murphy (1963) showed the life span of platelets to be reduced during heavy smoking. Two independent studies (Glynn et al., 1966; Hawkins, 1972) found platelet aggregation chronically increased in heavy smokers as compared to nonsmokers. Levine (1973) observed an acute effect of cigarette smoking on platelet aggregation in response to a standard aggregat-ing agent. The phenomenon was directly related to inhalation of tobacco smoke in a double blind controlled study.

Since the role of coagulation and thrombosis in atherogenesis is not yet clear, it is not possible to evaluate alterations in platelet functions as factors in atherogenesis. It appears likely, however, that these changes could be involved in the terminal occlusive episode of coronary heart disease.

Cellular Elements of Blood

Several studies have shown an increase in hematocrit, red cell count, and hemo-globin in cigarette smokers (Eisen and Hammond, 1956; Howell, 1970; Isager and Hagerup, 1971; Billimoria et al., 1975). This change is presumably related to blood carboxyhemoglobin and the consequent reduction in oxygen-carrying capacity of the blood, simulating a mild state of hypoxia. Although polycythemia predis-poses to thrombosis, the slight degree of polycythemia attained in smokers does not appear sufficient to account for the increased risk of coronary heart disease associated with cigarette smoking. No association of atherogenesis with poly-cythemia has been reported.

Cigarette smokers also show elevated leukocyte counts (Friedman et al., 1973; Corre et al., 1971; Billimoria et al., 1975) which are correlated more with in-halation than with degree of chronic bronchitis. The increase involves all types of leukocytes, and therefore is not due solely to an adrenal cortical effect. There is no known mechanism by which this change can be related directly to ath-erosclerosis. However, leukocytosis may be associated with increased endothelial permeability, which is an integral step in most current hypotheses of the patho-genesis of atherosclerosis. If any component of cigarette smoke alters endothelial permeability and induces local inflammatory reactions in the walls of arteries, this effect could provide a mechanism of the cigarette smoking effect.

Cardiac Effects

Bekheit and Fletcher (1976) reported that a few puffs of cigarette smoke increase the velocity of conduction in the heart and shorten the refractory period of the A-V node. They attribute this affect to adrenergic stimulation by nicotine. Cigarette smoke also increases the ventricular rate in atrial fibrillation and antagonizes the cholinergic effect of digitalis.

Hart et al. (1976) reported enhanced salivary antipyrine disappearance rate in smokers, presumed due to induction of the hepatic microsomal enzyme system. Since the liver is the primary source of lipoproteins and plays a major role in the metabolism of cholesterol and other lipids, there may be secondary effects on serum lipid and lipoprotein composition.

Immunologic Mechanisms

Becker and associates (1976) isolated and characterized a glycoprotein in tobacco which is highly antigenic. Both smokers and nonsmokers positive skin tests to the substance. An immunochemically similar material was present in cigarette smoke. This antigenic glycoprotein also is present in other plants of the same family as tobacco. Circulating immune complexes and antigen-antibody reactions may cause intimal damage and increase endothelial permeability.

Other Effects

Other miscellaneous effects on cigarette smoking also must be taken into account. For example, Higgins and Kjelsberg (1967) showed that smokers have thinner skin folds and weigh less than nonsmokers; and also have lower serum uric acid concentrations. Wehner et al. (1976) showed that cigarette smoking exposure increased the life span and decreased the average weight of rats. These effects seem to be in the direction of reducing rather than increasing risk of atherosclerotic disease.

Verdy et al. (1975) have reported an increased growth hormone level in cigarette smokers, which would be consistent with the hyperinsulinemia. However, there is no known association of growth hormone disturbances with atherogenesis.

Dales et al. (1974) reported that cigarette smokers have decreased creatinine and albumin concentrations.

Alexander et al. (1976) showed that serum carcinoembryonic antigen levels were higher in the blood of smokers than of nonsmokers.

Interactions With Other Variables

Another puzzling aspect of the relationship of cigarette smoking to atherogenesis is the interaction of smoking with other risk factors. Only a limited amount of data is available on the effects of cigarette smoking in persons with very low or no risk factors. Available data suggests that no effect on coronary heart disease is produced in their absence. Viel et al. (1968) found that cigarette smokers in Santiago, Chile had no more extensive lesions than did nonsmokers.

Keys (1970), in the "Seven Countries Study", found no association of cigarette smoking with coronary heart disease mortality in those countries with overall low coronary heart disease rates and correspondingly low levels of major risk factors, such as hypercholesterolemia and hypertension. Thus, is appears that cigarette smoking must be combined with moderately severe atherogenic factors in order to augment atherogenesis or the atherosclerotic diseases. It appears that cigarette smoking accelerates, but does not initiate, the formation of fibrous plaques.

Conclusion

Intensive study of the many variables in cigarette smokers other than the incidence of coronary heart disease, chronic obstructive pulmonary disease, and lung cancer has only recently begun. The above listing of reported alterations related to cigarette smoking undoubtedly represents only a few of the metabolic derangements that will be found in cigarette smokers. It will be important to confirm these observed changes and to search for more changes which also may serve as intervening variables in the effect of cigarette smoking on atherogenesis. It also will be valuable to examine experimental models of cigarette smoking inhalation to determine whether they develop similar alterations.

OXYGEN TRANSPORT AND SMOKING

John L. Gainer

Many have considered the possibility that oxygen is a factor in the initiation of atherosclerosis, particularly hypoxia. An extensive review and resulting hypothesis of this phenomenon are presented by Hueper (1944), who suggested that hypoxic injury to the vascular wall occurs and increases the wall permeability. Robertson (1968) proposed a biochemical mechanism to describe hypoxia-induced atherosclerosis, in which it is assumed that hypoxia causes an increase in the permeability of the endothelial lining, after which cholesterol and lipids can diffuse into the intima and media. Hypoxia is also presumed to inhibit the ability of these cells to emulsify and disperse cytoplasmic lipids, and the lipid micelles are thus transformed into globular fat.

A question which immediately comes to mind concerns the possible cause of hypoxia at the vascular wall. For example hypoxia is mentioned by Bredt (1969) as being suspected to be the precipitating cause that leads to persistent edema. However, he comments subsequently that it is not clear why this particular part of the sclerotic plaque should be deprived of oxygen, seeing that it is adjacent to blood rich in oxygen.

Oxygen reaches the vascular wall by diffusing from the red blood cell. Diffusion of any species through a solution is described by Fick's law which, in the case of oxygen diffusing through blood plasma, relates the flux of oxygen to the diffusivity of oxygen through plasma and the concentration difference of oxygen across the diffusion distance, or:

$$NO_2 = DO_{2-P} \left(\frac{PO_{2,RBC} - PO_{2,wall}}{L} \right),$$

where NO_2 = flux of oxygen to vascular wall,

DO_{2-P} = diffusivity of oxygen through plasma,

$PO_{2,RBC}$ = oxygen tension adjacent to red blood cell,

$PO_{2,wall}$ = oxygen tension at vascular wall, and

L = distance from red blood cell to wall.

Thus, the transport of oxygen can be decreased if the blood oxygen tension or the diffusivity is decreased, or if the distance is increased.

The blood oxygen tension can be reduced easily by subjecting the human or animal to an atmosphere lower in oxygen. Several publications by Helin and Lorenzen have also demonstrated that arteriosclerosis can be induced by exposing rabbits to daily periods of systemic hypoxia (Garborsch et al., 1969). In a similar experiment, K. Kjeldsen et al. (1968) were able to prevent formation of severe arteriosclerosis in rabbits fed cholesterol by exposing them to an oxygen-rich atmosphere. Carbon monoxide from smoking will react preferentially with the hemoglobin in the red blood cell, and, in effect, also reduce the oxygen level in the blood. Thus, carbon monoxide will also result in a decreased flux of oxygen to the vascular wall, and it has also been shown that atherosclerosis can be caused by increased carbon monoxide levels (Kjeldsen, 1969; Astrup, 1974).

The average distance of diffusion will increase if the hematocrit is decreased. Perhaps this is why it is so easy to produce atherosclerosis in rabbits fed a cholesterol diet. The atherosclerosis induced in rabbits fed a cholesterol diet may well be associated with mural hypoxia since the hematocrit of these animals decreases from 45% to 30% after 8 weeks on a hypercholesterol diet (Westerman et al., 1970). The last variable in the flux equation that might change, causing a decrease in the oxygen flux, is the diffusivity of oxygen through plasma.

We have studied oxygen diffusion in blood plasma for several years, and our first studies involved the effect of plasma protein levels on the diffusivity. The diffusivity of oxygen was found to decrease by about 60% as plasma albumin levels were increased, and this occurred over what is usually considered to be the normal physiologic range for human adults (2 – 4.5 g/100 ml) (Navari et al., 1970). Similar results were obtained for other experiments in which the concentration of γ-globulin was varied. Increased protein levels are not, however, the only means of causing decreased diffusivity of oxygen through plasma, and it now appears that many substances probably have similar effects (Gainer and Chisolm, 1973). For example, serum glucose levels also cause oxygen diffusivity decreases of around 25% between serum glucose levels of 100 and 250 mg/100 ml.

Both of the preceding observations, i.e., a decrease in the oxygen diffusivity due to increased plasma protein or glucose levels can be related to the possible etiology of atherosclerosis. It is well-known that atherosclerosis and diabetes are often associated with one another. Arteriosclerosis is also usually associated with aging, and, although the total protein content of the plasma varied little during aging,the levels of the globulins increase (Rafsky et al., 1952). This increase could result in a significant decrease of oxygen diffusivity with age (Chisolm et al., 1971), and atherosclerosis due to hypoxia if globulins exert a particularly significant effect of the diffusivity as we have found in vitro.

It is obvious that if there is an increased oxygen concentration in the plasma, or an increase in the diffusivity of oxygen through plasma, then the oxygen flux from the red blood cell to the vascular wall would be increased. As mentioned previously, some experimenters have caused regression of atherosclerosis by using an oxygen-rich atmosphere. It would appear to be much easier, though, to increase the oxygen flux by increasing the diffusivity of oxygen through plasma. This can be done by using a drug which increases oxygen transport. We have found that of all substances, the compounds which cause the greatest increases in the diffusivity of oxygen are the carotenoids, particularly crocetin (Chisolm and Gainer, 1974; Gainer and Jones, 1975).

We have previously shown that crocetin results in less severe atherosclerosis in experimental animals (Chisolm and Gainer, 1974; Gainer and Jones, 1975). In addition, we have shown that crocetin also causes a reduction in serum cholesterol and triglycerides (Gainer and Jones, 1975; Pool et al., 1976). Thus, it appears that crocetin may also be able to overcome the effects of carbon monoxide.

THE EVIDENCE FOR NICOTINE AS AN ETIOLOGICAL FACTOR IN CARDIO-VASCULAR DISEASE (CVD)

H. Schievelbein

Epidemiological studies show that cigarette smoking is a risk factor in CVD (U.S. Dept. HEW, 1974; WHO, 1975). Cigarette smoke consists of a mixture of several hundred compounds and theoretically every one of them may have an influence on the development of CVD. However, one of the most pharmacologically active compounds in tobacco smoke is nicotine. It is known that nicotine possesses a pronounced cardiovascular action and because of this property the question arises whether the alkaloid may participate in the development of CVD.

To consider this question, two presuppositions seem to be necessary: (1) atherosclerosis is a result of disturbed fat metabolism, and (2) inhalation of tobacco smoke is a risk factor in the etiology of atherosclerosis. CVD is mainly caused by sclerosis of coronary arteries and peripheral blood vessels.

The manifestations of CVD may have a chronic or an acute origin, and nicotine may have a chronic and has an established acute effect.

To influence physiologic mechanisms, nicotine has to be present in the body of the smoker in a concentration great enough to produce a pharmacologic action. This is the case and can be demonstrated by calculating the intake of nicotine statistically (Timm, 1974) and by measuring the nicotine concentration in the blood of smokers (Table 1).

Table 1. Blood levels of nicotine in cigarette smokers

Authors	Nicotine content (ng/ml)	Remarks	Methods
Schievelbein and Grundke (1968)	25	Whole venous blood mean of 6 smokers	Gas-liquid chromatography
Isaac and Rand (1972)	25	Plasma of venous blood, mean of 5 smokers	Gas-liquid chromatography
Langone et al. (1973)	up to 73	Maximal value in sera of about 240 smokers	Radio-immunoassay
Armitage et al. (1974)	30 - 40	Arterial whole blood, 4 smokers	Measurement of ^{14}C-labeled nicotine

Chronic Action of Nicotine

In Figure 1, the possible chronic cardiovascular actions of nicotine are demonstrated. The broken lines in the scheme indicate possible direct actions of nicotine without the mediation of catecholamines. There are no investigations in humans with respect to the chronic action of nicotine, and we will have to rely on animal experiments for resolution of this problem.

Acceleration of the development of atherosclerosis by nicotine may be a consequence of the effect of nicotine on fat metabolism. The release of catecholamines

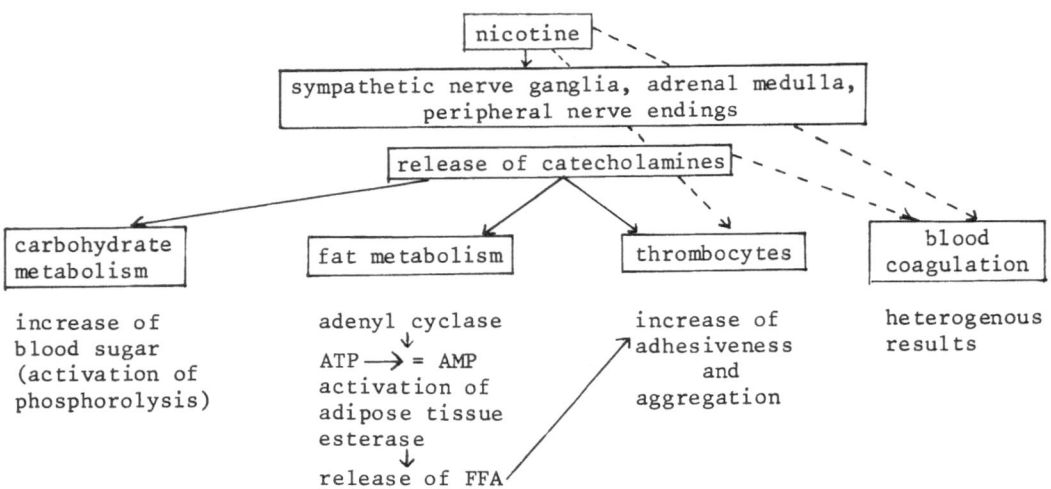

Figure 1. Possible chronic cardiovascular action of nicotine

by nicotine leads to an activation of adenyl cyclase and by this action to the formation of CAMP with the consequent release of free fatty acids by way of the activation of adipose tissue esterase. This action, together with an influence on the aggregation of blood platelets, may play a role in the development of CVD. To evaluate these possibilities, we performed a long-term experiment using rabbits (Schievelbein et al., 1970).

Up to the performance of this experiment, several authors tried to show the influence of nicotine on atherosclerosis in animals given an atherogenic diet. They found enhanced atherosclerosis under the influence of both atherogenic diet and nicotine (Wenzel and Beckloff, 1958). One of the purposes of our experiment was to recognize whether an experimental animal, liable to a high degree to develop a spontaneous atherosclerosis, can be induced to accelerate the development of atherosclerosis by administration of nicotine without atherogenic diet.

At the end of the experiment (20 months), all animals had severe atherosclerotic lesions in the aorta and in the coronary arteries, but there was no difference between the control and the experimental group. All hematologic and clinical-chemical variables showed no pathologic results.

In reviewing the results of these animal experiments, we can say that evidence has not been presented that nicotine alone is a causative factor in atherosclerosis.

Acute Action of Nicotine

As already mentioned, nicotine acts by release of catecholamines. The outstanding effects of these hormones are an augmentation of the contractile force of the myocardium, an increase of heart frequency, and an elevation of blood pressure. In Figure 2, the acute cardiovascular actions of nicotine are registered in detail. These effects can be demonstrated by application of nicotine experimentally.

The acute effects of nicotine can be demonstrated in patients with angina pectoris, who showed a decrease in the mean duration of exercise time before the onset of pain after smoking cigarettes with different nicotine contents (Aronow, 1973; Aronow et al., 1974).

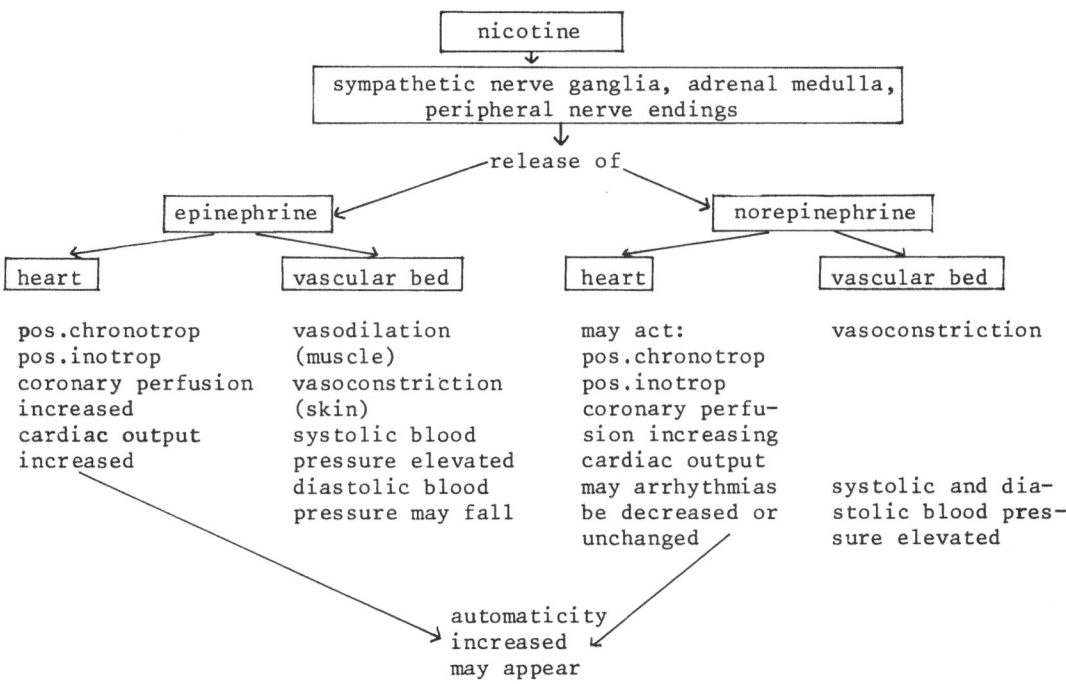

Figure 2. Acute cardiovascular actions of nicotine

Under normal conditions, coronary flow is greatly enhanced during O_2-consumption. In the case of sclerotic coronary arteries, coronary blood flow cannot be elevated. In this situation, the coronary insufficiency during intake of nicotine may occur and the onset of angina pectoris seems possible.

In a recent review of the Framingham study, Kannel stated that smoking has no association with angina. Therefore, it seems to him that smoking has a triggering effect in lethal coronary attacks.

Another effect of nicotine, which may contribute to acute actions of nicotine in CVD, is enhancing platelet aggregation. This we showed several years ago (Werle and Schievelbein, 1965), and it has been recently confirmed in a controlled double blind study, in which smoking one single cigarette increased the platelet response to a standard aggregating stimulus, namely ADP.

In summarizing the presented evidence, we conclude that at the utmost nicotine may act as an additional factor for the etiology of clinic and acute CVD. However, more evidence is needed, especially with respect to the action of nicotine in humans.

ABSTRACTS

DIABETIC ANGIOPATHIES. A REVIEW WITH NEW VIEWS

O.J. Pollak
Dover, Delaware/USA

The prevalent concept that diabetes mellitus predisposes to atherosclerosis, myocardial infarction, and thrombosis has to be revised. In spite of the usual dyslipemia in the diabetic patient the incidence of myocardial infarction is not significantly higher in patients with diabetes than in patients without it. The age at death is not higher for men and women who die of myocardial infarction and who had diabetes than for men and women without diabetes. The two conditions often coincide. However, non-atherosclerotic arterial disease is common in diabetics: (1) There are the capillary diseases, glomerulosclerosis, retinopathy, iridopathy, neuropathy, probably also papillary necrosis; (2) diabetic microangiopathy may be generalized or confined to one organ or tissue, as an early or late occurance in the life history of diabetes; (3) diabetic macroangiopathy is characterized by calcification. These calcifications are longitudinal, involving long segments, in contrast to the short-segmental stenoses caused by secondary calcium deposits in atheromata. The two types may coincide, as atherosclerosis and diabetes mellitus coincide. The calcinosis is caused by chronic or episodic acidosis. This has been proven experimentally. The two types of arterial calcification differ etiologically, biochemically, morphologically, radiologically, and clinically.

LARGE VESSEL DISEASE IN DIABETICS — ATHEROSCLEROSIS OR SPECIFIC DIABETIC ANGIOPATHY?

Knud Lundbak, Niels Juel Christensen, Thomas Ledet, and Bent Neubauer
Department of Medicine, Kommunehospitalet, Aarhus/Denmark

The following points will be discussed, suggesting that large vessel disease in diabetes is at least partly a specific angiopathy.
1. A study of 211 subjects demonstrated statistical correlations between glucose tolerance and linear calcification of leg arteries (quantitative) - not with spotty calcifications.
2. Linear calcifications in leg arteries of long-term diabetics result in reduced peak blood flow (Xenon 133. Tilted/untilted position).
3. Quantitative studies of small and large vessels in hearts from old and young long-term diabetics and controls revealed differences suggesting a specific element (diabetic cardiopathy).
4. In vitro studies of rabbit aortic medial cell cultures show cellular proliferation when the cultures are grown in media containing diabetic serum (rabbit or human serum).
5. A study of the noradrenalin content of the heart and large vessels demonstrate profound reduction in long term diabetics.
These findings, together with other evidence, especially epidemiological, point to the existence of a specific diabetic macroangiopathy.

INFLUENCE OF MEAL FREQUENCY ON HORMONE AND LIPID LEVELS IN NORMAL PERSONS AND INSULIN DEPENDENT DIABETICS

J. Terpstra, L.W. Hessel*, J. Seepers, and C.M. van Gent*
University Medical Center, *Gaubius Institute, Health Research Organization TNO, Leiden/The Netherlands

In an attempt to lower diurnal triglyceride levels by increasing meal frequency, groups of 4 persons (normal or diabetics) were studied under carefully controlled steady state conditions on a 65% carbohydrate diet. Glucose, insulin, cortisol, growth hormone, FFA, TG, cholesterol were measured after small intervals throughout 24 hours. On 3 meals per day (at 9.00, 13.00 and 17.00 hr) "fasting" TG levels increased by about 50 mg/dl between 4.00 and 9.00 hr, continued to rise till 15.00 hr and then gradually decreased in spite of the 17.00 hr meal. Insulin secretion was always largest after the 9.00 hr meal. Isocaloric change to 8 equal, equidistant meals resulted in highest TG levels at night and falling levels during the morning in spite of food intake. Integrated diurnal TG levels were not lower than on 3 meals.
Results in diabetics were similar but more variable.

THERMOGRAPHY OF THE FACE: AN EASY WAY FOR THE EARLY DIAGNOSE OF ARTERIO-CEREBRAL ARTERIOSCLEROSIS

J. Marriq
Hopital P. Desbief, Marseille/France

Anatomical and physiological basis: As the face is irrigated by branches of ophthalmic artery, itself branch of the internal carotid, when there is a stenosis or even hemodynamic troubles in the carotidian system, there is also troubles of the facial temperature; so, the picture of the face taken by a camera able to catch infra-red rays shows (by different colours) cold points in such or such places, according to the vasculo-cerebral lesion.
Clinical use: We have more than 350 cases of different facial thermographies and we will give, with examples, description of: normal picture, arterial stenosis, diffuse sclerosis and hemodynamic troubles. We have often completet thermography by arteriography, E.E.G. and other methods; so, we can compare the informations given by each of them.
Thermography is, for us, an easy and practical method to diagnose early vasculo-cerebral sclerosis and to overlook its evolution.

A QUALITATIVE OBSERVATION OF SERUM LIPOPROTEIN IN CEREBROVASCULAR DISORDERS

Shigeru Takamatsu, Kazuho Henmi, Seitoku Mizuno Mutsu Takamatsu, and Hideho Sugawara
Department of Pathologic Physiology, Institute of Cerebrovascular Disease, Hirosaki University School of Medicine, Hirosaki/Japan

The mid-band detected in disc electrophoresis of serum lipoportein is recently regarded as an indicator of abnormal lipid metabolism in atherosclerotic disorders. Because of close relation between cerebral infarction and atherosclerotic disorders it would be of interest to observe qualitatively the mid-bands in sera of cerebrovascular patients. In the normolipidemic subjects the mid-bands were detected in 66 of 98 patients and in 43 of 114 controls by Narayan's method, and found more frequently in patients with cerebral infarction, with abnormal ECG findings, and with impaired renal function than in patients with cerebral hemorrhage, with normal ECG findings, and with normal renal function. Although only a little attention has been attracted to serum lipid levels in cerebrovascular disorders up to this time, the results obtained show importance of further qualitative studies on serum lipoprotein in cerebrovascular patients with normal serum lipid levels.

AN EPIDEMIOLOGICAL STUDY ON CEREBRO-CARDIO VASCULAR ATTACK IN MASS SCREENING

Chikao Arai, Masatake Abe, Takeshi Kawasaki, Yoshinori Aizawa, Yoshihiro Kashiwakura, Yoshimasa Yabe, Motoharu Hasegawa, and Shozo Yoshimura
The first Department of Intern. Medicine, Jikei University School of Medicine, Tokyo/Japan
Tsutomu Komazawa and Chikio Hayashi
The Institute of Statistical Mathematics
Shinichi Yagi and Kiyoshi Nakayama
Faculty of Science & Technology, Sophia University, Tokyo/Japan
Shigehiro Kinoshita and Kenju Suzuki
Institute of Arteriosclerosis Association of Labour's Welfare and Health, Tokyo/Japan

Mass screening of arteriosclerosis was carried out in 420,000 subjects during the past eight years by means of urinaysis, serum cholesterol, blood pressure, ECG, eye ground and aortic pulse wave velocity (PWV). In 70,180 subjects, existance of attack was followed up by mail and 585 subjects in all who had an attack: angina pectoris (AG) 164, myocardial infarction (MI) 140, cerebral infarction (CI) 178, cerebral bleeding (CB) 69, subarachnoidal bleeding (SB) 34. The results obtained were as follow.
1. Percentage who were over Sheie II in eye ground was 29% in CB, 13% in CI. Who had ST-Tschange was 22% in AP, 22% in MI. Who were over 160 mm Hg in maximum pressure was 58% in CB, 48% in CI. Who were over 240 mg/dl in cholesterol was 12% in AP, 21% in MI. Who were over 9 m/sec in PWV was 26% in AP, 29% in MI, 39% in CB, 39% in CI.
2. According to the multidimensional analysis, AP was connected with cholesterol. MI was connected with ST-Tchange and PWV. CI was closely connected with blood pressure. CB was connected with blood pressure.

EFFECT OF CIGARETTE SMOKING ON UPTAKE OF 3-OLEIC AND ^{14}C-LINOLEIC ACID BY HUMAN ARTERIES IN VITRO

A.K. Horsch, A. Koch, C.C. Heuck, and H. Mörl
Medizinische Universitätsklinik, Heidelberg/BRD

The effect of cigarette smoke on arterial wall metabolism was studied in vitro using human serum of several donors before and after smoking (5 cigarettes in 1 hour) as incubation medium for human umbilical and femoral arteries (fibrous plaques). The incorporation of ^{3}H-oleic and ^{14}C-linoleic acid into the arteries was determined simultaneously. After 4 hours of incubation the lipids were extracted, separated on TLC and GLC and the respective radioactivity determined. The uptake of both labels per mg of tissue protein was increased in the "after smoking" incubation system for all arteries. While the distribution of the endogenous fatty acids in the serum was not influenced by smoking, the fatty acid fraction of the arteries incubated in the "after smoking" serum showed an increased breakdown of the labels, a higher proportion of radioactivity being recovered in the medium chain fatty acids. These findings suggest an effect of the substances of cigarette smoke present in or released into the serum after inhalation, on arterial wall fatty acid uptake and turnover.

SMOKING AND ATHEROSCLEROSIS

Hugo Kesteloot and Omer Van Houte
Department of Pathopysiology, Section Cardiology, St. Raphael University Clinic,
Leuven/Belgium

The differences between never smokers, cigarette smokers and ex-smokers have been
studied in a large male population group consisting of 42,804 subjects between 15
and 60 years old. Discriminant analysis has demonstrated that age, height and
weight, systolic and diastolic blood pressure, cholesterol, the presence of an
arcus senilis, the presence of a pathological Q wave in the electrocardiogram,
social class and a history of possible myocardial infarction (WHO criteria) are
significant independent discriminators between the smoking classes.
Contrary to electrocardiographic and anamnestic evidence of myocardial infarction,
a history of angina pectoris is not distributet differently to a significant
degree between non-smokers and cigarette smokers. Lung function tests (LFT) give
significantly lower values in cigarette smokers compared to other smoking classes.
The difference in LFT increases both with the duration of smoking and the amount
of cigarettes smoked. In heavy smokers 1 sec forced expiratory volume is 230 ml
lower than in never-smokers ($p < 0.001$).

II
Lipoproteins

STRUCTURE OF THE PLASMA LIPOPROTEINS - A REVIEW

Antonio M. Gotto and Richard L. Jackson

Introduction

The plasma lipoproteins are complexes of lipid and protein which appear as
spherical particles when viewed in the electron microscope with negative staining
(Forte and Nichols, 1972). There are four major classes of the plasma lipoproteins
(Table 1). They are the chylomicrons, the very low-density lipoproteins (VLDL),
the low-density lipoproteins (LDL), and the high-density lipoproteins (HDL). The
lipid composition of each of these families decreases from the chylomicrons to
the HDL and there is a concomitant decrease in the rate of flotation of each lipoprotein class (Table 1). The chylomicrons have an S_f or flotation rate greater
than 400, VLDL 20-400, and LDL between 0-20. The HDL do not float at density
1.063. In a recent review, Eisenberg and Levy (1975) have also pointed to the importance of an intermediate density lipoprotein (IDL) which is isolated between
the densities of 1.006 and 1.019 and which have an S_f of 12-20. Each lipoprotein
class is heterogeneous with respect to their protein and lipid compositions. At
present, there is no universally accepted nomenclature of the lipoprotein proteins

Table 1. Composition and properties of human plasma lipoproteins

Properties	Chylomicrons	VLDL	LDL	HDL
Density, g/ml	<0.95	0.95-1.006	1.006-1.063[a]	1.063-1.210
Molecular weight	>0.4 x 10^9	5-10 x 10^6	2.7-4.8 x 10^6	1.8-3.6 x 10^5
Major apoproteins	ApoB ApoC-I ApoC-II ApoC-III	ApoB ApoC-I ApoC-II ApoC-III ApoE	ApoB	ApoA-I ApoA-II
Minor apoproteins	ApoA-I ApoA-II	ApoA-I ApoA-II ApoD		ApoC-I ApoC-II ApoC-III ApoD ApoE
Major lipids	Triglyceride	Triglyceride	Cholesteryl esters Phospholipids	Phospholipids Cholesteryl esters
Minor lipids	Phospholipids	Phospholipids Cholesteryl esters	Free cholesterol Triglyceride	Free cholesterol

[a]This density range also contains an intermediate density lipoprotein (IDL) which
Eisenberg and Levy (1975) have referred to as a unique lipoprotein separate from
VLDL and LDL.

or apoproteins. In the present review, we have used the A, B, and C system of Alaupovic (1971). In this system, apoA refers to the apoproteins that are primarily, but not exclusively, found in HDL. ApoB is the major apoprotein of LDL, but also comprises about 35% of the protein of VLDL. ApoC represents a group of small proteins originally described in VLDL but which are also present in HDL. In addition, there is the "arginine-rich" protein and the "thin-line" protein. For a more complete review of the structure and properties of these proteins, the reader is referred to several recent reviews (Jackson et al., 1976; Scanu et al., 1975; Morrisett et al., 1975a). These apoproteins function not only in the transport of lipid but also serve as activators of various enzymes that are involved in the catabolism of the plasma lipoproteins. For example, apoA-I and apoC-I are activators of lecithin-cholesterol acyltransferase (Soutar et al., 1975; Fielding et al., 1972) while apoC-II activates lipoprotein lipase from adipose tissue (LaRosa et al., 1970). The overall structure of each lipoprotein is determined by lipid-lipid, protein-protein and by protein-lipid interaction. In the present review, we discuss the various models which have been proposed to account for the organization of the lipids and proteins in the plasma lipoproteins. In addition, evidence related to the mechanism of apoprotein-lipid interaction will be presented.

VLDL Structure

Our knowledge of VLDL structure and of specific lipid-protein interactions in the native lipoprotein is limited. Comparative lipid-binding studies indicate that apoC-III interacts more strongly with the polar lipids, especially with phosphatidylcholine and sphingomyelin than with neutral lipids such as triolein or cholesteryl oleate (Morrisett et al., 1975b). It is assumed that the protein and polar head groups of the phospholipids of the plasma VLDL are oriented toward the aqueous exterior of the particle. The waterinsoluble cholesteryl esters and triglycerides would be protected within an inner hydrophobic environment. Based on these assumptions, Morrisett et al. (1977) have proposed a model for VLDL as shown in Figure 1. In this model the protein and phospholipid, about 10% and 20% by weight, respectively, are localized together near the outer surface of the particle while the more abundant triglyceride constituents (about 50% by weight) are located inside the particle. The particle arrangement shown in Figure 1 permits access of lipoprotein lipase to the apoC-II activator protein and the access of LCAT to apoC-I for catabolism of the particle. The model also predicts that the rate of catabolism of the lipoprotein is influenced by the lipid structure. Information relevant to this prediction has come from studies with ^{13}C nuclear magnetic resonance (NMR) spectroscopy (Hamilton et al., 1974) and with electron spin resonance (ESR) spectroscopy (Morrisett et al., 1976). The principale behind these approaches is based on the fact that interactions between apoproteins and lipids and between lipids and lipids results in a restriction of the segmental and rotational mobility of the lipid constituents. The NMR studies (Hamilton et al., 1974) indicate that the lipid constituents of the VLDL are in liquid-like states and are quite mobile. However, as compared to lipids in organic solvents, the rotational segmental mobility of the lipids in VLDL is reduced. The NMR studies of VLDL indicate that the fatty acyl chains have a high degree of segmental and rotational motion. The segmental motion in VLDL is greater than that observed in LDL or HDL, but is less than that of pure cholesteryl oleate or in triolein. Morrisett et al. (1976) have attempted to relate the structural properties of VLDL to their physiologic and metabolic characteristics. These investigators have found that the fatty acyl chains in VLDL from individuals on a high polyunsaturated fat diet are significantly more mobile and less ordered than are those in the VLDL from subjects on a high saturated fat diet. Furthermore, in vitro experiments suggest that the mobility of microscopic fluidity of the lipids affects the rate of catabolism of the VLDL. Lipoprotein lipase was shown to hydrolyze the more fluid, unsaturated triglycerides at a faster rate than the more solid saturated analogues. Accordingly, the action of lipoprotein lipase on a heterogeneous lipid mixture such as VLDL would be expected to result in the release of more unsaturated fatty acid and in the production of a remnant particle

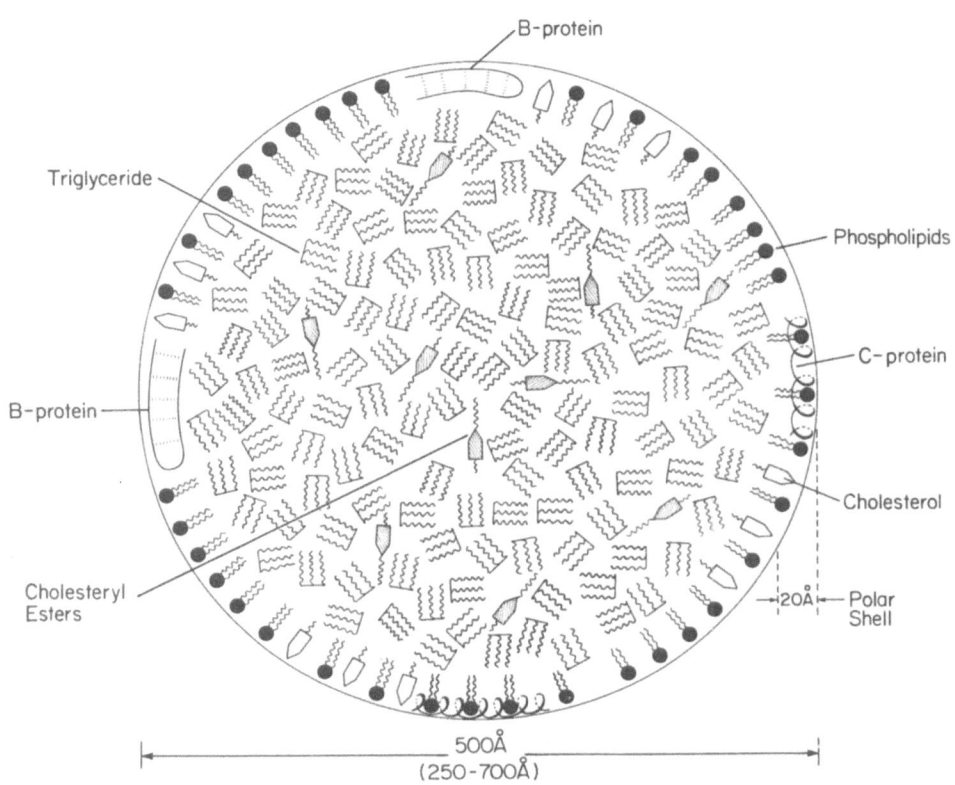

Figure 1. Schematic representation of a very low-density lipoprotein particle
as described by Morrisett et al. (1977). In this model, the polar head groups of
phospholipids, the hydroxyl group of cholesterol, and the protein are on the outside of the particle while the cholesteryl esters and triglycerides are on the
inside. In this model, the cholesteryl esters are placed randomly throughout the
particle

whose lipids are less mobile and less fluid than are those of the original intact
particle.

LDL Structure

The major apoprotein of LDL (apoB) has not been well-characterized because of its
poor solubilty in nondissociating systems. Most of our knowledge concerning lipid
protein interactions has been obtained by direct study of the native particle.
Based on x-ray scattering methods, Laggner et al. (1976) and Stuhrmann et al.
(1975) have assigned the protein of LDL to a polar shell near the periphery of
the particle. Aggerbeck et al. (1976) have assigned a surface location for selected phospholipids of LDL. These results were based on the accessibility of LDL
phospholipids to phospholipase A2. This enzyme hydrolyzes all the phosphatidylcholine, phosphatidylethanolamine and phosphatidylserine in LDL, producing a
particle which remains water-soluble. Phospholipase C cleaves all of the phos-
phoryl moieties from the phospholipids of LDL and results in a completely water-
soluble, diglyceride-enriched particle. These observations suggests that the hy-
drating effect of the phospholipids of LDL is not essential for the solubility of
the native lipoprotein. Approximately 60% of the phospholipids in LDL are rapidly
cleaved while the remaining 30% are cleaved more slowly. Such studies suggest
that about two-thirds of the phospholipid polar head groups of LDL are located
near the outside of the particle while the other 30% have a deeper location with-

179

in the lipoprotein or interact with other lipids or proteins to make them less accessible to cleavage.

Current evidence suggests that the cholesteryl esters which make up the major fraction of LDL lipids are structurally autonomous, occupying separate domains and not intimately associated with either the protein or the phospholipids. Deckelbaum et al. (1975) have shown that LDL undergoes a reversible thermal transition between 4° and 37°. This property is due to the cholesteryl esters. On heating from 4° to 37°, LDL gives an x-ray defraction pattern whose thermal behavior is indistinguishable from that of the cholesteryl esters isolated from LDL. Laggner et al. (1976) have suggested that the cholesteryl esters are organized as two separate concentric shells. One shell occupies the central core while the other occupies a space midway between the central core and the outer polar shell of protein and phospholipid (Fig. 2A). Based on interpretations of low angle x-ray scattering methods, Luzzati's group (Stuhrmann et al., 1975) has proposed that the apoprotein subunits of LDL occur on the surface as regularly spaced protrusions. While earlier studies had assigned protein to both surface and core positions in LDL, this interpretation does not seem consistent with the low angle x-ray scattering results. A model (Fig. 2B) based on NMR studies by Finer et al. (1975) places the lipid in LDL a trilayer structure with phospholipid in the outer and inner layers, with the cholesteryl esters sandwiched between the layers. The apoprotein is depicted as projecting outward from the surface.

HDL Structure

Before considering HDL structure, it is appropriate to discuss the determinants of apoprotein-lipid interactions. One key fact to recognize is that very little of the neutral lipids are bound by the apoprotein in the absence of phospholipid. This property has lead to the concept that the primary interaction between the apoprotein and lipid components occurs between the phospholipid and the apoprotein. Morrisett et al. (1977) have reviewed the important variables for the binding of apoprotein and phospholipid. These variables include the physical form of the phospholipid, lipid concentration, nature of the polar head group, length of the fatty acyl chain in each lipid, and temperature of the gel → liquid crystalline transition temperature. The phospholipid must be at or above the transition temperature for the melting of the fatty acyl chains in order for optimal binding of lipid to apoprotein to occur. As shown in Figure 3, there is a dramatic in-

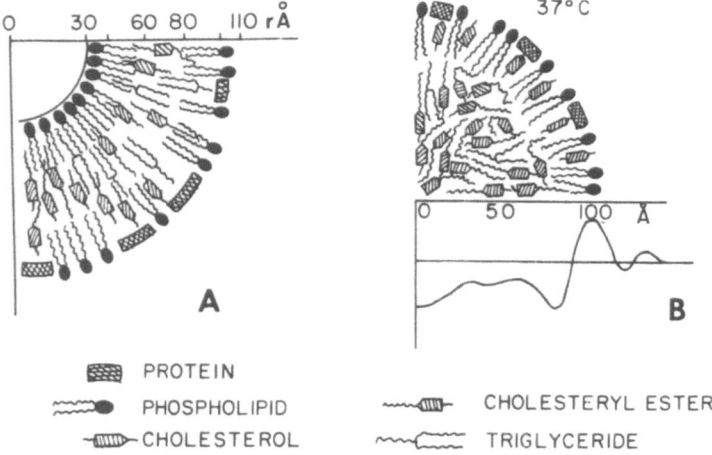

Figure 2. Schematic representation of LDL structure as described by: A. Laggner et al. (1976) and Finer et al. (1975)

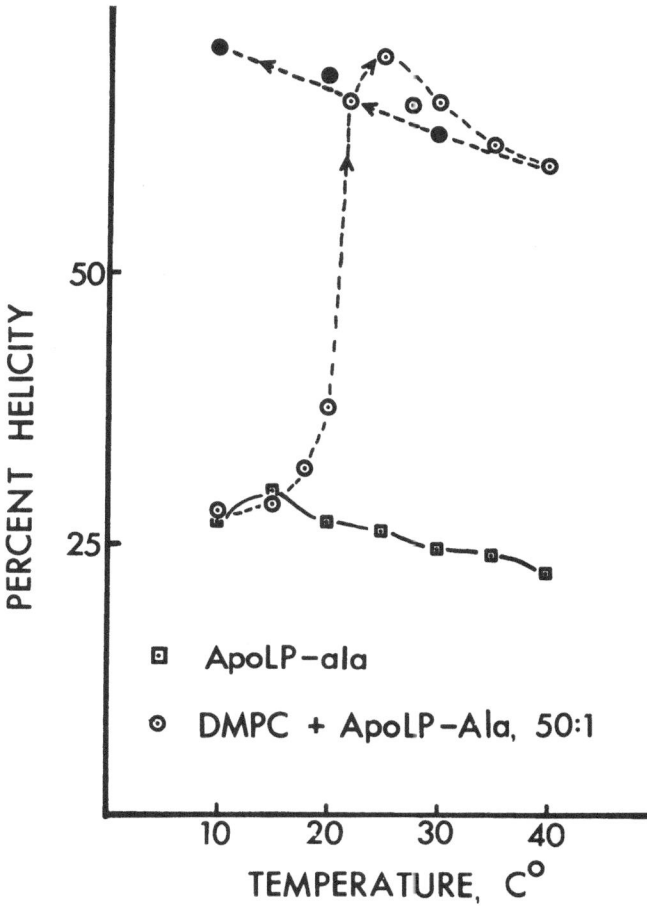

Figure 3. Temperature dependence of the α-helicity of apoC-III (apoAla) in the absence and presence of dimyristoyl phosphatidylcholine vesicles (Morrisett et al., 1975b)

crease in the content of α-helix conformation of apoC-III which coincides with the melting temperature of dimyristoyl phosphatidylcholine. Once the apoprotein-phospholipid complex is formed, it is not dissociated by cooling the complex below the transition temperature. The fact that all of the apoproteins show increases in α-helical conformation with phospholipid binding has led Segrest et al. (1974), Jackson et al. (1974a, 1975), and Assmann and Brewer (1974) to suggest that the α-helical conformation is itself involved in the lipid-protein interaction.

The amino acid sequences of four plasma lipoproteins, apoC-I (Jackson et al., 1974b; Shulman et al., 1975); apoC-III (Brewer et al., 1974); apoA-I (Baker et al., 1974); and apoA-II (Brewer et al., 1972) have been elucidated. In terms of their overall amino acid composition, the plasma apolipoproteins are not greatly different from other soluble proteins in their relative proportions of hydrophobic and hydrophilic amino acids. Inspection of the amino acid sequences per se does not immediately lead to an understanding of the mechanism whereby they interact with lipids. One structural feature that is apparent in the examination of the amino acid sequences is the frequency of ion pairs of oppositely charged amino acids which occur in a one:two or one:four sequence relationship in the apoproteins, i.e., Lys-Glu or Lys-Val-Ser-Glu. Examination of the sequence of apoA-I, the major protein of HDL and the largest to be sequenced to date, shows that there are 14 one:two and 22 one:four ion pairs (Table 2). An interesting feature of these ion pairs is that they tend to be located within helical segments of the protein. Such helical regions have been referred to as amphipathic helices as illustrated for apoC-I in Figure 4. Segrest et al (1974) and Jackson et al. (1975) have suggested that these amphipathic helical regions may represent the phospholipid bindung sites of the proteins. The structural features which must be present are oppositely charged ion pairs in one:two or one:four sequence relationship located within a helical region of the protein. There is a single methionine in apoC-I located at residue 38. Cyanogen bromide cleavage of the apo-protein produces a carboxyl-terminal fragment which does not bind phospholipid

Table 2. Abundance of zwitterionic pairs resulting from the 1:2 or 1:4 sequence relationship of oppositely carged amino acid side chains in the four human apo-lipoproteins sequenced to date, and four typical globular proteins which do not bind lipid[a]

Apoprotein	1:2 pairs	1:4 pairs	1:2 + 1:4 pairs[b]	Amino acid residues	Amino acid residues per 1:2 + 1:4 pairs
A-I	14	22	36	245	6.8
A-II	5	5	10	77	7.7
C-I	6	7	13	57	4.7
C-III	5	1	6	79	13.2
Subtilisin Carlsberg	1	0	1	274	274.0
Porcine elastase	3	1	4	240	60.0
Bovine chymotrypsinogen	4	1	5	245	49.0
Papaya papain	4	2	6	200	33.3

[a]Taken from Morrisett et al. (1977). [b]Not necessarily nonoverlapping.

and an amino-terminal fragment which does (Jackson et al., 1974a). Inspection of the helical regions of apoC-I shows that the NH_2-terminal segment contains two amphipathic segments while the COOH-terminal contains one. The reason for the designation amphipathic helix is that these regions have both a polar and a non-polar face. In other helical proteins which are not plasma apolipoproteins, the apolar face is more of an edge than a face. Each face of the amphipathic helix occupies fully 180° of a cylindrical helix. In addition to the polar face, there is a unique distribution of the charged amino acids. These zwitterionic pairs referred to above occupy a one:two or one:four sequence relationship. The topo-graphic distribution is such that there is an alternating occurrence of the basic and acidic amino acids. The acidic glutamic and aspartic residues are oriented to the center of the polar face, while the positively charged lysines and argi-nines are oriented toward the periphery or to the interface region between the nonpolar and polar faces. Based on this model, tryptophan at residue 41 would be located in a strongly acidic environment between two glutamic acid residues (Fig. 3). This prediction is consistent with fluorescence quenching experiments (Jackson et al., 1974a). Sigler et al. (1976) and Harding et al. (1976) have achieved the total synthesis of apoC-I using solid phase peptide synthesis meth-odologies. In addition to binding phospholipid, the synthetic protein activates LCAT; the activities of the synthetic and naturally occurring proteins were in-distinguishable. The relationship between the ability to activate LCAT and to bind phospholipid is currently under investigation.

While apoC-I represents a good example of amphipathic helices, similar regions have been found in all of the apoproteins for which the sequences are known. We postulate that the amphipathic helices represent the phospholipid binding sites of the apoproteins. Other evidence which supports the amphipathic helical theory has been obtained from the synthesis of specific fragments of apoC-III. The sequence of apoC-III is shown in Figure 5. It is predicted from model building experiments that the carboxyl-terminal regions of this protein should be rich in amphipathic helix while the amino-terminal region is not. This prediction is consistent with the experimental observation that the 40 residue amino-terminal fragment does not interact with the phospholipid while the carboxyl-terminal one does (Sparrow et al., 1973). Synthetic fragments corresponding to residues 61 – 79, 55 – 79, 48 – 79, and 41 – 79 have been prepared. Whereas the two shorter fragments do not bind phospholipid, the two longer ones interact with phospholipids forming isolatable complexes. If the amphipathic helical features of the plasma apopro-

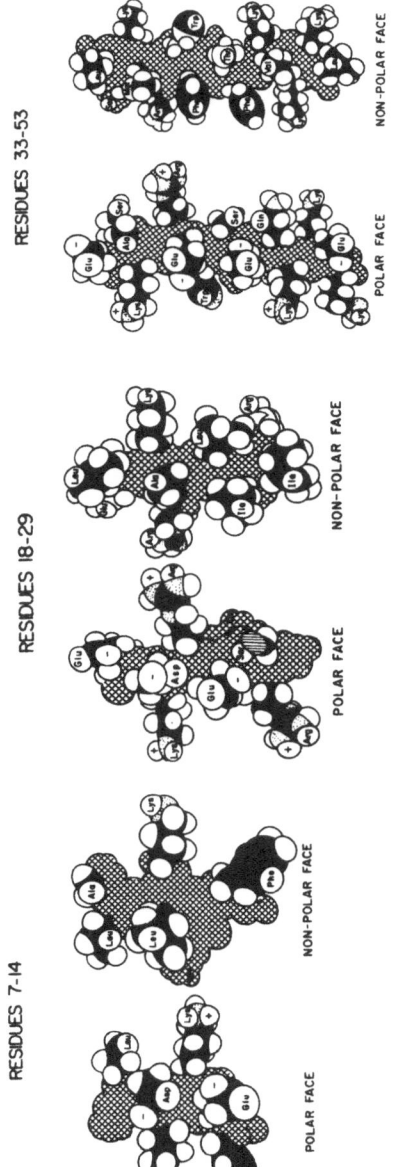

Figure 4. Space-filling models of amphipathic helical regions of apoC-I. Each region is shown with its axis oriented parallel to the plane and its NH$_2$-terminal end toward the top of page. Two views of each helix, rotated around the helix by 180°, are shown. Details of this model are found in the text and in Jackson et al. (1974a). NB: non-polar → nonpolar

proteins specify phospholipid binding, then it should be possible to synthesize peptides which exhibit the same amphipathic property. We have recently undertaken the synthesis of such peptides in order to test the amphipathic hypothesis and to assess the contribution of the hydrophobicity of the apoprotein to the phospholipid-binding phenomenon. Sparrow et al. (1975) have prepared a series of synthetic peptides which bear no relationship to any known sequence of the naturally occurring proteins other than the fact that they should contain an amphipathic helix. The sequences of three such peptides is shown in Figure 6. Synthetic peptide I, with 20 amino acid residues, has a predicted hydrophobicity index of 829. Peptide III is identical to peptide II except for the substitution of a tyrosine and tryptophan at residues 7 and 8 in place of the two alanines. This two amino acid substitution has increased the hydrophobicity index of peptide III to 1031. According to model binding studies, peptides I and II should contain the amphipathic helix but they do not bind phospholipid. Peptide III which contains the amphipathic helix but which has a hydrophobicity index of over 1000 actively binds phospholipid (Sparrow et al., 1975). It is interesting to compare the hydrophobicity of the synthetic peptides with that of the various regions of apoC-III. Residues 1 to 40 of this naturally occuring apoprotein have a predicted hydrophobicity index of 603. This part of the molecule did not contain the amphipathic helix and did not interact with lipid. The overall hydrophobicity index of apoC-III is 652. That part of apoC-III that did bind phospholipid, residues 41-79, had a hydrophobicity index of 904. For one particular region, 41-67, which was predicted to contain the amphipathic helix, the index was

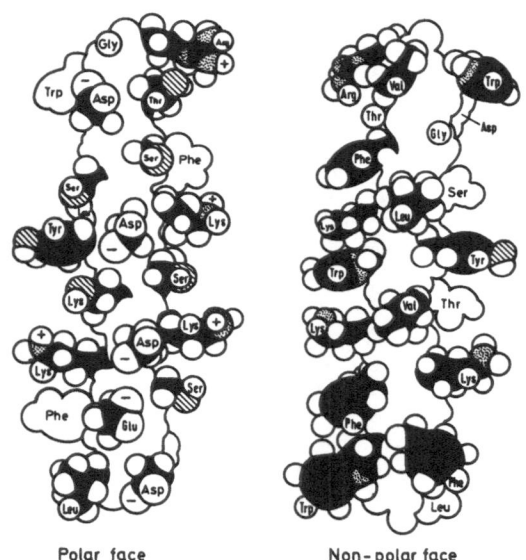

Polar face   Non-polar face

Apo lipoprotein C - III

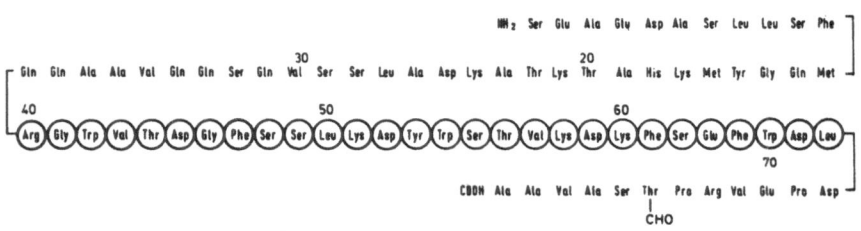

Figure 5. Amphipathic helical regions of apoC-III as described by Segrest et al. (1974)
NB: non-polar → nonpolar

184

Ala-Ser-Leu-Lys-Asp-Ser-Leu-Ser-Asp-Lys-Trp-Lys-Asp-Ser-Leu-Ser-Asp-Lys-Leu-Ser

I

Val-Ser-Ser-Leu-Lys-Asp-Ala-Ala-Ser-Ser-Leu-Lys-Asp-Ser-Phe-Ser

II

Val-Ser-Ser-Leu-Lys-Asp-Tyr-Trp-Ser-Ser-Leu-Lys-Asp-Ser-Phe-Ser

III

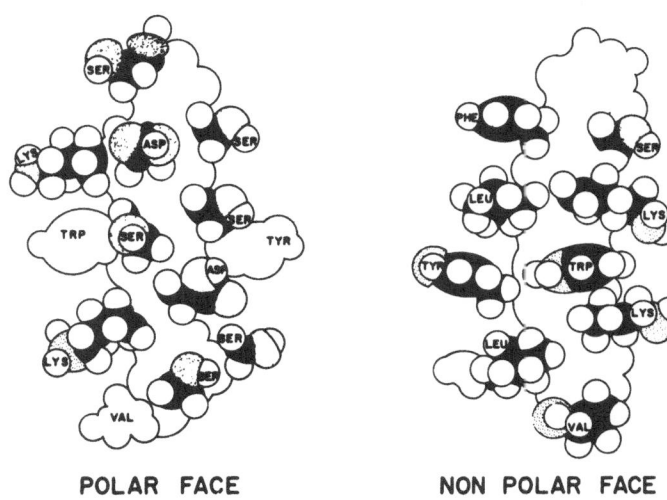

POLAR FACE   NON POLAR FACE

Figure 6. Amino acid sequence and space-filling models of synthetic model peptides
NB: non-polar → nonpolar

1039 which is very close to that of peptide III. Stoffel et al. (1974) have presented evidence from nuclear magnetic resonance spectroscopy which supports the importance of hydrophobic interactions between the protein and the phospholipid as a structural determinant of the plasma lipoproteins.

The current model for HDL structure is based primarily on low angel x-ray scattering studies and NMR. The protein and polar head groups have been assigned to an electron dense region of 12-15 Å or thickness on the surface of HDL. This region is thick enough to accommodate both the polar head groups of phospholipid and is also the approximate dimension of the thickness of an α-helix. Jackson et al. (1975) have proposed (Fig. 7) an HDL model in which the fatty acyl groups of the phospholipids are perpendicular to the axis of the helix of the protein. Packing of the chains would seem to be facilitated by the perpendicular arrangement. The cholesteryl esters are shown intercalated between the fatty acyl groups of the phospholipid and with their own fatty acids oriented toward the center of the particle. In this model, the protein is on the surface of HDL and interacts with the phospholipid by way of the amphipathic helices within the protein.

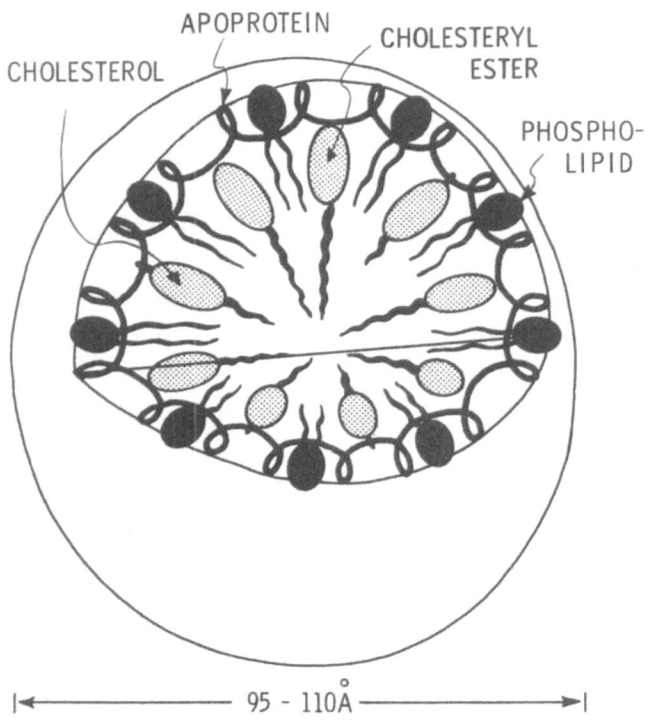

Figure 7. Schematic representation of HDL structure as described by Jackson et al. (1975)

Relationship of Lipoprotein Structure to Other Protein Structures

The concept of an amphipathic helix is not new, nor is it limited to the plasma apolipoproteins. For example, myoglobin contains eight interconnected sections of amphipathic α–helix. However, the difference between these helices and those of the apoproteins is that the hydrophobic face occupies only about 30%, rather than 50%, of their cylindrical surface. Therefore, they contain an apolar edge rather than an apolar side. In myoglobin, the stability and spatial interrelationship of the helices are controlled to a large extent by the heme moiety.

The lipid-binding sites on the apolipoproteins also appear to be fundamentally different from those of the proteins which contain well-defined pockets or crevices which can accommodate discrete ligands with a high degree of steric, electrostatic or hydrophobic specificity. This property is very well-illustrated by albumin (Fig. 8). Based on sequence analysis and model building, Brown (1976) has proposed that albumin contains three distinct domains. Each domain in turn has three helical segments which are localized in what is referred to as sub domains. The fatty acid binding site is formed when the three helical segments are arranged parallel to each other. About 30% of the cylindrical surface is hydrophobic and about 70% hydrophilic. With this arrangement, the three helical segments form a long groove into which a single fatty acid can fit. By contrast, when an apoprotein binds to a phospholipid vesicle, there is no such discrete pocket on the surface of the apoprotein to which the phospholipid binds. It is probably more correct to think in terms of the apoprotein initially presenting to the phospholipid a surface of appropriate polarity.

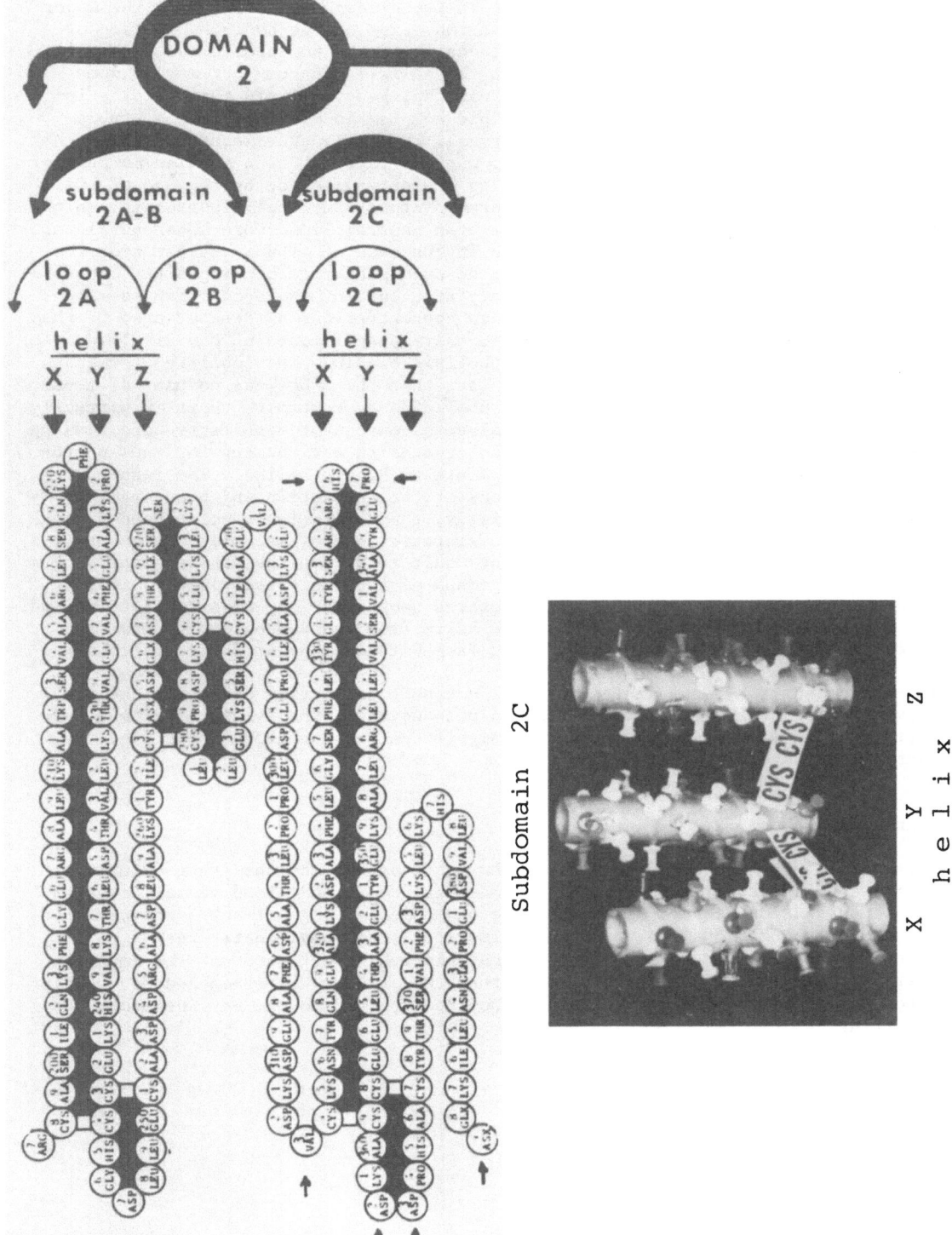

Figure 8. Schematic representation of the three domains of albumin as described by Brown (1976). Published with permission

Stoffel et al. (1974), and Assmann et al. (1974) failed to find any evidence for strong ionic interactions in native HDL. In the plasma apolipoproteins the major interaction is one between the nonpolar amino acids on the hydrophobic face of the amphipathic helix and the fatty acyl chains of the phospholipids. The role of the zwitterionic pairs of amino acids in the helix is unknown but may in some way initiate or orient the phospholipid binding. Neutral lipid must also be incorporated into the apoprotein-phospholipid complex in order to form a stable spherical lipoprotein particle. The physical, chemical determinants of this transformation are not well-established. One way this has been studied morphologically is by converting free cholesterol to cholesteryl ester by the use of LCAT. When this occurs, the vesicle is transformed into a spherical lipoprotein, which presumably is stabilized by the presence of a neutral lipid core. Whereas albumin possesses preformed binding sites, which in the case of albumin result from the presence of 17 disulfide cross-linkages, no such preformed binding sites occur in the apoproteins. Instead, the secondary structure of the apoprotein is relatively labile and is easily altered by low concentrations of denaturants. Of the four human apoproteins sequenced to date, only apoA-II contains one disulfide and even that is not essential for phospholipid binding. The lability of the apoprotein structure is illustrated by the fact that the α-helical content of these proteins is increased on binding to phospholipid. By contrast, there is virtually no detectable structural alteration in albumin consequent upon fatty acid binding. These differences indicate that the lipid creates an environment for the apoprotein which induces certain unordered segments to become helical. The induced helical segments are very like the regions of the apoprotein which interact strongly with phosphatidylcholine. Initially, the zwitterionic polar head groups of the vesicle may serve orient, by electrostatic mechanisms, the complementary ion pairs of amino acid. Such attractions would result in the displacement of bound water at the external polar head groups of the vesicles. Finally, it may be envisaged that the helical segment rotates about its long axis so as to remove the hydrophobic sites of the amphipathic helix from the aqueous bulk phase and to allow interaction of this hydrophobic face with the apolar fatty acyl chains.

In conclusion, the amphipathic theory is amenable to testing and while the final answer to its overall importance remains unanswerable, the evidence to date suggests that it may contribute in a very significant way to the structure of the plasma lipoproteins.

Acknowledgements

Part of the work presented in this review was developed by the Atherosclerosis, Lipids and Lipoproteins section of the National Heart and Blood Vessel Research and Demonstration Center, Baylor College of Medicine, a grant-supported research project of the National Heart and Lung Institute, National Institutes of Health, Grant No. HL 17269. R.L. Jackson is an Established Investigator of the American Heart Association. The authors wish to thank Ms. Brenda Wittenben and Ms. Debbie Mason for preparing the manuscript for publication and to Ms. Kay Shewmaker for preparing the Figures.

CELLULAR CATABOLISM OF SERUM LIPOPROTEINS

O. Stein, V. Ebin, H. Bar-On, and Y. Stein

During the past decade, attention has focused on the catabolism of the lipid and protein components of serum lipoproteins. In the rat (Roheim et al.; 1971) and probably also in the human, the high-density lipoproteins (HDL) are cleared from the circulation as complete particles. In the rat their half-life in the circulation is about 10 h and the main organ responsible for the removal of serum HDL is the liver (Roheim et al., 1971). With the help of radioautography, it was shown that the labeled protein is taken up by the parenchymal cells. Concentrations of radioautographic reaction over secondary lysosomes pointed to these organelles as the site of HDL catabolism (Rachmilewitz et al., 1972). The degration of serum very low-density lipoproteins proceeds in two stages — vascular and cellular and again the parenchymal cells of the liver were shown to be responsible for the cellular phase (Stein et al., 1974). Radioautography at the electron microscope level revealed that binding of the particles to the sinusoidal cell surface of hepatocytes precedes their interiorization. Concentrations of label found over secondary lysosomes provided support that the degradation of protein moiety of serum VLDL or rather remnant particles (Stein et al., 1974) is effected by lysosomal enzymes. Presently, the effect of chloroquine, an inhibitor of cathepsin B, on the degradation of serum lipcproteins in rat liver was studied in vivo and in liver homogenates. Chloroquine had no effect on the clearance from the circulation of ^{125}I labeled rat or human verly low-density lipoproteins or human low-density lipoproteins. Pretreatment with chloroquine for 3 h resulted in a 2–2.5-fold increase in ^{125}I very low-density lipoprotein recovered in the liver 45 min after injection of the homologcus and heterologous lipoproteins (Fig. 1). This effect was evident on both the ^{125}I protein and ^{125}I lipid moiety. Thirty minutes following injection of ^3H-cholesterol linoleate labeled very low-density lipoproteins, 70% of the injected label was recovered in the liver, of both control and cloroquine treated rats. Since the percent of label recovered in free cholesterol was 50% in the control and 20% in the experimental group, it was concluded that chloroquine has interfered with the hydrolysis of ^3H-cholesterol linoleate. ^{125}I human low-density lipoproteins were cleared from the circulation, but only 4% of the injected lipoprotein was recovered in the liver of control rats and not more than 10% after chloroquine treatment. Hence, while very low-density lipoprotein protein and cholesterol ester are catabolized in the liver, the catabolism of low-density lipoproteins occurs mainly in extrahepatic tissues (Sniderman et al., 1974). Using postnuclear liver supernatant, optimal degradation of various serum lipoproteins was found at pH 4.4 (Fig. 2), and chloroquine inhibited their degradation. Degradation of very low-density and low-density lipoproteins was completely inhibited at 0.05 M chloroquine, while less pronounced inhibition was seen with high-density lipoproteins, apolipoproteins and apolipoprotein AI. These results indicate that liver acid hydrolases in vivo participate in the degradation of serum lipoproteins.

EFFECT OF CHLOROQUINE ON RECOVERY OF
^{125}I-VLDL PROTEIN IN RAT LIVER

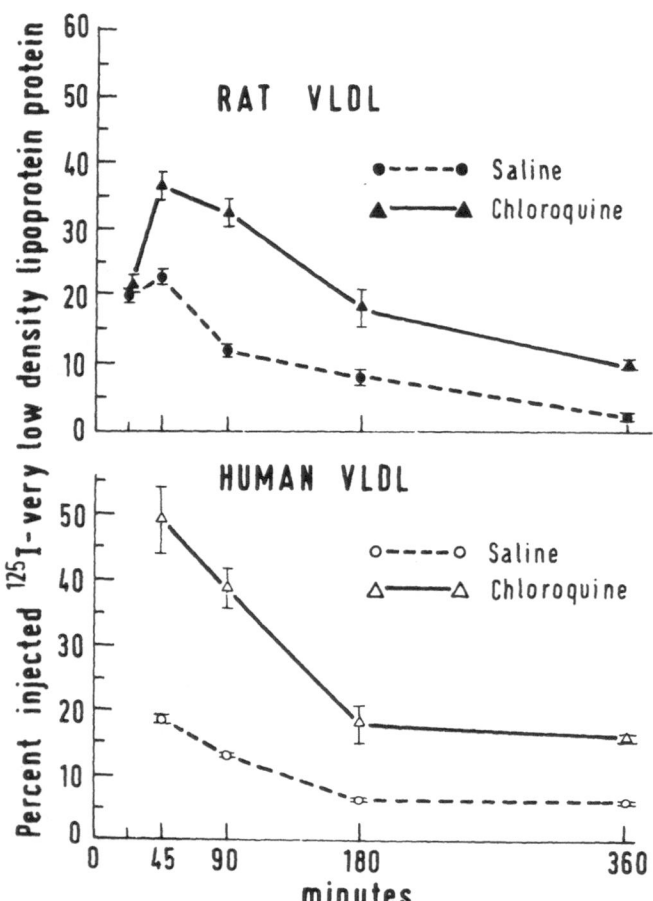

Figure 1. At time zero, the rats were injected i.p. with chloroquine (75 mg/kg b.w.) and 60 min thereafter were given a second injection of 50 mg/kg body weight. Labeled very low-density lipoproteins (100-300 μg protein and 10^6 counts/min of ^{125}I) were injected i.v. 2 h after the first dose of chloroquine, and the rats were killed by exsanguination 22 min - 6 h thereafter. In experiments that were terminated later than 45 min after lipoprotein injection, chloroquine (50 mg/kg b.w.) was readministered at 2 h intervals after the second chloroquine injection. Values are means ± SE of 5-6 determinations
NB: ^{125}I - very low density → ^{125}I very low-density

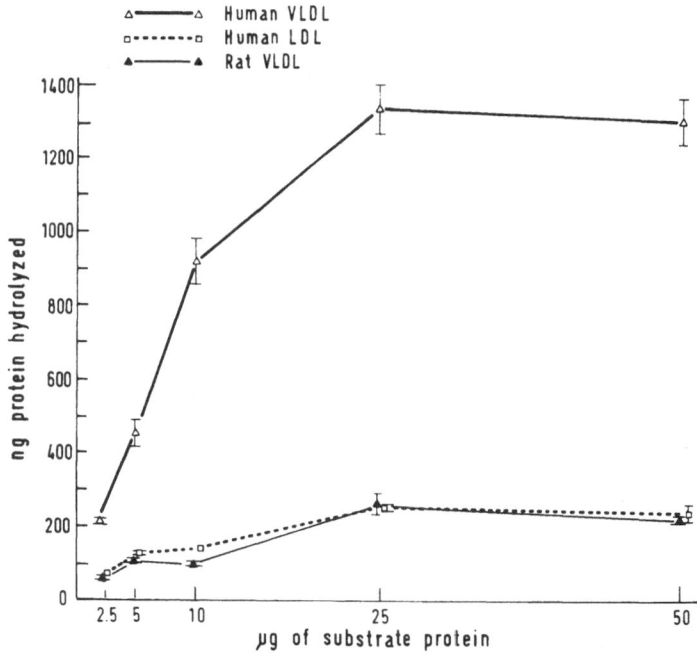

Figure 2. Livers were removed from fasted rats and 10% homogenates were prepared in distilled water containing 2 mM EDTA, pH 7.0, with a teflon pestle using 5 strokes. The homogenate was sonicated for 2 x 15 s at 0° and centrifuged for 10 min at 2000 x g. To study hydrolysis, the following system was used: 0.1 M sodium acetate buffer, pH 4.4, 17–100 µg of liver supernatant protein, 1 mM EDTA, 5 mM dithiotreitol, and up to 500 µg of lipoportein protein in a final volume of 0.2 mL. Incubations were carried out in air at 37° for 2 h. To terminate the incubation, 0.1 ml of 10% albumin was added followed by 2.0 ml of 15% TCA. Protein degradation was determined by measuring noniodine TCA soluble radioactivity as previously described (Bierman et al., 1974).

SYNTHESIS AND SECRETION OF PLASMA LIPOPROTEINS AND APO-LIPOPROTEINS*

Richard J. Havel and Robert L. Hamilton

Research during the past 20 years has shown that the plasma lipoproteins are synthesized in parenchymal cells of the liver and absorptive cells of the small intesteine. In the past 10 years, the structure of these macromolecular aggregates and the identification of their individual apoproteins have been the subject of increasing attention. However, the mechanism by which lipoproteins are assembled and the respective importance of the liver and intestine in the secretion of the individual apoprotein components remain largely unknown. Here we will summarize research in our laboratories[1] dealing with these questions in the rat and relate our findings to the situation in humans.

Lipoprotein Structure

It is now recognized that the major groups of plasma lipoproteins under normal conditions exist mainly as spherical particles in which nonpolar lipids (cholesteryl esters and triglycerides) are covered by a monolayer of polar lipids (primarily cholesterol and glycerophosphatides) together with specific apoproteins. This structure may be designated as *pseudomicellar* (Havel, 1975). Recently, it has become apparent that certain lipoproteins first observed in some human disorders have quite a different structure, here designated as *lamellar*, in which a single bilayer of polar lipid is associated with some of the proteins found in pseudomicellar lipoproteins. We first recognized this structure in the characteristic abnormal lipoproteins of cholestasis, often called "Lp-X". This particle is a spherical vesicle 400-600 Å in diameter, the wall of which is a bilayer composed of a 1:1 mixture of cholesterol and glycerophosphatides (Hamilton et al., 1971, 1974). A small amount of apoprotein is associated with the vesicle. The basic structure, therefore, is that of a unilamellar liposome-containing protein. A second lamellar lipoprotein has been observed together with the vesicle in individuals with genetically determined deficiency of lecithin-cholesterol acyltransferase (Torsvik et al., 1970; Forte et al., 1971), in some individuals with cholestasis (Hamilton et al., 1971; Forte et al., 1974; Utermann et al., 1974), and in cholesterol-fed guinea pigs (Sardet et al., 1972). This high-density lipoprotein (HDL) is a bilayer disc composed of polar lipids with a substantial apoprotein component.

During the past few years, we have obtained evidence that lamellar HDL occur normally as a secretory product of the liver. This observation has led to the hypothesis that formation of lamellar particles is an initial step in lipoprotein assembly and that their conversion to pseudomicellar lipoproteins provides the fundamental mechanism for packaging of the nonpolar lipids that are transported in extracellular compartments (Hamilton, 1972; Hamilton and Kayden, 1974).

*
The authors' personal research cited was supported by Arteriosclerosis SCOR Grant HL-14237 and Grant HL-24187 from the United States Public Health Service.

[1]Important contributions to this research have been made by Cheryl A. Alexander, Menahem Fainaru, Tünde E. Felker, Christopher J. Fielding, Katsumi Imaizumi, and Mary C. Williams.

Secretion of Lipoproteins by the Liver

The perfused rat liver secretes two major lipoproteins — triglyceride-rich, pseudomicellar very low-density lipoproteins (VLDL) and lamellar HDL (Hamilton et al., 1976). Little material accumulates in perfusates in the density range of low-density lipoproteins (LDL), in agreement with other evidence that LDL are a product of the catabolism of triglyceride-rich lipoproteins (Havel, 1975). VLDL in perfusates resemble the "nascent" VLDL that can be isolated from a Golgi apparatus-rich fraction of rat liver (Hamilton, 1972). Both the nascent and the newly secreted VLDL differ from plasma VLDL in certain surface components: the former have somewhat more phospholipids and less of the proteins of low molecular weight ("C" apoproteins) (Hamilton, 1972; Hamilton et al., 1976). Simple mixing of nascent VLDL with VLDL-free plasma or plasma HDL results in interchange of these surface components so that the apoprotein composition of the resulting VLDL closely resembles that of plasma VLDL (Hamilton, 1972). Thus, it seems that synthesis of VLDL is almost completed before they are secreted. By contrast, the HDL that accumulate in perfusates of rat liver differ drastically in structure and composition from those in blood plasma (Hamilton et al., 1976). When livers are perfused in the presence of 5,5'-dithionitrobenzoic acid (DTNB) to inhibit lecithin-cholesterol acyltransferase (LCAT) (which the liver also secretes), the HDL appear mainly as discs. When negatively stained preparations are examined by electron microscopy, the discoidal particles often form rouleaux. The individual particles have an average diameter of about 190 Å and a thickness of 46 Å, which is close to that of a bilayer of phospholipids containing cholesterol. The lipids are mainly glycerophosphatides and cholesterol, with very little nonpolar lipids. Most probably, the acyl chains at the edges of these bilayer discs are covered by the protein that constitutes about 35% of their mass.

Most plasma HDL in the rat are spherical, pseudomicellar particles, 90 – 120 Å in diameter, in which cholesteryl esters in the core comprise about 25% of the particle mass (Hamilton et al., 1976). The proportions of the protein components of discoidal and spherical HDL differ drastically. As will be more fully described later, the arginine-rich apoprotein (ARP) is the major protein component of perfusate HDL, whereas the A-I apoprotein (apo A-I) is the predominant protein of plasma HDL (Hamilton et al., 1976; Marsh, 1976; Felker et al., 1976). When livers are perfused without the LCAT inhibitor, both discoidal and spherical particles accumulate. The spherical particles are almost certainly produced by action of the enzyme upon the discoidal particles, because their component cholesterol and lecithin are an excellent substrate for LCAT (Hamilton et al., 1976). A model for conversion of lamellar to pseudomicellar HDL envisions the movement of the nonpolar cholesteryl ester product into the hydrocarbon domain of the bilayer, progressively spreading it to form an oily core surrounded by a monolayer of remaining polar lipids and the component apoproteins. This conversion consumes the major surface lipids of the discoidal particles which then may receive additional polar lipids by collision with the surfaces of cells or other lipoproteins. This model is consistent with the concept proposed by Glomset and Norum (1973) and by Schumaker and Adams (1969) that the function of LCAT is to "scavenge" surface lipids. Because the action of LCAT on plasma HDL is much slower, we have suggested that the "nascent" HDL accumulating in perfusates may be the "natural" substrate for the enzyme (Hamilton et al., 1976). The paucity of discoidal HDL in plasma then may simply reflect the rapid conversion to mature spherical HDL, which are known to have a life span of many hours. The presence of similar discoidal HDL in states of LCAT deficiency suggests that the same process of conversion of discs to spheres occurs normally in humans.

It should be emphasized that our studies have not proved that the liver actually secretes discoidal HDL because we have not yet succeeded in isolating them from subcellular fractions of liver. However, they are not solely the product of the ultracentrifugal procedure required to isolate them because identical structures can be seen by electron microscopy in negatively stained preparations of whole perfusates and in plasma of patients with cholestasis (Hamilton and Kayden, 1974; Hamilton, R.L., unpublished observations).

Assembly of Lipoproteins in the Liver

As already mentioned, formation of VLDL is largely completed before they are released into the circulation from the Golgi apparatus of the hepatocyte. Nascent VLDL are readily visualized by electron microscopy within tubules and vesicles of this organelle (Hamilton, 1972; Hamilton and Kayden, 1974). Similar particles are often evident within profiles of smooth endoplasmic reticulum, a compartment in which lipids are known to be synthesized (Stein and Stein, 1974). Occasionally, such particles are seen in ribosome-free portions of junctions between smooth and rough reticulum. Apoprotein components are synthesized on the ribosomes of the rough endoplasmic reticulum (Marsh, 1963), but the site at which these proteins join with the lipids to form a lipoprotein is unknown. In a study recently reported from our laboratory (Alexander et al., 1976), a major apoprotein component of VLDL, the B-apoprotein, was identified immunocytochemically with peroxidase-labeled specific antibody. B-apoprotein was present on the ribosomes of the rough reticulum and within its cisternae. It was also present on nascent VLDL in tubules and vesicles of the Golgi apparatus, but reaction product of peroxidase substrate could not be identified on the particles that resemble nascent VLDL in cisternae of typical smooth endoplasmic reticulum. However, the smooth-surfaced junctions between smooth and rough reticulum often contained intense deposits of the reaction product in the absence or presence of the particles. These observations led us to propose that triglyceride-rich particles, stabilized by phospholipids or by other proteins, are synthesized in the smooth reticulum and then are transported to a junction with the rough reticulum, where they receive their complement of B-apoprotein. Many secreted proteins are synthesized in a precursor form larger than the eventual product (Campbell, 1975). Possibly such a pro-B-apoprotein has increased water-solubility which facilitates its transport to the site of union with the triglyceride-rich lipid particle.

How the stabilized microdroplet of triglyceride is formed in the smooth endoplasmic reticulum is unknown. One plausible mechanism is analogous to the previouly described formation of a pseudomicellar plasma HDL from its lamellar precursor. Thus, regions of the bilayer membrane of the endoplasmic reticulum may be acted upon by the membrane-bound enzyme system that synthesizes triglycerides to create a pseudomicellar structure. Some apolipoproteins are able to sequester regions of liposomal membranes to form discoidal particles (Hauser et al., 1974), and it is therefore reasonable to propose that such sequestration also constitutes the earliest step in the formation of lipoproteins in the endoplasmic reticulum (Hamilton, 1972; Hamilton and Kayden, 1974). Sequestration could occur before, during, or after nonpolar lipids are inserted into the bilayer by the appropriate membrane-bound enzymes. ARP is an attractive candidate for the sequestering agent because it is a major apoprotein of both newly secreted VLDL and HDL (Hamilton et al., 1976; Marsh, 1976; Felker et al., 1976) as well as of discoidal plasma HDL (Utermann et al., 1974, 1975; Danielsson et al., 1975; Norum et al., 1975; Ostwald and Guo, 1975).

Hepatic Secretion of Apolipoproteins

Most, if not all, apolipoproteins exist in more than one of the major classes of plasma lipoproteins. Some of them may also exist in a lipid-poor state in plasma. These facts have complicated quantitative measurements of their secretion and catabolism. We have approached the problem of measurement of apolipoprotein secretion by devising specific quantitative radioimmunoassays. Although such assays are technically complex, they have certain advantages over other quantitative immunologic techniques. First, immunoreactivity of an apoprotein in different lipoproteins can be evaluated by testing its ability to displace the isolated labeled apoprotein from specific antibody. Second, the high sensitivity of the technique makes it possible to quantify secretion rates in small samples from perfused organs or incubated cells. Radioimmunoassays for ARP (Fainarv et al., 1976b) and apo A-I (Fainarv et al., 1976a) (the major apoproteins of HDL in perfusates and plasma, respectively) have been developed that detect all of these

molecules in the major lipoprotein classes of blood plasma. Sodium decyl sulfate
has been a valuable reagent in these assays. Unlike sodium dodecyl sulfate, sodium decyl sulfate does not precipitate serum proteins. In the case of A-I, inclusion of this detergent in the assay medium provides complete immunoreactively
of the protein in all major plasma lipoprotein classes. In the assay of ARP, it
stabilizes the radiolabeled protein and thus permits a single preparation to be
used for up to 3 weeks.

With these assays, the isolated, perfused liver from fed rats weighing about 350 g
has been shown to secrete ARP at an approximately constant rate of 500 μg per
hour for up to 6 hours (Felker et al., 1976). The rate of secretion of apo A-I
is less certain, because it falls during a 6-hour period of perfusion. Taking the
average rate, it amounts to about 60 μg per hour. These rates are not affected
by addition of LCAT inhibitor to the perfusate.

Most of the A-I is associated with HDL in perfusates, as it is in the plasma, but
ARP is contained in both VLDL and HDL (Felker et al., 1976). ARP is the major
protein of the discoidal HDL, accounting for about one-half of the total protein;
apo A-I accounts for only about 10%. By contrast, apo A-I comprises almost two-
thirds of the protein of plasma HDL, and ARP only about 10%.

In both perfusates and blood plasma, measurable amounts of A-I and ARP are also
present in proteins sedimenting at density of 1.21 g/ml. In plasma, about 5% of
A-I and 40% of ARP are in this lipoprotein-poor ultracentrifugal fraction, whereas respective values for perfusates, obtained in the presence or absence of LCAT-
inhibitor, are about 30% and 15% (Felker et al., 1976). When blood plasma is
subjected to chromatography on 10% agarose gel, eluted fractions containing VLDL
and HDL have considerably more ARP than VLDL and HDL separated by ultracentrifugation, and less than 5% of ARP is found in fractions containing the bulk of serum
proteins (Imaizumi, K., Fainuru, M., Havel, R.J., unpublished observations).
Comparison of ratios of ARP to cholesterol in VLDL and HDL obtained by gel filtration and by ultracentrifugation suggest that about 30% of the ARP present in VLDL
and 60% of that in HDL are dissociated by ultracentrifugation. Although similar
studies have not been conducted for ARP and A-I in perfusates, it is obviously
possible that the discoidal HDL may have lost one of their component apoproteins
during centrifugation. However, it should be emphasized that potential losses
during centrifugation cannot alter the general conclusion that ARP is the major
and apo A-I is a minor protein component of perfusate HDL.

Secretion of Apolipoproteins in Intestinal Lymph

Previous reports have indicated that chylomicrons from rat intestinal lymph contain appreciable amounts of a protein with characteristics of apo A-I (Windmueller
et al., 1973; Slickman and Kirsch, 1973). By quantitative radioimmunoassay, we
have found that apo A-I accounts for about 30% and ARP for about 5% of the protein
of chylomicrons (protein comprises about 0.6% of particle mass) (Imaizumi et al.,
1976). B-apoprotein comprises about 10% and C-apoproteins most of the remainder.

Earlier work (Windmueller et al., 1973; Havel et al., 1973) has shown that chylomicrons, like VLDL, take up C-apoproteins from HDL after they enter vascular
spaces. More recently, we have found that chylomicrons from rat lymph also rapidly take up large amounts of ARP upon exposure to blood plasma (Imaizumi et al.,
1976). The protein content of chylomicrons that have been incubated with VLDL-
free plasma increases from about 0.6 to more than 2% of particle mass. No increase in content of A-I occurs.

Transport of A-I and ARP has been measured in intestinal lymph for up to 72 h
(Imaizumi, K., Fainaru, M., Havel, R.J., unpublished observations). Transport of
A-I in fat-fed rats is on the order of 200 μg per hour and that of ARP is about
20 μg per hour. These rates are somewhat lower in animals fed glucose or fasted.
These studies do not by themselves establish the origin of these proteins. How-

ever, when considered in light of data of Windmueller et al. (1973) and of Glickman and Kirsch (1973) on incorporation of radioactive amino acids into proteins
of lymph chylomicrons, the tentative conclusion can be drawn that apo A-I is synthesized primarily in absorptive cells of the intestinal mucosa. Thus, these results, together with those on secretion rates from perfused liver, stronlgy suggest that in the rat the intestine is the major source of apo A-I whereas almost
all of the ARP is derived from the liver.

Summary and Conclusions

The results summarized here by no means provide a comprehensive picture of the
processes of synthesis, assembly, and secretion of plasma lipoproteins. Rather,
they constitute a progress report. It must be recognized that, whereas the fundamental processes of assembly and secretion of lipoproteins are likely to be
similar among mammals, important quantitative differences may well exist among
species. Presently, the following conclusions can be drawn for the rat.

1. Triglyceride-rich lipoproteins are secreted in an almost completed state from
the cells of origin in liver and gut. The lipid-rich particle arises from the
endoplasmic reticulum, possibly by enzymatic action upon lamellar complexes of
protein and phospholipid. The B-apoprotein may be added subsequent to formation
of the triglyceride-rich particle at the site at which the rough and smooth endoplasmic reticulum join.

2. HDL are secreted from the liver in a precursor form and appear in perfusates
as lamellar discs in which the protein is mainly ARP. This particle is a preferred substrate for LCAT, which converts it in the blood plasma to a typical
pseudomicellar lipoprotein with a core of cholesteryl esters. The apo A-I, which
in this process becomes the major protein of HDL, is probably derived to a large
extent from the small intestine. Thus, the origin of plasma HDL is likely to be
complex, with apoprotein elements arising from both liver and gut.

3. Both VLDL and chylomicrons are modified as soon as they enter vascular spaces.
For VLDL, this involves largely the addition of C-apoproteins from HDL. For
chylomicrons, it involves addition of both ARP and C-apoproteins, again probably
from HDL. Thus, the apoprotein content of chylomicrons in plasma comes to resem-
bel much more that of hepatogenous VLDL.

4. Quantitative analyses indicate that changes in apoprotein composition accompany ultracentrifugation of some lipoproteins. Apart from their importance
for our understanding of lipoprotein structures, these effects suggest caution
in the interpretation of metabolic data obtained with ultracentrifugally separated lipoproteins.

DYNAMICS OF LIPOPROTEIN INTERCONVERSION

Shlomo Eisenberg

It is now well-established that plasma low-density lipoprotein (LDL) is a final breakdown product of the metabolism of very low-density lipoprotein (VLDL). The process by which LDL is formed in the plasma compartment — the VLDL interconversion process — is mediated through the activity of the enzyme system lipoprotein lipase, and involves compositional, structural, and functional alterations of all major plasma lipoproteins. The purpose of the present discussion is to describe the many events which take place during lipoprotein interconversion and to present a hypothesis on possible molecular mechanisms of the process. Several reviews have been published lately on the structure and composition of lipoproteins (Eisenberg and Levy, 1975; Morrisett et al., 1975; Jackson et al., 1976; Eisenberg, 1976a). These subjects, therefore, will not be dealt with here.

Dynamics of Lipoprotein Interconversion

The initial event of the interconversion process is the interaction of triglyceride-rich lipoproteins (chylomicrons and VLDL) with endothelial-bound lipoprotein lipases. On the basis of tissue distribution of labeled fatty acids after the injection of lipoproteins labeled with triglyceride fatty acids (Olivecrona and Belfrage, 1965), it is generally accepted that chylomicrons and VLDL triglycerides are hydrolized predominantly by extrahepatic lipoprotein lipases. The extrahepatic enzyme, although similar in structure to the hepatic enzyme (Augustin et al., 1975), is of considerably different biological properties (LaRosa et al., 1972; Fielding, 1972; Krauss et al., 1973b, 1974). Most importantly, the extrahepatic enzyme is activated by apoprotein C-II (LaRosa et al., 1970; Krauss et al., 1973a), a major protein constituent of both chylomicron and VLDL particles (Shore and Shore, 1969; Brown et al., 1969; Albers and Scanu, 1971; Kostner and Holasek, 1972; Bersot et al., 1970; Koga et al., 1971). Thus, these two lipoproteins provide the enzyme with both substrate and activator in one single lipoprotein particle. Because of simple surface to volume considerations (Lossow et al., 1969; Sata et al., 1972; Eisenberg, 1976b), however, it must be assumed that apoproteins and surface lipid constituents — phospholipids and unesterified cholesterol — are removed from the lipoprotein concomitantly with the hydrolysis of triglycerides, a core constituent. Indeed, it can be calculated (see below) that as much as 60-80% of the phospholipids and unesterified cholesterol molecules present in intact VLDL particles are removed from the lipoprotein during the formation of LDL. The mechanism of removal of these lipids from VLDL and chylomicrons is yet obscure. In vitro studies (Eisenberg, 1975; Eisenberg and Schurr, 1976; Eisenberg, S., Schurr, D., Goldman, H., Olivecrona, T., unpublished observations) have suggested that one half or more of the glycerophosphatides — predominantly lecithin — are hydrolized to lysocompounds by the phospholipase activity of lipoprotein lipases of either hepatic (Zieve and Zieve, 1972; Pykalisto et al., 1974; Ehnholm et al., 1975) or extrahepatic (Eisenberg, 1975; Eisenberg and Schurr, 1976; Eisenberg, S., Schurr, D., Goldman, H., Olivecrona, T., unpublished observations; Pykalisto et al., 1974; Scow and Egelrud, 1976; Chajek, T., Eisenberg, S., unpublished observations) origin, and are removed from the lipoproteins. Phospholipids are removed from VLDL and chylomicrons also as intact molecules and can be found in high-density lipoproteins (Eisenberg, S., Schurr, D., Goldman, H., Olivecrona, T., unpublished observations; Chajek, T., Eisenberg, S., unpublished observations). Whether one of these two pathways predominates in vivo and in situ is unknown. Even less is known about the fate of unesterified cholesterol. Following abrupt initiation of lipolysis by the injection of heparin

to either humans or rats (LaRosa et al., 1971; Eisenberg, 1976b), the cholesterol content of HDL increases. Thus, some cholesterol seems to be transferred
to HDL. However, recent experiments have demonstrated an additional pathway of
removal of cholesterol from chylomicrons in the perfused mammary gland of lactating rats (Zinder et al., 1976). In this organ, a substantial amount of cholesterol can be found in the tissue and is presumably secreted with the milk.

The data cited above indicate that VLDL lipids are metabolized through several
pathways. Some are hydrolized to fatty acids and partial glycerides or lyso-
phosphatides; phospholipids and cholesterol may be transferred to other lipoproteins; and an unknown amount of lipids other than fatty acids and partial
glycerides may be taken up by tissue cells.

A divergent metabolic fate of apoB and apoC in VLDL was already demonstrated in
the first report on the metabolism of individual apoproteins in the human (Bilheimer et al., 1972). This observation has been confirmed since in humans (Bilheimer et al., 1972; Eisenberg et al., 1973, 1972a; Berman, M., Hall, M., Levy,
R.I., Eisenberg, S., Bilheimer, D.W., Phair, R.D., Goebel, R., unpublished observations; Phair et al., 1975; Sigurdson et al., 1975, 1976) and rats (Eisenberg
and Rachmilewitz, 1973a, 1973b; Faergeman et al., 1975; Fidge and Poulis, 1975).
The experiments, carried out in vivo and using VLDL labeled in its protein
moiety, have shown unequivocally that the apoB moiety of VLDL is a precursor of
the protein moiety of plasma LDL. Radioactive apoB leaving the VLDL density
range is first transferred to a lipoprotein of intermediate density, the IDL
(d 1.006 - 1.019 g/ml) and only later to LDL (Bilheimer et al., 1972). When heparin is injected in conjunction with the labeled VLDL (Eisenberg et al., 1973),
the formation of IDL particles is greatly enhanced. Particles indistinguishable
from IDL accumulate also in the VLDL density range, predominantly with the subfraction of S_f rate 20 - 60 (Eisenberg et al., 1973). Since labeled apoB appearance in the LDL density range (d 1.019 - 1.063 g/ml) is not significantly affected
by heparin injection, it has been suggested that the conversion of IDL to LDL may
be independent of the release of postheparin lipolytic activity into the circulation, at least in part. Alternatively, IDL particles may respond slower to the
enzyme.

The half-life time of apoB in the VLDL density range in humans is about 2 hours
(Berman, M., Hall, M., Levy, R.I., Eisenberg, S., Bilheimer, D.W., Phair, R.D.,
Goebel, R., unpublished observations), similar to that of VLDL triglycerides
(Quarfordt et al., 1970). In patients with hypertriglyceridemia (types I, III and
IV), the half-life time of apoB in VLDL is greatly delayed (Berman, M., Hall, M.,
Levy, R.I., Eisenberg, S., Bilheimer, D.W., Phair, R.D., Goebel, R., unpublished
observations). In rats, both the half-life time of apoB (Eisenberg and Rachmile-
witz, 1973a, 1973b; Faergeman et al., 1975; Fidge and Poulis, 1975) and triglyc-
erides (Harris and Harris, 1973) is considerably shorter, only a few minutes.

The studies on VLDL metabolism in rats (Eisenberg and Rachmilewitz, 1973a, 1973b;
Faergeman et al., 1975; Fidge and Poulis, 1975) have unmasked an additional pathway of metabolism of apoB in VLDL. The pathway, first described with radio-
iodinated VLDL (Eisenberg and Rachmilewitz, 1973a, 1973b) and subsequently confirmed by studies with VLDL labeled with amino acids (Faergeman et al., 1975),
consists of an extremely efficient mechanism of removal of VLDL intermediates
from the circulation, after their interaction with lipoprotein lipase at extrahepatic sites. Since about 90% of the VLDL apoB is removed from the circulation
and only 5 - 10% is converted to LDL (Eisenberg and Rachmilewitz, 1973a, 1973b;
Faergeman et al., 1975), this pathway provides a clue to the low levels of LDL
in the rat, in spite of an active VLDL apoB synthesis. In both studies, the liver
was shown to be the predominant site of degradation of the apoB-rich VLDL intermediate. A similar pathway may also operate in humans, especially with hyperlipoproteinemia (Berman, M., Hall, M., Levy, R.I., Eisenberg, S., Bilheimer, D.W.,
Phair, R.D., Goebel, R., unpublished observations). Electron microscopic study
of the rate liver after injection with labeled VLDL has demonstrated an initial
interaction of the lipoprotein with the hepatocyte cell membrane followed by

interiorization and catabolism (Stein et al., 1974). In analogy, it has been hypothesized that the liver is also the site of metabolism of IDL in humans (Eisenberg and Levy, 1975; Eisenberg, 1976a). In the human, however, the final breakdown product — the LDL — is released into the circulation, rather than being catabolized.

The metabolic fate of apoC is very different from that of apoB. ApoC molecules, either in VLDL or HDL, exchange rapidly between the lipoproteins, either in vivo or in vitro (Bilheimer et al., 1972; Eisenberg et al., 1973, 1972a; Bierman, M., Hall, M., Levy, R.I., Eisenberg, S., Bilheimer, D.W., Phair, R.D., Goebel, R., unpublished observations; Eisenberg and Rachmilewitz, 1975). During the degradation of chylomicrons and VLDL particles in vivo, apoC molecules are progressively removed from the particles and are transferred to HDL (Havel et al., 1973; Eisenberg et al., 1973). They recycle back from HDL to VLDL and chylomicrons when newly synthesized lipoproteins enter the circulation. The removal of apoC from VLDL is greatly enhanced following the injection of heparin to humans (Eisenberg et al., 1973) or rats (Eisenberg and Rachmilewitz, 1975) and this same process can be demonstrated in vitro following incubation of VLDL with lipoprotein lipase-rich plasma (Eisenberg and Rachmilewitz, 1975). It is the transfer of apoC from VLDL to HDL which explains the decreasing ratio of apoC to apoB found with VLDL density subfractions of increasing density and decreasing S_f rates (Eisenberg et al., 1972b).

The molecular basis of the transfer of apoC from VLDL particles during lipolysis is yet obscure. In an attempt to define better the determinants of apoC associations and dissociations with VLDL, we have recently studied the effects of lipolysis on apoC in VLDL using an incubation system devoid of plasma (Glangeaud et al., 1976). The study has demonstrated that apoC is removed from VLDL also when no known lipoprotein acceptors to apoC are present in the incubation system. Under these conditions, more than one-half of the apoC molecules were isolated with the buffer fraction of density greater than 1.21 g/ml, indicating that they were poorly lipidated, or even in a delipidated form. We have, moreover, observed that at any stage of lipolysis (measured as free fatty acids generation) the number of apoC molecules removed from VLDL in the absence of plasma was identical to that observed in the presence of plasma. *Therefore, we suggest that the process of removal of apoC during lipolysis of VLDL is solely dependent on the nature of the product lipoprotein form and is independent of the presence of an acceptor to apoC.*

Relatively little is known at the present time about the metabolic behavior of the arginine-rich protein, the ARP. This apoprotein normally present in VLDL in small amounts (Shore et al., 1974a; Shelburne and Quarfordt, 1974) is found in relatively high levels in lipoproteins isolated from cholesterol-fed animals (Shore et al., 1974b; Mahley et al., 1974, 1975) and in the abnormal lipoproteins found in the VLDL density range of patients with type III hyperlipoproteinemia (B-VLDL) (Havel and Kane, 1973; Utermann et al., 1975). It constitutes about 10% of total VLDL proteins in humans and 20 - 25% in rats. Because of poor labeling properties, the fate of ARP in humans has not been completely resolved in VLDL turnover studies. In rats, radioactivity associated with an apoprotein fraction enriched with the ARP (fraction VS-2) seems to decay from VLDL to HDL following the injection of labeled VLDL (Eisenberg and Rachmilewitz, 1973a, 1973b). About 30% of the protein present in this fraction disappear from VLDL during an in vitro induced lipolysis (Eisenberg and Rachmilewitz, 1975). A transfer of ARP from HDL to lower density lipoproteins has been described upon addition of lecithin:cholesterol acyltransferase (LCAT) to serum obtained from patients with familiar deficiency of this enzyme (Norum et al., 1975). Whether a similar shuttle of the ARP from high to lower density lipoproteins occurs also during the process of lipoprotein metabolism in normal humans or experimental animals is yet unknown (see, however, Dr. Havel's communication, present meeting).

A crucial question to the understanding of the lipoprotein interconversion process is related to the number of LDL particles originating from a single VLDL particle. To answer this question, the average mass of intact and postlipolysis VLDL particles and the exact composition of the two lipoproteins was determined using an in vitro incubation system (Eisenberg and Rachmilewitz, 1975). From these data, it was possible to calculate the absolute mass contribution of individual lipid and apoprotein constituents to the total mass of single particles. The results have confirmed the previous observations that phospholipids, cholesterol (predominantly unesterified) and apoC molecules are removed from VLDL during the lipolytic process. However, since the absolute mass contribution of apoB to postlipolysis VLDL particles was identical to that found in intact VLDL particles, it was concluded that *one and only one* product particle is produced from each precursor particle. Similar conclusions were reported also when the properties of human VLDL density subfractions were investigated (Eisenberg et al., 1973) and following injection of rat plasma VLDL to the supradiaphragmatic portion of the rat (Mjøs et al., 1975).

A better understanding of the effects of lipolysis on VLDL structure and function was achieved when an attempt was made to relate the observed compositional changes to the lipid core model of VLDL (Eisenberg, 1976b). In spite of a loss of about 80% of the triglycerides and 30% of the cholesteryl esters, the calculated core volume of intact and postlipolysis VLDL particles was similar to that of the calculated core lipid volumes. At the surface of the lipoproteins, the calculation yielded a remarkably constant concentration (molecules/unit of surface area) of all constituents, i.e., phospholipids, unesterified cholesterol, and total protein. This observation indicated that an almost perfect synchrony exists between the removal of core and surface constituents during lipolysis. However, whereas the general assembly of lipid and proteins in lipoproteins has not been changed during lipolysis, considerable changes were found to occur in the molar ratio of individual constituents within the various lipid and protein moieties. Thus, lipolysis caused a marked increase in the molar ratio of cholesteryl esters to triglycerides, and of sphingomyelin to lecithin at the core and surface of the lipoprotein, respectively. The most dramatic change, however, was found among the various apoprotein fractions. When expressed in molecular weight units of 10,000 daltons each, the concentration of apoB increased by almost 300% and that of the ARP, by 180%. In contrast, the concentration of apoC at the surface of postlipolysis VLDL particles was only 20% of that of the intact particle. These changes, depicted graphically in Figure 1, may be responsible for the changing biological behavior of the two lipoproteins, and in particular their interaction with lipoprotein lipase sites and tissue cells.

The Molecular Basis of Lipoprotein Interconversion: A Hypothesis

The basic process of lipoprotein interconversion is taking place at the site of interaction of VLDL with lipoprotein lipase. It is proposed that the interaction results in a stereotypic and predictable chain of events leading to transfer of lipids from the lipoprotein to the tissue and release of a partially degraded particle to the plasma space. This particle is smaller and heavier than the original particle, but is capable of reinteracting with lipoprotein lipases. After multiple interactions, an intermediate lipoprotein particle is formed, which is poor in apoC, contains all of the apoB present in the original particle, and is the precursor of LDL. The formation of the intermediate lipoprotein occurs predominantly in extrahepatic sites. The channeling of VLDL particles to these sites may be due to the abundance of apoC units at the VLDL surface coat. Other factors, such as size or lipid composition may contribute to the affinity of large VLDL particles toward extrahepatic lipoprotein lipase. Alternatively, all different particles interact with the enzyme; significant triglyceride hydrolysis, however, takes place only towards the large, apoC-II rich particles. The site of conversion of IDL to LDL is not known. It is attractive to speculate that this process occurs via an interaction of intermediate lipoprotein particles with tissue cells, predominantly in the liver (Eisenberg and Levy, 1975; Eisenberg, 1976a). According to this hypothesis, the relatively high concentration of apcB at the

INTACT VLDL   POST - LIPOLYSIS VLDL

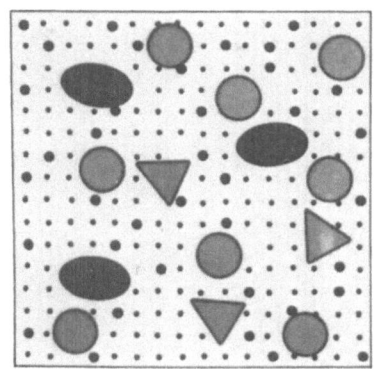   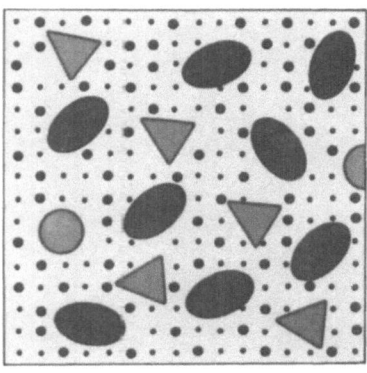

Figure 1. A schematic representation of the surface coat (25,000 Å²) of intact and postlipolysis VLDL particles. Lipid and apoprotein constituents are drawn at their actual calculated concentration at the surface, using 10,000 daltons as a molecular weight unit of all different apoproteins. Small dots = lecithin; large dots = sphingomyelin; circles = apoC; ovals = apoB; triangles = arginine-rich protein (ARP)

surface of the intermediate lipoprotein surface facilitates the interaction of the lipoprotein with the cell surface. This interaction results in further delipidation of the intermediate lipoprotein probably through the activity of the hepatic lipase. In spite of the different sites of interaction, hepatic and extrahepatic, it is assumed that the basic process of delipidation and deproteination (removal of apoproteins) from the intermediate lipoprotein is similar to that of VLDL. It is in the liver that the biological behavior of the intermediate lipoprotein differs between species: in rats, the particles are interiorized and catabolized; in humans, they are released to the circulation in the form of plasma LDL.

Any proposed molecular mechanism of the delipidation process must account for many different events that take place at the site of lipolysis. These include not only triglyceride hydrolysis but also removal of phospholipids, cholesterol, and apoproteins. Along this path, the integrity of the partially degraded particles is preserved, and the neutral lipid core of the lipoproteins is covered by an amphipatic surface coat. Thus, metabolism of surface constituents and rearrangement of both surface and core must occur concomitantly with hydrolysis of triglycerides and transfer of the hydrolytic products to the tissue cells.

We envision the initial event of the delipidation process as binding of the lipoprotein to the enzyme. At this stage, a portion of the lipoprotein surface coat, shown schematically in Figure 2, comes into contact with the endothelialbound enzyme. A specific lipid and protein configuration at the surface coat of the lipoprotein must be involved with this initial contact, most probably through apoC molecules. The presence of apoC, furthermore, activates the enzyme although the exact mode of the activiation process is yet unknown. Now lipolysis can start. We suggest that the enzyme acts on two substrates: triglycerides and glycerophosphatides, resulting in the production of free fatty acids, partial glycerides and lysophosphatide compounds. Some of these hydrolytic products may be removed from the lipolytic site by lateral diffusion in the surface coat monolayer, as

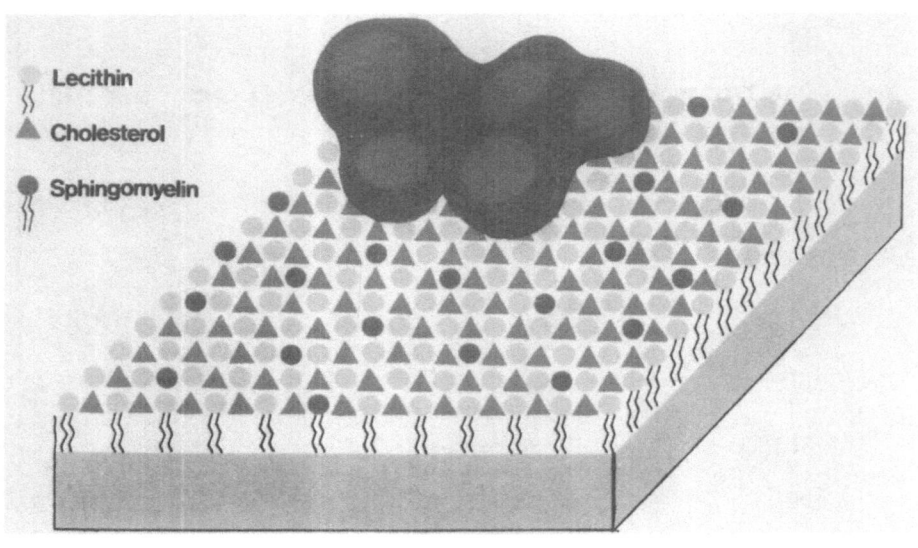

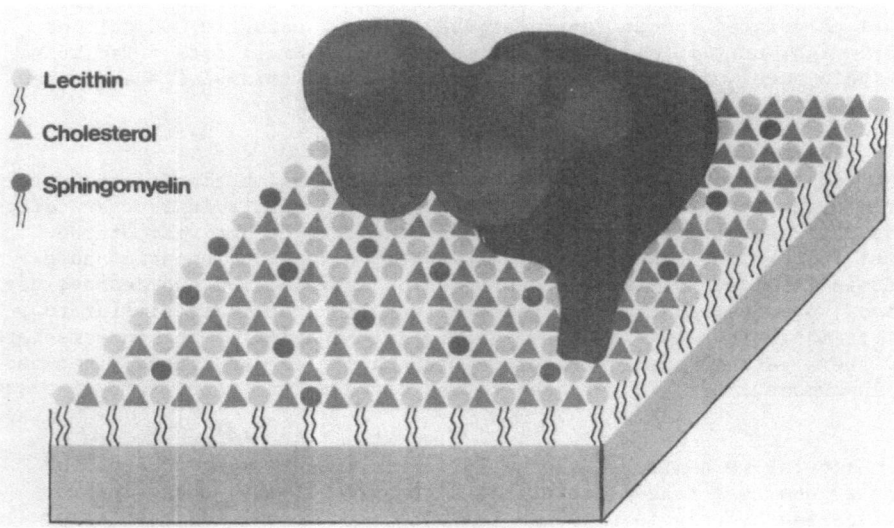

Figure 2. A schematic representation of a portion of the surface coat of intact VLDL, before interaction with lipoprotein lipase

suggested by Scow et al. (1976); others are removed by transfer to other plasma proteins and/or lipoproteins (i.e., albumin and high-density lipoproteins). However, regardless of the mode of removal of the hydrolytic products from the lipoprotein, the basic condition for the initiation of the removal process is a profound alteration of the lipoprotein — microenvironment at the site lipolyis. A diagrammatic illustration of a possible change of the lipoprotein surface coat at the site of lipolysis is shown in Figure 3. In the figure, we demonstrate several hypothetical changes occurring concomitantly: disappearance of phosphatidylcholine molecule, relative enrichment with sphingomyelin and unesterified cholesterol molecules, and accumulation of hydrolytic products. These changes may be difficult to demonstrate because of the small area involved with the interaction of the en-

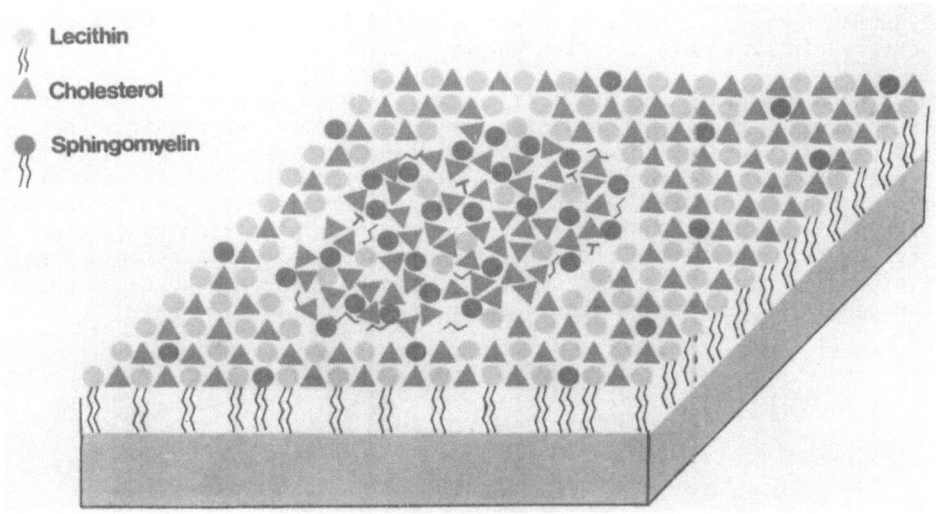

Figure 3. A schematic representation of possible derangement cf the surface coat of VLDL, at the site of interaction with lipoprotein lipase (see text)

zyme and the lipoprotein as compared to the total surface area of the lipoprotein. Nevertheless, they result in a drastic change of the properties of the surface monolayer of the lipoprotein at the site of interaction with the enzyme. An example of such change is the fluidity of the lipoprotein surface coat. Indeed, an experiment carried out recently in our laboratory has demonstrated a considerable decrease in the fluidity (increased apparent microviscosity) of postlipolysis VLDL, ans compared to the intact lipoprotein (Barenholtz, Y., Eisenberg, S., unpublished observations). It is this, or another change of the properties of the monolayer that is possibly responsible for the dissociation of protein molecules — predominantly apoC molecules — from the lipoprotein. The dissociation of apoprotein C is therefore an intrinsic feature of the lipolytic process, is solely dependent on the nature of the partially degraded lipoprotein, and is a consequence of the lipolytic process itself. In the presence of plasma, the dissociated apoC units associate themselves with HDL, probably due to surface interactions. In the absence of HDL, the apoC units are found in unassociated forms, predominantly in the plasma protein fraction of density greater than 1,21 g/ml. It is tempting to hypothesize further that some of the surplus surface constituents which accumulate at the site of lipolysis — in particular unesterified cholesterol and residual phospholipids — are removed along with apoC molecules, in the form of a small lipoprotein fragment. This hypothetical pathway provides a mechanism for the removal of surface lipids from the triglyceride-rich lipoproteins and is compatible with the general lipid-binding properties of apolipoproteins.

The sequence of events described above provides a molecular basis for the synchrony of removal of core and surface constituents from VLDL during lipolysis. An attractive feature of the hypothesis is its independence of factors other than the interaction between the lipoprotein and the enzyme. However, even more attractive is the possible role of this mechanism in regulating the degradation of triglyceride-rich lipoproteins. Since apoC units may serve as binders between lipoproteins and extrahepatic lipoprotein lipases, their removal will result in dissociation of the two and release of the partially degraded lipoprotein into the plasma space. This partially degraded lipoprotein contains less apoC than the original particle, but is still capable of reinteracting with lipoprotein lipases at extrahepatic sites. Only after multiple interactions, is an apoB-rich intermediate formed and channeled to liver cell surfaces. Since the activity of the hepatic enzyme is independent of the presence of apoC in lipoproteins, tri-glyceride hydrolysis may take place upon the interaction of the apoC-poor and apoB-rich intermediate with the enzyme.

The hypothesis presented above is compatible with many of the known events oc-curring during the interconversion process. It moreover predicts that the lipol-ysis process operates through autoregulation pathways, all of which are inherent in the specific features of the triglyceride-rich lipoproteins and of the proper-ties of the hepatic and extrahepatic lipoprotein lipase. Yet, it should be re-garded as a working hypothesis based predominantly on results obtained from in vitro experiments. It is thus that time has now come to test this hypothesis in vivo, and in particular with endothelial-bound enzymes, where the physiological process of lipoprotein interconversion is taking place.

LIPOPROTEIN METABOLISM IN TISSUE CULTURE

Y. Stein and O. Stein

In recent years we have used the tissue culture method to study interactions between cellular components of the arterial wall and serum lipoproteins (Bierman
et al., 1973, 1974; Stein et al., 1975, 1976; Stein and Stein, 1975a, 1975b,
1975c). Endothelium from human umbilical veins was cultured in vitro and the
cells were incubated with ^{125}I low and high-density lipoproteins isolated from
human plasma. The interaction can be divided into three stages, binding, uptake
and degradation, which are illustrated in Figure 1 (Stein and Stein, 1976). Human
LDL was bound, taken up, and degraded preferentially to human HDL. HDL reduced
markedly the uptake and degradation of LDL. These findings have two implications:

1. That the different levels of high-density lipoprotein encountered in normal
plasma of males and females could modulate differently the transendothelial transport of LDL and provide a possible explanation for the lesser incidence of atherosclerotic coronary artery disease in premenopausal females.

2. The second implication deals with the possible role of endothelial cells in
the in vivo degradation of LDL. On the basis of certain measurements and calculations, one can estimate that the total mass of endothelial in a normal adult of
70 kg averages about 270 g. Assuming a protein content of endothelium of 15%,
this will equal 40 g of endothelial protein. In culture, endothelial cells were
shown to degrade 16 - 24 µg of LDL protein/mg cell protein/day, when presented

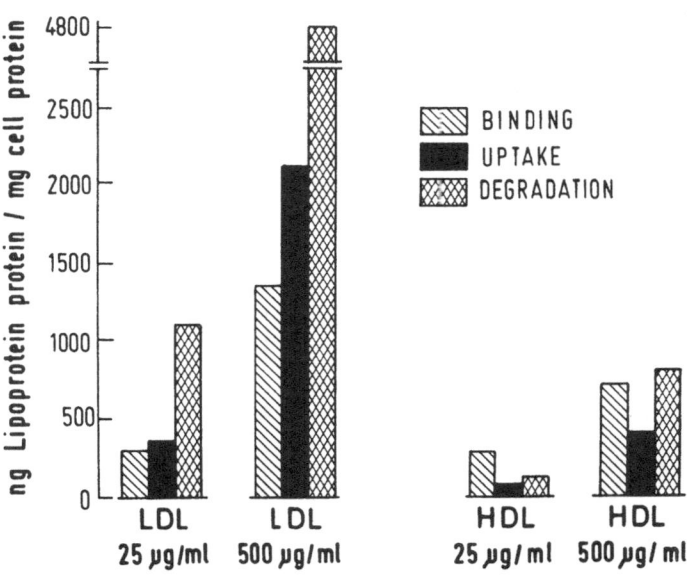

Figure 1. Interaction between endothelial cells and serum lipoprotein. Human
endothelial cells in culture were incubated for 6 h with ^{125}I LDL or ^{125}I HDL.
Binding was determined as trypsin releasable radioactivity, uptake as protein
radioactivity remaining in the cell pellet after trypsinization. Degradation was
measured by estimation of noniodine TCA soluble ^{125}I in the culture medium

with 600 µg of LDL protein/ml. Extrapolating these in vitro data to in vivo conditions, one can postulate that in a normal adult of 70 kg the total endothelial cell mass could degrade 0.64-0.96 g of LDL protein/day.

Enrichment and Depletion of Cultured Human Skin Fibroblasts and Rat Aortic Smooth Muscle Cells With Cholesterol and Cholesterol Ester

Under normal conditions, cellular cholesterol remains fairly constant, but accumulation of cholesterol ester in cells of mesenchymal origin is the hallmark of atherosclerosis. Presently, human skin fibroblasts and rat aortic smooth muscle cells in culture served as a model system to study intracellular cholesterol ester deposition in mesenchymal cells. Confluent cultures of human skin fibroblasts were exposed to homologous low-density lipoprotein alone and together with chloroquine. In the presence of low-density lipoprotein alone, even at half the circulating serum concentration, cellular-free cholesterol increased no more than 12%, while the increase in cholesterol ester ranged from 13 - 100% during 48 h of incubation. Addition of chloroquine to the culture medium containing low-density lipoprotein resulted in a very marked increase in cholesterol ester and the ratio of cellular esterified cholesterol to free cholesterol rose up to 2.2. (Fig. 2). The ultrastructural changes produced by LDL and chloroquine are illustrated in Figure 3 and consist of accumulation of particular and granular material in large membrane-bound vacuoles. Qualitatively similar results were obtained also with rat aortic smooth muscle cells (Table 1). In the presence of chloroquine and human low-density lipoprotein, there was a very significant accumulation of cholesterol ester. The magnitude of cholesterol ester accretion was inversely related to the cell density in the Petri dish, especially when cellular protein exceeded 2.0 mg. In both cell types the sum of uptake and degradation of ^{125}I low-density lipoprotein was enhanced in the presence of 20 µM chloroquine and at higher chloroquine concentrations (50 - 70 µM), the more pronounced inhibition of degradation resulted in the intracellular retention of undegraded protein.

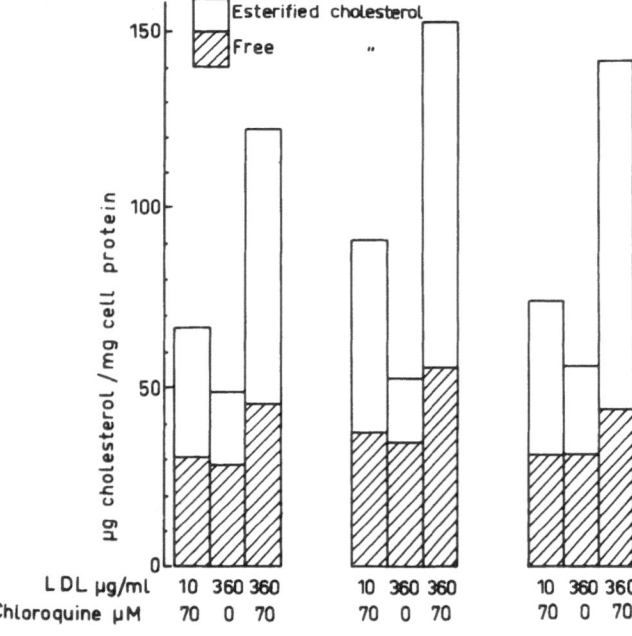

Figure 2. Effect of chloroquine on the accumulation of cholesterol and cholesterol ester in human skin fibroblasts in culture, during 48 h

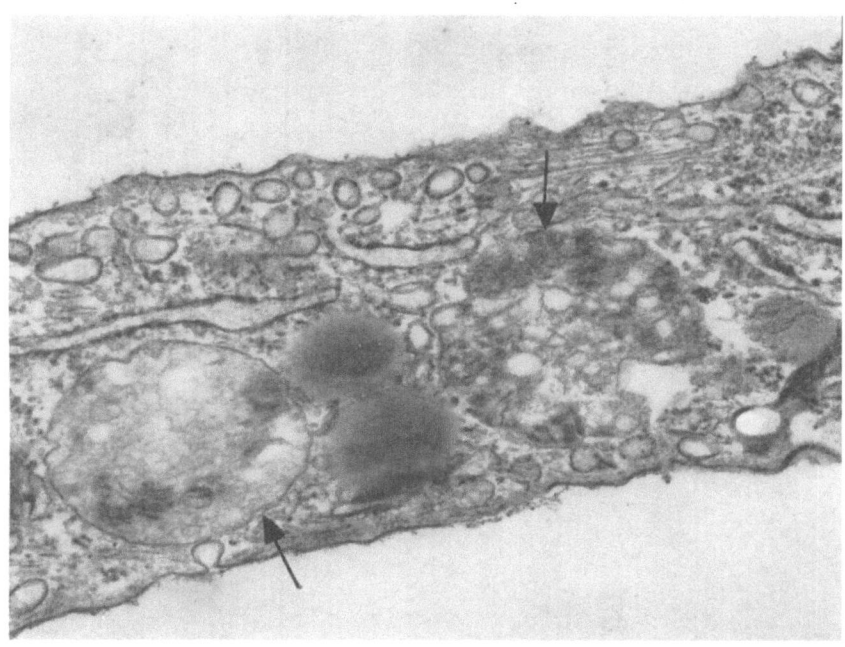

Figure 3. Electronmicrograph of a human skin fibroblast in culture exposed to LDL and chloroquine for 48 h. Note the presence of membrane-bounded vacuoles filled with material (arrows) and cytoplasmic lipid droplets (X 51,000)

Table 1. Cholesterol content of rat aortic smooth muscle cells treated with human low-density lipoprotein (LDL) and chloroquine for 2 and 4 days

Treatment, h	LDL protein µg/ml	Chloroquine µM	Cellular cholesterol µg/mg cell protein	
			Free	Ester
0	0	0	24.6	0.9
48	330	50	35.6	27.8
96	330	50	32.0	20.7

Upon removal of the chloroquine containing medium, there was a slight fall in the cellular cholesterol after 24 h incubation in a medium containing 10% fetal calf serum. Replacement of the fetal calf serum by lipoprotein deficient serum and a mixture of high-density apolipoprotein and sonicated sphingomyelin (Stein et al., 1976; Stein and Stein, 1973) increased very significantly the loss of total cholesterol from the cells. The morphologic counterpart of these events is shown in Figure 4. The present results provide an adequate and reproducible model system for the study of cholesterol accumulation in human mesenchymal cells, which is one of the basic changes in atheromatosis. The availability of choles-terol ester laden cells also provides a good system for the study of agents ac-tive in cholesterol removal.

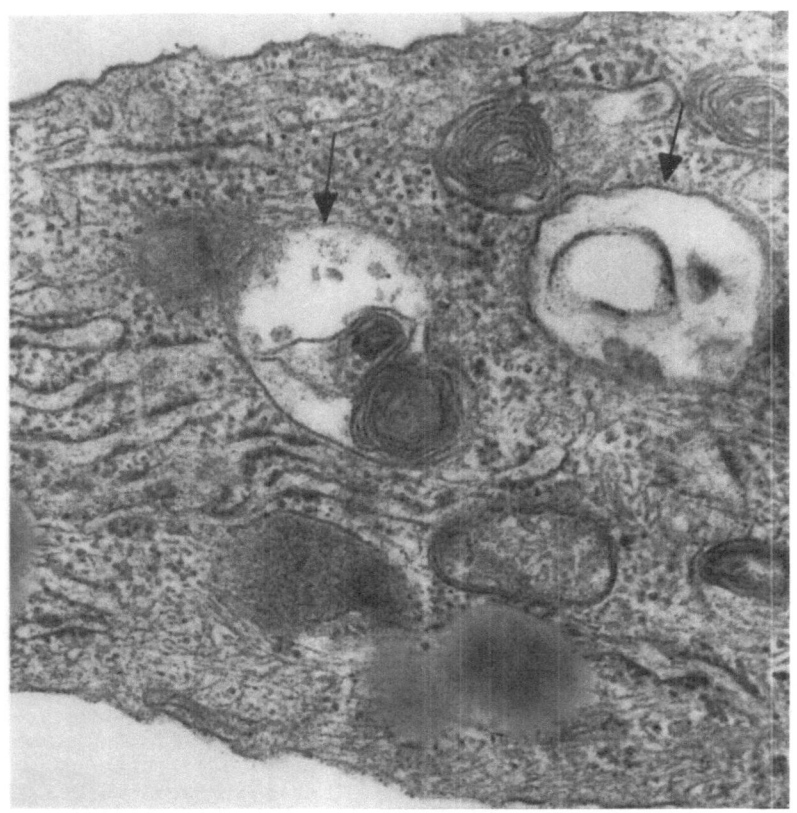

Figure 4. Electronmicrograph of a human skin fibroblast which had been enriched
with cholesterol ester by exposure to LDL and chloroquine for 48 h, and postin-
cubated with depleting medium for 24 h. Note the presence of membrane bound
vacuoles with little content, myelin figures, and cytoplasmic lipid droplets
(X 62,000)

CURRENT CONCEPTS OF HYPERLIPOPROTEINEMIA

Antonio M. Gotto, Jr.

Definitions

In discussing the current concepts of hyperlipoproteinemia, let me begin with the most basic definitions. First, the term *hyperlipidemia* is used to describe a condition in which the concentration of one or more of the plasma lipids, usually cholesterol or triglyceride, is elevated above normal limits. All definitions of hyperlipidemia are necessarily arbitrary. What is usually meant by a "normal" cholesterol or triglyceride, as reported from a clinical laboratory, is a statistical normal. This does not necessarily represent a safe or optimal or desirable level of the plasma lipid. Table 1 shows a list of arbitrarily chosen cutoff values for defining overt hyperlipidemia currently employed in the Lipid Clinic of The Methodist Hospital. There is no absolute cutoff point for either plasma cholesterol or triglyceride which divides the entire population into normal and abnormal groups.

Cholesterol and triglyceride concentrations are now routinely measured by autoanalyzer methods in most clinical laboratories. The fluorescence technique for determining triglyceride is one of high accuracy and precision. On the Technicon Autoanalyzer II, the Zak procedure was used with ferric chloride reagent for measuring cholesterol. On the Technicon Autoanalyzer II, the Lieberman-Burchardt reaction is used. The autoanalyzer II methodology gives cholesterol values that are slightly higher than the standard Abell-Kendall procedure. Determination of cholesterol in an unextracted sample, as employed in the SMA-12 procedure, may give a cholesterol value as much as 15 – 20% higher than the Abell-Kendall procedure.

Table 1. Cutoff values for defining overt hyperlipidemia[a] (from the Methodist Hospital Lipid Clinic

Age	Cholesterol	Triglycerides
1-9	200	120
10-19	205	140
20-29	210	140
30-39	240	150
40-49	265	160
>50	265	190

[a] These values should not necessarily be considered as safe ones. We do not know what a "normal" or "safe" cholesterol or triglyceride concentration is at the present time.

Hyperlipidemia as a diagnosis does not specify which of the families of plasma lipoproteins is elevated, although one can usually make a judicious guess. When the hyperlipidemia is defined in terms of a specific family or families of plasma lipoproteins, the term hyperlipoproteinemia then becomes appropriate. As with hyperlipidemia, the definition of hyperlipoproteinemia also is arbitrary as there are not clearly identifiable cutoff points for separating the lipoprotein concentrations of the population into normal and abnormal groups. Elevations of the plasma lipoproteins, thus arbitrarily defined, are classified on the basis of lipoprotein patterns or phenotypes. I would like to emphasize that an abnormal lipoprotein phenotype is not a disease. There are diseases or disorders to which I will make reference later which are associated with abnormal lipoprotein phenotypes. These include the familial or genetic hyperlipoproteinemias and the secondary hyperlipoproteinemias.

Historical Aspects

I would like to gave a brief historical summary that may help explain how we arrived at our present concept of the hyperlipoproteinemias. Medical knowledge of these disorders began in the 19th century with the anatomical observations of lipid deposits on the skin. One of the earliest such descriptions was reported in a publication of the Guy's Hospital of London in 1851 by Addison and Gull. They first used the term xanthoma to refer to fatty deposits on the skin. In this early period, the lesions were called xanthoma tuberosa, which very likely included tendinous xanthomas (those attached to tendons), tuberous xanthomas (unattached to tendons), and planar xanthomas (as occur in the palmar creases or around the eyelids). Another category of xanthomas was recognized on diabetics; they were called xanthoma diabeticorum. Subsequent observers discovered that these lesions occur also in nondiabetics as well as in diabetics who have turbid or lactesant plasma.

The next stage of development came with the introduction of methods for measuring concentrations of blood lipids and with the recognition of familial hyperlipoproteinemias. In some families, the disorder was primarily one of hypercholesterolemia, while in others, the triglycerides were elevated. One of the most significant developments was the discovery in 1929 of the plasma lipoproteins by Macheboeuf. In the late 1940's, the lipoproteins were studied extensively by Oncley and his group (1963) at Harvard and by Gofman and his colleagues (Jones et al., 1951) at the Donner Laboratory at Berkeley. Gofman's group (Jones et al., 1951) used primarily the analytic ultracentrifuge for their studies. They called attention to a high incidence of vascular disease in subjects with elevations of LDL and of VLDL. Clinical manifestions were becoming associated with the hypercholesterolemic and with the hypertriglyceridemic disorders. Dr. Ahrens and his colleagues (1961) at the Rockefeller University introduced a terminology of the fat-sensitive and carbohydrate-sensitive lipemias.

With the impetus of the work from Gofman's laboratory and with findings such as illustrated in Figure 1, that high levels of cholesterol are associated statistically with an increased frequency of early coronary artery disease, a controversy arose in the United States in the 1950's. The question was whether there was any advantage to measuring lipoproteins as contrasted to cholesterol concentration. One group of investigators on a national panel in the United States reached the conclusion that measurements of lipoprotein concentrations were no more useful than a simple determination of plasma cholesterol as a predictor of coronary atherosclerosis (Lewis et al., 1956). Doctor Gofman did not share this view (Gofman et al., 1956).

An important advance was made in the early 1960's by Hatch and Lees (1968) who introduced the use of albuminated buffer for the improved separation of lipoproteins on paper electrophoresis. Fredrickson et al. (1967) used this paper electrophoresis system for evolving a classification of the hyperlipoproteinemias which has been subsequently embodied by the World Health Organization (Beaumont

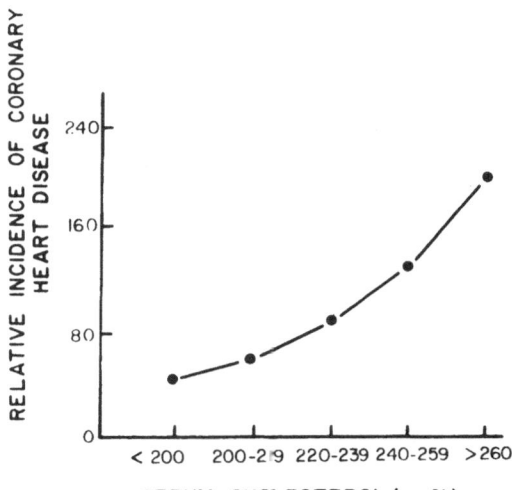

Figure 1. Relationship of serum cholesterol concentration to the relative incidence of coronary heart disease (from
the population studies of Ancel Keys)

et al., 1970). A sixth phenotype has been added to the original five. This is
the type IIb pattern in which there is both hypercholesterolemia and hypertriglyceridemia, with elevations of β- and pre-β-lipoproteins; in the original system of Fredrickson and Lees (1966), this pattern was called type III. As further
information has accumulated, the original definitions have been modified and
electrophoresis for the most part is used as a qualitative adjunct for the diagnosis. Recent improvements with agarose electrophoresis of lipoproteins may make
it possible to use this technique to quantify the individual classes by means of
densitomitry. Presently, individual lipoprotein classes are measured on the
basis of their cholesterol concentration, except for chylomicrons which are determined qualitatively. This procedure has been called lipoprotein quantification
or β-quantification and employs precipitation with heparin and manganese in conjunction with preparative ultracentrifugation and cholesterol measurements (Fredrickson et al., 1967).

Lipoprotein Phenotypes

Confusion has arisen from the use of the lipoprotein phenotypes, which are diagnosed simply from laboratory determinations (DHEW Publication, 1974), with specific inherited or genetic disorders of lipoprotein metabolism. There is not a one
to one correspondence between a lipoprotein phenotype and genotype. Thus, it becomes impossible to apply the Roman numeral system to the designation of the
genetic dyslipoproteinemias, since more than one given lipoprotein phenotype may
be found within an individual and kindred.

The major lipoprotein phenotypes are summarized in Table 2. Type I is defined as
fasting chylomicronemia with an absolute deficiency of adipose tissue lipoprotein
lipase or triglyceride lipase, type IIa by an increase in LDL or the β-lipoproteins, type IIb by an increase in LDL and VLDL, and type III by the presence of
floating β-lipoproteins. This last term refers to the occurrence in VLDL of lipoproteins which have β-mobility on electrophoresis. In type IV, there is an increase in VLDL or pre-β-lipoproteins, and in type V, there is chylomicronemia
with an increase in VLDL. Lipoprotein lipase from adipose tissue is present, but
may be diminished in activity. Secondary causes of hyperlipoproteinemia include
hypothyroidism, diabetes mellitus, the nephrotic syndrome, renal failure, alcoholism, obstructive liver disease, pancreatitis, dysglobulinemia, glycogen
storage disease, and porphyria.

Table 2. Hyperlipoproteinemia[a]. Characteristics of plasma lipoprotein phenotypes

Type	Definition	Cholesterol	Triglycerides	Plasma ratio (weight % of C/TG)[b]	Fasting chylomicrons	LDL[b]	VLDL[b]	HDL[b]
I	Hyperchylomicronemia with absolute deficiency of LPL[b] or PHLA[b]	Normal or ↑	Greatly ↑	<0.2	Present	Normal or ↓	Mildly ↑, normal or ↓	Absent
IIA	↑ LDL	↑	Normal	>1.5	Absent	↑	Normal or ↓	Normal
IIB	↑ LDL and ↑ VLDL	↑	↑	Variable	Absent	↑	↑	Normal
III	Floating[c] β-lipoprotein	↑	↑	Approximately 1 [d] [e]	Present may be ↑	d1.006–1.019↑ d1.019–1.063↓ [f]	↑ [c] [g]	Normal or ↓
IV	↑ VLDL	Normal or ↑	↑	Variable	Absent	↓ or normal	↑	Normal or ↓
V	Hyperchylomicronemia and ↑ VLDL LPL or PHLA present but reduced	Normal or ↑	Greatly ↑	>0.15 <0.60 TG/C >0.5	↑	↓ or normal	↑	Usually ↓

[a]Adapted from: (Gotto, 1974; Goldstein et al., 1973b; Fredrickson and Levy, 1972; Beaumont et al., 1970; Goldstein et al., 1976; Utermann et al., 1975; Fredrickson et al., 1975; Hazzard et al., 1972; Patsch et al., 1975).

[b]Abbreviations: LPL = Diacylglycerol; PHLA = Postheparin lipolytic activity; LDL = Low-density lipoprotein; VLDL = Very low-density lipoprotein; HDL = High-density lipoprotein; C = Cholesterol; TG = Triglyceride.

[c]"Floating" β-lipoproteins: indicates presence of an abnormal plasma lipoprotein of density <1.006 gram per ml with β-electrophoretic mobility in addition to pre-β migrating LP (Fredrickson and Levy, 1972).

[d]When the plasma triglyceride concentration is between 150 and 1,000 mgm/100 ml, a ratio of VLDL cholesterol to the plasma triglyceride concentration ≥0.30 is suggested to be diagnostic of type III Hyperlipoproteinemia (Fredrickson et al., 1975).

Table 2. Continued

Appearance of plasma	Genetic hyperlipidemia in which this phenotype may be present	Secondary disease that may cause this lipoprotein deficiency
"Cream" layer over a clear infranatant	Familial[h] lipoprotein lipase deficiency	Diabetic acidosis Hypothyroidism Dysglobulinemia Insulin dependent diabetes
Clear	Familial[i] hypercholesterolemia Familial[i] combined hyperlipidemia Polygenic[j] hypercholesterolemia	Hypothyroidism Dysglobulinemia Nephrosis Obstructive liver disease Dietary excess Autoimmune Cushing's disease Acute Intermittent porphyria
Usually turbid; may be also faint	Familial[i] broad-β disease	Secondary causes are rare as: Diabetes mellitus Autoimmune hyperlipoproteinemia Hypothyroidism Renal insufficiency
Usually turbid	Familial[i] hypertriglyceridemia Familial[i] combined hyperlipidemia	Diabetes mellitus Hypothyroidism Dysglobulinemia Obstructive liver disease

"Cream layer"	Familial[i] hypertriglyceridemia
	Familial[i] mixed or type V hyperlipidemia
	Familial[i] combined hyperlipidemia (rarely)
		Nephrotic syndrome
		Uremia
		Glycogen storage disease
		Alcoholism
		Pancreatitis
		Drugs:
		   Estrogens
		   Steroids
		   Other hormones

[e]VLDL Cholesterol/VLDL Triglycerides >0.42 is suggested to be diagnostic of type III in hypertriglyceridemic subjects (Hazzard et al., 1972).

[f]The lipoproteins of density 1.006-1.019 are called LDL$_1$. More recently, the term "intermediate density lipoprotein(s)" (IDL) has been employed for this density class. In the postabsorptive plasma of type III subjects, it is typically present in increased concentration and appears upon zonal ultracentrifugation in a density gradient as a distinct lipoprotein between VLDL and LDL$_2$ (d1.019-1.063) (Patsch et al., 1975).

[g]The VLDL "arginine-rich" protein (ApoE-III) in type III is missing one of its 3 polymorphic appearances, when using isoelectric focusing of this protein (deficiency of ApoE-III) (Utermann et al., 1975).

[h]Autosomal recessive mode of inheritance. [i]Autosomal dominant mode of inheritance.

[j]Polygenic mode of inheritance.

Inherited Hyperlipoproteinemia

Familial Lipoprotein Lipase Deficiency

The relationship between genetic hyperlipoproteinemias and lipoprotein phenotyping is a complex one. The genetic disorder called familial lipoprotein lipase deficiency is virtually always associated with type I phenotypic pattern. It occurs in children and is associated with abdominal pain, pancreatitis, eruptive xanthomas, fat sensitivity, and an absolute deficiency of lipoprotein lipase from adipose tissue. This activity is released into plasma after intravenous injection of heparin in normal subjects. Postheparin lipoprotein lipase has two major origins, hepatic and adipose tissue. The adipose tissue enzyme requires apoC-II for activation (Havel et al., 1973; LaRosa et al., 1970) and is inhibitied by protamine sulfate and high concentrations of salt. The hepatic enzyme does not show these characteristics and a test for inhibition with protamine sulfate or high concentrations of sodium chloride is required to distinguish between the two sources of activity. In familial lipoprotein lipase deficiency, the adipose tissue enzyme is absent, and this results in a type I lipoprotein phenotype.

Familial Hypercholesterolemia and Familial Combined Hyperlipidemia

Familial hypercholesterolemia has been known as a clinical entity for a number of years. In literature for the last ten years, this entity has been referred to as familial type II hyperlipoproteinemia. It affects all ages, is found in all parts of the world, is characterized by the presence of tendinous xanthomas, and is transmitted as a dominant trait. There is a devastatingly high incidence of early coronary artery disease, the average age of the first myocardial infarction being 40 – 45 years in males. The clinical hallmark of this disorder and particularly what distinguishes it from combined familial hyperlipidemia is an elevation of LDL from birth. Combined familial hyperlipidemia is also associated with premature coronary disease, but is not usually diagnosed biochemically until adulthood. Both inherited dyslipidemias appear to be transmitted as monogenic, dominant traits based on distributions of LDL or cholesterol in affected kindreds (Fredrickson and Levy, 1972; Goldstein et al., 1973a). In the Seattle study by Goldstein et al. of the distribution of hyperlipidemia in 164 survivors of myocardial infarctions, combined hyperlipidemia was the most common familial form of dyslipidemia, followed by familial hypertriglyceridemia (14% of total) and familial hypercholesterolemia (10% of total).

Goldstein and Brown (1975) have identified a cellular biochemical defect in the homozygotes of some kindreds with familial hypercholesterolemia. The studies, carried out with fibroblasts of homozygotes grown in tissue cultures, must be interpreted in light of the current state of knowledge concerning the cellular metabolism of LDL. LDL is thought to be irreversibly catabolized in peripheral tissues. While intracellular cholesterol is available for membrane synthesis, it must ultimately be transported back to the liver for excretion in the bile either as cholesterol or bile acid. A cell receptor that binds LDL is believed to regulate the uptake of this lipoprotein by peripheral tissues. Synthesis of the cell receptors for LDL may be regulated by the intracellular level of cholesterol so that when the cholesterol concentration rises, fewer receptors would be made. LDL is transported into the cell and taken up by lysozomes where it is then catabolized. Under ordinary conditions, when cells are grown in tissue culture, there is an inverse relationship between the concentration of LDL in the medium and the intracellular cholesterol synthesis (Rothblat, 1969; Bailey, 1966; Williams and Avigan, 1972). This relationship does not hold in fibroblasts from some subjects who are homozygotes for familial hypercholesterolemia. In such individuals, Brown and Goldstein (1974) have postulated that there is an absence of the LDL receptor. In the heterozygote state, approximately 40% of the normal receptors are present. Subsequent to the initial observations, kindreds with familial hypercholesterolemia have been identified in which homozygotes appear to have a defective rather than an absent receptor (Avigan et al., 1975; Breslow et al., 1975; Goldstein et al., 1975). Such homozygotes with a defective LDL receptor cannot be distinguished from the heterozygotes by the fibroblast markers. Free cholesterol in an ethanolic suspension can by-pass the LDL receptor mechanism. More polar sterol derivatives, such as 25-hydroxycholesterol and 7-ketocholesterol, are much more effective than cholesterol in suppressing HMG CoA reductase activity (Kandutsch and Chen, 1973, 1974; Brown and Goldstein, 1974).

Alternative explanations have been suggested to account for the biochemical defect in familial hypercholesterolemia. In one homozygous subject, the cells are reported to be defective in internalizing LDL but not in binding it (Stein et al., 1976). Fogelman et al. (1973, 1975) have inferred from studies with leukocytes of heterozygotes that the defect resides in an inappropriate loss of intracellular cholesterol. Because of the increased loss of cholesterol from the cell, there is a compensatory increase in intracellular level of HMG CoA reductase. Bilheimer et al. (1975) have provided evidence that some homozygotes may oversynthesize cholesterol or LDL. Regardless of the specific localization or identification of the biochemical lesion, the studies with homozygotes for familial hypercholesterolemia have been a great impetus for investigation of the regulation of cholesterol metabolism at the cellular level and in the whole organism.

Starzl et al. (1973) have described the results of performing a portal caval shunt operation in a homozygous child. After the surgery, the plasma cholesterol concentration decreased remarkably and the xanthomas disappeared. Angina pectoris was no longer present. A change in the ratio of glucagon to insulin was noted and it was postulated that this effect may be related to hypocholesterolemic phenomenon. Unfortunately, the experience with other patients has not yielded such spectular results and has not been effective enough to recommend that this procedure be applied.

Familial Broad-β Disease

The type III phenotype is characteristic of the primary or genetic hyperlipoproteinemia called familial broad-β disease. There is no absolutely specific diagnostic criterion for this genotype or phenotype. I have referred earlier to the occurrence in type III of an abnormal lipoprotein in the VLDL with β-electrophoretic mobility. The presence of the abnormal lipoprotein causes the VLDL to have a higher than usual content of cholesterol; this phenomenon has led to the suggestion of several criteria to diagnose broad-β disease (Fredrickson et al., 1975; Hazzard et al., 1972; Patsch et al., 1975). The designation floating β-lipoprotein is based on experiments in which VLDL is isolated in a single spin in a fixed angle head rotor at the plasma density of approximately 1.006 gm/cc (Fredrickson et al., 1967). If instead of this procedure, the plasma is spun in the zonal centrifuge, then the β-migrating component can be separated from the VLDL (Patsch et al., 1975). Under these conditions, floating β-lioprotein is not found in the VLDL. The remaining VLDL has pre-β, rather than β-mobility. The hallmark of broad-β disease is a remarkable increase in the concentration of the IDL fraction (density 1.006 to 1.019 gm/cc) which Patsch et al. (1975) have referred to as lipoprotein-III (LP-III). This phenomenon is illustrated in Figure 2. IDL contain apoB as the major apoprotein constituent (Shore and Shore, 1973), have less cholesterol and much more triglyceride and LDL, and are 210 to 350 Å in diameter (Patsch et al., 1976). Small amounts of IDL are present in other metabolic circumstances.

Another property of the VLDL in broad-β disease is an unusually high content of the arginine-rich protein (Shore and Shore, 1973; Havel and Kane, 1973). According to Utermann et al. (1974), one of the three polymorphic components of the arginine-rich protein of VLDL in broad-β disease is missing. These components are identified by isoelectric focusing of the protein. The significance of these various findings to the pathophysiology of the disorder remains to be determined.

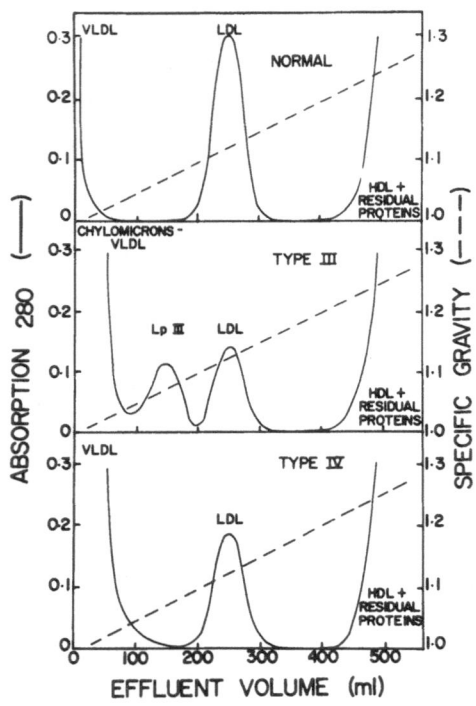

Figure 2. Distribution of plasma lipoproteins in the zonal ultracentrifuge
from a normal subject (upper panel), a
subject with type III phenotype (middle
panel), and a subject with a type IV
phenotype (Courtesy of Dr. Josef Patsch)

However, they are consistent with a defect in the following sequence: VLDL→IDL→
LDL, such that an abnormal quantity of IDL accumulates.

Familial Hypertriglyceridemia

The most common of the hyperlipoproteinemias encountered in the United States is
familial hypertriglyceridemia, often referred to as type IV or endogenous hypertriglyceridemia. Evidence exists for an oversynthesis of VLDL in some subjects
and for a decreased VLDL catabolism in others. In the Seattle study of Goldstein
et al. (1973b), the inheritance of familial hypertriglyceridemia was described
as monogenic. It seems likely that more than one type of mutation will be identified, since the subjects exhibit a variety of biochemical characteristics, such
as the concentration of LDL present. No biochemical markers have yet been identified. The type IV phenotype is at times inappropriately diagnosed because of confusion due to the presence of lipoprotein a[+] in a significant proportion of the
normal population (Albers et al., 1974; Simons et al., 1970). This lipoprotein
has pre-β mobility but does not float with VLDL, which has led it to be designated
as "sinking pre-β lipoprotein".

Weight reduction and alcohol restriction are efficacious in managing endogenous
hypertriglyceridemia. Disagreement exists as to whether or not carbohydrate restriction is necessary. The group of patients described by Ahrens et al. (1961)
as having carbohydrate-sensitive lipemia most likely manifested endogenous hypertriglyceridemia. However, not all patients with this hyperlipoproteinemia are excessively sensitive to dietary carbohydrate.

Since the type IV lipoprotein phenotype is so commonly encountered, I would like
to briefly share our own experience in its management (Gotto et al., 1976a, submitted for publication). Two hundred seventy-eight adult patients were identified
whose plasma lipid and lipoprotein concentrations were diagnostic of a type IV
phenotype. Secondary causes were excluded. One hundred three of these patients,
called group A, were followed over a period of 2 years with an average number of

clinic visits of three per year. At the initial visit, the patients were examined by a physician and instructed by a dietitian. On subsequent visits, the patient saw a physician or a dietitian or both. Group B represented patients with the same phenotype, but who came to The Methodist Hospital only on a yearly basis for a checkup. This group was given no personal dietary instruction and no consultation for the hyperlipoproteinemia. However, after they returned home, a copy of the diet booklet was mailed to the patient's physician with the recommendation that the patient follow it. Over the same 2-year period, Group A had a reduction in the mean plasma triglyceride from 381 mg% to 263 mg%. There was no significant change in triglyceride concentration of Group B. There was significant weight reduction in Group A, but not in Group B. Changes in the cholesterol concentration were not of statistical significance. This study illustrates the utility of regular dietary counseling in the treatment of endogenous hypertriglyceridemia and shows that triglyceride concentrations can be significantly changed over long periods of time through dietary intervention and weight reduction.

Familial Type V Hyperlipoproteinemia

The most appropriate trivial name for primary, or familial type V hyperlipoproteinemia seems to be type V. One study of familial type V did not find evidence for a monogenic inheritance (Fallot and Glueck, 1976). Affected family members may have either a type IV or a type V phenotype (Fredrickson and Levy, 1972). The association of both type V and familial hypertriglyceridemia with hyperuricemia remains an enigma, but a fascinating one. The relationship with glucose intolerance also has not been elucidated. A typical patient with primary type V is an adult with a diabetic glucose tolerance test, hyperuricemia and abdominal pain. The severity of the disorder is made worse by estrogens, obesity, and alcohol consumption. Acute hemorrhage pancreatitis is a potentially fatal outcome. While the mechanism of primary type V has not been worked out, Simons and Williams (1975) have obtained results which they interpret as indicating a block in the conversion of VLDL to LDL. The concentration of VLDL is increased while that of LDL is decreased in this disorder.

An Approach to Hyperlipoproteinemia

Decisions about hyperlipoproteinemia are summarized in Figure 3. The most important measurements are those of fasting plasma cholesterol and triglyceride. Valuable information can be obtained by the appearance of the serum. It is sometimes necessary to measure lipoproteins. The most convenient way of doing this is by electrophoresis. Lipoproteins should be measured if the level of cholesterol is considered borderline, e.g., 240 - 280 mg/dl, in order to determine the concentration of LDL cholesterol. Also, if both cholesterol and triglyceride are elevated, it is desirable to measure lipoproteins to determine whether there is an increase in LDL or if broad-β disease is present. Differentiation of primary versus secondary etiology requires medical evaluation. Whether the disorder is familial necessitates family screening. Finally, the consideration of treatment depends upon the phenotype, the condition of the patient, and the clinical and biochemical variables which are present. The most clear-cut indication for treating hyperlipoproteinemia is abdominal pain. We still do not have an answer as to whether or not treatment will reduce the risk of heart disease; this is a presumed but unproven benefit.

Continuous Relationship of Plasma Cholesterol and Triglyceride with Coronary Artery Disease

I would like to turn to the question of measuring lipoproteins versus cholesterol or triglyceride concentrations as indicators of coronary artery disease and to the significance of the absolute values for each lipid. We have recently com-

DECISIONS ABOUT HYPERLIPOPROTEINEMIA

1. What is the Type?

    a) Always do C, TG
    b) Always look at serum
    c) Sometimes do lipoproteins

2. Primary vs. Secondary

3. Is it Familial?

4. Treatment

    a) Diet   (1) calories
               (2) content
    b) Drugs

Figure 3. An approach to the work-up and treatment of the patient with hyperlipoproteinemia

pleted a study of 496 subjects evaluated for chest pain by coronary arteriography at The Methodist Hospital (Gotto et al., 1976b, submitted for publication). We define coronary artery disease based on three different degrees of coronary narrowing, namely 75%, 50%, and 25%. The reason for this approach was to include in the study patients with milder forms of coronary artery disease. A vessel with less than 25% narrowing was defined as being free of coronary artery disease. The extent of disease was measured on the basis of the total number of coronary vessels with 25% or greater stenosis. One hundred six of the patients had no coronary artery disease by these criteria, while 390 had 25% or greater occlusion of one or more major vessel. Mean age for the group with coronary artery disease was 55.7 years, and without disease, 49.4 years. Both cholesterol and triglyceride concentrations were significantly higher in the group with coronary artery disease, with p <0.001 in each group. The plasma lipids were divided into quartiles. For each quartile, representing an increase in cholesterol concentration, there was a significant increase in the percentage of patients with coronary artery disease. A similar phenomenon was seen when this type of analysis was applied to the concentrations of plasma triglyceride, although the differences were not as great as with cholesterol. In an analysis of cholesterol concentrations and the extent of coronary artery disease, the mean cholesterol concentration in males increased from 195 mg/dl in the group without coronary disease, to 219 mg/dl in the group with three-vessel disease, and to 223 mg/dl in the group with four-vessel disease. The comparable rise in females from no disease to three-vessel was 207 to 252. Triglyceride concentrations had a similar but less consistent relationship with a measure of the extensiveness of coronary artery disease. When quartile analysis was performed on combined cholesterol and triglyceride values, again there was a progressive increase in the percentage of patients having coronary artery disease from those with the lowest lipid levels to those with the highest lipid levels. The age corrected correlation coefficients between the number of vessels involved were 0.201 for cholesterol and 0.181 for triglyceride. These correlations were significant at a P value of less than 6×10^{-5}.

When patients were stratified according to lipoprotein phenotypes, no significant relationships were found between types II and IV, or between type II and IV and the normal groups with respect to frequency of coronary artery disease. The finding was the same whether the 25%, 50%, or 75% obstruction criterion was used. When comparing the extent of disease for patients, with and without hyperlipoproteinemia, there was a slight difference between the type IV and normals, but not between the type II and normals or between the type II and type IV groups. I wish to emphasize the point that many patients with severe coronary artery disease had lipid levels below the criteria for hyperlipidemia as defined by The Lipid Research Clinics and by most clinical laboratories. The fourth and highest quartile in our patients start from a cholesterol concentration of 236 mg/dl. We were unable to identify a critical cutoff point for either cholesterol or triglyceride levels which separated those with coronary artery disease and those without disease. In our population, we found a continuous relation between cholesterol and triglyceride levels and the frequency and extent of coronary disease. We concluded from this study that the use of arbitrary cutoff values to define hyperlipidemia or hyperlipoproteinemia may be misleading. In regard to coronary artery disease, a physician may find it of greater value to consider the actual plasma lipid levels in the management of the patient. Thus, we come full cycle to the recommendation of Lewis et al. as reported in 1956 concerning measurements of cholesterol versus lipoproteins as an indicator of coronary artery disease. Nonetheless, there is no doubt that the emphasis on plasma lipoproteins and on measurements of these macromolecules has been a great stimulus to investigations of their structure, of their metabolism, of their contribution to pathophysiology of the lipid transport disorders, and of atherosclerosis. While not recommended for screening purposes, determination of the lipoprotein phenotype in a given patient may be highly useful in the management of the dyslipoproteinemias.

WORKSHOP 6. Lipoproteins

Chairmen: A.M. Scanu, USA
C. Naito, Japan

Participants: P. Alaupovic, USA
G. Shipley, USA
D. Seidel, BRD
H. Peeters, Belgium
G. Assmann, BRD
A.M. Scanu, USA

ELECTROIMMUNOASSAYS OF SERUM APOLIPOPROTEINS IN NORMOLIPIDEMIC SUBJECTS AND PATIENTS WITH PRIMARY HYPERLIPOPROTEINEMIAS

Petar Alaupovic, Michael D. Curry, and Walter J. McConathy

A number of studies from this and other laboratories have demonstrated the protein heterogeneity of all major density lipoprotein classes of human serum (Alaupovic et al., 1972; Blum and Levy, 1975). These findings led to the concept (Alaupovic et al., 1972) of lipoprotein families as the fundamental physicochemical components of the serum lipoprotein system. The lipoprotein family concept is based on apolipoproteins as the only distinct chemical markers by which lipoproteins may be identified and differentiated. At the present time, this concept recognize the existence of five lipoprotein families, each of which is characterized by the exclusive presence of a single apolipoprotein: lipoprotein family A (LP-A) is characterized by the presence of apolipoprotein A (apoA or its constitutive A-I and A-II polypeptides), lipoprotein B (LP-B) by apolipoprotein B (apoB), lipoprotein C (LP-C) by apolipoprotein C (apoC or its constitutive C-I, C-II, and C-III polypeptides), lipoprotein D (LP-D) by apolipoprotein D (apoD or "thin-line" polypeptide), and lipoprotein E by apolipoprotein E (apoE or "arginine-rich" polypeptide).

To establish the concentration profiles of lipoprotein families in normolipidemic subjects and patients with familial hyperlipoproteinemias, we have developed electroimmunoassays ("rocket" electrophoresis) for quantification of A-I, A-II, apoB, C-I, C-II, C-III, apoD and apoE. Purified apolipoproteins were used to prepare monospecific antisera (Alaupovic et al., 1972; McConathy and Alaupovic, 1976; Curry et al., 1976b) and to standardize assays. All apolipoproteins were also estimated by radial immunodiffusion and apoB by radioimmunoassay. The electroimmunoassays were shown to be sensitive, specific, rapid (time required for the completion of assays is 5-8 hours), and precise (both the within- and between-assay coefficients of variation are 5-8%). The assays are applicable to measurement of apolipoproteins in whole serum and lipoprotein density classes. The results correlate well with those obtained by either radial immunodiffusion (correlation coefficients, r, for apolipoproteins varied between 0.85 and 0.90) or radioimmunoassay (the correlation coefficient, r, for apoB was 0.92). The detailed procedures for the quantification of individual apolipoproteins have been published (Curry et al., 1976b; Curry et al., 1976a; Curry et al., 1977).

Preliminary results of the electroimmunoassays of apolipoproteins in the whole serum of normolipidemic adult men and women are shown in Table 1. This first complete set of data on the human serum apolipoprotein concentrations represent mean values for both sexes. Due to limited number of samples analyzed, it has not yet been possible to establish the mean values of apolipoprotein levels for sexes and age groups. As expected, the apoA polypeptides (A-I, 143 mg/dl, and

Table 1. Concentrations of serum apolipoproteins of normolipidemic subjects and patients with familial hyperlipoproteinemias[a]

Phenotype	A-I	A-II	ApoB	C-I	C-II	C-III	ApoD	ApoE
				mg/dl				
Normals (n = 50)	[b] 143±20	78±18	110±20	7±2	4±2	14±3	10±3	10±3
Type I (n = 5)	54±17	28±12	72±16	———— Not determined ————				
Type IIa (n = 48)			200±27					
Type IIb (n = 40)			200±30			25±9		
Type III (n = 6)			[c]	18±4	9±2	24±5		27±8
Type IV (n = 58)			[c]					26±9
Type V (n = 3)			[c]	25±6	15±4	33±9		25±6

[a]Only concentrations significantly different than normal are shown (p <0.001).
[b]Data are based on 30 serum samples from women and 20 serum samples from men.
[c]ApoB levels are moderately elevated but not statistically significant.

A-II, 78 mg/dl) and apoB (110 mg/dl) represent the major and the apoC polypeptides (C-I, 7 mg/dl, C-II, 4 mg/dl, and C-III, 14 mg/dl), apoD (10 mg/dl) and apoE (10 mg/dl) the minor apolipoproteins. Although it has been observed that women tend to have higher levels of apoA and lower levels of apoB than men, these differences have not been statistically significant. There were no differences between sexes with respect to the concentrations of apoC, apoD, and apoE. However, additional data are needed for a more definite conclusion regarding the sex and age differences.

The average weight ratio of A-I/A-II in the whole serum is 1.8 and the corresponding molar ratio is close to unity. These results differ from those based on spectrophotometric estimation of column chromatographic eluates of A-I and A-II indicating a weight ratio of 3 and a molar ratio of 2. Our studies indicated (Curry et al., 1976a, 1977) an incomplete separation of A-I and A-II and the presence of apoD in the eluates from Sephadex column as the most probable explanation for this discrepancy. The C-I, C-II, and C-III polypeptides seem to occur in the whole serum in a molar ratio of 3:1:3.

Results shown in Table 1 indicate some significant differences in the serum apolipoprotein levels between hyperlipoproteinemic phenotypes. Patients with hyperchylomicronemia (type I) are characterized by significantly lower levels of A-I, A-II, and apoB than normals. Patients with type IIa hypercholesterolemia only have increased levels of apoB, whereas patients with type IIb have increased levels of both apoB and C-III. Apolipoprotein profile of patients with endogenous hypertriglyceridemia (type IV) is characterized by a significant increase in the concentration of C-III and a slight increase in the concentration of apoB when compared to normal. As a result of this disproportionate increase in C-III, the molar ratio of C-I/C-III is reduced in patients with type IV disease. Both the patients with type III and type V hyperlipoproteinemias have elevated concentrations of apoC polypeptides and apoE. The concentration of apoB is also higher than in normals. Since there is a proportionate increase in the levels of apoC polypeptides, the molar ratio of C-I/C-III remains close to unity. These results reveal the occurrence of four apolipoprotein profiles characteristic of patients with familial hyperlipoproteinemias. The first profile is characterized by decreased levels of A-I and A-II (type I), the second by increased level of apoB (type IIa), the third by increased level of C-III and reduced molar ratio of C-I/C-III (type IV), and the fourth by elevated concentrations of apoC polypeptides and apoE (types III and V). These studies suggest that apolipoproteins may be better markers than lipids for studying the genetic basis of familial hyperlipoproteinemias and that the electroimmunoassay of apolipoproteins is the most suitable immunologic procedure for screening studies of large population samples.

LIPID ORGANIZATION IN HUMAN PLASMA LOW-DENSITY LIPOPROTEINS

G. Graham Shipley, Richard J. Deckelbaum, David Atkinson, and Donald M. Small

Introduction

Although there is agreement concerning the low resolution structure of plasma high-density lipoprotein, until recently, there was conflicting evidence regarding the molecular organization of low-density lipoprotein (LDL). In this paper, we will describe the use of small angle x-ray scattering (SAXRS) and differential scanning calorimetry (DSC) to clarify the structural organization of the neutral lipid components, the cholesterol esters, and triglycerides in LDL.

Results and Discussion

Figure 1a shows DSC curves of LDL. Three endothermic transitions are observed on heating: (1) a broad reversible transition between 20-40°C (ΔH = 0.5 cal/g LDL lipid) which is not affected by cooling to -60°C, (2) an irreversible transition between 65-90°C (ΔH = 1.0 cal/g LDL protein), (3) following the irreversible

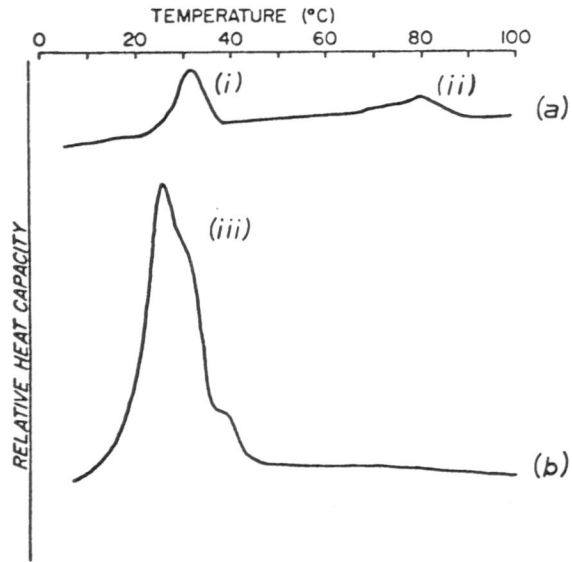

Figure 1. DSC heating curves of a single LDL sample. (a) 0-100°C; (b) 0-100°C after heating to 100°C and cooling to -60°C

high temperature transition and cooling to -60°C, a high enthalpy transition (ΔH ≃ 3 cal/g LDL lipid). On the basis of polarizing light microscopy and turbidity studies, we can define the irreversible transition centered at ~80°C as LDL denaturation with release of its cholesterol esters to form large oil droplets (Deckelbaum et al., 1975). The large enthalpy transition (5-45°C) following LDL denaturation is due mainly to the melting (crystal → liquid) of cholesterol ester crystals formed on cooling to -60°C (Deckelbaum et al., 1975).

Our early studies of the temperature-dependent small angle scattering of LDL, LDL cholesterol esters, and mixtures of pure cholesterol esters have demonstrated that the reversible transition (20-40°C) in LDL is due to a transition of its component cholesterol esters from a smectic-like structure to a more disordered liquid-like arrangement (Deckelbaum et al., 1975).

Our more recent studies have concentrated on (1) a more detailed analysis of the temperature-dependent SAXRS of LDL and (2) the influence of other molecular components of LDL on the reversible transition.

Temperature-Dependent SAXRS of LDL

The SAXRS profiles obtained from LDL at 10°C and 45°C are shown in Figures 2a and 2b, respectively. The series of scattering maxima at angles corresponding to $s < (1/40 \text{ Å}^{-1})$ are typical of the scattering from a quasi-spherical particle. The intense maximum at $s = 1/36 \text{ Å}^{-1}$ observed at 10°C is absent from the scattering profile from LDL at 45°C. The maxima in the scattering at $s < 1/40 \text{ Å}^{-1}$ are essentially identical at the two temperatures, demonstrating that the spherical morphology of LDL remains intact at 45°C. Although our early studies suggested that the presence of the $1/36 \text{ Å}^{-1}$ maximum is associated with an ordered smectic-

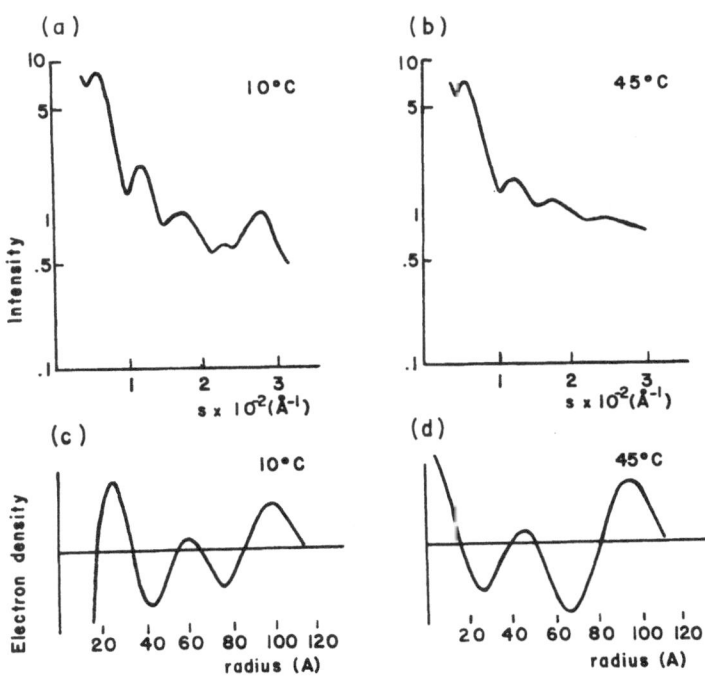

Figure 2. Microdensitometer traces of SAXRS curve of LDL at 10°C (a) and 45°C (b). Radial electron density distribution of LDL at 10°C (c) and 45°C (d) by Fourier transformation of the experimental data $(I^{1/2}(s))$

like arrangement of cholesterol esters in LDL (Deckelbaum et al., 1975), its precise origin is uncertain. This maximum may arise from either separate diffraction effects from organized microdomains of cholesterol ester in the core of the LDL particle or may be part of the fringe pattern due to the spherical morphology as "modified" by the internal organization of the particle. The electron density profiles calculated from the experimental data are shown in Figure 2c and 2d. The peak at ~ 100 Å arises from electron-rich surface-located phospholipid and protein. The electron density peaks at 30 and 60 Å in the profile for LDL at 10°C suggest a radial distribution of electron density in the core of the particle. The *trans*-form for LDL at 45°C showing a single peak at 40 Å indicates a change in the core organization.

Models of the molecular packing of the cholesterol esters within the core of LDL have been used to examine the origin of the scattering maximum at $1/36$ Å^{-1}, using as the starting point for cholesterol ester packing the crystal structure of cholesteryl myristate (Craven and de Titta, 1976) (Fig. 3a). The addition of four methylene groups to the myristate chain would not alter the chain packing provided an all-*trans* conformation is retained. The presence of *cis*-unsaturated double bonds in the hydrocarbon chains of the C_{18} cholesterol esters of LDL may, however, modify the crystal packing. Cholesterol esters in both the smectic and isotropic phase show a broad diffuse band at ~ 5 Å^{-1}, indicating a lack of short-range intermolecular order. For the smectic phase, this disorder of the cholesterol ester structure is simulated by a decrease in the length resulting from "melting" of both hydrocarbon regions. The overall length of the molecular pair of cholesterol esters is then approximately 38 Å, a value close to the dimension of 36 Å determined by the single diffraction line observed for LDL cholesterol esters in the smectic phase (Deckelbaum et al., 1975). The molecular packing is shown in Figure 3b.

At low resolution, the cholesterol ester molecule may be described by two electron density levels as shown in Figure 3c: (1) the two liquid hydrocarbon regions $\rho = 0.29$ e/Å^3 identical to that of the hydrocarbon region of a liquid crystalline phospholipid bilayer (Luzzati, 1968), (2) the fused steroid ring, $\rho = 0.42$ e/Å^3. These electron density levels are illustrated in Figure 3c.

Figure 3d shows the radial electron density distribution of a particle with two radial repeating units of cholesterol esters (the particle has a radius similar to that of native LDL, ~ 110 Å) and the scattering profile calculated for this distribution is shown in Figure 3e. The effect of the radially repeating structural organization within the particle is to produce a high relative intensity in the scattering fringe pattern at the angular region corresponding to the bilayer repeat spacing of 38 Å. The experimental scattering curve of LDL at 10°C exhibits a high relative intensity of only the fifth subsidary maximum at $1/36$ Å^{-1}, whereas the relative intensities of both the fourth ($1/50$ Å^{-1}) and the fifth ($1/38$ Å^{-1}) maxima are increased in the scattering curve for the model particle.

The high relative intensity of the fourth fringe in the calculated scattering curve arises from the electron density peaks approximately 50 Å apart (see Fig. 2c). Additional perturbations of the structure involving translation of the cholesterol ester pairs parallel to their long axis (Fig. 4a) remove these 50 Å correlations but still leave the organization dominated by the length of the molecular pair. The overlapping region of hydrocarbon chain and cholesterol moieties results in an average electron density higher than that of pure hydrocarbon. The overlapping sterol ring regions, however, produce an electron density distribution which contains only single peaks with 38 Å separation (Fig. 4b). This electron density profile radially oriented in a spherical particle of radius 110 Å (Fig. 4c) gives the scattering curve shown in Figure 4d. There is good qualitative agreement between the calculated scattering curve and the curve obtained from LDL at 10°C (cf. Fig. 2a).

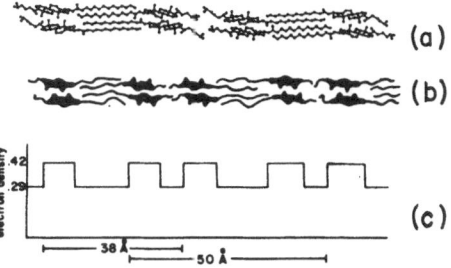

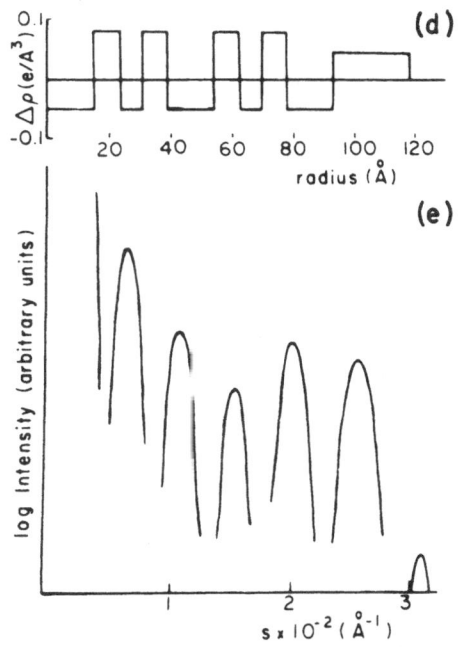

Figure 3. (a) Crystal packing of cholesteryl myristate (Craven and de Titta, 1976). (b) Schematic representation of the thermally perturbed structure with the hydrocarbon chains in a liquid-like conformation. (c) Electron density profile of the molecular packing shown in (b). (d) Model radial electron density distribution for a spherical particle containing two radially repeating bilayer units of cholesterol ester. The electron density peak at the surface of the particle (r = 93-118 Å) represents the location of the phospholipid polar groups and protein. (e) Calculated SAXRS curve (I(s) where s = 2 sin Θ/λ) from the model particle shown in (d)

The effect of the order → disorder transition was simulated by further lateral perturbations of the cholesterol ester packing resulting in an averaged, uniform electron density (Fig. 4e and 4f). With this uniform core electron density (Fig. 4g) the scattering curve shown in Figure 4h results. The fifth maximum now has a relative intensity lower than the fourth, in agreement with the experimental scattering curve from LDL at 45°C in which the fifth maximum is not observed (see Fig. 2b).

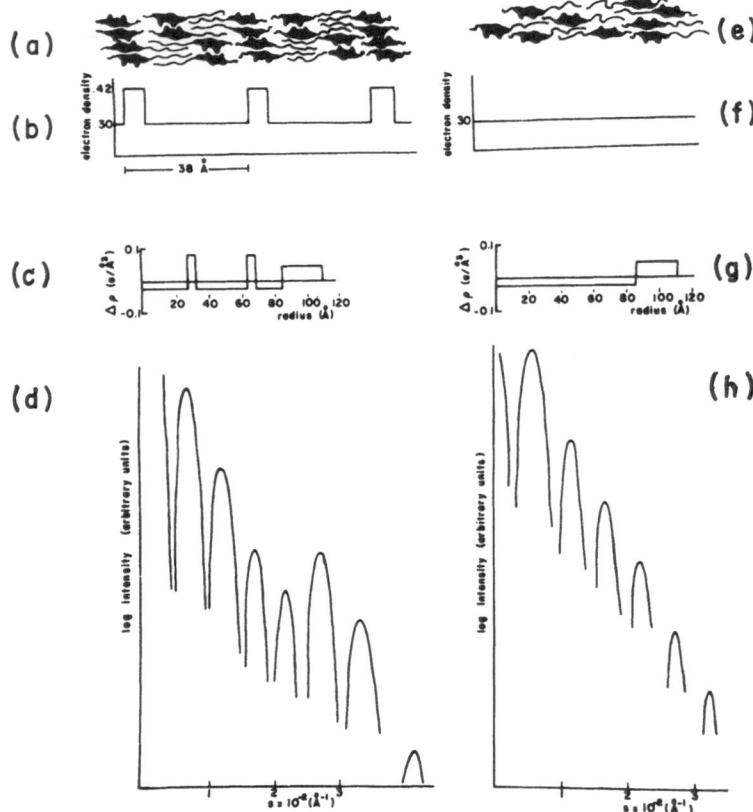

Figure 4. (a) Perturbation of the cholesterol ester arrangement shown in Figure 3b. (b) Electron density distribution of the molecular packing showing electron dense peaks separated by ~ 38 Å. (c) Radial electron density distribution for a particle containing two repeating cholesterol ester bilayers. (d) Calculated SAXRS curve from the particle shown in (c). (e) Further perturbation of the cholesterol ester packing in which there is no correlation in molecular position. (f) Uniform electron density distribution from model shown in (e). (g) Radial electron density distribution for a particle with uniform electron density in the core of the particle. (h) Calculated SAXRS curve from the model particle shown in (g)

The model calculations show that specific molecular arrangements of the cholesterol esters within the spherical particle will adequately account for the observed changes in both the scattering and electron density profiles of LDL (Fig. 2) and provide further evidence that the thermal transition in LDL between 20° and 40°C is related to changes in the structural organization of the cholesterol ester-rich core.

Influence of LDL Triglycerides on the Reversible Transition

Although multiple samples of LDL from a single donor showed an almost identical reversible transition by DSC, LDL taken from different individuals showed considerable variability (Deckelbaum et al., 1977). The mean onset temperature in 21 preparations was 17.3°C, the peak temperature 30.3°C, and the end temperature 41.0°C. As shown in Figure 5a, increasing amounts of LDL triglyceride relative to LDL cholesterol ester correlated with the peak transition temperature (r =

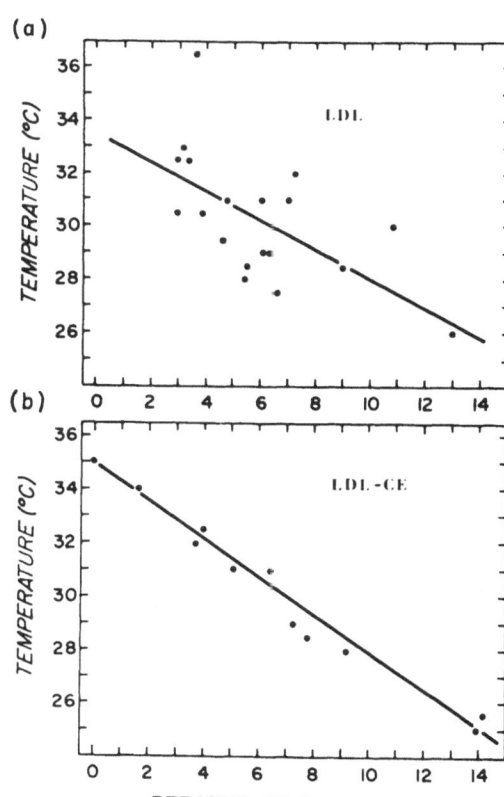

Figure 5. (a) Peak temperatures of
the calorimetric transitions of intact LDL plotted against wt % of
LDL triglyceride relative to cholesterol ester. (b) Transition temperatures of mixtures of extracted LDL
cholesterol esters containing varying
amounts of LDL triglyceride plotted
against wt % triglyceride in the
total mixture

– 0.61, p = .005). This relationship is mainly determined by the triglyceride
content of LDL since cholesterol ester content alone did not correlate with the
peak temperature. Triglyceride alone has a correlation coefficient of – 0.60
(p = .006), and there were no other significant compositional correlations (p <
.05).

The transition temperature of isolated individual LDL cholesterol esters showed
no relationship to the transition temperature obtained from its intact parent
LDL. However, increasing amounts of isolated LDL triglyceride progressively depressed the temperature of the smectic → liquid transition of isolated LDL cholesterol ester (Fig. 5b). The cholesterol ester smectic → cholesteric transition
enthalpy decreased with addition of small amounts of triglyceride and disappeared with mixtures containing greater than 3% triglyceride. Thus, the reversible
transition of intact LDL reflects the behavior of the two neutral lipids, cholesterol esters, and triglyceride in model systems with increasing amounts of triglyceride producing a disordering effect on the molecular organization of the
cholesterol ester-rich core of LDL.

Our data show that in intact LDL at 37°C, some individuals will have a fraction
of LDL cholesterol esters in a smectic-like state (Deckelbaum et al., 1975, 1977).
The physical state of the lipids in LDL may play an important role in the metabolism of the particle. For example, the fluidity of the lipid core may influence
the surface structure of LDL and alter its interaction with various tissues such
as the arterial wall (Stein and Stein, 1975), cell membrane receptors (Brown and
Goldstein, 1976), etc.

FORMATION AND STRUCTURAL PROPERTIES OF LIPOPROTEIN-X

D. Seidel

The liver ist the major site of synthesis of plasma lipoproteins and has central functions in lipoprotein catabolism. In recent years, studies from different laboratories have well documented the possibility for alterations of all plasma lipoprotein fractions in liver disease. Among all and with the only exception of familial LCAT deficiency, lipoprotein X formation is the most specific and unique abnormality. Before discussing problems and findings related to LP-X, some other features should briefly be mentioned.

Whereas a normal plasma lipoprotein pattern obtained by lipid electrophoresis on agarose shows distinct bands for β-, pre-β, and α-lipoproteins, the lipoprotein pattern of patients with severe liver dysfunction of any kind often shows the characteristic feature of only one lipoprotein band in β-position. However, this does not necessarily indicate a lack of very low-density lipoproteins normally migrating in pre-β-position, nor does it necessarily indicate a lack of the high-density lipoproteins normally migrating in α-position and standing for lipids. Very low-density lipoproteins are present in normal concentrations or sometimes elevated. The protein lipid composition and size of the compounds are close to normal, but this fraction displays β-mobility on agarose or paper electrophoresis, probably due to an abnormal apoprotein composition, i.e., a lack of apoC, which becomes apparent on PAGE patterns in 8 M urea (Fig. 1). Using ultracentrifugation and/or immunologic techniques instead of lipid electrophoresis, we found no significant changes in the concentration of apolipoprotein A, the major protein moiety of α- or high-density lipoproteins in patients with liver disease. However, in contrast to normal α-lipoproteins, this fraction revealed a pattern likely to indicate the presence of HDL in dissociated forms, showing primarily if not exclusively only apoA-I or apoA-II. ApoA-I in this situation is recovered in the d 1.21 g/ml bottom fraction. Since this fraction does not contain lipids in appreciable amounts, it may be concluded that apoA-I in this form is devoid

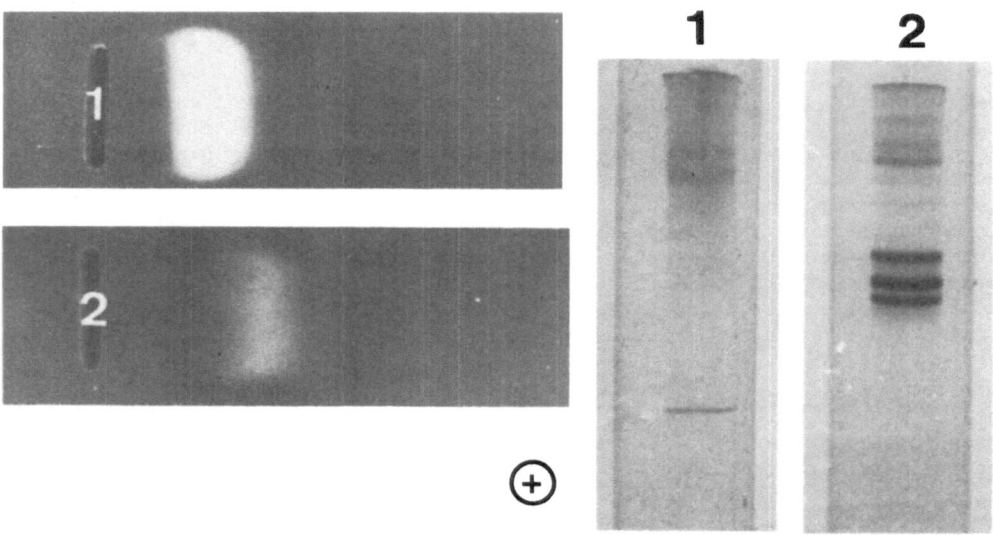

Figure 1. Agarose (1%) and polyacrylamide (8 M urea) electrophoresis of isolated VLDL obtained from a patient with liver disease (1) and of a control subject (2)

or almost devoid of lipids (Seidel et al., 1972b). Qualitatively but not quantitatively, the HDL pattern in liver disease therefore shows some similarity with that of Tangier disease (Seidel, 1977).

Plasma low-density lipoproteins in patients with biliary obstruction contain abnormally high levels of phospholipids and unesterified cholesterol, most of these lipids being present in the form of a distinct lipoprotein designated LP-X (Russ et al., 1956; Switzer, 1967; Seidel et al., 1969, 1970, 1972a; Picard and Veissière, 1970; Mills et al., 1969; Hamilton et al., 1971). The protein constituents of LP-X make up only 4-6% of the total lipoprotein weight (Fig. 2). Two main protein classes have been identified and separated: the apoX polypeptides which are either very closely related or identical with the apoC proteins and apoD, and a protein which is immunologically identical and very similar in chemical and physical properties to plasma albumin. Since albumin cannot be detected by immunologic methods in intact LP-X, it is assumed that its immunologic determinants are effectively masked in the native particles. By a similar argument, some of the apoX proteins, on the basis of their immunocreactivity in intact LP-X, are thought to be located on the surface of the lipoprotein. LP-X phospholipids are readily digested with phospholipase A_2, a fact which suggests that their polar head groups are exposed on the exterior of the lipoprotein particles. However, the structure of LP-X changes during the digestion, and some phospholipids which were originally protected may become exposed to the enzyme.

Electron micrographs of LP-X show round particles, 300 - 700 Å in diameter, having a strong tendency to aggregate and change shape. The most characteristic morphology is stacks of discs, each disc with a major axis 400 - 600 Å and a minor axis around 100 Å. Low-angle x-ray diffraction studies of LP-X suggest that this lipoprotein may exist as a vesicle, where a phospholipid and cholesterol bilayer separates internal and external water compartments (Hamilton et al., 1971). Various observations on related systems lend some support to this view of LP-X structure. Extensive chemical modification of LP-X protein with succinic anhydride does not affect the total structure of this lipoprotein (Jonas and Seidel, 1974). Although average succinylation of about 80% of the reactive groups on the protein changes markedly some properties of the lipoprotein, for example, electrophoretic mobility and immunologic reactivity, the overall structure remains the same as indicated by the electron micrographs, flotation, and sedimental properties. One conclusion from those studies might be that the specific protein components of LP-X are stabilized by their interaction with lipids and that succinylation is not sufficient in disrupting the protein-lipid interactions or changing the protein configuration to an extent that would be reflected in circular dichroism spectra or in the overall structure of LP-X. That this is probably the case is indicated by the contrasting behavior of many globular proteins upon extensive succinylation and by a similar behavior of normal plasma lipoproteins (Scanu el al., 1968). The finding that albumin, which is known to undergo marked structural changes upon succinylation in solution, does not dissociate from LP-X nor does it cause any apparent changes of the LP-X structure when succinylated in this lipoprotein poses several aspects as to the role and location of this protein in LP-X. It must either interact with the lipid phase or, assuming that LP-X is a vesicle, be located in the internal water compartment. The latter alternative appears more likely. Assuming that apoX has a relatively extended configuration on the surface of LP-X, it can be calculated that this protein component would cover about 30% of the particle (av. dia., 500 Å; av. area per amino acid residue 30 Å). From the preceding considerations, it is apparent that a significant portion of the LP-X surface consists of protein and that protein-protein interactions could play a role in interparticle interactions. However, the results of the succinylation study indicate that a marked increase of the negative surface charge, localized in the protein components which would be sufficient in disrupting globular subunit proteins, has no effect on the structure of LP-X, and suggest that protein-protein interactions may not be essential in promoting the characteristic LP-X stacked-disc structures. In this connection, recent studies from our laboratory in which LP-X was assembled in vitro are of interest. These studies also provided evidence for the origin of LP-X in cholestasis.

Density class	1.035 – 1.063 g/ml
S_f	14 – 16
Electrophoretic mobility	Agar cathode
	Agarose anode
Protein-lipid composition	6% Protein, 25% cholesterol, 3% triglycerides, 66% phospholipids
Proteins	Albumin; ApoC-I; C-II; C-III; apoD
Size and shape: Vesicle of ~⌀ 600 Å with a strong tendency to aggregate = 0,1 μm	

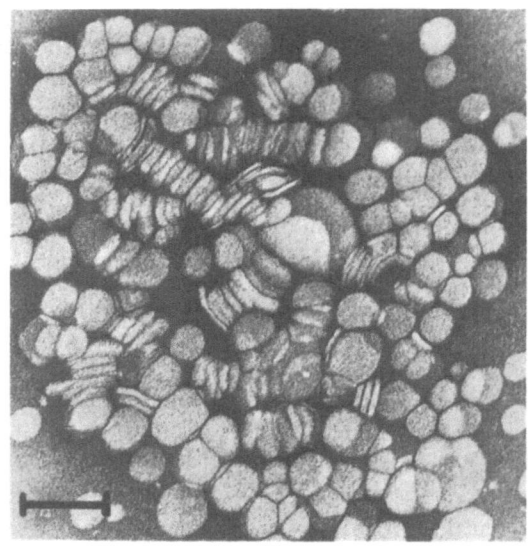

Figure 2. Characteristics of lipoprotein X isolated from the serum of a patient with extrahepatic biliary obstruction

It has been previously demonstrated that LP-X appears in appreciable amounts in dog and rat plasma within the first 24 h following surgical ligation of the common bile duct. The same time seems to be necessary for LP-X to appear in patients with extrahepatic biliary obstruction.

It was demonstrated that during extrahepatic biliary obstruction, bile passes from the bile ducts to the hepatic lymphatics, from there to the thoracic lymphatic duct, and finally into the blood stream (Popper, 1968).

It is also well-established that liver excreets lipids, predominantly phospholipids and unesterified cholesterol with the bile fluid. Thus, the lipid composition of LP-X isolated from serum shows great similarity to the lipids found in bile. Even the phosphatide distribution and phosphatide fatty acids of bile are almost identical to that of LP-X (Picard et al., 1972). These facts taken together strongly suggested a close relationship of bile lipids and LP-X. Human bile when submitted to agar or agarose electrophoresis reveals a lipoprotein band migrating toward the anode, which can be visualized by polyanion precipitation, as well as with a lipid stain or protein stain. Immunochemically albumin and immunoglobulins as well as other plasma proteins can be identified, but no immunoprecipitation reaction is obtained with antibodies to any of the major apolipoproteins apoA, apoB, apoC, and apoD. Under the electron microscope, it is not possible to detect any reproducible particular structures; occasionally, some lamellar structures are apparent. LP-X, however, with its characteristic structure under the electron microscope, or even more specifically with its typical migration toward the cathode on agar electrophoresis, cannot be detected in either native or water dialyzed bile. All bile lipids may be separated from bile in the form of an albumin lipid complex (designated bile LP). This complex shows a lipid composition very similar to LP-X but displays different physicochemical characteristics.

When bile, however, is incubated in vitro with either pure albumin or with total (LP-X negative) serum, LP-X is formed and may be isolated showing an electrophoretic behavior and other physicochemical characteristics similar to those found in the serum of patients suffering from cholestatic liver disease (Fig. 3). Addition of various amounts of isolated VLDL, LDL or HDL, as well as purified immunoglobulins to native bile does not result in LP-X formation (Manzato et al., 1976).

The amount of LP-X formed from bile after addition of albumin or serum depends to a high degree on the concentration of native bile, in particular on the concentration of bile lipoprotein, bile salts, and the amount of albumin added to the system. Comparison of LP-X formed by albumin alone (designated LP-X (alb)) or by serum (LP-X (ser)) with native LP-X revealed a very similar lipid composition (Fig. 4). Significant differences are apparent, however, in their protein moiety, and the structural properties as judged by electron microscopy and electrophoresis on agar gel. LP-X (alb) shows somewhat larger and more heterogenous particles on electromicrographs, it migrates further to the cathode on agar electrophoresis and is devoid of apoC and apoD. After in vitro incubation with HDL or VLDL, this material, as well as LP-X (ser), shows these apolipoproteins, the latter is almost indistinguishable from native LP-X. From these in vitro experi-

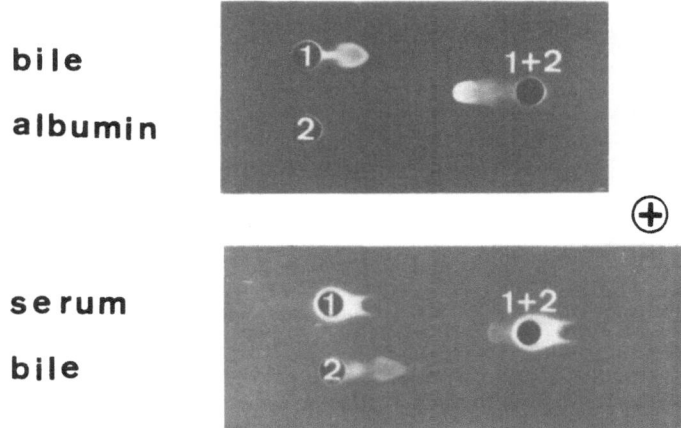

Figure 3. Agar gel (1%) electrophoresis of native bile, albumin, and LP-X negative serum before and after incubation of the fractions. In both cases LP-X can be visualized by its typical band migrating to the cathode after incubation

231

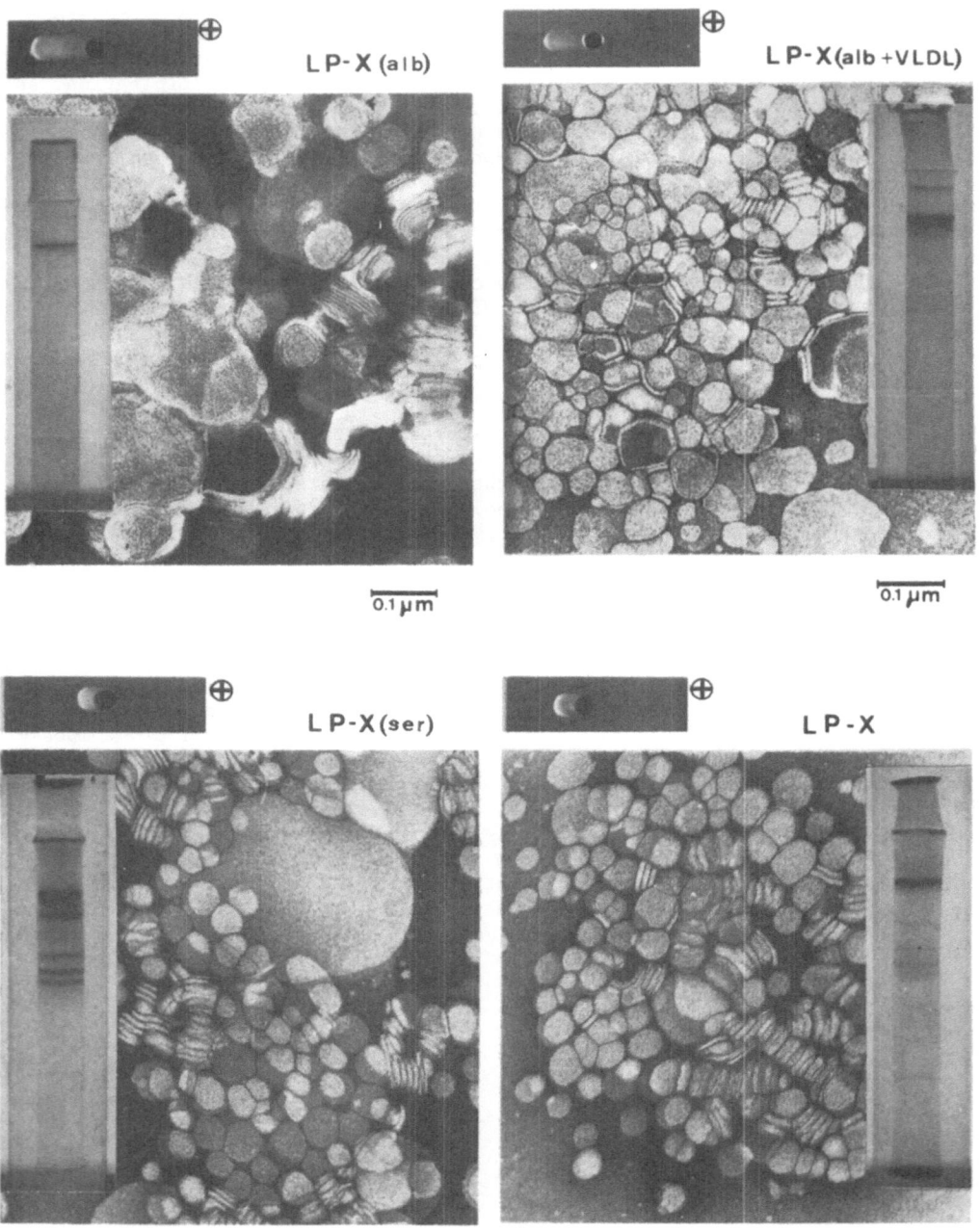

Figure 4. Electrophoretic (1% agar gel; polyacrylamide gel in 8 M urea) and
electron microscopic pattern of various forms of LP-X in comparison.
Although LP-X (alb) shows the features characteristic for LP-X, some structural
differences and differences in the apoX peptides are apparent in comparison to
LP-X (alb) after incubation with VLDL or with LP-X (ser) and native LP-X. (For
further description, also see the text)

ments, which are strongly supported by in vivo studies in dog, it seems evident that LP-X formation takes place when bile LP is converted into LP-X by the action of albumin in the proper ratio to bile salts. Thus albumin, rather than other apoX peptides, seems to be the key protein in LP-X formation and in maintaining the unique physicochemical characteristics of LP-X, although apoC and apoD, in addition, may have some stabilizing effect on the structure of this abnormal plasma lipoprotein.

ISOTHERMAL CALORIMETRIC STUDIES ON HUMAN HDL APOLIPOPROTEINS

H. Peeters and M. Rosseneu

Isothermal calorimetry measures the enthalpy change involved in a chemical reaction. When adapted to the microscale, it quantitates the amount of millijoules associated at a given temperature with the mixing and reassembly of biochemicals, i.e., in our case an apoprotein solution and a phospholipid dispersion. The extent of reassembly and the complex composition can be derived from density gradient ultracentrifugation experiment performed in parallel with the microcalorimetric measurements (Rosseneu et al., 1974).

The enthalpy changes ΔH measured at various lipid to protein ratios yield an enthalpy titration curve. The maximal enthalpy of binding ΔH_n, corresponding to the complex saturation, together with the complex composition, can be derived from the experimental data, provided the curve can be fitted to a simple theoretical model (Rosseneu et al., 1976b).

We should note that differential scanning calorimetry - such as used by Tall et al., (1975) - implies the determination of the transition temperature of lipids and lipid-protein complexes and thus covers a different field. But clearly the temperatures at which the isothermal microcalorimetric measurements are performed take into account the transition temperature of the lipid components and complexes involved. Measurements are mostly performed at temperatures above the transition point (at 28° for dimyristoylphosphatidylcholine (DMPC) and at 41° for sphingomyelin).

Figure 1a shows the binding of DMPC liposomes - obtained by sonication of the phospholipid until close-shelled vesicles - to the whole apoHDL, and to its major apoprotein constituents apoA-I and apoA-II. The enthalpy curve for apoHDL lies between the curves for isolated apoA-I and A-II proteins in agreement with the whole apoHDL containing two molecules of apoA-I for one molecule of apoA-I. The maximal enthalpy ΔH_m amounts to -210kcal/mol apoA-I, -220kcal/mol apoHDL, and to -230kcal/mol apoA-II. When recalculated per amino acid, this corresponds to -0.9kcal/residue for apoA-I and -1.5kcal/residue for apoA-II. This negative enthalpy change is favorable to binding and can, therefore, be considered as a driving force in the phospholipid binding process (Rosseneu et al., 1976a).

The enthalpy curve for apoA-I is characterized by an endothermal process at low phospholipid levels ($n \leq 50$) (Fig. 1a). We attribute this phenomenon to the disaggregation and conformational changes in the apoprotein induced by the binding of the first phospholipid molecules (Rosseneu et al., 1976a). The superposition upon the endothermal process of an exothermal binding process similar to that observed with apoA-II and apoHDL yields the sigmoidal-shaped curve. This was experimentally confirmed by preincubating apoA-I with 12 mol lysolecithin prior to binding DMPC. Figure 1b shows that the binding curve in this case presents the regular shape of a Langmuir isotherm. The endothermal process has disappeared and the difference $\Delta H'$ between the two curves at any phospholipid ratio represents the heat of conformational change of apoA-I and amounts to +30kcal/mol. Figure 1 agrees closely with that derived by Tall et al. (1977) from their differential scanning calorimetry data.

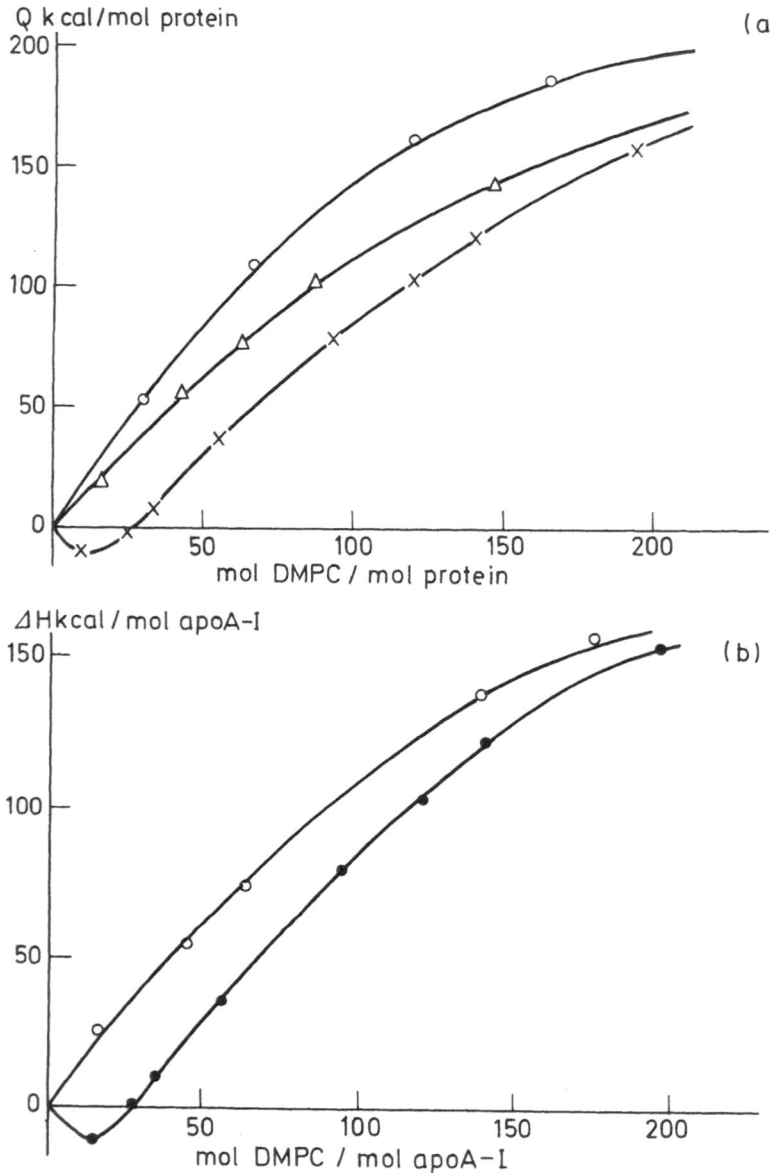

Figure 1. (a) Heat released on binding DMPC to apoA-I (×), apoA-II (•), and apoHDL (o). (b) Enthalpy change on binding DMPC to native apoA-I (•) and to apoA-I preincubated with 12 mol lysolecithin (o)

There is good evidence that the binding of apoA-I and apoA-II to phospholipids is primarily hydrophobic (Stoffel and Därr, 1976). In order to assess the contribution of ionic forces to complex formation, we investigated the ionization behavior of apoA-I and its complex with DMPC, and carried out both calorimetric and potentiometric titration on the native apoprotein and on the complex (Rosseneu et al., 1976c). Figure 2a shows the enthalpy titration curves for native apoA-I and the apo-I-DMPC in the basic pH range. The enthalpy change for the native apoprotein corresponds to the ionization of 21 lysines and seven tyrosines (Baker et al., 1975). In the complex, less groups are ionized in the pH range

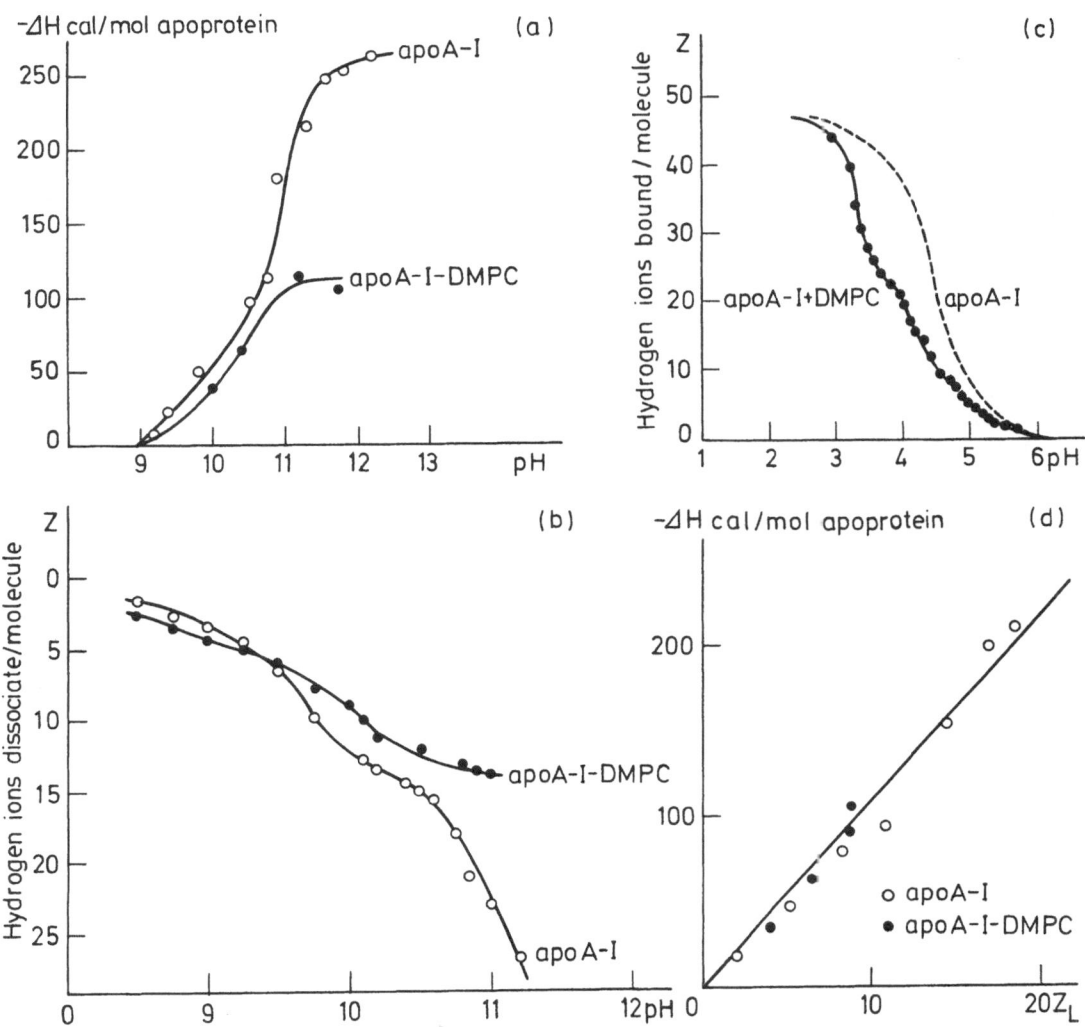

Figure 2. (a) Enthalpy titration curve in the basic pH range for native apoA-I
(×) and the apoA-I-DMPC complex (•). (b) Potentiometric titration curves of lysine
and tyrosine residues in the native apoA-I (o) and in the apoA-I-DMPC (•) complex.
(c) Potentiometric titration curves of the acidic residues in the apoA-I-DMPC complex and theoretical curve for apoA-I (pK = 4.4). (d) Enthalpy for lysine ionization in native apo-A (o) and in the apoA-I-DMPC complex (•)

9-12 accounting for the lower enthalpy change. The potentiometric titration
curves at basic and acidic pH's are shown in Figures 2b and 2c. In native
apoA-I, 14 lysines plus tyrosines titrate between pH 8.5 and 10.2 and ten more
groups titrate at higher pH. In the complex, only 14 groups ionize in this pH
range and their pK is shifted toward higher values. These differences account
for the lower ionization enthalpy observed for the complex. The titration curve
of the complex at acidic pH shows the contribution of two types of aspartic and
glutamic acid residues : 25 titrating with a pK of 4.4 and 21 titrating with an
abnormally low pK, all residues being titrated at pH ≤ 3.

In order to evaluate the respective lysine and tyrosine contribution, the tyrosine residues were titrated spectrophotometrically and substracted from the overall

235

ionization curve to yield the lysine contribution. It now appears that the enthalpy for lysine ionization (Fig. 2d) is the same in native apoA-I as in the
apoA-I-DMPC complex showing that the presence of phospholipids does not affect
the available lysine residues.

These results are summarized in Table 1 and show that under DMPC binding, the pK
of 21 carboxylic residues and ten lysines is shifted by about 1 pK U. This corresponds to a change in free energy $\Delta G = -0.2$ kcal/mol phospholipid (at complex
saturation n = 120) due to ionic binding which amounts to about 10% of the value
$\Delta G = -2.4$ kcal resulting from hydrophobic binding.

In conclusion, a pH change in the solutions of native apoA-I and of the apoA-I-
DMPC complex induces an enthalpy change which is larger for native apoA-I than
for the complex. This suggests that given amino acids are masked during the recombination of the apoprotein with a phospholipid. It was shown for apoA-I that
a set of lysine and acidic residues must be involved. These experiments also indicate that weak ionic interactions exist between phospholipid and aproprotein,
though hydrophobic forces are prevailing. In considering the apoprotein sequence,
the localization of the charged amino acids lysine, arginine, aspartic, and glutamic acid in a sequential arrangement susceptible to directly interact with the
phospholipid was attempted (Soetewey et al., 1976).

As ionic and hydrophobic forces are simultaneously involved in phospholipid binding, it is required that the reacting lysines and arginines should be located at
the level of an hydrophobic region. Only some of the charged residues meet with
that requisite and are shown in Figure 4. Similar results are obtained with apoA-
II, apoC-I, apoC-III and agree with the experimental titration data according to
which only part of the residues are directly involved in DMPC binding and create
the discrete binding sites (Peeters et al., 1976).

At the physiologic level, this kind of information might be related to the differences in the sphingomyelin to phosphatidylcholine ratio observed in HDL from
different hyperlipoproteinemic patients or from animals under different experimental diets in casu type II and type IV. Analogous data obtained after recombination of other phospholipids differing either in the acyl chain length or structure, e.g., dioleylphosphatidylcholine and myristoylsphingomyelin, will shed
more light on the selectivity of the phospholipid load of apoproteins.

We believe that the primary sequence is a determining factor for the type and
number of phospholipid molecules bound to the apoproteins while on the other
hand the fatty acid content of the phospholipids must contribute to the overall
lipid composition of the lipoprotein complex.

Table 1. Potentiometric and calorimetric titration of native apoA-I and of the
apo-I.DMPX complex. ΔH is expressed in kgcal/mol residue

Residue	ApoA-I			Apo-I + DMPC		
ASP-GLU	n = 48	pK = 4.4[a]	ΔH_T = 0-2[a]	n_1 = 25 n_2 = 21	pK_1 = 4.4 pK_2 = 3.25	
LYS	n_1 = 11 n_2 = 10	pK_1 = 9.6 pK_2 = 10.6	ΔH_T = -11 ΔH_T = -11	n_1 = 11	pK_1 = 9.6	ΔH_T = -11
TYR	n_1 = 3 n_2 = 4	pK_1 = 9.5 pK_2 = 11	ΔH_T = -6[a] ΔH_T = -6[a]	n_1 = 3 n_2 = 4	pK_1 = 10.5 pK_2 = 12.1	ΔH_T = -6[a] ΔH_T = -6[a]

[a]Taken from Ch. Tanford

236

ASP-GLU-PRO-GLN-SER-PRO

1 TRP-ASP-ARG-VAL-LYS-ASP-LEU-ALA-THR-VAL-TYR-VAL-ASP-VAL-LEU-LYS-ASP-SER-GLY-ARG-ASP-TYR
          10   20

VAL-SER-GLN
30

2 PHE-GLN-GLY-SER-ALA-LEU-GLY-LYS-GLN-LEU-ASN—LEU-LYS-LEU-LEU-TRP-ASP—ASP
                    40   50

VAL-THR-SER-THR-PHE

3 SER-LYS-LEU-ARG-GLN-GLU-LEU
                60

GLY-PRO-VAL-THR

4 GLU-GLU-TRP-PHE-ASN—ASP-LEU-GLN-GLU-LYS-LEU-ASN—LEU-GLU-LYS-GLU
             70   80

THR-GLY

5 GLU-LEU-ARG-GLN—GLU-MET-SER-LYS-ASP-LEU-GLU-GLU-VAL-LYS-ALA—LYS-VAL-GLN
                 90   100

PRO-TYR

6 LEU-ASP-ASP-PHE-GLN-LYS-LYS-TRP-GLN-GLU-MET—GLU-LEU-TYR-ARG-GLN-LYS-VAL
               110   120

GLU-PRO

7 LEU-ARG-ALA-GLU—LEU-GLN-GLU-GLY-ALA-ARG-GLN-LYS-LEU—HIS—GLU-LEU-GLN-GLU-LYS-LEU
               130   140

SER-PRO-LEU-GLY

8 GLU-GLU-MET-ARG-ASP-ARG-ALA-ARG—ALA-HIS—VAL-ASP-ALA-LEU-ARG—THR-HIS-LEU
           150   160

ALA-PRO-TYR-SER
170

9 ASP-GLU-LEU-ARG-GLN-ARG—LEU-ALA-ALA-ARG-LEU-GLU-ALA-LEU-LYS-GLU—ASN
                    180

GLY-ALA-GLY-ARG
190

10 LEU-ALA—GLU-TYR—HIS—ALA-LYS-ALA-THR-GLU—HIS-LEU-SER-THR-LEU-SER-GLU-LYS-ALA
               200   210

LYS-PRO-ALA

11 LEU-GLU-ASP-LEU-ARG—GLN-GLY-LEU
                    220

LEU-PRO-VAL

12 LEU-GLU-SER-PHE-LYS-VAL-SER-PHE-LEU-SER-ALA-LEU-GLU-GLU
               230

TYR-THR-LYS-LEU-ASN-THR-GLN
240   245

Figure 3. Lipid binding units in apoA-I. Helical regions are underlined and sequences interacting with lipids are outlined

237

HIGH-DENSITY LIPOPROTEIN ABNORMALITIES ASSOCIATED WITH DISEASE

Gerd Assmann

The purpose of this report is to briefly summarize recent advances in the understanding of high-density lipoprotein (HDL) structure and metabolism with special emphasis on certain metabolic and genetic derangements, in which structural alterations of HDL lead to metabolic abnormalities and vice versa.

In the quaternary structure of HDL, the major driving force in the binding of lipids to apoproteins is hydrophobic involving the nonpolar face of amphipathic helices and the carbon atoms of fatty acyl chains (Stoffel, 1976; Gotto et al., 1976; Assmann and Brewer, 1974). The major apoproteins of HDL, apoA-I and apoA-II, occur as integral constituents of these macromolecules, though the molecular basis of apoA-I - apoA-II interaction is not yet understood. It is reasonable to assume that a concentration balance of the A-apoproteins in normal plasma is determined by regulatory mechanisms in the biosynthesis of these apoproteins. In the degradation of human HDL, apoA-I and apoA-II decay at identical rates, indicating that most likely these macromolecules are catabolized as a structural entity (Levy et al., 1976).

The quantities and distribution patterns of apoproteins in plasma can be assessed by different methods. Results of quantitative determinations of A-apoproteins in whole serum have been obtained by different laboratories employing radial immunodiffusion, electroimmunoassays and radioimmunoassays (Schonfeld and Pfleger, 1974; Karlin et al., 1976; Mao et al., 1975; Assmann et al., 1977; Fainaru et al., 1975; Curry et al., 1976; Albers et al., 1976). As indicated in Table 1, there is still a considerable difference in the absolute apoA levels as determined by various laboratories. ApoA-I levels in serum differ between 100 and 154 mg %, and apoA-II levels differ between 35 and 83 mg %. More significantly, from a structural point of view, there is as yet no agreement on whether the molar ratio of apoA-I to apoA-II in plasma is approximately 2/1 as determined by radioimmunoassay (and chemical methods) or close to unity as assessed by electroimmunoassay. General agreement, however, exists that more than 90% of the A-apoproteins occurs in the density 1.063 - 1.21 class. There is some uncertainty on whether or not sex-related differences exist in values for apoA-I and apoA-II.

There are certain familial and acquired disorders in which HDL - cholesterol levels are relatively low and in which α-lipoproteins may exhibit abnormal electrophoretic properties (Table 2). The lipid abnormality in these disorders is accompanied by a relative deficiency in the A-apoproteins, the most pertinent example being Tangier disease. This disease is a rare autosomal disorder of plasma lipid transport which is clinically characterized by hepatosplenomegaly, large

Table 1. A-apoprotein concentrations in human serum

Reference	Method	ApoA-I (mg/dl)	ApoA-II (mg/dl)	A-I/A-II ratio (molar)
Schonfeld and Pfleger (1974)	Radioimmunoassay	100 (104)		
Starr et al. (1974)	Radioimmunoassay	102 (100)		
Assmann et al. (1977)	Radioimmunoassay	113 (124)	35 (41)	2/1
Albers et al. (1976)	Immunodiffusion	120 (149)		
Fainaru et al. (1975)	Radioimmunoassay	121		
Karlin et al. (1976)	Radioimmunoassay	13o (154)		
Curry et al. (1976)	Electroimmunoassay	143 (146)	78 (83)	

Table 2. Conditions with decreased HDL concentration

1. Tangier disease
2. Abetalipoproteinemia
3. Lcat deficiency
4. Familial hyperchylomicronemia
5. Hypertriglyceridemia (type IIV, IV, V)
6. Malnutrition
7. Gross hepatic failure
8. Dysglobulinemia
9. Carbohydrate feeding

orange-yellow tonsils, relapsing peripheral neuropathy, and widespread tissue storage of cholesteryl esters (Fredrickson et al., 1972). It has been demonstrated that patients with this disease have only small amounts of HDL in their plasma that are similar, but not identical, to normal lipoproteins of this density class (Lux et al., 1972).

In recent studies, we have determined, by radioimmunoassay and double immunoelectrophoresis, the total quantities and distributions of A-apoproteins in three adult patients affected with Tangier disease (Assmann et al., 1977). Compared with normal plasma, the total quantities of apoA-I and apoA-II in Tangier plasma were determined to be < 1% and 5-7%, respectively. In Tangier patients, approximately 90% of the apoprotein A-I sedimented when ultracentrifugations of plasma were carried out at density 1.21 g/ml KBr. By contrast, more than 85% of the apoA-II floated under those conditions. In normal plasma, approximately 90% of both apoproteins A-I and A-II is found in the 1.063-1.21 g/ml density fraction.

Fractionation of the Tangier 1.063 - 1.21 lipoproteins by agarose column chromatography revealed that only a relatively minor quantity of Tangier 'HDL' has the α-mobility normally associated with this density class. These lipoproteins, HDL_T, are spherical particles overlapping in size, only the smallest HDL particles found in normal plasma. ApoA-II, which usually comprises 30-35% of apoHDL, was the only apoprotein consistently demonstrated in HDL_T, while apoA-I is nearly or completely absent (Assmann, G., Herbert, P.N., Fredrickson, D.S., Forte, T., unpublished observations).

Whether this observed dissociation of A-apoproteins in Tangier plasma reflects an abnormality in primary structure causing a failure of apoA-I to be associated in normal HDL particles is as yet undetermined. A single aminc replacement in apoA-I or apoA-II, at a position important for specific protein-protein or protein-lipid interaction, conceivably may destroy the quaternary structure of HDL. Alternatively, a faulty regulation of apoprotein synthesis may result in the secretion of HDL subpopulations which are normally absent from plasma or masked in normal plasma by an overwhelming amount of other HDL.

Apparantly, both the absence of normal HDL and severe deficiency of apoA-I may secondarily affect lipoprotein interconversion, LCAT activity, and cellular cholesterol metabolism. Some of the implications of HDL deficiency as related to lipoprotein structure and observed in Tangier patients are summarized in Table 3 (Assmann, 1976). The storage of cholesteryl esters in tissues as the most prominent consequence of genetic HDL deficiency is currently best explained by ineffective 'sweeping' or removal of cholesterol (cholesteryl esters) from tissues or phagocytosis of abnormal HDL or chylomicron particles.

Tangier disease is not the only disorder in which a dissociation of apoA-I and apoA-II polypeptides occurs; genetic LCAT deficiency and liver disease are other examples. α-lipoproteins in the plasma of patients with LCAT deficiency are quantitatively reduced and have been separated into two subfractions by Sephadex

Table 3. Findings secondary to genetic HDL deficiency

1. C-apoproteins absent from 1.063-1.21 fraction
2. Total C-apoprotein content in plasma diminished
3. Size and composition of VLDL normal
4. 5-7-Fold increase of triglyceride in LDL at the expense of cholesteryl esters
5. Total LDL concentration 10-50% of normal
6. LCAT activity and extrahepatic lipase activity diminished

G-200 chromatography (Glomset and Norum, 1973). A major, large molecular weight
fraction, appearing mainly as 'stacked discs) or in rouleaux formation upon electron microscopy, is depleted of cholesteryl esters. A minor subfraction of
smaller molecular weight with particles 45-60 Å in diameter contains apoA-I as
the principal apoprotein. As in the case of Tangier disease, one might assume
that the tissue lipid abnormalities (corneal opacities, kidney failure, etc.) represent deposits of abnormal circulatory lipoproteins. Thus, Tangier disease and
LCAT deficiency are genetic disorders in which an apoprotein and/or lipid abnormality leads to perturbation of HDL structure with specific consequences.

We have recently observed a structural HDL abnormality in patients affected with
severe hepatocellular damage (hepatitis, cancer of the liver, etc.). Normally in
double immunoelectrophoresis, the reaction between HDL contained in native serum
and HDL antisera (which recognize both the presence of apoA-I and apoA-II) is
characterized by one, and not by two, rocket-shaped immunoprecipitates in α-electrophoretic position (Fig. 1). In certain patients with hepatocellular damage,
however, two precipitin lines, indicative of the formation of abnormal HDL subpopulations, can be observed (Fig. 2). When instead of HDL antisera, apoA-I and
apoA-II antisera were used to monitor for the presence of individual A-apoproteins in the native serum of these patients, the reaction of apoA-I was characterized by two precipitin lines resembling those obserced with whole HDL antiserum. The reaction of apoA-II, however, was characterized by only one precipitin
arc (the more slowly migrating arc in normal α-electrophoretic position).

Our results strongly suggest that a partial dissociation of the major A-apoproteins, as well as an abnormal spectrum of HDL subpopulations, exists in the plasma of these patients. Whether the observed structural HDL abnormality in liver
disease reflects a defect in the assembly of the major A-apoproteins, whether
the dissociation occurs in the plasma compartment or as a specific consequence
of disturbed catabolism is as yet unknown. The study of defects in HDL associated
with genetic or acquired disorders, however, is expected to shed further light on
the structural features and the metabolic role of these lipoproteins in human
plasma.

LIVER   DISEASE

NORMAL

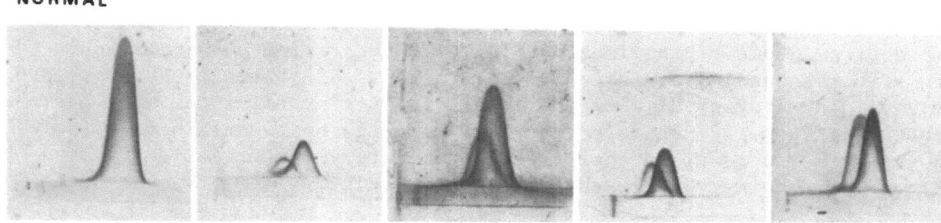

ANTI - HDL SERUM

Figure 1. Double immunoelectrophoresis (employing HDL antisera) of normal serum
(left) and serum obtained from patients with severe hepatocellular damage

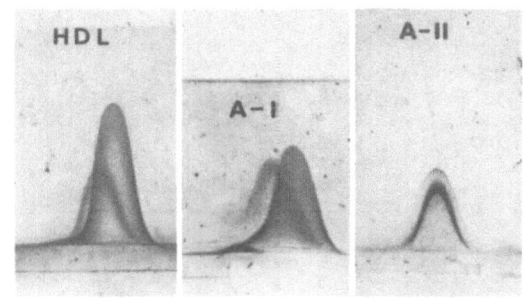

Figure 2. Double immunoelectrophoresis of serum of a patient affected with liver disease employing HDL antiserum (left), apoA-I antiserum (middle), and apoA-II antiserum (right)

ON THE ROLE OF APOLIPOPROTEIN A-I IN THE STRUCTURE OF SERUM HIGH-DENSITY LIPOPROTEINS (HDL)*

Mary C. Ritter and Angelo M. Scanu

Previous studies in this laboratory (Vitello and Scanu, 1976) and by Stone and Reynolds (1975) have established that the lipid-free human serum apolipoprotein (apoA-I) self-associated in aqueous solution. Preliminary observations also suggested a correlation between the binding of apoA-I to lipids and its state of association (Vitello et al., 1975). In order to explore this correlation further, we carried out a systematic investigation on the association in vitro of this apoprotein with HDL lipids (cholesterol, cholesteryl esters, phospholipids, and triglycerides) as a function of apoA-I concentration and lipid-protein weight ratios.

ApoA-I and HDL lipids were isolated from human serum HDL (Scanu, 1966; Scanu and Edelstein, 1971; Scanu et al., 1969; Lux et al., 1972), and were cosonicated to yield complexes which were separated from the unreacted components by ultracentrifugal techniques and gel permeation chromatography (Ritter and Scanu, 1976). We considered the lipid-protein complex as the product containing both protein and lipid, banding by ultracentrifugation or eluting on agarose columns in positions intermediate between those of the individual reactants.

Typical CsCl density gradient ultracentrifugation profiles of lipid-free apoA-I, free lipid, and the lipid-apoA-I complex obtained at an initial lipid-protein ratio of one are shown in Figure 1. The band corresponding to the lipid-free apoA-I has a peak density of 1.28 g/ml (Fig. 1C) in the same position as that occupied by apo-I in the absence of lipids (Fig. 1A). The band of the protein-free lipid is at top of the tube (Figs. 1C and 1D) and has the identical position as that of the lipids alone (Fig. 1B); in turn, the lipid-apoA-I complex has a peak hydrated density of 1.13 g/ml. This complex was found to be similar to native HDL3 in the broadness of its elution profile and in its lipid and protein composition (Figs. 1C and 1D).

---

*Operated by The University of Chicago for the United States Energy Research and Development Administration under Contract E(11-1)-69.

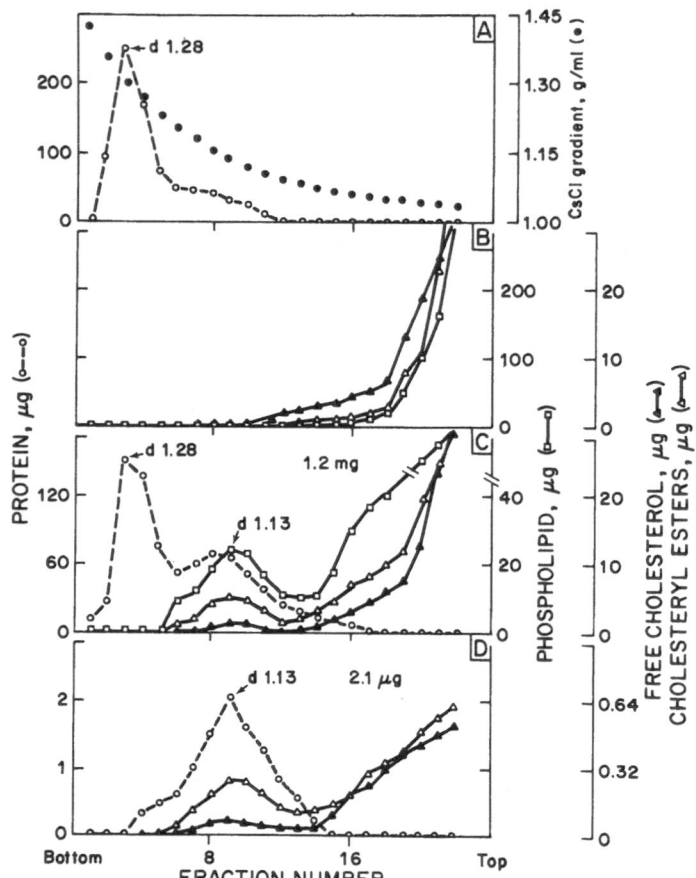

Figure 1. Profiles of apoA-I, lipid, and lipid-apoA-I complexes obtained by density gradient ultracentrifugation. The gradient extends from density 1.45 approximately to density 1.03 g/ml (from left to right). ApoA-I and/or HDL lipids were cosonicated in a total volume of 6.4 ml and centrifuged at 11° for 24 h at 38,000 rpm in a Spinco 40.3 rotor, followed by isophycnic density gradient ultracentrifugation, as already described (Ritter and Scanu, 1976). The numbers above the bands are the average density in g/ml.
(A) 1.2 mg sonicated apoA-I without lipids (the dotted line denotes a typical gradient observed after centrifugation).
(B) 1.2 mg sonicated HDL lipids without apoA-I.
(C) 1.2 mg apoA-I and HDL lipids at an initial lipid-protein weight ratio of one.
(D) 21 µg apoA-I and HDL lipids at an initial lipid-proteon weight ratio of one

The banding hydrated density of the lipid-protein complex formed varied with the initial lipid-apoA-I ratio (compare Figs. 1C and 1D with Table 3). In all instances studied, however, the lipid-apoA-I complex floated at a density of 1.063 -1.21 g/ml, and thus it was similar to native HDL in operational terms. We will refer to this reassembled complex as R-HDL, using the subscripts S (small) or L (large) to refer to the radius of the R-HDL particle (see Table 3).

242

Effect of ApoA-I Concentration

The reassembly of apoA-I was studied at different apoA-I concentrations, but at a constant ratio of protein to lipid, so that the effect of protein concentration on the yield and lipid-binding capacity of apoA-I could be determined. At a low concentration (0.1 μM), the incorporation of apoA-I into R-HDL reached almost 100% (Fig. 1D and Table 1). The parallel increase in the concentration of the reactants (i.e., apoA-I and lipids) caused a progressive decrease in the percentages of lipid and protein recovered in the complex, without affecting the lipid distribution of the complex (Table 1; compare Fig. 1C with Fig. 1D).

These results suggested a possible relationship between the state of association of the protein and its lipid-binding capability. We therefore determined the state of aggregation of apoA-I by gel filtration chromatography under our experimental conditions and then correlated the amount of each oligomeric form of apoA-I with the amount of apoA-I incorporated in R-HDL at different initial apoA-I concentrations at a lipid-protein ratio of one. The data in Table 2 indicate that the amount of apoA-I incorporated into R-HDL$_S$ (column 5) was proportional to the number of monomer-dimers in the initial lipid-protein mixtures (column 4); only at an initial apoA-I concentration of 0.1 μM was there a good correlation with the monomer of apoA-I in solution. The quantitative incorporation of monomer-dimers regardless of the experimental conditions examined indicates that R-HDL formation is irreversible and under kinetic control.

Effect of Initial Lipid-Protein Weight Ratio

In another series of experiments, we compared the properties of R-HDL as a function of varying lipid concentrations while keeping the amount of apoA-I constant. As shown in Figure 1, at a weight ratio of one, R-HDL$_S$ had a peak hydrated density of 1.13 g/ml and was well-resolved from lipid-free apoA-I and protein-free lipid. Under these experimental conditions, no other lipid-protein complexes

Table 1. Effect of apoA-I concentrations on yield and composition of the lipid-apoA-I complex isolated by CsCl density gradient ultracentrifugation

Analytical results	Initial molarity of apoA-I reacted with HDL lipids				
	0.1[a]	01	1.0	5.6	6.7
Lipid-free apoA-I, % weight	100	9	25	50	58
ApoA-I in complex, % weight	0	91	75	50	42
Lipid-apoA-I weight ratio in complex[b]	–	0.15	0.16	0.14	0.16
Cholesteryl esters-apoA-I in complex, molar ratio	–	5.0	5.2	5.0	5.3
Free cholesterol-apoA-I in complex, molar ratio	–	2.3	2.3	2.2	2.5

[a] ApoA-I only; no lipids.
[b] Based on yield of cholesteryl esters and free cholesterol.

Table 2. Relationship between oligomeric forms of apoA-I and amount of apoA-I incorporated in R-HDL$_S$ at different initial apoA-I concentrations at lipid-protein weight ratio of one

Molarity of apoA-I in initial solution	Molarity of apoA-I			
	In			In R-HDL$_S$
	Monomer[a]	Dimer[a] (no lipids)	Monomer + dimer[a]	
0.1	0.10	0.00	0.10	0.09
1.0	0.26	0.55	0.81	0.75
5.6	0.80	1.90	2.70	2.80
6.7	0.87	2.33	3.20	2.81

[a]From agarose column experiments.

were observed. The properties of this R-HDL$_S$ particle were similar to those of native human serum HDL$_3$ (Ritter and Scanu, 1976), except that the content of cholesteryl esters was significantly lower (see also Table 3).

When solution containing apoA-I were cosonicated with HDL lipids at lipid-protein ratios less than one, the hydrated density and lipid composition of the lipid-protein complexes formed were different from those obtained at the ratio of one. Compared to native HDL$_3$, these R-HDL$_S$ particles were impoverished in lipid (Table 3).

At lipid-protein ratios above one, CsCl density gradient ultracentrifugation poorly resolved a broad component, with general properties similar to those of R-HDL$_L$ (Table 3), from a light component which floated near the top of the tube and contained mostly lipid with a very small amount of protein. The latter component will be referred to as the lipid-rich particle. When the lipid-protein ratio was increased above six, both R-HDL$_L$ and the lipid-free apoA-I were no longer detected, whereas the lipid-rich particle became the predominant component. Gel permeation chromatographic studies corroborated the density gradient ultracentrifugal observations.

Solutions of apoA-I of varying concentrations were equilibrated in 4 ml of 0.02 M EDTA, pH 8.6, for 2 h at 4°, and then cosonicated with HDL lipids, when present, at an initial lipid-protein weight ratio of one in a total volume of 6.4 ml, as previously described (Ritter and Scanu, 1976). The sonicated mixtures were centrifuged at 11° for 24 h at a density of 1.006 g/ml, followed by CsCl density gradient ultracentrifugation (Ritter and Scanu, 1976). Lipid-free apoA-I and the lipid-apoA-I complex are the fractions shown in Figure 1.

The values in the subheading and in the second row of Table 1 are the molar concentrations in the first and fifth columns of this table. The data in the second and third columns were calculated by graphical integration of the elution profiles of apoA-I on agarose columns at each specified concentration. The area corresponding to the dimeric or monomeric forms of apoA-I was divided by the total area of the oligomeric forms of apoA-I, and the quotient was multiplied by the amount of apoA-I in the initial mixutre. The figures in the fourth column are the sum of the values in columns two and three. The conditions for the fractionation of apoA-I by agarose column chromatography were previously described (Ritter and Scanu, 1976). The molarity of apoA-I is expressed in terms of the molecular weight of the monomer.

ApoA-I was cosonicated at an initial concentration of 5.5 µM in a total volume of 6.4 ml and centrifuged at a density of 1.063 g/ml (Ritter and Scanu, 1976). The density 1.063 g/ml undernatants were then fractionated by CsCl density gradient ultracentrifugation, ultracentrifugal flotation at density 1.21 g/ml, or gel permeation chromatography (Ritter and Scanu, 1976). The lipid-rich particle was obtained from the floating material separated by ultracentrifugation at density 1.063 g/ml, as described previously (Ritter and Scanu, 1976). The apparent molecular weight and the hydrated density were obtained from the peak fraction of the lipid-protein complex eluted from agarose columns and CsCl density gradient ultracentrifugation, respectively (except where indicated). The lipoprotein size and composition of human serum HDL3, given in the last column, are calculated from data in the literature (Skipski et al., 1967; Hirz and Scanu, 1967; Scanu, 1971). The weight percent composition in protein, phospholipid, cholesteryl esters, and free cholesterol of the lipid-protein complex is given in parentheses; a value aof 5% triglycerides per particle is assumed.

Table 3. Relationship among lipid binding of apoA-I, lipoprotein size, and composition

	Initial lipid-apoA-I weight ratio								Control
		R-HDL$_S$				R-HDL$_L$		Lipid-rich particle	HDL$_3$
	0.2	0.50	0.67	1.00	2.00	4.00	6.00	4.00	
				Particles formed					
Apparent molecular weight, x 10	0.74	0.92	1.00	1.15	1.43	1.75	1.90	1.90	1.75[b]
Hydrated density, g/ml	1.21	1.16	1.14	1.13	1.12	1.11	1.11	<1.063	1.15[c]
Radius, Å	29.0	31.6	32.6	34.3	37.0	39.7	40.1	42.3[a]	39.2
Chemical composition				Moles per particle (weight %)					
Protein	2.0 (76.1)	2.2 (66.5)	2.2 (60.2)	2.3 (57)	2.8 (55.5)	2.9 (45.7)	3.1 (44.4)	0.7 (10.5)	3.4 (55)[d]
Phospholipid	13.6 (14.3)	23.7 (20)	34.5 (26.7)	39.5 (26.6)	55.2 (29.9)	95.9 (42.5)	105.1 (44.0)	156.0 (63.7)	51.9 (22.5)[d]
Cholesteryl esters	4.3 (3.8)	9.5 (6.7)	10.5 (6.2)	15.0 (8.5)	15.6 (7.1)	13.9 (5.2)	16.4 (5.1)	33.4 (11.4)	32.0 (11.7)[d]
Free cholesterol	1.3 (0.7)	4.5 (1.9)	5.2 (2.0)	8.5 (2.9)	10.9 (3.0)	9.5 (2.1)	9.8 (2.0)	4.2 (8.6)	13.0 (2.9)[d]

[a] Assuming a hydrated density of 1.00. [b] Hirz and Scanu (1967). [c] Scanu (1971).
[d] Skipski et al. (1967); the protein content of HDL3 was considered to be the equivalent weight of apoA-I.

245

Data Analysis

We analyzed the results obtained at varying initial lipid concentrations at a constant apoA-I concentration to determine how many different classes of HDL particles were reassembled, and whether the lipid composition of the particles was a reflection of apoprotein content (Table 3). The radius of the individual particles was calculated from the relationship

$$\frac{M \times 10^{24}}{d \times 6 \times 10^{23}} = \frac{4 \pi r^3}{3},$$

where M = apparent molucular weight of particle, d = hydrated density of particle, and r = radius of particle in Å. The value of r is only operational and is not necessarily a hydrodynamic parameter. Using the weight percent composition of the lipid-protein complex, and assuming a 5% content of triglycerides per particle, we calculated the number of molecules per particle for each component. The results indicated that R-HDL can be grouped into two classes: one with a radius of 31 ± 2.2 Å and 2 mol of apoA-I (R-HDL$_S$), and the other with a radius of 39 ± 1.5 Å and 3 mol of apoA-I (R-HDL$_L$). Thus, the size of the lipoprotein appears to be determined by the number of apoA-I molecules in each complex. A slight variation in size observed within each class was probably due to variations in lipid composition. A comparison of these data with those for native HDL$_3$ indicated that R-HDL$_S$, formed at lipid-protein ratios between one and two, contains protein and lipid in amounts comparable to those in HDL$_3$, except for cholesteryl esters which are present in about half the amount. The results also show that R-HDL$_L$, formed at lipid-protein ratios above two, contains more phospholipid than expected for an HDL particle. On the other hand, the lipid-rich particle obtained at a lipid-protein ratio of four appears not to be a lipoprotein, but most probably a lipid vesicle with apoA-I adsorbed to it.

In summary, apoA-I, when cosonicated with HDL lipids in vitro, forms HDL complexes with properties similar to those of native HDL. The reassembly process is kinetically driven and is dependent on the state of association of apoA-I in solution. These results, and the size dependence of the reassembled HDL particles on the number of apoA-I molecules incorporated therein, indicate that apoA-I has an essential role in the structure of human HDL.

Acknowledgements

This research was supported in part by funds from the United States Public Health Service, National Heart and Lund Institute, grant (HL-08727 and HL-15062) and from the Chicago Heart Association (A75-4).
M.C.R. was the recipient of Chicago and Illinois Heart Association Research Fellowship F72-3 and USPHS Postdoctoral Fellowship HL-53,817.
A.M.S. was the recipient of USPHS Research Career Development Award HL-24,876.

MOLECULAR PATHOLOGY OF SERUM LIPOPROTEINS

Jan J. Opplt, Robert C. Bahler and Marie A. Opplt
Cleveland Metropolitan General Hospital, Case Western Reserve University, Cleveland, OH/USA

The best known separation techniques for serum lipoproteins are the elctrophoretic and ultracentrifugal. The newest and until now, not very well understood, is the molecular filtration technique. This procedure has enabled us to study serum lipoproteins on a molecular basis. One hundred fifty-six physiologic and pathologic lipoprotein patterns, obtained from clinically normal subjects and patients with proven coronary disease has revealed eight standard fractions. Each one was characterized by its elution volume, electrophoretic mobility, chemical analyses, immunochemical properties, mean size of particles (by a laser-light scattering correlation technique), relative distribution of particles (by electron-microscopy) and by the pattern of corresponding apolipoproteins. For the further distinction of the molecular distribution of lipoproteins according to densities, we have also applied the micro-ultracentrifugation technique.
The major achievements gained by such study are related to the demonstration of associations of lipoproteins, differing in molecular size and density in each of the fractions obtained by molecular filtration. Relatively pure sub-classes of lipoproteins are alternating with "remnants" as seen in the molecular filtration patterns. This analytical system allows us to study the pathways of possible shifts or delays in lipoprotein metabolism in different standardized types of dyslipoproteinemia, with the relationship to the severity of the metabolic disorder.

FRACTIONATION OF LIPOPROTEIN DENSITY CLASSES ON IMMUNOSORBERS. EVIDENCE FOR THE LIPOPROTEIN HETEROGENEITY

Walter McConathy, Heinrich Wieland, and Petar Alaupovic
Lipoprotein Laboratory, Oklahoma Medical Research Foundation, Oklahoma City, OK/USA

To examine whether the already established apolipoprotein heterogeneity of major density classes reflects a corresponding lipoprotein heterogeneity, we have fractionated lipoprotein density classes by affinity chromatography on immunosorbers. Lipoproteins with $S_f > 12$, S_f 0-20 and HDL isolated from plasma of fasting, normolipemic subjects were fractionated on immunosorbers to A-I, ApoB, ApoC, ApoD, and ApoE ("arg-rich" polypeptide). The unretained and retained fractions were characterized by double diffusion, acidic and basic polyacrylamide gel elctrophoresis and protein analyses. It was concluded that lipoproteins with $S_f > 12$ consisted of a small amount of free LP-C and following association complexes: LP-B: LP-C:LP-E, LP-B:LP-C, LP-C:LP-E, LP-C:LP-D, LP-D and unknowns. Lipoproteins with S_f 0-12 contained predominantly LP-B (80%) and small amounts of LP-C, LP-D, LP-A, LP-B:LP-C and LP-B:LP-C:LP-E. Fractionation of HDL indicated a similar degree of complexity with LP-A as the predominant lipoprotein (60%). We conclude from this study that 1) major density classes consist of a mixture of lipoproteins in both free and associated forms, and 2) the view of major density classes as single physical-chemical entities is not tenable.

CHANGES IN VERY LOW DENSITY LIPOPROTEIN STRUCTURE AND TURNOVER IN CHOLESTEROL FED RABBITS AFTER ILEAL BYPASS

Alberico Catapano, Umberto Fox, Giancarlo Ghiselli, Cesare Sirtori, and Walter Montorsi
Center E. Grossi Paoletti and III Institute of Surgical Pathology, University of Milano, Milan/Italy

Structure and turnover of rabbit VLDL was investigated after cholesterol feeding and subsequent ileal bypass (Buchwald H., Surgery *58,* 22, 1965) in New Zealand male rabbits. Total cholesterol levels decreased to pre-operative levels within two months after surgery. VLDL lipid composition, at this point, resembled that of normal rabbits, while a significant decrease of B apoprotein was noted one and two months after surgery. Arginine rich protein was still evident at one month. Data on the turnover of I-125 labelled VLDL from and into bypassed rabbits will be presented, as well as quantitative and structural analysis of tissue lipids.

VERY LOW DENSITY LIPOPROTEIN (VLDL) B-PROTEIN KINETICS IN HYPERLIPIDAEMIA

P. Nestel, M. Reardon, and N. Fidge
Department of Clinical Science, The Australian National University, Canberra, A.C.T./Australia

The turnover of VLDL B-protein has been measured in subjects with normal or raised lipids (Type 2b and 4) by reinjecting autologous I^{125}-labelled VLDL. The specific activity of B-protein in several VLDL classes was measured over at least 3 days; the purity of VLDL B-protein was established by chromatography and electrophoresis. Reinjected S_f 20-400 VLDL conformed to 2-pool kinetics: mean turnover was 1739 mg/day; mass pool A was 25% higher than the intravascular VLDL B. S_f 20-400 and S_f 12-20 showed precursor-product kinetics but turnover in S_f 12-20 (monoexponential decay) was less than in S_f 20-400, showing that catabolism of VLDL B partly bypassed S_f 12-20. Reinjecting S_f 100-400 gave monoexponential decay; removal of S_f 12-100 was multiexponential and kinetics showed that only part was derived from S_f 100-400. Reinjecting S_f 12-60 labelled I^{131} together with S_f 60-400 (I^{125}) showed that VLDL "intermediate" was in S_f 12-60 rather than in S_f 12-20 range. Finally, VLDL 20-400 B-protein turnover was proportional to pool-size, suggesting overproduction of VLDL in Type 2b and 4 hyperlipoproteinaemia, though diminished removal was also suggested by flattening of the turnover versus pool size curve at high triglyceride levels.

ISOLATION OF LIPOPROTEIN A (LP-A) AND LIPOPROTEIN A-I (LP-A-I) BY IMMUNOSORPTION: EVIDENCE FOR THE LIPOPROTEIN HETEROGENEITY OF NORMAL HUMAN HDL

Alan Suenram and Petar Alaupovic
Lipoprotein Laboratory, Oklahoma Medical Research Foundation, Oklahoma City, OK/USA

To establish whether A-I and A-II polypeptides are assembled with other minor peptides of HDL into a single molecular complex or form separate lipoproteins, we have sequentially fractionated HDL on immunosorbers to individual apolipoproteins. Whole plasma was passed through an immunosorber to ApoD, and HDL were isolated by ultracentrifugation of ApoD-free plasma. Chromatography of HDL on an immunosorber to A-II resulted in retention of LP-A, the protein moiety of which only consisted of A-I and A-II. Since the unretained fraction still contained some

A-I, HDL were sequentially chromatographed on immunosorbers to ApoD, ApoC, albumin and A-II. The unretained fraction consisted only of a small amount of LP-A-I with A-I as the sole peptide. The LP-A was characterized by a protein/lipid ratio of 1.2, A-I/A-II molar ratio close to unity and a mol. wt. of 370,000. The protein/lipid ratio of LP-A-I was 0.33 with phospholipid as the main lipid component. These results show that 1) HDL is not composed of single physical-chemical entities, but separate lipoprotein families, 2) LP-A is the major and LP-A-I a minor lipoprotein of HDL and 3) A-I has a native ability to bind lipids.

CATABOLIC RATE AND FATE OF CANINE APOLIPOPROTEIN A-I

Tsuguhiko Nakai and Thomas F. Whayne, Jr.
Oklahoma Medical Research Foundation, Oklahoma City, OK/USA

The catabolic rate and fate of purified apolipoproteins has not been established. In this study, we investigated the catabolic rate and fate of apolipoprotein (Apo) A-I. Canine Apo A-I was chosen because lipoprotein family A is the major carrier of cholesterol in the dog and Apo A-I is its major constituent polypeptide. Apo A-I was purified by column chromatography of totally delipidated high density lipoprotein subfraction (HDL$_3$). The purified Apo A-I, molecular weight 28,000, had only one precipitin line to either anti-Apo A-I or anti-Apo HDL$_3$ serum. The complete amino acid composition and the 30 N-terminal amino acid sequence of canine Apo A-I were very close to those reported for human Apo A-I. Alanine was the C-terminal amino acid and aspartic acid was N-terminal. Apo A-I was iodinated by the iodine monochloride method of McFarlane and its catabolic rate and fate were investigated. The $T_{1/2}$ of ^{125}I-Apo A-I in HDL$_3$ was 3.33 $\pm$ 0.08 days and in plasma 3.52 $\pm$ 0.17 days, representing no significant difference. The disappearance curve of radioactivity recovered in density fractions d < 1.110 and d > 1.210 g/ml was the same as in HDL$_3$. This indicates that even though distribution of labeled Apo A-I occurs after injection of ^{125}I-Apo A-I, Apo A-I in each density class has an identical rate of catabolism. This adds further support to the concept of lipoprotein families, each with a unique metabolism to be expected throughout the entire lipoprotein density spectrum.

ABNORMALITIES OF THE LIPID TRANSPORT SYSTEM ACCOMPANYING HUMAN LIPOPROTEIN A (LP-A) DEFICIENCY (A VARIANT OF TANGIER DISEASE)

Anders Gustafson, Walter McConathy, Petar Alaupovic, Michael Curry, and Devaki Ganesan
University of Göteborg, Göteborg/Sweden and Oklahoma Medical Research Foundation, Oklahoma City, OK/USA

Further investigation of a patient with familial LP-A deficiency characterized by normal appearance of tonsils, diffuse planar xanthoma, and normal levels of cholesterol, have shown abnormalities of the lipid transport system not previously reported for the classical case of LP-A deficiency, Tagnier disease. In addition to elevated LDL$_1$, normal levels of LDL$_2$ and an absence of LP-A, the electroimmunoassay of apolipoproteins in serum demonstrated slightly elevated levels of ApoB, ApoC and ApoE ("arg-rich" polypeptide). ApoD and A-II were reduced and A-I was almost absent (1/2, 1/6 and 1/100 of normal levels, respectively). Though LP-A deficiency has an almost complete absence of HDL and A-I, the normal serum levels of ApoB, ApoC and ApoE demonstrate that they are synthesized independently of ApoA. In addition to the presence of an abnormal lipoprotein LP-A-II in LDL$_2$, the percent composition of LP-B was dissimilar to normal LP-B [TG = 26.0 vs 7.8; TC = 14.2 vs 38.2; PL = 19.2 vs 26.4; and ApoB = 40.6 vs 27.6 (abnormal B versus normal B)]. Fractionation of post-heparin lipases (PHL) demonstrated slightly reduced levels of triglyceride lipase and LPL$_{C-I}$ but significantly decreased levels of LPL$_{C-II}$ similar to the pattern seen in broad-β disease. The ratio of esterified/free cholesterol was normal. These results show that this variant of LP-A deficiency differs from Tangier disease.

CELLULAR AND SUBCELLULAR CATABOLIC SITE(S) OF CANINE APOLIPOPROTEIN A-I

Tsuguhiko Nakai and Thomas F. Whayne, Jr.
Oklahoma Medical Research Foundation, Oklahoma City, OK/USA

The definite cellular and subcellular site(s) and mechanisms involved in apolipoprotein catabolism have not been established. In this study, we investigated: 1) Cellular and subcellular distribution of apolipoprotein (Apo) after injection of ^{125}I-labeled canine Apo A-I into dogs, and 2) in vitro proteolysis of high density lipoprotein subfraction (HDL$_3$) by lysosomal enzymes. The liver took up 5 times more radioactivity than both kidneys and 20 times more than spleen. Highest subcellular fraction radioactivity was in lysosomes. In vitro analysis of isolated subcellular proteolytic activity was studied to explore this further. Due to decreased solubility of canine Apo A-I and Apo HDL$_3$ in the assay pH of 3.8, native canine HDL$_3$ (1.110 < d < 1.210 g/ml) was incubated with soluble fraction of canine liver lysosomes at pH 3.8. HDL$_3$ proteolysis by lysosomal acid proteases, measured as peptide and amino acid release by ninhydrin, followed hyperbolic curves; straight lines were obtained on Lineweaver-Burk plots. Incubation with other subcellular organelle fractions did not result in HDL$_3$ proteolysis. Iodoacetate (specific inhibitor for cathepsin B) inhibited HDL$_3$ proteolysis 100% and bovine albumin proteolysis 65%. Pepstatin (specific for cathepsin D) inhibited HDL$_3$ proteolysis 45% and bovine albumin proteolysis 70%. Our in vivo and in vitro data indicate that hepatic lysosomes from enzyme inhibition studies suggest that a specific lysosomal endopeptidase, cathepsin B, may play a key role in this proteolysis.

COMPARATIVE PROPERTIES OF THE HDL APOPROTEINS OF HUMAN AND NON-HUMAN PRIMATES

V. Blaton, M. Rosseneu, and H. Peeters
Simon Stevin Instituut, Brugge/Belgium

The HDL lipoproteins of human and non-human primates have a different sphingomyelin (S) and lecithin (L) content: this results in a S/L ratio of 0.2 in man and chimpanzee and of 0.07 in the baboon. The major apoproteins of high density lipoproteins (1.090 < d < 1.21) from baboons and chimpanzees under the same diet were fractionated of DEAE-cellulose, characterized by physical and chemical methods and compared to the human apoproteins. The chimpanzee has a monomeric apoA-I and a dimeric apoA-II very similar to man whereas the baboon has a monomeric apoA-II different from man in aminoacid composition. Differences in the reassembly of phospholipids were detected by spectrophotometry and ultracentrifugation. Changes in the secondary structure during relipidation were established by CD. The differences between the sphingomyelin and lecithin content and ratio are probably related to the differences in aminoacid composition and sequence.
From the comparative properties of the apoproteins in human and non-human primates a better insight into the validity of the animal model for the study of hyperlipoproteinemia and atherosclerosis in man is obtained.

INTERASSOCIATION OF HDL APOPROTEINS IN MAN AND BABOON

M. Rosseneu, F. Soetewey, J. Lievens, V. Blaton, H. Peeters
Simon Stevin Instituut Brugge/Belgium and W.V. Brown University of California,
San Diego, CA/USA

The enthalpy changes involved in the binding of synthetic dimyristoyl phosphatidylcholine (DMPC) to isolated HDL apoproteins from man and baboon have been measured by microcalorimetry. Human apoA-I and human apoA-II in its dimeric and monomeric form have been compared to apoA-I and monomeric apoA-II from the baboon.
The enthalpy changes are slightly lower for baboon apoA-I and apoA-II than for
their human counterpart though the stoichiometry of the complexes is very similar.
Apoprotein mixtures containing various ratios of human apoA-I together with either dimeric or monomeric human apoA-II were recombined with DMPC. The measured
enthalpy changes are higher than those expected for non-interacting mixtures and
the maximal association occurred at either an equimolar ratio of apoA-I to dimeric apoA-II or at a 1/2 ratio of apoA-I to monomeric apoA-II. Identical results
were obtained with baboon apoA-I/monomeric apoA-II mixtures, suggesting that
this type of association is a fundamental process in stabilization of the HDL molecule.
Based on these observations a mechanism for lipid/protein and protein/protein associations within the HDL will be presented.

SURFACE BINDING OF APO-LDL BY HUMAN LYMPHOCYTES

D. Reichl and N.B. Myant
Medical Research Council Lipid Metabolism Unit, Hammersmith Hospital, London/
England

Human lymphocytes were incubated for 2 h with radioiodinated human low-density
lipoproteins (LDL) at $4°C$. After incubation the cells were washed 8 times with
Eagle's Minimum Essential Medium (MEM). They were then incubated for 30 min at
$4°C$ in MEM or MEM containing 10 mg/ml of heparin. Alternatively, they were incubated with 0.12% trypsin for 2 min at $37°C$ to release surface-bound LDL. The
amount of surface-bound non-lipid radioactivity (presumed to be LDL protein) released by trypsin was several times that released by heparin cf MEM. Lymphocytes
from a patient with homozygous familial hypercholesterolaemia behaved in the
same way as lymphocytes from normal subjects. The effect of heparin on surface-
binding of LDL was examined by incubating lymphocytes in MEM (control cells) or
in MEM containing heparin (10 mg/ml) for 1 h at $4°C$. The cells were then washed
repeatedly and incubated for a further 2 h at $25°C$ in MEM containing radio-LDL
at various concentrations. Surface-bound LDL was measured at the end of the incubation. With control cells, surface-bound LDL/mg of cell protein was linearly
related to LDL concentration up to 300 µg of LDL protein/ml. With heparin-treated
cells, surface-binding of LDL was non-linear with respect to LDL concentration
and at all concentrations was less than that by control cells. We conclude that
lymphocytes possess high-capacity binding sites for LDL and that binding capacity is decreased by pre-treatment with heparin.

STUDY OF A POST PRANDIAL SERUM LIPOPROTEINS

Fumio Akuda, Kazunari Wada, Mitsuo Wada, and Junichi Mise
Department of Internal Medicine, Yamaguchi University School of Medicine,
Ube/Japan

In 91 human subjects aged 40 to 55 years, who underwent physical and laboratory
examinations frequently for five years, the effect of the diet on serum lipopro-

teins represented by PAGE disc or block electrophoretogram and lipoprotein precipitation technique was studied.

A high carbohydrate diet, particularly alcohol intake, induced hyper pre-beta lipoproteinemia. The frequency of hypo alpha lipoproteinemia was high in the hyper pre-beta lipoproteinemia accompanied with hypertriglyceridemia.

Post prandial triglyceride rich serum lipoproteins determined by lipoprotein precipitation technique remained at a high level on the ischemic heart diseases with sustained hypertriglyceridemia.

CABOXYL-TERMINAL AMINO ACIDS OF APOLIPOPROTEIN B, THE MAJOR PROTEIN MOIETY OF LOW DENSITY LIPOPROTEINS OF HUMAN PLASMA

Diana M. Lee, Douglas Lawrence, and Shuan Huang
Cardiovascular Research Program, Oklahoma Medical Research Foundation, Oklahoma City, OK/USA

Low density lipoproteins of d 1.019-1.053 g/ml (LDL_2) were isolated by phosphotungstate precipitation and ultracentrifugation. The albumin-free LDL_2 were delipidized. The apoLDL_2 were partially soluble in 6 M guanidine hydrochloride (GuCl) and Tris buffer at pH 8.3. The protein solution was chromatographed on Bio-Gel A-5m equilibrated with the same buffer system. The first peak, eluted at the void volume, was immunochemically reactive only with anti-LPB. The GuCl-insoluble protein became soluble in GuCl after treatment with reducing and alkylating agents and was also eluted at the void volume of Bio-Gel A-5m. The C-terminal amino acids of ApoB were studied by ^{3}H-labeling followed by 24 h acid hydrolysis or carboxypeptidase A of B (CPA or CPB) digestion. Amino acids were separated on an amino acid analyzer. Aliquots of the separated amino acids were removed and counted for radioactivity. Labeled amino acids were identified by amino acid analyzer utilizing two internal standards. The labeled amino acids were found to be leucine, serine and lysine. High voltage electrophoresis and paper chromatography were also employed to achieve better separation between serine and threonine resulting in radioactivity only on serine. Kinetic studies with CPA or CPB on unlabeled ApoB confirmed leucine, serine and lysine as the C-terminal amino acids of ApoB.

These results suggest that ApoB contains at least three non-identical polypeptides.

DIRECT MICRODETERMINATION OF β-LIPOPROTEIN CHOLESTEROL WITHOUT ULTRACENTRIFUGATION

C.C. Heuck, H. Raetzer, and G. Schlierf
Klinisches Institut für Herzinfarktforschung, Heidelberg/BRD

A newly developed procedure for the direct quantification of cholesterol concentrations in lipoproteins fractionated from 10 µl serum is compared with the classical method of ultracentrifugation. Serum lipoproteins are separated by electrophoresis on agarose at pH 8,6 and visualised by precipitation with dextran sulfate/$CaCl_2$.

The lipoprotein bands are scraped off and the agarose slices are hydrolysed with KOH. Cholesterol is extracted with heptane and quantitated by GLC. Correlation with ultracentrifugation: r = 0,97 for total cholesterol, r = 0,96 for β-cholesterol. Slightly higher values are obtained for VLDL/pre-β and HDL/α fractions by the micro procedure.

REGULATION OF CHOLESTEROL BIOSYNTHESIS IN RAT LIVER BY TWO DIFFERENT PLASMA LIPOPROTEINS

Michael Liersch, Christian C. Heuck, Giovanella Baggio, and Dietrich Seidel
Medical Clinic, University of Heidelberg, Heidelberg/BRD

The cause of increased hepatic cholesterol biosynthesis (HCB) in cholestasis is not yet clear. Since it was believed that plasma cholesterol is a powerful inhibitor of HCB and since it was shown that lipoproteins of lower density exert a negative feed-back on HCB we compared the effect of LP-X, the plasma-lipoprotein characterizing cholestatis and normal LDL on HCB in rat. Male Sprague-Dawley rats (160-180g) were infused intravenously from 8 a.m. to 10 p.m. with 0.9% NaCl (controls), LDL (25 mg cholesterin/100 g rat) or LP-X (24 mg cholesterin/100 g rat). The livers were removed and perfused. Cholesterol and fatty acid synthesis were measured by incorporation of tritiated water. Results: cholesterol synthesis (μatom ^{3}H/h/g dry weight $\pm$ S.E.): controls 17.9 $\pm$ 1.6 (n = 10); LDL 7.6 $\pm$ 2.1 (n = 5); LP-X 14.5 $\pm$ 2.9 (n = 6). Fatty acid synthesis: controls 23.3 $\pm$ 4.9; LDL 28.4 $\pm$ 10.1; LP-X 20.5 $\pm$ 6.3. Our results demonstrate that LDL in contrast to LP-X exerts a feed-back inhibition on HCB and suggest that not so much the level of plasma cholesterol is important for the regulation of HCB but rather the properties of the particles which transport cholesterol in plasma.

IN VITRO CHOLESTEROL ESTERIFICATION IN PATIENTS WITH TYPE II AND TYPE IV HYPERLIPOPROTEINAEMIA

Costas D. Moutafis and George E. Merikas.
University Medical Department, Hippokration Hospital, Athens/Greece

The study of cholesterol esterification (CEF) in hyperlipoproteinaemia could help in understanding the relationship between this reaction and the metabolism of lipoproteins.
Two normal subjects, two type IV and four type II (two hetero and two homozygotes) were studied.
Fasting serum was mixed with $4C^{14}$ cholesterol-albumin emulsion and incubated at 37°C for 11 hours. Six aliquots were taken at various intervals during the incubation, were mixed with DTNB and put in 4°C. Other aliquots were also mixed with DTNB after 5 hours incubation but were left at 37°C for up to 6 hours. The chol. ester sp. act. was determined in total serum in HDL, LDL and VLDL by ultracentrifugation, TLC and liquid scintillation counting.
CE sp. act. was rising in all fractions during the incubation. The total serum CE sp. act. and the rate of CEF was higher in normal and in type IV patients and lower in type II. In all subjects the CE sp. act. was higher in HDL, lower in LDL and intermediate in VLDL, but the ratio of CE sp. act. of HDL to LDL was falling during the incubation. Addition of DTNB during the incubation resulted in a fall of CE sp. act. of HDL whereas LDL and VLDL CE sp. act. continued rising until isotopic equilibrium was reached. This fall was faster in type IV. The study of the sp. act. curve suggests that CEF occurs in HDL and the newly formed CE exchange with the CE of LDL mainly via VLDL. It seems very likely that VLDL not only increases the rate of CEF but also participated in the exchange of CE between HDL and LDL.

METABOLIC COMPENSATION TO DIETARY CHOLESTEROL

A. Poyser and P. Nestel
Department of Clinical Science, The Australian National University, Canberra,
A.C.T./Australia

Dietary cholesterol (CH) contributes to serum CH level, though this depends on
compensating factors such as reduced CH synthesis and increased CH excretion.
This was tested in 8 subjects, 2 normocholesterolaemic and 6 hypercholesterolaemic, by comparing 2 levels of CH intake: 250 and 750 mg/day. Diets were standardized and high in polyunsaturated fats. CH absorption, synthesis (net balance),
endogenous excretion and bile acid excretion were measured by isotopic and chemical analysis of faecal sterols over periods of 8-14 weeks.
Two types of response were observed. 1. In the 2 normal and in 3 hypercholesterolaemic subjects, serum CH did not rise significantly with added 500 mg CH (as
egg yolk). Percent absorption of CH and bile acid excretion were unchanged. CH
synthesis was clearly reduced; CH re-excretion rose in some. These compensating
factors balanced increased absorption in all 5. In other normal subjects, compensation was complete even with 1g added CH. 2. In 3 hypercholesterolaemics, CH
synthesis was only minimally suppressed by higher CH intake. Though CH re-excretion rose, serum CH rose substantially.
Conclusions: 1. Moderate intake of CH need not raise serum CH if CH synthesis is
inhibited. 2. Increased CH re-excretion may follow rise in serum CH.

RELATIONSHIP OF BILE LIPIDS AND PLASMALIPOPROTEINS: A MODEL TO STUDY LIPID METABOLISM AND PROTEIN-LIPID-INTERACTION

Giovanella Baggio, Enzo Manzato, Renato Fellin, Heinrich Wieland, and
Dietrich Seidel
Medical Clinic, University of Heidelberg/BRD, and the University of Padova,
Padova/Italy

Evidence will be provided that bile lipids are organized in form of a lipoprotein (bile-LP) carrying albumin as major apoprotein and devoid of the normal apoproteins A,B,C,D and arginine rich peptide. The protein-lipid-composition of
bile-LP is similar to LP-X, the lipoprotein characterizing cholestasis, but the
two differ in major physicochemical and chemical properties. However, bile-LP
may be utilized as a precursor particle for complete in vitro formation of LP-X.
In vitro conversion of bile-LP to LP-X is independent of any active metabolic
process but dependent on certain physicochemical requirements primarily on the
kind and concentration of proteins and bile- or other acids in the system. Variation of the system results in differently composed and/or structured lipoprotein compounds, which may widely be used as models to study protein-lipid-inter-
action and the regulation of lipid metabolism.

CHARACTERIZATION OF TWO ELECTROPHORETIC POPULATIONS OF HUMANS VERY LOW DENSITY LIPOPROTEINS

A. Pagnan, R.J. Havel, and J.P. Kane
Cardiovascular Research Institute, University of California, San Francisco,
CA/USA and Clinica Medica II, University of Padova, Padova/Italy

By preparative agarose-gel electrophoresis, two populations of VLDL migrating in
pre-beta position as two distinct bands, were isolated in 5 subjects. The weight
ratio of cholesteryl esters (CE) to triglycerides (TG) is about 0.13 and 0.44 in
the fast and slow fractions, respectively. The protein moiety of the slower fraction is enriched in B apoprotein and arginine rich protein (ARP) at the expense
of the C apoprotein. By negative staining electron microscopy the mean diameter

of the slower fraction is about 60-100 A less than that of the faster fraction. The protein composition of particles isolated in the density range 1.006-1.019, intermediate density lipoprotein (IDL), resembles that of the slower VLDL fraction but IDL are still smaller and have an even higher ratio CE to TG. The slowly migrating VLDL variant, shares several features with the beta VLDL of primary dysbetalipoproteinemia, but beta VLDL have a ratio CE to TG and ARP to B apoprotein even higher than the slow pre-beta VLDL. In addition, upon isoelectric focussing gel electrophoresis of the apoproteins, both beta and pre-beta VLDL from patients with dysbetalipoproteinemia lack one or more of the multyple bands of ARP present in the two populations of "double pre-beta" VLDL.

THE TRANSPORT OF ESTERIFIED CHOLESTEROL IN PLASMA HIGH DENSITY LIPOPROTEINS

Philip Barter and Janice Lally
School of Medicine, Flinders University of South Australia, Australia

Previous studies have suggested that the pools of both esterified cholesterol (EC) and triglyceride in the plasma high density lippproteins (HDL) are kinetically heterogeneous. These present studies were performed to examine the kinetics of EC transport in plasma HDL using 2.5 kg male rabbits as a model.
Donor rabbits were injected iv with 1 mCi of ^{3}H-mevalonic acid and 12 hours later when the major proportion of the HDL cholesterol label was in the EC fraction, serum was obtained and the HDL isolated by ultracentrifugation. After dialysis, this labeled HDL was reinjected into recipient rabbits. Four separate experiments were performed in each of which the HDL from one donor animal was reinjected into two recipients. Serial blood samples were collected from each recipient and the HDL isolated. The HDL free cholesterol label disappeared rapidly with only 2-3% of the injected dose remaining after 15 minutes. Disappearence of the HDL EC label was slower and computer analysis indicated a biexponential decay with the slower turning over component possessing a T 1/2 of about 2 1/2 hours and the faster component a T 1/2 of about 30 minutes.
It is concluded that the transport of EC in the plasma HDL fits a two-pool model.

STUDIES INDICATING METABOLIC DIFFERENCES BETWEEN Lp(a+) AND Lp(a-) INDIVIDUALS

Gösta Dahlén and Kåre Berg
Laboratory of Clinical Chemistry, County Hospital, Boden/Sweden and
Institute of Medical Genetics, University of Oslo, Oslo/Norway

A series of 30 previously investigated and presumably healthy middleaged males from Northern Sweden has been studied. In an oral glucose tolerance test insulin mean value at 120 min was significantly lower in individuals possessing the Lp(a) antigen and high amounts of "true" pre-β_1-lipoprotein (with density 1.050-1.080 g/ml) than in those who were negative with respect to these lipoprotein phenomena. Fasting triglyceride and insulin levels at 60 min were significantly correlated in Lp(a-) but not in Lp(a+) individuals. The mean value for free thyroxine factor was significantly higher in the Lp(a-) than in the Lp(a+) group of persons.
Pooled data from 12 populations studied previously showed that the mean total cholesterol and "LDL-cholesterol" were significantly higher in Lp(a+) than in Lp(a-) individuals. On the other hand, the mean triglyceride level was found to be lower in Lp(a+) than in Lp(a-) individuals. This difference was highly significant in middle-aged and elderly people.
In view of the positive association found between presence of Lp(a) antigen/ pre-β_1-lipoprotein and atherosclerotic heart disease in several series studied, these differences may be of clinical importance.

DIFFERENCES BETWEEN RAT AND MAN IN THE FORMATION OF LOW DENSITY LIPOPROTEIN FROM VERY LOW DENSITY LIPOPROTEIN

N. Fidge and P. Poulis
Department of Clinical Science, The Australian National University, Canberra, A.C.T./Australia

Most plasma low density lipoprotein (LDL) in man is derived from very low density lipoprotein (VLDL). In order to test the rat as a model for investigating this pathway, ^{125}I or ^{14}C labelled VLDL were injected into rats and the specific radioactivities (SR) of the B apoprotein of VLDL, LDL_1 and LDL_2 determined at various time intervals thereafter.
The kinetics of VLDL B protein disappearance best fitted two exponential curves (T 1/2 10 min and 4 h). The turnover rate of VLDL B protein was 1.82 mg/Kg/h, compared to 0.7 mg/Kg/h in humans. The SR of LDL_2 peaked at between 30 and 60 min. Although the results suggested precursor-product relationships between VLDL and LDL_1 (S_f 12-20) no crossover of B protein SR occurred between VLDL and LDL_2 (S_f 0-12) at its peak SR and the proportion of LDL_2 derived from VLDL was calculated to be 35%. This data suggests that, unlike man, only a small proportion of VLDL B protein is converted to LDL_2 and about 1/3 of LDL_2 B protein is derived from plasma VLDL.
Studies on rat LDL show that this lipoprotein is richer in triglyceride (TG) than LDL_2 in man and we suggest that a TG rich LDL_1 (secreted by rat liver or intestine) is, like VLDL, converted to higher density LDL_2 in the plasma.

REGULATION OF LIPOPROTEIN SYNTHESIS IN ALCOHOLIC LIVER DISEASE

H.B. Stähelin, J.T. Locher, N. Thurnherr, and N. Gyr
Department of Internal Medicine, Kantonsspital, University of Basle, Basle/Switzerland

Chronic alcohol ingestion leads in man to an increased triglyceride (TGL) synthesis. The effect on the apo-protein synthesis is poorly understood. In order to explore this question lipoproteins were labeled in vivo with ^{75}Se-selenomethionine (SeM) in 7 subjects with chronic alcohol intake (I) and after 2-3 weeks of abstinence (II). The VLDL, IDL, LDL, and HDL were isolated by ultracentrifugation. The activity of the incorporated SeM and the apo-protein concentration of each fraction was determined. Plasma cholesterol and TGL were estimated.
The fraction of SeM incorporated in apo-VLD did not differ from study I to II (2.37 vs 2.35%). T_{max} (4.4 ± 1.9 vs 4.3 ± 1.6 h) and fractional turnover of VLD-SeM was similar in I and II (k_h-1 .15 ± .05 vs .17 ± 07). However, the apo-VLD concentration was higher (p < .01) in I compared to II (222 ± 166 vs 108 ± 94 mcg/ml plasma). Similarly the TGL were higher in I than in II (232 ± 123 vs 123 ± 70 mg/dl; p < .01). No significant changes were noted in the other fractions. The discrepancy between the unchanged incorporation of SeM (a measure of the de novo synthesis) and the estimated apo-VLD turnover (pool size x k) in I compared to II is best explained by a variable transfer of unlabeled apo-proteins to nascent VLDL. This mechanism would allow the transport of changing amounts of VLD-TGL with minor changes in the de novo apo-VLD synthesis.

FILTRATION OF CHYLOMICRONS AND THEIR REMNANTS BY THE LIVER

R. Fraser, A.G. Bosanquet, and W.A. Day
Department of Pathology, Christchurch Clinical School; Christchurch/New Zealand

The liver plays a central role in the metabolism of chylomicrons. Large chylomicrons are not metabolised by the liver, but remnant chylomicrons are. This indicates that the liver must "recognise" the remnant but not the chylomicron. The description by Wisse of pores of 100 nm in the endothelium separating the blood sinuses from the space of Disse and hepatocytes in rat livers is a possible site of recognition. Our hypothesis is that chylomicrons must be catabolised to less than 100 nm in diameter before they can contact liver cells because of the size limit imposed by these pores. Electron microscopy and isotope studies of the liver following the injection of chylomicrons and their remnants into the portal vein support this hypothesis. This sieving may have physiological importance, since during low dietary fat intake some chylomicrons may be small enough to contact liver cells, but during high fat intake most chylomicrons are too large to contact hepatocytes. They must first be stripped of much of their triglyceride by peripheral lipases and so reduced to smaller cholesterol-rich remnants. The liver filter may thus help explain partitioning in the metabolism of different dietary lipids and the effect of different quantities and types of dietary fats on cholesterol metabolism and even atherogenesis.

INTERMEDIATE DENSITY LIPOPROTEIN (IDL) APOLIPOPROTEIN B (APOB) CONCENTRATIONS IN NORMAL AND HYPERLIPIDEMIC (HLP) SUBJECTS

Pesach Segal and Paul Roheim
Metabolic Research Laboratory, The Chaim Sheba Medical Center,
Tel-Hashomer/Israel

ApoB was measured by quantitative immunoelectrophoresis and it's levels in IDL were estimated from the difference between ApoB concentrations in the ultracentrifugally separated 1.006 and 1.019 bottom fractions. The absolute amounts of IDL ApoB were similar in normals, and in patients with type II and type IV HLP. However it was considerably higher in patients with type III HLP, and in patients with type IV HLP who presented with milky serum and erruptive xanthoma. Normal subjects and type IV HLP patients had 13% of the 1.006 bottom ApoB in IDL, whereas type II HLP patients had only 7% in this fraction. Patients with type IV HLP who presented with erruptive xanthoma and treated by low CHO diet, had 30% of their 1.006 bottom ApoB in IDL. Type III HLP patients before treatment had 60% of their 1.006 bottom ApoB in IDL, and a low CHO diet reduced it to 36%. Type III HLP patients have an abnormally high IDL ApoB levels even when they become normolipemic on a low CHO diet.
Conclusions: 1) Type III HLP patients have an abnormal IDL, as well as VLDL, which can be detected even when they become normolipemic by dietary intervention. 2) Patients with milky serum and erruptive xanthoma, also have abnormally high IDL levels, inspite of the fact that they do not conform with the criteria of type III HLP.

LIPOPROTEIN ANALYSIS WITH ELECTROPHORESIS USING AN INTERNAL STANDARD

Tomojiro Seki, Takao Fujinami, Nagahiko Sakuma, Junichi Yokoi, Katsuhiko Hayashi, Sagami Nakano, and Reiji Higuchi
Central Laboratory of Clinical Pathology, Department of Internal Medicine,
Nagoya City University Medical School, Nagoya/Japan

For the purpose to estimate total lipids and lipoprotein constituents in serum, an internal standard was introduced to electrophoresis on agarose gel. The internal standard is dyed, carbamylated human serum albumin (DC-albumin) which has similar color to lipoprotein staining dye, Sudan black B, and faster mobility than albumin. DC-albumin was made a solution which was mixed with each serum sample with a definite ratio. The mixture was applied on agarose gel plate and separated in electic field. The plates were fixed and stained as usual and estimated by a densitometer at 570 nm. Reciprocal of percent density of DC-albumincorrelates significantly with total lipids content simultaneously determined by Fings's method (r = -0.91). Each lipoprotein fractions calculated by products of total lipids which estimated from reciprocal of DC-albumin and percent densities on electrophoresis were correlated significantly with those determined by quantitative ultracentrifugation. Thus, electrophorectogram can be used not only to estimate total lipids content but also to analyze lipoprotein constituents in serum quantitatively. This simple method is an useful tool for investigation on lipoprotein metabolism in clinical practice for atherosclerosis or other lipid metabolism disorders.

CHEMICAL COMPOSITION OF ULTRACENTRIFUGAL LIPOPROTEIN (U.C.) FRACTIONS IN DIFFERENT PICTURES OF HUMAN ATHEROSCLEROSIS

P. Avogaro, G. Cazzolato, G.C. Taroni, and F. Belussi
Regional General Hospital, Venice/Italy

Chemical composition of U.C. has been studied up to now only in post-infarction state. Data are here referred regarding, beside 37 post-infarcted men (M.I.), 23 patients with non-obstructive ischaemic heart disease (I.H.D.), 23 with atherosclerosis of inferior limbs (P.A.) and 23 affected by cerebrovascular disease (C.V.D.). M.I. group differed significantly from 52 controls in higher values of total-C, VLDL-C, LDL-C; I.H.D. in higher values of total-C, VLDL-C, LDL-C, total-TG, VLDL-TG, LDL-TG, HDL-TG; A.P. in higher values of VLDL-C, HDL-C, total-TG and VLDL-TG. No significative variations from controls have been recorded in C.V.D. In M.I., I.H.D. and P.A. nearly comparable frequencies of types IIA, IIB and IV have been found. Frequency of HL states in C.V.D. was minor than in controls.

Chairmen: D. Vesselinovitch, USA
          T. Nakashima, Japan

Participants: D. Vesselinovitch, USA
              H.Y.C. Wong, USA
              F. Numano, Japan
              W. Insull, USA
              F. Kuzuya, Japan
              M.G. Bond, USA
              N.D.M. Lehner, USA

REQUIREMENT FOR REGRESSION STUDIES IN ANIMAL MODELS

D. Vesselinovitch and Robert W. Wissler

Animal models serve as a rich source of information in the study and elucidation of atherosclerotic disease, in addition to epidemiological studies, tissue culture, and biochemical analyses. Experimental work on regression of atherosclerosis in animal models has an important role in the accumulation of data regarding effect and interrelationships among diet, hypocholesterolemic agents and other therapy in arresting or reversing this disease process.

One of the most persistent dogmas in medicine has been the conviction held by many that atherosclerotic disease cannot be reversed. Nevertheless, regression of spontaneous and experimental atherosclerosis has long been suspected. Only recently have some basic but crucial animal studies been able to verify this.

Since the early rabbit regression studies (Anitschkow, 1928), work has been done with chickens (Horlick and Katz, 1949; Wong et al., 1973), pigeons (Clarkson et al., 1971; St. Clair et al., 1972), dogs (Bevans et al., 1951; DePalma et al., 1968), squirrel monkeys-*Saimuri sciurea* (Maruffo and Portman, 1968), rhesus monkeys-*M. mulatta* (Armstrong et al., 1970; Tucker et al., 1971; Vesselinovitch et al., 1973; Stary, 1974; Wissler et al., 1975), cynomolgus-*M. fascicularis* (Armstrong and Megan, 1974), rats (Morrison et al., 1972), and swine (Daoud et al., 1974; Kim et al., 1975).

An overview of studies concerned with the reversal of atherosclerosis is presented in Table 1. Most of these experiments were planned with this objective in mind, while in others regression phenomena were observed in the course of other atherogenic studies. An attempt is made to divide the work into three groups according to the results obtained. The studies where reversal or arrest was observed are summarized in the first column. The second column presents the number of investigations with questionalbe regression, despite some changes in lesions suggestive of the regression. In the third column, studies with definitely negative results are given. It is evident that the negative studies are the least numerous. However, the largest number of unsuccessful studies is in rabbits. In this species, cessation of the atherogenic regimen and its substitution with a low-fat, low-cholesterol diet does not result in reversal of moderate or severe disease (Constantinides et al., 1960; Connor et al., 1966; Clarkson et al., 1971; Adams et al., 1973). A tendency in this species to store enormous quantities of cholesterol might be responsible for this kind of reaction. However, positive results were obtained when the feeding period was brief and most of the resulting lesions were mild (Bortz, 1968; Yusufi, 1974) or when combined therapy was employed (Wartmann et al., 1967; Vesselinovitch et al., 1968; Kjeldsen et al., 1969; Kramsch and Chan, 1975).

Table 1. Regression studies of atherosclerosis in animal studies (1928-1976)

	Successful	Intermediate	Unsuccessful
Total no. of studies	29	10	8
Total no. of advanced disease	9	3	1

Thus, the question is no longer if atherosclerosis can be arrested or reversed, but rather, where, when and how, and whether the changes in the lesions are an indication of regression, arrest or modification. Therefore, the questions to be answered are: in what species, in what part of the arterial tree, in what type of lesions, and with what kind of therapy can regression be achieved?

From studies done so far, it is obvious not only that atherosclerotic lesions appear to regress differently in different species, but also differently in various parts of the arterial tree. Already, Anitschkow (1928) has observed a differential regression rate between various portions of the aortic wall, and more recent observations have confirmed this (Stary, 1972). In all species there is an intricate relationship between the action-reaction phenomenon in the vessel wall, and the changes in this balance determine in which direction the atherosclerotic process will go. The aim of the studies concerned with reversal is to control which of these processes is predominant in the species under study.

The postulate of Horlick and Katz (1949) still holds true that there is a limit to the degree of atherosclerotic damage that can be repaired. Lesions of a certain age or makeup can disappear completely (Duff and McMillan, 1951); others can only undergo limited repair. Although a whole gamut of lesions is seen in humans, fatty streaks seldom result in complications of any significance (Tejada et al., 1968). On the other hand, the raised fibrous plaques or advanced arterial lesions, the true atheromas or so-called "human-type lesions", are frequently respondible for clinical complications.

However, the number of investigations concerned with the regression of moderate or severe human-type lesions is quite small (Table 1). The reason for the small number of studies is the fact that in certain species the induction of severe human-type lesions is not easy. It requires either prolonged dietary manipulation, alternating diets, or a combination of induction methods, such as diet combined with immunologic (Minick and Murphy, 1973) or mechanical injury (Baumgartner and Studer, 1966), or with x-irradiation (Vesselinovitch et al., 1968; Kirkpatrick, 1967; Lee et al., 1971), hypoxia (Kjeldsen et al., 1968; Helin and Lorenzen, 1969), or others. Whatever method or methods used, the evaluation of these so-called human lesions and documentation of their fate is of utmost importance for the treatment of human disease. However, to produce similar results in experimental animals different kinds of therapy will be needed depending on the species under study and the severity of the disease.

Table 2 summarizes the results of regression studies in our laboratory. By a combination of either low-fat, low-cholesterol diet, O_2 (100% 2 h/day) and 1% cholestyramine, or low-fat, low-cholesterol diet, O_2 and estrogen (1.332 mg estradiol benzoate, s.c.), we were able for a period of 10 weeks to arrest and reverse diet-induced moderate and severe disease in rabbits (Vesselinovitch and Wissler, 1968; Vesselinovitch et al., 1973). In rhesus monkeys, on the other hand, lesions induced by feeding a coconut oil, butterfat, and cholesterol diet for a period of 18 months were substantially reduced by a low-fat, low-cholesterol diet, either alone or in combination with drug N-y-phenylpropyl-N-benzyloxy acetamide (W-1372) (Vesselinovitch et al., 1974, 1976). Feeding the same atherogenic diet for a period of 12 months resulted in lesions which have shown evi-

Table 2. Regression studies in rabbits and rhesus monkeys

Rabbits

Marked reduction of lesions induced by diet

    Treatment:

        a) Diet, O_2, cholestyramine
        b) Diet, O_2, estrogen

Monkeys

Reduction of lesions induced by different kinds of diets

    Treatment:

        a) Low-fat, low-cholesterol diet
        b) Low-fat, low-cholesterol diet + W 1372
        c) Low-fat, low-cholesterol + cholestyramine
        d) Atherogenic diet + cholestyramine
        e) American "prudent-like" diet

Table 3. Objectives of reversal studies

To establish treatment of human disease by means of:

        a) Specific diet
        b) Drug therapy
        c) Surgery
        d) Physical exercise

To explore mechanisms underlying regression by studying:

        a) Lipid chemistry and metabolism
        b) Role of hormones
        c) Effect of O_2
        d) Role of enzymes

----

dence of regression by a low-fat, low-cholesterol diet, with or without a 2.5% cholestyramine. An interesting finding in these studies was that cholestyramine alone resulted in some regression even when the monkeys continued to be fed the atherogenic diet (Wissler et al., 1975).

Table 3 lists some of the problems and requirements for intensive study of regression in animal models. Standardization of a few induction methods, including time and animal species, is needed. One of the difficulties is the variability of induction methods. In animal studies, experimental results are only valid for the precise conditions under which the experiments were conducted, which makes comparison between various models difficult. If one looks at the bar graph (Fig. 1) which summarizes timetables of both induction and regression periods, one must be impressed by the variability in both periods. Judging from this bar graph, if the results are to be positive, the regression periods must be equal to or longer than the induction time, or a combination of therapeutic agents must be employed for treatment.

Another very real problem is our inability to induce uniform lesions. Although certain diets may result in predominantly characteristic lesions, none of the dietary fats studied so far ever induces lesions of only one type. A wide range of lesions can be seen for any particular diet (Wissler et al., 1976).

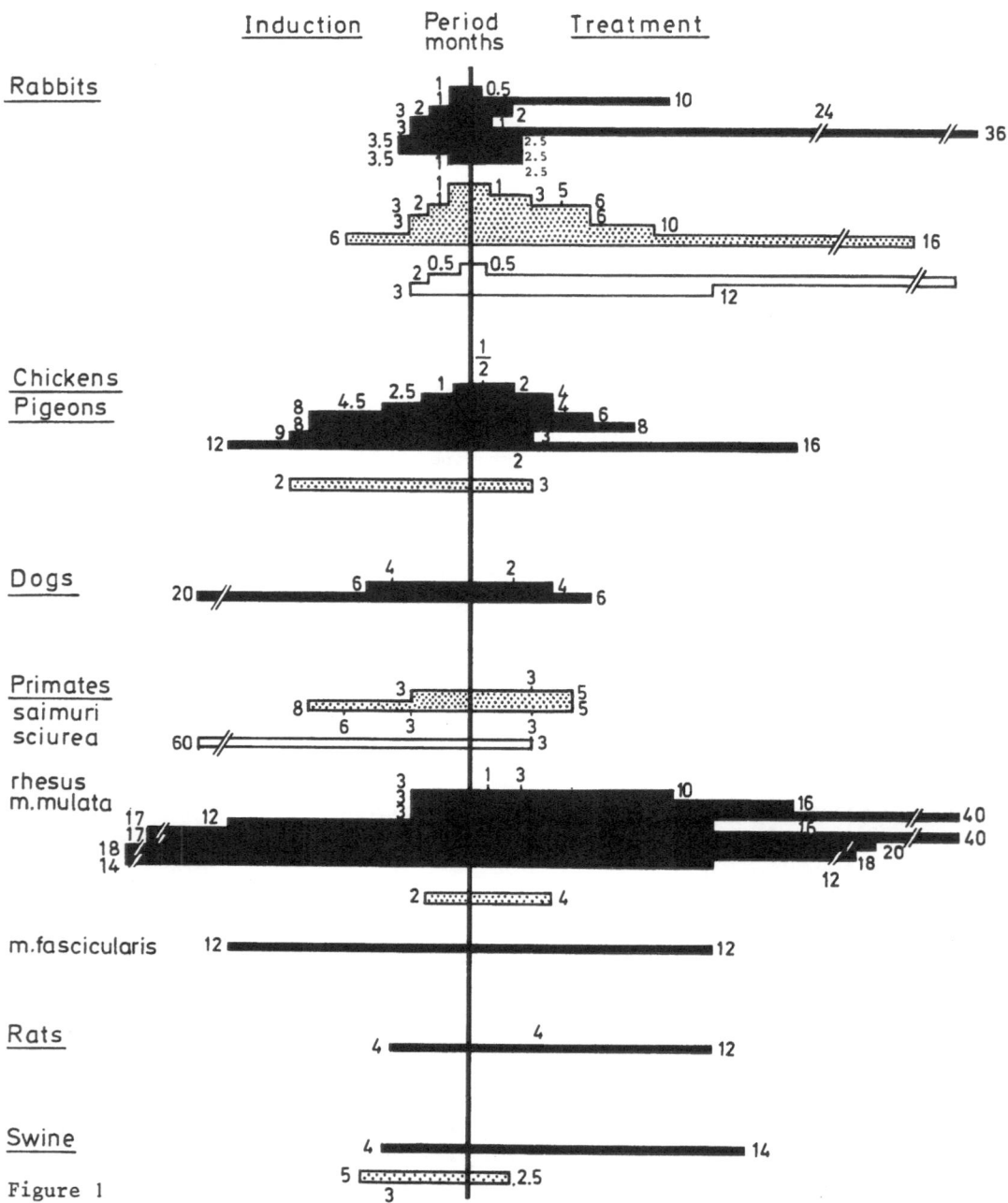

Figure 1

Another requirement for regression studies is standardization. This should be
done not only in a few induction methods but with a few treatment regimens and
most importantly for lesion components both during progression and regression.
For this purpose, morphometric and histochemical methods and controlled biochemistry can be employed. That is, microextraction of various lesion components
should be accompanied by morphologic identifications and measurements of the
particular part of the arterial wall or lesion. In addition, we need to develop
a quantitative, preferably computer-aided, method for measurement of lesions components. A number of investigators have recently developed a method for analyzing neuroanatomical data and similar systems should be developed for our purposes (Marx, 1976).

Another problem encountered in comparing regression studies is the variability of therapy employed. Although regression was achieved in a majority of the studies simply by cessation of the atherogenic regimen, specially prepared diets or combinations of diets with various hypocholesterolemic drugs or agents have also been widely used.

In addition, a more accurate study of the topography of lesions should be done. In this manner we would know the exact location of lesions in our control or reference groups and be able to study comparable locations for remnant lesions in treatment groups. This should prove helpful since it is still difficult to follow a single lesion (Buchwald, 1967; DePalma et al., 1972; Blankenhorn, 1975). It should also give us some insight into the activity of the different parts of the arterial wall and enable us to discover if the lesions which develop first also regress first or vice versa.

Last but not least, there is the problem of objective assessment of the results both in vivo and by postmortem evaluation. One needs to obtain as much clinical data as possible during the experimental period. The clinical results should than be related to the postmortem findings.

A careful gross evaluation of lesions by a combination of mappings, or semimicroscopic photography with point counting, or by using gross stainings is informative regarding topography, severity, and characteristics of lesions. Characterization and identification of lesion components and their modifications should be evaluated by using these methods, identification of lipids, collagen, elastin, glycosaminoglycans, calcium, and cell death can be established. Autoradiography gives information regarding the degree of cell proliferation as well as what type of cells are most actively involved. Histochemistry is, on the other hand, particularly useful in identification of cells in lesions. The importance of the tissue chemistry cannot be overestimated; a knowledge about all components and their relationships brings us a step closer to solving the mystery of this disease. Very few studies include all these approaches, although as pointed out by Claude Bernard (1957): "Phenomena of living beings must be considered as a homogenous whole as the effects vary with conditions but the underlying laws which control them do not."

The objectives of regression studies seem to be twofold: first, to establish treatment of human disease by means of (1) specific diets, (2) drug therapy of various agents which have been shown to have ameliorating effects, (3) surgery, as done by partial ilial by-pass or biliary diversion, or (4) either physical exercise, alone or in combination with the above therapy; second, to explore the mechanism underlying regression by (1) studying lipid metabolism and chemistry, (2) establishing the role of hormones, and (3) observing the effects of oxygen and (4) the role of enzymes (Table 3).

It may be concluded that although large numbers of problems concerning regression studies still exist, the present-day evidence is encouraging enough to justify continuing research in this field.

THE EFFECT OF STRENUOUS EXERCISE ON PLASMA LIPIDS AND ATHEROSCLEROSIS IN CHOLESTEROL-FED COCKERELS*

Harry Y.C. Wong and Frank B. Johnson

Several investigators have reported that physical exercise lowers blood cholesterol. Holloszy et al. (1964), Pohndorf (1957), Montoye et al. (1959), and Johnson and Wong (1961) have reported that physical training resulted in a significant reduction of serum cholesterol in men. Mann et al. (1955), Morris et al. (1953), and Schlessinger (1958) found that men engaged in physical work had lower plasma cholesterol. Animal studies by Kobernick et al. (1953), Myasnikov (1958), Link et al. (1972), Orma (1957), Warnock et al. (1957), and Wong et al. (1957) have shown that strenuous physical activity is an effective hypocholesterolemic factor of animals on a high-cholesterol diet. Recently, Wong et al. (1975) reported that physical exercise could reverse atherosclerosis in cockerels induced by and maintained on a high-cholesterol diet. Brown et al. (1956) have reported that physical exercise had no consistent influence on the pathogenesis of atherosclerosis in rabbits receiving low- or high-cholesterol regimens. It has been reported by McAllister et al. (1959) that exercised dogs had higher serum cholesterol and showed more atherosclerosis in all vessels, including the coronaries, than the sedentary animals.

The present study was undertaken to determine the effects of strenuous exercise on plasma lipids and its relationship to the degree, incidence, and severity of atherosclerosis of cockerels fed an atherogenic diet.

Materials and Methods

Day-old Hy-line cockerels were obtained from Heatwole Hatcheries in Harrisonburg, Virginia. They were placed in a brooder and fed starter-grower-mash and water ad lib. When 15 weeks old, they were placed in individual cages, and at the age of 35 weeks, they were divided into four groups of 11 - 15 birds each, as follows: (1) controls on plain mash, (2) controls with exercise, (3) atherogenic diet only, and (4) atherogenic diet with exercise. The atherogenic diet consisted of 2% cholesterol and 5% cottonseed oil added to starter-grower-mash. Exercise consisted of running approximately 750 yards in a circular treadmil, twice daily for 30 min, 5 consecutive days a week for 24 weeks. After fasting overnight, the body weight and blood samples of all birds were taken at the beginning of the experiment, and weekly thereafter. The blood samples were analyzed for total plasma cholesterol, phospholipids, and triglycerides according to the methods of Wong et al. (1965), Stewart and Hendry (1935), and Van Handel and Zilversmit (1957), respectively. After 24 weeks, these cockerels were sacrificed, and the heart and abdominal aorta were rapidly removed. The aortae were opened longitudinally to be grossly examined for the presence of atherosclerotic lesions by the method of Kath and Stamler (1963) and graded on a 0 - 4 scale. Histologic sections of the thoracic aortae and coronary arteries were made and stained by the oil red-0 method (Luna, 1968).

Results

The effect of strenuous exercise for 24 weeks on the body weights or normal and artherogenic-fed cockerels is summarized in Table 1. Our data indicate that exercise had no marked influence upon the body weight of any of the groups in the experiment. Table 2 depicts the influence of exercise on the plasma cholesterol of cockerels on plain mash or an atherogenic diet at the beginning and end of the study. There was no significant change in the plasma cholesterol of the non-exercised control birds. The controls on plain mash which were exercised showed a significant increase in plasma cholesterol when the final level was compared to its intital value ($p < .01$). Birds on an atherogenic regimen only showed a marked increase of plasma cholesterol when compared to the exercised or nonexercised control. The birds on an atherogenic diet which were exercised showed a significant decrease in the plasma cholesterol levels as compared to the non-exercised group ($p < .05$). Table 3 shows that the plasma phospholipid levels of

---

*
Supported by grants # H-2420, RRO8016 and 1-TG-2GM-05 010-01 (MARC) from the National Institutes of Health.

the birds on plain mash or on atherogenic regimen indicate a similar trend as the plasma cholesterol values. There were no significant differences between the two groups of controls on plain mash whether exercised of not. The group on an atherogenic diet only showed the highest level of plasma phospholipid. However, there was a marked decrease in the phospholipid value of the exercised cockerels when compared to the nonexercised group (p < .05). The initial triglyceride level of the various groups of birds at the beginning of this study was not significantly different, as indicated in Table 4. At the end of the study, there was no marked change in the triglyceride value of the nonexercised control group. The controls, which were exercised, showed a significant decrease from the initial level of 11.8 mg% to a final value of 7.3 (p < .01) and they were markedly lower when compared to the nonexercised group (p < .01). The triglyceride level of the atherogenic-fed group rose markedly from 13 mg% to 117 as opposed to the group fed a similar diet which were subjected to exercise increased from 12 to 52 mg%. The triglyceride value of the exercise group on a cholesterol diet was significantly reduced when compared to the similar nonexercised group (p < .02).

Table 5 shows that after 24 weeks, no gross lesions were observed in the thoracic aorta of the control birds on plain mash. One cockerel in the exercised control group had abdominal atherosclerosis. In the group fed an atherogenic diet, 14 of 15 birds had lesions of the thoracic aorta, with an average gross grading of 2.6, while 12 birds had abdominal atherosclerosis with an average gross grading of 2.0. Only two of 13 cockerels on an atherogenic regimen with exercise had thoracic lesions averaging 0.5, and only one bird in this group was observed to have abdominal lesion with an average grading of 0.05. The thoracic and abdominal atherosclerosis were significantly reduced by exercise. Microscopic examination of aorta showed no aortic lesions in the controls on plain mash, whether exercised or not, although one lesion was noticed grossly in the plain mash group which was exercised. All birds on an atherogenic diet had aortic lesions while two of 13 birds has lesions in the exercised group on a similar regimen. None of the controls on plain mash, whether exercised or not, had coronary lesions. In the nonexercised group fed an atherogenic diet, 13 of 15 birds had lesions while in a similarly fed group with exercise, only two of 13 cockerels had lesions.

Discussion

It is well-established that different types of exercise will alter the plasma lipids of humans and animals (Holloszy et al., 1964; Pohndorf, 1957; Montoye et al., 1959; Johnson and Wong, 1961; Mann et al., 1955; Morris et al., 1953; Schlessinger, 1958; Kobernick et al., 1953; Myasnikov, 1958; Link et al., 1972; Orma, 1957; Warnock et al., 1957; Wong et al., 1957, 1975). However, these experimental studies have conflicting results, especially with respect to whether plasma cholesterol can be reduced by physical activity (Brown et al., 1956; McAllister et al., 1959). The results presented in this study indicate that the plasma cholesterol, phospholipids, and triglyceride levels of cockerels on an atherogenic diet can be significantly lowered by exercise. In addition, there was a decreased incidence and severity of atherosclerosis of the thoracic and abdominal aorta as well as a decrease in the coronary atherogenesis of these birds as compared to the sedentary group. The plain mash group which was exercised had a markedly elevated final plasma cholesterol level when compared to its initial value. It was interesting to note that both exercised groups of cockerels had significantly lower initial cholesterol levels than their controls. We speculate that this difference in initial plasma cholesterol levels was due to the fact that these birds were exercised 5 days a week for 2 weeks on the treadmill in order to select the best runners for the experiment. Papadopoulos et al. (1969) reported that lower plasma cholesterol levels were found in the rats after 1 week of daily exercise. Carlson (1967) observed that the serum cholesterol value of old rats was much lower after strenuous exercise. Paris et al. (1971), using young rats, observed that there were no statistical differences of the plasma cholesterol between the exercised and nonexercised groups.

Table 1. The effect of strenous exercise on body weights of cockerels on plain mash or an atherogenic diet

Regimen	No. of cockerels	Initial body weight (g)	Final body weight (g)
Controls, plain mash	15	1798 ± 40[b]	1878 ± 40
Controls + exercise	11	1873 ± 73	1927 ± 83
Atherogenic diet[a]	15	1939 ± 40	1921 ± 45
Atherogenic diet + exercise	13	1867 ± 41	1975 ± 52

[a]2% cholesterol plus 5% cottonseed oil added to grower-starter-masch. [b]SEM.

Table 2. Influence of exercise on plasma cholesterol

Regimen	No. of cockerels	Initial mg%	Final mg%
Controls, plain mash	15	117 ± 3[b]	125 ± 5
Controls + exercise	11	97 ± 3	119 ± 4
Atherogenic diet[a]	15	114 ± 7	1421 ± 99
Atherogenic diet + exercise	13	96 ± 3	981 ± 106

[a]2% cholesterol plus 5% cottonseed oil added to starter-grower-mash. [b]SEM.

Table 3. Influence of exercise on plasma phospholipids

Regimen	No. of cockerels	Initial mg%	Final mg%
Controls, plain mash	15	184 ± 5	190 ± 7
Controls + exercise	11	199 ± 9	183 ± 4
Atherogenic diet[a]	15	195 ± 3	384 ± 40
Atherogenic diet + exercise	13	193 ± 6	295 ± 20

[a]2% cholesterol plus 5% cottonseed oil to starter-grower-mash. [b]SEM.

Table 4. Effect of exercise on plasma triglyceride levels

Regimen	No. of cockerels	Initial mg%	Final mg%
Controls, plain mash	15	11.3 ± 0.8[b]	10.6 ± 0.5
Controls + exercise	11	11.8 ± 0.8	7.3 ± 0.7
Atherogenic diet[a]	15	12.7 ± 0.8	117.2 ± 24
Atherogenic diet + exercise	13	11.8 ± 0.8	52.2 ± 10

[a]2% cholesterol plus 5% cottonseed oil added to starter-grower-mash. [b]SEM.

Table 5. Summary of exercise on gross and microscopic grading of aortic and coronary atherosclerosis

Regimen	No. of cockerels	Gross grading[a]						Microscopic grading			
		Thoracic			Abdominal			Aortic		Coronary	
		No. with lesions	%	Avg. lesions	No. with lesions	%	Avg. lesions	No. with lesions	%	No. with lesions	%
Controls, plain mash	15	0	0	0	0	0	0	0	0	0	0
Controls + exercise	11	0	0	0	1	10	0.01	0	0	0	0
Atherogenic diet[b]	15	14	94	2.6	12	79	2.0	15	100	13	87
Atherogenic diet + exercise	13	2	15	0.5	1	8	0.05	2	15	2	15

[a] Based on 0 – 4.

[b] 2% cholesterol plus 5% cottonseed oil added to starter-grower-mash.

The significant decrease of plasma triglyceride by exercise as compared to the controls on plain mash or on atherogenic diet indicates that physical activity has a marked effect on this lipid fraction. Similar results were reported by Papadopoulos and co-workers (1969) that strenuous exercise does lower the plasma triglyceride in rats.

Our results confirm the observation of Kontinnen and Nikkila (1964) who reported that there is a decrease of plasma triglyceride with exercise. Link et al. (1972) have noted that miniature pigs fed an atherogenic regimen developed elevated plasma lipids. There were no sex differences for plasma cholesterol, triglyceride, or total lipids. However, the exercised pigs had less atherosclerosis when compared to the sendentary group. Myasnikov (1958) reported that rabbits fed a high cholesterol diet and exercised to exhaustion on an electric treadmill had lower plasma cholesterol levels than the nonexercised. In addition, gross examination revealed that exercise lowered the development of aortic and coronary atherosclerosis. These data confirm our previous laboratory studies (Wong et al., 1972; Orimilikwe et al., 1977) that exercise is an effective factor in lowering the plasma cholesterol of atherogenic-fed cockerels. In addition, physical activity reduced the incidence and severity of lesions in the thoracic and abdominal aortae as well as in the coronary arteries. Data presented in this investigation appear to show that there is a direct relationship between the plasma cholesterol level to the pathogenesis of aortic and coronary atherosclerosis. Recently, Wong et al. (1975) reported that a possible mechanism by which exercise lowers aortic and coronary atherosclerosis in cholesterol-fed cockerels is that exercise decreases the collagen to elastin ratio. They observed that exercise had no effect on the C/E ratio of thoracic aortas of the control cockerels on plain mash. However, the ratio of the cholesterol-fed group with exercise was significantly lower than that of the nonexercised birds fed a similar regimen.

Summary

The effect of strenuous exercise was undertaken to determine its influence on body weight, plasma cholesterol, phospholipids, and triglyceride levels as well as aortic and coronary atherosclerosis of cholesterol-fed cockerels. Exercise consisted of running in a circular treadmill 750 yards, twice daily for 30 min, 5 consecutive days a week for 24 weeks. Data from our studies indicate that the plasma cholesterol concentration of exercised birds on plain mash was significantly higher than the nonexercised controls on a similar diet. However, there was a marked decrease of plasma cholesterol, phophoslipids, and triglyceride levels in the exercised cockerels fed a cholesterol regimen when compared to the nonexercised group. It was further observed that there was a significant reduction in incidence and severity of thoracic, abdominal aorta, and coronary atherosclerosis of cholesterol-fed chockerels which were exercised when compared to the nonexercised controls.

CHANGES OF CYCLIC NUCLEOTIDES IN THE REGRESSIVE COURSE OF EXPERIMENTAL ATHEROSCLEROSIS AND THEIR MODIFICATION BY SEX HORMONES AND PHTHALAZINOL

Fujio Numano

Recent studies on atherosclerosis have been highlighted in the pathophysiologic or metabolic changes of the cellular component of arterial walls or of atheromatous lesion, hoping to achieve the long-standing dream of preventing and regressing atherosclerosis.

A number of trials have been reported on how to prevent populations from the disaster of atherosclerosis and whether atheromatous lesions could be regressed quantitatively. Nowadays, it is generally accepted that atheromatous lesions can be favorablely modified of arrested (Armstrong, 1976; Armstrong et al., 1970; Wissler and Vesselinovitch, 1976; Vesselinovitch et al., 1976; Gresham, 1976). On the other hand, cyclic nucleotides have been focused upon as the intracellular second messenger of various hormones and amines to regulate the physiologic or pathophysiologic conditions of tissues (Sutherland, 1971), and their important role stimulate us to search for their effect on arterial walls in relation to atherogenesis or to regression of atherosclerosis. In my previous studies (Numano et al., 1976), it was found that cholesterol-induced atheromatous lesions were characterized by a high activity of cAMP phosphodiesterase (cAMPPDE), a degradating enzyme of cAMP, and with the low level of cAMP. The withdrawal of cholesterol was associated with the increased level of cAMP and the decreased activity of cAMPPDE in their lesions. These changes of cyclic nucleotides make us postulate that they represent a good parameter for evaluating the regression of atherosclerosis. This paper studies the in vitro and in vivo effect of sex hormones and a cAMPPDE inhibitor, phthalazinol (EG-626), on cyclic nucleotides in the aortic wall in the hope of getting a clue as to what and how cyclic nucleotides modify in the aortic wall to regress atheromatous lesions. Phthalazinol is aphthalazine derivative synthesized by Ishikawa and Shimamoto in 1973 as a potent cAMPPDE inhibitor (Shimamoto et al., 1975; Adachi and Numano, 1977) who also reported its preventive effect against experimentally induced atherosclerosis.

Materials and Methods

In vivo study: Twenty 6-month-old albino rabbits were fed 150 g daily of 1% cholesterol-containing diet (Oriental Yeast Co. Rc 5) for 15 weeks. After that, they were divided equally into four groups and fed 150 g per day of commercial diet for 10 weeks. During this period, every morning the first five rabbits were given a placebo capsule containing potato starch. The second five received a capsule of 10 mg/kg of EG-626, the third five were injected i.m. with 0.1 mg/kg of conjugated estrogens, premarine (Ayest Co.), and the last five with 1 mg/kg of progesterone (Teikoku Zoki Ltd.). The level of serum cholesterol was measured before the experiment and in the 15th and 25th week of the experiment by the method of Zak-Henly, and the level of plasma estradiol and progesterone in the last week by radioimmunoassay. Immediately after sacrifice, the aortae were removed and four pieces of 1 x 0.5 cm sections were taken from atheromatous lesions in the thoracic aorta. The section was divided into two parts. One was immediately fixed with 5% glutaraldehyde solution (pH 7.4) for histologic study. The other was frozen with dry ice for biochemical analysis. Samples of atheromatous lesions or media were carefully dissected and cAMP was measured with the Gilman's competitive protein binding assay and Lowry's quantitative histochemical method modified by us (Numano et al., 1976). The activity of cAMPPDE was also measured by the microassay methods modified by us, which was precisely described before (Numano et al., 1977). We measured four samples from different parts of each atheromatous lesion or media of thoracic aorta. In each sample, cAMP and cAMPPDE were measured three times. Thus, a total of 12 measurements were made from each part of the aorta and the average of these measurements represents the level of cAMP or the activity of cAMPPDE in each rabbit. The mean and standard error (SE) of five values thus obtained from five rabbits represent the value of that group.

In vitro study: six rabbits were used. Twenty-four pieces of aorta were cut 5 x 5 mm from each aorta and floated on Hank's medium (pH 7.5) for 15 min at 37°C. After that, every four pieces of aortas were incubated for 5 min in Hank's solution (pH 7.5) with 4 x 10^{-9}M of estradiol, 3.5 x 10^{-8}M of progesterone, or 5 x 10^{-4}M of phthalazinol or without medication as a control. After incubation, the contents of cAMP and the activity of cAMPPDE were measured and the average of four measurements represents the values in each treatment. The mean and standard errors of six values obtained from six rabbits represents the effect of sex hormones or phthalazinol on cyclic nucleotides in the aortic wall.

Results

In vivo study: Figure 1 shows the changes of the serum cholesterol levels in four groups. At the 15th week of cholesterol feeding, the level of cholesterol revealed more than 1000 mg/dl and after that, the level decreased rapidly to be within normal range at the 25th week. As shown in Table 1, rabbits injected premarin for 10 weeks revealed a statistically significant high level of estradiol, and in turn, a low level of progesterone in plasma. On the contrary, rabbits treated with progesterone showed a four or five times higher level of plasma progesterone. Table 2 summarizes the level of cAMP and the activity of cAMPPDE in each group. In atheroma, a statistically significant low level of cAMP and in turn a high activity of cAMPPDE were recognized in the rabbits treated with estrogen, compared with those in the atheroma of the aorta of placebo control rabbits. Conversely, in rabbits treated with EG-626, the level of cAMP in atheroma increased and the activities of cAMPPDE decreased but these changes were not statistically significant. In media, a statistically significant increase of cAMP was confirmed in this group. On the contrary, aortae of rabbits treated with progesterone did not exhibit any statistical change of cyclic nucleotides compared with those in placebo control rabbits. Histologic examination revealed a typical atheromatous lesion characterized by a large amount of foamy cells, fatty degeneration, necrotic foci, covered with a thin frail fibrosis cap in placebo control rabbits. On the other hand, in the rabbits treated with estrogen, collagenous fibers were occupying atheromatous lesions and foamy cells were decreasing in number and becoming smaller. The appearance of a large number of smooth muscles was the most characteristic feature of atheromatous lesions the the aorta of rabbits treated with EG-626 or progesterone.

In vitro study: Figure 2 shows the level of cAMP and the activity of cAMPPDE in the aorta of rabbits incubated in Hank's solution mixed with a sex hormone or EG-626 for 5 min. A statistically significant high level of cAMP was observed in the aorta incubated with a progesterone or phthalazinol solution, compared with that in the aorta incubated without medication. Aorta incubated in an estrogen solution exhibited a low level of cAMP without a statistically significant dif-

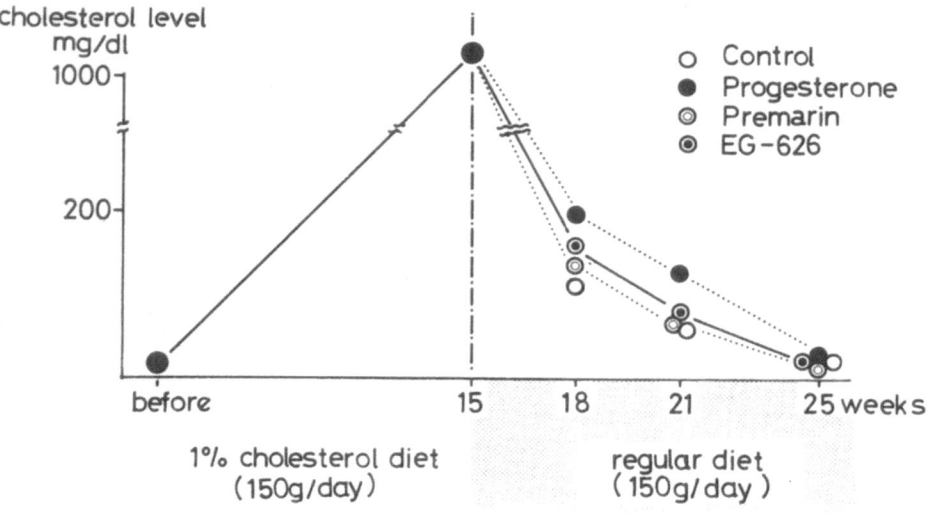

Figure 1. Plasma cholesterol level of rabbits in regressive course

Table 1. Plasma estrogen and progesterone level in rabbits in the 25th week of the experiment

Groups	Plasma estrogen level (Pg/ml)	Plasma progesterone level (ng/ml)
Placebo control	175.6 ± 17.7	1.40 ± 0.48
Premarin (0.1 mg/kg) treated group	336.0 ± 40.4^a	0.98 ± 0.24
Progesterone (1 mg/kg) treated group	180.0 ± 43.2	4.72 ± 0.10^a
EG-626 (10 mg/kg) treated group	180.0 ± 18.3	1.30 ± 0.20

Placebo vs. treated group.
[a] $P < 0.01$.

Table 2. Changes of cAMP and cAMPPDE activity in atheroma and media in aortic wall of rabbits treated with estrogen, progesterone, or EG-626 in regression

Aortic wall \\ Groups	Atheroma		Media	
	cAMP pmol/mg D.W.	cAMPPDE pmol/mg D.W./min.	cAMP pmol/mg D.W.	cAMPPDE pmol/mg D.W./min
Control	13.44 ± 2.11	9.81 ± 1.56	3.67 ± 0.38	7.80 ± 1.25
Estrogen 0.1 mg/kg	5.04 ± 1.05^a	15.80 ± 3.19^b	3.60 ± 0.22	12.92 ± 2.47^b
Progesterone 1 mg/kg	12.05 ± 1.50	10.21 ± 3.55	4.18 ± 0.25	10.57 ± 3.15
EG-626 10 mg/kg	18.46 ± 0.44	5.82 ± 2.16	5.03 ± 0.72	5.94 ± 2.40

[a] $P < 0.01$. [b] $P < 0.05$.

ference. On the contrary, cAMPPDE showed the highest activity in the aorta incubated in estrogen solution and a low activity in phthalazinol solution. However, there were no statistically significant differences between these groups and the control group.

Discussion

With the modern progress of scientific analysis, regression has been discussed as much from the qualitative as from the quantitative point of view. Armstrong et al., (1970) reported in his studies that coronary atheromatous lesions in rhesus monkeys improved by the withdrawl of cholesterol diet not only in size but

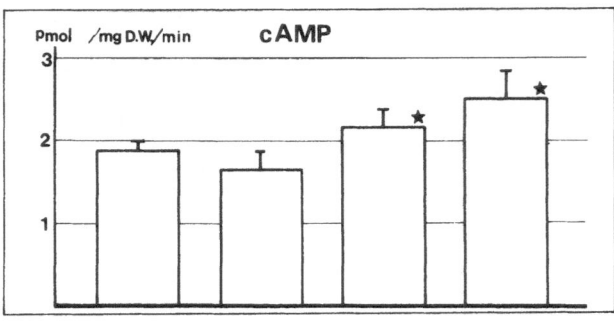

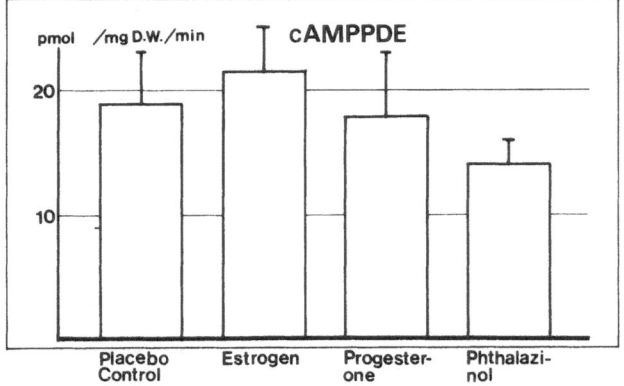

Figure 2. In vitro effect of estrogen, progesterone & phthalazinol on cAMP and cAMPPDE in aortic wall of rabbits. Placebo control vs. treated group. *P <0.05

also in histologic features characterized by a decrease in sudanophilic substances and fibrous healing. Daoud et al. (1976) pointed out in their regressive study that calcification could also be absorbed, paralled to the decrease in lesion size, in atheromatous lesions of swine which were produced by a combination of mechanical injury and a 4-month high-cholesterol diet and afterward regressed by a 14-month, regular mash diet. St. Clair et al. (1972) observed the striking decrease of cholesterol ester fraction in the aorta of pigeons in regression by changing a cholesterol diet into regular one. He viewed this as a chemical regression in atherosclerotic lesions. Fritz et al. (1976) also confirmed in their chemical analysis a decrease of cholesterol ester, phospholipid DNA synthesis in atheromatous lesions of swines in their regression. In my previous experimental study, (Numano et al., 1976), atheromatous lesions in the aorta of rabbits fed a cholesterol diet exhibited a remarkable increase in the activity of cAMPPDE and, in turn, a low level of cAMP. These characteristic changes of cyclic nucleotides were supposed to play an important role in the formation of foamy cells by decreased lipolysis, fibrosis by abnormal transformation, and calcification or necrosis by decreased metabolism of glucose or protein. By the withdrawal of cholesterol diet, these atheromatous lesions exhibited a regression characterized by the decrease in sudanophilic substances and an increase in collagenous and smooth muscle fibers; our microassay method confirmed the increase of the content of cAMP in these atheromatous lesions thus characterized.

These findings make us postulate that these changes in cyclic nucleotide may be a good parameter for evaluating the chemical regressive effect. From this point of view, both phthalazinol and progesterone seem to be helpful in initiating regression of atherosclerotic lesions. On the contrary, estrogen showed an accelerating effect of cAMPPDE activity in the aortic wall both in vivo and in vitro, developing a fibrosis in atheromatous lesions. These characteristic effects may render to its conflicting function of its atherogenetic and anti-atherogenetic process (Numano et al., 1971, 1972, 1973). Furthermore, from the regressive point of view, the physiologic effect of estrogen on cyclic nucleotide metabolism in the arterial wall seems to be unfavorable. However, these experimental studies on regression informed us of a fibrotic healing of atherosclerotic lesions as a consequence of regression by which further infiltration of lipid will be protected. These histologic features leave room for us to pursue in part the beneficial effect of estrogen for regression. Further studies will follow.

Summary

The effect of sex hormones and a new substance of a phthalazine derivative, phthalazinol, on cyclic nucleotides in the arterial wall was studied in vivo and in vitro on the regression of atherosclerosis. Rabbits fed a cholesterol diet for 15 weeks were treated with estrogen (0.1 mg/kg), progesterone (1 mg/kg), and phthalazinol (10 mg/kg) for 10 weeks under commercial diet. The content of cAMP and the activity of cAMPPDE in atheromatous lesions and media of aortic walls were measured by a microbiochemical method derived by us. At the same time, the in vitro effect of these hormones on cyclic nucleotides was also studied, using aortic walls of rabbits. Both phthalazinol and progesterone exhibited an effect which suppressed the activity of cAMPPDE and, in turn, increased the content of cAMP in accordance to the decrease of sudanophilic substances and increase of smooth muscles in atheromatous lesions. On the contrary, estrogen showed an effect which increased the activity of cAMPPDE and histologically accelerated fibrosis in atheromatous lesions.

MODEL OF ARTERIAL INJURY BY BALLOON DE-ENDOTHELIALIZATION: REAPPRAISAL, IMPROVEMENT, AND APPLICATION TO MEASUREMENT OF ENDOTHELIAL GROWTH

William Insull and Christopher C. Chidi

De-endothelialization of arteries by drawing an inflated balloon through the artery to squeeze the endothelium off the wall has been frequently employed since it's introduction by Baumgartner in 1963. It has proven particularly useful in the studies of factors influencing thrombogenesis by the arterial wall and more recently for the induction of smooth muscle cell proliferation, and when applied in conjunction with hyperlipidemia, for the production of experimental lesions of atherosclerosis (Baumgartner, 1973; Spaet et al., 1975; Ross and Glomset, 1973; Namm et al., 1973; Lee and Lee, 1975; Katocs et al., 1976). Investigators have observed additional changes in the artery wall including grossly visible and microscopic necrosis, calcification, and aneurysm formation, complications which may obscure and alter the effects of de-endothelialization. A critical evaluation of the production of these complications in relation to the techniques of manipulating the catheter and the balloon has not been published.

With the aim of acheiving uncomplicated de-endothelialization we have systematically evaluated the procedure as applied to the aorta of rabbits weighing 2.5 kg and using a 4 F embolectomy catheter. The ideal technique requires the size of the inflated balloon to match the size of the artery while exerting sufficient pressure to displace the endothelium without damaging the arterial wall by overdistention. To estimate the fit of the balloon and the aorta, we measured the diameter of the aorta of 31 rabbits fixed while perfused *in situ* at normal mean arterial pressure, 100 mm Hg. The diameter progressively decreased, being 3.8 mm at the level of the first intercostal artery, 3.1 at the superior mesenteric artery, 2.4 at the midabdominal segment, to 2.0 mm at the bifurcation into the iliac arteries. As the diameter of the fully inflated balloon was 9 mm, this difference in sizes causes significant distention to occur, and there appeared to be an obvious need to carefully adjust the balloon size by readjustment of inflation pressure to avoid over distention and permanent damage. We investigated the effects of different inflation pressures ranging from 480 to 750 mm Hg upon the occurrence of damage to the media and the production of complete de-endothelialization in ballooning the thoracic aorta of rabbits. The inflation pressure was constantly monitored by a recording strain-gauge manometer and was readjusted as needed to maintain the pressure of the value under test.

We observed, at increasing inflation pressures above 650 mm Hg, a progression of changes ranging from grossly visible scattered focal, sharply demarcated thinning of the arterial wall with replacement of the neointima by fibrous tissue, to gross circumferencial thinning and aneurysmal dilatation. At pressures decreasing below 550 mm Hg, there was progressively more incomplete de-endothelialization. This demonstrated that the pressure range of 550 - 650 mm Hg was optimal, producing grossly uncomplicated, complete de-endothelialization for the thoracic aorta of young adult rabbits. We have applied this procedure to the study of growth of endothelium.

Endothelial regeneration following de-endothelialization of the entire aorta of the rabbit occurs from the outgrowth of uninjured endothelium remaining at the lip of the ostium of each aortic branch. (Minick, C.R., Stemerman, M., unpublished studies) The regenerating endothelium forms islands of continuous sheets one cell thick which spread from each ostium centrifugally across the luminal surface. These islands are readily observed when the aortas are stained in vivo by Evans blue administered intravenously prior to sacrifice, the de-endothelialized luminal surfaces staining a deep blue while those possessing endothelium are unstained and remain white. The identification of these tissues was verified histologically with paraffin section microscopy, transmission electron microscopy, and scanning electron microscopy. The growth of endothelium can be determined by measuring the increasing dimensions of the islands in a series of animals sacrificed at intervals after de-endothelialization. We have measured the size of islands around the ostia of nine intercostal arteries in 29 animals sacrificed 1 - 30 days after de-endothelialization. The measurements were made from calibrated 35 mm color photographs of the aortic lining using a micrometer ocular at about 10 X magnification. The dimension of each endothelial island was measured along the island's radii from the lip of the intercostal ostium to the outer edge of the endothelial island. The dimensions of each island were measured along the rostral, lateral, and caudal radii. The regrowth of endothelium, after de-endothelialization, showed a fast rate for about 7 days, then abruptly a slow rate up to the end of observations on the 30th day. In order to better characterize the growth dynamics, curves were fitted to these data by the least squares calculation. The best fit was obtained by two successive geometric functions, one for the period days 0 - 7, and the second for days 7 - 30. The calculated rate of spread for the 1st day averaged 168 μm/day and on the 7th day 875 μm/day. In the phase of slow growth, the growth rate for the 8th day was 33 μm/day and decreased slightly to 29 μm/day by the 30th day. The abrupt slowing about the 7th day appears to be related to the advancing front of endothelial cells encountering smooth muscle cells in a fully developed confluent growth on the luminal surface of the de-endothelialization aorta.

The technique of de-endothelialization by balloon catheter, when refined to avoid gross damage to the arterial wall by careful inflation of the balloon, can provide quantitative data on the growth of endothelium and the interaction of endothelium with adjacent smooth muscle cells.

REVERSIBILITY OF ATHEROSCLEROSIS IN PYRIDOXINE-DEFICIENT MONKEYS

Fumio Kuzuya

Introduction

The author has reported on atherosclerosis in pyridoxine-deficient monkeys for the past several years (especially at the 6th international Congress of Gerontology). This atherosclerosis is widely involved from the aorta to the arterioles, and further, is seen in the aorta, iliac arteries, heart, kidneys, spleen, pancreas, testes, mesentery, brain, and other organs. As previously reported, its histologic changes are variable, quite similar to that in man. This paper is to report on the results of our dynamic experiment on the reversibility of atherosclerosis in pyridoxine-deficient monkeys.

Experimental Methods

The animals used were young *Macaca fuscata yakui*. The foods given were prepared as shown in Table 1, and were administered orally every day with vitamins. In the control 3 mg of pyridoxine per day was added.

Results

On feeding with the pyridoxine-deficient diet, the monkeys lost weight gradually. The control monkeys did not show an increase in body weight because the feeding was controlled. We do not have any experimental data as to whether there are any factors (quantitatively or qualitatively) deficient in the diet. Twelve months later, when they were fed with the control diet, their body weight increased rapidly. From the 3rd to 4th month on, the increase was very slow, reaching the growth curve of a normal monkey. These animals were autopsied at 2 months, 6 months, 12 months, and 24 months. The thymus showed the most significant change, recovering quite rapidly after pyridoxine was given. Thus, reversibility of the thymus weight is the most significant. No experimental proof was obtained whether the thymic function also recovered. Similarly, the spleen showed a de-

Table 1

Basal diet (compressed in tablets)

Sucrose	50	parts
Glucose	4	"
Vitamin-free casein	20	"
Cocorin	7	"
Cottonseed oil	3	"
McCollum salt	4	"
Polyethylenglycol (mol wet 6000)	4	"
Talc	8	"

Vitamins (as aqueous solution) per day

B_1-HCl	0.4	mg	Folic acid	100	γ
B_2	0.6	mg	Inositol	30	mg
Nicotinic acid	2	mg	Choline HCl	100	mg
PABA	5	mg	Pantothenic acid-Ca	2	mg
Biotin	10	γ	Vitamin A	3000	IU
B_{12}	1	γ	Vitamin D	300	IU
Vitamin C	25	mg	Vitamin K	50	γ

crease in weight on pyridoxine deficiency, but its extent was not as much as in the thymus, although the weight was increased on adding pyridoxine. The weight of the adrenals increased on the deficient diet, but interestingly, it returned close to that in the control group when pyridoxine was added.

The atherosclerotic changes in pyridoxine-deficient monkeys varied histologically, and the presence (+) or the absence (-) of the changes as recorded and shown in Table 2. The number of (+) decreased gradually on increasing the length of the recovery period. Even after 24 months of recovery, atherosclerotic changes remained in portions of the abdominal aorta, common iliac and renal arteries, but no atherosclerosis was present in other organs. This may indicate that reversibility varies among different organs. There seems to be some relations between the occurrence and its reversibility of the atherosclerotic changes. It is certain, however, that the frequency and severity of the atherosclerotic changes decrease on increasing the length of the recovery period such as 2 months, 6 months, 12 months, and 24 months. This indicates that there is some reversibility in a certain limit. Thus, it is certain that the atherosclerotic changes become gradually less in their distribution and severity. In respect to the distribution of lesions, the heart and spleen are most interesting among the various organs studied: namely, the coronary arteries and spleen arteries showed a very rapid recovery, specifically having a strong reversibility. Furthermore, arterioles in various organs also showed very rapid recoveries.

Summary and Discussion

In pyridoxine-deficient monkeys, the atherosclerotic changes distribute widely without loading high lipids, involving the large, middle and small arteries and the arterioles. In this instance, blood cholesterol does not usually elevate. Thus, it is important to recognize that loading of high lipids is not essential to produce atherosclerosis in monkeys. On the recovery experiments, the coronary arteries and spleen arteries showed very rapid disappearance of the changes, having a strong reversibility. In contrast, the changes existed for a relatively long period of time in the abdominal aorta, common iliac and renal arteries. Thus, it is assumed that the atherosclerotic changes induced by pyridoxine deficiency could recover within a certain limit. The monkeys used were extremely young, and thus were in the best condition for recovery. It is doubtful whether similar facts are to be obtained in aged monkeys.

A definite recognition of reversibility of atherosclerosis is difficult to be obtained clinically, but there has been much experimental evidence. Some experiments were done on rabbits by Leary, MacMillan, Bradgdon, Pollak, Charkravarti, Friedman, Miller, Constantinides and others.

Friedman et al. reported that an excess at cholesterol and other fats disappeared rapidly from the fragment of atherosclerotic aorta transported into the eye of normal rabbit. The experiments on young roosters were done by Pick et al. Wills et al. recognized reversibility of atherosclerosis in guinea pigs, Kendall et al. in dogs. Taylor et al. obtained the evidence for reversibility of atherosclerosis in man; cholesterol plaques were thought to be absorbed as a foreign body. Rustein et al. found that the aortic cells in tissue culture medium picked up cholesterol or β-lipoproteins from the medium, and that cholesterol in the cells disappeared soon after cholesterol was removed from the medium. Almost all these data were obtained in experimental atherosclerosis induced by an excess fat loading. The author, however, recognized similar facts in monkeys, and further recognized the reversibility of fibrous plaques induced by not administering excess fat loading. Moses stated that atherosclerosis produced experimentally recovered at least in a period longer than that needed to produce it. However, he does not have any experimental proof for his statement. The author's data may be the experimental evidence for his statement.

Table 2

Group	No.	Sex	Exper. periods month (Def.)	Exper. periods month (Cont.)	Serum cholest. mg/dl	A G	Aorta Thorac	Aorta Abd	Common Iliac	Coronary	Kideny Large artery	Kideny V.aff V.eff	Spleen Large artery	Spleen Central	Cerebrals Basiral	Cerebrals Intracereb.
Deficiency	1	♂	10				+	+	+	+	+	–	+	+	+	–
	2	♂	10				–	+	+	+	+	–	–	+	–	–
	3	♀♂	12		192	0.39	+	+	+	+	+	+	+	+	–	–
	4	♂	14		113	0.68	–	+	+	+	+	+	+	+	+	+
	5	♂	15		141	0.67	–	+	+	+	+	+	+	+	–	+
	6	♀	16		100	0.71	+	+	+	+	+	+	+	+	+	+
Control	1	♂	12		121	1.09	–	–	–	–	–	–	–	–	–	–
	2	♀	15		134	1.00	–	–	–	–	–	–	–	–	–	–
	3	♀	15		153	0.91	–	–	–	–	–	–	–	–	–	–
Recovery	1	♂	12	2	121	1.00	–	+	+	–	+	–	–	+	+	–
	2	♂	12	6	114	0.99	–	+	+	–	+	–	–	+	–	–
	3	♂	12	12	97	2.69	–	+	–	–	+	–	–	–	–	–
	4	♀	14	24	92	1.10	–	+	+	–	+	–	–	–	–	–

Conclusion

Atherosclerosis induced experimentally in pyridoxine-deficient monkeys can be reversed, and a long period of time is necessary for its recovery. The speed of its recovery varies among different organs as seen in the occurrence of the atherosclerotic changes, and especially the coronary arteries, spleen arteries and arterioles in various organs have a strong reversibility.

REGRESSION OF ATHEROSCLEROSIS AT PLASMA CHOLESTEROL CONCENTRATIONS ACHIEVABLE IN MAN *

M. Gene Bond, Bill C. Bullock, Noel D.M. Lehner, and Thomas B. Clarkson

There is now some agreement that regression of diet-induced atherosclerosis does occur in the aorta and coronary arteries of nonhuman primates when these animals are maintained at low plasma cholesterol concentrations (137 - 175 mg/dl) (Armstrong et al., 1971; Tucker et al., 1971; Eggen et al., 1974; Vesselinovitch et al., 1976). Less clear, however, is the course of development of atherosclerosis at plasma concentrations which are realistically attainable by treatment of human hyperlipidemic patients. Specifically, will reducing plasma cholesterol concentrations from 300 to 200 mg/dl result in reduced extensiveness or severity of those arterial lesions thought to be (1) the early lesions of atherosclerosis, i.e., the fatty streak and (2) the typical lesions of atherosclerosis, i.e., the fatty and fibrous plaques?

We have obtained experimental data that bear on these questions by designing an experiment using a nonhuman primate model of atherosclerosis (54 rhesus monkeys). All animals were fed an atherogenic diet containing 1.0 mg cholesterol/kcal for 19 months to induce atherosclerosis. At the end of this induction period, the animals were divided equally into three groups with the conscious bias of equalizing total plasma cholesterol concentrations among the groups. Group 1 was killed at the end of the 19 month induction period for baseline studies of the extent and severity of atherosclerosis. Groups 2 and 3 were maintained by dietary manipulation for an additional 24 months at mean plasma cholesterol concentrations of either 300 mg/dl (group 2) to be comparable to untreated hyperlipidemic patients or at 200 mg/dl (group 3) to be comparable to hyperlipidemic patients properly managed by diet and/or drug therapy. The findings in the aorta of these animals are the basis of this report.

All animals were anesthesized and killed by exsanguination. The aortas were removed, opened longitudinally along the ventral midline and separated into thoracic and abdominal segments just superior to the origin of the celiac artery. Each segment was divided longitudinally into a right and left side. One-half was processed for chemical analysis of the constituents of the arterial wall and the contralateral side for gross and microscopic evaluation. The arteries were fixed flat in 10% buffered formalin and stained overnight with Sudan IV in dilute isopropanol for gross demonstration of lipids. Thoracic and abdominal aortas were evaluated by two observers for the percentage of intimal surface involved with four distinct types of lesions: (1) fatty streaks, seen as flat, red areas, (2) diffuse intimal thickening, flat, white areas (DIT), (3) fatty plaques, elevated, red staining areas, and (4) fibrous plaques, elevated non-Sudan staining "pearly" areas.

---

*This study was supported by Grant HL14164 from the National Heart and Lung Institute.

The intimal surfaces of the thoracic aortas of group 1 animals were involved primarily with sudanophilic areas, that is, fatty streaks (72%) and fatty plaques (16%) with only small amounts of DIT (2%) and fibrous plaque (2%) (Table 1). Total surface area involved with elevated lesions (fatty plaque + fibrous plaque) in this group was 18%. Thoracic aortas from group 2 (average plasma cholesterol of 300 mg/dl) contained primarily sudanophilic areas with fatty streaks affecting 50% of the intima and fatty plaques affecting 16%. DIT occupied 15% of the intimal surface in this group and total plaque 21%.

Thoracic aortas from animals in group 3 (average plasma cholesterol of 200 mg/dl) had markedly less aortic sudanophilia, with fatty streaks decreasing to 16% and fatty plaques to 2% of the intimal surface. The extensiveness of fibrous plaque was about the same in groups 2 and 3, 6% and 7%, respectively; however, DIT increased in group 3 when compared to group 2, affecting 50% of the intimal surface. The extensiveness of total plaque was 9% in group 3 compared to 21% in group 2, a decrease significant at the 7% confidence level.

There were similar findings among the abdominal aortas. The extensiveness of atherosclerosis among the baseline group 1 animals was 29% fatty streak and 29% fatty plaque (Table 2). The extent of total plaque was 42% of the intimal surface and DIT 8%. By comparison, the extensiveness of atherosclerosis among group 2 was 13% fatty streaks, 20% fatty plaques, and 43% total plaques. Diffuse intimal thickening involved 34% of the intimal surface. Group 3 when compared to group 2 contained fewer fatty streaks (4%) and substantially fewer fatty plaques (1%). DIT, fibrous plaque, and the amount of total plaques were about the same for both groups.

Compared to animals maintained at mean serum cholesterol concentrations of 300 mg/dl, animals maintained at 200 mg/dl had less stainable lipid in both aortic segments, more diffuse intimal thickening, and less total plaque in the thoracic aorta, about the same amount of fibrous plaque in both segments and about the same amounts of diffuse intimal thickening and total plaque in the abdominal aorta. These findings are consistent with the notion that fatty streaks in the thoracic aorta may have a fate different from that of fatty streaks in the abdominal aorta of rhesus monkeys maintained at plasma cholesterol concentrations roughly similar to those of people.

Table 1. Extent of lesions of the thoracic aorta[a]

Group	N	Fatty streak	DIT[b]	Fatty plaque	Fibrous plaque	Total plaque[c]
1	18	72 ±6	2 ±1	16 ±5	2 ±1	18 ±6
2	18	50 ±6	15 ±3	16 ±5	6 ±3	21 ±6
3	18	16 4	50 ±8	2 ±1	7 ±2	9 ±3
Differences p <		2>3 (0.001)	3>2 (0.001)	2>3 (0.01)	NS	2>3 (0.07)

[a]Expressed as percent of intimal surface affected by four types of lesions considered (mean ± SEM).

[b]DIT, diffuse intimal thickening.

[c]Total plaque is fatty plaque plus fibrous plaque.

Table 2. Extent of lesions of the abdominal aorta[a]

Group	N	Fatty streak	DIT[b]	Fatty plaque	Fibrous plaque	Total plaque[c]
1	18	29 ±5	8 ±4	29 ±4	13 ±5	42 ±8
2	18	13 ±5	34 ±7	20 ±6	22 ±7	43 ±7
3	18	4 ±2	43 ±9	1 ±1	36 ±8	37 ±8
Differences p <		2>3 (0.07)	NS	2>3 (0.005)	NS	NS

[a]Expressed as percent of intimal surface affected by four types of lesions considered (mean ± SEM).

[b]DIT, diffuse intimal thickening.

[c]Total plaque is fatty streak plus fibrous plaque.

This study would suggest that lowering serum cholesterol from 300 to 200 mg/dl resulted in a reduced amount of lipid in the aortic intima; however, it did not reduce the surface area involved with fibrous plaques in either the thoracic or abdominal segments. Furthermore, total surface area involved with raised lesions, i.e., plaques, was not reduced in the abdominal aortas of those animals maintained at the lower serum cholesterol concentration, although they may have been less thick. These observations are consistent with those made previously on pigeons suggesting that plaques change in composition and pathologic character but do not likely disappear (Clarkson et al., 1973).

AORTIC ATHEROSCLEROSIS OF PRIMATES*

Noel D.M. Lehner, William D. Wagner, Bill C. Bullock, and M. Gene Bond

Evaluation of animals for use in studies of atherosclerosis has been on ongoing activity at our institution for a number of years, with some emphasis being given to primate species during the past 10 years. These evaluations have included studies of both naturally occurring and induced atherosclerosis, characterization of plasma lipoproteins, and studies of lipid metabolism. The purpose of this paper is to present our observations on diet-induced aortic atherosclerosis of nonhuman primates and to compare these lesions with those found in human beings. These observations include information on the characteristics, distribution, and extent of aortic lesions in nine species of monkeys as well as their aortic cholesterol and calcium concentrations.

The monkeys in this study were limited to young adult males and included four South American species (*Saimiri sciureus, Lagothrix sp., Ateles sp., Cebus albi-*

*Studies reported in this paper were supported in large part by Grant HL14164 from the National Heart and Lung Institute.

frons), four Asian species (*Macaca mulatta, Macaca nemestrina, Macaca arctoides,* and *Macaca fascicularis*), and one African species (*Cercopithecus aethiops*). These animals were subjects in several separate studies. Descriptions of experimental conditions and methods were included in previous reports and will only be described briefly (Lofland et al., 1968; Bullock et al., 1969, 1975; Pucak et al., 1973; Wagner and Clarkson, 1975).

The monkeys were fed atherogenic diets for periods of time which ranged from 36 to 42 months, except for the Cebus (24 months) and Ateles monkeys (49 months). All of the monkeys except Ateles were fed the same diet which contained 1 mg of cholesterol/kcal (composition g/100 g) - nonfat dry milk solids 30.0, wheat flour 20.0, casein 13.0, lard 25.0, applesauce 7.3, vitamin mixture 2.2, USP XIV salt mixture 2.0, and cholesterol 0.5. The Lagothrix were fed the above diet for 30 months and then liquid diets containing up to 1 mg of cholesterol/kcal for 12 additional months. The Ateles were fed a diet composed of commercial monkey chow 74.5, butter 12.5, coconut oil 12.5, and cholesterol 0.5 for 38 months, followed by a diet similar to that fed the other monkeys, except for equal parts of butter and coconut oil instead of lard, for 11 more months.

Human aortas were obtained from consecutive autopsy cases. The only selection criteria were that the subjects be male Caucasians without a history of hypertension, diabetes mellitus, or syphilis.

Methods for grading aortic atherosclerosis varied somewhat in different studies. Aortas from humans, Saimiri, Cercopithecus, Lagothrix, and *M. arctoides* were evaluated unstained. Those of Ateles, *M. fascicularis*, *M. mulatta*, and *M. nemestrina* were graded after being stained with Sudan IV. Cebus aortas were graded after staining with a water-soluble blue dye. The extensiveness of atherosclerosis was expressed as the percentage of the total intimal surface affected with fatty streaks (flat, white to yellow flecks or streaks in unstained arteries or sudanophilic areas in Sudan IV stained preparations), plaques (raised, white to yellow areas in unstained or raised sudanophilic or nonsudanophilic areas in stained aortas), or complicated plaques (raised areas affected with hemorrhage, thrombus, ulceration, or mineralization).

Aortic calcium concentrations were determined by atomic absorption spectrophotometric analysis of acidic extracts of the arteries (Wagner and Clarkson, 1975). Aortic cholesterol concentrations were determined by extracting the lipid with chloroform methanol, separating the cholesterol and esterified cholesterol fractions by thin layer chromatography, and determining their concentrations by the method of Block et al. (1966).

Duration of the atherogenic regimen, serum cholesterol concentration, and amount of aortic atherosclerosis of the nine monkey species are listed in Table 1. The extensiveness of lesions observed in human aortas from individuals ranging in age from the 2nd to the 8th decade are listed in Table 2. Data obtained from control animals are listed as compositive values since each species was quite similar. Lesions in control animals were usually limited to slight amounts of fatty streak. The degrees of hypercholesterolemia induced by the atherogenic diets were somewhat lower in the South American species and in *C. aethiops* when compared to the macaques. Based upon the extensiveness of raised lesions, the severity of atherosclerosis was also less in these animals. The most extensive lesions present in the South American species were fatty streaks, although Saimiri and Lagothrix had up to one-fourth of their thoracic or abdominal aortas affected with raised lesions. Based upon the type and extensiveness of lesions present, the aortas of the South American species were comparable to those of humans in the 3rd and 4th decades.

The macaques, as a group, had the highest serum cholesterol concentration and the greatest surface area of aorta containing plaques of any of the monkeys examined. Almost the entire intimal surfaces of the aortas of *M. arctoides, M. fascicularis,* and *M. nemestrina* were affected with raised lesions while the aortas of

Table 1. Duration of atherogenic regimen, serum cholesterol concentration and extensiveness of aortic atherosclerosis in nine species of monkeys[a]

Species	Dura-tion months	N	Serum choles-terol mg/dl	Aortic seg-ment	Fatty streaks % of	Raised lesions Total intimal	Raised lesions Complicated surface
Control[b]			–	T[c]	8±2[d]	<1	0
				A	4±1	<1	0
Saimiri sciureus	42	8	474±54	T	64±8	25±9	<1
				A	68±9	14±7	1±1
Lagothrix sp.	42	3	144±11	T	40±13	18±16	0
				A	38±17	27±18	0
Cebus albifrons	24	4	461	T	45	0	0
				A	34	0	0
Ateles sp.	49	4	334±15	T	30	0	0
				A	0	10	0
Macaca arctoides	42	4	698±33	T	8±4	79±13	2±1
				A	1±1	93±5	0
Macaca nemestrina	36	6	810±55	T	0	82±8	4±2
				A	2±2	70±15	3±2
Macaca mulatta	38	20	627±29	T	44±9	32±7	0
				A	18±6	67±7	1±1
Macaca fascicularis	36	7	701±47	T	13±6	80±10	3±3
				A	1±1	95±3	1±1
Cercopithecus aethiops	42	4	479±27	T	38±3	26±9	0
				A	36±9	49±7	1±1

[a]Adapted in part from Bullock et al. (1969, 1975), Wagner and Clarkson (1975), and Pucak et al. (1973).

[b]Control values are averages derived from control or commercial chow-fed *S. sciureus*, *M. arctoides*, *M. nemestrina*, *M. fascicularis*, and *C. aethiops*.

[c]T – thoracic aorta, A – abdominal aorta.

[d]Values listed as mean or mean ± SEM.

M. mulatta were affected a little less severely. The plaques in the three former species were even more extensive than those observed in the aortas of human beings through the 8th decade of life; however, the amount of complicated lesions, principally mineralization, was much less than that observed in the aortas of humans.

Atherosclerotic plaques in the aortas of *C. aethiops* were more focal and less extensive than those of the macaques. With the exception of complicated lesions, the type, distribution, and extensiveness of lesions in the aortas of *C. aethiops* were comparable to those in aortas of humans in the 6th decade.

The atherosclerotic lesions of the various primate species had many histologic features in common and included a wide spectrum of characteristics. The predomi-

Table 2. Age and extensiveness of aortic atherosclerosis in humans from the 2nd to the 8th decade[a]

Age in years	N	Aortic segment	Fatty streaks % of		Raised lesions	
					Total intimal	Complicated surface
10-19	5	T[b]	6±4[c]		<1	0
		A	7±5		<1	0
20-29	5	T	6±3		0	0
		A	14±9		1±1	0
30 39	5	T	61±14		3±1	0
		A	39±10		19±4	0
40-49	5	T	44±11		18±13	2±6
		A	41±10		34±14	13±6
50-59	5	T	48±14		32±16	5±5
		A	43±7		45±5	15±5
60-69	5	T	43±12		41±15	19±14
		A	19±9		66±17	47±14
70-79	5	T	41±1		43±9	14±6
		A	29±8		61±12	44±14

[a]Adapted in part from Wagner and Clarkson (1975).

[b]T - thoracic aorta, A - abdominal aorta.

[c]Values listed as mean ± SEM.

nance of some features of lesions tended to differentiate some species from others. The microscopic appearance of fatty streak lesions were very similar in all species. Characteristically, these lesions consisted of slight cellular thickenings of the intima with abundant intracellular lipid. The raised lesions of Ateles and Lagothrix were composed primarily of smooth muscle cells which contained only small amounts of lipid. A few lesions in these animals had a relatively acellular lipid core subjacent to a cap-like layer of smooth muscle cells. Aortic plaques of Saimiri were variable in histologic appearance. Some lesions contained lipid cores with smooth muscle cell caps, while others were predominantly composed of foam cells. Other lesions in these same animals were highly cellular and contained abundant connective tissue elements.

Raised lesions in the macaques presented a continuum of characteristics, from lipid poor fibrous lesions to large foam cell lesions rich in lipid, or mixtures of these elements. Atheroma with fibromuscular caps, lipid cores containing sterol clefts, and mineralization were features which were also commonly seen in the lesions from these animals. Many of the lesions had a multilayered appearance with alternating bands of connective tissue elements and pools of lipid or foam cells. Masses of lipid were often associated with the intima-media junction but were also found at various depths within the intima. Mineralization when present was associated with pools of lipid regardless of their depth in the lesion. Foam cells were found in the lesions of all species but appeared to be a larger component of the lesions of *M. mulatta*, *M. nemestrina*, and *M. fascicularis* than *M. arctoides*. The lesions of *M. arctoides* characteristically were smooth muscle thickenings with more numerous finely dispersed elastic fibers and collagen when compared to the other species. Foci of mineralization appeared to be more frequent in *M. arctoides, M. fascicularis,* and in the thoracic aorta of *M. nemestrina* than in *M. mulatta.*

The characteristics of aortic plaques of *C. aethiops* were less variable than those of the macaques. With some consistency, these lesions had a pool of lipid material usually containing abundant sterol clefts at the intima-media junction which was partially surrounded by a layer of collagen. The most superficial part of the lesions consisted of a fibromuscular cap. Extensive mineralization was present in the larger lesions, in association with the pools of lipid material.

Aortic cholesterol and calcium concentrations of the monkeys are listed in Table 3 and for humans in Table 4. The aortic cholesterol concentrations of the monkeys

Table 3. Aortic calcium and cholesterol concentrations of nine species of cholesterol - fed monkeys[a]

Species	Aortic segment	Aortic cholesterol			Aortic calcium mg/gm wet wt
		Total mg/gm wet wt	Free	Ester	
Control[b]	T[c]	2.2[d]	1.7±0.1	0.5±0.1	0.9±0.2
	A	1.9	1.6±0.2	0.3±0.1	0.4±0.1
Saimiri sciureus	T	8.4	6.0±1.0	2.4±0.4	2.6±0.4
	A	4.4	2.8±0.3	1.6±0.4	1.3±0.3
Lagothrix sp.	T	1.6	1.1±0.1	0.5±0.2	0.5±0.1
	A	4.2	2.2±0.4	2.0±0.9	0.8±0.2
Cebus albifrons	T	7.5	–	–	–
	A	3.4	–	–	–
Ateles sp.	T	3.0	1.9	1.1	–
	A	2.8	2.0	0.8	–
Macaca arctoides	T	12.0	6.0±1.6	6.0±1.9	4.3±1.8
	A	18.6	8.4±1.2	10.2±2.6	4.8±1.7
Macaca nemestrina	T	15.7	7.0±0.6	8.7±0.8	3.3±1.0
	A	15.5	5.8±0.7	9.7±1.6	1.0±0.3
Macaca mulatta	T	7.4	3.9±0.4	3.5±0.4	0.3±0.1
	A	12.1	6.1±0.6	6.0±0.7	0.6±0.1
Macaca fascicularis	T	16.2	8.8±1.7	7.4±1.2	3.8±1.8
	A	19.5	9.3+1.1	10.2±1.0	4.7±2.0
Cercopithecus aethiops	T	18.9	14.1±3.7	4.8±1.5	4.7±2.8
	A	20.7	12.7±3.8	8.0±1.8	4.2±1.5

[a] Adapted in part from Lofland et al. (1968), Wagner and Clarkson (1975), and Pucak et al. (1973).

[b] Control values are averages derived from control or commercial chow-fed *S. sciureus, M. arctoides, M. nemestrina, M. fascicularis,* and *C. aethiops.*

[c] T - thoracic aorta, A - abdominal aorta.

[d] Values listed as mean or mean ± SEM.

Table 4. Aortic calcium and cholesterol concentration of humans from the 2nd to the 8th decade[a]

Age in years	Aortic segment	Aortic cholesterol Total	Free mg/gm wet wt	Ester	Aortic calcium mg/gm wet wt
10-19	T[b]	2.3	1.7±0.5[c]	0.6±0.3	0.4±0.0
	A	2.4	1.5±0.2	0.9±0.3	0.3±0.1
20-29	T	2.1	1.3±0.2	0.8±0.2	0.6±0.1
	A	2.8	1.5±0.2	1.3±0.4	0.5±0.1
30-39	T	5.5	3.0±0.9	2.5±0.6	2.1±0.4
	A	7.7	3.5±0.9	4.2±1.5	1.3±0.3
40-49	T	9.1	4.6±1.1	4.5±1.5	4.3±0.7
	A	18.3	8.3±2.3	10.0±3.6	31.2±16.8
50-59	T	13.1	6.1±1.8	7.0±2.9	3.8±0.7
	A	16.6	7.1±2.2	9.5±2.6	23.8±17.2
60-69	T	23.4	13.1±5.1	10.3±3.5	8.6±2.6
	A	24.6	13.2±1.9	11.4±2.4	15.1±6.7
70-79	T	18.8	8.3±0.9	10.5±2.7	23.9±13.5
	A	38.5	18.5±4.4	20.0±3.0	24.7±10.2

[a]Adapted in part from Wagner and Clarkson (1975).

[b]T - thoracic aorta, A - abdominal aorta.

[c]Values list as mean ± SEM.

followed, for the most part, the extensiveness and severity of the lesions present. The South American species as a group had lower concentrations of aortic cholesterol than the other monkeys, with greater proportions of free cholesterol than cholesterol ester, and relatively low calcium concentrations. The concentrations of cholesterol and calcium in the aortas of these monkeys were similar to those of human aortas through the 4th decade.

The aortas of the four species of macaques and C. aethiops contained considerable concentrations of cholesterol. These monkeys tended to have greater concentrations of cholesterol in the abdominal aorta than in the thoracic, and in the case of the macaques, comparable or greater amounts of cholesterol ester than free cholesterol. With the exceptions of M. mulatta and the abdominal segment of M. nemestrina, these monkeys had large amounts of aortic calcium. The aortic cholesterol and calcium concentrations of C. aethiops equaled or exceeded those of the macaques even though the lesions in this species were not quite as extensive. The aortic cholesterol and calcium concentrations of C. aethiops and the macaques were comparable to the aortas of humans in the 5th and 6th decades.

MODERATE HYPERCHOLESTEROLEMIA IN THE RABBIT: CHOLESTEROL IN ATHEROSCLEROTIC AND NON-ATHEROSCLEROTIC AORTIC REGIONS

G.K. Hansson, A. Bylock, R. Brattsand, S. Björkerud, and G. Bondjers
Department of Medicine I, University of Göteborg, Göteborg/Sweden

In hypercholesterolemia, atherosclerotic lesions (AL) preferentially develop in regions with defective (high-injury) endothelium (HI). The present study was undertaken to investigate if there are any differences in cholesterol content between regions with intact (low-injury) endothelium (LI), HI regions, and AL. Rabbits were kept for 1 1/2 y. on various, individually stable serum cholesterol (S-C), 40-700 mg%. By a dye exclusion test the aortas were divided into AL, HI and LI regions. In these, unesterified (CA) and esterified (CE) cholesterol was determined. In LI regions, CA was constant in animals with S-C up to 400 mg%. Above 400 mg%, CA increased with increasing S-C. In HI regions a continuous increase of CA was observed with increasing S-C. CA showed the same increase in the AL of hypercholesterolemic rabbits. CE increased with increasing S-C in all types of regions. In HI, CA and CE were of the same magnitude as in AL, but significantly lower in LI. The discrepancy in CA content between LI and HI regions can be related to the intact endothelium as a barrier to cholesterol accumulation in the tissue. Thus, in HI regions there is an accumulation of cholesterol. This remains in AL; there is however no further increase of cholesterol when all structural properties of the lesion have been adopted. This suggests that accumulation of cholesterol may be a consequence of endothelial defects preceding the development of the atherosclerotic lesion.

PRODUCTION AND REGRESSION OF HYPERLIPIDEMIA AND EXPERIMENTAL ATHEROSCLEROSIS IN BEAGLE DOGS. EFFECTS OF DEXTROTHY-ROXINE

Rajiva Nandan, Jerry D. Fisher, James M. Mahoney, and Charles E. Ganote
Baxter Laboratories Inc. Morton Grove, IL/USA

Beagle dogs fed a thiouracil-free semisynthetic diet containing hydrogenated coconut oil and cholesterol (SS diet) develop hyperlipidemia and severe atherosclerosis. The effects of regression diet and dextrohyroxine (D-T4) therapy on these changes were studied. Twenty beagle dogs, 24 $\pm$ 6 months old, were initially fed the SS diet for 13 months. The animals were then divided into the following groups and maintained on their respective diets for 12 additional months. Group I, two male (M) and three female (F), were fed the SS diet alone. Group II (one M, four F) received the SS diet plus a single daily oral dose of D-T4 (0.1 mg/kg body weight). Group III (two M, three F) was reverted to regression diet feeding of purina dog meal. Group IV (two M, three F) was reverted to feeding of purina dog meal plus a single daily oral dose of D-T4 (0.1 mg/kg body weight). Untreated control (group V, two M, one F) received purina dog meal during the entire study. Group I developed marked elevation of serum lipids and severe atherosclerosis in large and small arteries. Lesions contained intimal and medial fibrofatty infiltration, formation of new IEM, calcification, extracellular polysaccharide, capillary spaces, edematous media and vascularization. Arterial lesions in groups II, III, and IV contained fibrous subintimal plaque with full thickness medial scarring (healed plaque). Medial involvement in the coronary arteries of group IV was significantly less severe than group I at $p < 0.05$, and group II at $p < 0.10$. Serum cholesterol in group IV was lower than group I at $p < 0.05$. Hyperlipidemia and atherosclerosis produced by the SS diet feeding was regressed by regression diet and simultaneous D-T4 therapy.

LONG-TERM EFFECTS OF CHOLESTEROL-FREE FAT MIXTURES RICH IN LAURIC, MYRISTIC OR PALMITIC ACID ON ATHEROSCLEROSIS IN THE RABBIT

René O. Vles, Jack J. Gottenbos, Willem G. Timmer, and Pieter L. van Pijpen
Unilever Research, Vlaardingen/The Netherlands

Male Dutch belted rabbits were fed for 22 months cholesterol-free semisynthetic regimens providing 40 per cent dietary energy from fat. The experimental fats consisted of various amounts of lauric, myristic or palmitic acid mixed with safflower seed oil fatty acids or oleic and linoleic acid. These fatty acid mixtures were randomly esterified with glycerol. Serum cholesterol, degree of aorta atherosclerosis and histopathology served as the main criteria. Replacement of saturated fatty acids by substantial amounts of linoleic acid largely prevented the hypercholesterolemic and atherogenic effects of the experimental diets. Incidence and severity of atherosclerosis decreased with increasing levels of dietary linoleic acid. Lauric, myristic and palmitic acid appeared to be equally atherogenic in dietary fat mixtures containing 40 per cent saturated fatty acids, 55 per cent oleic and 5 per cent linoleic acid. Microscopical examination of the aortas revealed advanced atherosclerosis which showed various features of the lesions observed in man.

EFFECTS OF GLUCOSAMINE ON CHOLESTEROL-INDUCED ATHEROSCLEROSIS IN RABBITS

Steen Stender and Poul Astrup
Department of Clinical Chemistry, Rigshospitalet, Copenhagen/Denmark

It has been claimed that heparin given intravenously counteracts the development of atherosclerosis in man. The effect of heparin's absorbable subunit glucosamine on experimental atherosclerosis was therefore investigated. 1% of glucosamine was added to a cholesterol-enriched diet in a group of 12 rabbits while the control group of 12 rabbits did not have glucosamine added to their cholesterol-enriched diet. The amount of cholesterol in the diet was individually adjusted so that all rabbits experienced the same level of serum cholesterol throughout the experimental period of 12 weeks. Although glucosamine did not affect the concentration response of serum cholesterol to dietary cholesterol, it did cause a reduction in the concentration value of aortic cholesterol, an increase in the wet weight of the inner aorta and an increase in the ratio of linoleic acid to oleic acid in the fatty acids of the cholesterol esters in serum, liver and inner aorta.

THE EFFECT OF A NEW PYRIDO-/1,2a/ PYRIMIDINE DERIVATE, CHINOIN-123, ON THE DEVELOPMENT OF AORTIC ATHEROMATOSIS IN RABBITS AFTER SHORT-TERM CHOLESTEROL FEEDING

Gyula Sebestyén, Zoltán Mészáros, István Hermecz, Márta Kovács, and Sándor Virág
Research Centre, Chinoin Pharmaceuticals Ltd., Budapest

It is hardly possible to demonstrate in the individual animal any consistent connections between, on the one hand, the hypercholesterolemic curves in relation to time, and, on the ohter hand, the enhanced cholesterol content of the aorta. After inducing an initial phase of cholesterol-influx (= hypercholesterolaemia), even varying intensity, triggers off in the aortic wall a process which causes increasing quantities of cholesterol to be deposited more or less regardless of the serum cholesterol concentration.
The effect of Chinoin-123, a pyrido-/1,2a/ pyrimidine derivate has been investi-

gated in rabbits after the phase of initial cholesterol-influx in order to reveal the efficacy of the compound on the cholesterol deposition in the aortic wall.

ATHEROMATOSIS OF THE RABBIT CAROTID ARTERY: I-AN IRRADIATION INDUCED EXPERIMENTAL MODEL

C.Th. Smit Sibinga, J. v.d. Meulen, and H.B. Lamberts
Coag. Laboratories, Department of Radiopathology, University Hospital Groningen/ Netherlands

The rabbit carotid artery is very resistant to atheromatous lesions in hypercholesterolaemia. Even very high serum cholesterol levels do not result in the formation of atheromatous plaques, unless the hypercholesterolaemia persists for several months. Only when the vessel wall has been damaged, lipid will infiltrate and be deposited. Rabbits were kept on a diet 1 week before and 4 weeks after irradiation. One carotid artery was irradiated upon (single dose 2000 R, dose rate 120 R/min), the other one being lead shielded from the X-rays. The rabbits were killed for histological examination of the carotid art.- the non-irradiated one being the control to the irradiated one, stained with o.r.O, Verhoeff, h.e. Group I: no diet, no irradiation (n=6). Group II: 0.5% chol. diet, irradiation (n=9), Group IV: 0.5% chol. diet, irradiation (n=14). Results: lipid analysis of the serum shows in the 0.5% chol. group II and IV a remarkable increase in lipid, mainly due to an increase in esterified chol. The carotid art. of the non-irradiated group III showed no signs of lipid infiltration or deposition. The carotid art. of the irradiated chol. fed group IV showed a definite deposition of lipid throughout the whole wall of the artery, with plaque formation at the intimal site. It is shown that only the combined loading effect of chol. and irradiation induced damage causes atheromatous lesions.

EVALUATION OF ANIMAL FOR ANTI-ATHEROSCLEROSIS DRUG RESEARCH

C.E. Day, W.W. Stafford, K.P. Chapman, C.M. Schmidt, and P.E. Schurr
The Upjohn Company, Kalamazoo, MI/USA

Twenty-four different strains of small laboratory animals were examined for macroscopic aortic atherosclerosis and hypercholesterolaria (elevated arterial cholesterol) after 8 to 12 weeks on an atherogenic diet containing cholesterol. Each of the strains was chosen for its small size and ready availability which make it suitable for screening large numbers of compounds for anti-atherosclerosis activity. In the rat different forms of arterial injury, such as vitamin D toxicity or intravenous infusions of vasoactive amines and enzymes, were tested in conjunction with the atherogenic diet for their effect on hypercholesterolaria.
No macroscopic atherosclerosis was seen in any of the rodent strains including genetically diabetic, obese, or hypercholesterolemic mice. In the 10 inbred strains of mice aortic cholesterol levels were elevated only slightly on the atherogenic diet. Only slight hypercholesterolaria could be induced in rats by chemical injury of the aorta in vivo. Rabbits, pigeons, chickens, and quail all exhibited macroscopic atherosclerosis and hypercholesterolaria and the incidence and severity of fatty streaks were greatest in male, SEA, Japanese quail. Of the 24 strains of animals, SEA Japanese quail were the best model to use in a large scale screening program to detect pharmacologic agents that prevent or reverse atherosclerosis.

LOSS OF ENDOTHELIAL CELLS IN RABBIT AORTA FOLLOWING SHORT-TERM CHOLESTEROL FEEDING

Leif Jørgensen
Institute of Medical Biology, University of Tromsø, Tromsø/Norway

Endothelial cells are continuously lost at certain predilection sites where also atherosclerotic lesions tend to develop. In order to see whether short-term cholesterol feeding influences this process, 16 rabbits were fed 2% cholesterol in the diet whereas 9 rabbits served as controls. In the cholesterolfed animals light, scanning, and transmission electron microscopy showed increased alterations and loss of endothelial cells in areas of irregular intimal fold pattern. This pattern probably reflects eddies of flow. The cells appeared to have been peeled off in single or sheets and to form brigdelike structures which probably indicate endothelial injury.
Platelets occurred in association with the altered endothelial cells and the denuded areas, but rather infrequently.
Increased focal endothelial destruction could be one of the initiating events in the development of atherosclerotic lesions.

INTER-INDIVIDUAL VARIATIONS IN METABOLISM OF CHOLESTEROL STUDIED IN RABBITS DURING NORMAL AND CHOLESTEROL-ENRICHED DIETS

Steen Stender
Department of Clinical Chemistry, Rigshospitalet, Blegdamsvej 9, DK-2100 Copenhagen, Denmark

Metabolism of cholesterol in 8 normocholesterolaemic rabbits (40 mg/dl) was investigated, based on the specific activity of cholesterol in serum measured during a period of 3 months after an intravenous injection of labeled cholesterol. The average daily output of cholesterol synthesized in the body during this period was within the range of 100 mg to 200 mg. The concentration of cholesterol in serum was increased to 800 mg/dl for all the rabbits and maintained at that level for 4 months by adding to the diet an individually adjusted amount of cholesterol - 100 mg/day in the most "cholesterol-sensitive" animal, 1000 mg/day in the most "cholesterol-resistant" animal. With a new injection of labeled cholesterol, the cholesterol metabolism was reinvestigated and for each individual compared with the metabolism before the cholesterol-feeding. The average daily output of cholesterol, absorbed and synthesized during the hypercholesterolaemic period was within the range of 150 mg to 750 mg.

DIETARY ENDOGENOUS AND EXOGENOUS HYPERCHOLESTEROLAEMIA IN YOUNG ♂ BABOONS

R. Zschocke, G. Hofrichter, A.V. Ginocchio, and A.N. Howard
Research Laboratories Klinge, Munich/BRD, Consultox Laboratories, London and Department of Medicine University of Cambridge, England

Serum total cholesterol (STC) analysis, lipoprotein electrophoresis (LEP) on agarose using Fat Red 7B and prep. ultracentrifugation (UC) were used to study serum lipoproteins (LP) in young ♂ baboons (5/group) given the following three dietary regimens for at least four weeks: (1) normal monkey chow (protein 14%, fat 2.5%), (2) a high protein (24%) & fat (7%), low cholesterol diet, (3) a high cholesterol (2%) & fat (12.5%), low protein (12%) diet. STC, LDL-TC & total LP were respectively (mg/100 ml): (1) 108,36,521; (2) 143,53,653; (3) 230,96,849. All LEP patterns were remarkably similar to human, the stainable β-LP increasing from 64% (diets 1 & 2) to 75% with diet (3). In contrast, quantitative analysis of UC fractions showed HDL predominating with diets (1) & (2). Only with diet (3) was a typically human pattern (LDL > HDL) obtained. VLDL was low in all groups. Another major difference between diets (2) and (3) was a marked increase in HDL-TC only in the latter group (1:59.2, 2:42.0, 3:118). These two hypercholesterol-aemic diets provide different models for the study of endogenous and exogenous hypercholesterolaemia. The effects of clofibrate, nicotinic acid, cholestyramine and a new hypocholesterolaemic 1,3-diaryloxipropanol-(2) derivative were also studied. Differing results obtained with each model provided valuable information on possible mechanisms of drug action.

EFFECT OF CEREBRAL PHOSPHOLIPIDS ON ATHEROSCLEROSIS-INDUCED MODIFI-CATIONS IN GLUCOSE METABOLISM OF RABBIT AORTAS

Marco Prosdocimi, Gino Toffano, Alberta Leon, Laura Caparrotta, and Giuliana Fassina
Chair of Pharmacology and Pharmacognosy, Padua University, Padova/Italy

Regression and inhibition of experimental atherosclerosis by i.v. phospholipids have been shown. Accordingly, we studied the effect of ox cerebral phospholipids (BC-PL): highly purified, containing long chain polyunsaturated fatty acids, in rabbits fed 45 days with atherogenic diet (D). BC-PL were injected i.v. 100 mg/Kg/day. Biochemical and haematological changes were compared in the two treated groups (D,BC-PL) and in controls (C). The atherogenic diet induced increase in cholesterol, triglycerides total lipids and β/α-lipoprotein was not statistical-ly different in the two groups (D,BC-PL). In aortas from rabbits fed atherogenic diet (D), glycogen increased while glucose, lactate and pyruvate decreased when compared with the controls (C).
Reversal of two parameters was induced by BC-PL treatment: it reduced the glyco-gen increase and restored pyruvate to control values. Reversal of the above pa-rameters on arterial wall, without lowering serum cholesterol, has to be pointed out.

EFFECT OF BOVINE BRAIN PHOSPHOLIPIDS ON CHOLESTEROL-INDUCED MODIFI-CATIONS IN MOUSE BRAIN

Gino Toffano, Alberta Leon, Daniela Benvegnù, and Elena Boarato
Research Laboratories of FIDIA Pharmacology, Abano Terme/Italy

Mice under (Thomas' atherogenic) cholesterol-supplemented diet for 40 days showed changes in behavioral pattern, that is, decreased spontaneous motor activ-ity and decreased capacity to avoid a painful electrical stimulus, accompanied with decrease in both cerebral catecholamine and cAMP content. The cerebral gly-colytic pathway was also modified leading to decrease of glycogen, glucose, lac-tate and pyruvate content. Furthermore the glycogen/glucose and lactate/pyruvate ratios increased.
Endovenous treatment with sonicated dispersions of bovine brain phospholipids (100 mg/kg) initiated 20 days after the diet, induced changes in all the above parameters. Data suggest an atherogenic diet-induced anoxic state which leads to an impairement of cerebral aminergic activity.

THE EFFECT OF AGING, INCREASED CHOLESTEROL INTAKE, AND SEX DIFFERENCES ON SERUM LIPID CONCENTRATION AND LIPOPROTEIN PATTERNS OF SPONTANEOUSLY HYPERTENSIVE RATS (SHR) AND NORMOTENSIVE RATS (NTR)

Herbert K. Naito, Lena A. Lewis, and Irvine H. Page
Divison of Research and Laboratory Medicine, Cleveland Clinic Foundation, Cleveland, OH/USA

These studies were made to determine whether the serum lipid-lipoprotein distribution of the rat is altered by aging, increased cholesterol intake or by hypertension, and if so whether the changes are sex related. Five-week old SHR or NTR were fed either a basal chow, Purina, or a 2% cholesterol-supplemented-Purina chow diet for 60 weeks. Changes in serum lipid levels in NTR and SHR of various ages were similar. The increase in serum triglyceride and phospholipid levels of old females of both strains and both diet groups was greater than in the males. Increase in serum cholesterol level in all groups was minimal. When the elevation of blood pressure of the SHR was prevented or treated by Apresoline HC1, the observed hyperlipidemia disappeared. The major serum lipoprotein fraction of all groups of rats at all ages, 5 to 60 weeks, was α-lipoprotein and its predominance was not altered by aging of the rats, cholesterol content of the diet, sex, or hypertension. Aging caused some diffused intimal thickening in both strains of rats. Cholesterol feeding did not greatly enhance this process. The old SHR all developed diffused intimal thickening of the thoracic aorta with occassional focal areas of foam cells, particularly in the old female rat. However, there were no instances in which gross atherosclerotic lesions were seen in any of the treatment groups. This finding might help explain the reason for the resistance of this animal species to the development of atherosclerosis.

FORCED DIETARY METHOD PRODUCING ATHEROSCLEROSIS IN RABBITS AND THE EFFECT OF CHINOIN-123

Gábor Lusztig, Árpád Hesz, Ferenc Schneider, László Mák, József Lesznyák, István Hermetz, and Sándor Virág
Institute of Pathology, Research Laboratory, County Hospital Kecskemét, CHINOIN-Pharmaceutics, Budapest/Hungary

Authors' aim was by using an effective diet, to get serum and histologic changes in rabbits during a short period, characteristic of atherosclerosis. A diet of 15 ml sour-cream + 1 g cholesterol + 3000 IU Vitamine D_3 given daily proved to be effective. Hyperlipoproteinemia appeared in serum after 10 days treatment and atheromatous plaques in the aortic wall of rabbits after 12-16 days.
Investigating the influence of CHINOIN-123 on number and volume of mast-cells of aorta-adventitia in forced hyperlipemia, it was stated, that our diet did not control serum-cholesterol and total-lipid level. Still number and volume of mast-cells increase strongly and by influence of CHINOIN-123 it decreases significantly. The function of mast-cells represent a part of the general mesenchymal reaction, CHINOIN-123 influencing above all the mesenchyma of the vessel-wall.

STUDIES ON EXPERIMENTAL ATHEROSCLEROSIS.
SERUM LIPIDS, EXOGENOUSLY AND ENDOGENOUSLY INDUCED CATECHOLAMINE VALUES, AND HISTOLOGICAL CHANGES IN RABBITS WITH EXPERIMENTALLY INDUCED ATHEROSCLEROSIS

Kenshi Nishino, Nagao Kajiwara, Yoshihiko Satoh, Tadashi Murota, Akio Koike, Hiroshi Yagi, Masao Itoh, Shinobu Suzuki, Noboru Yokoyama, Kazuo Masubuchi, Toru Yamazaki, and Michinobu Hatano
The 2nd Department of Internal Medicine, Nihon University School of Medicine, Department of Cardiology, Surugadai Nihon University Hospital, Tokyo/Japan

The effects of hypertension on the development of atherosclerosis were investigated in rabbits. The control group was fed a basal diet, while the atherosclerosis group received a diet containing cholesterol. Part of the cholesterol group was divided in to three subgroups in which hypertension was induced: (1) a Goldblatt group (2) a group in which the carotid artery was constricted, and (3) a group administered catecholamine exogenously. Total cholesterol, triglyceride, free fatty acid, and catecholamine values were determined and histological changes were observed. Serum lipid values were greater in both the hypertensive and normotensive groups than in the control group, but no significance between the two cholesterol-fed groups. Catecholamine concentration was higher in the hypertensive group than in the other groups. Atherosclerotic changes were more pronounced in the hypertensive group than in the other groups.

A COMPARISON OF HYPOCHOLESTEROLEMIC ACTIVITY OF β-SITOSTEROL AND β-SITOSTANOL IN RATS

Michihiro Sugano, Ikuo Ideda, and Hidekazu Morioka
Laboratory of Nutrition Chemistry, Kyushu University School of Agriculture, Fukuoka/Japan

We have previously reported that hydrogenation of the phytosterol mixture from corn oil intensifies its hypocholesterolemic property. The present study deals with the comparison of cholesterol-lowering activity of β-sitosterol(S) and β-sitostanol(HS). These preparations were fed at different levels (0.5-1.0%) to young male Wistar rats for 2-4 weeks with (0.5-1.0%) or without cholesterol. HS never influenced on the food intake, growth and weight of organs. Also, no diarrhea was observed. In combination with cholesterol, HS showed significantly greater activity in lowering plasma cholesterol levels; the concentration of cholesterol of rats fed equal amounts of cholesterol and HS was equal to or below that of rats fed no cholesterol. Elevation of plasma triglyceride due to feeding S was in no way observed with HS. However, for prevention of the accumulation of cholesterol and triglyceride in liver after feeding cholesterol, both S and HS showed similar abilities. The stanol further stimulated the fecal recovery of cholesterol. The rate of intestinal absorption of dietary HS was markedly lower, irrespective of the presence or absence of cholesterol in the diet, than that of S, and thus the deposition into plasma and liver lipid fractions was negligibly small.

WORKSHOP 8. Cholesterol Metabolism

Chairmen: D.S. Goodman, USA
          Y. Yamamura, Japan

Participants: A.K. Bhattacharyya, USA
              H.S. Sodhi, USA
              N. Takeuchi, Japan
              T.A. Miettinen, Finland
              K. Hellström, Sweden
              D.S. Goodman, USA

CHOLESTEROL METABOLISM IN HIGH- AND LOW-RESPONDING RHESUS MONKEYS*

Ashim K. Bhattacharyya and Douglas A. Eggen

The response of serum cholesterol to dietary cholesterol varies not only among species of animals but also among individuals of the same species. The rhesus monkey is no exception to this phenomenon (Eggen, 1976). Thus, when we fed a high-cholesterol diet which provided saturated fat at 40% of calories and cholesterol at 1 mg/kcal to 36 young male rhesus monkeys, they developed hypercholesterolemia with serum cholesterol levels distributed essentially normally but with large variability. The mean serum cholesterol for the 36 animals was 431 ± 137 (S.D.) mg/dl, whereas the mean for individual animals ranged from 151 to 721 mg/dl.

The mechanism(s) underlying this large differential response of the serum cholesterol to dietary cholesterol could reside in any of the several aspects of cholesterol metabolism, either singly or in combination. These include (1) intestinal absorption of cholesterol, (2) biosynthesis of cholesterol in liver or intestine or both, (3) fecal excretion of neutral or acidic steroids or both, and (4) the distribution of total body cholesterol among various tissues. In order to determine which of these aspects may be responsible for the large variability in serum cholesterol levels, we studied cholesterol absorption and whole-body cholesterol metabolism in groups of rhesus monkeys selected to have widely differing response of serum cholesterol to high-cholesterol diet.

Methods

From the 36 animals referred to above, the six with highest serum cholesterol (range 567-721 mg/dl, mean 619 mg/dl) and six with lowest (range 151-230 mg/dl, mean 199 mg/dl) were selected for the study and were referred to here as the high-responding (HI) and the low-responding (LO) animals, respectively. We studied the whole-body cholesterol metabolism using isotopic balance and isotopic kinetic analysis techniques (Hellman et al., 1957; Goodman et al., 1973) in five each of these HI and LO animals while they were fed a high-cholesterol diet for a period of 11 1/2 months and then fed a basal, low-fat, essentially cholesterol-free diet (Eggen, 1976. Eight months after beginning the high-cholesterol diet, a tracer dose of $4-^{14}C$ cholesterol was given intravenously to each animal. The specific activity of serum cholesterol was determined at varying intervals for 3 1/2 months, and the serum cholesterol specific activity decay curve was analyzed according to the three-pool model of Goodman et al. (1973). Three 5-day samples

*Supported by Grant HL08974 from the National Heart and Lung Institute, National Institutes of Health, Bethesda, MD.

of feces were collected at 2-week intervals beginning 9 weeks after the intravenous dose of radioactive cholesterol. The neutral and acidic steroids were extracted (Miettinen et al., Grundy et al., 1965), and the endogenous component (that derived from sources in isotopic equilibrium with serum cholesterol) was determined by the isotopic balance method of Hellman et al. (1957). Total fecal neutral steroid was determined by combined thin layer and gas-liquid chromatography (Miettinen et al., 1965). Cholesterol absorption was calculated using method I of Quantao et al. (1971) in which unabsorbed dietary cholesterol is obtained by subtracting the fecal endogenous neutral steroid fraction from the fecal total neutral steroids.

The animals were returned to the basal diet 3 1/2 months after the intravenous tracer dose of $4\text{-}^{14}C$ cholesterol and 5 months later, each animal was fed a meal containing tracer doses of $4\text{-}^{14}C$ cholesterol and ^3H β-sitosterol. Feces collected as a single pool for the following 8 days was analyzed for the determination of absorption of cholesterol according to the method of Borgstrom (1969).

Twelve months after return to the basal diet, the isotopic balance and isotopic kinetic studies were repeated as described above.

Results and Discussion

Serum Cholesterol

The mean serum cholesterol concentrations in HI and LO animals are presented in Table 1. Because of the way they were selected, the mean serum cholesterol was several fold greater in the HI (697 mg/dl) than in the LO group (256 mg/dl) during the high-cholesterol dietary period. Both during the initial basal diet period and, after stabilization, following return to basal diet, the serum cholesterol levels were significantly (p <0.02) greater in the HI (139 and 137 mg/dl) than in the LO group (96 and 94 mg/dl). The time required to attain the steady basal level was much greater in the HI group (7-14 weeks) than in the LO group (2-3 weeks).

Intestinal Absorption of Cholesterol

The mean percent absorption of cholesterol was statistically significantly greater in the HI group compared with the LO group whether the animals were fed the high-cholesterol diet or the cholesterol-free basal diet (Table 2).

As for possible mechanisms underlying this difference in absorption, we measured free and esterified cholesterol content and specific activity of free and esterified cholesterol in plasma chylomicrons of four low-responding and six high-responding animals 4 hours after feeding a meal by gavage containing labele choles-

Table 1. Mean serum cholesterol concentrations in high- and low-responding rhesus monkeys

Group (N)	Initial	High-cholesterol diet		Basal diet		
		0-12 wks.	13-50 wks.	2 wks.	8 wks.	52-76 wks.
		mg/dl ± SEM				
High (5)	139 ± 11	619 ± 27	697 ± 36	294 ± 33	155 ± 19	137 ± 12
Low (5)	96 ± 5	199 ± 14	256 ± 32	110 ± 6	88 ± 6	94 ± 12

Table 2. Mean intestinal absorption of cholesterol in high- and low-responding rhesus monkeys

Group (N)	High-cholesterol diet		Basal diet
High (5)	52.9	a	59.7
	b		b
Low (5)	45.4	c	46.2

[a] Significant difference between adjacent means, p <0.05.

[b] Significant difference between adjacent means, p <0.01.

[c] Not significant.

terol. The mean free and esterified cholesterol content of the plasma chylomicrons were significantly higher (p <0.05) in the HI group than in the LO group (1.8 vs. 1.0 mg%, respectively for free cholesterol and 4.8 vs. 2.5 mg%, respectively for esterified cholesterol). Specific activity of free cholesterol was higher in the HI group (4732 dpm/mg) than in the LO group (3443 dpm/mg); however, specific activity of esterified cholesterol was similar in HI and LO groups (2527 and 2547 dpm/mg, respectively). These results suggested that the uptake of cholesterol by the intestinal mucosal cells and the incorporation of cholesterol into chylomicrons in the intestinal mucosa was higher in the HI than in the LO group.

Body Pools of Cholesterol

The mean sizes of the exchangeable pools of cholesterol as determined by computer analysis of the serum cholesterol specific activity decay according to the three-pool model (Goodman et al., 1973) are presented in Table 3. On basal diet, the total exchangeable pool was similar in HI and LO groups, about 750 mg/kg body wt. On high-cholesterol diet, all exchangeable pools (except M_2) expanded in both HI and LO groups, but the increases were much greater in the HI than in the LO group. The total exchangeable pool of cholesterol was greater in the HI than in the LO group by about 700 mg/kg body wt.

The percentage of the increase in the total pool that appeared in the rapidly exchangeable pool (M_1) was approximately 50% for both groups. Further, the fraction of the increase in the total pool that appeared in either the plasma pool (M_1p) or the tissue component (M_{1T}) of the rapidly exchangeable pool was also similar in the two groups (about 24%). Thus, it appears that the increase in the total body pool of cholesterol that occurred on feeding high cholesterol was similarly distributed among the various exchangeable pools in HI and LO groups.

Fecal Excretion of Neutral and Acidic Steroids

The isotopic balance data presented in Table 4 show that the mean rates of excretion of both neutral and acidic steroids were similar in HI and LO groups during the basal diet period. On feeding the high-cholesterol diet, the bile acid excretion was higher in the HI than in the LO group; however, the increase in rate of excretion of neutral steroids, although high as compared to basal diet period in both groups, was similar in the two groups. It appears, therefore, that the high-responders failed to increase neutral sterol excretion enough to compensate for the increase in the cholesterol input. Whether factors other than the increased reabsorption of endogenous neutral sterols (such as biliary composition or volume) may be involved is not yet known.

Table 3. The distribution of cholesterol in the different exchangeable body pools of 5 high- and 5 low-responding rhesus monkeys

Pool	High-cholesterol diet		Basal diet	
	High-responders	Low-responders	High-responders	Low-responders
	mg/kg body wt.			
M_{1P} [a]	251 [d]	92	50 [e]	35
M_{1T} [b]	367 [d]	196	152	141
M_1	618 [d]	288	202	176
M_2 [c]	237	152	254	218
M_3 [c]	794 [e]	512	312	336
Total	1649 [d]	952	768	730

[a] Total plasma pool, plasma cholesterol in mg/ml x total plasma volume calculated as 36 ml/kg body wt (Altman and Dittman, 1974).

[b] Cholesterol pool of tissues comprising pool 1, i.e., $M_{1T} = M_1 - M_{1P}$.

[c] Minimum estimates assuming no synthesis in pools M_2 or M_3 and no direct excretion from these two pools.

[d] Significant difference between adjacent means, $p < 0.01$.

[e] Significant difference between adjacent means, $p < 0.05$.

Table 4. Mean daily fecal excretion of endogenous neutral sterols and bile acids in 5 high- and 5 low-responding rhesus monkeys

Fecal fraction	High-cholesterol diet		Basal diet	
	High-responders	Low-responders	High-responders	Low-responders
	mg/kg body wt.			
Endogenous neutral sterols	12.2	13.1	3.8	4.6
Bile acids	11.3 [a]	7.0	3.8	3.8
Total steroids	23.5 [b]	20.1	7.6	8.4

[a] Significant difference between adjacent means, $p < 0.01$.

[b] Significant difference between adjacent means, $p < 0.05$.

On the basal diet, the mean production rate of cholesterol in the pool M_1 (that is, the rate at which cholesterol appears in the pool) was about 10.7 mg/day/kg body wt for both groups. On the high-cholesterol diet, die production rate (which by definition includes absorbed cholesterol (Goodman et al., 1973) was high in both groups but was significantly higher in the HI (29.4 mg/day/kg) than the LO group (23.1 mg/day/kg), partly because of the increased absorption of cholesterol in the high-responders (Table 2).

To explore the potential differences in the rates of biosynthesis of cholesterol in HI and LO groups, we studied the relative rates of total body cholesterol synthesis in both groups using the "desmosterol suppression" technique of Bricker et al. (1972). While the animals were at steady state while being fed a diet providing a moderate amount of cholesterol (150 μg/kcal), we added triparanol to the diet (0.05%) for 28 days and followed the plasma concentration of cholesterol and desmosterol (Fig. 1). Triparanol feeding caused a decrease in plasma cholesterol and an increase in plasma desmosterol concentrations in both groups. The mean plasma desmosterol concentrations in HI and LO groups were 9.8 and 23.0 mg%, respectively after feeding triparanol for 28 days. From Figure 1, it is also evident that the rate of increase in plasma desmosterol concentration was much greater in the LO than in the HI group. This indicates that in those tissues in which desmosterol exchanges with that in plasma, the rate of synthesis of cholesterol is greater in the LO group than in the HI group. Since liver is one such tissue, and since it is known that cholesterol biosynthesis in the liver is regulated by cholesterol absorbed from the intestine, it might be expected that the greater absorption in the HI group would cause a greater feedback inhibition of

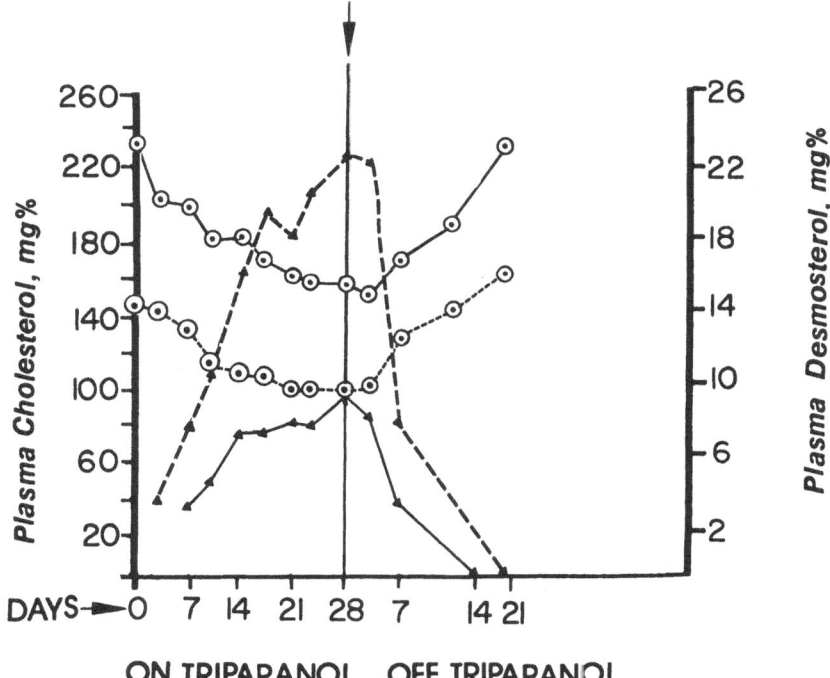

Figure 1. The mean plasma cholesterol (circled dots) and desmosterol (triangles) concentrations in five high-responding (solid lines) and four low-responding (broken lines) rhesus monkeys fed triparanol along with a moderately high-cholesterol diet (0.15 mg cholesterol per kcal per day). At arrow, the drug was withdrawn

hepatic cholesterol synthesis. Similar measurements of relative rates of synthesis on cholesterol-free diet have not yet been completed.

Summary

Rhesus monkeys with the highest response of serum cholesterol during feeding of a high-fat, high-cholesterol diet also have a higher mean serum cholesterol level on the basal, cholesterol-free diet. During both dietary periods, the percentage intestinal absorption of cholesterol is higher in the high- than in the low-responding group. The results also suggest that the uptake of cholesterol by the intestinal mucosal cells and incorporation of cholesterol into chylomicrons in the intestinal mucosa was greater in the HI than in the LO group. The increase in cholesterol content of the body due to cholesterol feeding is distributed similarly in the high- and low-responding groups. During a moderate intake of dietary cholesterol, the high-responding group has an appreciably lower rate of synthesis of cholesterol than the low-responding group. This may be a result of greater inhibition of hepatic cholesterol synthesis due to high cholesterol absorption. Thus, the results obtained to date indicate that differences in intestinal absorption of cholesterol is one factor involved in producing the large differences in the response of serum cholesterol to dietary cholesterol among animals.

RELATIONSHIPS BETWEEN METABOLISM OF CHOLESTEROL AND THE TURNOVER OF PLASMA LIPOPROTEINS

H.S. Sodhi, B.J. Kudchodkar, D.T. Mason, and N. Borhani

While there is some literature on the correlations between the metabolism of plasma triglycerides and the metabolism of plasma lipoproteins, the metabolism of endogenous cholesterol has not, in general, been related to the metabolism of lipoproteins. Studies done in our laboratories indicated to us that synthesis and catabolism of endogenous cholesterol as well as the esterification of plasma-free cholesterol were signficantly greater in hypertriglyceridemic patients than in those with normal plasma triglycerides and comparable levels of plasma cholesterol (Sodhi and Kudchodkar, 1973a, 1973b; Sodhi 1974; Kudchodkar and Sodhi, 1976). Since plasma triglycerides by themselves are unlikely to cause these changes in cholesterol metabolism (Sodhi and Kudchodkar, 1974a), we reasoned that the observed correlations in man must be mediated through the state of lipoprotein metabolism associated with hypertriglyceridemia (Sodhi and Kudchodkar, 1973c). The bulk of available evidence indicated that hypertriglyceridemia in man was generally associated with increased synthesis and turnover of plasma very low-density lipoproteins (VLDL). (Reaven et al., 1965; Nestel and Whyte, 1968; Nikkila und Kekki, 1971; Brunzell et al., 1973; Kaye and Galton, 1975; Sigurdsson et al., 1976; Kudchodkar and Sodhi, 1976; Nestel, 1976). We should, however, recognize that the method used in the laboratories of Havel (Havel et al., 1970) and of Carlson (Boberg et al., 1972) produced data which did not fully agree with the results obtained by most other methods. The latter, however, were in good agreement with each other (Brunzell et al., 1976).

We therefore postulated that the hepatic synthesis of cholesterol was coupled to the hepatic synthesis and secretion of new plasma lipoproteins, especially the VLDL (Sodhi and Kudchodkar, 1973c; Sodhi, 1975). We also suggested that the cholesterol derived from the degradation of plasma lipoproteins is not reused for synthesis of new plasma lipoproteins but that it was preferentially excreted in the bile (Fig. 1).

298

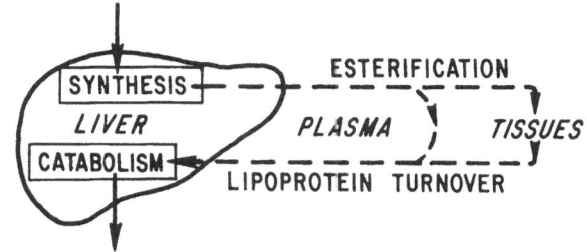

Figure 1. Sodhi and Kudchodkar's model for metabolism of hepatic cholesterol

Although there is no a priori reason for *obligatory* realtionships between the turnover of endogenous cholesterol and the metabolism of plasma lipoproteins, it would be difficult to explain the correspondence such as the following, without postulating relationships between them.

1. Metabolic changes apparently limited to the turnover rates of plasma lipoproteins are associated with significant changes in the total production of endogenous cholesterol.
2. Tissues which synthesize plasma lipoproteins (i.e., the liver and the intestines) synthesize more than 90% of the total endogenous chclesterol (Dietschy and Wilson, 1970).
3. Liver is the major component of pool A of cholesterol (Goodman and Noble, 1968), and as can be seen in Figure 2, the entry into and the exit from pool A bear direct relationships to the entry into and the exit from the hepatic pool of free cholesterol. Estimated amounts of free cholesterol incorporated by liver into plasma lipoproteins are of the same order of magnitude as the amounts of new cholesterol entering the liver pool (Kudchodkar and Sodhi, 1976; Fig. 3).
4. The hepatic secretion of free cholesterol into plasma lipoproteins is in turn similar to the amounts of free cholesterol esterified in plasma (Kudchodkar and Sodhi, 1976).

These observations favor the existence of relationships between the turnover of plasma lipoproteins, hepatic synthesis of cholesterol, and esterification of plasma-free cholesterol. Direct experimental evidence in support of these suggestions is provided by the work of Goh and Heimberg (1973). They demonstrated

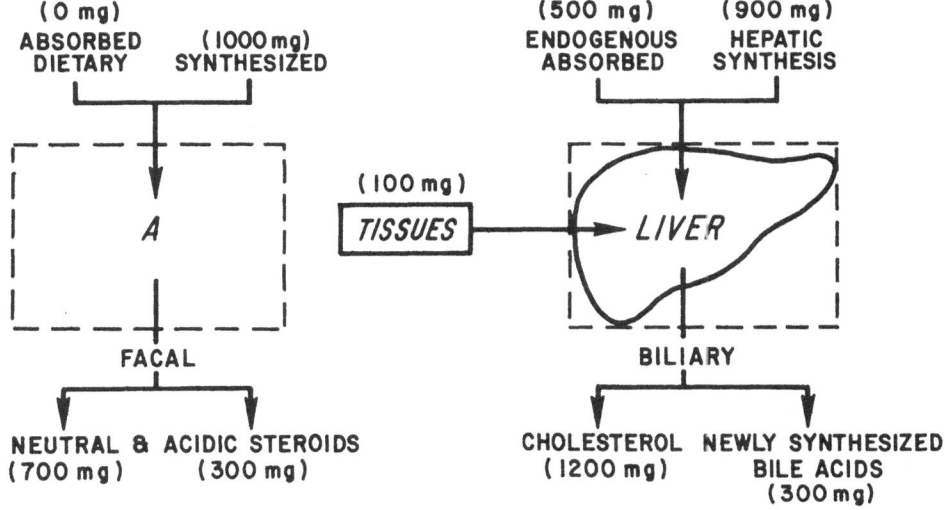

Figure 2. Relationships of input and output of cholesterol between pool A and liver

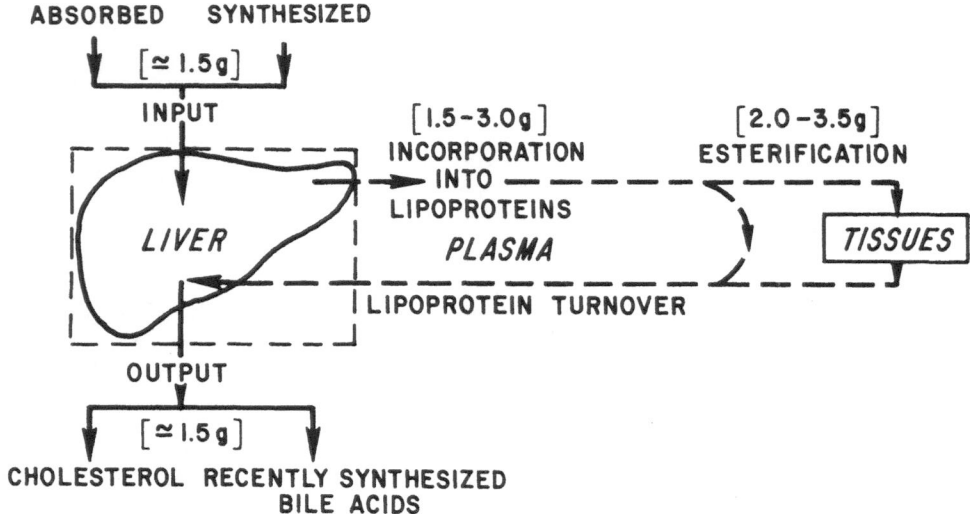

Figure 3. Estimates of the amounts of cholesterol (per day) channeled into various pathways

that hepatic synthesis of cholesterol was increased when synthesis of lipoproteins was enhanced by perfusing the rat liver with increasing amounts of free fatty acids.

Clinical studies carried out in a number of laboratories provide confirmation of our initial observations (Sodhi and Kudchodkar, 1974b; Kudchodkar and Sodhi, 1976).

Increases in endogenous synthesis of cholesterol (Miettinen, 1971a; Miller et al., 1976), in esterification of plasma-free cholesterol (Nestel, 1970; Fabien et al., 1973; Wallentin, 1976), in biliary and fecal excretion of metabolites of endogenous cholesterol (Nestel and Hunter, 1974; Simons and Myant, 1975), and in hepatic synthesis of bile acids (Kottke, 1969; Einarsson and Hellstrom, 1972) have all been documented in patients with elevated plasma triglycerides. However, it is worth emphasizing that the hypothesis relates metabolism of cholesterol to the turnover rates of plasma lipoproteins, although the observations related the former only to the levels of plasma triglycerides. Indeed, some of the hypertriglyceridemic subjects failed to show the changes in cholesterol metabolism (Grundy, 1975; Smith et al., 1976) observed by us.

The experimental and clinical observations on obesity also provide additional evidence in support of this hypothesis. Work of Robertson et al. (1973) in rats, and of Olefsky et al. (1974) in man, clearly indicated that there is an increase in hepatic synthesis and secretion of triglycerides and VLDL in obesity. These in turn are associated with increases in synthesis of cholesterol (Nestel et al., 1973; Miettinen, 1971b), turnover of endogenous cholesterol (Nestel et al., 1969, 1973; Smith et al., 1976), and increases in the esterification of plasma-free cholesterol (Nestel and Monger, 1967; Nestel, 1970; Akanuma et al., 1973). Restriction in caloric intake is associated with prompt decreases in plasma triglycerides, endogenous synthesis of cholesterol, and esterification of plasma-free cholesterol; all probably secondary to a reduction in the hepatic synthesis and secretion of plasma VLDL (Sodhi and Kudchodkar, 1975). Similarly, drugs*

---

*These effects of the drugs are often associated with mobilization of tissue cholesterol and its attendant effects on the excretion of fecal metabolites of endogenous cholesterol (Sodhi et al., 1973).

(cholestyramine, colestipol) which increase turnover of plasma VLDL (Angelin et al., 1976) are associated with increased synthesis of endogenous cholesterol (Grundy et al., 1971; Nazir et al., 1972), increased esterification of plasma-free cholesterol (Clifton-Bligh et al., 1974), and increased catabolism of endogenous cholesterol (Grundy et al., 1971; Nazir et al., 1972). Conversely, clofibrate which reduces the turnover of plasma VLDL decreases endogenous synthesis and esterification of plasma-free cholesterol (Sodhi et al., 1971).

These observations provide considerable support to some aspects of our model (Sodhi and Kudchodkar, 1973c), while data in support of other apsects are not yet available. Our suggestions that hepatic synthesis of cholesterol, biliary excretion of cholesterol and its metabolites, and esterification of plasma-free cholesterol are all related to the hepatic synthesis, and turnover of plasma lipoproteins appear well-substantiated, while there is still some uncertainty about the definition of anabolic and catabolic pools of hepatic cholesterol (Sodhi and Kudchodkar, 1973c).

STUDIES ON THE MECHANISM OF DEVELOPMENT OF HYPERCHOLESTEROLEMIA: EFFECT OF AGING AND GENETIC FACTORS IN ANIMAL MODELS

Nozomu Takeuchi

It was shown by the in vitro experiments using serum lipoproteins labeled with radioactive cholesterol that the isolated rat hepatocytes removed ester cholesterol from serum LDL, VLDL, and chylomicrons efficiently (Fig. 1). But cholesterol concentrations of VLDL and chylomicrons in peripheral blood are usually lower than that of LDL. So, the serum cholesterol removed by the liver in vivo is considered to be derived considerably from LDL cholesterol. The uptake of cholesterol by the hepatocytes seems to be specific for serum LDL, because the

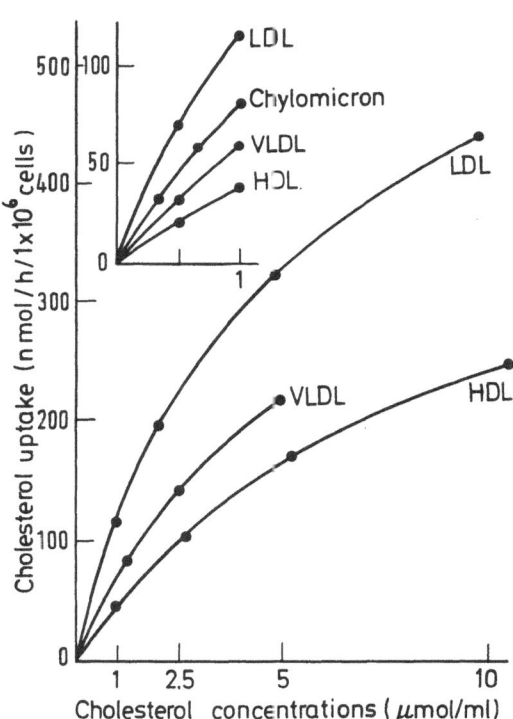

Figure 1. Uptake of cholesterol by isolated hepatocytes from various lipoprotein fractions

uptake from LDL was inhibited by the addition of nonlabeled LDL but was not affected by serum albumin at a ten times higher concentration than serum LDL (Fig.
2). Consequently, apoB protein which is contained in these three serum lipoproteins (Eisenberg and Levy, 1975; Jackson et al., 1976) probably plays an important role in the transfer of the cholesterol moiety from lipoproteins to hepatocytes through the membrane receptors.

Inhibition of cholesterol synthesis by a negative feedback control of high-cholesterol diet was impaired in aged rats (Takeuchi et al., 1976d). Moreover, the induction of the synthesis by glucose feeding after long-term fasting was also decreased (Takeuchi et al., 1976d). The uptake of cholesterol by the isolated hepatocytes from such aged animals was proved to be impaired as compared with that
from young rats. From the experiments of the distribution of labeled cholesterol
orally ingested into hepatic subcellular fractions, it was suggested that the
intracellular transport of exogenous cholesterol to microsomes or mitochondria
was reduced in old rats. When the hepatic microsomes from young rats were incubated with cytosol from old rats instead of that from young rats, cholesterol
synthesis in the microsomes was markedly decreased (Takeuchi et al., 1975). On
the other hand, cholesterol synthesis of old microsomes was increased by the incubation with young cytosol (Takeuchi et al., 1975). Thus, the inducible activity
in cytosol fraction to cholesterol synthesis of hepatic microsomes was also impaired in old rats. Therefore, cytosol carrier proteins of sterols or their precursors and membrane receptors on hepatocytes seemed to be reduced together with
enzyme systems for cholesterol metabolism as aging advanced. The combination of
these functional changes by aging causes the impairment of cholesterol metabolism
such as the elevation of serum cholesterol concentration.

It was found that the long-term treatment of an antioxidant agent up to 12 months
prevented the progress of these enzyme retardations concomitantly with the decreased lipid peroxide in the subcellular organelles (Takeuchi et al., 1976c)
which has been considered to affect the functional changes of the membrane bound
enzymes (Wills, 1971; Grinna, 1976). The elevation of serum lipid concentrations
by aging was also prevented in the rats treated by antioxidant (Takeuchi et al.,
1976c). By contrast, antioxidant-deficient rats which accumulated a large amount

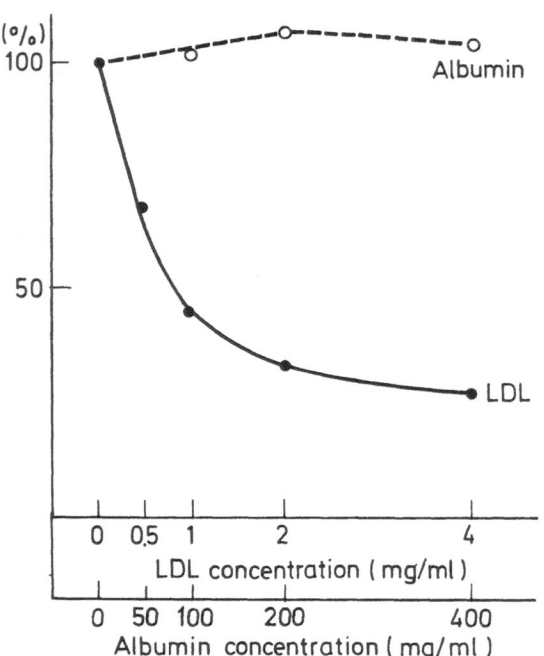

Figure 2. Effect of addition of
LDL or albumin to incubation medium
on the uptake of labeled cholesterol
from LDL

of lipid peroxide in the subcellular organelles, as well as serum, showed impaired activities of the metabolic enzymes of cholesterol in the liver, and resulted in the hyperresponse of serum cholesterol concentration to dietary cholesterol as observed in the aged (Takeuchi et al., 1976b).

Hyperresponsiveness of serum cholesterol which occasionally is found in some animals appeared to be an inheritable defect in animals and to be derived from the reduced removal rate of serum cholesterol (Takeuchi et al., 1976a). Neither hepatic cholesterol synthesis nor intestinal absorption of dietary cholesterol is considered to participate in the development of hyperresponsiveness of serum cholesterol in the rat (Takeuchi et al., 1976a). The uptake of serum cholesterol by the isolated hepatocytes in vitro was decreased in such animals (Table 1). Therefor, decreased hepatic removal rate of serum cholesterol by the reduced uptake by the hepatocytes from serum lipoproteins should be an important factor in the modulation of serum cholesterol concentration. Such functional changes have to cause the delay of the clearance of serum cholesterol to affect the synthesis and excretion of cholesterol and bile acids and successively to induce the tendency of elevation of serum cholesterol level. A negative feedback control of cholesterol synthesis has been considered to be conducted by the increased uptake of cholesterol by the cells or the assimilation of ester cholesterol in the cells (Dietschy and Wilson, 1970). Reduced uptake of serum cholesterol by the liver should result in the increase of cholesterol synthesis because of the reduction of feedback control (Brown and Goldstein, 1976). However, bile acid metabolism has to influence the cholesterol metabolism in the liver (Miettinen, 1973). Feeding of a large amount of cholesterol increased the biliary excretion of chenodeoxycholic acid, which accerelated the fecal excretion of secondary bile acids and enhanced the turnover rate of cholesterol and bile acids (Beher et al., 1970). The increase of endogenous cholesterol synthesis enhanced the formation of cholic acid (Uchida et al., 1975). It has been well-documented that increase of HMG Co A reductase activity induced by diets is very rapidly inactivated (Edwards and Gould, 1974; Kirsten and Watson, 1974). Such a rapid decrease of cholesterol synthesis might have some relationship to the metabolic pathway of bile acids. Hydroxy- or keto-compounds of cholesterol have been proved to have the strong inhibitory activities of cholesterol synthesis, which probably have something to do with a negative feedback control (Kandutsch and Chen, 1974; Brown and Goldstein, 1974). Administration of chenodeoxycholic acid or its secondary bile acids to the rats fed a cholesterol supplemented diet did not affect the serum cholesterol level. But cholic acid or deoxycholic acid administration markedly elevated serum cholesterol concentration. Cholic acid or deoxycholic acid is reabsorbed well and enlarges the pool size of bile acid and induces the increase of the serum cholesterol level (Uchida et al., 1975).

It was observed that oral glucose administration after long-term fasting stimulated the hepatic cholesterol synthesis and simultaneously the catabolic reactions of cholesterol (Takeuchi et al., 1974). Thus, marked enhancement of the synthesis did not always influence the serum cholesterol concentration (Fig. 3).

Table 1. Uptake of cholesterol by isolated hepatocytes from hyper- and hyporesponded rats

Animal groups	Serum cholesterol after cholesterol diet (mg/100 ml)	Percent uptake of cholesterol (Percent/h/10^6 cells)	Net amount of cholesterol uptake (n mol/h/10^6 cells)
Hyporesponder	80.8 ± 3.52 [a]	2.28 ± 0.12	46.18 ± 2.32
Hyperresponder	301.3 ± 39.1	1.17 ± 0.08	23.57 ± 1.60
P	<0.001	<0.01	<0.01

[a] 4 rats $\bar{x}$ ± SEM.

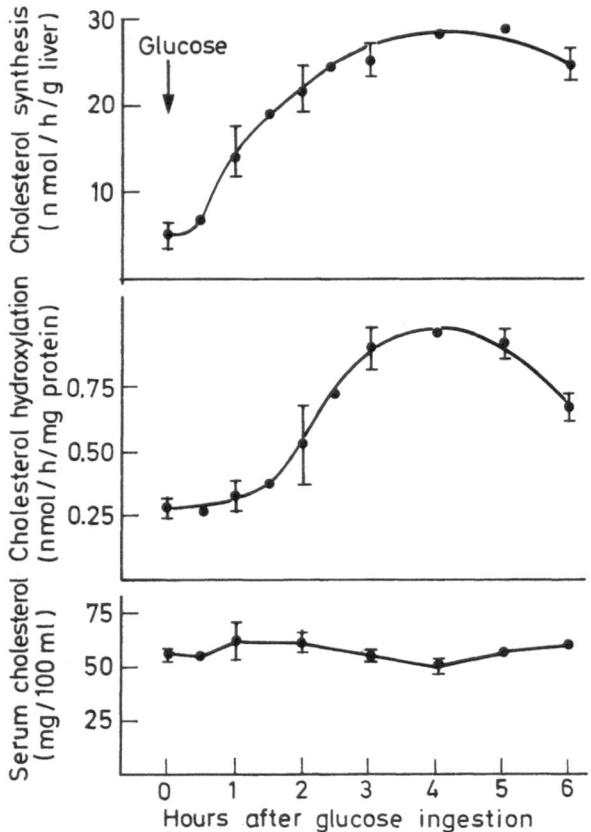

Figure 3. Effect of glucose ingestion on hepatic cholesterogenis, 7 α-hydroxylation of cholesterol and serum cholesterol level

Even a wide diurnal fluctuation of HMG Co A reductase activity did not affect the serum cholesterol concentration. Intrahepatic anabolic and catabolic processes of cholesterol metabolism are very intimately interacted through bile acid metabolism in the liver.

From our present experimental results, it is concluded that the defect of receptors on hepatocyte membrane (Bachorik et al., 1976) in hyperresponded or aged animals decreases the uptake of cholesterol to the cells from serum lipoproteins and causes the delay of clearance of serum cholesterol to elevate the concentration of serum cholesterol. Synthesis and excretion of bile acids from cholesterol of peripheral circulation might be reduced successively. However, cholesterol synthesis in the liver, which is expected to be enhanced by the reduced uptake of serum cholesterol, might be modulated by the catabolic products of cholesterol, because endogenously synthesized cholesterol is mainly metabolized to cholic acid, which consequently enlarges the pool size of bile acids by the intestinal reabsorption of bile acid and reduces the synthetic rate of cholesterol secondarily.

Tatu A. Miettinen

Quantitation of cholesterol production takes place with fecal steroid analysis (Grundy et al., 1965; Miettinen et al., 1965) or with kinetic analysis of serum cholesterol specific activity data with a two-pool or a three-pool model (Goodman et al., 1973; Samuel et al., 1972). The kinetic methods require that cholesterol production and removal take place in and from rapidly exchangeable pool 1.

Kinetic Analysis of Cholesterol Metabolism with ^{14}C-Mevalonate, ^{3}H-Water, and ^{3}H-Cholesterol

Computer analysis of the data obtained from serum and fecal steroids and from water after administration of ^{14}C-mevalonate and ^{3}H-water or ^{14}H-cholesterol to

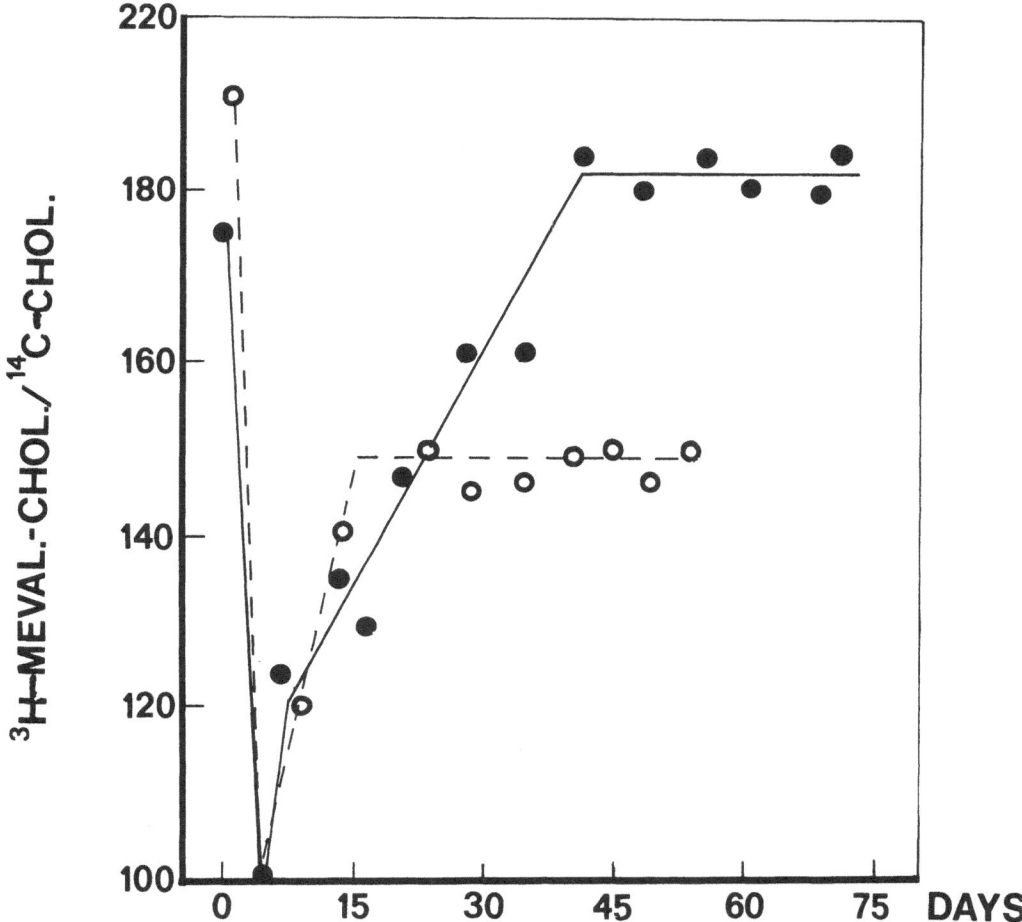

Figure 1. Ratio of serum ^{3}H-cholesterol/^{14}C-cholesterol after an intravenous injection of a ^{3}H-mevalonate-^{14}C-cholesterol mixture to a human subject. The lowest point of the ratio, occurring usually on the 4th day after the injection, is indicated by 100 to which all other values are related. o = first study; ● = second study, 1 year later when the body weight had been increased by 8 kg. The plateau value of the ratio, occurring 2-4 weeks after the injection, correlated positively (r = 0.815) with the relative body weight in nine studies performed on five subjects

man indicated, however, that cholesterol was not solely synthesized in rapidly exchangeable pool. As a matter of fact, the computer solution revealed that in normolipidemic nonobese subjects about 35% of cholesterol was produced in slowly exchangeable pool(s). A positive correlation of the pool 2 synthesis with total body fat suggested that adipose tissue had contributed to this production (Kekki et al., 1977).

A deviation of the serum ^{3}H- and ^{14}C-cholesterol specific activity time curves during 2-4 weeks after an intravenous administration of ^{14}C-cholesterol and ^{3}H-mevalonate suggested that mevalonate-derived cholesterol had released to the blood from some slowly turning over pool(s). The magnitude of this deviation appeared to correlate with the degree of obesity (r = 0.815 between the relative body weight and the deviation shown in Fig. 1), again suggesting a causal role of the adipose tissue in the cholesterol synthesis in slowly exchangeable cholesterol pool(s).

Squalene, Methyl Sterols, and Cholesterol in Different Human Tissues

Cholesterol precursor analyses were performed in different tissues so as to reveal the possible site of pool 2 synthesis (Miettinen, 1976). In adipose tissue, the squalene concentration was extremely high (Table 2), an observation found also by others (Liu et al., 1976). Renal squalene was not very high while the overall squalene pool of skeletal muscle appears to be fairly large owing to large muscle mass. Lanosterol and other methyl sterols were present in negligible amounts only (Table 1). A marked weight reduction after a jejunoileal by-pass of obese subjects was associated with a transient increase of both cholesterol and squalene in adipose tissue during the first postoperative year (Miettinen, 1976). Even though the fecal steroid data showed the overall cholesterol synthesis to be permanently increased by 1-2 g/day, the increase in adipocyte cholesterol and squalene was probably not due to enhanced local synthesis but was more likely caused by a rapid shrinkage of fat cells. This was apparently followed by a gradual mobilization of retained cholesterol and squalene after the rapid weight redcution had ceased.

Table 1. Squalene and sterol contents of different human tissues

Tissue	Squalene	Lanosterol	Dimethylsterol	Cholesterol
		μg/100 g		
1 Spleen	80	55	16	414
2 Aorta	126	159	38	1426
3 Lung	167	20	2	276
4 Kidney	270	35	13	233
5 Gut	451	56	32	200
6 Heart	487	38	24	97
7 Liver	578	341	72	295
8 Muscle	856	18	4	55
9 Fat	23.8	219	92	110
10 Fat 0	18.3	–	–	120
11 3 Mo	21.6	–	–	146
12 6 Mo	31.9	–	–	163
13 12 Mo	28.7	–	–	130
14 24 Mo	22.7	–	–	91

1-9 autopsy material; averages of four cases. 10-14 average values of seven overweight subjects obtained from needle biopsy specimens before and 3-24 months after a jejunoileal by-pass operation. Precursor sterols of cholesterol, lanosterol, and dimethylsterol could not be measured from the small needle biopsy samples. Squalene of fat tissue is expressed in mg/100 g [6].

Table 2. Cholesterol synthesis in vitro in human adipose biopsies

Precursors	Product, % of total		
	Squalene	Lanosterol	Cholesterol
^{14}C acetate	90	7	3
^{3}H mevalonate	85	7	8
Lipid dropled	82	6	7
Membranes	3	1	1
^{3}H mevalonate [a]	100	100	100
Serum	0.2	2.5	89.9
Fat cells	99.8	97.5	10.1
^{14}C acetate [b]	38 [c]	-	44 [c]
^{3}H mevalonate	61	-	98

Adipose biopsies were incubated for 3 h, precursor concentrations of acetate and mevalonate being 2 mM. Lanosterol includes all the methyl sterol precursors of cholesterol.

[a] Incubated with human adipose tissue for 3 h. Adipocytes isolated and reincubated with human serum for 3 h. Radioactivity analyzed from cells and medium. (Tilvis, R., Miettinen, T.A., Kovanen, P., unpublished observations).

[b] Biopsies obtained before and 3 – 7 days after a 75 caloric diet; averages as % of controls from five subjects.

[c] Statistically significant (P <0.05) change.

Synthesis of Squalene and Cholesterol in Adipose Tissue

Incubation of human adipose tissue with labeled acetate and mevalonate (Tilvis, R., Miettinen, T.A., Kovanen, P., unpublished data) showed only a small amount of cholesterol to be made, the major incorporation of the labels taking place, in contrast to earlier studies (Schreibman and Dell, 1975), into squalene, less so than into methyl sterols (Table). From 90 – 97% of the synthesized squalene, methyl sterols, and cholesterol were found in lipid droplets of adipocytes. Thus, newly formed squalene was apparently trapped and diluted by the large squalene pool, allowing only a small amount of the labels to be converted to cholesterol. Since the newly formed squalene may not have been homogeneously mixed with the unlabeled squalene during the incubation period, the specific activity of the squalene converted to methyl sterols and further to cholesterol is not known. Accordingly, cholesterol synthesis in terms of µg/g of adipose tissue cannot be measured accurately with in vitro studies. The use of the specific activities of the initial precursor labels gives too low that of squalene too high values. Incubations of fat biopsies obtained before and 3 – 7 days after a 75 calorie diet revealed that the synthesis of both squalene and cholesterol was reduced by about 60% from acetate, less significantly from mevalonate. This suggests that total fast inhibits cholesterol synthesis at an early stage probably at HMG CoA reductase. Addition of different lipoproteins into the medium showed that newly formed adipose squalene was not exchanged with or released into the medium even though newly synthesized radioactive methyl sterols and especially cholesterol were significantly released (or exchanged) from the fat tissue. This took place in an increasing order of magnitude by VLDL, LDL, and HDL.

The results indicate that in view of a marked dilution of cholesterol precursors in different steps, but at the squalene step in particular, adipose tissue cholesterol synthesis in vitro is actually higher than has been realized at the moment and may significantly contribute to the obesity-induced increase in cholesterol synthesis. Active squalene production indicates that the large adipose tissue squalene pool could have been formed by local synthesis. No evidence was obtained that newly formed squalene was released from adipocytes. In contrast, it is equilibrated with and slowly "released" from the large squalene pool and converted slowly to cholesterol which in turn is diluted with the cholesterol (belongs to the slowly exchangeable cholesterol pool) of the adipocyte and ultimately released slowly into the blood stream probably with the aid of HDL. This can be hypothesized to be the mechanism by which adipose tissue contributes to pool 2 synthesis of cholesterol (Fig. 2). From among the other tissues, the kidneys are known to strongly retain nonsaponifiable material formed from mevalonate (Penttilä and Miettinen, 1968; Hellstrom et al., 1973) and muscle tissue, with its large mass and fairly high squalene content, may have a similar action.

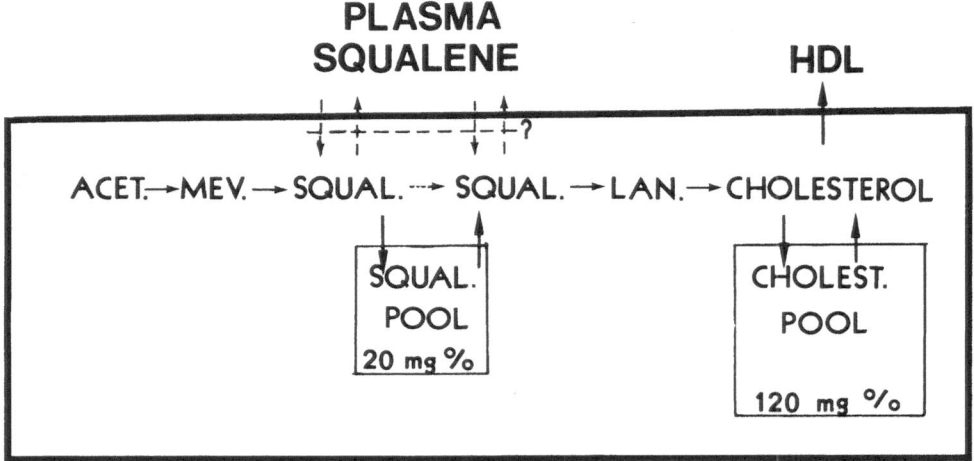

Figure 2. Proposed cholesterol synthesis in human adipocyte. Mixing of newly formed squalene and cholesterol with the respective adipocyte pools makes reliable measurement of cholesterol synthesis difficult and markedly retards appearance of precursors as cholesterol into plasma probably with the aid of high-density lipoprotein (HDL). This retardation could contribute to the increase of the ratio illustrated in Figure 1, provided the injected ^{3}H-mevalonate is taken up by the adipose tissue. As compared to squalene, the diluting effect of other precursor sterols (illustrated by LAN.) of cholesterol is less significant

BILE ACID METABOLISM UNDER BASAL AND EXPERIMENTAL CONDITIONS IN NORMO- AND HYPERLIPIDEMIC SUBJECTS

Kjell Hellström

Cholesterol is synthesized in most tissues but mainly eliminated in feces as bile acids (BA) and neutral steroids. The central role of BA in cholesterol metabolism has focused interest on mechanisms regulating BA metabolism. Much of our work during the past years has been aimed at characterizing BA kinetics in patients with various forms of hyperlipoproteinemia (HLP). These studies conducted under both basal and experimental conditions are summarized in this paper.

Material and Methods

The patients (35-67 years of age) were those consecutively admitted because of primary HLP. Not included in the study were subjects with diseases known to interfere with lipoprotein (LP) metabolism as well as those addicted to alcohol and narcotics. All patients were hospitalized during the investigations. The diet was strictly standardized and of natural type. HLP was classified according to the recommendations of WHO. BA kinetics were studied as originally described by Lindstedt (1957). Neutral steroids were determined with GLC. Details about the procedures and methods used have been reported earlier (Hellström and Einarsson, 1976).

Results

Basal Conditions

Bile acid kinetics were studied under basal conditions in altogether 15 normolipidemic subjects and in 17 patients with type IIa, in 12 patients with type IIb, and in 27 patients with type IV LP pattern. A few patients with HLP type IIa suffered from heterozygous familial hypercholesterolemia (FH). None was homozygous.

The values (means ± SEM) encountered for the formation of cholic acid (C) and chenodeoxycholic acid (CD) are demonstrated in Figure 1. The combined BA production was within the normal range in HLP type IIa and type IIb but abnormally high in HLP type IV. This group was very heterogenous and BA synthesis was quantitatively normal in one-third of the patients. The total BA pool was normal in HLP type IIa and type IIb and above normal in part of the patients with type IV LP pattern. The BA fractional turnover rate was essentially the same in the controls and the hyperlipidemic patients.

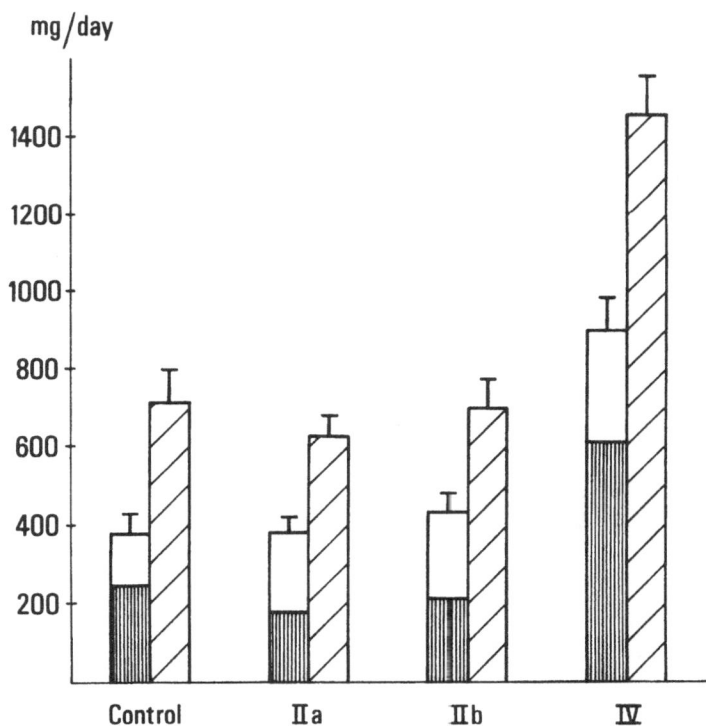

Figure 1. Synthesis of bile acids (⊞cholic acid, ☐ cehnodeoxycholic acid) and net steroid balance (▨) in patients with varius types of hyperlipoproteinemia

Although quantitatively normal, BA synthesis was still defective in HLP type II. Thus, the ratio between the amounts of C and CD produced averaged two in the controls and only about one in patients with the type IIa and type IIb pattern. This finding was higly significant and encountered in most patients irrespective of sex, age, and body weight. A different pattern was recorded in HLP type IV. Due to a high production of C, the C/CD ratio of BA synthesis was above normal in most cases. The net steroid balance (defined as BA production plus fecal excretion of neutral steroids minus cholesterol intake) was within the normal range in HLP types IIa and IIb and abnormally high in 50% of the patients with the type IV LP pattern.

Experimental Conditions

Subgroups of the patients studied under basal conditions were reinvestigated after being treated with hypolipidemic drugs for several months. At the time of the second steady, the serum lipids had in general decreased and long since reached a new steady state. The results from these investigations are summarized in Figure 2.

Treatment with cholestyramine resulted in a marked elevation of the BA formation in HLP type II. This increase was mainly due to a stimulated synthesis of C, whereby the C/CD ratio of the BA synthesized turned to normal. The C/CD ratio was initially high in the patients with the type IV pattern. It tended to decrease during cholestyramine treatment as the biosynthesis of CD increased more than that of C.

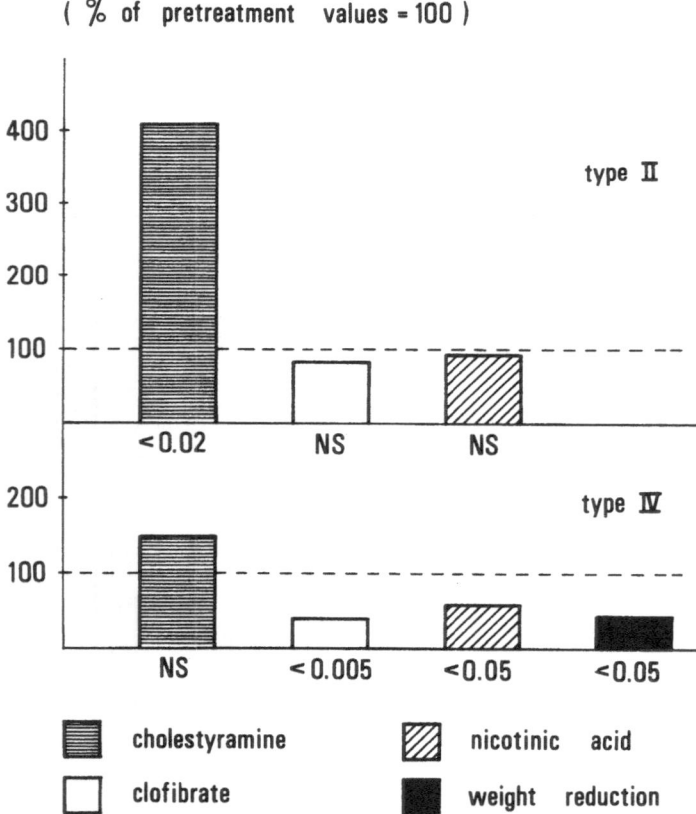

Figure 2. Bile acid formation during therapy (% of pretreatment values = 100) in patients with hyperlipoproteinemia type II and type IV

Bile acid kinetics were also studied in patients treated with clofibrate and nicotinic acid. The response to therapy was almost identical with both drugs (Fig. 2). Whereas no significant effects were observed in HLP type II, the total BA formation in type IV decreased by about 50%. A similar reduction in BA formation was also observed in five type IV patients who had lost 5-10 kg in body weight.

Discussion

A major part of the plasma VLDL is produced in the liver. As apoprotein and cholesterol originally located in VLDL can be recovered in LDL, it appears to be a precursor-product relationship between these two types of particles (Sodhi, 1975; Eisenberg and Levy, 1975; Felts and Rudel, 1975). Hepatic cholesterol used in the formation of both VLDL and BA is synthesized locally and in addition obtained by degradation of LPs. Several lines of evidence indicate a lack of total equilibrium between the "synthetic" and "degradation" pools of cholesterol in the liver (Sodhi, 1975). Experiments in rats (Mitropoulus et al., 1974) also suggest that newly synthesized cholesterol is transformed to a proportionally higher extent into C than into CD. However, whether this observation has any bearing on human subjects is not known.

With the possible exception of homozygous FH (not studied in the current investigation), the type IIa LP pattern is in general associated with a subnormal formation of C and a reduced FCR (fractional catabolic rate) of LDL (Langer et al., 1975; Sigurdsson et al., 1976). Upon treatment with cholestyramine, the formation of BA shows a significant increase and the C/CD ratio of BA synthesized turns to normal. These changes are mostly associated with a drop in the plasma LDL level, an effect possibly due to acceleration of the LDL FCR (Levy and Langer, 1973). Simultaneously with the decrease of the plasma LDL concentration, there is a reciprocal elevation of the plasma VLDL level. Recent findings in our laboratory (Angelin, B., Einarsson, K., Hellström, K., Leijd, B., unpublished observations) indicate that this phenomenon is related to an elevated formation of plasma Tg (VLDL). The combined evidence from these studies with cholestyramine strongly indicate that the metabolism of VLDL, LDL, and BA is integrated.

Further support for a close interrelationship between the turnover of LPs and BA was gained in the studies with the patients suffering from HLP type IV. Under basal conditions, many of them have an elevated formation of BA (and an increased C/CD ratio), Tg, and VLDL. Hellström and Einarsson, 1976). During treatment with clofibrate and nicotinic acid the BA formation decreases by about 50%. Similar results were also observed upon weight reduction. As these regimens primarily may act by inhibition of the FFA turnover and the formation of Tg and VLDL, it appears that the reduced formation of BA reflects corresponding changes in the turnover of LPs.

CHOLESTEROL TURNOVER AND METABOLISM IN NORMAL AND HYPERLIPIDEMIC HUMANS

DeWitt S. Goodman, Frank R. Smith, Robert P. Noble, and Ralph B. Dell

The turnover of plasma cholesterol has been studied extensively in recent years to provide information about the metabolism of cholesterol in normal subjects and in patients with hyperlipidemia and with obesity. In 1968, we reported (Goodman and Noble, 1968) that the plasma cholesterol specific radioactivity time curves obtained in experiments of about 10 weeks duration could be resolved into two exponential functions and, hence, that the turnover of plasma cholesterol conformed to a simple two-pool model. This model has been used extensively in many laboratories to study cholesterol turnover. In 1970, Samuel and Perl reported that in some patients the slow slope of the plasma decay curve deviated from monoexponential behavior after approximately 20-25 weeks. This suggested that a multicompartmental model of more than two pools was necessary to describe the long-term turnover of plasma cholesterol in man. The turnover of plasma cholesterol was subsequently studied by us for periods of 32-41 weeks in six subjects, and, in each subject, the best description of the turnover curve was found to be provided by a three-pool rather than a two-pool model (Goodman et al., 1973).

Long-term studies of the turnover of plasma cholesterol were then carried out in 24 subjects (Smith et al., 1976). Eight subjects were normolipidemic, six had hypercholesterolemia alone, eight had hypercholesterolemia and hypertriglyceridemia, and two had hypertriglyceridemia alone. Ten of the hyperlipidemic patients had a definite familial lipid disorder. In all subjects in this heterogeneous study population (except one for whom complete data were not available), the same three-pool model (Fig. 1) gave the best fit for the data. The parameters of the three-pool model found in normal subjects were compared with the model parameters found in the patients with the different kinds of hyperlipidemia. In addition, single and multiple regression analyses were conducted to explore the relationships between the model parameters and various physiologic variables, including age, body size, and serum lipid concentrations.

Significant differences between groups or correlations with serum lipid levels were seen for several parameters of the three-pool model (Smith et al., 1976). The production rate (PR) in normal subjects was not significantly different from that found in patients with hypercholesterolemia, with or without hyperglyceridemia. The major determinant of cholesterol PR was overall body size, expressed either as total body weight or as surface area. The correlations between PR and indices of adiposity (percent ideal weight and excess weight), although statistically significant, were much weaker in this nonobese population (Fig. 2). Cholesterol PR, after adjustment for body size variation, was not correlated with the serum cholesterol concentration but was weakly ($p<0.05$) correlated with the triglyceride concentration. When the two patients with very high triglyceride concentrations were excluded, however, no correlation between adjusted PR and triglyceride level was observed. We believe that hypertriglyceridemic patients represent a heterogeneous population in which a large proportion do not show increased cholesterol PR. Methods for identifying different subsets of patients within this heterogeneous population remain to be developed.

The size of the rapidly exchangeable pool 1 (M_1) was correlated with all body size variables but most strongly with excess weight. After adjusting for the effects of body size, M_1 was also correlated with the serum concentrations of both cholesterol and triglyceride. Major differences were found with regard to pools 2 and 3. The size of pool 2 (M_2), the pool which consists of cholesterol which equilibrates at an intermediate rate with plasma cholesterol, was correlated neither with any of the indices of body size or adiposity, nor with the levels of either serum cholesterol or triglyceride. In contrast, all estimates of M_3, the size of the most slowly turning over pool 3, were significantly correlated with indices of adiposity (both percent of ideal weight and excess weight),

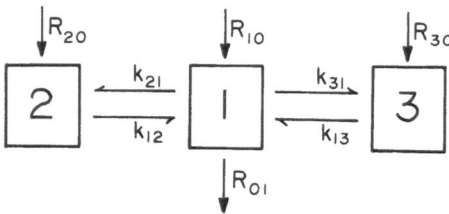

Figure 1. Three-pool model of cholesterol turnover in man (see Goodman et al., 1973 and Smith et al., 1976 for definition and discussion of symbols)

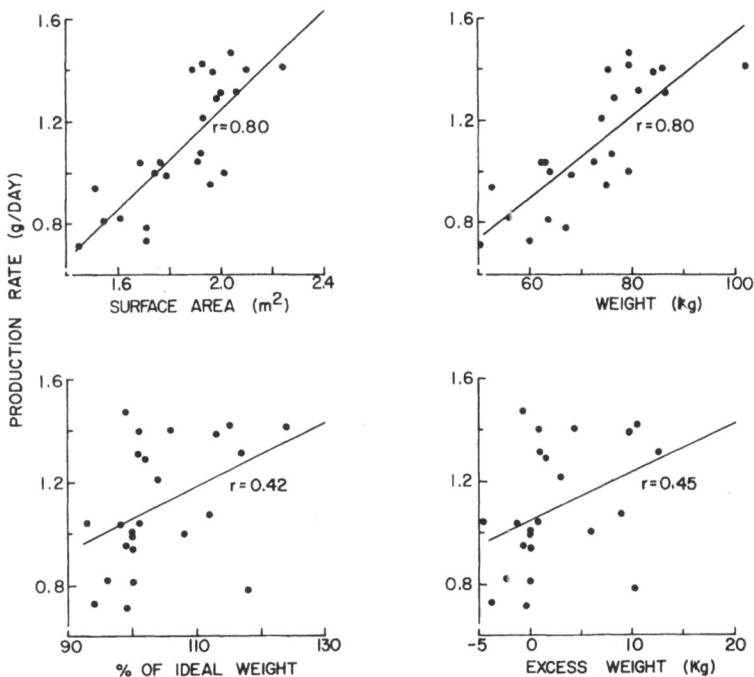

Figure 2. Correlations between cholesterol production rate and indices of body size. Surface area and total body weight were used as indices of overall body size; percent of ideal weight and excess weight represent indices of adipositas

but not of overall body size, and with the serum cholesterol concentration. The positive correlation between M_3 and adiposity is consistent with the finding that adipose tissue cholesterol appears to be an important part of pool 3. Schreibman and Dell (1975) have reported recently turnover studies of both plasma and adipocyte cholesterol, of 10-20 weeks duration, that were carried out in six subjects. For each subject, a three-pool model was fit simultaneously to both plasma and adipocyte specific activity time curves. In five of the six subjects, the kinetics of adipocyte cholesterol closely fit that of the slowly turning over pool 3, indicating that adipose tissue cholesterol comprises an important part of this compartment. The results also indicated that adipose tissue cholesterol synthesis contributes very little, if at all, to the enhanced cholesterol synthesis of obesity.

The observed correlation between the size of pool 3 (M_3) and the serum cholesterol concentration (Fig. 3) suggests that the kinetic analysis used can provide a method for estimating the size of patholigic accumulations of cholesterol in slowly equilibrating tissue sites. If this is true, it may be possible to study the effects of therapy (e.g., lipid lowering drugs) on the amount of cholesterol in tissue pools by repeating long-term studies of cholesterol turnover after a period of therapy in specific patients. Studies directed towards this question are in progress in our research clinic.

In the completed studies described above, the long-term turnover of plasma cholesterol was determined by injecting labeled cholesterol intravenously and then sampling plasma at 34-40 different times during an approximately 35-40 week period. This technique is inconvenient for both patient and investigator and does not guarantee sampling times that allow the most accurate parameter estimates of the three-pool model. Accordingly, studies are in progress to try to assess the optimal sampling times and the minimal sampling frequency needed to estimate the parameters of the three-pool model. We have deceloped a procedure that uses our

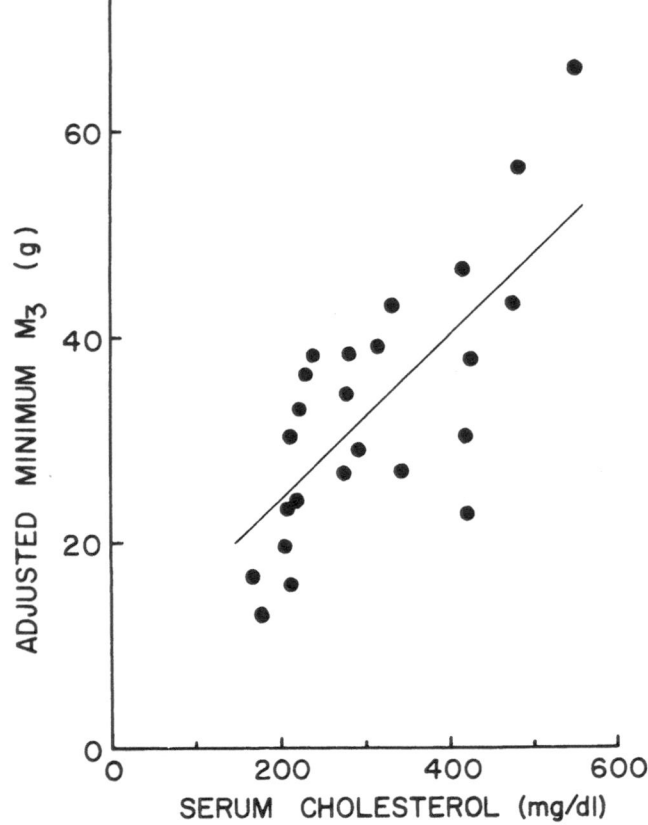

Figure 3. Relationship between minimum M_3, adjusted for effects of excess weight, and the concentration of serum cholesterol (r = 0.70). (Reprinted from Smith et al., 1976 with permission from the publishers)

accumulated information on long-term turnover to predict sampling times that minimize the sum of squared coefficients of variation of the parameter estimates. The best theoretical strategy for a total of 36 samples is to sample at six times, collecting six samples at each time (Dell et al., 1974). A pilot study has been carried out using this "optimal" strategy, as well as the usual sampling strategy, in five normal subjects. The first three sampling times were chosen from prior information and were the same for all subjects. In each subject, prior information was combined with the data at the first three times to choose the fourth time; the fifth and sixth times were chosen similarly. The model parameter estimates given by this procedure were not significantly different from estimates for the same individual given by the usual sampling strategy. However, the residual error of the data at the six times about their best fit was smaller than that of the data at the 36 times. The interpretation of these findings is not entirely clear, since the apparent increase in precision may reflect mainly the existence of significant day-to-day biological variation. Further studies with normal subjects and with patients with hyperlipidemia are in progress in order to try to evaluate more fully the potential usefulness of the proposed simplified sampling strategy.

DIFFERENCES IN THE HEPATIC METABOLISM BETWEEN THE ENDOGENOUS AND PARTICULATE CHOLESTEROL INJECTED IV IN ALCOHOLIC SALINE

Harbhajan S. Sodhi, Bhalchandra J. Kudchodkar, Antone F. Salel, and Dean T. Mason
Cardiovascular Medicine, UC Davis, CA/USA

In view of its use in determining the synthesis and absorption of cholesterol, we compared the hepatic metabolism of particulate cholesterol (PC) with that of endogenous (hepatic) cholesterol (EHC) in dogs given simultaneous injections into the portal vein of C^{14}-mevalonate and H^3-cholesterol suspended in alcoholic saline. In addition to the differences shown in the Fig. the following were seen. All of the PC was excreted in bile as bile acids (BA), whereas only 20% of the EHC was excreted as BA at 15 min. However, its excretion as BA also increased to 80% by 90 min. Esterification of PC in the liver was much less and in plasma was much greater than the esterification of EHC. The total biliary excretion of EHC was significantly less than that of PC during the first 180 min, however, the quantitative significance of such differences will have to be evaluated for each type of the determinations in which PC is used.

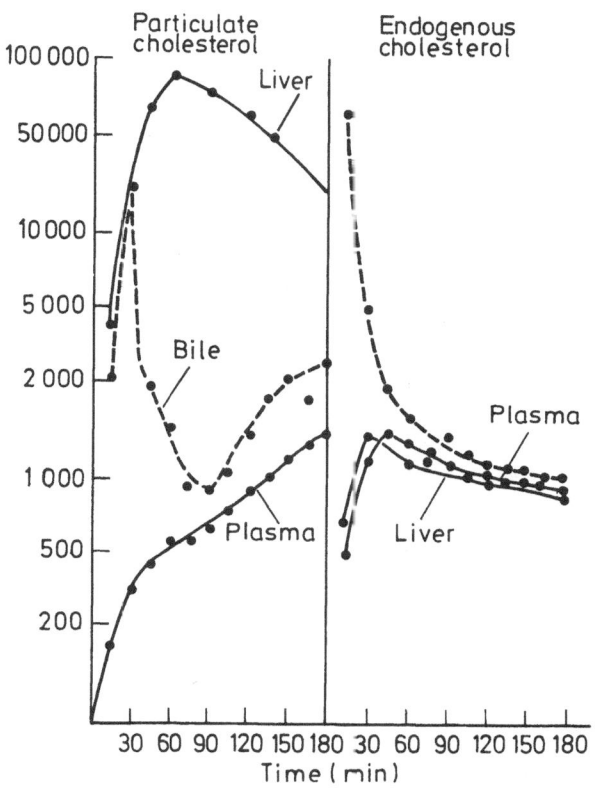

A NEW METHOD FOR DETERMINATION OF LECITHIN CHOLESTEROL ACYLTRANSFERASE (LCAT)

U. Klör, H. Jäger, A. Popp, and H. Ditschuneit
Division of Metabolism, Department of Medicine, University of Ulm, Ulm/BRD

Despite its importance for lipid metabolism studies the measurement of plasma LCAT activity has not yet found widespread application because of the complexity of the assay methods currently used. Therefore, a simple assay method was developed using the decrement of plasma free cholesterol (FC) as parameter for the enzyme activity. Plasma FC levels were measured in 20 min intervals up to 1 h during incubation at 37^oC by a new enzymatic method (Boehringer, Mannheim). The precision of the FC determination was better than 0.8%. The day to day variation of the LCAT assay itself was less than 7% over several months. Plasma pH and incubation temperature were found to be critical for reproducibility. On comparison of the present method with that of Stokke and Norum (1971) and with that using gas chromatographic determination of FC good agreement was observed. LCAT values expressed as %FC esterified per ml plasma/h were 5.9±1.1 and 4.8±1.5 in

50 normal males and females of different age, respectively. In terms of nmoles FC esterified per ml/h the respective figures were 82±15 and 68±19. Both kinds of data correspond well with those established for normals by the method of Stokke and Norum.

LECITIN:CHOLESTEROL ACYL TRANSFER (LCAT) RATE IN SUBJECTS WITH NORMAL AND ELEVATED LIPOPROTEIN CONCENTRATIONS

Lars Wallentin
Institution of Internal Medicine and Clinical Research Centre, Linköping University, Medical School, Linköping/Sweden

Lecithin:cholesterol acyltransferase takes part in the catabolism of lipoproteins in plasma. Therefore LCAT rate, mainly according to Stokke-Norum, and lipoprotein concentrations were measured in plasma from subjects with normal and elevated lipid concentrations.
In the normolipidemic group LCAT rate was skewly distributed with mean 93 (60-145, n=80) μmol/1/h. LCAT rate correlated positively with VLDL and LDL but not with HDL concentration. By multiple regression log LCAT rate could be predicted (r=0.80) from log triglyceride and unesterified cholesterol concentration. In all types of hyperlipoproteinemia mean LCAT rate was elevated – IIa 121 (80-175, n=36), IIb 151 (118-192, n=5), III 176 (129-214, n=4), IV 181 (113-270, n=42) and V 286 (212-340, n=3) μmol/1/h. In type IV individual LCAT rate could be predicted according to the regression equation of the normolipidemic group while half of the individuals with type IIa had lower LCAT rate than predicted.
Conclusion: Rate of LCAT in plasma reflected individual rate of cholesterol turnover. In almost all subjects with type IV there was an increased cholesterol turnover and production rate. In half of the subjects with type IIa there was a decrease of relative elimination rate of cholesterol while production rate was normal or high.

ACTIVATION OF PLASMA LECITHIN:CHOLESTEROL ACYLTRANSFERASE DURING ALIMENTARY LIPEMIA

Herbert G. Rose and Joseph Juliano
Department of Medicine, VA Hospital, Bronx, NY/USA

Removal of chylomicron and very-low-density lipoprotein (VLDL) unesterified cholesterol (UC) and lecithin (PC) during lipolysis has been suggested as the physiologic role of plasma acyltransferase (LCAT). To test this hypothesis LCAT has been measured in 8 normal subjects while postabsorptive and following ingestion of a high-fat test meal. Activity was assayed by determination of reduction of UC concentration during a 3 hour incubation. Plasma triglycerides, chylomicrons, and VLDL increased at 2.5 hours, peaked at 5 hours, were receding at 7.5 hours and normalized at 10 hours. In contrast, LCAT did not elevate until 5 hours, reaching a broad plateau which was maintained up to 10 hours. The mean maximal individual increase was 37.2±13.3 (SD)%. Enzyme activity correlated best with changes in high-density lipoprotein (HDL) composition. HDL-2 protein, free and ester cholesterol (EC) and PC were elevated at 5-10 hours, while HDL-3 PC and UC increased at 7.5-10 hours. Very-high-density lipoproteins showed reductions in all components. EC/UC ratios fell in all lipoproteins. Kinetic studies during lipemia indicated changes in primary substrate pool sizes. Conclusions: 1) Dietary fat provokes an elevation of plasma LCAT which is temporally related to the clearance phase. 2) HDL show associated compositional changes in substrate and product lipids, perhaps reflecting appearance of lipolytic remnants, which suggest enhanced susceptibility to enzymic transacylation.

INCREASED LECITHIN:CHOLESTEROL ACYL TRANSFER (LCAT) RATE DURING AN EXCESS OF LECITHIN IN PLASMA IN VIVO AND IN VITRO

Lars Wallentin
Institution of Internal Medicine and Clinical Research Centre, Linköping University, Medical School, Linköping/Sweden

Lecithin:cholesterol acyltransferase takes part in the catabolism of triglyceride (TG) rich lipoproteins in plasma but little is known about changes of LCAT rate during lipid metabolism in normal subjects. Therefore LCAT rate was measured, mainly according to Stokke-Norum, in plasma from healthy subjects before and after addition of fat solutions in vivo and in vitro.
After fat ingestion there was an increase of LCAT rate simultaneous with an increase of phospholipid (PL) but not simultaneous with the increase of TG concentration in plasma. When TG concentration was normal after 8 hours LCAT rate and PL concentration were still raised. In vitro addition of isolated chylomicrons to plasma did not change LCAT rate. In vitro addition of either a PL stabilized TG emulsion or a PL emulsion caused an increase of LCAT rate. After intravenous infusion of the PL emulsion in healthy subjects there was also an increase of LCAT rate. The same increase of PL concentration in plasma caused about 3 times greater increase of LCAT rate in vivo than in vitro.
The increase of LCAT rate after fat ingestion might be explained by a temporary excess of lecithin in plasma lipoproteins after hydrolysis of TG. Elimination of an excess lecithin (and cholesterol) by LCAT might be necessary for catabolism of TG rich lipoproteins.

PHOSPHATIDYLCHOLINE SUBSTRATE SPECIFICITY OF LECITHIN-CHOLESTEROL-ACTYLTRANSFERASE

Gerd Assmann, Gerd Schmitz, Dac Lekim, and Kurt Oette
Universitätskliniken Köln, Klinische Chemie, Köln/BRD

LCAT was purified appr. 5000 fold from lipoprotein-free plasma, using a combination of ultracentrifugation, hydroxylapatite- and dextran blue 2000 sepharose 4B affinity chromatography. As demonstrated by immunodiffusion and radioimmunoassay, the final preparation was free of apoprotein A-I. Five different phosphatidylcholine (PC) preparations, chemically synthesized with stearic- or linoleic acid in α-position and ^3H or ^{14}C labeled oleic, linoleic or linolenic acid in β-position have been employed to obtain defined PC-cholesterol single bilayer vesicles as substrates. In addition, the use of double labeled PC-cholesterol bilayer vesicles establishes whether or not these substrates are utilized on an equimolar basis in the transesterification reaction. This was found to be dependent upon the purity of the enzyme preparation. The rate of transacylation varied with the heterogeneous acyl donors in α- and β-position, with 1-stearoyl-2-oleoyl-PC and 1,2 linoloyl-PC being the most effective substrates. Both activation and inhibition of transesterification by apoprotein A-I could be observed, depending on the different PC acyl donors used. It is concluded that transesterification may depend on the segmental mobility of unsaturated fatty acids and hydrophobic interaction between PC and the LCAT enzyme.

THE EFFECT OF PHOSPHOLIPID COMPOSITION OF HIGH DENSITY LIPOPROTEINS (HDL) ON LECITHIN:CHOLESTEROL ACTYLTRANSFERASE (LCAT) REACTION

Shinji Yokoyama, Yasuo Akanuma, and Naomi Hojo
Institute for Adult Diseases, Asahi Life Foundation, Tokyo/Japan

The reaction of partially-purified LCAT with heat-inactivated human plasma was accelerated by the addition of dipalmitoyl lecithin (DPL), but not by that of

dilinoleoyl lecithin (DLL) in vitro. Both of these lecithins were incorporated
into HDL coupled to Sepharose from respective sonicated dispersion, but the incorporation of the former was more prominent than that of the latter. More enzymes were bound to HDL-Sepharose complexes which had been pretreated with DPL
than to those untreated or pretreated with DLL. The enzyme activity which was
bound to HDL-Sepharose increased in parallel with the amount of DPL incorporated
into HDL-Sepharose; however, the bound enzyme activity did not increase with the
amount of incorporated DLL. Both of these lecithins were demonstrated to be substrate of LCAT reaction in HDL-Sepharose. The relative reactivity of the enzyme
was higher in DPL than in DLL. It may be indicated that the amounts and fatty
acid compositions of the lecithin present in HDL affect the LCAT-binding to
HDL, and that the catalytic reaction of the enzyme depends on the amount of the
enzyme bound to HDL.

RELATIONSHIP OF CHOLESTEROL METABOLISM WITH BODY WEIGHT AND PLASMA TRIGLYCERIDES

Harbhajan S. Sodhi, Bhalchandra J. Kudchodkar, Antone F. Salel, and Dean T.
Mason
Cardiovascular Medicine, UC Davis, CA/USA

To elucidate the correlations of cholesterol metabolism (CM) with body weight
(BW) and hypertriglyceridemia further, most published data on cholesterol balance studies ($\approx$150) were pooled and analyzed with the help of computers. Cholesterol Synthesis (CS) showed an excellent correlation (n=132; r=0.65;
p<0.00001) with BW. Similar relationships between BW and cholesterol turnover
(r=0.7); endogenous cholesterol secreted into GI tract (r=0.62), fecal neutral
steroids of endogenous origin (FNS)(r=0.65) and fecal bile acids (FBA)(r=0.57)
were seen. To exclude the influence of BW from the correlations of CM with
plasma triglycerides (PT), the values of CM were expressed "per kg BW". Correlation of CS per kg/BW with PT concentration was highly significant (n=106; r=0.34;
p<0.0004). Similar relationships between PT and total of endogenous fecal steroids (r=0.32; p<0.0006), FNS (r=0.2, p<0.040) and FBA (r=0.44; p<0.00001) when
expressed as kg/BW were seen. As postulated by us earlier it is not the BW or
hypertriglyceridemia per se which influence the CM but in all likelihood it is
the hepatic synthesis and secretion of VLDL in both of these conditions which
mediates their correlations with different parameters of cholesterol metabolism.

PLASMA LECITHIN:CHOLESTEROL ACYLTRANSFERASE (LCAT) ACTIVITIES IN FAMILIAL TYPE II HYPERLIPOPROTEINEMIA

Yasuo Akanuma, Shinji Yokoyama, and Yasuhiko Iwasaki
Brd. Department of Internal Medicine, Tokyo University, Tokyo/Japan

Plasma LCAT activities in familial type II hyperlipoproteinemias were measured
using inactivated ^{3}H-cholesterol-containing plasma. ^{3}H-cholesterol sol was first
incubated with LDL-Sepharose, then labelled LDL-Sepharose was incubated with
heat-inactivated plasma, and the labelled plasma was used as a substrate after
separating from LDL-Sepharose. VLDL and LDL containing no LCAT were removed by
ultracentrifugation at d=1.063. The infranatant contained all the enzyme activities present in original fresh plasma. This fraction (d>1.063) was dialyzed
against Tris-NaCl buffer and the enzyme activity was determined by Glomset and
Wright method.
Free cholesterol (FC) contents of d>1.063 of type II patients were not raised
significantly compared with those of controls. The relative content of FC of
d>1.063 in incubation mixture was only 0.8--2.2%. LCAT activities of normal controls and type IV hyperlipoproteinemias were significantly correlated with their
plasma FC concentrations. LCAT levels of type II were raised significantly com-

pared with those of controls. However, the relative amount of LCAT to plasma FC was smaller than normals or type IV, suggesting lower fractional cholesterol esterification in plasma in type II.

HEMOPERFUSION IN HEPATIC COMA. BEHAVIOUR OF TOTAL CHOLESTEROL (TC), ESTERIFIED CHOLESTEROL (EC), FREE CHOLESTEROL CONCENTRATIONS AND LECITHIN:CHOLESTEROL ACYLTRANSFERASE ACTIVITY

A. Weizel, P. Czygan, and E. Ast
Department of Medicine, University of Heidelberg, Heidelberg/BRD

Previous studies with Amberlite hemoperfusion had shown changes in lipid levels during treatment. The 8 patients in this study had hemoperfusion in hepatic coma with activated charcoal. The mean lipid levels before perfusion were significantly below normal (TC 81.2±57.6, CE 47.1±50.6, FC 34.1±12.8 mg/100 ml). Mean LCAT activity was also low with 12.1 umol/1/h.
Hemoperfusion with charcoal did not alter the concentration of TC, CE, FC or the LCAT activity.

INTERCONVERSION OF LIPOPROTEINS IN TANGIER DISEASE

Gerd Assmann, Gerd Schmitz, Klaus Adler, Herbert Heckers, and Kurt Oette
Universitätskliniken Köln, Klinische Chemie, Köln/BRD

Four cases of Tangier disease have been observed in three kindred. The distribution and quantity of residual A apoproteins have been determined by radioimmunoassay; apo A-I is almost exclusively confined to the D>1.25 region, devoid of most lipid as demonstrated by immunoprecipitation and delipidation, and amounting to <0.5% of apo A-I in normal plasma. Since the absence of normal HDL might severely affect lipoprotein interconversion and lipolysis, VLDL catabolism and LCAT activity have been investigated in vitro. The initial rate of LCAT activity in Tangier plasma as determined by gas chromatography and radioassay were subnormal. Addition of apoprotein A-I or isolated normal human lipoproteins resulted in a concentration dependent increase of the initial rate of esterification. As shown by incubation of Tangier plasma with labeled phosphatidylcholine, the LCAT reaction products cholesteryl ester and lysolecithin were mostly confined to the LDL and the 1.21 ultracentrifugal bottom fraction, respectively. The conversion of I-125 VLDL to LDL was associated with a relative enrichment of C-apoproteins in Tangier LDL, while HDL_T was incapable of integrating C-apoproteins into its structure. The findings suggest that HDL is necessary for regular LCAT activity and normal conversion of triglyceride-rich lipoproteins to LDL. In the absence of HDL, abnormal cholesteryl ester-rich remnants of lipoproteins accumulate which may give rise to intracellular cholesteryl ester storage in these patients.

DISPOSITION OF NEWLY SYNTHESIZED CHOLESTEROL IN THE LIVER OF RAT

Harbhajan S. Sodhi, Bhalchandra J. Kudchodkar, Antone F. Salel, and Dean T. Mason
Cardiovascular Medicine, UC Davis, CA/USA

Hepatic secretion of cholesterol into plasma and into bile (as cholesterol or bile acids) are the two major pathways open for recently synthesized cholesterol in the liver. To determine the relative importance of these pathways anestetized rats with bile duct cannulae were used. After injections of radioactive DL-mevalonate into portal veins, the radioactivity in liver, bile and blood cholesterol was determined at intervals. At 30 minutes the hepatic cholesterol had

14.5±1.7% of the injected dose, which decreased to 11.8±1.7% at 60 minutes. Assuming the total radioactivity lost from the hepatic cholesterol between 30 and 60 minutes as 100, <2.0% was recovered in the bile collected during that interval, suggesting that >98% of the newly synthesized hepatic cholesterol was secreted into the circulation. However, most (82%) of it had already left the circulation for extra hepatic tissues and the increase in circulating radioactive cholesterol between 30-60 minutes was only 16%.

If the bile cholesterol or bile acids are not derived from newly synthesized hepatic cholesterol, these data are in accord with the two pool model suggested by us for hepatic metabolism of cholesterol (Sodhi, H.S. and B.J. Kudchodkar; Lancet 1:513, 1973).

ROLE OF HDL ON LDL CONCENTRATION AFTER CHOLESTEROL ADMINISTRATION IN MAN

T. Yasugi, E. Sasa, T. Kinoshita, M. Harada, S. Kobari, K. Sugita, T. Knno, M. Iijima, M. Hatano, and K. Oshima
Department of Medicine, Nihon University, School of Medicine, Tokyo/Japan

Human male subjects with serum cholesterol level between 120-200 mg% were subdivided into two groups; the 1st group: serum HDL levels were lower than normal level, the 2nd group: HDL level within the normal level. Six eggs daily (chol. content approx. 1.5 g) were administered to the subjects for 7 days. Then, serum levels of HDL, LDL, VLDL, TC, PL and TG were determined before and after the administration. Result & conclusion: In the 1st group in which serum cholesterol level increased approximately 20 mg% by the eggs administration, the LDL level did not change significantly. On the contrary, the HDL level increased significantly. In the 2nd group in which serum cholesterol level increased approximately 30 mg%, the LDL level increased significantly while the HDL level did not increase. Above results suggest that increase of the LDL concentration under high cholesterol diet might be affected by the HDL concentration of the subject. Then, it may be concluded that dietary cholesterol might play the important role to stimulate the production of HDL in the subject with low HDL level and might be included in the cholesterol bearing LDL in the subject with average level of HDL.

SERUM CHOLESTEROL BINDING RESERVE AND REGULATION OF ATHEROGENESIS

S.L. Hsia, Yu-Sheng Chao, and Harold Haines
Department of Dermatology and Biochemistry, University of Miami School of Medicine, Miami, FL/USA

We recently reported that serum cholesterol binding reserve (SCBR)(the amount of exogenous cholesterol which a serum can solubilize in addition to its cholesterol content) is lower among patients with premature myocardial infarction than controls (Lancet 1975 ii 1000). In further studies, we identified two serum lipoprotein subfractions which solubilized exogenous cholesterol: SFV from very low density lipoprotein, and SFH from high density lipoprotein. Preliminary examination of SFV by electron microscope revealed discrete particles approximately 40-60 nm in diameter. After solubilization of cholesterol, the particles appeared larger in size. Extraction of SFV with hexane diminished its cholesterol-solubilizing capability, which could be restored by recombination with lipids removed by hexane. The amount of exogenous cholesterol solubilized by SFV and SFH accounted for more than 80% of the SCBR. These results suggest that SCBR is an indirect measurement of SFV and SFH, which may facilitate the egress of cholesterol from the vessel wall, thus retarding atherogenesis.

COMPLEX FORMATION OF LECITHINE WITH CATECHOLAMINE, WITH SPECIAL REFERENCE TO CONTRACTION OF SMOOTH MUSCLE IN AORTA BY CATHECOLAMINE

Fumio Kuzuya, Noboru Yoshimine, and Kunio Mori
The Third Department of Internal Medicine, Nagova University, School of Medicine, ShowaKu, Nagoya/Japan

Authors reported already that lecithine combined with adrenaline in vitro and plateletes aggregation induced by adrenaline was inhibited when the adrenaline was preincubated with lecithine (Jap. Circ. J. 38:579, 1974). On this paper, authors investigated that noradrenaline or dopamine, also, may combined with lecithine. Authors observed radioactivity of 14-C-noradrenaline or 14-C-dopamine on phospholipid-band with thinlayerchromatography and did not find them on the other band. Furthermore, it was found that the contraction of smooth muscle in aorta from rabbits by addition of noradrenaline in Magunus Tube was inhibited when noradrenaline was preincubated with lecithine for 60 minutes at 37ºC. This inhibitory action of lecithine was dependent on dosis among the catecholamine and lecithine reciprocally. The certain dosis of lecithine was able to inhibit perfectly the contraction of smooth muscle by noradrenaline.

RELATIONSHIP BETWEEN THE METABOLIC PATHWAY OF VLDL ⁀O LDL AND THE MOVEMENT OF FFA ON THE ADIPOSE TISSUE IN RATS

Seiichiro Yamasaki*, Masato Ageta*, Noboru Kimura, Hironori Toshima, Seiki Nanbu, Sumito Kariya, Haruo Mae, Takahiko Kamogawa, and Dairo Arakawa
The Third Department of Internal Medicine and Clinical Laboratory*, Kurume University, School of Medicine, Kurume/Japan

The purpose of this experimental study is to define the relationship between the triglyceride and the free fatty acid on lipoprotein metabolism. The relationship between the movement of very low density lipoprotein-triglyceride (VLDL-TG) and the movement of free fatty acid (FFA) on the adipose tissue were determined in spontaneously hypertensive rats. The rats were divided into two groups according to the load with or without 20% glucose solution. The synthesis and the utilization of VLDL-TG were determined using ^{14}C-palmitic acid and ^{3}H-glycine. Before and after the isolation of the portal vein and the proper hepatic artery in each group, the incorporation of ^{14}C-palmitic acid into VLDL-TG and FFA on the adipose tissue were analysed.

WORKSHOP 9. Hormones, Lipoprotein Lipase and Atherosclerosis

Chairmen: H. Greten, BRD
H. Orimo, Japan

Participants: H. Greten, BRD
J. Augustin, BRD
T. Olivecrona, Sweden
A. Noma, Japan
C. Ehnholm, Finland
J. Brunzell, USA
H. Orimo, Japan

HORMONES, LIPOPROTEIN LIPASE AND ATHEROSCLEROSIS

H. Greten

Almost 35 years ago, it was first observed that the intravenous injection of the mucopolysaccharide heparin in animals with post-prandial lipemic plasma caused the clearing of plasma within a few minutes. During recent years, it became evident that the heparin-releasable intravascular lipolytic activity is of great significance for the catabolism of circulating plasma triglycerides and that post-heparin lipolytic activity (PHLA) is a heterogenous system of lipolytic enzymes. PHLA consists of at least two triglyceride lipases with different molecular properties and different sites of origin, namely hepatic triglyceride lipase (H-TGL) and extra-hepatic triglyceride lipase or lipoprotein lipase (LPL). Both enzymes have recently been purified and characterized. Antibodies against these lipolytic enzymes have been produced which led to specific immunochemical methods for selective measurement of H-TGL and LPL. Other methods based on separation by column chromatography or salt inhibition were also developed. The pathogenesis of primary or secondary lipid hypertriglyceridemias has only partly been elucidated yet. There are results which indicate that increased synthesis of triglyceride-transporting lipoproteins may be responsible for this metabolic rearrangement. On the other hand, there is growing evidence for the possibility that hypertriglyceridemia may also be caused by delayed catabolism of macromolecules in plasma. The clinical relevance of these metabolic diseases in relationship to coronary heart disease, peripheral occlusive atherosclerotic disease, cerebral vascular disease, and gastroenterologic manifestations has been documented in many clinical trials. It is the purpose of this symposium to summarize new information which is now available both on the molecular properties and the clinical relevance of lipoprotein lipase.

MOLECULAR ASPECTS OF HEPATIC TRIGLYCERIDE LIPASE AND LIPOPROTEIN LIPASE FROM HUMAN POST-HEPARIN PLASMA

J. Augustin, H. Freeze, and W.V. Brown

The intravascular catabolism and degradation of triglyceride-rich lipoproteins is correlated with glycerol ester hydrolizing activities, which are assumed to reside on the luminal surface of the capillary endothelial cells. One of these enzymes, lipoprotein lipase (LPL), has been found in several tissue homogenates, including adipose tissue, heart and mammary gland (Korn, 1955) as well as milk (Quigley et al., 1958). LPL is released from its membrane site by high molecular weight polyanions, in particular sulfated polysaccharides (Robinson, 1970). Shortly after intravenous heparin injection the activity is detectable in the plasma compartment. In recent years it has been demonstrated that postheparin lipolytic activities (PHLA) represent at least two major triglyceride hydrolyzing enzymes with a variety of others being present (La Rosa et al., 1972; Ehnholm et al., 1973; Greten et al., 1973). One of these is by kinetic criteria identical to LPL, the second is hepatic in origin and differs from LPL in not requiring a cofactor for full activity. In addition the hepatic triglyceride lipase (HTGL) is resistant to high salt concentrations and protamine in the assay medium (Ehnholm et al., 1973). However, although after heparin injection HTGL is released earlier and in larger quantities into the blood stream than LPL, exhibits greater stability and remains active much longer within the vascular bed. The physiological role of this enzyme is still questionable (Brown et al., 1976), particularly since the liver removes only a small portion of the triglyceride moiety of circulating lipoproteins (Stein et al., 1969). On the other hand it has been shown that triglyceride-rich lipoproteins, especially large chylomicrons, are a preferred substrate for HTGL (Augustin et al., 1976). Thus, the enzyme would be synthesized in the liver cells, transported to the capillary wall, actively secreted or directly attached to the circulating lipoproteins, and hydrolysis would occur mainly in extra hepatic areas. In the postalimentary state HTGL would be present in the whole plasma compartment to provide rapid chylomicron clearance. Finally the small triglyceride-poor remnants could be actively transported into the space of Disse, where the degradation of the particels could be completed.

Although there is strong evidence that the enzymes are located at the surface of endothelial cells, besides their prompt appearance in heparin-containing perfusates, histochemical data have demonstrated that lipolysis of adherent chylomicra may occur at this location (Blanchette-Mackie and Scow, 1971), neither the mode of interaction between lipases and lipoproteins nor their binding to specific receptor sites and their release by heparin is known. Therefore the investigation of the molecular properties of both enzymes may lead to a better understanding of intravascular triglyceride metabolism. Heparin-Sepharose affinity chromatography has been widely used for the isolation of LPL from adipose tissue (Bensadoun et al., 1974) and milk (Egelrud and Olivecrona, 1972). HTGL and LPL from human postheparin plasma were also shown to bind to this material (Boberg et al., 1974). Besides, several advantages, i.e. no delipidation, rapid chromatography of large quantities on small columns, highly purified activities in one step, this method, using the different affinities of HTGL and LPL for heparin, provides the only possibility so far for separate isolation of both enzymes. Subsequent purification procedures may be varied.

In our laboratory affinity chromatography with Concanavalin A-Sepharose was successfully used to further purify HTGL and LPL. At this stage several preparations were already homogenous by different criteria, some still being slightly contaminated. Therefore a third purification step was introduced for both activities, which are rather unstable under these conditions. Especially LPL possessed an extremely short half-life (Augustin et al., 1976). Although both enzymes were purified more than 32,000-fold with a specific activity exceeding 3000 micromoles FFA release per h/mg enzyme protein (Augustin et al., 1974) this yield may be low compared with the native enzyme, since the preparations represent active and possibly partially or totally inactivated material. Isoelectric focusing was applied as the third step in the purification of HTGL whereas this procedure yielded only small residual LPL activity. Therefore the latter enzyme was subjected to a second heparin-Sepharose column with sufficient recovery.

Postheparin plasma was obtained 15 min after intravenous injection of 60 units per kg bodyweight sodium heparin from healthy young males and females. There is no considerable increase in activity after the injection of larger heparin doses. Total recovery after all purification steps varied for both enzymes between 15% and 20%. Since the amount of protein was in the range of 1.5 mg/l plasma for HTGL and 0.5 mg/l for LPL, totally releasable enzyme protein does not exceed 20 and 7 mg respectively in a 70-kg volunteer. Tissues like heart and liver contain several times as much LPL and HTGL in intracellular, i.e., nonreleasable compartments (Anrinsen et al., 1952; Assmann et al., 1973).

The purification scheme yields highly purified enzymes which, in contrast to other procedures (Fielding et al., 1974) does not change the properties of the activities; they still bind to matrix-supported heparin, they are not activated by heparin being present in the assay medium; LPL is inhibited by protamine and 1 molar NaCl.

The amino acid composition of both 9 glycoproteins is close to being identical and reveals no uncommon distributions. All amino acids were present and there was a slight preponderance of acidic residues. Since the polarity index was 50% for both enzymes, a nonrandom spatial distribution at the active site has to be postulated. This would guarantee polar and apolar regions, allowing the enzymes to act at hydrophobic-hydrophilic interfaces. Hydrophilic areas are also provided by the large carbohydrate moiety, totalling about 13% for LPL and 16.5% for HTGL (Augostin et al., 1975).

Molecular weight determinations by gel filtration and SDS polyacrylamide gel electrophoresis are comparable with values obtained for LPL from other species. Apparently LPL does not form dimers in a native state in plasma, whereas disaggregation of HTGL occurs only after prolonged exposure to the salt (Ehnholm et al., 1974). Gelfiltration experiments had to be performed in high salt and high sugar concentrations to prevent the enzymes from binding to the gel and because of stability problems. Under these conditions, aggregation and dimerization may be prevented, but under physiological conditions dimerization of human plasma LPL obviously was not present. DTT reduction as well as performic acid oxydation of the enzyme proteins reveals preparations with the original molecular weight, the existence of smaller subunits being rather unlikely. Both enzymes seem to exist in a rather simple peptide chain, only one amino- and one carboxy -terminal amino acid could be detected. Other terminal residues however may be blocked by sugar chains. After tryptic digestion for 24 h usually 26 to 28 peptides were developed. These peptides were identical for both enzymes in size, migration, and staining intensity.

Where as some of these peptides migrated a considerable distance during electrophoresis, others did not move at all. Some of these seem to consist mainly of apolar amino acids and may be part of the active site of the activities.

Since none of the analytical methods mentioned resulted in a difference between the two enzymes, it has to be concluded that the protein moiety of HTGL and LPL with a molecular weight of about 58,000 D is almost if not completely identical. Only sequencing of the peptides would finally prove this, but adequate methods are not available for these small amounts of enzyme protein. Antibodies could be developed against both enzymes with selective precipitation and inhibition. Most recently, sufficient assays with enzyme antibody precipitation of one of the lipases were introduced for enzyme quantification (Greten et al., 1976; Huttunen et al., 1975). Other antibodies cross reacted and precipitated both activities, which would be expected for identical peptide chains. The selective reaction may be due to the carbohydrate moiety of both enzymes, which differs considerably between HTGL and LPL. Circulating glycoproteins in the plasma compartment usually contain fucose in large quantities, the importance of this finding being still unclear. In the HTGL and LPL glycoproteins no fucose could be detected. This finding indicates that the membrane is the site where the action of postheparin plasma lipases takes place. In recent years it has often been postulated that a physiologically occurring mucopolysaccharide may release the enzymes from their binding sites at the capillary wall into the circulation. This would explain secondary hyperlipoproteinemias in some cases of lupus erythematodes with elevated antiheparin γ-globulin titers (Glueck et al., 1969). In postalimentary hyperlipemia the secretion of such a compound would lead to a subsequent increase in intravascular lipase activity, thus, the membrane-bound enzymes would be converted to circulating glycoproteins. This hypothesis might help to explain the rather uncommon carbohydrate pattern found for HTGL and LPL.

Our results as well as others (Fielding et al., 1974; Iverius and Ostlund Lund-quist, 1976) demonstrate that the enzymes in their final state of purification consist of a considerable amount of carbohydrates but it is unlikely that any heparin is bound as a prosthetic group although the activities bind to immobilized heparin in vitro. This binding could be due to electrostatic interactions, high sodium chloride concentrations result in complete release of the enzymes but do also change the confirmational state of both glycoproteins (Ehnholm et al., 1974) which might inhibit association of lipases and heparin. This type of release is probably unimportant under physiological conditions.

Besides heparin the enzymes bind to several other polysaccharides (Olivecrona et al., 1976) some of them being structural elements of the capillary endothelial wall. They may also be involved in the formation of specific enzyme receptors, allowing the activities to interact with triglyceride-rich lipoproteins at the surface of the cells or intraluminally. The affinity of the enzymes for their substrates is evidently high since even in the presence of heparin in the extraction medium of LPL from acetone ether powders floatation of enzyme substrate complexes can be used for enzyme purification (Ehnholm et al., 1975). Therefore it cannot be excluded that lipoproteins are able to displace the activities from their binding sites. In this case initial degradation of large chylomicrons and VLDL would occur at least in part within the plasma compartment. Properties of enzyme receptors may also vary between different tissues. Rather low affinity for the enzymes would facilitate intravascular enzyme substrate formation high affinity would result in receptor-enzyme-substrate complexes with lipolysis in or on the capillary membrane. The former possibility is more likely for the liver-HTGL-receptors since despite the considerable lipolytic potential of this organ only minor hydrolysis of lipoprotein triglycerides occurs at this site. The latter type of receptors may exist in adipose tissue.

A model of lipase binding to these receptors must explain the ability of heparin to release the enzymes into the plasma compartment.

As already pointed out the formation of the heparin-enzyme complex is unlikely, the glycoproteins do not contain any heparin even if affinity chromatography on heparin-Sepharose which might remove this mucopolysaccharide, is not used in the purification procedure. The activities could be detached from the surface proteoglycane receptors either by induction of the confirmational change of the enzymes or by direct competition between heparin and the enzymes for the binding sites. Both mechanisms clearly have to be further evaluated although heparin does not interfere with the catalytic reaction of purified lipases. These results favor the latter possibility.

In summary, HTGL and LPL consist of similar or even identical polypeptide cores, the differences being found in the carbohydrate moiety. Thus these lipases can be classified as isoenzymes.

THE INTERACTIONS OF LIPOPROTEIN LIPASES WITH COFACTOR PROTEINS LIPID SUBSTRATE, AND CERTAIN SULFATED POLYSACCHARIDES *

Thomas Olivecrona and Gunilla Bengtsson

Lipases hydrolyze glycerol esters at lipid water interphases (Verger and de Haas, 1976). Whereas most other lipases act more efficiently on plain emulsified lipids than on lipoproteins (chylomicra or VLDL), the reverse is true for lipoprotein lipases. This is because these triglyceride-rich lipoproteins have on their sur-

*This work was supported by the Swedish Medical Research Council (13X-00727).

face a cofactor protein which enhances the activity of lipoprotein lipases (Havel et al., 1973). In vivo, lipoprotein lipases act on these lipoproteins at the luminal surface of the capillary endothelium in certain extrahepatic tissues (Scow et al., 1976). It follows that they must have a binding affinity for some component of the endothelial cell surface (Olivecrona et al., 1976a). Thus, in addition to its active site (about which little is known), a lipoprotein lipase presumably has sites at which it can interact with (and bind to) endothelial surface, lipid substrate, and cofactor protein.

The interaction of lipoprotein lipases with cofactor protein is rather specific; thus, most workers find that of the human apolipoproteins only C 2 enhances the activity of lipoprotein lipases (Havel et al., 1973). In contrast, this apolipoprotein does not enhance the activity of other lipases. The effect of cofactor protein is seen mainly with long-chain triglycerides as substrate, whereas short-chain triglycerides (Egelrud and Olivecrona, 1973) and 1-(3)-monoglycerides (Egelrud and Olivecrona, 1973; Fielding, 1970; Twu et al., 1976) are rapidly hydrolyzed also in the absence of cofactor protein, although the same active site on the enzyme is involved (Twu et al., 1976). If the cofactor protein exerts its effect through direct interaction with the enzyme, one might expect a species specificity. Most previous studies had been carried out with human serum as the source of cofactor protein, and we decided to attempt to purify such proteins from a quite different animal. The hen was chosen since its lipoprotein lipase(s) had been previously studied (Korn and Quigley, 1957) and can rather easily be purified (Egelrud, 1973). From egg yolk lipoproteins (which are similar to hen blood VLDL), we have obtained two peptide fractions which markedly enhance lipoprotein lipase activity (Bengtsson, G., Olivecrona, T., unpublished observations). One of these peptides (T1) has a molecular weight of about 9000, the other (T2) of about 5000. Both of them enhance the activity of lipoprotein lipases from several different animals. However, the cofactor proteins from egg yolk gave a markedly higher stimulation of hen (postheparin plasma) lipoprotein lipase than human HDL did, whereas with bovine milk lipoprotein lipase, the reverse was true, i.e., human HDL caused a more marked stimulation than either of the egg yolk cofactor proteins did. Further studies showed that several of the kinetic characteristics of the reaction differed depending on the source of cofactor proteins, as well as the source of the enzyme. One distinguishing property of lipoprotein lipases is that their activity is inhibited by high salt concentrations. This inhibition occurred at different salt concentrations and to different extents depending on the (source of the) cofactor proteins used. Fielding and Fielding (1976) have shown that high salt concentrations abolish the stimulation of rat postheparin plasma lipoprotein lipase activity by rat VLDL proteins. Similar results were obtained in our experiments with human serum and human HDL, but the two cofactor proteins from egg yolk VLDL both caused stimulation of enzyme activity also at high salt concentration. Thus, salt did not abolish the interaction of these cofactor proteins with the enzyme but made it somewhat less productive. At 0.66 M NaCl, human HDL did not enhance the activity of the bovine milk lipoprotein lipase. However, when increasing amounts of HDL were added to a system containing almost optimal amounts of T2 at this salt concentration, a progressive decrease in the enzyme activity occurred. Thus, HDL could compete with T2 also under conditions when HDL alone had no effect on the enzyme activity. These studies strongly suggest that the cofactor proteins enhance the activity through direct interaction with the enzyme. The degree of stimulation depends on the nature of the enzyme and the cofactor ("how well they fit") as well as on environmental factors (e.g., the salt concentration).

Lipoprotein lipases bind to lipid emulsions. This binding does not require cofactor protein and also occurs at high salt concentrations (Fielding and Fielding, 1976). The binding is probably by hydrophobic interaction, as has been elegantly shown for pancreatic phospholipase A2 (Verger and de Haas, 1976; Verger et al., 1973). Addition of detergents (e.g., deoxycholate) detaches the enzyme from the lipid surface to the solution (Fielding, 1970) and inhibits hydrolysis of long-chain triglycerides by the enzyme. In contrast, the activity against monoglycerides is not inhibited by similar concentrations of deoxycholate (Egelrud, 1973), suggesting that the effect of this detergent is on the binding of the enzyme to emulsified lipid, not on the active site of the enzyme. Our work with bovine milk lipoprotein lipase has given additional evidence for detergent binding. Deoxycholate markedly increases the solubility of this enzyme at low salt concentrations and also stabilizes the enzyme activity. On agarose gel electrophoresis at alkaline pH, this enzyme does not move, or moves slowly toward the cathode. However, if deoxycholate is added to the buffer, the enzyme moves rapidly toward the anode. This is best explained by formation of negatively charged, soluble enzyme-deoxycholate complexes. It is likely that the enzyme has a hydrophcbic site at which it can bind to emulsified lipid substrates. This same site may also interact with detergents to form soluble enzyme-detergent complexes.

A third very interesting interaction of lipoprotein lipases is with heparin and some related molecules. The original observation was that intravenous injection of heparin releases the enzyme into the circulating blood. More recent studies have shown that lipoprotein lipases from many different sources bind tightly to heparin-Sepharose. Together with professor Lindahl and his group in Uppsala, we

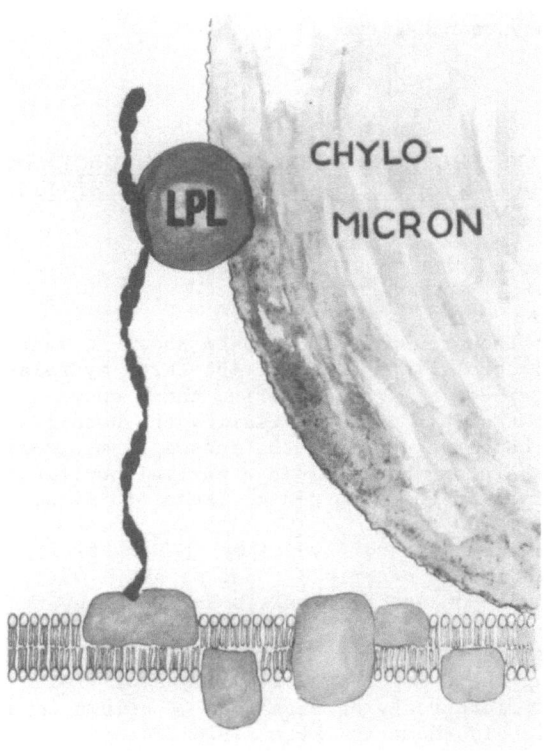

Figure 1. A model for the interaction of lipoprotein lipase with a substrate lipoprotein at the capillary endothelium. A two-dimensional view of the plasma membrane of an endothelial cell. The solid bodies represent integral membrane proteins partly embedded in the lipid matrix. Some of these proteins carry polysaccharide chains which extend out from the membrane. It is suggested that certain periferal membrane proteins, e.g. lipoprotein lipase, are bound to these polysaccharides by electrostatic interaction. A chylomicron has bound to the plasma membrane, and the lipase molecule has moved to the substrate by lateral diffusion in the membrane of the protein moiety of the proteoglycan. Note that the enzyme may be attached to the polysaccharide at a considerable distance out from the membrane, which may facilitate its interaction with the substrate lipoprotein. This interaction is probably hydrophobic. Presumably, several lipase molecules gather around one chylomicron

327

are presently investigating what structural features a polysaccharide must have to interact with lipoprotein lipase (Olivecrona et al., 1976a). One very interesting result of these studies is that heparan sulfate can bind the enzyme. Heparan sulfate is a surface component on endothelial cells (Buonassisi, 1973) and on many other mammalian cells. Thus, both heparan sulfate and lipoprotein lipases are present at the endothelial cell surface and they have a high affinity for each other. On this basis we have suggested (Havel et al., 1973; Olivecrona et al., 1976b) that lipoprotein lipases may be held in place at the capillary endothelium through interaction with heparan sulfate (Fig. 1).

If we had isolated a lipoprotein lipase without knowing of its specialized properties, we would probably have considered it a rather uninteresting enzyme which was fairly active against short-chain triglycerides and against 1-(3)-monoglycerides but had low activity against long-chain triglycerides. However, interaction with cofactor protein enhances the activity several fold against long-chain triglycerides and makes the lipoprotein lipases efficient in their physiologic function – the hydrolysis of triglycerides in plasma lipoproteins; and the ability of these enzymes to bind tightly to heparan sulfate (and some related compounds) may serve to hold them in place at their physiologic site of action – the capillary endothelium.

PURIFIED MONOACYLGLYCEROL HYDROLASE FROM HUMAN POST-HEPARIN PLASMA: CHARACTERISTICS AND ROLE IN THE REACTION CATALYZED BY LIPOPROTEIN LIPASE

Akio Noma

Postheparin plasma has been shown to contain lipoprotein lipase, hepatic triacylglycerol lipase, monoacylglycerol hydrolase, phospholipase, and so on. On the basis of several criteria, these enzymes are considered to be different from one another. In order to clarify the detailed properties of these enzymes, it is necessary to purify the enzyme from others. Along this line, recent work in our laboratory has yielded a partial purification of monoacylglycerol hydrolase from human postheparin plasma (Noma and Kita, 1976).

Monoacylglycerol hydrolase (MGH) activity assays were carried out by the method previously described (Noma et al., 1974), using ^{3}H-glyceryl mono-oleate emulsified in the presence of triton X-100 as substrate.

Partially purified MGH was isolated from the plasma samples by a procedure including the removal of triacylglycerol lipase-substrate complex followed by affinity chromatography on Sepharose 4B column covalently bound heparin, as described previously (Noma and Kita, 1976).

As shown in Table 1 the total activity for MGH of human postheparin plasma is approximately 12 times of triacylglycerol lipase (TGL). Although Nilsson-Ehle and Belfrage (1972) reported no measurable TGL activity in their final infranatant after five treatments with Intralipid, the present results showed that approximately 18% of TGL activity remained in the final infranatant. After affinity chromatography, however, almost no measurable TGL activity was detected in the combined fraction. As described by Greten et al. (1972), MGH activity eluted from the heparin-Sepharose column with that of TGL. Then, it is necessary to separate these two enzyme activities before the application on the column. The present results show that the final specific activity of MGH is more than 5.7 μmol of fatty acids released per mg protein per min, representing a 535-fold purification from postheparin plasma.

Table 1. Purification of monoacylglycerol hydrolase from human postheparin plasma

	Protein (mg)	Monoacylglycerol hydrolase				Triacylglycerol lipase		Ratio MGH/TGL
		Total activity (u)	Specific activity (u/mg)	Purification (fold)	Yield (%)	Total activity (u)	Yield (%)	
Postheparin plasma (9 ml)	646.2	6931.8	10.7	1	100	572.4	100	12.1
Intralipid treatment	636.5	5864.3	9.2	0.9	84.6	107.0	18.7	54.8
Affinity chromatography								
Peak fraction (5 ml)	0.063	361.4	5736.5	535	5.2	a	a	
Combined fraction (15 ml)	0.225	946.8	4208.0	392	13.7	2.9	0.5	326.5

aNot measurable.

The MGH activity was significantly inhibited by bile salts at low concentrations and the inhibition increased progressively with increasing concentration of them.

The effects of sodium chloride and protamine sulfate, effective inhibitors of lipoprotein lipase, on the activity of the purified MGH are illustrated in Figure 1. Control experiments in which sodium chloride or protamine sulfate were added into the assay system showed slight and constant inhibitions in spite of their concentrations. MGH activity was also assayed after preincubation of the enzyme preparation for 30 min at 37° C with various concentrations of sodium chloride and protamine sulfate. Maximal inhibition of the enzyme activity was approximately 70% at 0.3 M NaCl, and the activity rose progressively as the NaCl concentration was increased above 0.5 M. On the other hand, the enzyme activity declined more than 80% as protamine concentration was increased to 200 μg/ml, and did not rise with higher concentrations employed. In view of the present results, similar inhibitions by sodium chloride have been described for hepatic TGL and those by protamine sulfate for extrahepatic TGL. Putting these facts together, it is clear that the pattern of response of MGH to changing concentrations of sodium chloride and protamine sulfate is different for either TGL activities from the two tissues.

The present study was also designed to help elucidate a second problem, i.e., the roles of MGH in the reaction catalyzed by lipoprotein lipase. This preliminary experiment, is however, at present still under investigation.

The effect of serum on the MGH activity is shown in Figure 2. Two types of experiments were undertaken. Preincubations of various amounts of serum with either the enzyme or the substrate were carried out. The enzyme activity assays then followed. In either case, the enzyme activity was inhibited progressively with increasing amounts of serum added. However, in the case of preincubation with enzyme, the inhibitions were slighter than those with substrate.

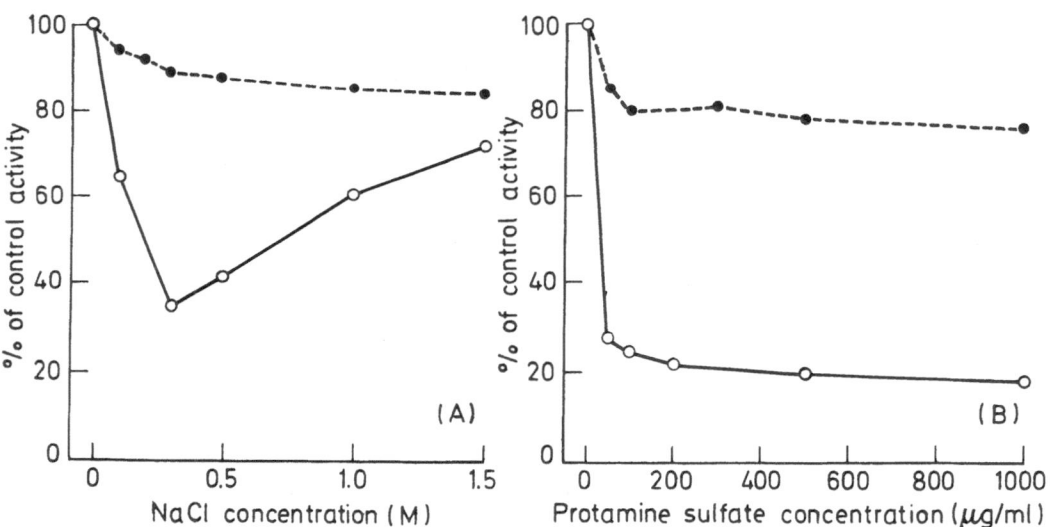

Figure 1. Effects of (A) sodium chloride and (B) protamine sulfate on the activity of the purified monoacylglycerol hydrolase. ●-----●, control experiments in which NaCl or protamine sulfate added to the assay system; o———o, preincubation experiments in which the enzyme was preincubated for 30 min at 37°C with NaCl or protamine sulfate at concentrations indicated on the abscissa. After the preincubation, the inhibitor concentration was adjusted to 0.3 M NaCl or 200 μg/ml protamine sulfate, substrate was added, and incubation was continued for 60 min at 37°C for the assay of enzyme activity

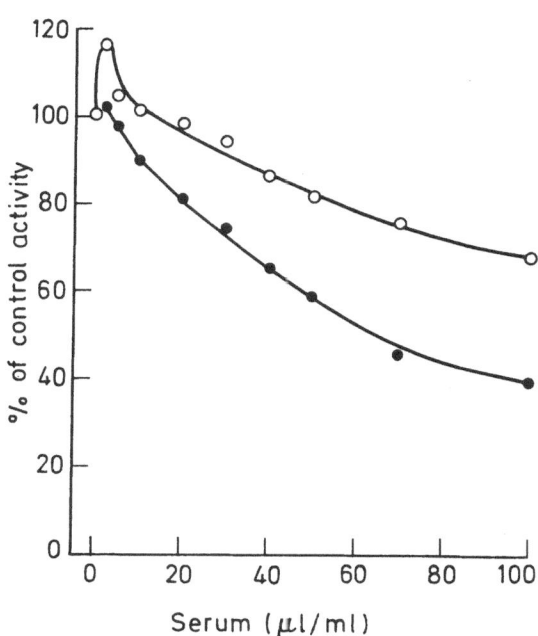

Figure 2. Effects of serum on the activity of the purified monoacylglycerol hydrolase. o———o, serum was preincubated with the enzyme at 37°C for 5 min; ●———●, serum was preincubated with the substrate at 37°C for 5 min

Subsequently, the effects of C-apolipoproteins on the MGH activity were investigated. Since the effects of apoLp-Ser and -Glu are similar to that of apoLp-Ala, Figure 3 shows the effects of apoLp-Ala, preincubated with either the enzyme or the substrate, on the MGH activity. The enzyme activity was activated in the case of preincubation of the apolipoprotein with the enzyme, whereas without effect with the substrate. These results suggest that serum component(s), by which the MGH activity is inhibited, is (are) not C-apolipoproteins. It is at present unknown and further studies are needed. The monoacylglycerol-apolipoprotein complex was as active as monoacylglycerol alone for the substrate of MGH. The possibility of monoacylglycerol forming a complex with apoLp-Ala has been suggested by Brown and Baginsky (1974). The present results also suggest that the MGH-apolipoprotein complex reacts as the activated form of MGH.

Adding 100 µg/ml of apoLp-Ala at 20 min after starting the reaction, the time-course of enzyme activity was entirely without effect. This result leads us to consider that the binding force of apoLp-Ala with monoacylglycerol is stronger than that with MGH. However, since the affinity is related to the amounts of components, further studies are necessary to determine the strength of the binding force of apoLp-Ala with monoacylglycerol or MGH.

In the absence of apoLp-Ala, the MGH activity was slightly inhibited with increasing amounts of triacylglycerol in the assay system. This inhibition, however, became smaller in the presence of the apolipoprotein.

In summary, MGH could also act as one of the blocking agents for the apoLp-Ala inhibition of lipoprotein lipase activity by forming a complex with apoLp-Ala. The monoacylglycerol-apoLp-Ala complex was the active substrate for MGH, and the MGH-apoLp-Ala complex reacted as the activated form of MGH.

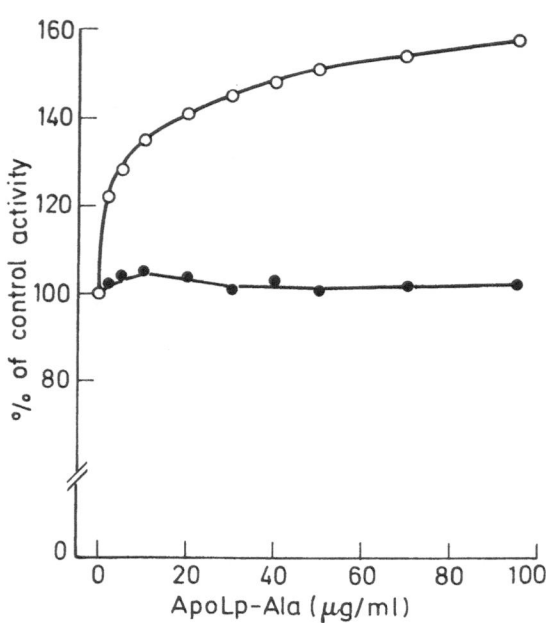

Figure 3. Effects of apoLp-Ala on the activity of the purified monoacylglycerol hydrolase. o————o, apoLp-Ala was preincubated with the enzyme at 37°C for 5 min; •————•, apoLp-Ala was preincubated with the substrate at 37°C for 5 min

MEASUREMENT OF POST-HEPARIN PLASMA LIPOPROTEIN LIPASE AND HEPATIC TRIGLYCERIDE LIPASE ACTIVITIES AND THEIR RELATION TO PLASMA TRIGLYCERIDE METABOLISM

C. Ehnholm, J.K. Huttunen, P.K.J. Kinnunen, and E.A. Nikkilä

Several methods have been used to estimate the removal capacity for serum triglycerides. The fractional removal rate of triglycerides can be measured after intravenous administration of triglyceride emulsions (Rössner, 1974) or after in vivo or in vitro labeling of the protein or lipid moiety of endogenous very low-density lipoproteins (VLDL) (Farguhar et al., 1965). The results obtained by these methods are influenced by the pool size of circulating VLDL and may, therefore, give a more or less erroneous estimate of the removal efficiency. An indirect approach for the characterization of the removal mechanisms involves estimation of the activity of lipoprotein lipase (LPL), an enzyme responsible for the assimilation of lipoprotein triglyceride in peripheral tissues.

Lipoprotein lipase is released into the circulation after intravenous administration of heparin (Korn, 1959). Postheparin plasma contains several lipolytic enzymes which contribute to the total postheparin lipolytic activity (PHLA). Thus, the triglyceride hydrolase activity consists of at least two enzymes, lipoprotein lipase and a second triglyceride lipase, hepatic lipase (HL), originating from the liver (La Rosa et al., 1972; Ehnholm et al., 1974; Hamilton, 1964; Assmann et al., 1973; Greten et al., 1974).

Selective Measurement of Postheparin Plasma LPL and HL

Several methods have been developed for selective measurement of LPL and HL activity in postheparin plasma. The two enzymes can be separated by affinity chromatography on Sepharose containing covalently bound heparin (Ehnholm et al., 1974), and a quantitative assay system using small heparin-Sepharose columns has been described by Boberg and his associates (1975a). This method is reproducible but time-consuming and may result in underestimation of lipoprotein lipase activity, Another assay procedure takes advantage of the fact that under appropriate conditions LPL is inhibited by protamine sulfate, whereas HL is not (Krauss et al., 1974).

We have developed and validated an immunochemical method which is based on the determination of LPL under optimal conditions (0.1 M NaCl, serum addition) after immunoprecipitation of HL (Huttunen et al., 1975a). HL is measured under conditions (1.0 M NaCl, no serum addition) where LPl is totally inhibited. High concentrations of VLDL and LDL do not interfere with the measurement, making the method suitable for studies in patients with different hyperlipidemias. Comparison of the immunochemical procedure with the protamine sulfate inhibition method described by Krauss et el. (1974) suggest that, in general, the two assay systems measure the same enzyme activities (Fig. 1). The slightly higher absolute levels obtained by the immunochemical method may depend on the different substrate preparations used in the two assay procedures.

Postheparin Plasma Lipases and Lipoprotein Metabolism

The results of postheparin LPL measurements in normal subjects strongly support the idea that hydrolysis of VLDL by LPL forms a rate-limiting step in VLDL catabolism (Huttunen et al., 1976a). Thus, a definite negative correlation exists in healthy normolipidemic males and females between plasma triglyceride concentration and the activity of postheparin plasma LPL (Fig. 2). The activity of LPL is higher in females than in males in all age groups studied. These results are in good agreement with the observation that normal females have higher fractional removal rate of endogenous VLDL than males (Nikkilä and Kekki, 1971). A decrease

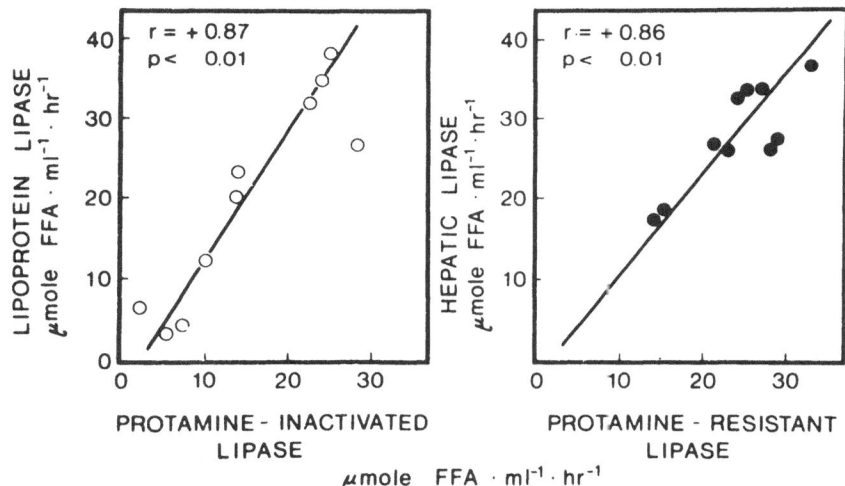

Figure 1. Comparison of the immunochemical assay method (Huttunen et al., 1975a) with the protamine inactivation procedure. Postheparin plasma samples from ten subjects were assayed for hepatic lipase and lipoprotein lipase activity with the immunochemical method and for protamine-resistant and protamine-inactivated lipase activities with the method of Krauss et al. (1974).

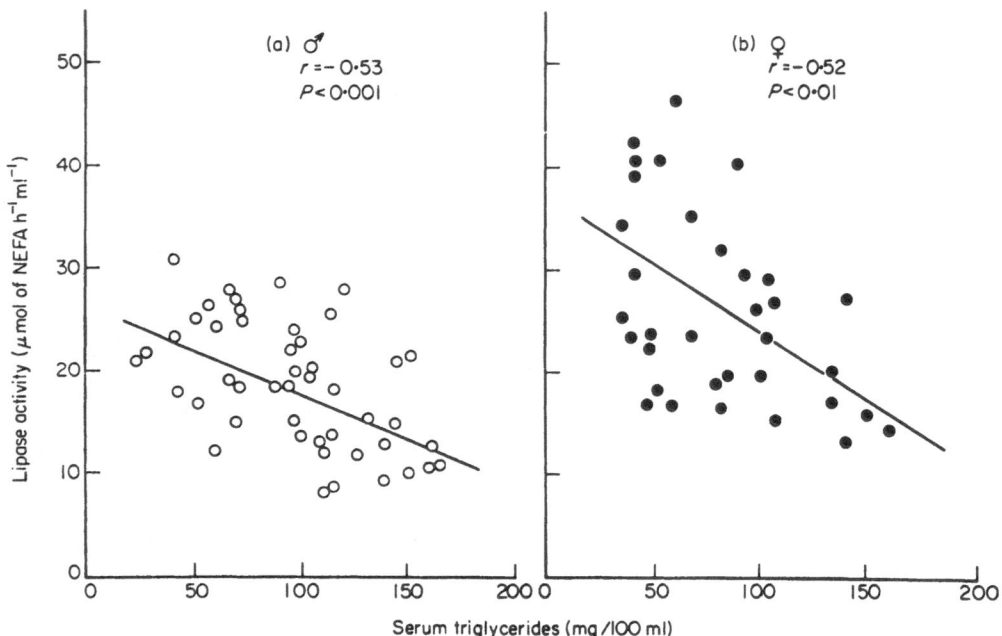

Figure 2. Relationship between the basal concentration of serum triglycerides and the activity of postheparin plasma lipoprotein lipase in healthy males (a) and females (b) (Huttunen et al., 1976a)

in LPL activity with age, consistent with the age-related increase of serum triglyceride level, is observed in both sexes. Finally, a positive correlation is found between the activity of LPL and fractional removal rate of endogenous triglycerides (Huttunen et al., 1976a) and between the activity of LPL and the removal rate of intravenously administered lipid emulsion (Huttunen et al., 1975b), observations which further support the important role of LPL in triglyceride clearance and in determining the plasma triglyceride level in normal subjects.

Low activity of postheparin plasma LPL has consistently been seen in type I hyperlipoproteinemia (Krauss et al., 1974; Greten et al., 1976) and in most subjects with type V abnormality (Krauss et al., 1974; Huttunen et al., 1976a; Greten et al., 1976). In contrast to the results of Krauss et al. (1974), we have found that the average postheparin plasma LPL activity is also subnormal in patients with IIb and IV hyperlipoproteinemia, although only few show a more severe deficiency of the enzyme (Huttunen et al., 1976a). Upon treatment of these patients with clofibrate (Nikkilä et al., 1976a), the activity of postheparin plasma LPL consistently increases (Fig. 3). Similar results have been reported by Boberg et al. (1975b) using a different assay method. However, despite the increase of the enzyme activity to normal range or even above, many of the subjects remained hypertriglyceridemic during the treatment. Thus, the basic abnormality in these patients seems to be increased hepatic production of VLDL resulting in hypertriglyceridemia inspite of adequate removal. If VLDL production is strongly increased, even an improved peripheral removal system (such as during clofibrate treatment) will not compensate for the VLDL secretion.

Measurement of postheparin plasma LPL activity in diabetic hypertriglyceridemia has further emphasized the importance of LPL and VLDL disposal (Nikkilä et al., 1976b). The mean postheparin plasma LPL activity is decreased by almost 50% in patients with untreated ketotic diabetes and by 20% in untreated mild to moderate nonketotic early onset diabetes. Insulin treatment of ketotic diabetes rapidly increased the activity of LPL with concomitant decrease in plasma triglycerides (Fig. 4). In normolipemic patients with adult onset diabetes, the activity of

334

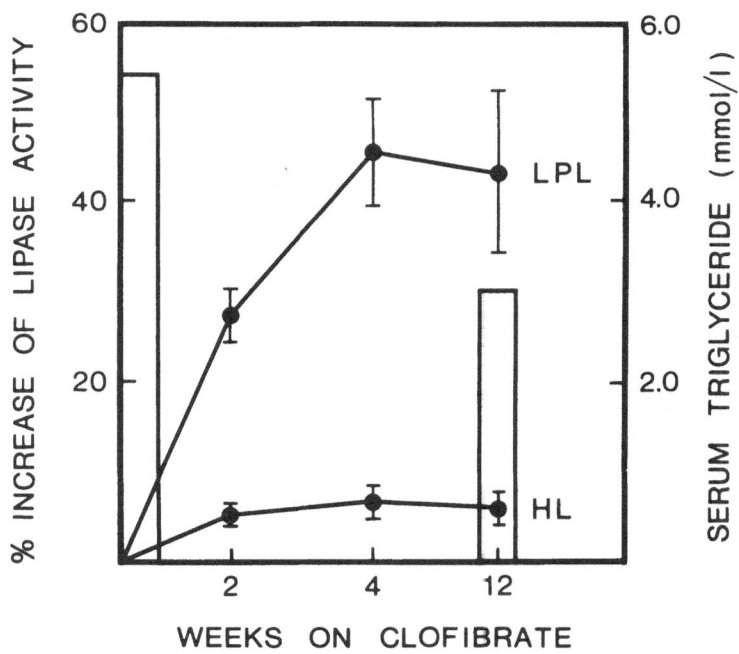

Figure 3. Effect of clofibrate treatment (2 g/day) on fasting serum triglycerides
and on postheparin plasma lipoprotein lipase activity in 17 subjects with primary
hypertriglyceridemia (Nikkilä et al., 1976a)

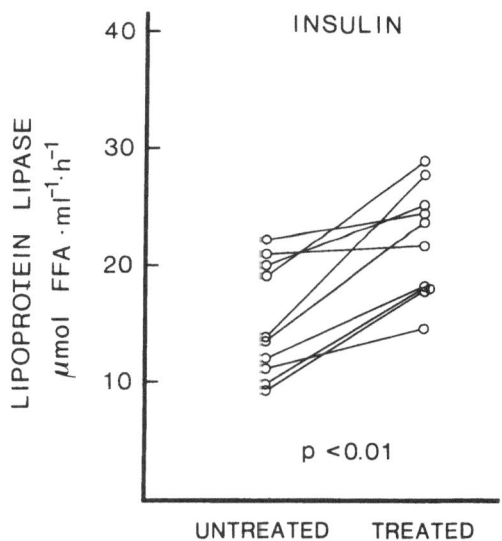

Figure 4. Effect of insulin treatment on the activity of postheparin plasma lipoprotein lipase in ten ketotic insulin-deficient diabetic patients. The patients
were studied during ketosis and after an interval of 10 - 20 days during which
period their diabetes had been brought under control by insulin (Boberg et al.,
1975b)

LPL is normal whereas in those with hypertriglyceridemia a slightly lowered enzyme level is observed.

The role of postheparin plasma HL in lipoprotein metabolism is currently unknown. The enzyme is active toward both phospholipids and triglycerides as shown in in vitro experiments (Ehnholm et al., 1975b) and by the parallel changes of the activities of HL and phospholipase A, in vivo (Ehnholm et al., 1975a). In contrast to postheparin plasma LPL, the activity of HL is higher in males than in females and does not correlate with age (Huttunen et al., 1976a). Furthermore, no relationship was found between the activity of postheparin HL and the level of serum triglycerides in healthy normolipidemic subjects.

The activity of postheparin plasma HL is normal in type I, IIb, III, and V hyperlipoproteinemia (Krauss et al., 1974; Huttunen et al., 1976a; Greten et al., 1976). On the other hand, low activity of HL has frequently been encountered in diseases characterized by high serum cholesterol concentration. Thus, the activity of HL was found to be low in many, although not in all patients with heterozygous familial hypercholesterolemia (Nikkilä et al., 1976c). Low activity has also been reported in hypothyroidism (Krauss et al., 1974), in liver diseases (Bolzano et al., 1975; Sauer et al., 1976), and in chronic uremia (Huttunen et al., 1976b), all conditions associated with secondary hypercholesterolemia. Clofibrate treatment does not influence the activity of HL (Nikkilä et al., 1976a), whereas an increase of the enzyme activity has been consistently observed during administration of oxandrolone, an anabolic steroid used for lowering of serum triglycerides (Ehnholm et al., 1975b).

Conclusions

Selective measurements of postheparin plasma lipoprotein lipase and hepatic lipase in normal subjects and in patients with primary and secondary hyperlipoproteinemias indicate that the activity of postheparin plasma LPL reflects the removal capacity for lipoprotein triglyceride. The results presented strongly suggest that the cause of hypertriglyceridemia in type I hyperlipoproteinemia, in many subjects with type V hyperlipoproteinemia, and in patients with diabetic hypetriglyceridemia is low activity of LPL. The majority of subjects with type IIb and IV hyperlipoproteinemia have normal or slightly lowered LPL activity, suggesting that increased production rather than deficient removal of VLDL is the cause of their hypertriglyceridemia.

The role of postheparin hepatic lipase in lipoprotein metabolism is as yet unknown. Originally purified as a triglyceride lipase, this enzyme also hydrolyzes monoglycerides, phospholipids, and long-chain acyl-CoA-thiol esters. Whether this enzyme in vivo functions as phospholipase or triglyceride hydrolase or both is still an open question.

HORMONAL REGULATION OF HUMAN ADIPOSE TISSUE LIPOPROTEIN LIPASE

John D. Brunzell and Andrew P. Goldberg*

Introduction

The intravenous injection of heparin releases a variety of lipolytic activities into the plasma that are active against a variety of substrates including triglycerides (TG), monoglycerides, and phospholipids (Biale and Shafrir, 1969; Vogel et al., 1971). Lipoprotein lipase (LPL), the rate-limiting enzyme in the removal of TG from plasma lipoproteins (LP) (Robinson, 1963, 1970), is present in many

---

*The authors are indebted to Ms. Julianne Carlen, Ms. Martha Kimura, and Mr. Howard Beiter for their technical assistance.

tissues (Robinson, 1970; La Rosa et al., 1972; Pykälistö et al., 1974); therefore, its activity is estimated indirectly as postheparin lipolytic activity (PHLA) (Robinson, 1970; Korn, 1959). Recent evidence suggests that postheparin triglyceride lipase activity (PHTGLA) is composed of several enzymes including a hepatic triglyceride lipase (TGL) that contributes significantly to PHLA (La Rosa et al., 1972; Krauss et al., 1974; Ehnholm et al., 1974a, 1974). Hepatic TGL can be differentiated from LPL by immunochemical methods (Huttunen et al., 1975) and affinity chromatography on Sepharose (Ehnholm et al., 1974b) and does not require C-apolipoproteins for activation (Ehnholm et al., 1974a). LPL, which is present in many tissues, may also be heterogeneous in requiring different apolipoprotein activators (Ganesan et al., 1975). The importance of either one or several TGLs in the removal of TG from plasma LP in man is suggested by the association of marked hypertriglyceridemia with decreased PHLA (Havel and Gordon, 1960) and low adipose tissue LPL (Harlan et al., 1962) in familial LPL deficiency. However, the exact mode of action and the regulation of these TGLs has not been established.

Evidence suggests that adipose tissue is an important site of action of LPL and a major organ in the removal of TG from plasma LPs (Robinson, 1970; Bezman et al., 1962; Blanchette-Mackie and Scow, 1971). Therefore, the activity of LPL in adipose tissue has been extensively studied in animals, particularly the rat (Robinson, 1970). Several investigators have proposed models of the synthesis, activation, and secretion of LPL in rat adipose tissue (Cryer et al., 1974; Nilsson-Ehle et al., 1976). Nilsson-Ehle et al. (1976) suggest that an enzyme in the adipocyte is activated and secreted as an extracellular enzyme and that this site of activation and secretion is the site of hormonal regulation (Garfinkel et al., 1976). These same investigators have also suggested that the elution of LPL activity from fat cells by heparin is at the site of hormonal regulation (Nilsson-Ehle et al., 1976).

The role of various hormones in the regulation of human adipose tissue LPL has not been studied extensively. Therefore, in this study, the activity of LPL was measured directly in subcutaneous biopsies of buttock adipose tissue in patients under various metabolic conditions and compared to the activity of the enzyme in normal control subjects. Thus, evidence is provided that human adipose tissue LPL is regulated by multiple hormones.

Methods

Patient Selection

The patients selected were normal subjects or those with untreated diabetes, hypothyroidism, or chronic renal failure receiving maintenance hemodialysis. In addition, patients with primary, familial LPL deficiency were studied and compared to patients with primary endogenous hypertriglyceridemia. Patients with other secondary forms of hypertriglyceridemia or broad beta disease and patients receiving drugs known to affect lipid metabolism were excluded.

Chemical Determinations

Adipose tissue LPL was measured as previously described (Pykälistö et al., 1975a, 1976). Briefly, 100 - 200 mg of adipose tissue were obtained by needle aspiration from subcutaneous buttock tissue. One piece of adipose tissue was fixed and frozen for the determination of cell diameter and cell volume by the method of Goldrick (1967). The other piece was incubated in Krebs-Ringer phosphate buffer in the presence of heparin (2 u/ml). This medium releases the "heparin-elutable" enzyme from adipose tissue. The enzyme activity was then incubated with a $1-14C-$ labeled triolein substrate and the LPL activity expressed as the nmol/min of free fatty acid produced by 10^6 fat cells during a 45-min incubation with heparin. One milliunit (mU) of enzymic activity represents the production of one nmol of free fatty acid/ml/min. The fasting activity of adipose tissue LPL was measured in the morning after a 12-hour overnight fast. Postprandial LPL activity was determined 6 hours after high-carbohydrate (85% dextrose, 15% protein) formula feeding at 1, 2, and 5 hours after the initial biopsy. This provided an assessment of the effect of feeding on adipose tissue LPL activity. Preliminary experiments have demonstrated no significant difference between fasting LPL activity and the activity measured 1, 2, or 3 hours postprandially.

Results and Discussion

Fasting adipose tissue LPL activity in normal male subjects was similar to that found in normal, premenopausal female subjects (Table 1). Persson (1973a, 1973b) found similar results, but Nilsson-Ehle (1974) has reported that females have higher levels of LPL than males. The reason for this disagreement is not apparent. When these normal females were studied after 14 days of ethinyl estradiol (1 mg/kg/day), there was no significant change in adipose tissue LPL levels.

In two patients with primary, familial LPL deficiency, the fasting level of adipose tissue LPL was essentially zero. LPL activity in patients with endogenous hypertriglyceridemia was not different from normal males (Table 1). The postprandial activity of adipose tissue LPL was higher than the fasting level both in normal males and in males with primary endogenous hypertriglyceridemia. However, there was an inverse relationship between the fasting level of adipose tissue LPL and the postprandial change both in the normal individuals (r = -0.76) and in the hypertriglyceridemic individuals (r = -0.94). Thus, the lower the fasting level of adipose tissue LPL, the greater the increase with feeding. Those patients with high fasting LPL activity actually had lower postprandial levels of LPL (Fig. 1A). Since there was no difference in the fasting activity of LPL or in the response of LPL to feeding in either the normal or the hypertriglyceridemic subjects, they will be considered together (Fig. 1A, r = -0.90).

Table 1. Adipose tissue LPL

	n [a]	Fasting [b]	n	Postprandial [b]
Normal male	19	3.37 ± 2.58	8	4.70 ± 2.94
Normal female	(12)	3.84 ± 2.39		
Normal female + estrogen	(12)	4.61 ± 4.39		
Primary LPL deficiency	2 (1)	0.04 ± 0.17 [c]		
Endogenous hypertriglyceridemia	15	3.32 ± 3.69	5	4.42 ± 1.89
Untreated diabetes mellitus	8 (1)	0.98 ± 0.47 [c d]	5	1.36 ± 0.67 [c]
Treated diabetes mellitus	5 (1)	3.46 ± 3.01		
Hypothyroid	5	1.54 ± 0.93 [c d]		
Treated hypothyroid	5	3.71 ± 2.26		
Hemodialysis: normal TG	10	3.01 ± 2.49	9	3.96 ± 2.03
Hemodialysis: ↑ TG	15	1.50 ± 0.82 [c d]	9	2.24 ± 1.04 [c d]

[a] Number of females in parentheses.

[b] mU/10^6 cells (mean ± SD).

[c] Significantly lower than normal.

[d] Significantly different from treated or matched group.

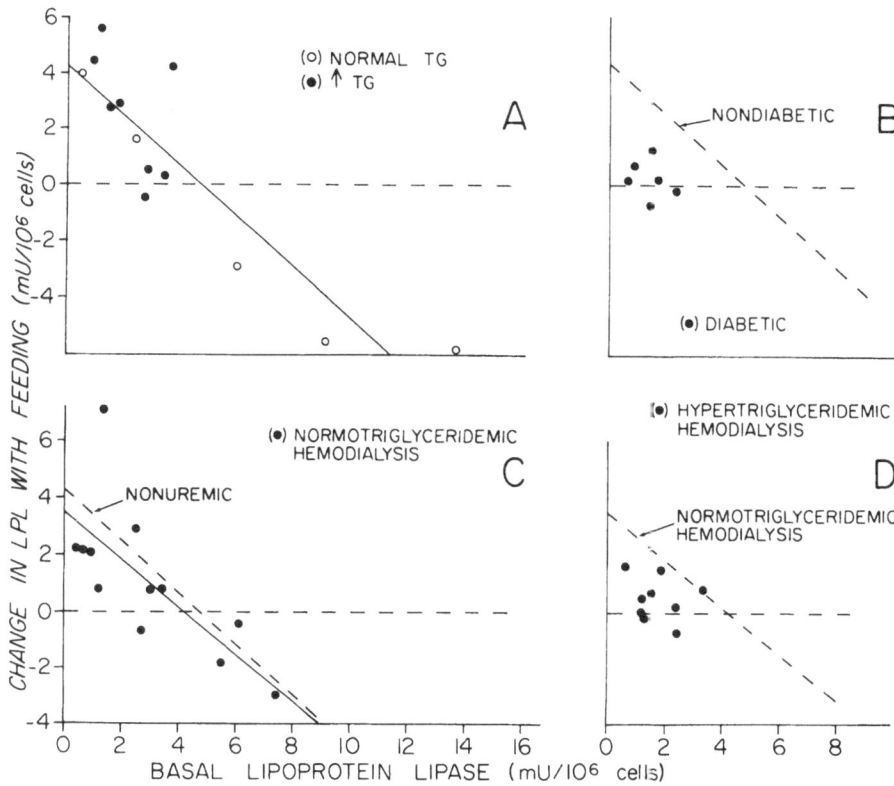

Figure 1. Comparison of basal (fasting) heparin elutable adipose tissue LPL with the postprandial increment in LPL in:

A. Normal and hypertriglyceridemic subjects;
B. Uncontrolled diabetic subjects; dashed line from data in 1A;
C. Normotriglyceridemic subjects on hemodialysis; dashed line from data in 1A;
D. Hypertriglyceridemic subjects on hemodialysis; dashed line from data in 1C

The role of insulin in the regulation of human adipose tissue LPL is apparent in diabetic subjects with untreated fasting hyperglycemia and insulin deficiency. These subjects are characterized by both lower fasting levels of adipose tissue LPL (Pykälistö et al., 1975b) and the failure to increase the enzyme postprandially (Pykälistö et al., 1975b) (Table 1, Fig. 1B). When these untreated diabetics with fasting hyperglycemia were treated with either insulin or an oral sulfonyl-urea for at least 3 months, fasting LPL levels returned to normal and plasma TG levels decreased (Pykälistö et al., 1975b). Furthermore, in normal subjects and in those with fasting hyperglycemia, the postprandial (6-h) percent change in heparin elutable LPL activity is a function of the relative insulin response above the fasting level (percent increase) during the first 2 hours of feeding (r = 0.71, p < 0.01, n = 12, Fig. 2).

Patients with primary hypothyroidism who have increased thyroid-stimulating hormone (TSH) levels and decreased thyroxine levels, also have low fasting LPL levels (Pykälistö et al., 1976; Persson, 1973a). Following treatment with thyroxine (for more than 3 months), there was a decrease in plasma TG levels that was associated with an increase in fasting adipose tissue LPL levels into the normal range (Pykälistö et al., 1976) (Table 1). Whether the abnormality in LPL was due to: (1) suppression of the activity of the enzyme by high TSH levels (Pykälistö, 1970), (2) a lack of thyroid hormone, or (3) these two factors acting simultaneously by different mechanisms, could not be answered by studies in these patients.

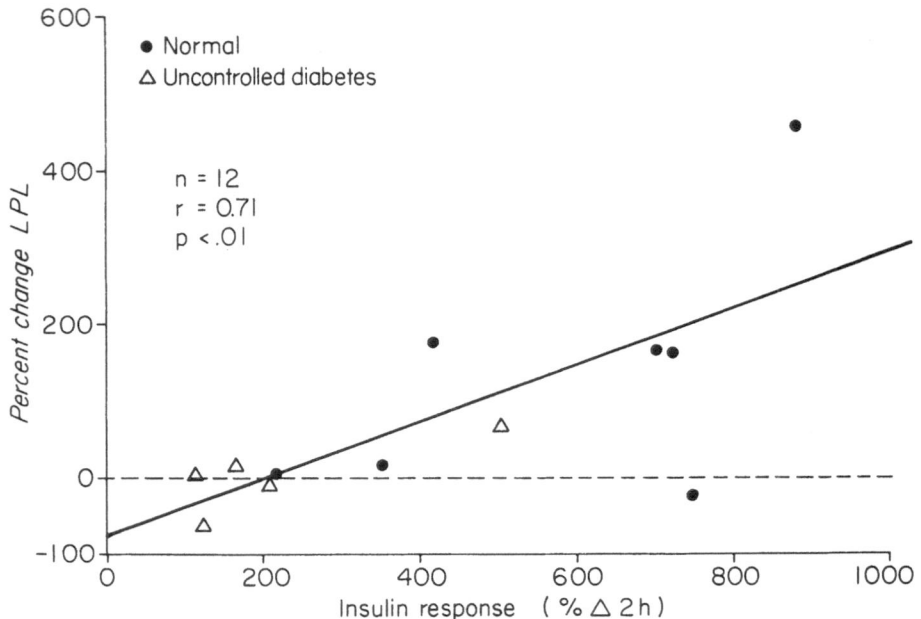

Figure 2. Relationship between the postprandial increment in LPL and the 2-hour insulin response to the feeding in untreated diabetics and normal subjects

Many patients with chronic renal failure who receive maintenance hemodialysis have elevated serum TG levels. When both the fasting and the postprandial activity of adipose tissue LPL are compared in normotriglyceridemic dialysis and nonuremic control patients, they are not different (Table 1, Fig. 1C) (Goldberg et al., 1976). In contrast, those hemodialysis patients with elevated serum TG levels have both low fasting and postprandial adipose tissue LPL levels (Table 1, Fig. 1D). While the diabetic individuals may have failed to increase LPL with feeding due to a lack of insulin secretion, the hypertriglyceridemic hemodialysis patients secreted normal amounts of insulin, yet did not increase adipose tissue LPL postprandially. Although in the normotriglyceridemic hemodialysis patients the fasting activity of LPL was a significant function of relative body weight as measured by Metropolitan Life Insurance tables, no such relationship existed in the hypertriglyceridemia dialysis patients (Fig. 3). A similar relationship has been previously reported in nonuremic patients with varying degrees of obesity (Nilsson-Ehle, 1974); however, it did not exist in the normal controls in this study. Hemodialysis patients have multiple hormonal abnormalities and an increased prevalence of many common secondary causes of hypertriglyceridemia, such as hypothyroidism, diabetes mellitus, and anabolic steroid therapy (Feldman and Singer, 1974). When the patients with these secondary causes of hypertriglyceridemia were excluded from a large dialysis population (Brunzell et al., 1975), it was found that the degree of hypertriglyceridemia appeared to correlate with the degree of vitamin D deficiency produced by the chronic renal failure. That is, utilizing multiple regression analysis, TG levels were an inverse function of the parathyroid hormone concentration and calcium concentration ($r = -0.42$, $n = 37$, $p < 0.01$).*

Extensive studies in rats have also suggested that adipose tissue LPL is regulated by insulin (Robinson, 1970; Garfinkel et al., 1976; Cryer et al., 1976; Schnatz and Williams, 1963) (a decrease in activity with decreased insulin levels and an increase in activity with increased insulin levels). Thus, in this case, regulation appears to be similar to that observed in humans (Pykälistö et al.,

---

*Unpublished observations: Baylink, D., Sherrard, D., and Brunzell, J.

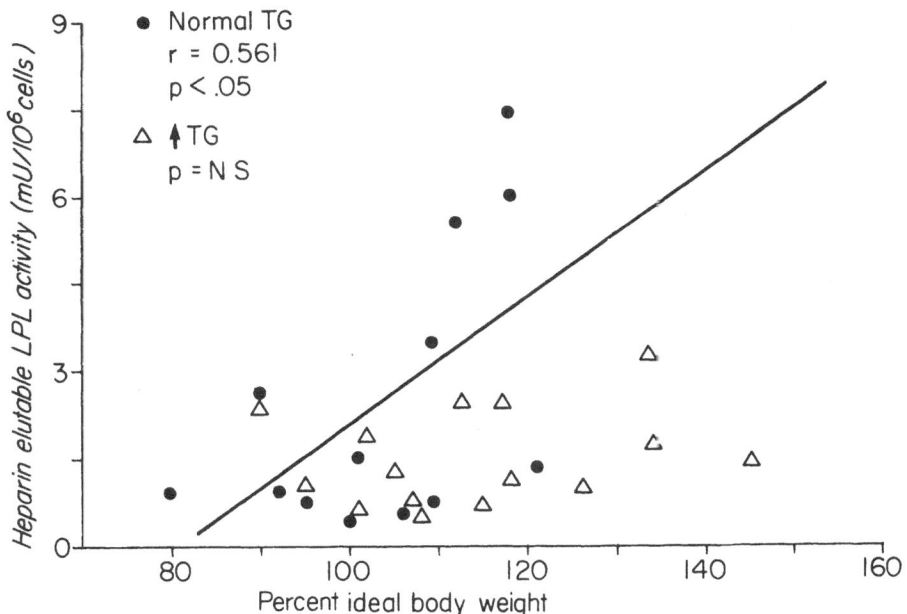

Figure 3. Comparison of the fasting activity of LPL with relative weight in normo-triglyceridemic and hypertriglyceridemic subjects on hemodialysis

1975b). However, marked species differences can be demonstrated with the alterations of other hormonal states. For example, while the fasting level of adipose tissue LPL is low in hypothyroid men (Pykälistö et al., 1976), it is either unchanged or high in hypothyroid rats (Shafrir and Biale, 1971). Adipose tissue LPL is unchanged in the human female treated with estrogen (Applebaum et al., 1976), while it is markedly decreased in the estrogen-treated rat (Hamosh and Hamosh, 1975). And finally, while the fasting level of adipose tissue LPL is decreased in uremic humans who are hypertriglyceridemic while on maintenance hemodialysis (Goldberg et al., 1976), it is either unchanged or high in hypertriglyceridemic uremic rats (Bagdale et al., 1976).

Therefore, human adipose tissue LPL, as measured by that activity eluted from adipose tissue with heparin, is regulated by multiple hormones. Insulin appears to be important for maintaining both normal basal and fed LPL levels. The treatment of diabetes mellitus with insulin increases low fasting LPL levels into the normal range. In patients with varying insulin secretion, the postprandial increase in LPL is a function of the insulin response during the early period of feeding. The decrease in adipose tissue LPL in hypothyroidism may be due to either low thyroxine levels or high TSH levels. These abnormalities return to normal with thyroxine therapy. In hypertriglyceridemic hemodialysis patients, the decrease in adipose tissue LPL levels in the fed and fasted state, despite appropriate insulin secretion, suggests that some factor inhibits LPL. Whether this is hormonally related to the inverse correlation between TG levels and parathyroid hormone and calcium concentrations is yet unknown.

POST-HEPARIN TRIGLYCERIDE LIPASE ACTIVITY (PHTGLA) IN DIABETIC RATS

Hajime Orimo, Tadazumi Nakano, and Akio Noma

I would like to briefly summarize our preliminary data on the postheparin triglyceride lipase activity (PHTGLA) in rats with experimental diabetes.
Experimental diabetes was produced in rats by i.v. injection of 80 mg/kg of streptozotocin. Serum glucose, triglyceride, and nonesterified fatty acid in these diabetic rats were markedly higher than in the control rats. PHTGLA was measured by using 14C triolein as a substrate according to the method of Schotz et al. (1970) with minor modifications. Selective measurement of hepatic and extrahepatic triglyceride lipase activities in rat postheparin plasma was performed by using protamine sulfate according to the method of Krauss et al. (1973). It was found that the total PHTGLA 10 min after the single i.v. injection of 200 U/kg of heparin was significantly smaller in the diabetic than in the control rats. Furthermore, protamine-inhibited (extrahepatic) PHTGLA was significantly smaller in the diabetic than in the control rats.

On the other hand, protamine-resistant (hepatic) PHTGLA in the diabetic rats was not significantly different from that in the control rats. Subsequently, PHTGLA after the repeated i.v. injection of 200 U/kg of heparin was measured in the diabetic rats.

As shown in Figure 1, total PHTGLA 10 min after each injection of heparin was significantly smaller in the diabetic than in the control rats. Protamine-resistant (hepatic) PHTGLA in the diabetic rats was not different from the control rats. On the other hand protamine-inhibited (extrahepatic) PHTGLA was significantly smaller in the diabetic than in the control rats. These results suggest that the decrease in PHTGLA in the diabetic rats is mainly due to the fall in the protamine-inhibited (extrahepatic) PHTGLA. It is possible that the reduced PHTGLA in the diabetic rats 10 min after the first injection of heparin may be due to the smaller pool size of PHTGLA or the disturbance in the mobilization of PHTGLA from the capillary endothelium.

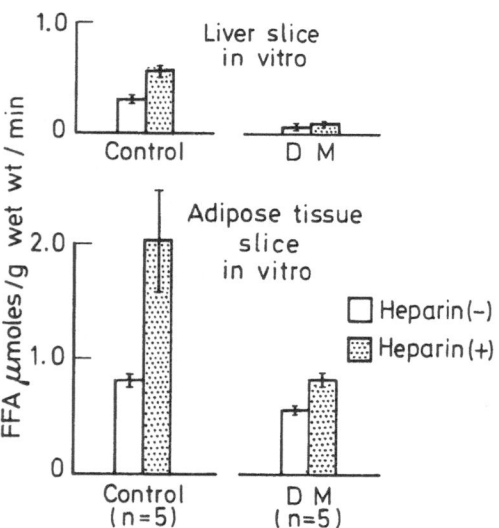

Figure 1. Postheparin triglyceride lipase activity in diabetic rats. PHTGLA after the repeated i.v. injection of 200 U/kg of heparin was measured in the diabetic rats. Total and protamine-inhibited PHTGLA 10 min after each injection of heparin was significantly smaller in the diabetic than in the control rats. PHTGLA was expressed as μmol of free fatty acid/ml/min

On the other hand, it is tempting to speculate that the decreased PHTGLA in the diabetic rats after the repeated injection of heparin may reflect the disturbance of PHTGLA mobilization from the adipose tissue.

In order to examine this possibility, we have subsequently studied the effect of heparin in vitro on the release of triglyceride lipase from the adipose tissue of the diabetic rats.

Five hundred mg of epididymal adipose tissue obtained from diabetic or control rats was incubated in vitro with or without 10 U of heparin at 37°C for 1 h, and the release of triglyceride lipase from the adipose tissue into the medium was measured.

As shown in Figure 2, heparin-stimulated release of triglyceride lipase from the adipose tissue in vitro was significantly smaller in the diabetic than in the control rats. These results suggest the possibility that either the synthesis or the mobilization of triglyceride lipase from the adipose tissue is disturbed in diabetic rats.

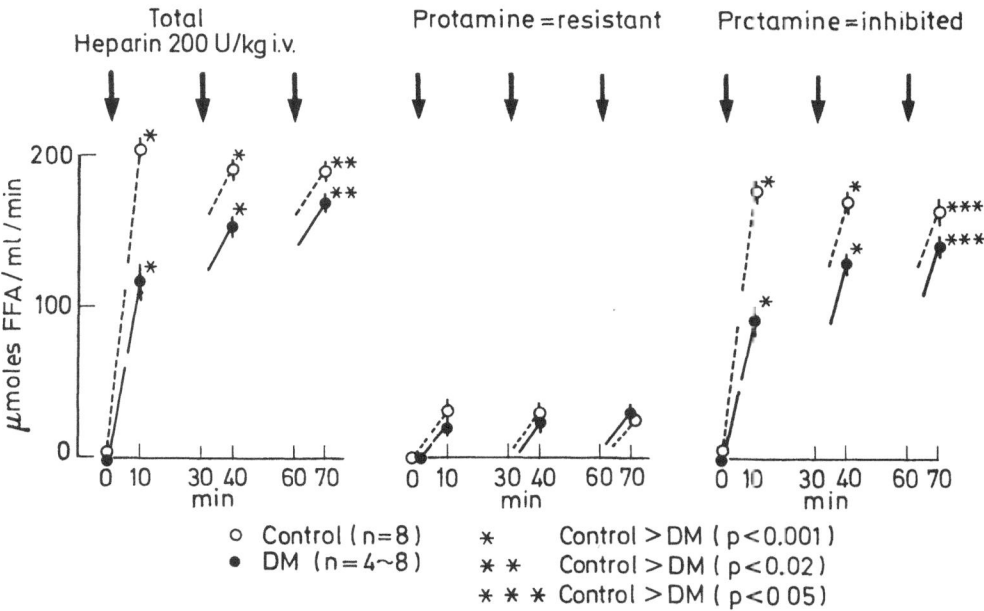

Figure 2. Triglyceride lipase activity in diabetic rats. Effect of heparin on triglyceride lipase from rat liver and adipose tissue slices in vitro. Heparin-stimulated release of triglyceride lipase from adipose tissue in vitro was significantly smaller in the diabetic than in the control rats. Triglyceride lipase activities were expressed as μmol of free fatty acid/g wet wt/min

PURIFICATION OF LIPOLIPIN FROM HUMAN ATHEROSCLEROTIC INTIMA AND THE KINETICS OF INHIBITION OF BOVINE MILK LIPOPROTEIN LIPASE

Premanand V. Wagh, and Thomas Olivecrona
VA Hospital, Little Rock, AR/USA, and Department of Chemistry, Umeå University, Umeå/Sweden

Intimal tissue from human atherosclerotic aortae was collected by the "Dermatome Procedure" (Atherosclerosis, 20:533, 1974). The tissue was extracted with 5 mM Tris·HCl buffer containing O.3 M NaCl and 1 mM EDTA, pH 7.4. Ammonium sulfate precipitate between 40-80% saturation obtained from the extract was fractionated on a DEAE-cellulose column and the effluent was monitored for lipoprotein lipase (LPL) inhibition employing purified bovine milk LPL. The substrate used was an emulsion of purified olive oil and tritiated triolein. Human serum was the source of activator of the substrate. The inhibitor was eluted within the same ionic concentration (0.16 - 0.18 M NaCl) as that required for porcine intimal glycoprotein (Biochemistry, 11:4222, 1972 Adv. Exptl. Med. Biol., 52:281, 1975). The inhibitor was further purified by preparative isoelectric focusing. Lipolipin electrofocused at 4·3 - 4·4 pI. The purified preparation inhibited both the basal and the serum stimulated LPL activity at various concentration of the inhibitor. The inhibition was non-competitive with respect to either added triglyceride or serum. Lipolipin did not inhibit the lipolytic activity of purified hog pancreatic lipase. These studies indicate that lipolipin interacts with the enzyme-activator complex preventing the hydrolysis of triglyceride. (Supported by Veterans Administration Research Funds, Project 9166-01 and the Med. Faculty, Umeå.)

HYDROLYSES OF TRIGLYCERIDES IN CHYLOMICRONS, VERY LOW- AND LOW-DENSITY LIPOPROTEINS BY C-I ACTIVATED LIPOPROTEIN LIPASE FROM NORMAL HUMAN POST-HEPARIN PLASMA

Diana M. Lee, Devaki Ganesan, and Helen Bass
Cardiovascular Research Program, Oklahoma Medical Research Foundation, Oklahoma City, OK/USA

C-I activated lipoprotein lipase (LPL_{C-I}) was isolated from normolipidemic human post-heparin plasma (PHP) by a method involving substrate-enzyme complex formation, $Ca_3(PO_4)_2$ gel chromatography and gel filtration on Sephadex G-100. This procedure yielded 35,000 fold purification of the enzyme. LPL_{C-I} was tested for its ability to hydrolyze triglycerides (TG) in chylomicrons (CM, $S_f > 400$), VLDL (S_f 20-400) and LDL_1(S_f 12-20) from human plasma. Results showed that CM-TG were the preferred substrates to TG in VLDL and LDL_1. The hydrolytic rates for CM-TG rich in C_{16} and C_{18-1} fatty acids (FA) (donors taking dairy cream and corn oil respectively) were 20 times greater than those rich in C_{18-2} (donors taking safflower oil), 100 times greater than those for TG in VLDL and LDL_1 and 10 times greater than those for triolein emulsion (TE) and C-I. LPL_{C-I} hydrolyzed CM-TG rich in C_{16} and C_{18-1} FA at a much higher rate than PHP, whereas the opposite was true for the CM-TG rich in C_{18-2}. The explanation for preferential hydrolysis of CM by LPL_{C-I} was probably due to an optimal C-I/TG (0.19/100 wt/wt) ratio exhibited by CM. It was found with TE, the optimal activation concentrations of C-I/TG were 0.06-0.68/100. VLDL and LDL_1 had C-I/TG ratios (2.3/100 and 5-7/100 respectively) far from the optimum range. These data support the earlier reports that in Type I hyperlipoproteinemics the accumulation of CM is due to deficiency of LPL_{C-I}.

DIVERGENT RESPONSE OF EXTRA-HEPATIC AND HEPATIC POST-HEPARIN-LIPO-LYTIC-ACTIVITY (PHLA) TO A LOW-FAT, HIGH-CARBOHYDRATE, ISOCALORIC, ELEMENTAL DIET IN NORMAL AND HYPERTRIGLYCERIDEMIC HUMANS

F. Damgaard-Pedersen, H. Meinertz, and O. Faergeman
Department of Clinical Chemistry and Departments of Medicine B & P., Rigsspitalet,
University of Copenhagen, Copenhagen/Denmark

An elemental diet ("Vivasorb"), supplying less than 1% of calories as fat, efficiently lowered plasma triglycerides in 3 subjects with exogenous (low total
PHLA) and in 2 subjects with exogenous-endogenous (normal total PHLA) hypertriglyceridemia. The same diet slightly elevated triglycerides in 5 normal subjects.
In all 3 groups, cholesterol decreased. In all 3 groups moreover, extra-hepatic
PHLA (inhibited by 1 M NaCl) was markedly decreased in all subjects (mean =
65.7%), whereas hepatic PHLA (not inhibited by 1 M NaCl) increased or remained
unchanged (mean increase = 58.3%). The rate of clearing from plasma of intravenously injected "Intralipid" was related to extra-hepatic PHLA by a hyperbolic
function (r = 0.72, determined by least squares technic). This study support the
concept that lipoprotein lipase, as reflected in extra-hepatic PHLA, is rate
limiting in the early steps of triglyceride-rich lipoprotein catabolism. The
function and control of the hepatic lipase remain undefined but may be quite different.

EFFECT OF ESTROGEN ON POST-HEPARIN LIPOLYTIC ACTIVITY: SELECTIVE DECLINE IN HEPATIC TRIGLYCERIDE LIPASE

Deborah Applebaum, Andrew Goldberg, Olavi Pykälisto, and William Hazzard
Northewest Lipid Research Clinic, University of Washington, Seattle, WA/USA

Estrogens cause a modest rise in triglyceride (TG) and a marked decrease in postheparin lipolytic activity (PHLA) which do not correlate (r = −.359, N.S.). One
possible explanation for this discrepancy is a selective decline in one of the
activities in PHLA, hepatic TG lipase (HTGL) or extra-hepatic lipoprotein lipase
(LPL). This possibility was explored by measuring both HTGL and LPL in postheparin plasma from 13 normal women before and after 2 weeks of ethinyl estradiol
(1 μg/kg/d). HTGL and LPL activities were determined after separation by heparin-
Sepharose chromatography and following selective inhibition with specific antibodies to post-heparin HTGL and milk LPL. Estrogen uniformly depressed HTGL
whether measured by column (−68±10%, p <.001) or by antibody (−63±11%, p <.001).
LPL showed no significant change by column (−22±28%) or antibody (−3±42%). Direct
measurement of adipose tissue LPL from buttock fat biopsies also showed no significant change in heparin-elutable (+64±164%) or acetone-ether extracted (+21±77%)
activities. The change in HTGL correlated with the change in PHLA (r = .939,
p <.01) but, like PHLA, did not correlate (r = −.352, N.S.) with the increase in
TG during estrogen (+44±30 mg%). The decrease in PHLA during estrogen thus results from a selective decline in HTGL which does not appear to mediate the
hypertriglyceridemia induced by estrogen in human subjects.

UPTAKE OF CHYLOMICRON REMNANT PARTICLES BY ISOLATED LIVER CELLS

Trevor Redgrave and Nicholas Vakakis
Department of Physiology, University of Melbourne, Victoria/Australia

The cholesterol of primary intestinal lipoproteins is removed from the plasma
after most of the lipoprotein triacylglycerol has been removed by the action of
lipoprotein lipase in peripheral tissues. In this study the uptake by isolated
liver cells of chylomicron particles and their remnants has been compared. Remnants isolated from the serum of hepatectomised rats were taken up by isolated

liver cells in physiologically significant amounts whereas intact chylomicrons were taken up to a much smaller extent. Uptake of remnants was independent of serum proteins and was independent of cellular respiration. The Q-10 of the uptake process was 1.4, and the Arrhenius plot showed an abrupt change in slope at 20°, indicating that the physical state of membrane or particle lipid influences uptake. Physiological concentrations of insulin, glucagon, thyroxine, prostaglandin, heparin and pancreozymin did not affect the uptake process.

EFFECT OF POST-HEPARIN SERUM ON THE UPTAKE OF CHYLOMICRON-CHOLESTEROL AND ITS INHIBITIORY MECHANISM OF CHOLESTEROL BIOSYNTHESIS IN ISOLATED HEPATOCYTES OF RATS

Chikayuki Naito, Tamio Teramoto, and Kodo Okada
The First Department of Internal Medicine, Faculty of Medicine, University of Tokyo, Tokyo/Japan

When the hepatocytes were incubated with ^{14}C-cholesterol-labeled chylomicron in the medium containing either "post-heparin" (PH) or "normal" (N) rat serum, ^{14}C-cholesterol was taken up almost equally by hepatocytes. However, while cholesterol ester ratio in the cells did not significantly decrease with the incubation time in the PH serum group, the ratio decreased significantly with the time in the N serum group. This effect of PH serum on the esterification of cholesterol may be due to the simultaneous uptake of fatty acids, because an increment of free fatty acid concentration of N serum by an addition of oleic acid-albumin complex kept the ester ratio in the cells higher with the time as in the case of PH serum group. The cholesterol ester ratio in the incubation medium unchanged during the experimental period. Two hour-preincubation of isolated hepatocytes in the medium containing "cold" chylomicron caused the inhibition of cholesterol biosynthesis from ^{14}C-acetate when the medium contained PH serum, but not when the medium contained N serum. These results suggested that the feedback inhibition of cholesterol biosynthesis in hepatocytes by intestinal lipoprotein might have been caused by the esterified cholesterol, rather than free one. Because the inhibition appeared after the short period incubation, it is also suggested that the inhibition may be allosteric.

A LIPOPROTEIN LIPASE STABILIZING FACTOR OF BOVINE MILK

Israel Posner and Darío Bermudez
Departamento de Biología Celular, Escuela de Biología, Facultad de Ciencias, Universidad Central de Venezuela, Caracas/Venezuela

Lipoprotein lipase (LPL), a key enzyme in lipoprotein metabolism, is highly unstable. For example, from 60 - 95% of LPL activity of post-heparin plasma (PHP), heart or adipose tissue extracts may be lost in one hour at 37°C, but only 18 - 25% of bovine milk LPL activity is lost under these conditions. We attribute this fact to the presence of a stabilizing factor (SF) in the milk. Indeed a partially purified factor with stabilization properties has been prepared from LPL-free bovine milk. The addition of this factor to rat PHP, heart or adipose tissue extracts results in 2 - 3 fold increases in LPL activities and in its presence only about 20% of enzyme activities are lost during a one hour incubation at 37°C. SF is non-dialyzable it may be precipitated with ammonium sulfate, it loses its stabilizing properties in 15 minutes at 100°C, but it is stable for several hours at 42°C. Further purification and characterization of this factor are in progress.

PREPARATION AND ACTIVATION OF HIGHLY PURIFIED LIPOPROTEIN LIPASE FROM BOVINE MILK

Ann-Margret Östlund-Lindqvist, Per-Henrik Iverius, and Peter Lindqvist
Department of Medical and Physiological Chemistry, University of Uppsala,
Biomedicum, Uppsala/Sweden

Lipoprotein lipase of very high purity was isolated from bovine milk by affinity
chromatography on heparin-Sepharose, adsorption to C_γ-alumina hydroxide gel and
intervent dilution chromatography on heparin-Sepharose. Chemical analysis indicates that the enzyme is a glycoprotein containing 8% carbohydrate. The monomer
molecular weight determined under reducing conditions in 6.6 M guanidine HCl by
sedimentation equilibrium ultracentrifugation and analytical gel chromatography,
is close to 50,000.
The effects of C-apolipoproteins from very low density human lipoproteins on the
enzyme activity was studied using a triglyceride phospholipid emulsion (Intralipid) as substrate. No activity was recorded with the substrate alone and apo-
CII was the only C-peptide that activated the enzyme. Maximal activity required
a sufficient concentration of activator and an optimal ratio between activator
and substrate. At substrate excess, the enzyme activity was reduced by about 50%
or less depending on the concentration of activator employed. Under these conditions, however, appropriate additions of apo-CI or apo-CIII restored part of the
lost activity. Interaction studies on LPL, activator and substrate indicate that
the activator as well as the enzyme was bound to the substrate.

THE EFFECT OF ALBUMIN AND IONIC STRENGTH ON PURIFIED PLASMA LIPO-PROTEIN LIPASE

Jan Augustin, Gerald Klose, and Heiner Greten
Klinisches Institut für Herzinfarktforschung an der Medizinischen Universitätsklinik, Heidelberg/BRD

Plasma lipoprotein lipase (LPL) was measured by two different methods: (1) Human
post-heparin plasma LPL was isolated by affinity chromatography on heparin-
Sepharose 4B and (2) LPL activity was determined after selective precipitation of
the other major lipolytic activity in plasma, hepatic triglyceride lipase (H-TGL)
by means of specific enzyme antibodies. With both methods the following optimal
assay conditions were obtained when an artificial radioactive triolein emulsion
was used as substrate: in a final volume of 220 µl the assay consisted of (a)
8.47 mM triglyceride (TG), (b) 0.2 M Tris-HCl, pH 8.2, (c) 0.15 M NaCl, (d) 20 µg
isolated apoprotein C II or 20 µg pre-heparin plasma as cofactor. With purified
plasma LPL as enzyme source it was found that activation of LPL by apoprotein C II
only occurred in the presence of albumin with an optimal concentration of 1 mg
albumin/mg TG. Lack of albumin resulted in only 15% of maximal activity with C II.
Furthermore, the well-known inhibitory effect of high NaCl concentration on LPL
could only be demonstrated in the presence of albumin. The interaction of purified LPL with plasma proteins and ions will be discussed.

STIMULATION OF A LIPOPROTEIN LIPASE ACTIVITY FROM HUMAN ADIPOSE TISSUE BY APOLIPOPROTEIN C-III

Hans Lithell, Jonas Boberg, Ann-Margret Östlund-Lindqvist, and Ivàn Håkansson
Department of Geriatrics, University of Uppsala, Uppsala/Sweden

A method for quantitation of lipoprotein lipase activity (LPLA) in human adipose
tissue (HAT) has been developed. A soybean oil-phospholipid emulsion (labelled
with ^{3}H-trioleate) was used in a reaction medium comprising glycine-NaOH buffer,
apolipoprotein C-II (or serum) as activator, heparin and albumin. By using

glycine-NaOH buffer a good stability of enzyme activity was achieved during long time incubation. Heparin usually inhibits LPLA in concentrations above 10 IU/ml. However, in the present assay a heparin concentration of 100 IU/ml caused 2.5 times greater LPLA extraction from HAT than 1 IU/ml. In addition, when apolipoprotein C-II was omitted from the assay a triglyceride lipase activity was still present. Both apolipoprotein C-II activated and non-activated HAT lipolytic activity were similarly inhibited by protamine sulfate and NaCl. Apolipoprotein C-III caused inhibition of apolipoprotein C-II activated LPLA. Apolipoprotein C-II non-activated HAT lipolytic activity, however, was stimulated by low concentrations of apolipoprotein C-III and was inhibited by high concentrations. Evidence will be presented that this probably depends on the presence of small quantities of C-II.

IS DECREASED LIPOPROTEIN LIPASE C-II IN TYPE III HYPERLIPOPROTEINEMIA A CAUSE OR AN EFFECT OF INCREASED APOLIPOPROTEIN E?

D. Ganesan, H.B. Bass, and W.J. McConathy
Cardiovascular Research Program and Lipoprotein Laboratory, Oklahoma Medical Research Foundation, Oklahoma City, OK/USA

We have shown that post-heparin plasma (PHP) lipoprotein lipase C-II (LPL_{C-II}) in Type III hyperlipoproteinemia is decreased in lipolytic activity, protein concentration and its ability to hydrolyze triglyceride (TG) in VLDL was impaired (10 - 20% of control). Increased apolipoprotein E (ApoE, "arg-rich" polypeptide) levels in VLDL and serum of these patients have also been reported. Therefore, effect of ApoE (0-90 µg/ml assay mixture) on highly purified LPL_{C-I} (C-I activated) and LPL_{C-II} from PHP of normal controls were tested in assay mixtures containing 14C-triolein emulsified in Triton X-100 or lecithin. ApoE had no effect on the LPLs by itself but when added to LPLs fully activated by C-I or C-II, an inhibition (20% of control lipolytic activities at 10 µg conc.) was observed. ApoE inhibition, unlike that of C-III, was not dependent on TG conc. or emulsifier. Since decreased LPL_{C-II} and increased ApoE levels characterize the biochemical abnormality in Type III patients, three possible mechanisms could be involved:1) inhibition of LPL_{C-II} by increased levels of ApoE,2) deficiency of LPL_{C-II}, and 3) the two former possibilities co-exist independently but mutually aggravate the condition further. Although LPL_{C-I} was also inhibited in vitro by ApoE, LPL_{C-I} was normal in Type III. On the basis of these findings, second and/or third alternative seems more likely.

HYDROLYSIS OF NORMAL AND "ABNORMAL" CHYLOMICRONS WITH PURIFIED PLASMA HEPATIC TRIGLYCERIDE LIPASE AND LIPOPROTEIN LIPASE

Jan Augustin, Robert Geursen, Heinrich Wieland, and Heiner Greten
Klinisches Institut für Herzinfarktforschung an der Medizinischen Universitäts-klinik, Heidelberg/BRD

This study was performed to evaluate in vitro a possible substrate preference for plasma hepatic triglyceride lipase (H-TGL7 and lipoprotein lipase (LPL). Chylomicrons from both normals and a patient with Type III hyperlipoproteinemia were isolated by ultracentrifugation and subjected to gel chromatography on Biogel P 2. Two major fractions with Sf values > 2,000 (fraction A) and Sf values 400 - 2,000 (fraction B) were obtained. The apoprotein composition of fraction A which had a triglyceride/protein ratio of 2,000/65 and of fraction B with a ratio of 2,000/138 was quantitatively determined by disc gel electrophoresis in tetramethylurea. These fractions were incubated with highly purified plasma H-TGL and LPL. It could be shown that (1) physiological albumin concentrations were required for full activity, (2) Vmax for H-TGL with fraction A was 3.3, Km 0.9, and for LPL 1.56 and 0.23 respectively, (3) the values for fraction B were Vmax =

2.32 and Km = 1.2 for H-TGL, 2.2 and 0.61 for LPL, (4) the chylomicron fraction A of the Type III patient was neither hydrolyzed by H-TGL nor by LPL. Hydrolysis of fraction B yielded for both enzymes lower Vmax with no change in Km compared with fraction B from normals. The mechanism of this release and its consequence for hyperlipoproteinemia will be discussed.

THE RELATIONSHIP BETWEEN THE CONCENTRATION OF STEROID HORMONES AND LIPOPROTEINS IN PLASMA OF PATIENTS WITH CORONARY ATHEROSCLEROSIS AND IN HEALTHY SUBJECTS

Elena N. Gerasimova
Biochemical Laboratory, A.L. Myasnikov Institute of Cardiology AMS USSR, Moscow/
USSR

In coronary atherosclerosis patients with different types of hyperlipoproteinemia and in men at the age of 49 - 59 without ischaemic heart disease the comparative investigation of androgenes, estrogenes and cortisol content in plasma was carried out. The hormones were determined by the radioimmunoassay with the use of Sorin kits. It was found that the changes in the content of steroid hormones were correlated with the differences in the content of triglycerides (Tg), cholesterol (Ch), Ch of a lipoproteins, percentage of pre-β-and α-lipoproteins in plasma. At the same time the changes of lipid composition of α-lipoproteins (Tg, Ch, Ch-esters lecithin, lysolecithin) were found. The results showed that the differences in the concentration of steroid hormones are related to plasma lipoprotein spectrum.

STIMULATORY EFFECT OF ACTH ON CARNITINE METABOLISM IN ATHEROSCLEROSIS

Masaru Maebashi, Norimitsu Kawamura, and Mitsuo Satoh
The 2nd Department of Internal Medicine, Tohoku University, School of Medicine, Sendai/Japan

To examine whether carnitine is involved in the pathogenesis of atherosclerosis, urinary excretion of carnitine and serum carnitine level were measured in normal subjects and in patients with atherosclerosis and other abnormal lipid metabolism. The patients had serum carnitine level and urinary excretion close to those of normal subjects. After administration of ACTH, the quantitative differences in the carnitine level and the excretion were apparent between in normal subjects and in the patients. In response to ACTH, the excretion and the serum level increased highly on the day of the administration in normal subjects, probably due to an enhanced adrenocortical activity. In the patients, the excretion increased slightly on the 1st day and reached a maximum on the 2nd day. These changes were associated with enhanced lipolysis, and there was a significant correlation between carnitine excretion and serum lipids concentrations. These evidences suggest that delayed incorporation of carnitine into lipid metabolism after lipolytic stimulation may be one of the possible explanation for the etiology of atherosclerosis.

Collagen, Elastin, Mucopolysaccharides in Atherosclerosis

Chairmen: W.H. Hauss, BRD
         M. Nakamura, Japan

Participants: W.H. Hauss, BRD
             B. Radhakrishnamurthy, USA
             J.P. Lindner, BRD
             S. Glagov, USA

INFLUENCE OF MUSCULAR TRAINING ON ARTERIAL WALL CELL REACTION

W.H. Hauss

In the last 15 years, we demonstrated in animal models and in human arteriosclerosis by several methods, especially by investigations with ^{3}H-thymidine and
^{35}S-sulfate, that atherogenic or sclerogenic factors induce immediately, regularly and promptly a reaction of the arterial wall cells, being a part of the mesenchymal system (Hauss et al., 1968; Hauss, 1973, 1976a, 1976b). Most important in
this reaction are proliferation and acceleration of metabolic processes of the
arterial wall cells. We suggest that this reaction of the arterial wall cells induced by "risk factors" is the first, a regular, and a fundamental step in the
development of the arteriosclerotic process.

Arterial hypertension, being one of the most important sclerogenic factors, induces cell proliferation in intima, media, and adventitia of rats' aortas
(Fig. 1). The incorporation rates of ^{35}S-sulfate into the sulfomucopolysaccha-
rides (SMPS) of aortic wall cells are considerably higher in hypertensive rats
than in normotensives (Fig. 2). All atherogenic, sclerogenic, risk, and stress
factors studies (the names in this case mean the same thing) induced acceleration of cell proliferation and metabolism in the arterial wall.

We live in an Olympic year. Since thousands of years, sportive life is thought
to be healthy. But convincing evidence that muscular exercise is keeping away
diseases, especially preventing arteriosclerosis, is lacking. In animal experiments, we studied the effect of muscular exercise on the reaction of the arterial wall cells.

	Normal	Acute hypertension (1 hour)	Chronic hypertension (weeks)
Intima	3	14	59
Media	12	136	235
Adventitia	4	218	255
Total	19	368	549

Figure 1. Cell reduplication in the aortic wall induced by hypertension. (Number
of labeled cells in 100 microscopic fields)

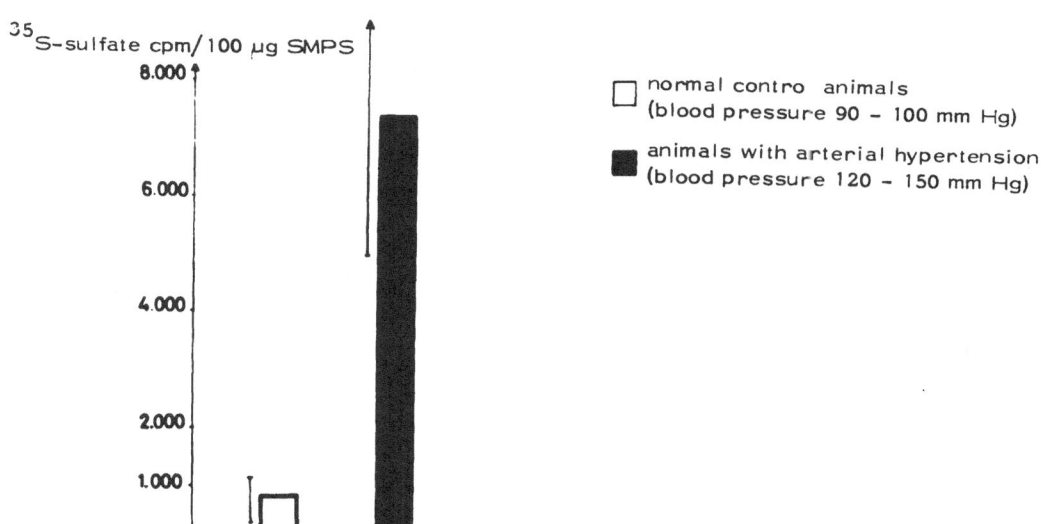

Figure 2. Influence of arterial blood pressure on the metabolism of arterial wall cells. (Incorporation of ^{35}S-sulfate into the sulfumucopolysaccharides of rats' aortas)

Animal Materials and Arrangement of Experiments

Three groups of 7-17 Wistar male rats of equal age, with a body weight of 140-160 g, were kept under constant conditions.

The first group was a control group (group I, Fig. 3). The second group was damaged by muscular stress, running 2 days, 6 hours a day in an activity wheel (5 turns/min), and by one toxin injection (1 ml staphylolysin i.p., Behring

	Animal group	1st-6th week	6th week			
			1st day	2nd day	3rd day	4th day
I	Control animals untrained without toxin without running stress				^{35}S-sulfate injection	†
II	Control animals untrained with toxin with running stress		6 h running stress	6 h running stress	1 x toxin injection then ^{35}S-sulfate injection	†
III	Experimental animals trained[a] with toxin with running stress	3x1/2 h-3x5 h running	6 h running stress	6 h running stress	1 x toxin injection then ^{35}S-sulfate injection	†

[a]Training in activity wheels (5 turns/min) on 3 days per week with 1 day intermission

Figure 3. Experimental arrangement of the research program

Werke)(group II, Fig. 3). Some of the animals in group II died in the nights after running stress days. The third group was stressed in the 6th week in the same way as group II, after being trained by 5 weeks running in the activity wheel 3 days/week, 1/2 hour daily in the 1st week, 1 hour in the 2nd, 2 hours in the 3rd, 4 hours in the 4th, and 5 hours in the 5th week. Each day of training was at least followed by one day of rest (group III, Fig. 3). The effect of stress and preceding training was studied by measuring the synthesis of SMPS in the aorta of the rats, injecting 1 mC ^{35}S-sulfate i.p., 24 hours before sacrificing the animals (Fig. 3).

Results and Discussion

Running stress and toxin injection induce a big reaction in the arterial wall cells of untrained animals (group II), raising the uptake of ^{35}S-sulfate into the SMPS nearly threefold, while the same damage in trained animals (group III) did not much alter the metabolism (Fig. 4).

Figure 5 shows the measured incorporation rates and the statistical evaluation. There is a significant difference between the second and the first group but not between the third and the first group, though groups II and III were damaged in the same ways.

The stress effect of hypoxemia combined with muscular overstraining could also be eliminated by training (Hauss et al., 1969). However, we did not yet succeed in eliminating the effect of high blood pressure in rats with renal hypertension, but probably the training had not been long enough in these experiments.

Our experiments show that muscular training can protect or adapt the arterial wall cells against the pathogenic influence of overstraining, toxin, and hypoxemia. It works obviously unspecifically. We are going on to study the problem of the training effect.

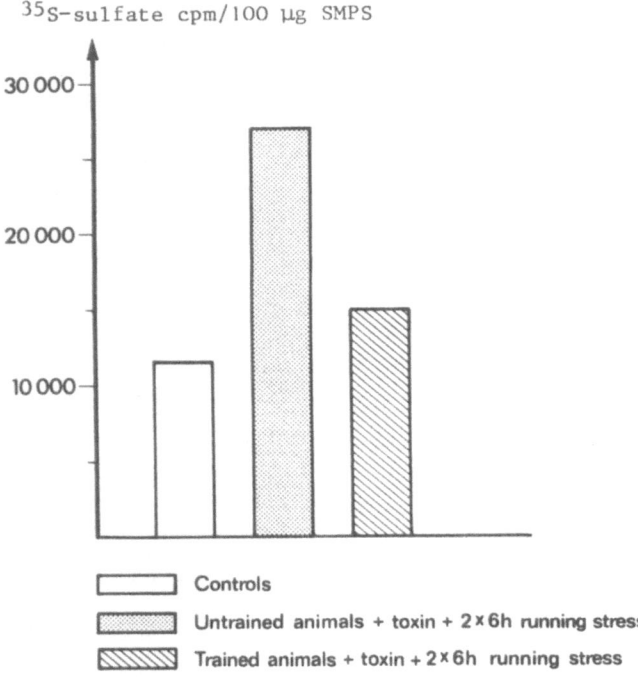

^{35}S-sulfate cpm/100 µg SMPS

Controls

Untrained animals + toxin + 2×6h running stress

Trained animals + toxin + 2×6h running stress

Figure 4. Changes in mesenchymal metabolism in aortas of rats in untrained animals and in trained animals after damaging by combination of running stress and toxin injection. (^{35}S-sulfate incorporation into the SMPS of aorta)

Animal group	Incorporation of ^{35}S-sulfate in SMPS $\bar{x} \pm$ SEM	Comparison of groups	t value	p	Statistical difference: significant = + not significant = □
I	Control animals untrained without toxin without running stress n=7	10661,43 ±1865,86				
II	Control animals untrained with running stress with toxin n=11	28890,09 ±6354,90	II/I	<5,49	0,001	+
III	Experimental animals trained with running stress with toxin n=	14080,00 ±6393,14	III/I	>1,34	0,05	□

Figure 5. Statistical evaluation of findings

Summary

In former studies we have shown that arterial hypertension, muscular exercise, infectious diseases, and bacterial toxins induce cell proliferation in the intima, media, and adventitia of rats' aortas (demonstrated by ^{3}H-thymidine labeling) and acceleration of wall cells' metabolism, demonstrated by measuring the incorporation rate of ^{35}S-sulfate. Muscular exercise is considered to prevent diseases especially arteriosclerosis, but convincing evidence is lacking. We studied this problem in an animal model.

While running stress and toxin injection in Wistar rats induced a big reaction in the arterial wall cells of untrained animals, raising the uptake of ^{35}S-sulfate into the SMPS nearly threefold, the same damage in trained animals did not alter the metabolism significantly. The preceding muscular training has obviously protected or adapted the arterial wall cells against stressors. We suggest that these animal experiments can provide information about the preventive quality of human sport.

COMPLEX CARBOHYDRATES OF ARTERIAL WALL CONNECTIVE TISSUE*

B. Radhakrishnamurthy, G.S. Berenson, and E.R. Dalferes, Jr.

The role of connective tissue of the arterial wall is often overlooked in the consideration of the development of atherosclerosis. In part, this may be due to overemphasis in one area, cholesterol and lipid deposition, yet it is not clear whether the role of lipids is primary or secondary. Virchow, as early as 1856, suggested that atherosclerosis was caused primarily by nonspecific injury and

*Supported by funds from the National Heart and Lung Institute of the USPHS (HL 02942) and the Specialized Center of Research-Arteriosclerosis (HL 15103).

that lipid deposition was a secondary phenomena. It is interesting that current observations are suggesting a mechanism(s), for these phenomena (Wagner and Clarkson, 1973; Ross and Glomset, 1976).

The integrity of the cardiovascular structures depends upon the molecular organization of its connective tissue components. Of particular interest are carbohydrate macromolecules, glycosaminoglycans (GAG), proteoglycans (PG), and glycoproteins (GP). Fairly extensive studies on the GAG of the arterial wall carried out by several investigators have been extensively reviewed (Berenson et al., 1971). Although the exact role of GAG in the development of vascular lesions is not clearly understood, it has been shown that under certain conditions GAG form insoluble complexes with serum lipoproteins, may deposit in the arterial wall, and contribute to the development of atherosclerotic lesions (Cornwell and Kruger, 1961; Srinivasan et al., 1970, 1975).

Although abundant information is available on the GAG of the arterial wall, little is known about PG, the native state in which GAG occur in the tissue. We (Ehrlich et al., 1975) have recently isolated a chondroitin sulfate (CS)-dermatan sulfate (DS) PG from bovine aorta by extraction with 3.1 M $MgCl_2$ by the procedure of Sajdera and Hascall (1969). The chemical and physical properties of the PG were studied after purification and fractionation by CsCl density gradient centrifugation (Table 1). The molecular weight of the PG was 72,000, unlike cartilage PG which ranged from 2 - 6 x 10^6 (Mathews and Lozaityte, 1958). Whether the aorta PG aggregates with hyaluronic acid (HA) and "link protein" is not known (Hascall and Heinegard, 1974).

Table 1. Composition of glycosaminoglycans from bovine aorta after 3.0 M $MgCl_2$ extraction by hydrolysis with elastase and collagenase

Hydrolysis	HA[a]	HS	CS-A	DS
	(mg UA/gdry defatted tissue)			
Elastase (in the presence of protease inhibitor)	180	360	30	90
Collagenase	130	–[b]	180	20
Control	–	–	25	–

[a]HA: hyaluronic acid; HS: heparan sulfate; CS-A: chondroitin 4-sulfate; CS-C: chondroitin 6-sulfate; DS: dermatan sulfate; UA: uronic acid.
[b]Not detected within 5%.

Dissociative solvents cannot completely extract all proteoglycans from aorta as they can from cartilage. This suggests that some of the PG in aorta may be associated with fibrous proteins of the tissue and are somewhat difficult to extract. In an attempt to understand the nature of 3.0 M $MgCl_2$ nonextractable PG, the residual tissue after extraction was selectively hydrolyzed by collagenase and elastase, and GAG were isolated from the hydrolyzates, characterized, and quantitated (Table 2). Since the elastase preparations contain nonspecific proteolytic activity, nonspecific proteases were inhibited by soybean trypsin inhibitor (Walford and Kickhöfen, 1962). The residual tissue contained a considerable amount of HA which could be extracted by digestion of the tissue with both enzymes. Heparan sulfate (HS) in the tissue was selectively obtained by elastase hydrolysis but not by collagenase. A greater amount of DS was solubilized by elastase than by collagenase. Collagenase, on the other hand, solubilized more CS than elastase. These findings suggest that in bovine aorta HS and DS, at

Table 2. Properties of proteoglycans from bovine aorta

Properties	3.0 M MgCl$_2$ extracted PG	Elastase solubilized PG
Chemical composition:	(% of dry weight)	
Hexuronic acid	21	18
GlcUA:IdUA[a]	14:1	100% GlcUA
Hexosamine	28	20
GalN:GlcN	20:1	100 GlcN
Total sulfate	10	7
N-sulfate	–	3
Protein	12	15
GAG composition		
CS-C:CS-A:DS	56:20:7	–
HS	–	100% HS
Molecular weight	72,000[b]	64,000[c]

[a] GlcUA: glucuronic acid; IdUA: iduronic acid; GalN: galactosamine; GlcN: glucosamine; for other abbreviations refer to Table 1.

[b] Determined by sedimentation velocity.

[c] Determined by gel filtration on Sephadex G-200.

least in part, are firmly bound to elastin and CS to collagen. Possibly, GAG are entrapped in the network of collagen and elastin fibers, or the sulfate groups of GAG react with collagen and elastin through Ca^{++}, forming stable complexes.

A HS proteoglycan has recently been isolated from bovine aorta by a sequential digestion of the tissue with 0.15 M NaCl, collagenase, and then elastase. The elastase-solubilized HS PG was purified by CM cellulose chromatography, CsCl density gradient centrifugation, and gel filtration on Sephadex G-200. The chemical and physical properties of the PG are reported in Table 2. Like CS-DS PG, this PG is also a low molecular weight substance. It would be interesting to study the contribution of the protein moiety to biological properties of HS, for example, anticoagulant activity and lipoprotein lipase-releasing activity.

Another important group of carbohydrate macromolecules of the connective tissue are GP. These show much of the properties of proteins but contain covalently bound sialic acid, hexosamines, and neutral sugars. Our laboratory first presented evidence of GP presence in the arterial wall by isolating these proteins from bovine aorta (Berenson and Fishkin, 1962; Radhakrishnamurthy et al., 1964). These GP are soluble in water, can be easily extracted from tissue by 0.15 M NaCl, and precipitated by (NH$_4$)$_2$ SO$_4$ at pH 4.0. Studies by high resolution gel electrophoresis suggested that a family of these proteins are present in cardiovascular connective tissue and vary from individual to individual suggesting an individuality of these proteins in aorta (Berenson et al., 1966). GP isolated from aortas of human, bovine, and ovine identical twins showed identical electrophoretic bands whereas those from nonidentical twins were considerably different (Srinivasan et al., 1971). These GP are highly antigenic and are capable of producing antibodies when injected into rabbits. Other studies to understand the biological role of GP suggested that multiple enzymatic activities such as esterase, phosphatase, and glucuronidase occur in the GP preparations (Dugan et al.,

1967). Wagh (1974) reported that a GP preparation from pig intima inhibited lipoprotein lipase activity from postheparin dog plasma, suggesting an important role for the aorta GP in lipid metabolism.

The chemistry of arterial wall GP is somewhat unique in that these GP contain covalently bound glucose without having hydroxyproline or hydroxylysine as a constituent amino acid. Structures of glycopeptides from highly purified GP were studied (Radhakrishnamurthy and Berenson, 1966, 1973). Each has two different glycopeptides — one has commonly occurring Asp-Glc NH_2 linkage and the other, which contains glucose, has Ser-Gal linkage.

Since studies of GP from aorta are of recent origin, little is known about the changes of specific GP in atherosclerosis although several investigators have reported changes in sugar composition of the aorta (Berenson et al., 1971). Studies now in progress in our laboratory suggest certain changes in the sugar composition of the GP from atherosclerotic lesions (Table 3). Although lesser amounts of total GP were obtained from fatty streaks than from controls and fibrous plaques, relatively smaller amounts of sugars are present in fibrous plaques than in other tissues. Figure 1 illustrates gel electrophoretic patterns of GP from the lesions. Both qualitative and quantitative changes in GP in lesions may be observed. It is, however, premature to interpret these observations other than to note that marked changes are occurring in soluble glycoproteins in atherosclerotic lesions.

These studies indicate a very complex nature of the connective tissue composition of the arterial wall. Further appreciation of the importance of these macromolecules in normal tissue is needed to understand their role in the disease process.

Table 3. Carbohydrate composition of glycoproteins (GP)[a] from human atherosclerotic lesions and normal intima

Lesion[b]		Total GP mg/g tissue	Carbohydrate composition			
			Total hexoses	Sialic acid	Hexosamine	Fucose
Fibrous plaques	I	1.74	37.0	51.4	40.5	5.7
	II	1.83	32.3	46.1	38.9	5.0
Fatty streaks	I	0.65	86.6	143.2	101.5	7.2
	II	0.35	119.8	160.3	236.4	12.9
	III	0.41	65.4	88.3	109.9	11.6
Normal intima	I	1.25	91.9	165.2	266.0	12.0
	II	1.47	77.1	127.4	165.8	7.4

[a]Glycoproteins were isolated by a previously described procedure (Walford and Kickhöfen, 1961).

[b]Tissues were pooled for replicate isolations.

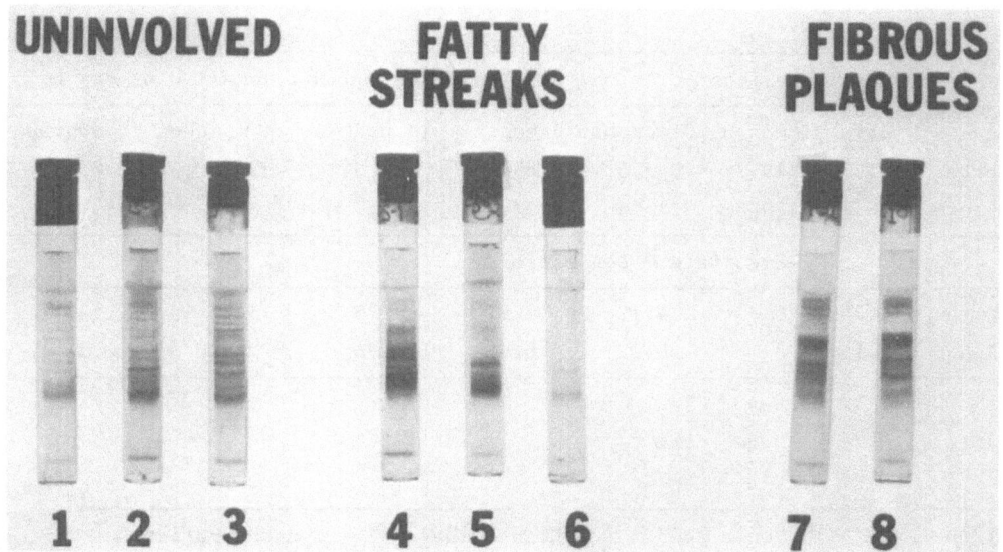

Figure 1. Polyacrylamide gel electrophoretic patterns of glycoproteins from human atherosclerotic lesions and uninvolved intima. Coomassie blue stain. Numbers refer to separate isolations. Both qualitative and quantitative differences are apparent

NEW RESULTS ON GAG AND COLLAGEN IN ATHEROSCLEROSIS

J. Lindner, K. Grasedyck, and B. Schütte

Specified stains demonstrate glycosaminoglycans (GAG) in examples (not in press) in the arterial (vascular) intima and media around the elastic network, often enhanced below the lamina elastica interna. The increased intensity of these widely validated GAG stains is often correlated with an increased labeling in autoradiograms — also of human atherosclerotic arteries (biopsy materials) — in, around, and between the arterial smooth muscle cells within the first 2 hours after the start of in vitro (or experimental in vivo) incorporation of the best suited radioactive-labeled precursors ($35S$-sulfate is most frequently used for review, see Lindner, 1969). The $35S$-sulfate incorporation rates and the specific activities of sulfated GAG decline exponentially during maturation and additionally, at a higher age, the DNA content, but only in certain life periods of rats (as of humans). But both GAG metabolic parameters ($35S$-sulfate incorporation and specific activities) decline only partially in relation to the DNA content of aorta (as compared to skin; Table 1).

The same is mostly true in progressive stages or lesions of atherosclerosis. The aorta shows (in comparison to skin, but also to rib cartilage) the highest $35S$-sulfate incorporation rate in relation to the DNA content because smooth muscle cells constitute more than 90% of the total cell content of rat aorta and, therefore, partly possess a higher GAG synthesis capacity than chondro- or fibroblasts (Lindner, 1972).

Results with rats are similar to those with humans. This comparison between ageing and atherosclerosis is important! Table 2 shows the significant increase of the total hydroxyproline contents of the aorta from 3 – 18-month-old rats (also until the 3rd year as in ageing human arteries) in contrast to the skin and the

Table 1

	35S-sulfate incorporation, rat (in vitro 0.1 µCi; cpm/100 mg dry wt						
Age	9 days	1 month	3 months	6 months	12 months	24 months	36 months
Aorta	2701.2	1219.7	963.5	787.1	445.8	337.4	323.6
Skin	6630.1	4439.3	3115.1	1217.4	1218.7	1185.6	1197.4
	35S-sulfate — DNA ratio						
Aorta	4.30		4.12	3.91	3.75	3.71	2.22
Skin	1.11		0.92	0.98	0.94	0.89	0.85

Table 2

Organ rat	Uronic acid (mg/g dry wt)			Hexosamine (mg/g dry wt)			Hydroxyproline (mg/g dry wt)		
Months	3	6	18	3	6	18	3	6	18
Aorta	3.51	2.69	3.58	3.15	2.74	3.27	51.26	52.84	63.16
Skin	1.28	0.93	0.91	2.14	2.16	1.62	109.83	109.83	98.56
Liver	1.16	0.65	1.08	1.62	1.99	2.32	0.69	0.64	1.08

Underlined values: $p < 0.01$, 3 – 18 months.

liver. The hexosamine contents of skin decrease, those of the liver increase significantly; the uronic acid contents of the skin also decrease with ageing; but not the uronic acid contents of the rat aorta (Table 2).

The fact is very important, especially since the uronic acid and hexosamine contents significantly decline in relation to the DNA content in the aorta as in orhter organs. Furthermore, the ^{3}H-thymidine incorporation rates related to the DNA content decrease in aorta, skin, and liver with ageing (Table 3). That means that the uronic acid and hexosamine contents, as well as the ^{3}H-thymidine incorporation rates, are reduced in relation to the single cell with ageing. That finally means that the productivities of the older connective tissue cells of connective as well as of parenchymatous organs are diminished with ageing.

Table 3

Organ rat	Uronic acid DNA			Hexosamine DNA			^{3}H-thymidine DNA		
Months	3	6	18	3	6	18	3	16	18
Aorta	0.564	0.505	0.479	0.504	0.514	0.437	6.35	3.89	2.71
Skin	0.287	0.226	0.173	0.480	0.525	0.308	7.74	7.98	2.79
Liver	0.114	0.044	0.104	0.158	0.133	0.224	0.43	0.27	0.18

Underlined values: $p < 0.01$, 3 – 18 months.

Table 4

Organ rat	Uronic acid Hydroxyproline			Hexosamine Hydroxyproline		
Months	3	6	18	3	6	18
Aorta	0.049	0.050	0.056	0.061	0.052	<u>0.052</u>
Skin	0.012	0.008	0.009	0.019	0.019	0.016

Underlined values: $p < 0.01$, 3 - 18 months.

Table 4 shows no alteration in the uronic acid-hydroxyproline ratio, while the hexosamine-hydroxyproline ratio only declines significantly in the aorta of 3 - 18-month-old rats! The importance and consequences of these findings, especially for the onset and progression of atherosclerosis in the course of life, should be discussed. The same is true for the significant decline of the hexosamine-hydroxyproline ratio of the human aorta, for the reduction of the hexosamine content, and for the significant increase of the hydroxyproline content with ageing, as is to be found, for example, in advanced and complicated stages of human atherosclerosis (these and the following Figs. are not in press). We found in fresh atherosclerotic edema plaques of human aorta a higher hexosamine content than the uronic acid content in any age group! These findings depend on the increased serum glycoprotein content in edema plaques as compared to morphologically unchanged parts of the same human aorta. The serum albumin content is higher in intima than in media and higher than the globulin content in every atherosclerotic stage. These are results of quantitative assays of native tissue sections, carried out with the so-called ring test dilution method. The uronic acid and hydroxyproline contents increase during the development of atheroma and decrease partly in complicated lesions, but the uronic acid, hexosamine, and elastin contents mostly decrease, while the collagen contents increase.

The special arterial function of GAG synthesis is highest in fresh atherosclerotic edematous plaques, also in older age groups, compared with unchanged parts of the same human aorta. The values are higher in the intima than in the media. The oxygen consumption runs parallelly. The GAG synthesis increases immediately in fresh atherosclerotic lesions with enhanced serum content by disturbed permeability as the first arterial reaction to every kind of injury (Lindner et al., 1967).

Disturbances, mostly enhancements of the proteoglycan and of the GAG metabolism respectively are the first immediate and very sensitive reactions of the arterial wall to the manifold and various irritations and injuries. The first part of this uniform immediate reaction seems to be the increase of the ^{35}S-sulfate incorporation rates and the enhanced synthesis of sulfated GAG. This has been proved by many authors (for review, see Lindner, 1974). But we do not know exactly if the synthesis of the sulfate-free hyaluronic acid (HA) is also increased. Buddecke and Kresse (1973) found that HA has the highest turnover rates of the GAG in calf aorta. The turnover rates of the following three sulfated GAG were lower, decreasing in the order dermatant sulfate (DS), heparan sulfate (HS), and chondroitin sulfate (CS).

At present, it is not precisely clear whether an increase of GAG breakdown occurs earlier than the enhancement of GAG synthesis, e.g., in inflammation and other pathologic (or immediate!) reactions of several connective tissues. In most cases, an increase of degradation occurs in the beginning, followed immediately by an enhanced synthesis. It thereby yields a higher turnover level than before (for review, see Lindner, 1972b). But the GAG degrading enzymes have been insufficiently investigated in the different stages, lesions, and processes of atherosclerosis — often with contradictory results due to the different relations. The best point of reference for enzyme activities is the cell content, especially in tissues with homogenous (e.g. cartilage) or nearly homogenous (e.g. rat aorta) cell populations (Lindner, 1974). GAG and collagen-degrading enzymes decrease moderately in relation to the cell content at a higher age. The same is true for GAG and collagen synthesis enzyme activities (e.g., sulfotransferases, PPH and PLH). But some authors found an increase of some GAG-degrading enzymes and some unspecific proteolytic enzyme activities in cattle aorta (Kresse et al., 1974) and the same result as in cartilage of guinea pigs (Silberberg et al., 1970) and rats or in some other connective tissues of rats (Lindner, 1972a). It is, therefore, important to point out: 1) the differences between species and 2) the possibilities of increase, decrease, or constancy of cell performances during the life course in the investigation of atherosclerosis.

Regarding the synergistic collagen breakdown and using the collagen peptidase as an indicator enzyme, we again found the highest enzyme activity in the smooth muscle tissues of esophagus and intestinum compared to other kinds of connective tissues and organs (Lindner et al., 1971). The highest turnover rates and ^{3}H-thymidine labeling indices of smooth muscle cells are postnatally in the gut and much lower in arteries (with differences) decreasing during maturation. The cell content of aorta seems to be nearly constant during the life of man, rat, and mouse until the senium. Then the cell contents decrease in the aorta as in other connective tissues (Lindner, 1972a, b, 1974). The PPH activity of the aorta, partly used as indicator enzyme for collagen synthesis, is highest in early age, in the phase of early growth, and declines significantly with maturation and ageing, when the aorta and body weight increase (Table 5). The collagen turnover is again highest in the smooth muscle cell organs, the esophagus and aorta (in this order), in comparison to skin (and other organs), especially during the 1st to 12th month of life (rats). At the time, we differentiated four collagen types. The usual and simple (mainly distributed) collagen type I (of bone, skin, tendons, and other connective tissues, arterial ones included) possesses two identical $\alpha 1$ (I) chains and one nonidentical $\alpha 2$ chain. Collagen type II is the typical cartilage collagen, with three identical $\alpha 1$ (II) chains. Collagen type III is composed of three identical $\alpha 1$ (III) chains and collagen type IV (the basement membrane collagen, divided into three subgroups until now) is composed of three identical $\alpha 1$ (IV) chains. Collagen type III is typical of cardiovascular tissues, of embryonic and postembryonic new formation of connective tissues (= repair), also in arteries, and is identical with reticulin. The collagen type IV is typical of the several kinds of basement membranes of capillaries, epithelia, etc., with composition differences, also in ageing, larger arteries included.

The summary of own results and the literature is: the synthesis, degradation, total contents, and turnover of GAG and collagen increase in early and mostly decrease in advanced atherosclerotic lesions, while their half-life times are to the contrary! The total content of insoluble collagen increases in advanced atherosclerotic lesions, whereas the elastin content decreases! Progressive lesions show generally similar metabolic rates as aged arterial connective tissues, partly dependent on the decreased cell content. The functionally adequate high synthesis, degradation, and turnover rates of GAG and collagen decrease, and their half-life times increase with ageing as in advanced atherosclerotic lesions. But the water contents remain more or less constant during these metabolic processes of the connective tissue macromolecules of the aorta as of some other connective tissue organs of man or rat with ageing (Table 6) (Kewitsch, 1977). That is important and in opposition to earlier opinions (for review, see Lindner, 1972b).

Summary

The best validated histochemical stain methods localize, but do not sufficiently quantify and specify the several GAG. Increased intensities of GAG stains in fresh early atherosclerotic lesions can depend on enhanced GAG contents but also

Table 5

Age	Body weight (g)	Aorta weight (g)	PPH activity	
5 weeks	93.18 ± 7.44	0.111 ± 0.021	25.0 ± 6.2	
4 months	378.30 ± 17.76	0.254 ± 0.025	9.8 ± 1.3	$p < 0.01$
25 months	450.83 ± 51.05	0.315 ± 0.063	4.5 ± 0.7	$p < 0.01$

PPH activity of rat aorta at different ages (dpm x 10^{-3}/mg N); similar results were obtained when the PPH activity was related to the protein content, but also on intestinal smooth muscle tissue (compared to the heart).

Age	1.5	12	23 months
Intestine	1931.4 ± 480.1	811.6 ± 542.6	445.5 ± 245.4
Heart	1435.4 ± 530.9	1212.2 ± 338.9	855.1 ± 141.0 (dpm/mg protein)

Table 6. Water content (%)

Age (months)	3		6		12		18		22	31
Rat	♂	♀	♂	♀	♂	♀	♂	♀	♀	♀
Aorta	69.7	68.3	72.1	72.2	66.4	67.3	65.1	70.9	64.1	
Back skin	62.1	60.3	60.5	62.4	56.7	54.2	56.0	61.2	57.6	43.4
Rib. cart.	45.8	33.0	44.9	38.6	36.4	46.8	51.7	41.5	42.3	40.0
Xiph. cart.	55.3	52.5	51.4	46.8	46.0	57.9	61.8	48.3		

Age (years) Human	Aorta ♂	♀	Skin ♂	♀	Xiph. cart. ♂	♀
0 - 15	74.24	74.68	70.08	69.14		69.07
16 - 49	74.32	75.57	68.75	7.55	66.40	62.79
50 - 64	74.22	73.27	68.45	62.42	62.87	57.79
65 - 69	70.99	73.56	68.00	70.42	63.53	63.15
70 - 74	73.16		71.78		62.25	
75 - 79	72.02	73.78	66.99	69.12	61.44	59.01
80 - 84	70.79	74.78	68.60	69.92	63.22	61.70
85 - 89	72.88	73.58	68.65		56.53	

on alterations of their polymerization and sulfatation patterns, on changed macromolecular structures, organizations, and interactions of the GAG and proteoglycans, especially in the case of decomposition and increased degradation with decrease of bindings of proteoglycans and GAG with proteins, lipoproteins, phospholipids, and other macromolecules in early as well as in advanced atherosclerotic lesions. In all these cases, more anionic groups of GAG become available for reactions with cationic stains. Their intensifications are sometimes correlated with increased GAG breakdown, localized histochemically in smooth muscle cells, e.g., by indicator enzymes like β-glucuronidase, with enhanced activities quantified by biochemical analysis (especially in early lesions), like hexosaminidase, and also other key enzymes of GAG degradation.

The increased intensity of GAG stains is often correlated with the enhanced ^{35}S-sulfate incorporation, synthesis, and turnover rates of GAG, localized auto-radiographically in and around smooth muscle cells, especially quantified by usual methods, and with fractionation of sulfated (and nonsulfated) GAG.

These anabolic processes of GAG metabolism are enhanced more in earlier and less in advanced atherosclerotic lesions, are higher in the intima (than in the media), and highest in fresh edema plaques in every age group, running parallelly to the content of serum components. The GAG metabolism of the arterial wall shows the first, immediate, and most sensitive reaction to any arterial irritation, influence, injury etc., followed secondarily by disturbed collagen, elastin, lipid, and coagulation metabolism. The initial part of this first reaction of the disturbed GAG metabolism seems to be an enhanced catabolism, followed immediately by an increased synthesis of GAG. Their concentration can, therefore, be reduced in early and enhanced in advanced atherosclerotic lesions and finally reduced again in comparison to the increased collagen (and decreased elastin) content in complicated lesions.

FUNCTIONAL RELATIONS AMONG CELLS AND FIBERS OF THE AORTIC MEDIA: MICROANATOMIC AND BIOSYNTHETIC FINDINGS *

Seymour Glagov, John M. Clark, Donald Y.M. Leung, and Martin B. Mathews

Decreasing distensibility of the aorta with increasing intraluminal pressure was first observed nearly a century ago. Investigators have since used increasingly standardized preparations and refined measuring methods to provide precise quantitative data with regard to the relative roles of elastin, collagen, and smooth muscle cells in determining the shape of the distensibility curves under both static and dynamic conditions. Morphologic studies and measurements of rabbit aortas fixed while distended over a range of pressures permitted us to develop an initial three-dimensional picture of aortic medial structural organization consistent with its static mechanical properties. At distending pressures well below diastolic values, elastin fibers are wavy, collagen fibers seem to be distributed randomly, and cells appear to be disposed more or less radially between the wavy elastin lamellae. With increasing pressure, a different pattern emerged as the fibers straightened. At physiologic pressures, elastin appeared as a more or less circumferentially oriented network whose component fibers condensed at regular intervals across the wall to form relatively compact straight lamellae. Collagen fibers appeared to be oriented circumferentially among the elastin fibers. The aorta was most distensible at low pressures when elastin fibers were being straightened, became less distensible as collagen fibers became oriented in the direction of stretch, and was least distensible at and above systolic pressures when most of the relatively inextensible collagen fibers were drawn taught.

Though the precise nature of attachment and interconnection among aortic medial components was not entirely clear, the intimate association of similarly oriented fibers of different elastic modulus within a continuous matrix can be expected to provide definite adaptive advantages. These include a media of relatively high tensile strength (collagen) in the presence of an extensible network of elastin for distributing stresses uniformly and minimizing the propaga-

---

*The work was supported in part by grants HL 5654 and HL 17648-IHD-SCOR of the USPHS, and by a grant-in-aid from the Fenger Memorial Research Fund at the University of Chicago. The work by Drs. J.M. Clark and D.Y.M. Leung was done during the tenure of Medical Scientists Training Program Traineeships (PHS Training Grant 5 TO5 GMO1939, NIGMS).

tion of structural flaws. In such a system, regulation of the relative proportions of collagen, elastin, and cells could determine the compliance of the media in relation to segmental mechanical stimuli. Finally, the thickness of the
aortic layers in comparable locations was found to be remarkably independent of
species and the number of layers across the media in adult mammals was shown to
be proportional to radius. This finding indicated that the accretion of medial
layers represented an orderly stepwise adaptation of mammalian aortar to the increased tangential stress associated with increased size.

Our most recent microanatomic studies of aortas fixed *in situ* by controlled pressure perfusion have been enhanced by the application of scanning electron microscopy (SEM) to freeze fractured vessels. Several new concepts of medial organization and adaptive modeling have emerged and place increased emphasis on the
smooth muscle cell. At physiologic pressures, smooth muscle cells are elongated,
fusiform, parallel elements with adjacent cells closely overlapping and very
nearly parallel to their adjacent elastin lamellae. Carefully oriented thin
transverse sections (i.e., radial sections perpendicular to the direction of
flow) reveal that aortic elastin "lamellae" actually consist of two populations
of elastin bars, one on each side of a cell layer. The lamellae themselves are
sets of interconnected bars which are very well-demonstrated by SEM, especially
when cells and collagen have been removed by autoclaving. In addition, in such
preparations, groups of branching bars with slightly different orientations can
be perceived as one examines superimposed layers by looking through the wall.
Tangential or oblique sections of intact walls reveal that each of these slightly different branching elastin bar systems bracket similarly oriented groups of
parallel cells which form subgroups within each call layer. These subgroups are
emphasized in longitudinal sections (i.e., radial sections through the wall in
the direction of flow), and we have called them *musculoelastic fascicles*, for
they appear to be distributed in accordance with presumed medial patterns of
stress.

Collagen appears in two organizational forms: as relatively large undulating
bundles, mainly between the successive elastin-cell-elastin modules which make
up the aortic media and in more pervasive sheets of fibers often closely associated with basal lamina. The interlamellar bundles are coils of large pitch within which adjacent fibrils often have similar orientation and show morphologic
evidence of coordinated function. Bands of adjacent fibrils are aligned with one
another and with intervening microfibrils. Microfibrils also appear to form a
diffuse and continuous lattice over the surface of collagen bundles, elastin
bars, and basal lamina surfaces. The more diffuse sheets of collagen fibrils are
also oriented over the surfaces of smooth muscle cells and are seen to penetrate
the basal lamina. The functional significance of an extensive collagen-basal
lamina-microfibrillar matrix is suggested by two findings. First, the cellular
subgroups or fascicles delineated by their associated elastin systems are also
invested by a common underlying sleeve of basal lamina in which collagen fibrils
often fill gaps among cells. Secondly, where smooth muscle cell dense bodies are
in close contact with elastin, the basal lamina is thickened, the cell membrane
is more dense, and small fibrils are visible darkening the clear zone of the
basal lamina. When such sites were stressed by hyperdistention, cell projections
terminating in dense bodies were drawn out and remained attached to the elastin.
Hyperdistention followed by collapse before fixation caused these junctions to
spread apart. These consistently contained basal lamina, collagen fibrils, and
microfibrils oriented in parallel with the myofilaments passing through the related dense body. We may, therefore, conclude, for the time being, that for each
musculoelastic fascicle, mechanical coupling among cells and between cells and
elastin is accomplished by way of the diffuse basal lamina-collagen-microfibril-
lar net and its focal cell to elastin reinforcement at peripheral dense bodies.

Thus, the immediately apparent structural layers of aortic medial organization
have proced on further analysis to be elastin-cell-elastin modules with intervening collagen bundles (Fig. 1). Within these nodules, the actual unit of structure and function appears to be the relatively compact cellular subgroup and its

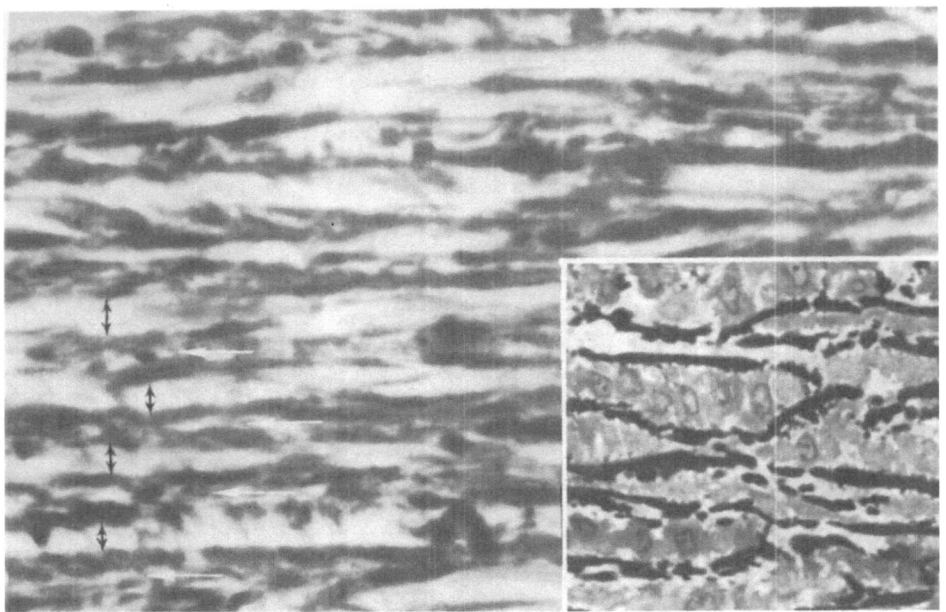

Figure 1. Transverse section of thoracic aortic media of an adult pig. The vessel was fixed while distended by an intraluminal pressure of 100 mm Hg. The media is composed of smooth muscle cell layers bounded on each side by elastin bars. These elastin-cell-elastin modules (black vertical arrows) are separated by bundles of collagen fibers (horizontal white arrows). Each of the cell layers is composed of subgroups, which are better seen on longitudinal or oblique sections (insert)

encompassing elastin system. The more extensive basal lamina-collagen net provides cohesion and mechanical coupling among the cells and between the cells and elastin. Under normal conditions, the size, shape, orientation, and number of aortic musculoelastic fascicles appears to be related to vessel geometry. Fascicles are shortest and most numerous about curves and branches where vessels are changing direction and cells are elongated in the direction of stress. In straight aortic segments, away from branches, especially in small animals, single fascicles are longer and may encircle the entire wall.

These anatomical considerations provide strong documentation for the common sense supposition that the organization, composition, and modeling of arotic medial connective tissues normally correspond to the mechanical stresses imposed on smooth muscle cells by distending pressure, blood flow, and vessel geometry. Direct evidence that mechanical stresses may normally regulate fibrous protein synthesis by smooth muscle cell is not so strong. Two new studies from our laboratories have recently provided some useful quantitative data in this regard. The first is a comparison of the chemical composition of the ascending aorta (AA) with that of the pulmonary trunk (PT) in growing rabbits. These vessel segments are nearly identical in length, radius, and dry weight at birth. Length and radius remain the same for the segments during growth, but the dry weight of the AA increases much more rapidly than that of the PT as pressure rises in the systemic circulation and falls in the pulmonic. Absolute quantities of elastin, collagen, and DNA are also the same for the two segments at birth, but by 2 months the AA contains five times as much elastin and twice as much collagen as the PT. DNA content increases in both vessels but at the same rate for each. Thus, the average synthesis per cell of fibrous protein, especially of elastin, is far greater in the AA than in the PT. This difference in cell response corresponds closely to the progressive divergence in estimated total tension for the two vessels during growth. These data suggest that cell proliferation in these segments during growth is independent of medial tension but that each cell is capable of a wide range of synthetic response which may be elicited by medial stress.

In the second study, rabbit aortic smooth muscle cells were cultured on purified elastin membranes prepared by autoclaving slices of bovine aorta. The cells remained attached to the membranes which were then subjected to cyclic stretching or agitated without stretching by means of a special motor assembly coupled to an incubator. Each experiment was conducted with a stationary control. Stretching or agitation was carried out for 2 days; radioactive precursors were then added and the experiments continued for 8 additional hours. Protein and collagen synthesis was measured by [^{14}C]-proline incorporation into proline and hydroxyproline. Mucopolysaccharide synthesis was measured by [^{3}H]-acetate incorporation into several fractions. DNA synthesis was measured by incorporation of [^{3}H]-thymidine. The cyclically stretched preparations incorporated [^{14}C]-proline into protein three to five times more rapidly and into hydroxyproline four to five times more rapidly than did stationary controls, but there was no difference in [^{3}H]-thymidine incorporation into DNA. Cells subjected to agitation without stretching incorporated [^{14}C]-proline into protein only one and one-fifth to two times more rapidly and into hydroxyproline only one and one-fifth to one and one-half times more rapidly than did stationary cultures but resulted in a nearly twofold increase in [^{3}H]-thymidine uptake. Synthesis of type I and type III collagen was increased to the same degree by stretching. Incorporation of [^{3}H]-acetate into hyalaronate and chondroitin-6-sulfate was increased threefold by stretching as compared to controls but there was no effect of stretching on incorporation into chondroitin-4-sulfate or dermatan sulfate. Agitation caused no significant difference in incorporation into any of these fractions as compared to stationary controls. These data provide direct evidence that cells can indeed respond to mechanical stimulation by synthesizing structural proteins.

In summary then, aortic medial cells and fibers are normally organized into distinct functional subunits which we have called musculoelastic fascicles. These are oriented, distributed, and their components apparently synthesized in conformity with the level and presumed distribution of mechanical stresses. In culture, aortic smooth muscle responds to mechanical stimulation with increased matrix component synthesis. All of these interesting avenues merit further detailed exploration. Characterization of the effects of amplitude, frequency, and wave form of mechanical stresses on arterial architecture and on the proliferative and synthetic capacity of smooth muscle cells in vivo and in vitro should provide a basis for quantitating medial adaptations to mechanical requirements under a variety of hormonal and metabolic conditions. Such data could help clarify the nature of medial connective tissue changes with accompany arterial disease and aging and could help to illuminate the relative significance of cell proliferation, fibrogenesis, and connective tissue organization and modeling in the development and regression of atherosclerotic plaques.

ABSTRACTS

EFFECTS OF VITAMIN C ON COLLAGEN AND ELASTIC CONCENTRATIONS OF AORTAE AND CORONARY ARTERIES OF MINIATURE PIGS FED AN ATHEROGENIC DIET

Harry Y.C. Wong, Stephen W. Chan, Eugene Miller, and Theodore R. Farber
Department of Physiology, Howard University, College of Medicine, and Food and
Drug Administration Division of Toxicology, Washington, WA/USA

We have studied the effects of large doses of Vitamin C on hydroxyproline concentrations (HP) on collagen (C) and elastin (E) changes in the aortae (A) and coronary arteries (CA) of pigs fed an atherogenic diet (AD) consisting of 6% cholesterol + 15% lard added to stock ration (SR). After 105 days the following were
obtained: 1. Vit. C had no marked effect on C, E or the ratio of collagen to
elastin (C/E) of the thoracic or abdominal aorta; and 2. In the CA, there were
no significant changes in the HP of collagen in any of the groups. The HP of E
was significantly lower in the AD + Vit. C group when compared to the group on an
AD only or the group on SR + Vit. C. The C/E ratio showed that there were no
marked differences in the control groups. The ratio of the AD + Vit. C pigs was
the highest of all the groups, and it was significantly increased when compared
to the group on AD only. The C/E ratio of the SR + Vit. C group was elevated as
compared to the AD group. Conclusion: The administration of Vit. C increased the
C/E ratio of the CA of pigs on an AD diet when compared to the AD controls which
suggests increase rigidity of the arteries. Based on the results of this study,
the impact of Vit. C on the pathogenesis of atherosclerosis should be further
investigated. (Supported by NIH grants #RRO8016 and 1-TO-2-GM-05010-01 (MARC)).

EFFECT OF PAPAIN ON ACID MUCOPOLYSACCHARIDES AND CHOLESTEROL CONTENTS OF AORTA AND RENAL PAPILLA IN RAT

Gosuke Inoue, Hyoei Yasuda, and Masaki Yoshikawa
Department of Geriatrics, Faculty of Medicine, University of Tokyo, Tokyo/Japan

Male Wister rats weighing 200-250 g were injected intraperitoneally with 1-3 mg/
0.1 kg body weight of papain in a 0.03 M cysteine solution. After 24 hours, the
aorta and the kidneys were obtained and analysed for acid mucopolysaccharides and
cholesterol contents of aortic wall and the renal papilla.
Insoluble collagen was employed as reference base. Significant decrease in acid
mucopolysaccharides and the rather large loss of cholesterol have been observed
by papain treatment in both tissues. Analysis of acid mucopolysaccharides composition revealed that not only chondroitin sulfates but also hyaluronic acid
were decreased by papain injection.
The results suggest that changes in acid mucopolysaccharides contents and compositions may affect the binding capacity of lipoprotein, resulting decreased concentration of cholesterol in these regions.

INTERACTION OF COLLAGEN TYPES WITH PLATELETS AND TRANSFORMATION OF COLLAGEN TYPE SYNTHESIS IN HUMAN ATHEROSCLEROSIS

Steffen Gay and Leopold Balleisen
Max-Planck-Institut für Biochemie München/Martinsried and I. Medizinische Universitätsklinik, München/BRD

Recent studies have established that connective tissue contains several chemically and genetically distinct collagens. Using immunohistochemical methods with

isolated typespecific antibodies the distribution of type I and type III collagens was investigated. Type III is mainly located in the subendothelium layer and in the media. Comparative investigations on the influence of collagen types I, II and III on the aggregation of human platelets demonstrate, that collagen type III is a particularly potent inducer of platelet aggregation. The results indicate, that in endothelial lesions the uncovered type III comes contact with blood platelets, resulting in a local platelet aggregation. Further studies demonstrated, that in early stages of intima fibrosis in atherosclerosis the fibrotic plaques contain mainly type III. This type III collagen predominates in those areas where lipids are deposited. In contrast, older atherosclerotic scars contain mainly type I collagen, probably because of the increased rate of type I synthesis.

COMPOSITIONAL DIFFERENCE OF ACIDIC GLYCOSAMINOGLYCANS IN ARTERIAL TISSUES: THEIR PHYSIOLOGICAL PROPERTIES AGAINST ATHEROSCLEROSIS

Koji Nakazawa and Katsumi Murata
Department of Medicine and Physical Therapy, University of Tokyo School of Medicine, Tokyo/Japan

Difference of the composition of acidic glycosaminoglycans (AGAG) in the intima, media and adventitia of human and bovine aortae was estimated by enzymatic analyses with chondroitinases and hyaluronidase, together with electrophoretic characterization and other chemical analyses. Their physiological properties were measured as follows: For anticoagulant activity by thrombelastography and partial thrombin time in occasion; for antithrombogenic property by thrombus formation time and thrombus weight. Analytical data indicated that the three layers contain chondroitin 4-sulfate, chondroitin 6-sulfate, dermatan sulfate (DS), heparan sulfates (HS) and hyaluronic acid. The proportion of DS and HS was increased in order from the intima to the adventitia.
The anticoagulant and anti-thrombogenic properties of the aortic AGAG clearly indicated that the AGAG in the adventitia posses the highest potency among three layers. The higher activity of the AGAG is considered to relate with greater proportion of HS and DS. Increased physiological properties of the AGAG in venous tissue were similarly related with increased amounts of DS and HS. The present results indicated that certain AGAG in vessel wall play a role in the process of atherosclerosis based on their anticoagulant and anti-atherosclerotic functions.

ACIDIC GLYCOSAMINOGLYCANS IN HUMAN CEREBRAL ARTERIAL TISSUE

Katsumi Murata and Koji Nakazawa
Department of Medicine and Physical Therapy, University of Tokyo School of Medicine, Tokyo/Japan

A stroke has been reported as the main disease with the highest mortality caused by vascular lesions in Japan. By multiple functions, vascular acidic glycosaminoglycans (AGAG) were indicated to play a role in atherosclerotic process. The constitution of the AGAG, therefore, in human cerebral arteries was studied using 45 samples by the electrophoretic characterization before and after enzymatic digestion with chondroitinase. The AGAG in coronary arteries were included in the study. The composition of chondroitin sulfate (CS) isomers was determined qualitatively based on the disaccharide subunits of CS chains after the depolymerization. The data indicated that AGAG in these arteries were composed of C-4S, C-6S, dermatan sulfate (DS), heparan sulfate (HS) and hyaluronic acid (HA). The proportions of the AGAG, however, were different between the vessels. The AGAG in cerebral arteries were distributed at higher proportion of HS and DS than those in coronary arteries. Existence of oversulfated CS and undersulfated CS in the cerebral AGAG was evidenced enzymatically. In addition, the presence of HA was detected by electrophoretic and enzymatic separations. Distribution of the individual

AGAG in cerebral arteries was also investigated on the basis of molecular weight by gel filtration on a Sephadex column. The possible role of the cerebral AGAG will be discussed in relation with the process of atherosclerosis.

INCREASED COLLAGEN BIOSYNTHESIS IN BLOOD VESSELS OF BRAIN AND OTHER TISSUES OF HYPERTENSIVE RAT

Akira Ooshima and Sidney Udenfriend
Department of Pathology, Faculty of Medicine, Kyoto University, Kyoto/Japan

We have already demonstrated that collagen biosynthesis is elevated in a large artery (aorta) and in arteries of medium caliber (mesenteric arteries) of DOCA-salt and spontaneously hypertensive rats.
We further showed that treatment with antihypertensive drugs (chlorothiazide or reserpine) can prevent or diminish this increase in vascular collagen biosynthesis induced by hypertension. Collagen metobolism was investigated using several parameters of collagen biosynthesis (prolyl hydroxylase activity, total collagen content and the incorporation of ^{14}C-proline into total protein and collagen).
A marked increase in collagen biosynthesis was observed in the brain microvessels, pial artery, basilar artery, circle of Willis and testicular artery of the hypertensive rat. When an antihypertensive drug (reserpine) was administered prior to the onset of hypertension, the increased collagen biosynthesis was prevented. The present findings indicate that there is increased collagen biosynthesis in arterioles and small arteries in the periphery and in the central nervous system of DOCA-salt hypertensive rat and provide an early biochemical indication that fibrogenesis is involved in the production of hypertensive vascular damage (arteriosclerosis).

OCCURRENCE OF TYPE I AND TYPE III COLLAGEN IN NORMAL AND ATHEROSCLEROTIC HUMAN AORTAS

J. Rauterberg and S.S. Allam
Institut für Arterioskleroseforschung (Leiter: Prof. Dr. W.H. Hauss), Münster/BRD

Media and intima of normal and atherosclerotic human aortas were separated and extracted with 8 M urea to remove non-collagenous materials. Collagen could completely be solubilized by cyanogen bromide cleavage, leaving almost pure elastin in the insoluble residue. The resulting mixture of CB-peptides of type I and type III collagen was characterized by polyacrylamide gel electrophoresis.
The collagen in the intima of non-atherosclerotic aortas exhibits a slightly higher proportion of type III than that in the media. As well in the plaques as in the "healthy" surrounding regions of atherosclerotic aortas the total amount of collagen in the intimal layer is increased, whereas the proportion of type III collagen is significantly decreased. On the other hand, the proportion of type III collagen in the media remains unchanged during the atherogenic process.

RELATIONSHIP OF SERUM AMPS AND OF URINE AMPS TO AGE, GLUCOSE TOLERANCE AND AORTIC ARCH CALCIFICATION — STUDIES ON METABOLISM AND EXCRETION OF ACID MUCOPOLYSACCHARIDE IN ARTERIOSCLEROSIS

Takemichi Kanazawa, Tokuya Komatsu, Masahiro Izawa, Toshio Terata, Hideki Mori, Kozi Shibutani, and Vasaburo Oike
2nd Department of Internal Medicine, Hirosaki University School of Medicine (Director; Prof. Y. Oike) Hirosaki/Japan
Hirobumi Metoki and Hisao Ito
Reimeikyo Rehabilitation Hospital (Director; K. Onodera) and Tetsuro Matsui Health Administration Center of Hirosaki University, Hirosaki/Japan

A) Acid mucopolysaccharides (AMPS) in serum and 24-hour urine were measured on 156 cases to investigate the relationship between AMPS and arteriosclerosis. 1) The relationship of the serum AMPS concentration was the same as that of "the young > the aged", "non diabetics ≤ diabetics" and "aortic arch calcification (AAC) (-)≑AAC(+)". 2) The relationship of the 24-hour urine AMPS amount was the same as that of "the young > the aged", "non-diabetics ≑ diabetics" and "AAC(-) ≥AAC(+)". B) Five hundred ml of 20% glucose solution was administered to 128 cases, and 500 ml of water to 13 healthy persons. The AMPS in serum and urine were measured hourly. 1) The patterns of hourly changes of serum as well as of urine AMPS by glucose administration were different from those by water administration. 2) Also, among age level, glucose tolerance and AAC there was found a difference in the pattern of hourly changes of serum as well as of urine AMPS by glucose administration. C) Summary: Age, glucose tolerance and aortic arch calcification have been understood by many investigators as similar factors related to arteriosclerosis. However, from the point of view of metabolism and excretion of AMPS, these three items should be understood as factors related to arteriosclerosis which are different from each other.

CEREBRAL ATHEROSCLEROSIS IN JAPANESE. 5. RELATIONSHIPS BETWEEN ESTERIFIED CHOLESTEROL AND GLYCOSAMINOGLYCANS

Motoomi Nakamura, Yasuhide Nakashima, Katsumi Imaizumi, Hideo Kanaide, and Yutaka Kikuchi
Research Institute of Angiocardiology and Cardiovascular Clinic, Kyushu University Medical School, Fukuoka/Japan

Concentrations of various lipids and glycosaminoglycans (GAG) in the intima of the grossly normal and atherosclerotic cerebral arteries were compared with those of the aorta and coronary arteries. The lowest percentage of esterified cholesterol (EC) in total cholesterol and of chondroitin sulfate-4/6 (CS-4/6) in total GAG, the highest percentage of heparan sulfate (HS) in total GAG are the characteristic feature of the normal intimas of the cerebral artery when compared with those in the aorta and coronary artery. In the cerebral arterial intimas, there was a significant positive correlation between contents of EC(Log EC) and percentage of CS-4/6 but not in the aorta and/or coronary artery. The positive correlation between EC and dermatan sulfate was statistically significant in the aorta and cerebral arteries. To examine the binding capacity of GAG to plasma LDL or HDL, CS and HS were purified from the aorta and cerebral arteries. The binding capacity of CS or HS to plasma HDL was negligible, and of CS to LDL was greater than that of HS in both arteries. The CS from the cerebral arteries which contained DS in greater percentage and CS-4-S in lower percentage in total purified CS, showed a greater binding capacity to LDL when compared with that from the aorta. These result may suggest that DS binds strongly LDL or CS-4-S inhibits the binding of GAG to LDL.

ISOLATION OF A HEPARAN SULFATE PROTEOGLYCAN FROM BOVINE AORTA

Bhandaru Radhakrishnamurthy, Harold Ruiz, and Gerald Berenson
Louisiana State University Medical Center, New Orleans LA/USA

Carbohydrate-protein macromolecules of connective tissues are important in maintenance and structural integrity of cardiovascular (C-V) structures and play a
major role in the pathogenesis of atherosclerosis. Although a great deal of information is available on glycosaminoglycans (GAG) from C-V tissues, little is
known of proteoglycans, GAG in the native state linked to protein. In earlier
studies we isolated and characterized a chondroitin sulfate-dermatan sulfate
proteoglycan from bovine aorta by 3.0 M $MgCl_2$. We have now isolated another,
heparan sulfate (HS) proteoglycan from bovine aorta by a sequential extraction.
Bovine aorta was extracted with 0.15 M NaCl to remove soluble proteoglycans. The
residual tissue was digested with collagenase to solubilize collagen-bound proteoglycans and then hydrolyzed by a highly purified preparation of elastase. The
elastase digest was resolved on a CM-cellulose column into one major and two
minor fractions. The major fraction containing HS proteoglycan was further purified by ultracentrifugation and gel chromatography. The proteoglycan contains
15% protein; 18% uronic acid; 20% hexosamine as glucosamine; a sulfate to hexosamine ratio of 0.76. The amino acid composition shows large amounts of glutamic
acid, aspartic acid, glycine, and alanine, in addition to serine and threonine.
A molecular weight of 60,000 - 70,000 was estimated by gel chromatography. These
studies suggest that HS proteoglycan is firmly bound to elastin in the aorta and
that the HS proteoglycan may play an important role in disease involving elastin
in C-V structures.

TOPOCHEMICAL STUDIES ON GLYCOSAMINOGLYCANS AND LIPIDS IN HUMAN AORTA. A SEVEN LAYERS ASSAY

Moysés A. Hodara
Department of Atherosclerosis Research, Rua Garibaldi, Porto Alegre/Brazil

Eleven 18 to 45 years old males thoracic descending aortas were sliced on a cryo-
mat and grade I atherosclerotic tissue (or posterior wall when grossly normal)
compared with non-atherosclerotic sites (or anterior wall). Results were: 1.
Total acid GAGs decrease from intima to outer media (45-15 to 10-2 μMol uronic
acid/g DDW); 2. Hybrid chondroitin sulfate-dermatan sulfate relative values
continuously decrease from intima to outer media (80-50 to 60-20%), opposite to
heparan sulfate (HS); 3. Concentration of total acid GAGs is usually larger in
atherosclerotic tissue (or posterior wall). Sometimes it is highest in inner
media (layer 2), specially HS; 4. This finding was detected also in non-atherosclerotic sites and was present in four cases with low total lipids values of
layer 2; 5. Hyaluronic acid was strikingly low in eight young cases (less than
2 μMol uronic acid/g DDW) and showed higher values in middle age (37, 37 and 45
years old males); 6. Phospholipids values are highest in intima and mid media
and total cholesterol and triglycerides are higher in intima and decrease continuously towards outer media; 7. Total lipids curves when only layers 3 to 7 are
considered are similar both in atherosclerotic and non-atherosclerotic sites
(50-20 mg/g DDW).

GLYCOSOAMINOGLYCANS COLLAGEN AND ELASTIN OF HUMAN ARTERIAL WALL IN THE COURSE OF DIABETES MELLITUS

Jeremiasz J. Tomaszewski and Janusz A. Hanzlik
Research Center and Medical Department, Medical Academy, Lublin/Poland

The content of glycosoaminoglycans, collagen and elastin in the intima-media layer of aorta in 16 persons died of vascular complications in the course of diabetes mellitus was investigated. As a control the same determinations were performed in 10 patients who died of another couses without any atherosclerotic changes in aorta wall.
In comparison with the control in the group of diabetes increase of hyaluronic acid and decrease of Ch-4-S have been observed. The total GAG content and another their fractions remained unchanged. In the investigated group essential decrease in soluble collagen and increase of insoluble collagen fraction have been stated. Similarely the content of elastin was increased in diabetic aortas as in comparison with the control group.
The results showed that the composition of intima-media of diabetic arterial all indicated essential differences in comparison with unchanged aortic tissue and with these observed in the course of physiological aging.

ULTRASTRUCTURAL STUDIES ON THE HUMAN FETAL AORTA. MORPHOLOGICAL INDICATIONS OF ENDOTHELIAL ELASTOGENESIS

Henrik Klem Thomsen
Department of Clinical Chemistry, Rigshospitalet, Copenhagen/Denmark, and Department of Pathology, Sundby Hospital, Copenhagen/Denmark

The aortas of ten human fetuses of gestation age two to five months obtained by legal abortion were examined. Within minutes after removal from the uterus the aortas were fixed from the adventitial side of the vessel wall by immersion in cold fixative.
The endothelial cells contained abundant narrow cisternas of rough-surfaced endoplasmic reticulum. Small aggregates of young elastic tissue were seen throughout the subendothelial space in close contact with the endothelial basement membrane. The elastic aggregates coalesced to join the internal elastic membrane. Subsequently, the luminal border of the membrane appeared serrated, while the border against media, where no "young" elastic tissue was seen, was quite smooth. Thus, in contrast to earlier investigations, this study indicate, that the fetal, human endothelial cells participate in the formation of the aortic internal elastic membrane.

THE DETERMINATION OF MEDIAL TISSUE ELASTIN OF HUMAN AORTA APPLYING MICROSPECTROPHOTOMETER — WITH REFERENCE TO ATHEROSCLEROSIS AND WALL ELASTICITY (PULSE WAVE VELOCITY, PWV)

Masatake Abe, Takeshi Kawasaki, Yoshinori Aizawa, Yoshihiro Kashiwakura, Chikao Arai, Yoshimasa Yabe, Motoharu Hasegawa, Akiji Tsuzuku and Shozo Yoshimura
The 1st Department of Internal Medicine, Jikei University School of Medicine, Tokyo/Japan
Tsutomu Komazawa and Chikio Hayashi
The Institute of Statistical Mathematics
Shinichi Yagi and Kiyoshi Nakayama
Faculty of Science and Technology, Sophia University, Tokyo/Japan
Shigehiro Kinoshita and Kokichi Takeuchi
The Institute of Arteriosclerosis, Association of Labour's Welfare and Health, Tokyo/Japan

Pathophysiological disorders of medial elastic tissue is inevitable to atherosclerosis. The purpose of this study is to determine the medial elastin by microspectrophotometric procedure (MSP method) and to define the relationship between elastin, wall elasticity and pathological findings of intima in human aorta. (Materials & Method) Aortae were obtained from 70 subjects in which PWV had been measured antemortem. Medial elastin content of the thoracic aorta was determined by MSP method, on the basis of the maximum extinction of the elastin, stained by resorcin-fuchsin is at 590 mμ. The pathological findings of intima such as non-fibrotic thickening (NFT), diffuse fibrotic thickening (DFT), atheromatous plaque (ATP) and calcification (CAL) were examined by the point counting method. (Result)

	NFT	DFT	ATP (-)	ATP (+)	CAL (-)	CAL (+)	PWV m/sec 8>	PWV m/sec 9<	PWV m/sec 7>	PWV m/sec 8	PWV m/sec 9<
Elastin (v/v%)	31.0	24.0	32<	30>	28<	27>	28<	27>			
Atheromatous plaque(%)									0	20-30	31-90

HUMAN AORTIC ELASTIN WITH CHANGES DURING ATHEROGENESIS

Katuhiko Tokita, Kuniaki Kanno, and Kyuhei Ikeda
The 1st Department of Internal Medicine, Tohoku University of Medicine, Sendai/Japan

Elastin was isolated from human thoracic aorta and was incubated with human low density lipoprotein. Elastin from sclerotic area was proved to uptake much more cholesterol than elastin from non-sclerotic area. The incubated elastin was further fractionated on the column of Sephadex G 100. The chromatogram showed two peaks, fraction A with larger molecular weight and fraction B with smaller molecular weight. The ratio of fraction A was higher in the elastin from sclerotic area comparing with the elastin from non-sclerotic area. It was evident that combined cholesterol was mostly co-exist with fraction A and not fraction B. In conclusion, the affinity of elastin from the sclerotic area with cholesterol might be based on the increased ratio of fraction A in such elastin preparations.

HUMAN AORTA ELASTASE. PURIFICATION, PROPERTIES AND EFFECT OF AGE AND ATHEROSCLEROSIS

L. Robert, W. Hornebeck and J.C. Derouette
Laboratoire Biochimie du Tissu Conjonctif, Faculté Médicine Université Paris-Val de Marne, Créteil/France

A procedure was described for the isolation and purification of a new elastinolytic enzyme from pig and human aortas (FEBS Letters 58, 66, 1975). It has a molecular weight of 23500 daltons, is inhibited by DFP and crossreacts with a rabbit antiserum to pig pancreatic elastase. It differs however from this enzyme by its reaction to various synthetic and natural specific substrates (K-elastin, succinyl-Triala-p. nitrophenyl ester) and inhibitors (α_1-antitrypsin and α_2-macroglobulin).

Using a new technique to quantify elastase on K-elastin gels, we have shown that such an elastinolytic activity is present in the adventitia, the media and the intima of human aortas (C.R. Acad. Sci. 278, 3251, 1974). This activity increases with age and with the degree of the arteriosclerosis. These two factors are independant and additive and could explain the fragmentation and lysis of the elastic fibers with age and its acceleration in atherosclerosis.

EFFECT OF ELASTASE ON SERUM AND AORTIC LIPOPROTEINS IN CHOLESTEROL-FED RABBITS

Tomio Kametani, Kosei Ueda, Toshihiro Haba, Seigo Ito, Junji Koizumi, Masayuki Oota, Susumu Miyamoto, Hiroshi Mabuchi, and Ryoyu Takeda
The 2nd Department of Internal Medicine, Kanazawa University, Kanazawa/Japan

The influence of elastase on serum and aortic lipoproteins in 1% cholesterol-fed rabbits was investigated. Elastase was injected (4 mg/rabbit/day) i.m. into 8 cholesterol-fed rabbits for 12 weeks. Marked hypercholesterolemia and atherosclerosis were produced by cholesterol-feeding. The serum cholesterol, VLDL-cholesterol levels and VLDL-apoproteins were significantly lower in elastase-treated rabbits than in the control rabbits (P 0.05). The mean triglyceride and LDL-cholesterol levels were lower in elastase-treated rabbits, but statistically insignificant. VLDL- and LDL-cholesterol contents in the aortic intima and media significantly increased in the cholesterol-fed rabbits. However, elastase produced no definite changes in the VLDL- and LDL-cholesterol contents of the aorta. These data suggest that elastase may reduce the hypercholesterolemia through the decrease of VLDL-cholesterol level, but may not produce a definite effect on atherogenesis in the severe hypercholesterolemic rabbits produced by 1% cholesterol-feeding.

III
Regression of Atherosclerosis

ANIMAL MODELS OF REGRESSION

R.W. Wissler and D. Vesselinovitch

Introduction

In this brief review, some of the current evidence that advanced atherosclerotic plaques in various species can undergo substantial regression will be considered. We will attempt to compare and contrast the various animal models that have been utilized in these types of studies. The main objective will be to provide a useful appraisal of the advantages and the disadvantages of each model.

By way of introduction, Table 1 gives a brief summary of some of the evidence that supports the assumption that atherosclerosis is at least partially reversible in human subjects. This has not generally been considered to be possible because this chronic disease process develops over a long period of time and is characterized by pathologic changes that are generally considered to be irreversible, i.e., *collagen-rich scar tissue* encapsulating a large area of *necrosis* and often accompanied by *calcification*. Can these plaques really undergo regression?

This table offers a selected list of some of the best-documented reports that have given some hope that these advanced plaques may be substantially reduced.

For the purposes of this presentation, I have divided these studies into three categories, i.e., epidemiological studies, autopsy studies, and clinical studies. In the epidemiological studies (Brozek et al., 1946; Malmros, 1950; Strøm and Jensen, 1951), the evidence, although often poorly controlled and circumstantial, indicates that populations which undergo remarkable changes in food consumption — especially of foods rich in cholesterol and animal fats — also undergo a large and often fairly prompt change in the attack rate from atherosclerosis-produced heart attacks and ischemic cerebral vascular attacks. Some of the most convincing of these studies come from experiences during and following World War II in Russia, Sweden, and Norway.

Table 1. Is human atherosclerosis reversible?

A. Epidemiological evidence
    1. Brozek et al. (1946)
    2. Malmros (1950)
    3. Strøm and Jensen (1951)

B. Autopsy studies
    1. Aschoff (1924)
    2. Beitzke (1928)
    3. Vartiainen and Kanerva (1947)
    4. Wilens (1947)
    5. Rivin and Dimitroff (1954)
    6. London et al. (1961)

C. Clinical studies
    1. Buchwald (1967); Buchwald et al. (1974)
    2. Zelis et al. (1970)
    3. Blankenhorn (1975)

The major problems with interpreting these epidemiological results stem from and are reflected by two questions:

1. Are the decreased ischemic episodes the result of decrease in the size of atherosclerotic plaques or rather are they the result of a decrease in complications of the plaques, i.e., thrombosis, platelet emboli, etc.?
2. Are the documented decreases in attack rates really related to factors other than decreased dietary cholesterol, fat, and calories or are these drops in heart attacks and brain strokes related to other changes such as decreases in hypertension, cigarette consumption, and a less sedentary state, all of which may also accompany the times of food shortage?

The autopsy studies, also often poorly controlled, help to document that the plaques really do change for the better — i.e., they become smaller and flatter and smoother. The observations referred to in Table 1 come largely from Germany following World War I (Aschoff, 1924; Beitzke, 1928), Russia following World War II (Vartiainen and Kanerva, 1947), and from the United States of America where patients with chronic wasting disease (Wilens, 1947) or cancer patients treated with estrogens have been studied (Riven and Dimitroff, 1954; London et al., 1961). They all offer positive evidence that plaques probably change for the better during periods of nutritional limitation and that this reparative or regressive process may be aided by estrogen therapy.

More recently, promising preliminary evidence has been offered from clinical studies in the USA. Dr. Henry Buchwald and his colleagues at the University of Minnesota have offered evidence, based on improvements in the signs and symptoms of ischemia (Buchwald, 1967) and also on evaluations of sequential arteriograms (Buchwald et al., 1974) that some individuals whose serum cholesterol has been reduced by "partial ileal bypass" exhibit a decrease in plaque size and improved cardiovascular or peripheral vascular function. Others appear to show a lack of progression of plaques.

Similar results, as far as function is concerned, have been described by the group at the Clinical Center of the National Heart, Lung and Blood Institute in the USA (Zelis et al., 1970).

David Blankenhorn and his co-workers at the University of Southern California and California Institute of Technology have also begun to describe studies, some based on subjective evaluation of coronary arteriograms by panels of radiologists and some based on much more objective evaluations of peripheral plaques. Some of these patients show rather striking evidence of plaque regression (Blankenhorn, 1975).

These results, although not conclusive, tend to reinforce each other indicating that in at least some individuals, atherosclerosis is partially reversible even with relatively brief periods of therapy.

Table 2 summarizes the limitations of studies of regression of atherosclerosis in human subjects. Several points are evident as one reviews the results of the studies referred to above.

In general, one has the impression that the prospective studies of small groups of patients utilizing methods of quantitation of plaque size using sequential observations offer the most promise for yielding the most definitive evidence of plaque regression in human subjects.

It also seems likely that more vigorous therapy with much greater lowering of the serum cholesterol will be necessary as compared to the cholesterol lowering achieved in the mass clinical trials that are now recorded.

Furthermore, one can look forward to the development of safer and more objective techniques to evaluate plaque size in the patient. Hopefully some of these approaches will be noninvasive.

Table 2. Limitations of studies of regression in human subjects

---

1. Epidemilogical studies yield only circumstantial evidence:
   a) Positive results may not be the result of regression of atherosclerosis.
   b) Control groups are difficult to establish.

2. Retrospective autopsy studies are not adequate:
   a) Control groups are difficult to establish.
   b) Treatment and control groups may not be comparable.
   c) Population may not be representative.
   d) Morphometry often is not possible retrospectively.

3. Large prospective clinical trials are expensive and often not conclusive:
   a) Investigators are difficult to convince that cholesterol must be lowered to 150 mg%.
   b) Autopsy studies are usually not feasible.

4. Studies based on sequential arteriography and/or improvement of function:
   a) Are usually limited to individuals with especially severe lesions who have had ischemic episodes.
   b) Technology is not yet perfected (risky and somewhat subjective).

Animal Models

The major recent advances that I want to discuss today are made possible by the development of more adequate and more easily utilized animal models of advanced atherosclerosis. Some of the advantages this approach offers are listed in Table 3. Several of these advantages will be illustrated in the papers that follow this one in the proceedings.

The components of the advanced atherosclerotic lesion as they relate to the process of regression are illustrated in Figure 1. The most important components are those that fill up space and thus contribute to the size of the plaque (Wissler, 1976). These consist of the "necrotic center" from which the plaque derives its name — usually filled with cell debris, cholesterol crystals, and cholesterol esters and adjacent calcium. The second important group of components are often referred to as the "fibrous cap." It consists of a variable number of intimally located, proliferated arterial smooth muscle cells, collagen (and other extracellular products of these multifunctional mesenchymal cells, i.e., elastin and glycosaminoglycans), extracellular and intracellular lipids, and variable numbers of foam cells.

Figure 2 illustrates that these two anatomical parts of the plaque are the ones most likely to be responsible for clinical effects:

Table 3. Advantages of regression studies in experimental models of advanced disease

---

1. Controlled prospective studies are possible and relatively inexpensive.

2. Definitive studies are relatively quickly accomplished.

3. Various treatment regimens can be compared directly.

4. Morphometry is feasible and can be done under almost ideal circumstances:
   a) Antemortem and postmortem arteriography can be compared.
   b) Chemical and morphological measurements can be compared.

5. Components of the lesions can be evaluated independently.

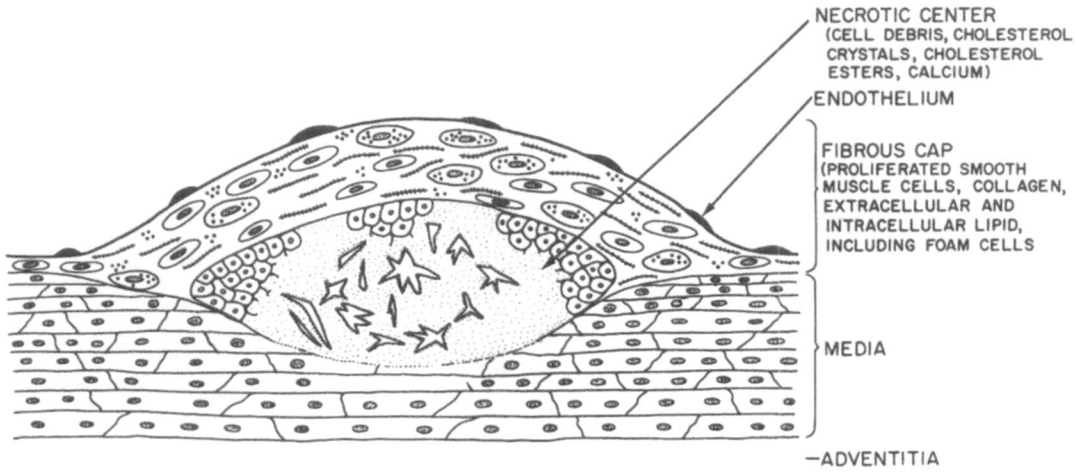

Figure 1. Diagram of an atherosclerotic plaque (after P. Constantinides)

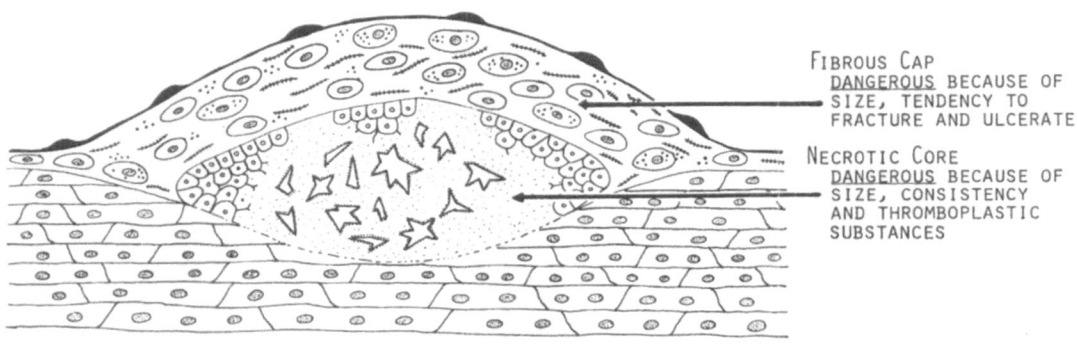

Figure 2. Relation of plaque components to clinical effects

1. The fibrous cap produces clinical effects because it can become very bulky and because it can fracture or rupture leading to "ulceration" of the plaque.
2. The *necrotic* atheromatous core is dangerous, not only because it contributes to the "space occupying" character of the plaque but because its soft, grumous character weakens the arterial wall, and because it is filled with substances that can favor thrombosis, contribute to emboli directly, attract platelets, etc.

Figure 3 presents a diagram of a regressing plaque. It indicates that one can expect beneficial clinical effects if the plaque is modified by therapy (or by unplanned environmental or planned preventive medicine intervention) in such a way as to decrease the size of the fibrous cap to make it smaller and firmer and more condensed, even if the collagen and cells are not decreased, or even if they are increased in concentration and even if the necrotic core is still there but is substantially smaller. Actually in many of the models studied, if the interval of therapy is long enough, the necrotic core is essentially eliminated and most of the residual lipid is associated with the thickened and sometimes reduplicated internal elastic membranes as indicated in this figure by the very heavy interrupted line. These changes, along with a relatively healthy endothelium, remarkably decrease the chances for stenosis, fibrous cap fracture, ulceration, and thrombosis.

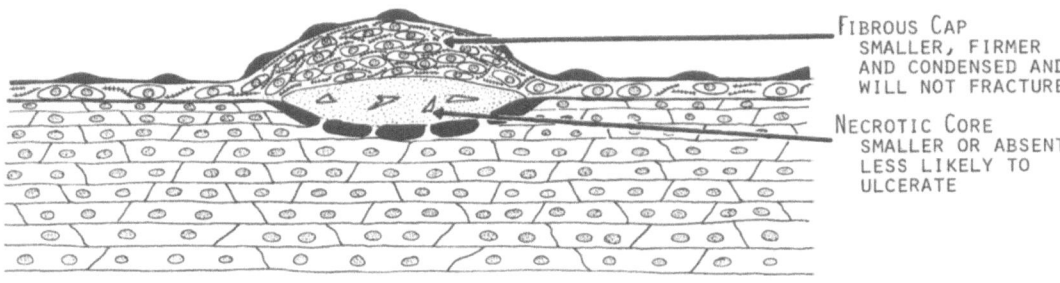

Figure 3. Benefits of plaque regression in elimentating clinical effects

The models of "severe" atherosclerosis in experimental animals that have been used with more or less success in regression studies are represented by a few examples listed in Table 4 by the person, usually the first author; although we must hasten to add that in many instances other well-known investigators were co-authors. As you can see, positive studies have been reported in dogs, fowl (chickens and pigeons), rabbits, macaques (especially rhesus and cynomolgus), and swine. All of these examples have been selected because, insofar as we could judge, these were all studies in which a substantial number of the animals had lesions that would fit the diagram of an advanced atherosclerotic plaque (Fig.1).

The following tables list the advantages and disadvantages of each of these models.

The dog (Table 5) is a "time-honored" experimental animal, especillay valued by surgeons and physiologists. The graphic and positive studies and the well-docu-mented results of Bevans et al. (1951) established it as a highly suitable model of advanced disease for regression studies. The Table lists its drawbacks as a model for regression studies. They include the substantial differences in its circulatory system relative to primates and swine. For example, it has a remark-ably different coronary circulation (Brooks et al., 1976). It also has an unusual-ly low serum cholesterol and a preponderance of its cholesterol serum carried in high-density lipoproteins that behave like low-density lipoproteins (Robers et al., 1975). It has a high relative resistance to development of advanced athero-

Table 4. Examples of regression of "severe" artherosclerosis in animals

A. Dogs
    1. Bevans et al. (1951)
    2. De Palma et al. (1968)

B. Fowl
    1. Horlick and Katz (1949)
    2. Clarkson et al. (1971)

C. Rabbits
    1. Anitschkow (1928)
    2. Vesselinovitch and Wissler (1968)

D. Macaques (rhesus and cynomolgus)
    1. Armstrong et al. (1970)
    2. Vesselinovitch et al. (1973)
    3. Bond et al. (1976)

E. Swine
    1. Daoud et al. (1974)

sclerosis (De Palma et al., 1968). It is also relatively difficult to obtain uniform, disease-free animals.

The fowl, (Table 6) of which the chicken (Katz and Stamler, 1953; Horlick and Katz, 1949) and pigeon (Clarkson et al., 1959; Clarkson and Lofland, 1961; Clarkson et al., 1971) are most utilized, has been adopted for many experimental studies because of the advantages listed in the left hand column of this table — especially size, cost, and ease of producing hypercholesterolemia and atheromatous lesions. But here again, there appear to be substantial drawbacks (listed in the right column), including an unusual lipid and cholesterol metabolism with cholesterol storage disease, the character of the plaques which rarely become advanced and complex under the conditions they have been used, the widespread small artery involvement, and the rather striking differences in arterial tree anatomy and atherosclerosis topography as compared to primates. It may be that some of the newer examples of models in fowl such as the Japanese quail will be free from some of these drawbacks.

The rabbit (Table 7) is probably the best-established and most widely used model (Anitschkow, 1913; Anitschkow, 1928; Vesselinovitch and Wissler, 1968; Vesselinovitch et al., 1974) and has the obvious advantages listed in the left column of the table but also has disturbing disadvantages (right column). It can, however,

Table 5. The dog as a model for atherosclerosis regression

Advantages	Disadvantages
1. Relatively available and inexpensive	1. Cardiovascular system not similar to human
2. Available in various sizes and shapes	2. Lipid and cholesterol metabolism differ from human
3. Considerable cardiovascular experience on which to build	3. Severe atherosclerosis difficult as compared to primates
4. Severe atherosclerosis can be produced with diet and thyroid depression	4. Uniform, disease-free dogs difficult to obtain and expensive

Table 6. Fowl as a model for atherosclerosis regression

Advantages	Disadvantages
1. Size and cost favorable for large studies	1. Lipid and cholesterol metabolism differ from human-nonmammal
2. Very susceptible to hypercholesterolemia	2. Arterial lesions are seldom similar to human plaque; rarely advanced and complex
3. Arterial lesions develop quickly	3. Often complicated by cholesterol storage in RES
4. Useful for genetic studies	4. Distribution of lesions in both large and small arteries
5. Interesting relation of plaques to topography	4. Anatomically different from humans

be made to develop much more "human-like" lesions as has been well-demonstrated by Constantinides (1965), Minick and Murphy (1973), Stemerman (1973), etc.

The macaque model of advanced atherosclerosis (Table 8) has attained prominence recently, largely because of the pioneering studies of Taylor et al. (1962, 1963, 1963), who showed that very severe stenosing and ulcerating atherosclerotic lesions leading to ischemic disease can be produced rather consistently in rhesus monkeys. It was used in the excellent studies of Armstrong et al. (1970), Armstrong and Warner (1971), and Armstrong and Megan (1972, 1973) at the University of Iowa who have demonstrated that substantial regression of lesions — many of which we think can be classified as advanced atherosclerosis — can be produced by the relatively simple expedient of reducing the serum cholesterol to baseline values (below 150 mg%) for many months. Our experience with this model has been similar (Vesselinovitch et al., 1973, 1976) and it appears that additional promising results are being reported by others (Bond et al., 1976).

The disadvantages of this model that I have listed are substantial but they can all be overcome. The short supply of the rhesus should be remedied in the USA by a rather large breeding program being initiated and supported by the National Institutes of Health.

Table 7. The rabbit as a model for atherosclerosis regression

Advantages	Disadvantages[a]
1. Size and cost favorable for large studies	1. Lipid and cholesterol metabolism differ from human
2. Very susceptible to hypercholesterolemia	2. Arterial lesions are seldom similar to human plaque
3. Develops arterial lesions quickly	3. Topography different from human atherosclerosis
	4. Often complicated by cholesterol storage in RES
	5. Lesions are very resistant to regression

[a]Most of these can be overcome by induction with a less elevated cholesterol level especially when this is combined with endothelial cell injury.

Table 8. Macaque monkey model for atherosclerosis regression

Advantages	Disadvantages
1. Advanced atherosclerosis relatively easy to produce; histogenesis and lesion components similar to humans	1. Expensive, hard to handle and hard to procure
2. Anatomy, physiology and biochemistry similar to human	2. Uniform, disease-free, adult animals in short supply
3. Studies thus far indicate that substantial regression can be obtained in relatively short time	3. Require special facilities and expert personnel
4. Size, lesion distribution, nutritional requirements favorable for study	

Finally, as indicated in Table 9, the swine model now appears to be emerging as a particularly advantageous model for those who are prepared to exploit it and who can develop the fairly extensive, but not particularly expensive facilities it requires (Florentin and Nam, 1968; Scott et al., 1972). Those who are able to develop these facilities and who take the necessary steps to accelerate the development of advanced disease can, we believe, expect the advantages listed in the left column. The two papers published recently in the Archives of Pathology and Laboratory Medicine by Daoud et al. (1974, 1976) and Fritz et al. (1976) of the Albany Medical College group led by Wilbur Thomas, give ample evidence of the ways that this model can be utilized for regression studies. They were able to produce rather advanced plaques rather quickly and consistently by utilizing balloon catheter injury plus diet. This group is to be complimented especially for the development of evidence that the important phenomena of smooth muscle cell proliferation and accumulation in the fibrous cap can be rather remarkably slowed down by a low-fat, low-cholesterol diet. They also have presented preliminary evidence that calcium as well as fat and cholesterol is reduced substantially in the advanced lesions during regression.

This model has great promise, we believe, for further study because so many of its features lend themselves to the kinds of studies medical scientists, including cardiovascular surgeons, internists, physiologists, and pathologists like to carry out in people and which can be done so much more readily for research and demonstration purposes in swine.

If time and space permitted, we would have illustrated a few of the results from our own recent and ongoing studies of regression of fairly severe atherosclerosis in rabbits and primates. These include gross, microscopic, ultrastructural, morphometric observations coordinated with chemical and metabolic measurements. Instead we will close with brief reference to the types of microscopic changes that Dr. Vesselinovitch and I have been observing during regression.

In our studies in male rabbits (Vesselinovitch and Wissler, 1968; Vesselinovitch et al., 1974) we have found a remarkable decrease in lesion size and morphologic complexity that we were able to induce rather promptly by means of administration of increased amounts of ambient O_2 combined with a low-cholesterol, low-fat diet and estrogen or cholestyramine therapy. The lesions from the treated animals showed a remarkable decrease in size, disappearance of lipid, decrease in cel-

Table 9. The swine as a model for atherosclerosis regression

Advantages	Disadvantages
1. Anatomy, physiology and biochemistry similar to human	1. Large, expensive and hard to handle
2. Arterial plaques seem to resemble human lesions	2. Advanced plaques difficult to produce without special manipulation
3. Large size permits measurements limited in other species a) arteriography b) open heart surgery c) measurements of cardiac function	
4. Lesions produced by diet plus balloon catheter are remarkable similar to advanced human plaques	
5. Regression can be followed quantitatively with sequential arteriography	
6. Pure-bred lines are plentiful	

Table 10. Problems to be considered regarding regression of atherosclerosis in animal models

---

1. How can one most easily and safely accelerate regression of advanced plaques?

2. What are the cellular and chemical, including enzymatic, mechanisms by which plaque regression is instituted?

3. What lesion components can be expected to regress and under what conditions — cells, cell mitosis, lipid, cholesterol, collagen, elastin, glycosamino-glycans and calcium?

---

lularity, and condensation of fiber proteins. Extracellular lipid predominated in the regressed lesions. The most evidence of regression was seen in those rabbits that were treated with a low-fat, low-cholesterol ration combined with daily treatments with ambient oxygen and either estrogen or cholestyramine.

More recently, we have been studying the even more advanced rhesus monkey lesions induced by coconut oil-butter oil and cholesterol-enriched ration. These lesions can be observed to become very much smaller and lose most of their necrotic lipid-rich core, their extracellular and intracellular lipid, and to condense and thin out their "fibrous cap.". When the animals are treated with a low-fat, low-cholesterol ration (Vesselinovitch et al., 1973, 1976), they improve even more when cholestyramine is added to this therapeutic diet (Wissler et al., 1975).

The regression seen in the aortas and coronary arteries of rhesus monkeys following combined cholestyramine and low-fat, low-cholesterol feeding can easily be appreciated and are being quantitated in a number of ways, both morphometrically and biochemically.

We feel that the era of prevention and regression of advanced atherosclerosis is just beginning (Wissler and Vesselinovitch, 1976). Some of the problems that should be addressed and hopefully solved soon using the large number of available animal models and the ongoing human clinical studies with sequential arteriography are listed in Table 10. Some of them will be addressed in the following chapters of this book. They include:

1. How can one most easily and safely accelarate regression in advanced plaques in man and experimental models?
2. What are the cellular, chemical, and enzymic mechanisms by which plaque regression is instituted?
3. What lesion components can be expected to regress and under what conditions — cells, cell mitosis, lipid, collagen, elastin, glycosaminoglycans, and calcium?

Acknowledgements

The studies from this laboratory referred to in this manuscript were supported in part by:
USPHS HL 15062, HE 2174, HL 6894, HL 2174, HL 6894, HL 14934 and by the Louis A. Block Fund of the University of Chicago. The authors are grateful for the help of Judy Johnson, William Johnson, and Bob Pisciotta.

METHODS TO ACCELERATE REGRESSION

K.T. Lee, A.S. Daoud, and Y.S. Kwak

In recent years, several studies have shown that diet-induced proliferative uncomplicated atherosclerotic lesions regress after removal of the dietary stimulus
Such regression has been reported in monkeys (Armstrong et al., 1970; Tucker et
al., 1971; Vesselinovitch et al., 1973), chickens (Pick et al., 1952; Horlick and
Katz, 1949), pigeons (Clarkson et al., 1971; St. Clair et al., 1972), and dogs
(Bevans et al., 1951; De Palma et al., 1970). In rabbits, however, regression of
artherosclerotic lesions appears to occur only when lesions are produced by cholesterol feeding for a short period (Bortz, 1968). No appreciable regression of
artherosclerotic lesions has been reported in rabbits when cholesterol was fed
for a long period (Friedman and Byers, 1963; Prior and Ziegler, 1965). In many
instances, withdrawal of the dietary stimulus was followed by further progression of the disease (Constantinides, 1965).

The possibility for regression of advanced necrotic lesions with their complications, such as calcification, hemorrhage, and thrombosis has not yet been completely documented except for some swine lesions which will be described in this
report and perhaps for some lesions in nonhuman primates. The mechanisms of regression are still obscure. The only factors that have been extensively studied
in many experiments are those concerning lipids (Friedman and Byers, 1963;
Armstrong and Megan, 1972; Eggen et al., 1974). No data are available on the number of cells in the lesions and their proliferative activity prior to and following regression except in our swine study. There are no adequate quantitative
studies of the effect of regression on other components of the lesions such as
collagen, elastic tissue, and glycosaminoglycans, or on the activity of the cells
in the synthesis of these components.

This morning, I would like to present my talk in two parts. In the first part of
my talk, I shall present a study from our laboratory that was designed to investigate whether advanced complicated atherosclerotic lesions in young swine
can be made to regress by dietary means alone.

Feeding a high-fat, high-cholesterol diet to swine results in the development of
some advanced atherosclerotic lesions but only after a prolonged period of feeding, which makes regression studies of such lesions unduly expensive and time-
consuming. We have reported in previous studies that complicated atherosclerotic
lesions can be produced rapidly in swine by a combination of atherogenic diet and
various types of injuries to the artery (Lee et al., 1971; Nam et al., 1973).
In this experiment, we used a combination of a high-fat, high-cholesterol diet
and mechanical injury.

Injury was induced by scraping the endothelium of the abdominal aorta by an inflated balloon inserted via a femoral artery. This mechanical injury apparently
produces only minimal damage to the underlying tissue. After anesthesia, a nick
was made in a femoral artery and a 5F Fogarty arterial embolectomy catheter was
introduced and passed into the abdominal aorta. The balloon at the end of the
catheter was inflated with 1.5-2.0 ml of saline and was pulled back and forth in
the abdominal aorta several times. The balloon was then emptied and withdrawn.

Forty miniature male swine were ballooned and divided into four groups, two
baseline and two regression groups. In the baseline groups, 16 swine (group 1)
were fed a high cholesterol diet for 4 months and sacrificed at the end of this
period together with four swine (group 2) fed a mash diet for the same period of

time to serve as their controls. In the regression groups, 14 swine (group 3) were fed a high-cholesterol diet (HC diet) for 4 months then shifted to a mash diet for 14 months. They were sacrificed at the end of this period, together with three swine (group 4) that were fed a mash diet for 18 months to serve as their controls.

At the initiation of the experiment, the serum cholesterol levels of the various groups were around 70 mg/dl. These levels rose in 2 months in the animals fed the high-cholesterol diet to over 800 mg/dl. When the animals in the regression group were shifted to a mash diet, their cholesterol levels came down quickly to values similar to those of their mash controls and at the end of the experiment, there was no difference between the two groups.

After the sacrifice, the abdominal aorta was divided longitudinally into two halves; one for chemical analyses and the other for morphologic studies. Chemical analyses performed include DNA synthesis by ^{3}H-thymidine, protein synthesis by ^{14}C-leucine, and collagen synthesis by ^{14}C-proline. Measurements were made of cholesterol, cholesterol esters, triglyceride, and phospholipids in lesion and nonlesion areas. ^{3}H-thymidine autoradiography was also carried out to demonstrate the location of proliferating cells.

On gross examination, the aorta from the HC diet-baseline animals (group 1) showed focal raised lesions distributed throughout the entire abdominal aorta. These varied in size from a few mm to over 1 cm in the greatest dimension, and were elevated up to 2 mm above the intimal surface. Sudanophilic staining of the intima was sometimes focal, sometimes diffuse. The mean percentage of the surface area stained with Sudan IV was 20%, which is significantly greater (P <.005) than that of all other groups (Table 1).

The aortas of the other three groups, including the "regression group" (group 3), were grossly similar and showed, in general, smooth intimal surface with occasional focal raised lesions and little or no sudanophilia.

Table 1. Summary of results: regression study

Parameter studies	Group 1	Group 2	Group 3	Group 4
No. of animals	16	4	14	3
Av. % of surface involvement	20.8%	<1.0%	3.2%	<1.0%
Av. thickness of lesion [a]	0.41 mm	0.15 mm	0.26 mm	0.26 mm
Av. thickness of media	0.64 mm	0.63 mm	0.89 mm	1.03 mm
Ration, lesion/media	65%	20%	28.5%	25%
Segments examined	203	105	391	91
Animals with atheroma	14	...	1	...
Segments with atheroma	50	...	1	...
Atheromas	73	...	1	...
Animals with thrombus	3	...	...	...
Segments with thrombus	4	...	...	...
Segments with hemorrhage	1	...	...	...
Animals with calcification	11	...	13	1
Segments with calcification	28	...	48	5
% of labeled cells [b]	1.36%	Not done	0.07%	Not done

[a] HC baseline (group 1) > regression (group 3)- P <.005.
 HC baseline (group 1) > mash baseline (group 2)- P <.005.

[b] HC baseline (group 1) > regression (group 3)- P <.005.

On microscopic examination, HC diet-baseline group (group 1) revealed a spectrum ranging from normal intima to very advanced complicated lesions (Fig. 1). The mean lesion thickness for the 203 sections examined was 410 μm, or 65% of the mean thickness of the adjacent media. Proliferative foam cell lesions were abundant, being present in all animals and virtually in all sections examined. They were usually raised above the intimal surface and were composed of a mixture of foam cells and spindle-shaped cells. In many instances, such lesions displayed a fibrous cap at the luminal surface. Not infrequently, the foam cell lesions extended into the upper part of the media. Autoradiography revealed varying numbers of labeled nuclei, which were most prevalent in the fibrous cap.

Necrotic atheromatous lesions with or without calcification, hemorrhage into the plaque, and thrombosis were present in approximately 25% of the segments examined (50 of 230) in the HC diet-baseline group (group 1), with some of the segments showing more than one lesion. The total number of necrotic atheromas found in this group was 73, and these were found in 14 of the 16 aortas studied (Table 1). Oil red O-stained frozen sections showed extensive intracellular and extracellular lipid accumulations in the necrotic center and a lesser degree in the fibrous cap. Over one-third of the necrotic atheromas (28 of 73) showed calcification (Table 1). The calcium deposits were usually extensive and in many instances occupied one-half of the area of the atheroma. Four necrotic atheromas disclosed complicating thrombi, and one showed hemorrhage into the plaque. ^{3}H-thymidine autoradiography showed many labeled cells. In the six necrotic atheromas present in radioautographic sections, there were 201 labeled nuclei among 14,700 cells, or a labeling index of 1.36% $\pm$ .0019.

The histologic pictures of the two matched control groups (group 2 and 4) and of the regression group (group 3) were similar to each other. Varying degrees of intimal thickening were present. A mean intimal thickening of the various groups was as follows: group 1, 410 μm, group 2, 150 μm, group 3, 260 μm, and group 4, 260 μm, or 65%, 22%, 28%, and 25% of the thickness of the media, respectively. In general, the intimal surface was flat with a few small "bumps." The cells were largely fusiform in shape with an occasional small accumulation of foam cells at the base of the lesions. These were more abundant in the regression

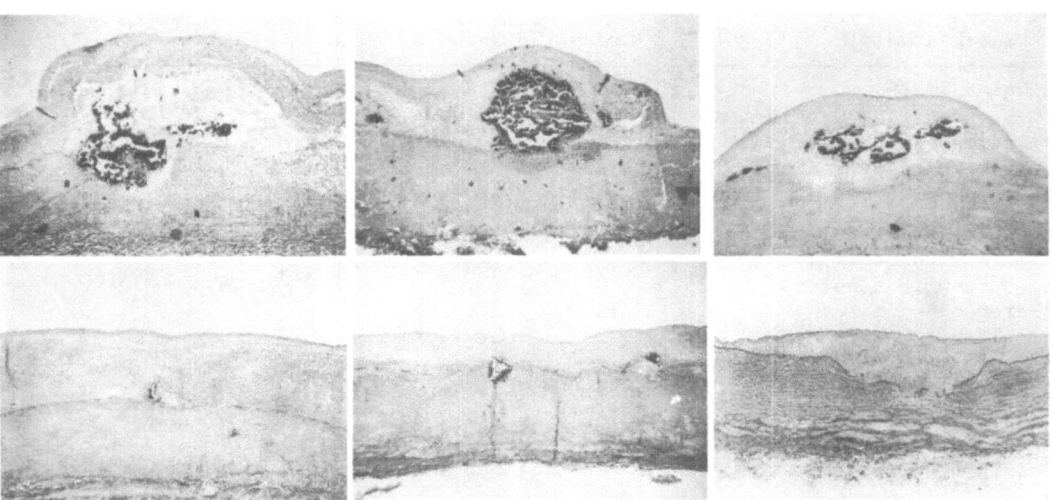

Figure 1. In the upper half are raised complicated atheromas from the baseline group (group 1). There are necrosis, fibrous cap, calcification, and medial involvement.
In the lower half are representative lesions from the regression group (group 3). They are smaller, flat, and fibrotic without necrosis and little calcification

group than in the two mash groups. Histochemically, there was apparently more collagen deposition in the regression group than in the mash groups and in the baseline group. The autoradiography showed only occasional labeled cells, and these appeared similarly distributed in all three groups and were much less frequent than in the basline group. In the six autoradiographic sections from the regression group matched with the six atheromas from the baseline group there were ten labeled nuclei among 12,380 cells counted, or a label index of 0.08% ± 0.001.

Atheromas were absent in the two mash groups, and only one small questionable area of necrosis was observed in the regression group. No hemorrhage in the plaque or thrombosis was seen in any of the sections examined. Calcification was absent in sections from animals on a mash diet that were killed at 4 months, but was present in those from the two HC diet groups. The frequency of calcification in the regression group was as great as in the HC diet-baseline group (Table 1), but the areas of calcification were much smaller.

In summary, complicated necrotic atherosclerotic lesions in the aorta of swine produced by an atherogenic diet plus mechanical injury were common in the HC diet-baseline group. Fourteen months after the withdrawal of a high cholesterol diet the thickness of the lesions was significantly less than that of the baseline group with remodeling of the intimal surface to become smooth. Necrosis, hemorrhage, and thrombosis were virtually absent. The number of calcified areas was the same but the areas of calcifications were much smaller in the regression group. The lesions in the regression group were less cellular as evidenced by the DNA concentration. There was slowing of proliferation as indicated by decrease in DNA synthesis. There was also significant depletion of cholesterol, cholesterylester, and phospholipids. There was no difference in the amount of triglyceride and protein synthesis. Studies on collagen synthesis have not been completed as yet. This study showed that advanced atherosclerotic lesions in swine regress with restoration and remodeling of the arterial wall 14 months after the withdrawal of the dietary stimulus.

The second part of my presentation is concerned with drug regimens that were used to accelerate the regression of atherosclerotic lesions. We have chosen and tested a number of drugs that are supposed to alter the metabolism of the arterial wall, as the means to accelerate the regression in rabbits and swine. This is an ongoing study in our laboratory and I shall present the portions of the study that are completed thus far in rabbits.

There have been many studies utilizing various drugs in animal models to learn if the course of experimental atherosclerosis can be modified by these therapeutic agents. Corticosteroids (Bailey and Butler, 1966), estrogen (Wolinsky, 1972; Rhee et al., 1974; Numano et al., 1972), pyridinilcarbamate (Numano et al., 1972; Shimamoto and Numano, 1969; Shimamoto et al., 1972), colchicine (Hollander et al., 1974; Lee et al., 1976), penicillamine (Hollander et al., 1974), acetytsalicylic acid (Hollander et al., 1974), and heparin (Rowsell et al., 1965) have been most widely tested aside from hypocholesterolemic drugs. Their effects appear to be different in different species of animals.

In the past 3 years we have mainly focused our attention on drugs interfering with metabolic events that may lead to the development of atherosclerosis.

Our working hypothesis of atherosclerosis is presented in Figure 2. Various insults, physical, chemical, and biological, act singly or in combination on the arterial wall. The injured artery further progresses toward accumulation of lipids and degeneration and proliferation of smooth muscle cells. Finally, the diseased artery becomes complicated with fibrosis, necrosis, and calcification.

For the prevention and regression of atherosclerosis, a reasonable approach would be the removal of causative factors or blocking the disease processes that lead to atherosclerosis by appropriate therapeutic agents.

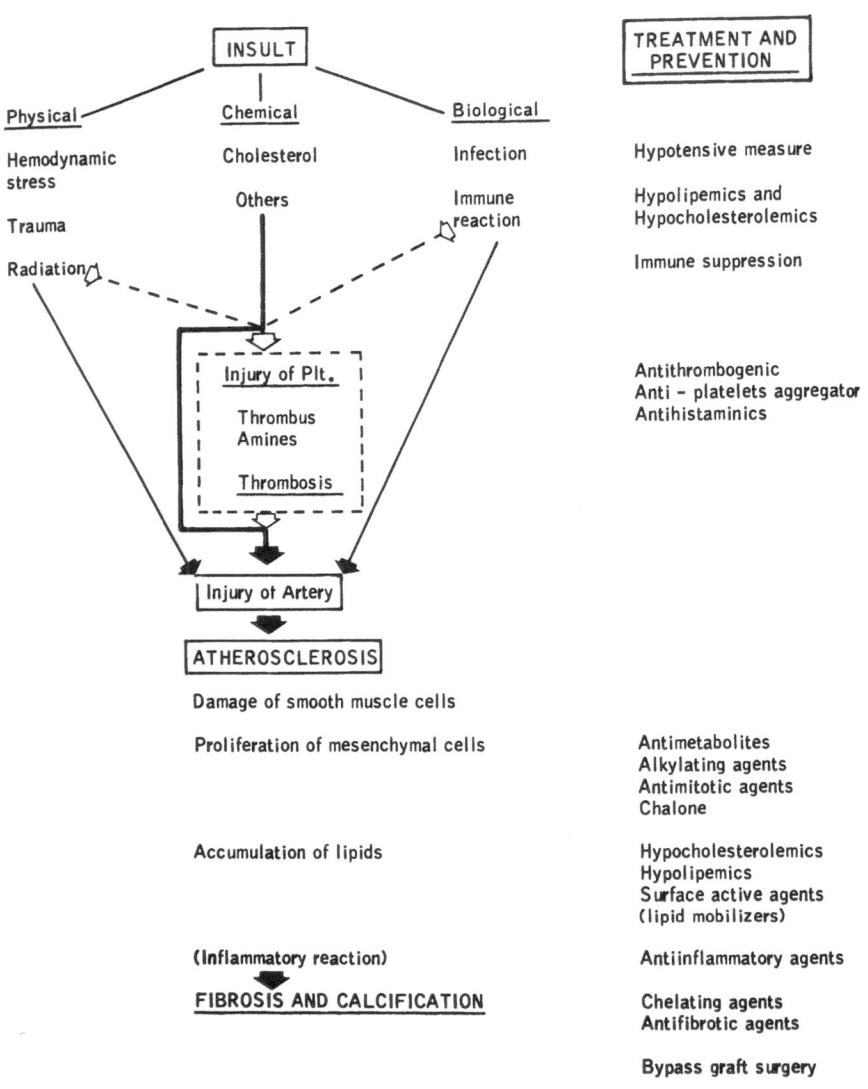

INSULT

TREATMENT AND PREVENTION

Physical   Chemical   Biological

Hemodynamic   Cholesterol   Infection   Hypotensive measure
stress
                  Others   Immune   Hypolipemics and
Trauma   reaction   Hypocholesterolemics

Radiation   Immune suppression

Injury of Plt.

Thrombus   Antithrombogenic
Amines   Anti - platelets aggregator
                                                       Antihistaminics
Thrombosis

Injury of Artery

ATHEROSCLEROSIS

Damage of smooth muscle cells

Proliferation of mesenchymal cells   Antimetabolites
                                                       Alkylating agents
                                                       Antimitotic agents
                                                       Chalone

Accumulation of lipids   Hypocholesterolemics
                                                       Hypolipemics
                                                       Surface active agents
                                                       (lipid mobilizers)

(Inflammatory reaction)   Antiinflammatory agents

FIBROSIS AND CALCIFICATION   Chelating agents
                                                       Antifibrotic agents

                                                       Bypass graft surgery

Figure 2. Working hypothesis of atherogenesis and prevention and treatment of atherosclerosis

Drugs tested for our studies were selected from the scheme shown in Figure 2. We have found that certain antimetabolites, namely, mercaptopurine and hydroxyurea, retarded the progression of cholesterol-induced atherosclerosis in rabbits (Kwak et al., 1976). The study with antimetabolites has two-fold interest. The anti-metabolites, in general, have known specific inhibitory action on the biosynthe-sis of nucleic acids or proteins. Therefore, by using these agents as a metabolic probe we can gain some insight into the proposed atherogenesis. And if these drugs are found to be effective on experimental atherosclerosis in both progres-sion and regression phases, we may be able to utilize this information to find better and safer means of treatment of human disease in the future.

The data I will be presenting this morning from these drug studies are based on the results obtained on the effects of the antimetabolites mercaptopurine and hydroxyurea, and a platelet-aggregation inhibitor, pyridinolcarbamate, that were tested as means to promote regression in a simple model of atherosclerosis in rabbits.

Table 2. Methods and experimental design

		Methods diet	
Cholesterol diet (C)		rabbit pellet	93 g/day
		cholesterol	1 g
		peanut oil	6 g
Pellet diet (P)		rabbit pellet	100 g/day

Experimental design

Group		Induction		Treatment	
		Diet	Duration	Diet drug	Duration
Control	(7)[a]	P	9mos		
Baseline	(15)	C	2mos		
Pellet alone	(8)	C	2mos	P	7mos
MP + pellet	(8)	C	2mos	P + MP (5 mg/day)	7mos
U-OH + pellet	(7)	C	2mos	P + U-OH (50 mg/day)	7mos
PDC + pellet	(8)	C	2mos	P + PDC (50 mg/day)	7mos

[a]Number of animals.

Materials and experimental designs of the current study were presented in Table 2. Six groups, each consisting of 7-15 male, New Zealand white rabbits weighing 2.5 ± 0.3 kg, were used to study the effects of three drugs mentioned above which are two antimetabolites and pyridinolcarbamate on the regression of cholesterol-induced atherosclerosis in rabbits.

For the induction of atherosclerotic lesions in rabbits, the cholesterol-containing diet was fed for 2 months. Daily ration of this diet contained 1 gm of cholesterol, 6 gm of peanut oil, and 93 gm of commercial rabbit pellets. Except for the control group which was fed the pellet diet throughout the entire experimental period of 9 months, all remaining five groups were fed the cholesterol diet for 2 months. At the end of 2 months of cholesterol feeding, the baseline group was killed and percent of the area of the aorta involved by atherosclerosis by planimetry, and cholesterol concentrations of serum and other tissues were measured. Then, the diet was changed to the pellet diet for the remaining four groups (under the dotted line in Table 2) and continued for the next 7 months. Each of the three groups was given one of the drugs, mercaptopurine (MP), hydroxyurea (U-OH), or pyridinilcarbamate (PDC) until they were killed after 7 months of drug treatment. One group was given no drugs and designated as the "pellet-alone" group.

The results of the drug-induced regression in these rabbits after 7 months of drug treatment are shown in Table 3. In this table, percent of the areas of the aortas involved by atherosclerotic lesions and the types of lesions observed in the aorta are presented. Also presented in this table are the cholesterol concentrations in the aorta, liver, and serum. In the control rabbits fed the pellet diet alone for the entire experimental period of 9 months, only 1.1% of the surface of the aorta was involved by atherosclerotic lesions which were mostly overlying spontaneous medial calcification. In the baseline group which was killed after 2 months of cholesterol feeding, 65.8% of the aorta was involved by lesions which were mainly foam cell lesions.

In the pellet-alone group, the extent of the lesions increased significantly from the baseline values (P < .05) and also the type of lesions changed from fibrous to atheromatous lesions, in spite of the fact that this group was fed the pellet diet without cholesterol for as long as 7 months. In all three groups, the mean

Table 3. Area of aortic atherosclerosis, cholesterol concentrations of serum, aorta and liver, and types of lesion

Group	Aortic lesion area (%)	Cholesterol			Types of lesion
		Aorta (mg/g)	Liver (mg/g)	Serum (mg/100 ml)	
Control	1.1 ± 0.5	1.2 ± 0.04	2.4 ± 0.06	30 ± 2.9	Medial calcification
Baseline	65.8 ± 5.5	17.6 ± 3.7	37.7 ± 3.7	2092 ± 126	Foam cell lesion (A)
Pellet alone (8)	89.0 ± 3.7^a	29.7 ± 3.9^a	2.9 ± 0.2^a	34 ± 9.7^a	Atheromatous lesion (B)
MP + pellet (8)	42.0 ± 11.5^b	14.3 ± 3.9^b	2.8 ± 0.1	27 ± 4.4	Mixture of A and B
U-OH + pellet (7)	54.3 ± 13.1^b	24.0 ± 5.6	3.1 ± 0.3	25 ± 5.2	Mixture of A and B
PDC + pellet (8)	48.0 ± 12.7^b	20.2 ± 5.4	2.8 ± 0.4	29 ± 3.1	Mixture of A and B

[a] Significantly different from baseline group (P <.05).

[b] Significantly different from pellet group (P <.01).

surface areas involved by lesions were reduced significantly as compared to the pellet-alone group (P <.01). The aortic cholesterol concentration was significantly reduced only in the mercaptopurine group as compared to the pellet-alone group. It was not significantly different in the other two drug groups. Cholesterol concentrations in the serum and various tissues other than the aorta returned to normal within 4 months of pellet feeding. The growth curves were similar in all groups, indicating that the drugs we used did not affect the growth rate of these rabbits.

Figure 3 represents a composite sketch of the surface areas of the aortas involved by atherosclerotic lesions in the pellet-alone group and in all three drug groups after 7 months of drug treatment. It is interesting to note that in the pellet-alone group the entire surfaces of all seven aortas were invariably involved by rather extensive atherosclerotic disease. In the three drug-treated groups approximately one-half or two-thirds of the aortas were almost free of significant atherosclerotic lesions. It appeared that some animals showed significant regression after the drug treatment and some did not.

In conclusion, this study showed that all three drugs tested, mercaptopurine, hydroxyurea, and pyridinolcarbamate, accelerated regression to a significant degree of cholesterol-induced atherosclerosis in some of the rabbits studied. The pellet-alone group showed significant progression of aortic atherosclerotic lesions even after the cessation of cholesterol feeding. The cholesterol concentrations in the serum and liver returned to normal level after 4 months of the pellet diet. The simple rabbit model used in the current study appears to be suitable for testing drugs that may promote regression of atherosclerotic lesions.

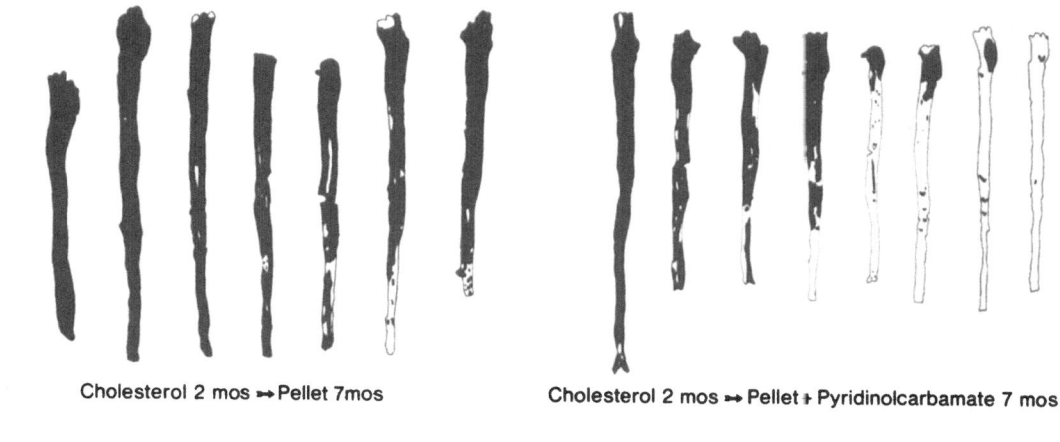

Cholesterol 2 mos ↠ Pellet 7mos

Cholesterol 2 mos ↠ Pellet + Pyridinolcarbamate 7 mos

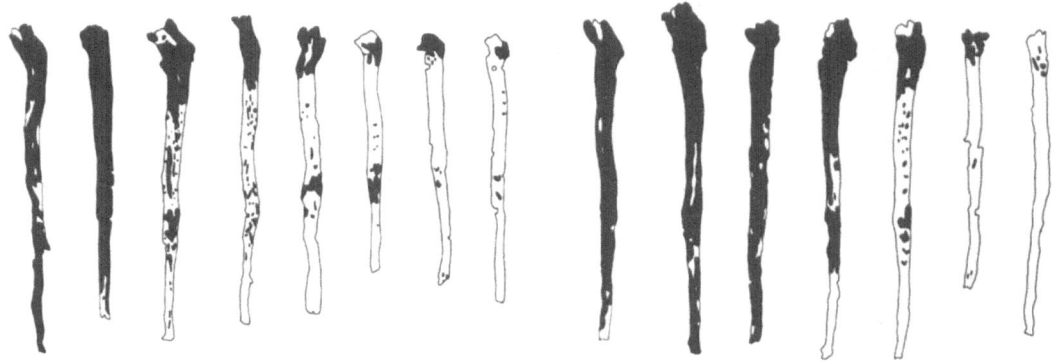

Cholesterol 2 mos ↠ Pellet + Mercaptopurine 7 mos

Cholesterol 2 mos ↠ Pellet + Hydroxyurea 7 mos

Figure 3. Composite sketch of areas of aortas involved by atherosclerotic lesions in four groups of rabbits

393

THE MECHANISM OF ATHEROSCLEROSIS REGRESSION

H.C. Stary, D.A. Eggen and J.P. Strong

Introduction

Anitschkow, not long after he had produced lesions experimentally by adding cholesterol to the diet, studied the possibility that atherosclerosis can regress.
In 1928, 15 years after the publication of his initial experiments, he reported
that lipid can be removed from atherosclerotic lesions by the removal of cholesterol from the diet (Anitschkow, 1928). In later years, the subject of regression
by dietary means received little attention and was studied only sporadically.

Interest in the dietary treatment of atherosclerosis developed when epidemiological studies reported a decreased incidence of the clinical sequelae of atherosclerosis after the period of inadequate nutrition, in particular with respect
to fats, that existed in Europe during and immediately after the Second World War.
These studies were reviewed extensively by Malmros (1950). Additional evidence,
recently reviewed by Keys (1975), suggested that populations with diets low in
fat had a lower prevalence of the sequelae of atherosclerosis than did those with
diets high in animal fat. Clincial trials aimed at preventing coronary heart
disease and other complications of atherosclerosis by lowering the amount of
animal fat in the diet were begun in the fifties and were generally encouraging,
although some produced controversial results (Dayton and Pearce, 1969).

Experimental studies to determine whether or not diet-induced arterial lesions
could be reversed by dietary means had not been pursued to any great extent before 1970. In 1969, McMillan and Hough (1969), reported at the American Heart
Association's annual meeting that only a fraction of 1% of grants from governmental and private agencies in support of arteriosclerosis research was concerned
with regression.

Interest in experimental studies on regression had a sudden rebirth at about
that time, stimulated perhaps by the earlier clinical diet trials. The numerous
morphologic studies of the past 7 years were spearheaded by the studies of Armstrong and colleagues (1969, 1970), who showed unequivocally that obstructive
atherosclerotic lesions induced in the coronary arteries of rhesus monkeys could
be markedly reduced in size by lowering the serum cholesterol to a range of 130-
150 mg/dl.

Recently, Wissler and co-workers (1975) showed that regression can be achieved
by treatment with cholestyramine, even in animals eating a high-cholesterol diet.
Wissler and Vesselinovitch (1976) have reviewed human and experimental studies
on regression and Armstrong (1976) reviewed those having particular reference
to rhesus and cynomolgus monkeys.

Today, the fact is well-established that a decrease in serum cholesterol results
in a decrease not only of the lipid component but also in the size of experimental atherosclerotic lesions. That finding is of fundamental importance, even
though the low serum cholesterol level needed for regression is not easily attained in humans. Experimental studies have also shown, however, that advanced
lesions do not disappear but are retained as fibrous residuals. Although the extent that residual lesions might precipitate clinical events is unknown, future
experimental studies will likely focus on minimizing the development of residual
lesions. Attempts to prevent such lesions would be benefited by information about
the regression mechanism. We have therefore used time-sequence studies to inves-

tigate the mechanism whereby atherosclerotic lesions are resolved. We have intensively evaluated the removal of cells that accumulated in the intima during the hypercholesterolemic period and have observed the disappearance of necrotic debris and the fate of lipid inclusions in arterial smooth muscle cells and macrophages.

Experimental Design

Our data on the mechanism of regression are from two successive experiments on regression of early atherosclerotic lesions in rhesus monkeys, summarized in Tables 1 and 2. Both experiments were identical with respect to diets during progression and regression and in the period of lesion induction. The experiments varied only in the number of weeks during which animals were given low-cholesterol food to induce lesion regression.

In the first experiment, we induced lesions by feeding the animals a high-cholesterol diet for 12 weeks. We then changed the diet to low-cholesterol and killed groups of animals after 2, 3, 16, 32, 40, and 64 weeks. The detailed experimental design, the response of serum and aortic lipids, and gross and microscopic findings in the aorta have been reported for the first study (Stary, 1972; Eggen et al., 1974; Stary, 1974b; Kokatnur et al., 1975; Strong et al., 1976). Later, we examined more closely the early and late stages of lesion regression. In this second experiment, groups of monkeys were given the high-cholesterol diet for 12 weeks and killed 4, 8, 12, 24, and 128 weeks after the change to the low-cholesterol diet. In addition, the two studies included control monkeys that received a low-cholesterol diet only. Control monkeys were divided into four groups, and separate groups were killed 14, 52, 76, and 140 weeks after the start of the experiment.

Methods

All 64 animals were male rhesus monkeys (*Macaca mulatta*), adolescents or young adults at the start of the experiment. We estimated their ages by body weight and dentition (Hurme, 1960). The importer had conditioned the animals on a low-cholesterol diet for 6 – 8 weeks after they arrived from India. From the time of their arrival at our laboratory until the start of the experiment, the animals received a research animal laboratory diet that has a low content of fat and cholesterol.

The high-cholesterol diet consisted of the research animal laboratory diet supplemented with butter and beef tallow (3:1), casein, cholesterol, vitamins, and

Table 1. Ranges of serum cholesterol values for control monkeys that received only the low-cholesterol diet for various periods

Experimental group (code)	Number of animals in group	Time maintained on low-cholesterol diet (weeks)	Mean serum cholesterol[a] (mg/dl)
0/14	3	14	140–155
0/52	2	52	115–125
0/76	3	76	110–135
0/140	3	140	140–165

[a]Mean of all determinations made in each animal.

Table 2. Ranges of serum cholesterol values in monkeys during the period on the high-cholesterol diet, and after receiving a low-cholesterol regression diet for various time periods

Experimental group (code)	Number of animals in group	High-cholesterol diet (Progression period)		Low-cholesterol diet (Regression period)	
		Duration (weeks)	Mean serum cholesterol[a] (mg/dl)	Duration (weeks)	Terminal serum cholesterol (mg/dl)
12/0	5	12	340–530	0	–
12/2	6	12	360–530	2	145–250
12/3	2	12	290–550	3	120–135
12/4	4	12	280–540	4	140–255
12/8	5	12	290–640	8	145–200
12/12	5	12	230–560	12	125–195
12/16	2	12	380–490	16	135–140
12/24	5	12	300–610	24	110–175
12/32	6	12	350–550	32	95–115
12/40	2	12	430–470	40	110–125
12/64	6	12	360–550	64	95–130
12/128	5	12	310–590	128	105–155

water. The diet contained 1 mg of cholesterol per calorie, or 0.37% cholesterol by weight. Food was offered once a day in a quantity just sufficient to maintain normal body growth.

We took serum samples at one-to four-week intervals throughout the study, determining the serum total cholesterol levels on all samples by the method of Abell et al. (1952).

We stripped the intima from the left half of the aorta by fine dissection under magnification, also stripping a portion of the media along with the intima. The dissected intima media was minced and extracted by the Folch procedure (Folch et al., 1951). We determined the total cholesterol (after saponification) and free cholesterol by gas-liquid chromatography. We separated cholesterol esters by thin layer chromatography and determined the fatty acids esterified to cholesterol by gas-liquid chromatography.

Tritiated thymidine was injected in a dose of 0.5 micro C/g of body weight. Most monkeys received one i.v. injection, 1 h before being killed. Some monkeys received an additional i.v. injection 8 h before being killed. We prepared radioautographs of the entire length of the aorta by a method described previously (Stary and McMillan, 1970).

Tissue taken for electron microscopy from the coronary artery consisted of consecutive cross sections of the left main stem, the bifurcation of the main stem into the left anterior descending and circumflex branches, and the proximal left anterior descending branch. We took aortic tissue from three standard sites in the thoracic and from one standard site in the abdominal segment. The tissues were fixed in two changes of buffered osmium tetroxide, dehydrated in graded alcohols, and embedded in the epoxy resin maraglas. From each tissue block semithin sections were prepared, stained with Paragon multiple stain, and examined with the light microscope. Areas of interest were fine-sectioned with a diamond knife, stained with lead citrate and uranyl acetate, and examined with the electron microscope.

Results

Normocholesterolemic Control Animals

The mean value of all serum cholesterol determinations was calculated for each control animal; the ranges of these mean values in each group are given in Table 1. The four groups of control animals had been maintained in our laboratory for various periods, the age of the groups varying from young-adult to mature-adult at the end of the experiment. None was very young or very old. No increase in the serum cholesterol values occurred with increasing age.

We previously reported in detail on normal coronary artery ultrastructure, with particular reference to the intima of the main coronary bifurcation (Stary and Strong, 1976a, 1976b). The present description is of both coronary arteries and of the aorta.

The intima had, independent of age, extensive segments of nonatherosclerotic thickening that varied according to location. Intimal thickening occurred either as cushions at arterial forks and around the mouths of branch vessels, or as diffuse thickening. Intimal thickening contained two types of intimal smooth muscle cells. Myofilament-rich smooth muscle cells, resembling medial smooth muscle cells, were the more frequent cell type. Less frequent were rER-rich smooth muscle cells, which differed from myofilament-rich cells by the presence of abundant rough-surfaced endoplasmic reticulum. The rER-rich smooth muscle cells were more frequent in the upper intima, an area usually rich in ground substance. In addition to smooth muscle cells, the intima contained infrequent isolated macrophages adjacent to the endothelial basement membrane.

Evidence of cell injury was present in both types of intimal smooth muscle cells and in medial smooth muscle. More cells in old than in young animals showed signs of injury. Injury was noted either as edematous swelling of peripheral cell processes in which intracytoplasmic structures were dissolved and the basement membrane was lost, or as a more diffuse conversion of cytoplasmic components into complex multilaminated bodies, presumably autophagosomes. Edematous swelling of isolated cell processes was more frequent. Cell processes with degenerative change frequently were separated from the main body of the cell and disintegrated in the interstitial space. Interstitial debris was the result of the ongoing process of injury and disintegration. Debris accumulated mainly in older animals, and it was more abundant in the media than in the intima. Although necrosis of smooth muscle cells was not seen in control animals, death of the infrequent intimal macrophages did occur.

Lipid inclusions occurred in the cytoplasm of some intimal and medial smooth muscle cells. When present, inclusions were small, multiple, homogeneous, and more often in close association with smooth-surfaced endoplasmic reticulum and other organelles at the center, rather than at the periphery, of the cells. Macrophages with lipid inclusions occurred as infrequent single cells in the intima near the endothelium.

Hypercholesterolemic Animals With Progressing Lesions

When the high-cholesterol diet was given, the serum cholesterol level increased rapidly during the first 4 weeks and more slowly thereafter. In experiments in which we fed animals the high-cholesterol diet for 40 – 50 weeks, we found that the serum cholesterol reached an unsteady plateau after 12 – 15 weeks (Stary, 1972; Eggen, 1976). Table 2 shows the range within each experimental group of the mean serum total cholesterol for each animal during the 12-week progression period.

The high-cholesterol diet induces focal intimal lesions in coronary arteries and somewhat more extensive lesions in the aorta. Lesions consisted of an increased number of cells in the intima, massive accumulation of intracellular lipid in smooth muscle cells (resulting in oblong myogenic foam cells) (Fig. 1), and in

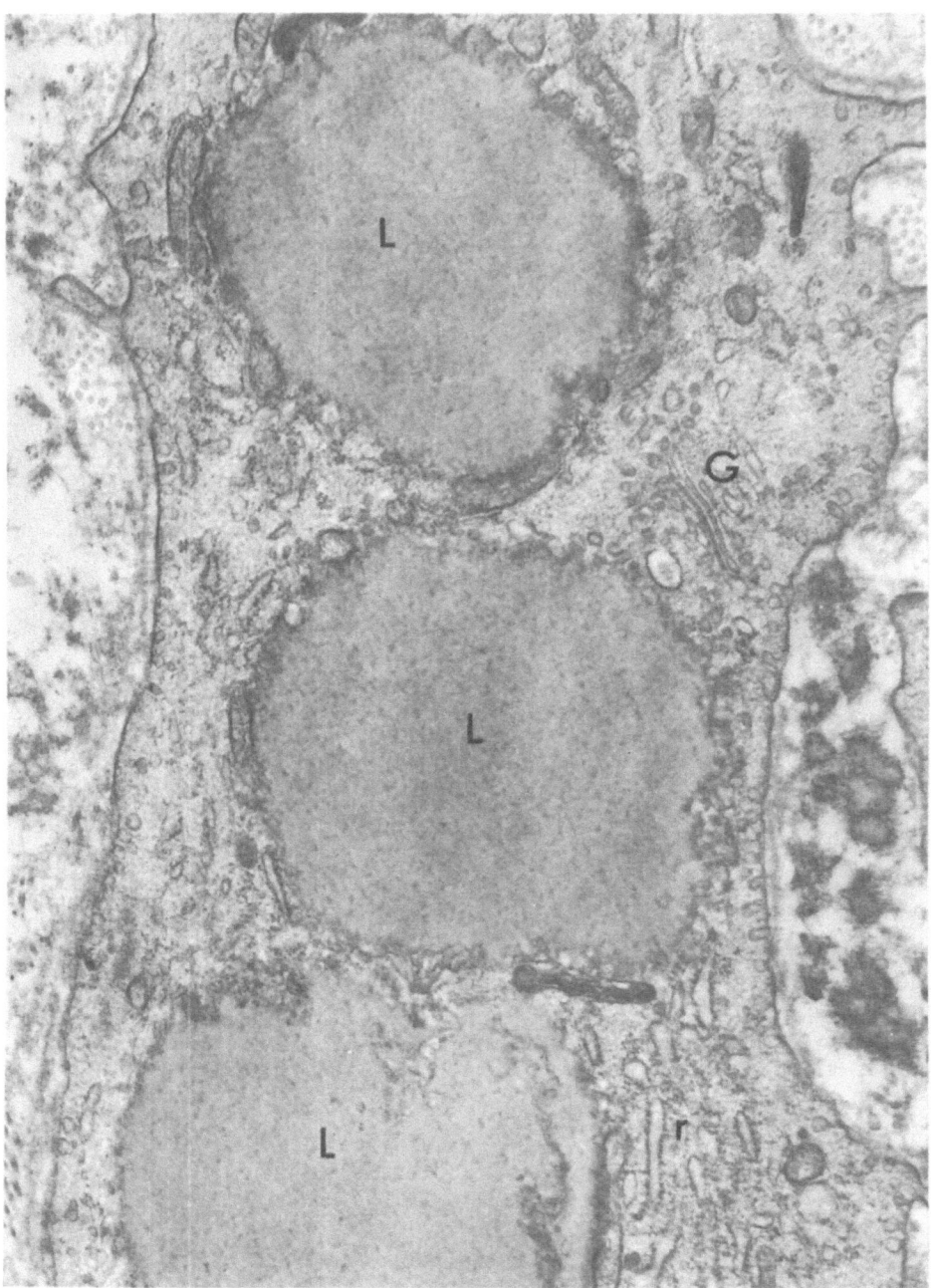

Figure 1. An intimal rER-rich smooth muscle cell in a lesion in the distal thoracic aorta. From a monkey killed after receiving a high-cholesterol diet for 12 weeks and then a low-cholesterol diet for 8 weeks. The mean serum cholesterol level during the 12 weeks on the high-cholesterol diet was 640 mg/dl; it had decreased to 200 mg/dl when the animal was killed. Lipid inclusions (L) are without a limiting membrane. Golgi complex (G); rough-surfaced endoplasmic reticulum (r) (Rhesus No. 130; X 31000)

macrophages (resulting in round foam cells). Radioautographs of the aorta in tritiated thymidine-labeled animals indicated that the increase in the number of cells resulted from proliferation of intimal macrophages and smooth muscle cells. These cell types labeled at a high rate in segments of the aorta having lesions (Stary and McMillan, 1970; Stary, 1974a, 1974b).

Cell injury and cell death were frequent in lesions. Death was more frequent in foam cells derived from macrophages than in smooth muscle cells. The morphologic criteria for certain cell death were dissolution of the plasma membrane and release of cell organelles and intracellular lipid inclusions into the extracellular space. A large number of lipid inclusions or of autophagosomes was the feature most frequently associated with cell death. Nevertheless, some smooth muscle cells and some macrophages without autophagosomes and with little or no lipid were also necrotic. Neutrophil and eosinophil granulocytes occured infrequently as single cells near the necrotic intimal cells and were themselves sometimes necrotic.

Debris from necrotic cells accumulated faster than it was removed, and pools of debris formed at the base of the intima. The internal elastic lamina acted as a barrier between intima and media, but, at points at which the lamina had gaps, debris from intimal pools extended into the adjacent media.

Animals With Regressing Atherosclerotic Lesions

The decline in serum cholesterol levels after the change from the high- to the low-cholesterol diet is shown in Table 2. Most animals regained normal levels within 4 - 8 weeks after diet change; however, in a few animals the serum cholesterol levels decreased either more rapidly or more slowly.

The most striking indication of regression was decreased cellularity of lesions, which resulted almost entirely from a decrease in the number of macrophage-derived foam cells. That number had decreased after 16 weeks. Twenty-four weeks after diet change, and at later periods, we saw only infrequent, single macrophage-derived foam cells in the intima. While the number of intact foam cells was diminishing, necrotic foam cells were always present, indicating that the return to normal cellularity resulted from their death. Intimal smooth muscle cells of these early atherosclerotic lesions were rarely necrotic after the serum cholesterol level had returned to normal. An explanation for the difference in the rate of death of smooth muscle cells and macrophages might be that, after the immediate cause of cell injury — that is, hypercholesterolemia — was removed, cell survival came to depend on the difference in the life span of cells. Thus, the accumulated macrophages, which are thought to have a limited life span, died over a period of several months, whereas smooth muscle cells, which have a much longer life span, survived.

We counted the labeled cells in some of the aortic radioautographs of the 38 monkeys injected with tritiated thymidine. Preliminary results (Stary, 1974b) indicate that the rate of proliferation of endothelial cells and smooth muscle cells, which increased during the hypercholesterolemic period, returned to normal levels after the serum cholesterol was lowered. By 16 weeks after change to the low-cholesterol diet labeling had decreased, and after 40 weeks it had returned to a normal level. Macrophages ceased to label before most of these cells had disappeared from the lesions.

Debris from necrotic cells, accumulated at the base of the intima during lesion progression, remained stable during the early part of regression. Twenty-four weeks after change to the low-cholesterol diet, the size of these pools of debris decreased coincident with the disappearance of most macrophage-derived foam cells and thus with the cessation of cell death. Pools of debris continued to decrease in extent. Sixty-four weeks after diet change, we saw only a minimal amount of debris in animals that had had the highest serum cholesterol elevation during the hypercholesterolemic period. No residual debris was present after 128 weeks. Debris disappeared first from the upper, and then from the lower intima. We presume that finely fragmented debris moved toward the adventitia and was carried away by adventitial lymphatics.

We determined the aortic cholesterol in the intima media preparation of 48 of the 64 monkeys in the two regression experiments. Results for the first study have been reported (Eggen et al., 1974; Strong et al., 1976). Results of the second study extend and confirm those reported for the first. Free an, to a greater extent, esterified cholesterol increased in the aortic intima media while the animals were receiving the high-cholesterol diet and for 4 - 8 weeks after return to the low-cholesterol diet. Most of the accumulated free and esterified cholesterol had disappeared by 24 - 32 weeks after diet change, coinciding with the disappearance of most macrophage-derived foam cells and with a decrease in the size of intimal pools of debris. The remainder of the cholesterol increment disappeared more slowly, until, after 64 weeks, the aortic free and ester fractions were essentially equal to those of the control animals.

The lipid inclusions of smooth muscle cells gradually decreased in size, although small residual inclusions that differed in morphology from the original inclusions remained in the cytoplasm. While lipid had accumulated in cells during the hypercholesterolemic period, the periphery of lipid inclusions was usually without a limiting membrane (Fig. 1). During the initial period of regression, most lipid inclusions continued to be without a peripheral membrane, although they progressively decreased in size. A double-contoured limiting membrane developed slowly and enveloped small residual inclusions during the late phases of regression. While lipid inclusions were decreasing in size, and as a limiting membrane was developing, minute osmiophilic granules and smooth-surfaced vesicles accumulated at the periphery of the inclusions (Fig. 2). Residual inclusions appeared to have a certain stability, because many were still present in intimal smooth muscle cells after 128 weeks. Residual inclusions probably represent remnants that are difficult to digest and are removed at an extremely slow rate. Some remnants might be insoluble. Some residual inclusions in smooth muscle cells were removed by a pathway other than that by which the bulk of the lipid accmulated by endocytosis was removed. The pathway involved the separation from the cell, and disintegration of cell processes containing inclusions.

The lipid inclusions of macrophage-derived foam cells that survived into the regression periods also had characteristic changes. Lipid particles, accumulated by endocytosis during the hypercholesterolemic period, had fused to form intracytoplasmic droplets. Although some droplets became partially enclosed by membrane initially, most were not membrane-bound. After lowering of the serum cholesterol level, all inclusions became rapidly enclosed by double-contoured membranes. New layers of membrane continued to appear until lipid droplets were converted into multilaminated structures (Fig. 3). The size of the lipid droplets decreased progressively while changing into multilaminated structures. The size of the resulting lipid-membrane complexes was not much smaller than that of inclusions during the progression phase. Sometimes, fusion of multilaminated structures created giant lipid-membrane complexes in the cytoplasm of regressing foam cells. Multilaminated structures were released into the interstitial space as foam cells became necrotic.

Smooth muscle cells and macrophages showed similarities and differences in the metabolism of lipid inclusions. Although lipid inclusions of both cell types developed membranes, the rate at which, and the extent to which, this development occurred was not the same. Membranes developed more rapidly around the inclusions of macrophage-derived foam cells than around the inclusions of smooth muscle cells. In smooth muscle cells, membrane-lipid complexes were small, the residuals of originally large lipid droplets that had decreased in size, probably through exocytosis of lipid particles. Macrophage-derived foam cells, on the other hand, retained large membrane complexes, indicating that, although its nature had changed, exocytosis of lipid from foam cells might not have occurred.

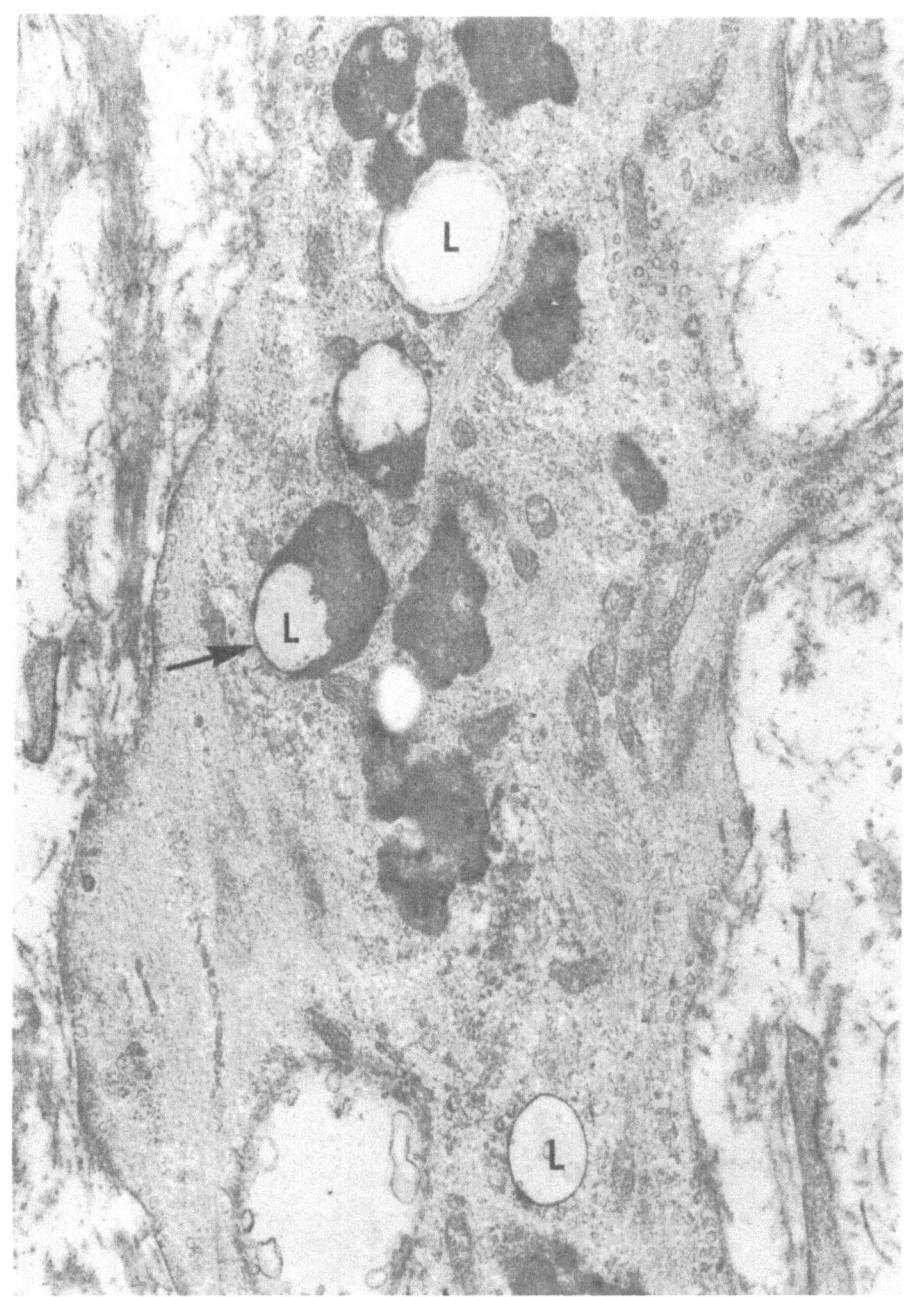

Figure 2. An intimal smooth muscle cell in a residual lesion in the distal thoracic aorta. From a monkey killed after receiving a high-cholesterol diet for 12
weeks and then a low-cholesterol diet for 128 weeks. Mean serum cholesterol level
was 590 mg/dl during the 12 weeks on the high-cholesterol diet. Normocholesterolemia (170 mg/dl) returned 12 weeks after diet reversal. In the late phase of regression, the lipid inclusions of smooth muscle cells differ from those seen in
progressing lesions. (Compare with smooth muscle cell in Fig. 1). Inclusions are
smaller and consist of lipid droplets (L) enclosed by one or more fine membranes
(arrow). Some inclusions consist entirely of fine multilaminated membranes
(Rhesus No. 121; X 22000)

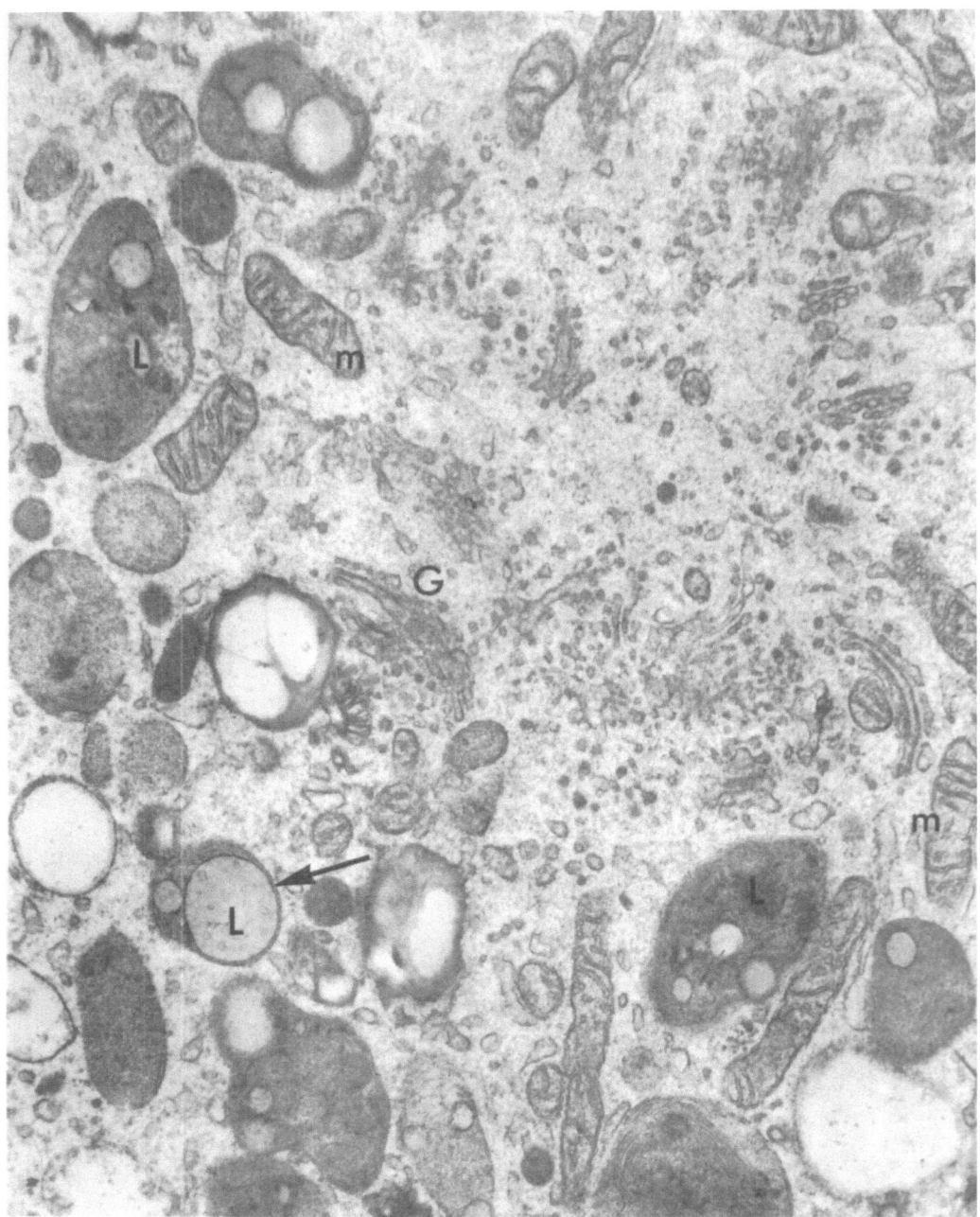

Figure 3. A macrophage-derived foam cell in a regressing atherosclerotic lesion in the distal thoracic aorta. From a monkey killed after receiving a high-cholesterol diet for 12 weeks and then a low-cholesterol diet for 16 weeks. Mean serum cholesterol level during the 12 weeks on the high-cholesterol diet was 490 mg/dl. Normocholesterolemia (150 mg/dl) returned 2 weeks after diet reversal. Macrophage-derived foam cells in regressing lesions differ from those in progressing lesions: lipid droplets (L) are enclosed by a double contoured membrane (arrow) or have converted into multilaminated lipid—membrane complexes. Golgi complex (G), mitochondria (m) (Rhesus No. 61; X 24000)

The Golgi complex was hyperplastic, particularly in macrophages, but also in smooth muscle cells with lipid inclusions. Cells with lipid also contained smooth vesicles that seemed to fuse with the periphery of lipid inclusions. In smooth muscle cells, vesicles were associated with the decrease in the size of the inclusions and with the formation of double-contoured membranes around residual inclusions. In macrophages, vesicles were associated with the conversion of inclusions into multilaminated structures. Smooth vesicles were derived from the hyperplastic Golgi complex and from endoplasmic reticulum. Smooth vesicles formed by the Golgi complex and by certain portions of the endoplasmic reticulum carry hydrolytic enzymes (Novikoff, 1973) and represent primary lysosomes. Fusion of vesicles with lipid inclusions represents the formation of secondary lysosomes. Both the small residual membrane-lipid complexes in smooth muscle cells and the larger multilaminated structures in foam cells are considered to represent secondary lysosomes.

Conclusions

The results of our experiments are summarized in parts I–IV of Figure 4.

I: The coronary artery and aortic intima of normocholesterolemic monkeys contained intimal smooth muscle cells that formed one or more cell layers in certain segments. Proliferation of intimal cells was low, but it was somewhat higher in segments of the intima with layers of intimal smooth muscle cells (cushions). Intimal smooth muscle cells were of two types: myofilament-rich smooth muscle cells containing mainly myofilaments, and rER-rich cells containing abundant rough-surfaced endoplasmic reticulum and few myofilaments. Lipid inclusions in smooth muscle cells were either absent or small and infrequent, and there was no extracellular lipid. The intima also contained rare, single, macrophages.

II: In hypercholesterolemic animals, proliferation of intimal smooth muscle cells and intimal macrophages increased, and, although numerous macrophages and smooth muscle cells were necrotic, the overall number of cells progressively became greater. Under our experimental conditions, the increase in macrophage-derived cells was greater than the increase in the number of smooth muscle cells. Lipid droplets accumulated in the cytoplasm of macrophages (resulting in round foam cells) and in smooth muscle cells (resulting in oblong myogenic foam cells). The Golgi complex and smooth vesicles associated with degradation of inclusions were hyperplastic. However, degradation of lipid droplets did not keep pace with their rapid intracytoplasmic accumulation. Most of the lipid droplets were without limiting membranes.

III: After substitution of low-cholesterol food for the high-cholesterol diet and return of high serum cholesterol to low levels, increased cell proliferation in the intima returned to normal levels. Intracytoplasmic lipid droplets in smooth muscle cells and in macrophages decreased in size progressively. In macrophages, decrease in size of droplets was associated with rapid conversion of droplets to multilaminated lipid-membrane complexes (secondary lysosomes). These accmulated in the cells and were released into the extracellular space only as macrophages became necrotic. In smooth muscle cells, conversion of lipid droplets into lipid-membrane complexes was less striking and less rapid, and intracytoplasmic retention occurred to a smaller degree. Although macrophages died, death of smooth muscle cells was rare after serum cholesterol reduction.

IV: Sixty-four weeks after return to low-cholesterol food, macrophages and macrophage-derived foam cells were either absent or rare and the bulk of the extracellular debris derived from cells that had become necrotic had disappeared. Lipid droplets in the cytoplasm of smooth muscle cells were infrequent and small; more frequent were small lipid-membrane complexes (secondary lysosomes) that remained as the residuals of larger lipid droplets and as evidence of former intimal lesions. Small lipid-membrane complexes in intimal smooth muscle cells were still present 128 weeks after return to low-cholesterol food.

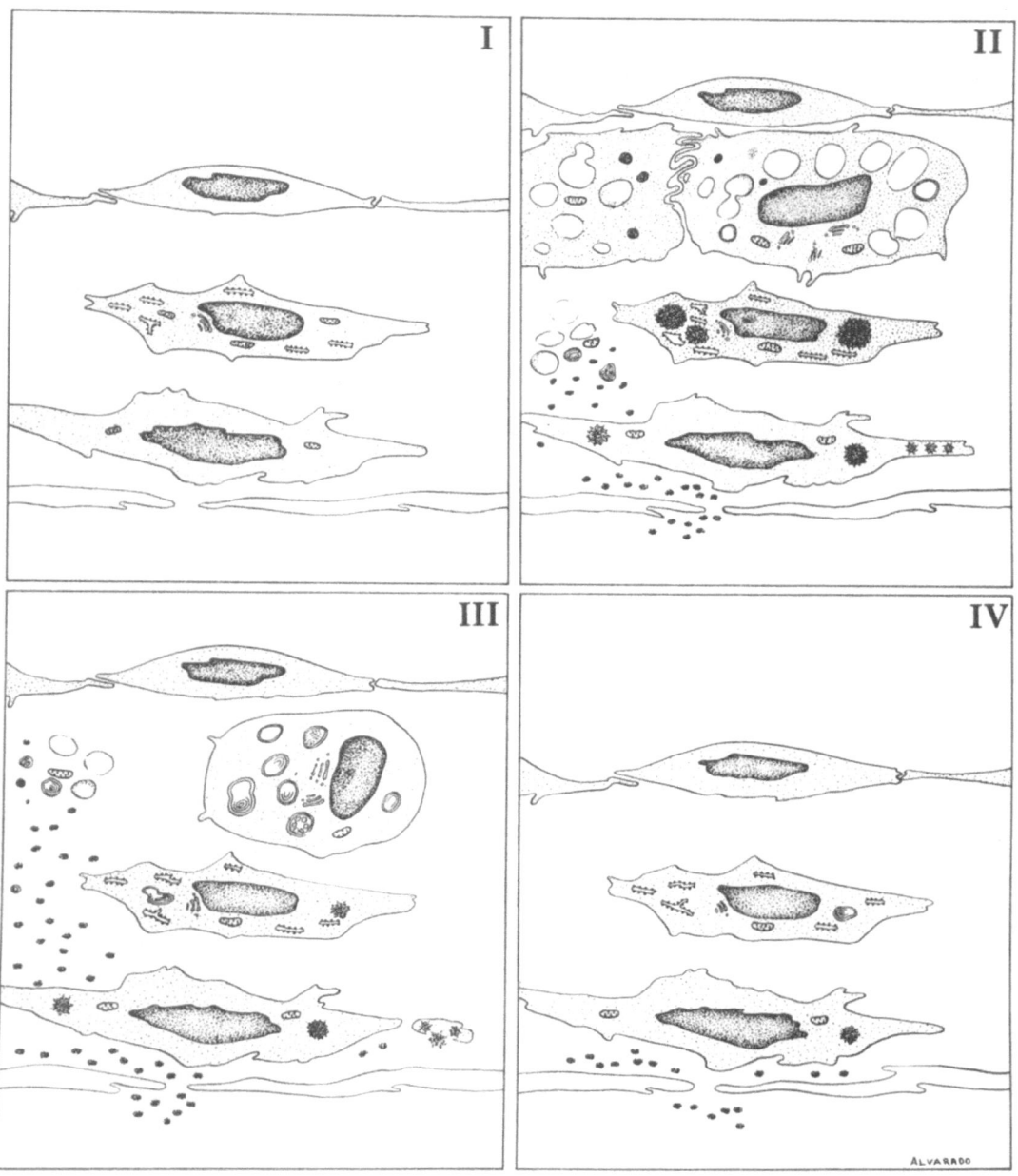

Figure 4. Schematic drawings summarizing the main ultrastructural features (I) of intimal thickening in normocholesterolemic control animals; (II) of progressing lesions in hypercholesterolemic animals; (III) of lesions in the early phase of regression; (IV) of residual lesions in the late phase of regression. For clarity, elastic and collagen fibers and mucopolysaccharide ground substance have been omitted from the drawings. Refer to the conclusions in the text for detailed descriptions

CONNECTIVE TISSUE CHANGES IN REGRESSION

Mark L. Armstrong

Arteries are endothelium-lined connective tissue tubes whose intima media contains chiefly smooth muscle cells. The atherosclerotic response of the arterial tubes involves endothelial changes (Shimamoto, 1974) and increases in the intimal cell population (Stary, 1974) with associated connective tissue changes. The response includes increased permeability to lipid, accumulation of intimal lipid in both intracellular and extracellular sites, and the formation of an intimal fibrous stroma that eventually attains plaque density. When experimentally induced atherosclerosis regresses, the resolution of the lesions involves decreases in the mass and labeling index of myointimal cells (Stary, 1972), depletion of lipid (Armstrong and Megan, 1972) and (the focus of this paper) changes in the connective tissue.

Connective tissue is a collective term, a "set" of cell products which belong together through interrelated biological functions. In the intima media of arteries, the set includes collagen, elastin with its associated microfibrillar protein, and assorted glycoproteins and proteoglycans. In postnatal life, the arterial cells continue to have the potential to elaborate an ordered array of these components of connective tissue according to metabolic need, e.g., that of growth. If a regression regimen is subsequently introduced, evidences of late repair and remodeling may appear. But the qualitative difference between the growth response and the injury response is not always clear, particularly if maturation and senescence are considered phases of growth. The increased bulk of connective tissue found in atherosclerosis is, with exceptions to be noted, rather similar to that found in the original artery. In unequivocal regression, the dimensions of the enlarged connective tissue mass are reduced. Two questions are posed about this change:
1. Is the connective tissue present in regression different in amount from that found in atherosclerosis?
2. What qualitative changes occur in the connective tissue?

Collagen Changes

Since mammalian collagen is used as biological patching material quite generally (Gillman, 1968), a much simpler model than the injured artery may serve as one illustration of the fate of response collagen. The subdermal carrageenan granuloma (van Robertson and Schwartz, 1953) is such a model. There is a proliferative reaction to an extracellular irritant with growth and regression phases (Perez-Tamayo, 1970) and the formation of new collagen (Jackson, 1957). If the concentration of collagen in the granuloma is plotted against tissue weight during growth and regression (Fig. 1), it is evident that collagen concentration increases during growth and sharply increases during regression. A third phase in late regression in which concentration falls is at least suggested by the data; it is noted because the same late decrease in regression is seen in arterial data. The total content of collagen in the granuloma contrasts sharply with the concentration, showing a steep rise during growth, a plateau during early regression, followed in turn by a precipitous decline (Fig. 2). Thus, a simple system in which the cell population is changing and collagen is used projects separate information when shown by collagen concentration and by total collagen content.

When atherosclerosis was experimentally induced in nonhuman primates by diet, and then a regression regimen substituted (Armstrong and Megan, 1975), the con-

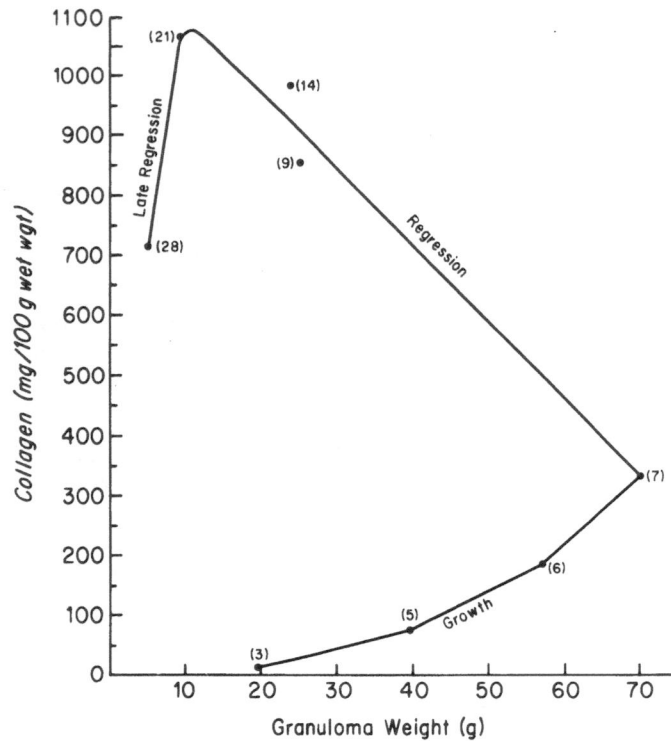

Figure 1. Carrageenan granuloma. Collagen concentration
plotted in terms of concurrent tissue weight. Numbers
in parenthesis indicate day
of experiment. Data from
Jackson, 1957

centration of collagen in the aorta (from the left subclavian artery to the
iliac bifurcation) was higher in regression than in atherosclerosis at three
separate regression intervals (Table 1): collagen became a more prominent part
of the arterial wall in regression than in experimental atherosclerosis. As in
the instance of the granuloma, these values for concentration cannot be taken to
show that collagen is greater in total amount. In this study, the aorta was also
measured *in situ* for length, and when collagen was expressed per unit length,
collagen decreased during regression (Table 1). Branch arteries of both elastic
and muscular types tended to show the same overall pattern (Armstrong and Megan,
1975).

If we plot aortic collagen concentration and the intima media weight measurements as was done for the carrageenan granuloma (Fig. 1), the curves are quite

Table 1. Aortic collagen

	Concentration[a]	Content[b]
Control	187 ± 12	3.04 ± 0.19
Atherosclerosis	180 ± 18	5.83 ± 0.49
Regression		
2 months	297 ± 13	5.19 ± 0.86
6 months	338 ± 18	5.07 ± 0.26
20 months	310 ± 7	4.89 ± 0.30

[a] mg/g dry weight.

[b] mg/cm length of artery.

All values are means ± SE.

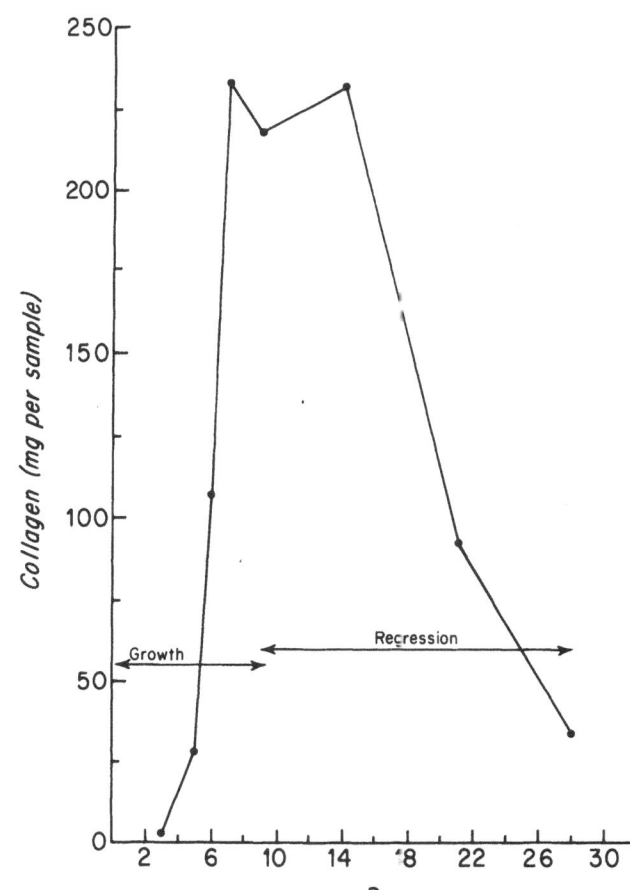

Figure 2. Carrageenan granuloma. Total collagen content. Sequential data points are those found at the experimental times shown in Figure 1. Calculated from Jackson, 1957

similar (Fig. 3). Corresponding to granuloma growth, lesion growth occurs during atherogenic challenge with a rise in collagen concentration; the subsequent regression phase is accompanied by a further rise in collagen concentration, and in a late regression phase, collagen declines more rapidly than intima media weight.

The changes in aortic intima media collagen content in atherosclerosis and regression (Table 1) would not be expected to follow the extreme trends seen in granuloma collagen content (Fig. 2). There is, nonetheless, the same evidence of loss of excess collagen during regression of experimental atherosclerosis, although it is attenuated. Thus two systems, the granuloma and the arterial wall, show broad similarities in collagen synthesis and utilization. The differences between the systems are almost excessively numerous: that any loss of arterial collagen would be perceptible during the regression of aortic atherosclerosis was unanticipated; that the behavior of collagen in so complex a system as experimental atherosclerosis resembled that of the short-lived granuloma model probably attests to generalities in collagen metabolism that are detectable over a very wide range of rates of resolution from injury, and in diverse tissues and types of injury.

The mass data on arterial collagen loss in the arterial wall during regression are not well-explained without invoking a mechanism for collagen breakdown. Collagenolytic activity has been described in experimental atherosclerosis in some settings (Linder, 1974), but collagenases or their surrogates have not been measured in regression. If collagenase-like activity exists, it may operate at a low level. Adequate lytic activity need not be readily measurable above the

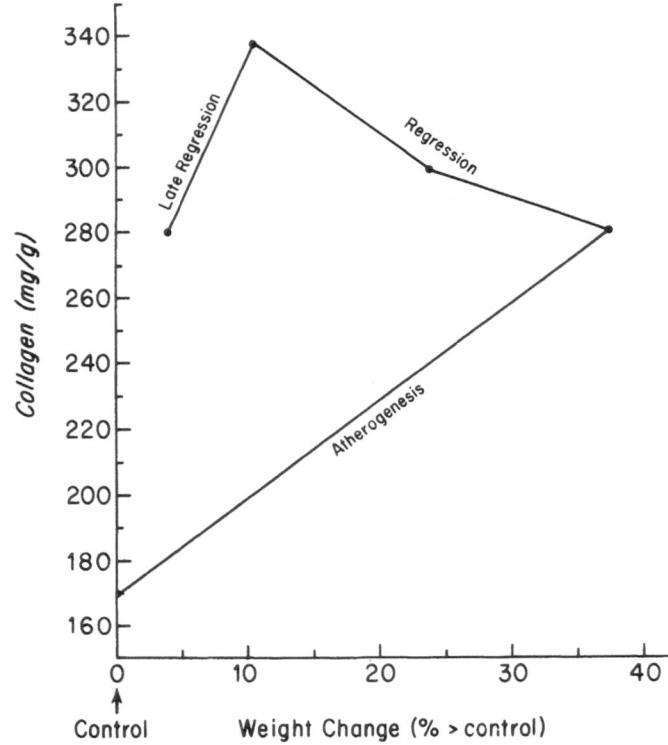

Figure 3. Collagen concentration in intima media of monkeys plotted in terms of concurrent tissue weight. Total experimental time was 37 months. Data from Armstrong and Megan, 1975

hypothetic levels required by collagen-containing tissue to respond to morphogenetic demands, and yet, as fibrogenic stimuli are reduced, be sufficient to cause a net loss of collagen from the artery.

The genetic type of collagen in the atherosclerotic plaque in man has been reported to be largely type I rather than type III (McCullagh, 1975). The preponderant collagen in the media is apparently type III synthesized by smooth muscle cells (Ross and Glomset, 1976). The distinction has been underscored by the suggestion that the major source of collagen in human atherosclerosis is an intimal fibroblast-like mesenchymal cell (McCullagh, 1975). It is certain that much work will be reported on these provocative points in the immediate future. Which of the collagen types is dominant in the lesions of induced atherosclerosis in nonhuman primates has not at this point been established, nor has it been shown which type of collagen is the more susceptible to depletion during regression regimens.

Elastin Changes

Morphologic evidence of fragmentation and loss of elastic fibers of the media is a major feature of experimental and human atherosclerosis (Taylor, 1965; Moon and Rinehart, 1952). Focal destruction of architectural elastin in experimental atherosclerosis may involve the total thickness of the wall (Armstrong and Megan, 1974b). These morphologic trends would be expected to lower elastin levels. Biochemical evidence of reduced elastin has been occasionally reported in atherosclerosis (Pernis and Clerici, 1957; Radhakrishnamurthy et al., 1975). Perhaps more often the concentration (and the content) in experimental atherosclerosis is reported as rising (Kramsch et al., 1973b; Armstrong and Megan, 1975) or not changing (Vesselinovitch et al., 1976). Atherogenic regimens that are similar except for the type of fat or carbohydrate may cause differing amounts of intimal fibrogenesis (Wissler et al., 1962; Armstrong et al., 1976); regulation of the proportions of collagen and elastin synthesized has been attributed to mechanical stress (Rodbard, 1974), but whether any difference in control exists among experimental dietary regimens compatible with health (e.g., not deficient in ascorbate or copper) has not been established.

Since new elastic fibers are seen in experimental lesions and architectural medial elastic fibers are destroyed, it seems plausible to conclude that the findings of unchanged elastin levels and elevated elastin in atherosclerosis are both reflections of the net change of synthesis and destruction of elastin. When elastin is increased in experimental atherosclerosis in the nonhuman primate, it tends to fall in regression (Table 2). When elastin is not elevated, suggesting smaller amounts in atherosclerotic tissue, it is not reduced in regression (Vesselinovitch et al., 1976). Taken together, the two observations seem to indicate that the elastin lost in regression is repair elastin. The morphologic evidence of moderately developed elastic fibers in the intima of atherosclerotic arteries has not correlated closely with increases in biochemically determined elastin. It may be that young, poorly stained elastin is what is found in large amounts in some studies of atherosclerosis, and that it is this elastin which subsequently decreases during regression. If collagen and elastin content are compared during regression in a primate species susceptible to rather marked atherosclerosis with medial damage (Armstrong and Megan, 1975), collagen content falls progressively (with an overall significant change) below atherosclerotic values, but elastin drops more sharply, leveling off near, or when significant medial damage has occurred in atherosclerosis, below control values. These regression data are compatible with other data suggesting that the turnover of new arterial elastin may in fact be more rapid than collagen in the aorta, but with a relatively constant mass ratio between the two fibrous proteins as polymerization advances during normal biosynthesis.

Analyses of elastin in atherosclerotic plaques have shown polar amino acids not found in elastin from other sites (Kramsch et al., 1971). The issue of whether this is possibly a true alteration in elastin composition (Kramsch and Hollander, 1973a) or an indication of a difficulty separable companion molecule (Keeley and Partridge, 1974) lies outside our inquiry. However, it is most pertinent to ask whether this significant change, which involves impressive evidence of increased binding of calcium and lipid to elastin, is altered in regression. The data available suggest that lipid isolated with the crude elastin pellet shows retarded or no depletion after 16 months of dietary regression (Wagner and Clarkson, 1973). Linked with these considerations of elastin behavior are unresolved questions about the role of the elastin-associated microfibrillar glycoprotein (Ross and Bornstein, 1970) in regression.

Table 2. Aortic elastin

	Concentration[a]	Content[b]
Control	374 ± 16	6.06 ± 0.06
Atherosclerosis	457 ± 12	9.43 ± 0.22
Regression		
2 months	320 ± 19	5.47 ± 0.70
6 months	245 ± 16	3.68 ± 0.34
20 months	284 ± 10	4.23 ± 0.40

[a]mg/g dry weight.

[b]mg/cm length of artery.

All values are means ± SE.

The Interfibrillar Matrix

The arterial collagen-elastin framework has a more intimate architecture containing protein-sugar complexes, the glycoproteins and proteoglycans. A number of functional and architectural roles have been defined for extracellular glycoproteins (Berenson et al., 1966; Franzblau et al., 1973; Robert et al., 1974). The morphology of the arterial proteoglycans has recently been clarified (Wight and Ross, 1975a). Although their total contribution to arterial mass is not great, the proteoglycans from a network of polygonal granules connected with filaments throughout the interfibrillar space, and they invest collagen and elastin. In atherosclerosis, proteoglycans become morphologically prominent in lesion areas before biochemical changes in the fibrous protein content of the artery are detectable (Armstrong, M.L., Megan, M.B., unpublished observations). The proteoglycan matrix may help control lesion formation in directing the course of newly formed fibrous protein (Fig. 4), thus functioning as one determinant of extracel-

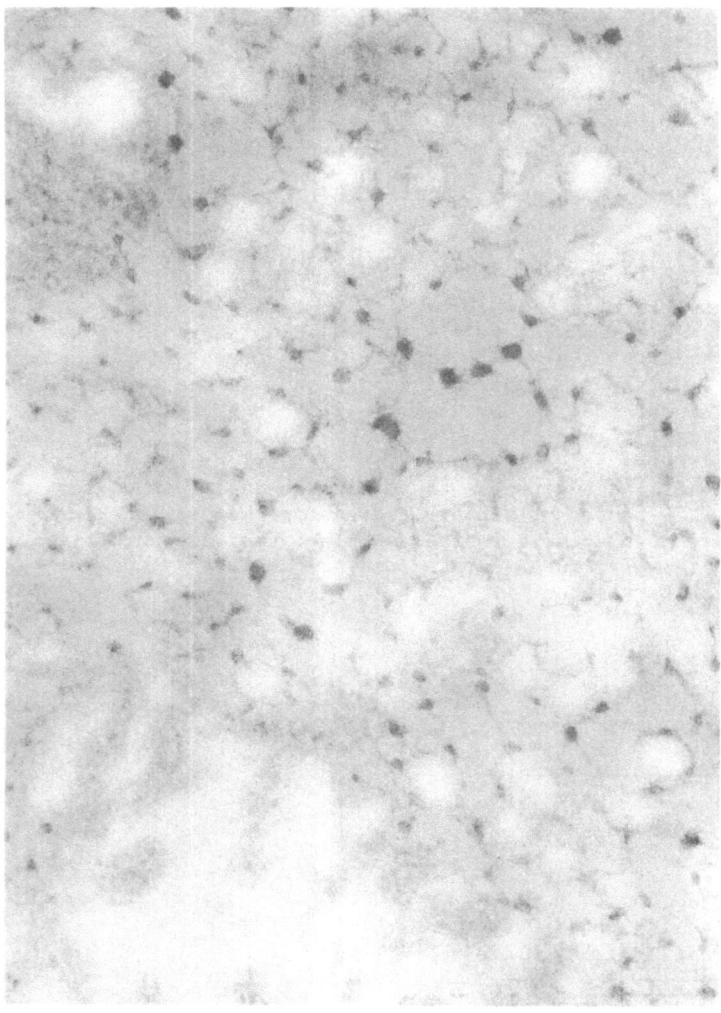

Figure 4. Proteoglycan matrix spacing new fibers in the intima. Matrix granules with filamentous interconnections occupy the interfibrillar space and surround small collagen fibers seen mainly in cross section. Ruthernium red and uranyl acetate (X 106,000)

lular architecture, and may also maintain tissue turgor within the artery (Wight and Ross, 1975a).

The visualized proteoglycan matrix increases as atherosclerotic lesions increase. The chemically determined total glycosaminoglycan concentration decreases as lesions become more fibrotic (Curran and Crane, 1962; Smith, 1965; Stevens et al., 1976), but considered in terms of surface area of the vessel rather than by unit weight total, glycosaminoglycans may show a marked increase with lesion severity (Stevens et al., 1976), in keeping with the morphologic picture of an expanded proteoglycan matrix. It is nonetheless probable that in some densely fibrotic, complicated lesions, the available matrix space is restricted, and the absolute amount of proteoglycans is reduced.

In the smaller lesions of regression, the proteoglycan matrix does not seem to change much from its appearance in atherosclerosis. This lack of change would be compatible with an absolute decrease within the lesions after regression, and would fit intima inner media data in which no total change per unit weight in glycosaminoglycans was found in regression (Radhakrishnamurthy et al., 1975).

It is not known whether the protein-glycosaminoglycan matrix assists or retards lipid depletion in regression. The mechanism of lipid depletion from the intima is poorly understood (Kokatnur et al., 1975). It is evident that significant distances of the extracellular space must be traversed by lipid for regress to occur. Is the interfibrillar matrix, a presumed site of lipid trapping by several postulated mechanisms in atherosclerosis (Iverius, 1971, 1973), a shuttle system in concert with lipoprotein during regression?

The arterial proteoglycans contain mixtures of individual glycosaminoglycans (Wight and Ross, 1975a; Eisenstein et al., 1975) which vary as to species (Engel, 1971) and to the responses among species to atherogenic regimens (Helin et al., 1970; Seethanathan and Kurup, 1971; Saxena and Nagchaudhuri, 1969). Perhaps as a generality, increases in chondroitin sulfates and dermatan sulfate may be considered delayed responses (Helin et al., 1970) and increases in hyaluronic acid an acute response (Saxena and Nagchaudhuri, 1969; von Berlepsch and Studer, 1969) to arterial injury leading to atherosclerosis. The major glycosaminoglycan synthesized in vitro by the artery of the nonhuman primate is dermatan sulfate (Wight and Ross, 1975b), and this glycosaminoglycan is present in greatest concentration in normal, atherosclerotic, and regressed monkeys (Radhakrishnamurthy et al., 1975). The greatest relative changes following regression in atherosclerotic rhesus monkeys were a decrease in chondroitin-6 sulfate and a rise in hyaluronic acid (Radhakrishnamurthy et al., 1975)[*].

In experimental regression, the glycosaminoglycan composition of the proteoglycans thus shows some evidence of change. Whether the glycoproteins, which tend to be increased as a class in atherosclerosis (Anastassiades et al., 1972; Wagh et al., 1973), are altered quantitatively or qualitatively seems not to have been evaluated. It is of interest that the intima becomes more PAS-positive and less alcianophilic as regression continues, but the nature of this chromatic change has not been defined in ultrastructural or biochemical terms.

Basement Membrane of Endothelium

This complex connective tissue product of the endothelium (Kefalides and Denduchis, 1969; Liepkalns et al., 1975; Jaffee et al., 1976) becomes thickened in atherosclerosis and seems to remain so after many months of regression. The

---

[*]In man, the condroitin sulfates and dermatan sulfate both rise in cerebral atherosclerosis (Nakamura et al., 1968) , and dermatan sulfate shows a variable relationship to tissue weight in aortic atherosclerosis (Buddeke, 1962; Klynstra et al., 1967; Kumar et al., 1967). There are no human regression data.

thickening is presumed to be a nonspecific response to injury (Vracko and Benditt, 1970). Whether transfer of intracellular lipid to extracellular subendothelial sites during regression tends to perpetuate this change throughout generations of endothelial cells is not known.

Dystrophic and Metaplastic Changes in Connective Tissue

Collagen Changes

A significant amount of the excess collagen synthesized in atherosclerosis remains as a permanent feature of the regressed artery. It becomes more Van Gieson positive, more dense, and not infrequently undergoes hyaline transformation. This residual collagen may also show dystrophic calcification.

Calcification often tends to persist in regression. Its occurrence in atherosclerosis has been largely linked to calcification of the internal elastic membrane, but calcification at or near other elastic membranes in the media have been found as a result of atherosclerosis or ageing and studied extensively (Yu, 1974). A link between calcium and lipid binding (Kramsch et al., 1974) has been mentioned, and an ingenious theory of calcium binding that makes the elastin molecule susceptible to lipid uptake (Urry, 1971) should be noted; it should be further noted that the mechanisms and even the precise sites of the calcifying process in arterial tissue are under continuing evaluation (Kim, 1976). In a manner comparable to cartilage calcification (Ali et al., 1970), it has been proposed that the primary mechanism of calcification in vascular tissue occurs by matrix vesicle transformation. These vesicles form from cell budding, may occur especially in areas of high cell turnover associated with elevated tissue lipids, and sometimes line the edges of elastic fibers. There are occasional instances in which the matrix vesicle hypothesis may explain calcification without the need of invoking calcium capture by elastin at sites where elastin is apparently absent. In many instances of early mineralization, however, the process is occurring in the proximity of elastin sites and matrix vesicles are not observed. It has been shown morphologically and chemically that acid mucopolysaccharides are increased in areas of ongoing calcification, but that acid mucopolysaccharides are destroyed at calcifying sites (Wusterman et al., 1972). These data fit the universal observation of dense alcianophilic material at calcifying sites as evidence of increased acid mucopolysaccharides, and the limited ultrastructural information that proteoglycan areas surrounding small calcifying sites show an apparent loss of material (Armstrong, M.L., Megan, M.B., unpublished data).

In regression from atherosclerosis that is induced by diet but greatly accentuated by a single endothelial denudation (Daoud et al., 1976), the amount of calcium is less by morphologic evaluation than in atherosclerosis. In atherosclerosis induced in nonhuman primates by diet, the story is more complex. Calcification was greater during regression than in atherosclerosis in monkeys whose regression diet had a high content of sugar (which may influence the tendency of connective tissue to calcify) (Armstrong and Megan, 1974a). Other morphologic aspects of resolution during regression were unaffected. A current study in the same nonhuman primate species (*M. mulatta*) is nondecisive as to the course of calcification. Another primate species (*M. fascicularis*) that was fed commercial laboratory chow during regression showed dystrophic changes not seen in atherosclerosis, including calcification, and rarely progression of calcification to bone (Armstrong and Megan, 1974b). It is, therefore, not possible to project a general expectation as to whether calcification will be diminished or exacerbated during successful regression regimens as judged by enlargement of the arterial lumen.

Overview of Connective Tissue Changes

Current information on the alteration of connective tissue after the regression of experimental atherosclerosis has an interim status that future studies are certain to modify. The present evidence is strong that excess collagen tends to be lost from the artery during regression, even while the residual intimal collagen becomes more dense and invulnerable to depletion. In some studies, there occurs a loss of elastin as well; there is reason to believe that the elastin lost in regression has no architectural function, in contrast to the architectural elastin that is destroyed in atherosclerosis. The specific roles of the protein polysaccharides and the glycoproteins have not been clarified in the regression phenomenon. Dystrophic changes in the fibrous proteins are not improved in all atherosclerosis——regression sequences, and in some sequences are made worse.

ANGIOGRAPHIC EVIDENCE OF ATHEROSCLEROSIS REGRESSION IN MAN

David H. Blankenhorn

Introduction

The natural history of human atherosclerosis can be studied from serial angiograms. This has been done in femoral artery by Knight et al. (1972), Tillgren (1965), Chilvers et al. (1974), Kuthan et al. (1971), Coran and Warren (1966), and DePalma et al. (1970); in coronary artery by Kimbiris et al. (1974), Nash et al. (1974), Gensini et al. (1974), Rosch et al. (1974), Henderson and Rowe (1973), Bemis et al. (1973), Knight et al. (1972), and Cohn et al. (1975). The angiographic response of atherosclerotic lesions to blood lipid lowering therapy has also been studied. Knight et al. (1972) evaluated ileal by-pass; Cohn et al. (1975) evaluated clofibrate therapy. In aggregate, these authors have studied femoral artery progress in 908 patients for a total of 2728 patient years and coronary artery progress in 374 patients for a total of 823 patient years. DePalma et al. (1970) report one patient with femoral atherosclerosis improvement. Knight et al. (1972) report three patients with coronary lesion improvement. Gensini et al. (1974) report two additional patients with coronary improvement. Atherosclerotic lesions in all other patients remained unchanged or became worse. The general picture emerging from these studies is of slow, steady lesion progression, little influenced by therapy.

The studies just reviewed all employed standard diagnostic angiographic procedures. The usual goal of standard diagnostic angiography is to provide information about the general distribution of blood flow through a vascular bed. This precludes exact definition of vessel wall pathology because injection and filming procedures do not allow this during simultaneous overview of many vessels. A similar problem occurs in landscape photography; when a broad expanse is to be recorded, fine details of a specific object in this landscape cannot be shown on the same photograph.

In 1971, my co-workers and I began development of angiographic procedures specifically providing high definition and high resolution of small sections of major blood vessel walls. The factors involved in angiography are: (1) factors in the angiographic procedure: catheterization of the patient, injection of contrast media, timing of films, (2) factors involved in the x-ray equipment: the character of the x-ray tube and generator, type of film changer, type of film, development conditions, and (3) factors involved in film interpretation. We introduced major modifications into film reading and relatively smaller changes into the other aspects of angiography. Each vascular bed presents unique problems and our procedure is now most advanced in femoral artery.

At the Third International Atherosclerosis Symposium in West Berlin, I presented a preliminary report of the prevalence and distribution of lesions in femoral atherosclerosis of 28 hyperlipoproteinemic patients. Repeat angiograms have now been obtained and analyzed in 25 of these patients. In the interval between angiograms, which averaged 13 months, they were treated with lipid-lowering drugs and diet. Changes in atherosclerosis have been observed and evaluated relative to blood lipid level change and hyperlipoproteinemic type. Cerebral and coronary angiography was not performed in these patients and we have no direct information about these circulatory beds. The relationship of change in cerebral and coronary vessels to femoral artery change is not known.

A second angiographic study now in progress will provide information as to coronary and femoral atherosclerosis interrelations. Patients in this second study have not been selected because of hyperlipoproteinemia, but rather on the basis of premature atherosclerosis manifest by myocardial infarction between ages 40 and 49 (Blankenhorn, 1976; Sanmarco et al., 1976). Patients in the second study have also shown femoral atherosclerosis regression and three examples are shown (Figure 1). The remainder of this presentation will present data on the 25 hyperlipoproteinemic patients who have had a complete analysis of femoral atherosclerosis change during 13 months of lipid lowering.

Materials and Methods

Patients and Patient Management

The 25 hyperlipoproteinemic patients reported here were referred to the Los Angeles County-University of Southern California Medical Center's Cardiac Lipid Clinic for therapy, as a rule because of inadequate response to therapy or difficulty in compliance to diet. Sixteen patients were asymptomatic, nine had a history of previous myocardial infarction or angina pectoris, but only one had claudication. Twelve patients had type IV hyperlipoproteinemia (type IV) and 13 had type II hyperlipoproteinemia (type II) as determined by total blood cholesterol and triglyceride (DHEW Publ. 75-628, 1944) and lipoprotein electrophoresis on cellulose acetate (Chin and Blankenhorn, 1968). All patients were euthyroid with normal liver function. Patients were seen at monthly intervals by a physician and nutritionist. Sitting blood pressure and smoking habits were recorded. Fasting blood lipids and uric acid were determined monthly. Intravenous glucose tolerance testing was performed by the method of Wahlberg (1966) during hospitalization before each angiogram. These data are presented in Table 1, which also shows "risk factor" levels between angiograms.

National Heart and Lung Institute hyperlipoproteinemic type specific diet therapy was prescribed and diet compliance estimated. Diets were modified to reduce sodium intake to 1 g/day if diastolic blood pressure exceeded 90 mm Hg. Weight loss was prescribed for patients above ideal body weight. Eight type IV patients were treated with clofibrate. Additional therapy to reduce lipid level in clofibrate-treated patients was: neomycin sulfate for clofibrate-associated increase in low-density lipoprotein (Nichols et al., 1968), one patient; insulin for adult onset diabetes, one patient. Four type IV patients were treated with tibric acid. Seven type II patients were treated with clofibrate plus neomycin sulfate, six with clofibrate alone. Prescribed drug dosage in all patients was: clofibrate 2 g/day, neomycin sulfate 2 g/day, and tibric acid 1 g/day. Blood pressure lowering agents were: hydrochlorothiazide, eight patients; hydrochlorothiazide plus methyldopa, one patient; and reserpine, one patient. In all patients, therapy had been initiated prior to first angiogram and was continued without change until the next angiogram.

Radiographic Technique, Clinical

The average interval between angiograms was 13 months. Patients were admitted to the University of Southern California's Clinical Research Center and taken off all medication except insulin 72 hours prior to angiography. Written informed consent was obtained by a protocol approved by the University's Human Research Committee.

For angiography, patients were positioned supine on the x-ray table with the foot stabilized by soft restraints to an angle of 45°. Scout films were taken with exposure factors chosen by thigh size and film densities measured with a spot densitometer. Background tissue densities of second angiograms were matched to those of first angiograms by adjusting kV. X-ray source to film distance was 40 inches and patients were positioned identically for both examinations. Twenty

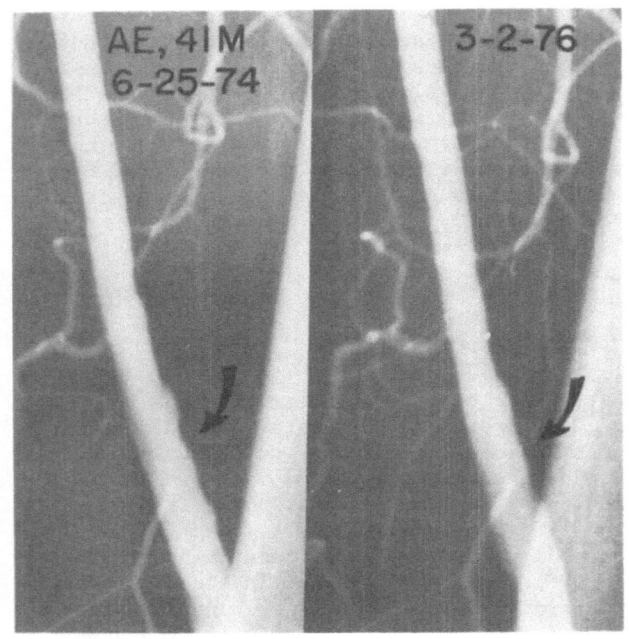

Figure 1a

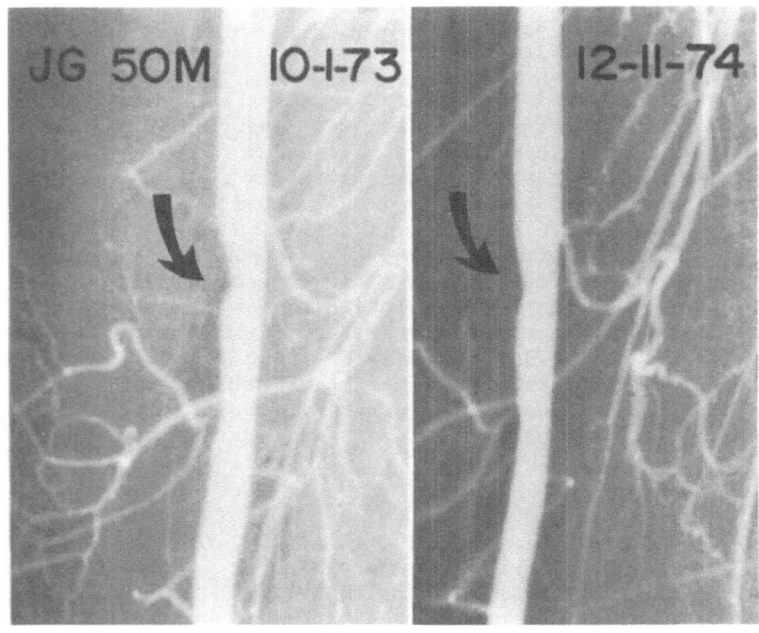

Figure 1b

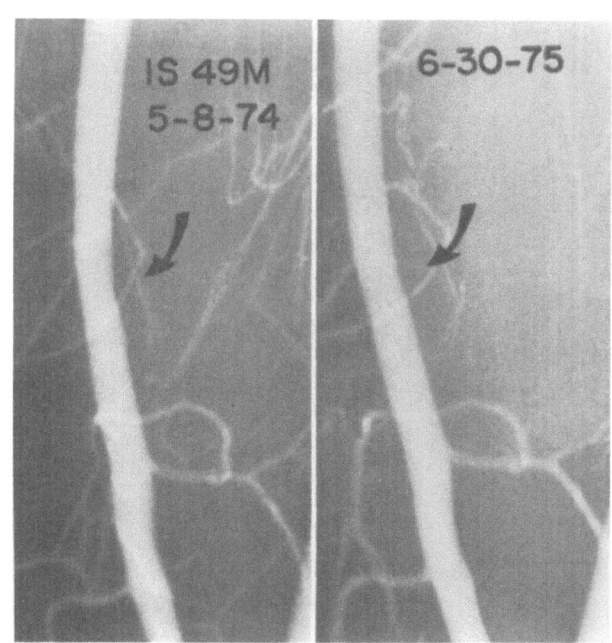

Figure 1c

Figure 1a-c. Three examples of femoral atherosclerosis regression. The date of each angiogram is indicated. The first film of each pair indicates the patient's initials, sex, and age

cm^3 of meglumine diatrizoate were injected through an 18 gauge needle and four films were taken during the first second after contrast injection. Fifteen to 18 more films were taken two per second. All films exceeded 4.3 cm^3 per second of 35% iodine-containing medium found diagnostic for femoral radiography by Lindbom (1950). An electrocardiogram was recorded and marked by a radiation exposure detector at the time of each film. There were no complications from angiography. All analyzed films were exposed late in diastole and met three criteria: (1) Complete filling of the area of interest with contrast media which extended from at least 15 cm above Hunter's canal to the popliteal space, (2) no evidence of flow separation, and (3) the film was one of three consecutive films with unchanged luminal contours.

Computer Image Dissector Procedures and Data Analysis

The image dissector, a DICOMED D-57* was used to sample film density every 52.7 μm along scan lines spaced at 52.7 μm. Densities were converted to numbers 0 - 255. A computer determination of atherosclerosis was calculated from measures of contrast shadow density variability between vessel edges and roughness of vessel shadow edges. The computing procedures used for this atherosclerosis determination were developed by autopsy x-ray studies of human cadavers described previously (Blankenhorn, 1976; Crawford et al., 1977). These autopsy studies indicate that computer determined atherosclerosis is correlated $r = 0.86$, $p < 0.001$ with what trained observers see when vessels have been opened for inspection (Crawford et al., 1977), but is more precise (Crawford et al., 1974).

Computer determined atherosclerosis was used to derive two statistics for each patient; atherosclerosis over age and atherosclerosis percent change per month.

*DICOMED Corp., Minneapolis, MN 55431.

Table 1. Clinical characteristics of patients

Patient No.	Age	Sex	% Ideal body weight[a]	Chol.[b]	Trig.[b]	Glucose K[c]	Uric acid[b]	Blood pressure[d] Systolic	Blood pressure[d] Diastolic	Smoking level[e]	Phenotype
1	50	M	102	277	109	2.10	5.6	153	100	0	II
2	56	F	95	351	63	1.19	4.3	117	65	0	II
3	37	M	135	343	1189	1.16	8.3	144	85	40	IV
4	39	M	99	323	60	1.11	4.8	119	80	25	II
5	29	M	107	260	171	1.28	7.1	140	88	40	II
6	39	M	130	309	1444	.42	4.4	133	83	10	IV
7	54	F	182	285	227	.22	6.8	151	100	0	IV
8	48	M	98	463	349	1.75	6.4	114	76	0	II
9	49	F	118	289	616	.66	6.0	117	78	0	IV
10	38	M	95	252	240	1.10	7.3	133	83	0	IV
11	32	M	139	454	2756	.87	5.5	117	81	0	IV
12	47	M	103	217	168	.90	7.8	122	73	0	IV
13	52	M	147	284	386	.74	7.8	131	89	0	IV
14	62	F	134	214	198	1.24	4.7	119	78	0	IV
15	22	M	88	293	.76	.96	4.9	114	72	20	II
16	65	M	92	325	124	.79	5.3	118	66	0	II
17	38	M	105	216	71	1.20	5.9	121	80	0	II
18	50	M	108	272	152	.82	7.8	121	78	0	IV
19	36	M	106	209	109	1.43	5.5	120	78	20	II
20	48	M	113	282	128	.68	6.7	115	74	0	II
21	48	M	119	257	145	.96	6.5	123	82	0	II
22	50	M	122	242	208	.82	6.3	138	80	30	IV
23	36	M	104	196	83	1.65	4.7	105	67	0	II
24	62	F	139	267	89	1.19	5.8	128	86	10	II
25	50	F	104	270	298	1.13	7.6	134	87	0	IV

[a] Statistical Bulletin, Metropolitan Life Insurance Company, 40: No. 3, Nov/Dec, 1959.

[b] mg% determined monthly, average value between angiogram #1 and angiogram #2.

[c] Glucose disappearance rate, 25 g IV glucose tolerance (Wahlberg, 1965). Average of two determinations, one before each angiogram.

[d] mm Hg determined monthly, average value between angiogram #1 and angiogram #2.

[e] Cigarettes per day, average between angiogram #1 and angiogram #2.

$$\frac{\text{atherosclerosis}}{\text{age}} = \frac{\text{atherosclerosis at angiogram } \#1}{\text{age (in years) at angiogram } \#1}$$

$$\text{atherosclerosis percent change per month} =$$

$$\frac{\text{atherosclerosis at angiogram } \#2 - \text{atherosclerosis at angiogram } \#1 \times 100}{\text{atherosclerosis at angiogram } \#1 \times \text{months between angiograms}}$$

Atherosclerosis over age is an estimate of the rate at which atherosclerosis has accumulated during the life of each patient prior to the first angiogram. Atherosclerosis percent change per month expresses the rate of change in the period of therapy between angiograms. If change is in the direction of lesion regression, this has has a negative sign.

In addition to computing the statistics described above, we compared atherosclerosis change as measured by computer with a visual determination of atherosclerosis change by four human readers "blind" as to the sequence of angiograms (Barndt et al., 1977). The correlation between computer determined atherosclerosis percent change and change in visually determined atherosclerosis area was $r = 0.68$, $p < 0.001$.

Results

Patients in Table 1 are numbers in rank order of lesion change. Patient #1 showed greatest lesion progression; patient #25 showed greatest lesion regression. Patients #14, #15, and #16 showed essentially no change in lesions.

Average values for atherosclerosis over age and atherosclerosis percent change per month are shown in Table 2. Prior to the first angiogram, the average rate of atherosclerosis accumulation, as estimated by atherosclerosis over age at the first angiogram, did not differ in the two types. During the therapy interval, the average rate of atherosclerosis percent change per month did not differ in the two types and this rate did not differ significantly from zero in either type. In summary, group averages did not demonstrate a difference in the behavior of atherosclerosis in the two types before or during therapy. However, it is important to note the marked variation in individual response of atherosclerosis during therapy. This occurred because some patients were changing in the direction of lesion progression, while others changed in the direction of lesion regression resulting in group means approaching zero.

Atherosclerosis percent change per month for each patient was considered in relation to that patient's age, sex, severity of preexisting atherosclerosis, atherosclerosis over age, glucose tolerance, obesity, average level of blood cholesterol, blood triglyceride, smoking, and blood pressure between angiograms. When

Table 2. Atherosclerosis over age at first angiogram and atherosclerosis change per month between angiograms

	Atherosclerosis over age	Atherosclerosis % change per month
Type II	15.7 ± 1.4[a]	-0.62 ± 0.36[a]
Type IV	13.9 ± 1.0	0.14 ± 0.42
	NS	NS

[a]SEM.

Table 3. Stepwise regression in type IV patients. Atherosclerosis % change per month versus clinical attributes listed in text

Multiple correlation = 0.846

Standard error of estimate = 0.871

Variables in equation

Variable	Coefficient	F ratio
Constant term	1.723	
Blood triglyceride	0.002	22.4[a]
Atherosclerosis over age	-0.196	6.0[b]

Analysis of variance

	Degrees of freedom	Mean square	F ratio
Regression	2	8.606	11.3
Residual	9	0.759	

[a]Significant at the 0.01 level.

[b]Significant at the 0.05 level.

patients of both types were considered simultaneously, blood cholesterol level, $r = 0.55$, $p < 0.01$ and blood triglyceride level, $r = 0.58$, $p < 0.01$, were significant single correlates. When type IV patients were considered alone, blood cholesterol, $r = 0.64$, $p < 0.01$ and blood triglyceride, $r = 0.72$, $p < 0.01$, were significant single correlates. When type II patients were considered alone, no significant correlates were found.

Stepwise regression of all variates listed above in type IV patients indicated that blood triglyceride level and atherosclerosis over age were significant as joint predictors of atherosclerosis percent change per month with a multiple correlation of 0.85 as shown in Table 3. The standard error of estimate was 0.87 and the regression equation was significant at the 0.01 level.

Discussion

When the direction and rate of atherosclerosis change can be determined frequently one means to compare therapies will be to measure changes in direction and rate during treatment with various agents. We are currently exploring this possibility in an animal model. In patients I report here, only one estimate of atherosclerosis change direction and rate was obtained by comparing two angiograms. For this, and additional reasons discussed later, I have confined this discussion to correlation with risk factor status determined between angiograms. When atherosclerosis change percent per month was correlated with risk factor level during the period between angiograms, a highly significant correlation with both blood cholesterol and blood triglyceride level was found. These variates were highly correlated with each other.

When hyperlipoproteinemic types were considered separately, the significant correlates with risk factor level were all found in type IV. I consider that the two hyperlipoproteinemic types were matched in regards to atherosclerosis accumulation before our experiment began because atherosclerosis over age did not differ significantly in the two types. The statistic, atherosclerosis over age, assumes a lifetime linear increase in atherosclerosis, and therefore has an inherent element of uncertainty. However, it seems as reasonable a basis for matching groups for studies of atherosclerosis as short-term estimates of risk factor level now widely accepted. Because significant correlates with risk factor level and atherosclerosis change rate were confined to type IV, I suggest that arterial wall responses in the two hyperlipoproteinemic types may differ.

The relationship between blood triglyceride level and atherosclerosis over age in type IV expressed in Table 3 is that change in the direction of lesion regression was most rapid in those with low blood triglyceride levels. Additionally, when the blood triglyceride effect has been taken into account, those who have accumulated atherosclerosis most rapidly show most rapid lesion regression. The multiple correlation coefficient between atherosclerosis percent change per month and these two variates considered simultaneously was $r = 0.85$. Therefore, in these 12 patients, 71% of the variability associated with atherosclerosis percent change per month appears attributable to these two factors. A correlation of this magnitude lends support to the rationale for lowering blood triglyceride level in type IV hyperlipoproteinemia, but clearly requires confirmation in additional patients.

This study, which was a pilot to examine the possibility of using femoral angiography for atherosclerosis evaluation in hyperlipoproteinemic patients, included too few subjects and employed too many types of therapy to allow judgement regarding the efficacy of individual drugs and diet. However, it is important to note that the magnitude of lipid lowering we have achieved was not greater than in a previous study where serial femoral angiograms showed no change in atherosclerosis (Knight et al., 1972). Differences in radiographic techniques allowing recognition of smaller lesion change in our study appear to be an important reason for this different result.

Acknowledgement

Members of the University of Southern California's Specialized Center of Research in Atherosclerosis Program who made a major contribution to this work are: Drs. Robert Barndt, Jr., Samuel H. Brooks, H.P. Chin, Donald W. Crawford, Miguel E. Sanmarco, Ronald H. Selvester, Tibor K. Zemplenyi, and Mr. Robert Selzer.

ENHANCEMENT OF REGRESSION OF HUMAN ATHEROSCLEROSIS

— With Antagonists of Thromboxane A$_2$, One of Local Risk Factors of the Plaque —

Takio Shimamoto

Introduction and a Short Historical Review

Recent epidemiological research on risk factors (Stamler et al., 1974), pioneered by Paul D. White and Ancel Keys, has contributed greatly toward the elucidation of risk factors, and various risk factors such as hypercholesterolemia, hypertension, cigarette smoking, etc., which lead to the progression of atherosclerosis, have been clearly identified. Following the discovery of such factors, various attempts toward their elimination have been successfully mode, particularly after the successful identification of individual cholesterol-bearing lipoproteins such as HDL, LDL, VLDL, chylomicron, etc. by Donald S. Fredrickson and his collaborators (Levy and Stone, 1974).

Besides the removal of such risk factors, the author has tried to open a new therapeutic approach and, since 1963, he (Shimamoto, 1963, 1969) has found substances capable of directly modifying local factors in and around the atheromatous lesions to prevent the further progress and to enhance the regression of atherosclerosis.

The regression of atheromatous lesions has long been known to occur to some limited extent in experimental animals; however, no drug was known to enhance the regression until 1965, when the First International Symposium on Atherosclerosis was held in Athens. At that meeting, the author (Shimamoto et al., 1968) published a paper on the enhancing effect of pyridinolcarbamate on regression of atheromatous lesions of cholesterol-fed rabbits and, at the same time, on the clinical effect of this compound on an angiographic and clinical improvement of femoropopliteal atherosclerosis of man. However, at that time, the regression of human atherosclerosis was not known and that of experimental atherosclerosis of this animal species, rabbits, had commonly been believed by the majority of European and American specialists not to occur even after the withdrawal of cholesterol feeding, but rather to progress further, so that it was hard for the author from the Far East to be understood by the audience of the Athens' symposium on the effect of pyridinolcarbamate.

We introduced pyridinolcarbamate as the most potent inhibitor of the edematous arterial reaction of rabbit aorta, but at the time the rabbit aorta contracting substance (RCS) (Piper and Vane, 1969) and thromboxane A$_2$ (Hamberg et al., 1975), the active agent of RCS as well as the most potent substance inducing the edematous arterial reaction, were not known. We also did not know at that time that pyridinolcarbamate shows a potent thromboxane A$_2$-antagonistic effect (Fig. 1).

However, in the lectures of the Fourth International Symposium on Atherosclerosis (1976) the paper of D.H. Blankenhorn (Beckenbach et al., 1974; Blankenhorn, 1975) has clearly shown the unmistakable regressive change of femoral atherosclerosis of hypercholesterolemic patients induced by dietary treatment by his image-scientific angiologic technique and the paper of the same symposium by K.T. Lee has also clearly shown a definite enhancing effect of pyridinolcarbamate on regression of atherosclerosis in his atherosclerotic rabbits produced by cholesterol and peanut oil added to their food.

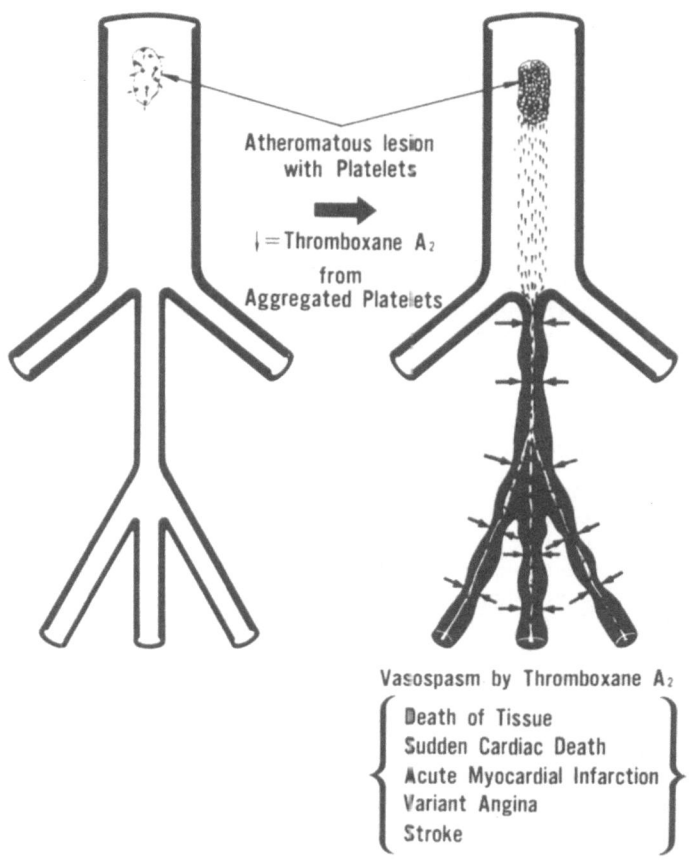

Atheromatous lesion
with Platelets

↓ = Thromboxane A₂
from
Aggregated Platelets

Vasospasm by Thromboxane A₂

Death of Tissue
Sudden Cardiac Death
Acute Myocardial Infarction
Variant Angina
Stroke

Figure 1. The sticking, aggregating, and possible release of active substances of platelets on atheromatous lesions are the common phenomena and the repetitious release of small amounts of thromboxane A_2 may be inevitable inhibiting the solubilization and release of stored lipids of intimal cells (left).
The number of platelets stuck and the amount of thromboxane A_2 released would become large enough; the vasospastic constriction of downstream arteries is inevitable (right)

Since 1964, pyridinolcarbamate has been widely tested clinically by world scientists using modern clinical pharmacologic techniques as summarized by the author (Shimamoto, 1973, 1975a, 1975b, 1975c; Shimamoto and Numano, 1974) and among the reports of these investigations there are a great many with positive results as well as one (Walton et al., 1973) with negative results.

Recently, a potent endogenous substance, thromboxane A_2 was discovered by Hamberg et al. (1975) and has been implicated as a trigger (Neeldeman et al., 1976; Kolata, 1975; Ellis et al., 1976; Nijkamp et al., 1976) of fatal events such as stroke, myocardial infarction, and sudden cardiac death (Fig. 1) of patients suffering from advanced atherosclerosis. In addition, its potent inhibitory effect on lipid metabolism (Kolata, 1975), inhibiting the mobilization of lipid from adipocytes, has been revealed. Furthermore, a similar inhibitory effect of thromboxane A_2 is suspected by the author to be present in intimal cells appearing in atheromatous lesions and to inhibit the release of cholesterol from the lesions and the repair process, because platelet sticking, invading, aggregating, and destruction are triggering phenomena of the local production of thromboxane A2 and also a well-known common phenomena of every atheromatous lesion. For such reasons, thromboxane A_2 is undoubtedly not only one of the potent endogenous atherogenic and thrombogenic substances, but also the aggravating substance of atheromatous lesions as well. The mild but highly specific thromboxane A_2-antagonistic property of pyridinolcarbamate has recently been discovered by the author and in addition, a roughly ten times more potent, highly specific, and nontoxic thromboxane A_2-antagonist, phthalazinol (7-ethoxycarbonyl-6,8-dimethyl-4-hydroxymethyl-1(2H)-phthalazine), was synthesized by the author under the collaboration with M. Ishikawa (Fig. 2).

In this paper, the author first introduced how the clinical effect of an anti-atherosclerotic substance like pyridinolcarbamate has been evaluated as to its effect on regression of atherosclerosis of man, and secondly, the author also reports the preliminary results on the experimental and clinical effects of a new and more potent antithromboxane A_2 compound, phthalazinol.

Clinical Application of Pyridinolcarbamate and Its Results Obtained During the Past 12 Years

This compound (Shimamoto, 1969, 1973, 1975a; Shimamoto and Numano, 1974) lowers neither the serum cholesterol level, nor the β- or pre-β-lipoprotein level, but prevents the acute entry of plasma proteins including β- and pre-β-lipoprotein into the subendothelial space of the arterial wall, which is induced by various substances such as angiotensin II, bradykinin, cigarette smoking, or traumatization. In addition, the removal of oil red-O positive lipid and cholesterol from the atheromatous lesions has been shown to be significantly enhanced by pyridinolcarbamate in its therapeutic doses in atherosclerotic rabbits. Furthermore, platelet aggregability has been shown to be reduced and primary as well as secondary platelet aggregation induced by ADP and arachidonic acid have been inhibited by this compound (Shimamoto, 1975b). Moreover, this substance is the first drug to be used as a platelet drug before the application of aspirin in the history of medicine.

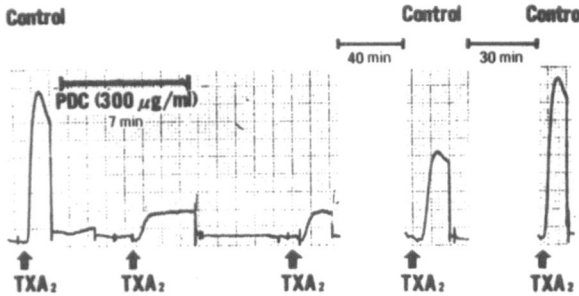

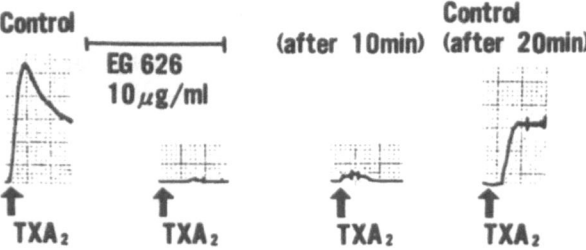

Figure 2. Antagonistic effect of pyridinolcarbamate (300 µg/ml) and phthalazinol (10 µg/ml) in vitro on rabbit aorta, contracting effect of thromboxane A_2 (35 mg in terms of angiotensin II). The method described by Bilis et al. (1976) was used in this experiment.

In order to see the enhancing effect of pyridinolcarbamate on regressive processes of human atherosclerosis, a well-controlled, clinical pharmacologic trial is required.

After several open studies, the author published a paper (Shimanoto et al., 1970) on the clinical pharmacologic evaluation of pyridinolcarbamate in the treatment of arteriosclerosis obliterans in 24 patients by a double blind crossover trial of a relatively short time treatment of 10 weeks regimen, starting in October, 1967 and lasting until the cold season in Tokyo. The careful analysis revealed a statistically significant therapeutic effect of pyridinolcarbamate over placebo, and this paper was published in the journals of the Western world (Shimamoto et al., 1970). Successively, many papers from abroad were published with positive results in the treatment with this compared of cerebral, coronary, and peripheral atherosclerosis as summarized by the author (Shimamoto, 1972, 1975c). There was also a paper with negative results (Walton et al., 1973). A double blind crossover clinical trial of much shorter regimen of 8 weeks was started in March of 1970, lasting until the warm season by Walton et al. (1973) in their 33 patients. They reported that they could not obtain a definite drug effect, but rather a seasonal variation effect.

Concerning the length of time of the treatment, the author emphasized the importance of a much longer period of time than 10 weeks in the treatment of human atherosclerosis as evidenced by animal experiments and at the same time, the importance of angiologic evaluation.

For such a purpose, Terry et al. (1975) performed a double blind trial of 2 years regimen with angiologic evaluation in their 38 male and female patients with an average age of 61.7 ± 9.0 years suffering from advanced arteriosclerosis obliterance of their arteries of the lower extremities in the hospital of New York Medical College.

Among them, 38 patients finished the 2-year regimens of either placebo or pyridinolcarbamate treatment. Namely, one group of 16 patients finished 2 years of placebo treatment while another group of 22 patients finished a 2-year pyridinolcarbamate regimen, with both groups being sex- and age-matched. Angiologic photographs were taken each year of the placebo or pyridinolcarbamate treatment, and the angiologic findings were compared over the 2-year period. Among the 16 patients of the age- and sex-matched placebo control group, angiologic analysis revealed a definite progresseion of atherosclerotic changes in 15 out of the 16 cases during the 2 years of their observation. They had already recognized the same general trend of the progression of atherosclerotic changes of the arteries of the lower extremities among quite a number of other patients of the same age. The other age- and sex-matched 22 patients were treated with pyridinolcarbamate in a daily dose of 2 g for 2 years, and the angiologic analysis exhibited a progression of atherosclerotic change in only three patients and the remaining 19 patients exhibited no progression (Table 1).

In addition, after the initial double blind trial, they continued the observation under open study, and they added that, following the initial 2-year period, 16 out of 18 patients treated with pyridinolcarbamate did not progress during another 2-year period. It may be of particular significance that three patients, who during the 2-year double blind period of the study had been previously treated with placebo, when switched to pyridinolcarbamate, did not show progression of atherosclerosis during the subsequent 27 months. These differences are again statistically significant at a level of $P < 0.001$.

Such evidence may show the presence of an enhancing effect of pyridinolcarbamate on the regression of atherosclerotic lesions found in atherosclerotic rabbits and also in man because the nonprogression of atherosclerotic changes in the classic angiographic demonstration may mean the stabilized condition of atherosclerotic lesions, not only a simple prevention on the progression, but also the balanced dynamic condition of the progression of atherosclerotic lesions counter-

Table 1. Angiographc evaluation of pyridinolcarbamate treatment of patients with advanced occulusive atherosclerosis of lower extremities. A double blind trial (by Terry et al., 1975)

	Nonprogression	Progression	Total number of patients
Placebo	1	15	16
Pyridinolcarbamate	19[a]	3	22
			38 cases

[a]Pyridinolcarbamate VS placebo p <0.001.

acted by enhanced regressive processes. Thus, they reported a statistically significant preventive effect of pyridinolcarbamate against the progression of human femoral atherosclerosis (P <0.001).

It may also be true that the satisfactory improvement of atherosclerotic lesions could result in an effective increase in the nutritional blood flow in the peripheral circulation of the affected arterial segment in some way, although a limited amount of the increase in the nutritional flow may be possible by adequate vasodilation without any change of the atheromatous lesions. In order to confirm such an effect of pyridinolcarbamate, the following double blind trial has been started in 154 patients suffering from ischemic gangrene due to atherosclerosis of the lower legs by Mishima et al. (1975).

In the treatment of ischemic ulcer due to atherosclerosis, sympathectomy or vasodilators, nicotinic acid or its derivatives, have been applied. Needless to say. the cure of ulcer is highly related to the improvement of local circulation and the amputation of the affected extremity is inevitable for quite a number of patients. As shown in Table 2, the curative effect of pyridinolcarbamate, a nonvasodilator, with its daily 1.5 g regimen, has been compared with that of a potent vasodilator, inositol niacinate, with its 1.2 g regimen in 154 patients with atherosclerotic ulcer in their legs under the generalized Wilcoxon twosample, double blind test. Two groups, age- and sex-matched, underwent the trial with 79 patients receiving pyridinolcarbamate in a daily dose of 1.5 g and the remaining 74 patients receiving inositol niacinate in a daily dose of 1.2 g. The evaluation was done at the end of 6 weeks of treatment and as shown in Table 2, improvement is counted in 54 (68.4%) cases of the pyridinolcarbamate group and 36 (48.6%) cases of the inositol niacinate group. A statistically significantly better response of the lesions to the treatment was obtained in the pyridinolcarbamate group as compared with the inositol niacinate group (P = 0.0006) (Table 2). It is worthwhile to note the marked vasodilative effect of inositol niacinate, while pyridinolcarbamate has almost no vasodilative effect, so that the effects of pyridinolcarbamate on regression of atherosclerotic lesions is reasonably thought to have participated in the cure of the ulcer. In the treatment of ischemic gangrene, numerous papers showing the therapeutic efficacy of pyridinolcarbamate have already been published.

In addition, in the treatment of 105 patients suffering from arteriosclerosis obliterans with a marked intermittent claudication, Atsumi et al. (1974) reported a statistically significant lower incidence of death due to myocardial infarction and stroke in a pyridinolcarbamate group of 60 cases than that of age-, sex-, and severity-matched 45 patients treated by other drugs in their observation of 4 years of long-term treatment.

In accordance with this report, Kato et al. (1975) reconfirmed the improvement of prognosis of postapoplectic patients by a long-term treatment with pyridinol-

Table 2. A multiclinical double blind trial on pyridinolcarbamate and inositol niacinate in the ischemic ulcer due to chronic arterial occlusion (Mishima et al., 1976)

Drug / Effect	Failure −	Poor ±	Fair +	Good ⧺	Excellent ⧻	Total number of patients
Pyridinol-carbamate	11	14	8	18	28	79
Inositol niacinate	19	19	11	17	8	74
						153 cases

A higly significant difference between 2 drug groups matched in sex, age, localization and severity of symptoms, is noted by the Wilcoxon 2-sample test (to = 3.449, P = 0.0006).
The improving rate is definitely higher in the pyridinolcarbanate group +19.7% difference with 95% confidence interval of +3.1 to +36.3%.

carbamate in their 4 years of controlled clinical observation of 35 male and female patients hospitalized in their hospital during the entire observation period. They reported that the 4-year survival rate is statistically significantly increased, and the recurrence of stroke was statistically significantly reduced and the electrocardiographic findings and the ophthalmoscopic findings of eyeground were also statistically significantly improved in the drug group as compared with the placebo group.

Discussion

In the clinical evaluation of the regression of atheromatous plaque, the direct demonstration of atheromatous plaque by image-scientific angiographic technique is useful in a certain limited arterial segment like the femoral artery as shown by Beckenbach et al. (1974) and Blankenhorn (1975). However, the technique is not commonly available, so that the confirmation of at least nonprogressive by ordinary angiologic techniques may be the proof of regression of atherosclerosis as shown by Terry et al. (1975), because they have shown, during 2 years by classic angiologic demonstration, that femoral atherosclerosis with clinical symptoms in men with an age of around 60 years progressed in almost all patients.

Under such conditions, the enhancement of regression by drug therapy is counteracted by progression-promoting factors of the atheromatous lesions, so that a simple prevention of progression is not realistic and for the realization of angiologic nonprogression, a powerful enhancing effect of the treatment on regressive processes seems essential.

The increase in nutritional blood flow in peripheral irrigating tissues of affected arteries is also an indirect but a definite proof of regression of atherosclerosis and the cure of atherosclerotic gangrene by medication in at least over 60% of the patients may be a necessary response for a regression-promoting drug treatment.

Needless to say, the prognosis of patients should be improved, when a certain drug shows an enhancement of regression, which is true of pyridinolcarbamate as shown by Atsumi et al. (1974) in their patients suffering from atherosclerotic disease of their extremities and also by Kato et al. (1975) in the 4 years of controlled clinical observation of their postapoplectic patients.

The above-mentioned clinical results of pyridinolcarbamate treatment including many other clinical pharmacologic observations may show the presence of the same enhancing effect on regression of human atheromatous lesions of pyridinolcarbamate as has been shown by us in rabbit's atheromatous lesions and has been reconfirmed by Lee, et al. Pyridinolcarbamate has been shown to enhance the activity of glycolytic enzymes and TCA-cycle enzymes by Numano et al. (1973) and the mitochondrial oxidation of cholesterol by Kritchevsky and Tepper (1971).

Particularly, pyridinolcarbamate has a quite specific thromboxane A_2-antagonistic effect, which eliminates the most powerful local risk factor, thromboxane A_2, from the atheromatous plaque.

Such evidence may encourage the search for more and more effective drugs, attacking directly the powerful local risk factors like thromboxane A_2, in and around the atheromatous lesions in the treatment of atherosclerosis, besides the effort in eliminating the so-called risk factors.

Prevention of Myocardial Infarction and Stroke. A Novel Trial With a Potent Antithromboxane A_2 Substance, Phthalazinol

Platelet drugs have been tested for their prevention of the recurrence of attack among survivors from myocardial infarction. Among them, aspirin has shown a preventive effect to some extent (Majerus, 1976). The inhibotory effect of aspirin-like compounds on platelet aggregation has been shown to come from the inhibition of the synthesis of prostaglandin endoperoxides, which are the precursor of prostaglandins, the essential autacoids of life, and at the same time the precursor of thromboxane A_2.

In order to counteract such an effect of thromboxane A_2, the simple inhibition of the biosynthesis of such potent and important autacoids, prostaglandins, may certainly encounter quite hazardous side effects including the prolongation of bleeding time, because the synthesis of many vasoconstrictive prostaglandins such as PGA_1, PGE_1, PGE_2, and $PGF_2\alpha$ could be impaired at the same time. It is also conceivable that the limited antithrombotic effectiveness of aspirin might be due to the concomitant inhibition of the production of PGE_1, which might act as an inhibitor of platelet aggregation.

For such reasons, a specific thromboxane A_2-antagonist is required in order to prevent more effectively and more safely the disasters, such as stroke, heart attack, and sudden cardiac death (Fig. 3).

Phthalazinol is effective in concentration of 1 μg in vitro and is effective in vivo as a thromboxane A_2 antagonist. The oral application induces the appearance of this compound in sufficient effective concentration in the blood of man and animals. Phthalazinol inhibits the primary and also secondary human platelet aggregation induced by arachidonic acid as well as thromboxane A_2 in low concentrations such as 2.5 - 10 μg/ml. This compound, in a dose of 0.1 - 1.0 mg per kg given intravenously, also significantly inhibited cerebral thrombosis in rats of Furlow and Bass (1974) induced by intracarotid injection of sodium arachidonate and in its daily oral administration of 12.5 - 50 mg significantly prevented the cerebral hemorrhage of spotaneously hypertensive rats of the stroke-prone strain of Matsuzaki (Shimamoto et al., 1975), which were kept on 1% salt water for 5 weeks, despite the fact that the high blood pressure of the animals was not significantly lowered by phthalazinol. The cerebral hemorrhage of spontaneously hypertensive rats has been shown to result from vasospasm, so that the antithromboxane A_2 activity of phthalazinol may have eliminated or prevented the vasospasm resulting in the prevention of cerebral hemorrhage (Fig. 4).

The fall in cAMP induced by thromboxane A_2 is believed to come from the inhibitory effect of thromboxane A_2 on adenyl cyclase and has been implicated as one of the possible causes of platelet aggregation. Phthalazinol (Shimamoto et al., 1975)

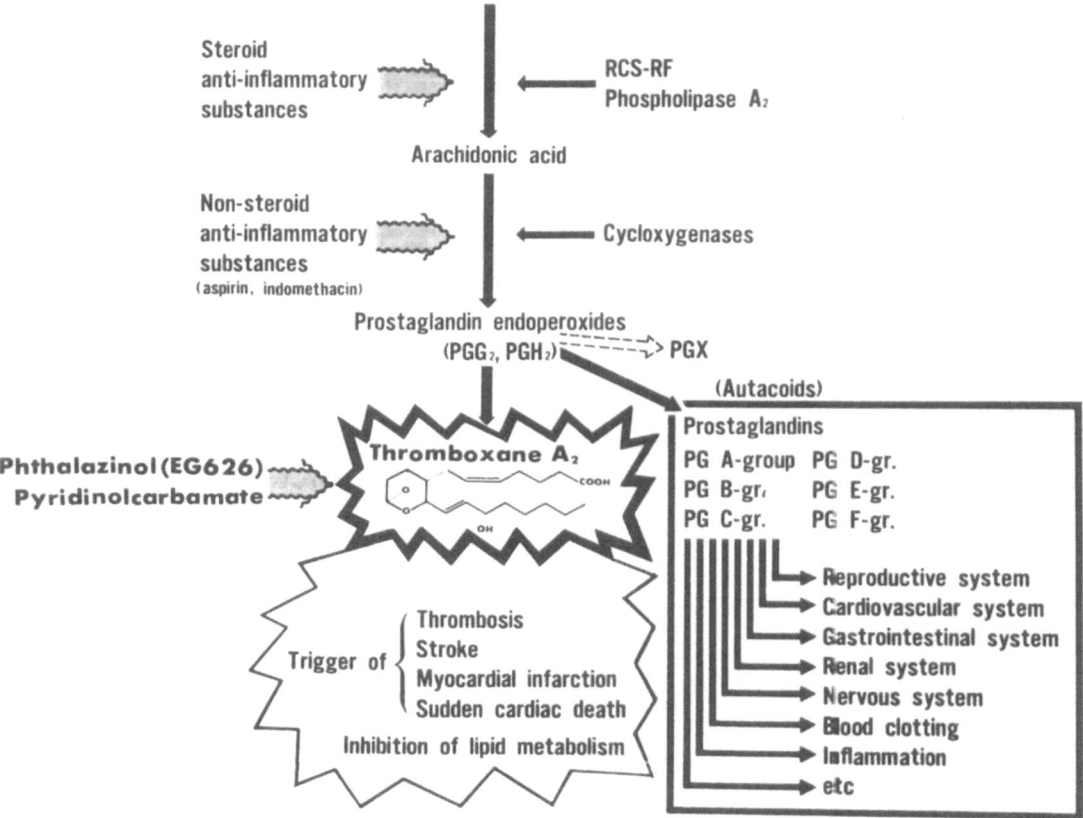

Figure 3. Steroid anti-inflammatory substances have been shown to prevent atherosclerosis of cholesterol-fed animals, but they are not available to man because of toxicity, and nonsteroid anti-inflammatory agents such as aspirin, have also been known to have a slight antiatherosclerotic effect but at the same time, side effects such as the prolongation of bleeding time. Furthermore, both agents inhibit prostaglandin biosynthesis so widely, sacrificing the important production of "autacoids" as shown in this Figure.
On the other hand, the target of thromboxane A2-antagonists like pyridinolcarbamate and phthalazinol is extremely restricted, so that effective doses as an antiatherosclerotic and antithrombotic drug are available to man without such side effects

shows the most potent inhibiting effect on cAMP phosphodiesterase in human platelets, endothelial cells, and vascular smooth muscle cells, and also shows a mild inhibitory effect on cAMP phosphodiesterase in nerve cells, skeletal and cardiac muscle, and skin, and also shows an inhibitory effect on cGMP phosphodiesterase in various tissues. However, its potency in inhibiting cAMP phosphodiesterases is more potent than that on cGMP in various tissues. For instance, the cAMP content of spinal fluid of patients suffering from amyotrophic lateral sclerosis exhibited a significant increase in a dose-dependent manner by oral administration of phthalazinol by Brooks et al. (1976), but the cGMP level did not show any change. Needless to say, the precursor of cAMP is ATP, which is increased by pyridinolcarbamate in the wall of arteries of experimental animals shown by the author in his unpublished study. In particular, the potent thromboxane A2 antagonistic effect of phthalazinol led us to begin the experiment to observe its antiatherosclerotic effect.

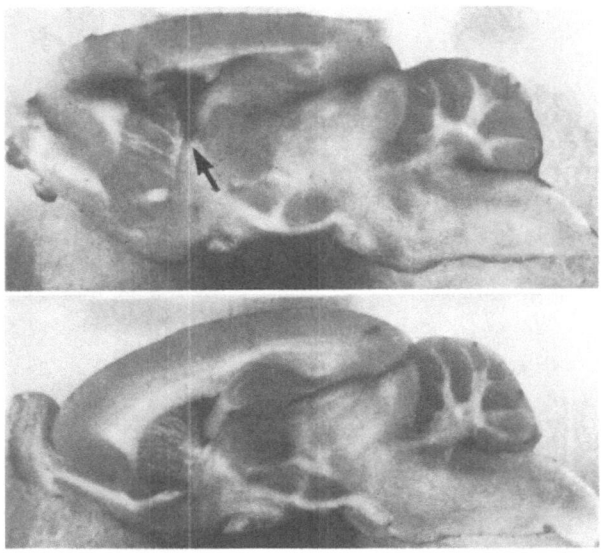

Figure 4. Spontaneously hypertensive rats (the stroke-prone rats) were kept on 1% salt water for 5 weeks and all of the placebo control group exhibited a cerebral hemorrhage, while the animals of the group treated with phthalazinol exhibited a dose-dependent preventive effect against the hemorrhage and the group treated daily with 50 mg of phthalazinol was perfectly free from the hemorrhage
Above: Cerebral hemorrhage ↑ of the spontaneously hypertensive rat of stroke-prone strain of the placebo control group
Below: No hemorrhage of the spontaneously hypertensive rat of stroke-prone strain of the treated group with phthalazinol (50 mg/kg, p.p., per day)

Thromboxane A$_2$-Antagonist, Phthalazinol, in Experimental Atherosclerosis

Phthalazinol has been tested for its preventive effect on atherosclerosis of cholesterol-fed rabbits. The method used has been the same technique as described elsewhere (Shimamoto, 1969). The 20 male rabbits were divided into the placebo and phthalazinol groups of the same number of animals and all rabbits received 1% cholesterol pellet. The rabbits of the placebo group received daily a capsule containing potato starch and the rabbits of phthalazinol group received daily a capsule with phthalazinol in a dose of 1 mg per kg for 15 weeks. Two animals of the placebo group were lost by accident, but the remaining 18 animals finished the regimens. Thereafter, the entire group of animals was sacrificed and histologic and chemical analyses were performed.

As shown in Figure 5 the blood cholesterol level was elevated in both groups without any significant difference; however, the appearance of aortic fatty streak involvement and the content of cholesterol in the aortas exhibited a statistically significant difference between the two groups, with the treated animals exhibiting less appearance of aortic fatty streaks regardless of the serum cholesterol level of the individual animals and a lower amount of cholesterol in the aortas.

This type of experiment was repeated three times and the preventive effect on fatty streak involvement has been repeatedly shown using a daily dose of 1 10 mg/kg of phthalazinol.

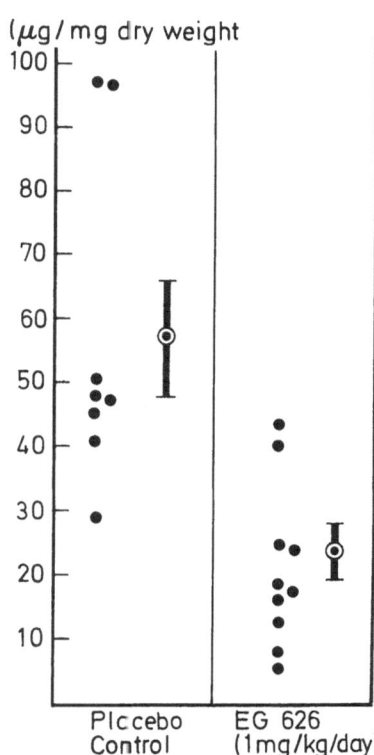

Figure 5. Cholesterol content of aortic wall.
[a]p <0.01

An Enhancing Effect of Thromboxane A$_2$-Antagonist, Phthalazinol, on Regression of Atheromatous Lesions of Rabbits

The daily administration of this compound in a dose of 10 mg per kg to atherosclerotic rabbits produced by balloon injury plus a mild hypercholesterolemia has
shown to enhance significantly the removal of stainable fat (oil red-O) and to
also enhance the replacement of foamy cells with regenerated matured smooth muscle cells (Numano et al., 1976) (Fig. 6). In addition in atherosclerotic rabbits,
produced by daily administration of 1% cholesterol pellet and peanut oil for 15
weeks, treatment with 20 mg of phthalazinol again exhibited a definite enhancing
effect on the elimination of cholesterol from the lesions and the replacement of
foamy lesions with regenerated matured smooth muscle cells after 15 – 30 weeks of
the treatment (Tables 3 and 4). It is important to note that the difference in
regressive changes of the drug group and the placebo control group was much more
pronounced in animals which received a 30 week-regimen than those which received
a 15 week-regimen, showing the importance of long-term treatment in this kind of
drug therapy.

Discussion

In adipocytes, cAMP has been believed to be a regulatory factor in the uptake or
release of lipids since reported by Butcher et al. (1968). Namely, cAMP-lowering
hormones induced the increased uptake of lipids from environmental fluid and the
cAMP-elevating hormones induced the increase of release of lipids from adipocytes.
In addition, thromboxane A$_2$ is a powerful inhibitor of adenylcyclase of adipocytes
according to Groman and his associates and inhibits the release of lipids from
the cells (Kolata, 1975), so that the definite enhancing effect of phthalazinol,
a potent antithromboxane A$_2$ substance and at the same time, cAMP phosphodiesterase
inhibiting agent, on the elimination of cholesterol with stainable lipids from
atheromatous lesions may possibly suggest the presence of the similar metabolic

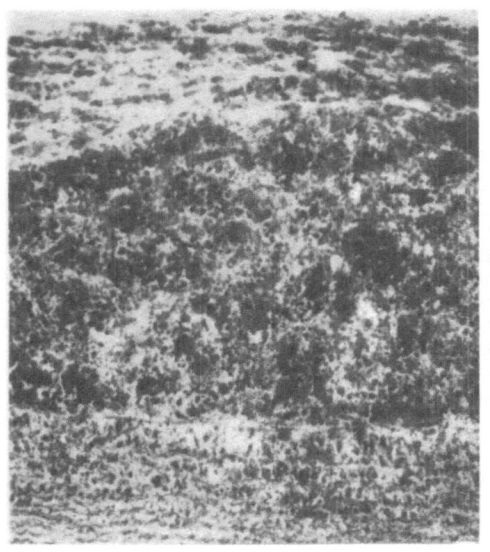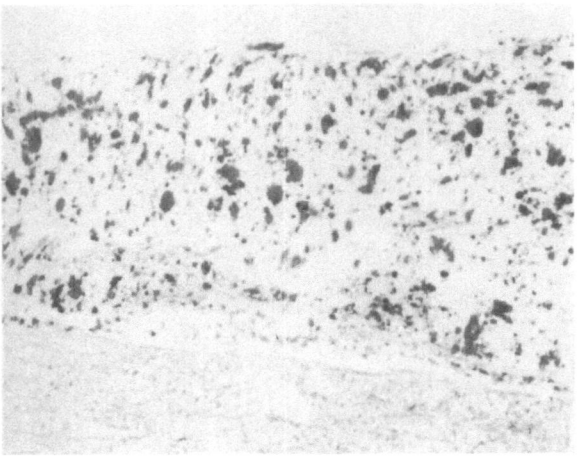

Figure 6. Oil red-O staining of atheroma of rabbits treated by placebo (at right) and phthalazinol 20 mg/kg p.o. 15 weeks (at left)

Table 3. Enhancing effect of phthalazinol in the removal of cholesterol from aortic atheromatous lesions

	15 Weeks treatment			30 Weeks treatment		
Treatment (Number of animals)	Placebo group (6)	EG-626 group (20mg/kg/day 15 weeks) (7)	Signif- icance	Placebo group (10)	EG-626 group (20mg/kg/day 30 weeks) (12)	Signif- icance
Cholesterol content of aortas (μg/mg DW)	24.0±7.3	14.8±6.4	N.S.	27.9±7.5	8.9±3.9[a]	P <0.05

Placebo control gr. vs phthalazinol gr.

[a] P <0.05, N.S. not significant.

process of lipid in foamy cells of atheromatous foci as in the case of adipo-cytes. Not only the denuded endothelium, but also the endothelial cells covering atheromatous lesions themselves show a tendency to stick to platelets and might produce thromboxane A_2 by various stresses. Thromboxane A_2 may undoubtedly par-ticipate in the acceleration of entry of plasma substance including LDL and VLDL and the accumulation of lipid in intimal cells resulting in their change to foam cells.

Besides the highly potent inhibitory effect of platelet aggregation of phthalazi-nol, its inhibitory effect on the increased phagocytic activity of hyperreactive endothelial cells covering atheroma (Shimamoto, 1975b) may possibly be one of the important factors in its enhancing effect on the regression of atherosclerosis, because the hyperreactive endothelial cells (Shimamoto, 1975b) highly actively

Table 4. Histologic findings (ratings) of aortas of rabbits treated either by placebo or by phthalazinol

Treatment (Number of animals)	15 Weeks treatment			30 Weeks treatment		
	Placebo group (6)	EG-626 group (20mg/kg/day 15 weeks) (7)	Signif-icance	Placebo group (10)	EG-626 group (20mg/kg/day 30 weeks) (12)	Signif-icance
Lipid in atheroma	3.02±0.16	2.38±0.17[a]	P <0.05	2.28±0.16	1.51±0.15[b]	P <0.01
Foam cell	1.50±0.21	0.71±0.13[b]	P <0.01	0.65±0.10	0.33±0.05[b]	P <0.01
Smooth muscle	1.18±0.18	1.83±0.21[a]	P <0.05	0.48±0.09	0.92±0.08[b]	P <0.01
Elastic fiber	1.63±0.15	2.14±0.20	N.S.	1.21±0.09	1.53±0.08[a]	P <0.05
Collagen fiber	2.77±0.16	2.50±0.16	N.S.	3.12±0.07	2.39±0.04[b]	P <0.01
Necrotic foci	0.83±0.20	0.66±0.19	N.S.	1.53±0.16	0.73±0.08[b]	P <0.01

Placebo control gr. vs phthalazinol gr.

[a] P 0.05. [b] P 0.01, N.S. not significant.

transport plasma protein including LDL, VLDL, and fibronogen through endothelial cytoplasm from the blood stream to the subendothelial space, especially in progressing atheromatous lesions as evidenced by immunofluorescent studies of the author (Shimamoto, 1972).

Clinical Application of Phthalazinol in Man

Clinical studies of phthalazinol have been underway since 1973, mainly under open study and the clinical results are quite encouraging in the prevention of stroke or myocardial infarction and in the treatment of patients suffering from transient ischemic attacks, postapoplectic disorders, diabetic retinopathy, propranolol resistant variant form of angina pectoris of Prinzmetal (singly or combined with propranolol), intractable angina pectoris (singly or combined with propranolol), impending myocardial infarction (combined with propranolol), diabetic gangrene, gangrene due to Bürger's disease, venous thrombosis, and other thromboembolic diseases and, in addition, a mild but definitely favorable result has been obtained in the treatment with phthalazinol of patients suffering from senile dementia (Shimamoto et al., 1976), cerebellar ataxia (Shimamoto et al., 1976), and parkinsonism presumably because of its mild cAMP-increasing effect.

It is also important to note that it has become possible to classify angina pectoris into "thromboxane A2 angina" and "β-adrenergic angina" according to its response to such specific antagonists, phthalazinol and propranolol. Needless to say, thromboxane A2 angina is much more dangerous than β-adrenergic angina, although the latter may possibly also involve in some cases a small amount of successive release of thromboxane A2 after foregoint release of β-adrenergic hormones.

In this paper, a clinical study on atherosclerotic ulcer is described.

Application of Phthalazinol in the Treatment of Atherosclerotic Ulcer

Preliminary observations on the effect of phthalazinol have been performed in
each of 12 male and one female patients aged 49 – 78 years suffering from atherosclerotic ulcers, which were resistant to vasodilators and were accompanied by
severe rest pains for the past 1 – 6 months. The compound is rapidly absorbed by
the gastrointestinal tract and appears in the blood in a concentration of 4 – 40
μg/ml 30 min 2 h after oral administration and is rapidly excreted into the
urine and the half-life is roughly 3 hours. In the patients suffering from
ischemic gangrene of finger, toe, and feet, a striking curative effect on the
ulcers has been obtained by phthalazinol in a daily dose of 600~900 mg in all
patients and a dramatically favorable effect on the rest pains started as early
as 3 days afther the initiation of treatment in all 10 patients, and about 1 week
thereafter, the local pains almost completely disappeared. The curative response
of gangrenous ulcers started quite rapidly and the cure and epidermization were
definitely accerelated in all cases under phthalazinol treatment, although the
double blind trial is needed to confirm this evidence and is now under was
(Fig. 7).

There were almost no side effects, no prolongation of bleeding time, and no
gastrointestinal side effects not only in patients suffering from atherosclerotic
gangrene but also in all patients having received phthalazinol through today.

Discussion

In atherosclerotic ulcer, the rest pain, especially severe at night, responded
poorly to analgetica as shown in the case histories of these patients and commonly continued weeks and months, so that the striking effect of phthalazinol
is higly impressive. The intractable rest pain of patients suffering from athero-

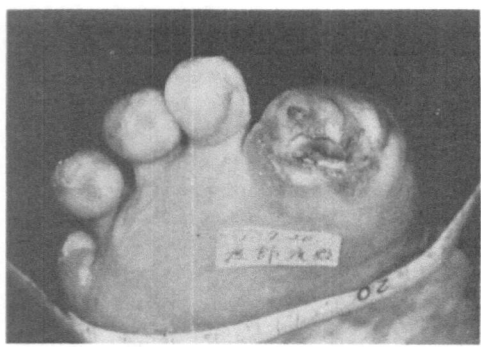

Figure 7. a) Ischemic gangrene due to
atherosclerosis of 60-year old male
patient (before the treatment)

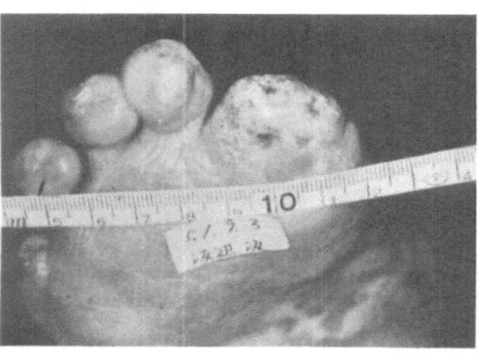

Figure 7. b) Cure by epidermization by
45 days of phthalazinol treatment
(600 mg/day) (Dr. Y. Sawada)

sclerotic gangrene may come from vasospasm, which is induced by the appearance of thromboxane A_2 and may be eliminated by the thromboxane A_2-angatonistic effect of phthalazinol. Phthalazinol has also a potent cAMP phosphodiesterase inhibiting effect, but the vasodilative effect appears in its high concentration of over 10^{-4} g/ml in vitro, and also clinically, no vasodilative effect has been recognized. Phthalazinol exhibited a definite enhancing effect on experimental atherosclerosis induced by balloon injury (Shimamoto et al., 1975) and cholesterol feeding as described in the previous section, so that such an enhancing effect on human atherosclerosis may be reasonably involved in its curative effect as in the case of another thromboxane A_2-antagonist, pyridinolcarbamate.

Clinical applications of phthalazinol have just begun in various fields including atherosclerotic disorders such as cerebral, coronary, and peripheral atherosclerosis under the open and double blind trials. The favorable effect on intractable angina pectoris, Prinzmetal type of angina pectoris, impending myocardial infarction, transient ischemic attack, and diabetic retinopathy is quite impressive in its open study. The preliminary observations are encouraging in the prevention and treatment of morbid conditions presumed to come from the appearance of thromboxane A_2 and also a lack of sufficient production of intracellular cAMP. Such an effort seems to open a new field in the therapy of various diseases including atherosclerosis.

Summary

The introduction of the image-scientific technique in angiography by Beckenbach et al. (1974) and Blankenhorn (1975) has enabled us to recognize the regressive change of human femoral atherosclerosis induced by a dietary treatment among patients taking customarily high-fat and high-cholesterol American diets.

Two thromboxane A_2-antagonists, a mild one, pyridinolcarbamate, and a potent one, phthalazinol, have been used in the treatment of atherosclerosis and the results obtained have been summerized in this paper.

A double blind trial with 2 years of a daily 2 g regimen of pyridinolcarbamate has been performed by Terry et al. (1975) in 38 patients suffering from advanced atherosclerotic disease in the lower extremities, from which they have shown angiographically a highly significant curative effect of pyridinolcarbamate, indicating the antiatherosclerotic effect of this drug in man, as has also been shown in animals. This compound in a daily 1.5 g administration has also been shown by Mishima et al. (1975) by their generalized Wilcoxon two-sample of double blind test in 154 patients to show a definite curative effect on ischemic gangrene due to atherosclerosis by an increase in the mutritional flow of the lesions presumably due to the regressive change of atherosclerosis of the irrigating arteries. A statistically significant improvement of prognosis of patients suffering from arteriosclerosis obliterans and of postapoplectic patients has been shown by a long-term treatment of patients with pyridinolcarbamate ($1 \sim 1.5$ g daily) for 4 years by Atsumi et al. (1974) and Kato et al. (1975), respectively, and they showed a significantly smaller incidence of stroke or myocardial infarction in the group treated with pyridinolcarbamate as compared with other drugs. The above-mentioned facts may show the ability of regression of human atherosclerosis at least to some extent either by removal of risk factors or by a drug like pyridinolcarbamate.

Phthalazinol shows a ten times more potent antithromboxane A_2 activity than pyridinolcarbamate and at the same time a cAMP phosphodiesterase inhibiting activity differing from pyridinolcarbamate. This compound, given intravenously in a dose of $0.1 \sim 1$ mg/kg, has been shown to prevent experimental cerebral thrombosis in rats induced by an intracarotid injection of arachidonate according to Furlow and Bass (1974), but the prolongation of bleeding time, as with aspirin, was not recognized. It is to be noted that phthalazinol in its daily oral administration of $12.5 - 50$ mg per kg prevented cerebral hemorrhage of spontaneously hypertensive rats kept on 1% salt water. The preventive effect of phthalazinol (in a daily dose of 1 mg per kg) against experimental atherosclerosis and the enhancing effect of this compound (in a daily dose of 10 - 20 mg per kg) on the regression of established atherosclerosis in rabbits are similar to, but more potent than, pyridinolcarbamate.

It is interesting to note that the common pharmacologic effect of pyridinolcarbamate and phthalazinol is the antithromboxane A_2-antagonistic effect.

Early clinical studies with daily doses of 300 - 1200 mog of phthalazinol have exhibited a promising result in the treatment of various atherosclerotic disorders and the such highly specific antagonistic effects on thromboxane A_2 of phthalazinol has made it possible to classify angina pectoris into thromboxane A_2 angina and β-adrenergic angina. The promising results of phthalazinol in the prevention of stroke and heart attack may urgently request world-wide research on this kind of thromboxane A_2-antagonistic drug treatment in the prevention of the most tragic disaster of the present world.

Notwithstanding, the utilization of a thromboxane A_2-antagonist like phthalazinol or pyridinolcarbamate may nevertheless contribute to the elimination of one of the most drastic endogenous risk factors in and around the atheromatous plaque, thromboxane A_2, and may certainly enhance the regression of human atherosclerosis.

WORKSHOP 11: Nutritional Factors and Atherosclerosis

Chairmen: D. Kritchevsky, USA
          Y. Goto, Japan

Participants: D. Kritchevsky, USA
              S. Nanbu, Japan
              P.J. Nestel, Australia
              K.K. Carroll, Canada
              C. Sirtori, Italy

INFLUENCE OF ALL NUTRIENTS ON ATHEROSCLEROSIS*

David Kritchevsky

Until recently most of the data regarding diet and atherosclerosis have been concerned with lipids, but now there is a growing awareness that all components of the diet may affect serum lipids, and, in turn, atherosclerosis. The variable response to cholesterol feeding observed within species may be attributable, in part, to other components of the diet.

It is well-established that dietary cholesterol leads to atherosclerosis in susceptible animal species such as the rabbit or chick. In a cholesterol-containing diet saturated fat is more atherogenic than unsaturated fat (Kritchevsky et al., 1956; Kritchevsky and Tepper, 1965). This difference also persists in rabbits fed a cholesterol-free, semipurified diet (Lambert et al., 1958; Malmros and Wigand, 1959). One dietary oil which exhibits an anomalous effect (considering its iodine value) is peanut oil. Peanut oil is atherogenic for rats (Gresham and Howard, 1960), monkeys (Vesselinovitch et al., 1974), and rabbits (Kritchevsky et al., 1971). Interesterification of this oil, a process which alters the triglyceride structure but not its iodine value, reduces its atherogenicity for rabbits (Kritchevsky et al., 1973a).

Ignatowski (1909) hypothesized that animal protein was the dietary factor responsible for atherosclerosis. He fed meat and other animal products to rabbits and caused atherosclerosis, but because the diet also contained cholesterol, it was assumed that the observed lesions were due to that sterol. However, subsequent research has shown that, when fed with cholesterol, casein is more atherogenic than soy protein (Meeker and Kesten, 1940). The level of dietary protein may also exert a unique effect with high (30%) levels of dietary protein being more atherogenic than low levels (8%) (Lofland et al., 1966; Strong and McGill, 1967). Carroll and Hamilton (1975) have shown that, in general, animal protein is more cholesteremic for rabbits than vegetable protein. Thus, a casein-dextrose diet is considerably more cholesteremic than a soy protein-dextrose diet (200 vs. 70 mg/dl), but substitution of potato starch for dextrose brings serum cholesterol levels of rabbits fed either protein into the normal range (40 - 50 mg/dl).

In semipurified diets containing 40% carbohydrate, 25% casein, 15% fiber, and 14% hydrogenated coconut oil, sucrose and fructose are more atherogenic than is glucose. This difference has been demonstrated in rabbits (Kritchevsky et al., 1968, 1973b), vervet monkeys (Kritchevsky et al., 1974a), and baboons (Kritchevsky et al., 1974b).

---

*Supported, in part, by USPHS research grants HL-03299 and HL-5209 and Research Career Award HL-00734 from the National Institute of Heart and Lung Diseases.

Table 1. Interaction of dietary components with regard to cholesteremia and atherosclerosis

Component	Effects
Fat	
	Cholesterol-containing diet
	Saturated > unsaturated
	Peanut oil inordinately atherogenic
	Reduced by interesterification
	Semipurified diet
	Saturated > unsaturated
	Peanut oil > corn oil
Protein	
	High > moderate
	Animal > vegetable
	Equivalent with proper carbohydrate, fiber
Carbohydrate	
	Sucrose, fructose > glucose
Fiber	
	Cellulose > alfalfa, wheat straw (rabbits)
	Pectin > bran (man)

The type of fiber present in the diet may also exert an effect. In semipurified diets containing the same sources of fat and carbohydrate, wheat straw has been shown to be significantly less cholesteremic and atherogenic than either cellulose or cellophane (Moore, 1967). In man, pectin has been shown to exert a hypocholesteremic effect (Jenkins et al., 1975) but bran has not (Truswell and Kay, 1976).

When rabbits were fed semipurified diets containing either casein or soy protein and cellulose, the former was the much more atherogenic protein. Substitution of alfalfa for cellulose reduced cholesteremia and atherosclerosis in rabbits fed either protein. Serum cholesterol levels in the casein-alfalfa-fed rabbits were somewhat higher than those in the soy-alfalfa-fed group, but atherosclerosis in the two groups was comparable (Story et al., 1976).

The foregoint data are summarized in Table 1. They illustrate the importance of interaction of dietary components in the development of cholesteremia and atherosclerosis.

INFLUENCE OF DIET FACTORS ON PLASMA LIPIDS IN ISCHEMIC HEART DISEASE

S. Nanbu, N. Kimura, H. Toshima, M. Ageta, S. Kariya, H. Mae, and T. Kamogawa

The present studies were undertaken to investigate the characteristics in ischemic heart disease (IHD) of the lipid composition of lipoprotein fractions rather than of the plasma lipids themselves.

The traditional diet in Japan is characterized by high-carbohydrate intake, especially from rice, which was 62% of total calories in 1973. Though fat intake has gradually increased up to 21% of calories, it is still low when compared whith the diets of Europeans and Americans. It is not likely that dietary factors, especially the percentage of calories derived from saturated fatty acids, strongly affect the plasma lipids concerned with atherosclerosis. In this study, the subjects had similar nutritional backgrounds.

On the other hand, the results from our population survey revealed that a low-protein intake was one of the important risk factors for cardiovascular disease in Japan (Kimura et al., 1972). Based on these findings, we have used the low-caloric diet with comparatively high-protein intake for therapy for prevention of cardiovascular disease.

High plasma triglyceride (TG) levels are sharply decreased in patients fed the diet for 4 weeks. These decreased levels are clearly proportional to the initial levels (R = 0.975, N = 165). It is suggested that diet factors, which are mainly excess claories from carbohydrate in Japan, strongly affect plasma TG levels, even when there is an underlying genetic predisposition. On the other hand, high plasma cholesterol (TCh) levels are also decreased by the diet, but the decreased levels are not as well-correlated with the initial levels as are TG levels (R = 0.676, N = 160).

Diet factors do not only affect plasma lipid levels but also induce abnormal distribution of plasma lipids in lipoprotein (LP) fractions. Though the relation-ship between plasma TCh and TCh in low-density lipoprotein (LDL) (which carries two-thirds of the plasma TCh) is fairly well-correlated before the diet therapy (R = 0.785, N = 44), there is some variation when these parameters are compared in the same subjects after 4 weeks of the diet therapy (R = 0.886, N = 44). There are two kinds of behavior of LDL-TCh toward the process which improves the cor-relation between plasma TCh and LDL-TCh caused by restriction of dietary factors. One increases in LDL-TCh without an increase in plasma TCh by the diet; the other decreases it with a decrease in plasma TCh. It is clearly shown that there is no significant difference between the initial lipid levels and the changing rate from initial level of plasma TG in these two groups. Group A which has LDL-TCh increased by the diet is characterized by a high ratio of TCh to TG in very low-density lipoprotein (VLDL). Namely, there is a relatively high TCh compared to TG in VLDL. It is interesting that after diet therapy this ratio is significantly decreased to the ratio found in group B.

Conceivably, what is more important, determination of lipid composition in LP and response to the restriction of diet makes it possible to clarify a charac-teristic of IHD manifested through plasma lipids. I have tried to select the subjects in this study following basic criteria and to divide the subjects into subgroups according to the response of their LP lipids to diet. First, the plasma TG level is under 117 mg/100 ml at 4 weeks of the diet therapy. We are using this level as the upper limit when there is no influence of the diet factors on plasma lipids. Second, relative body weight was under 120% at 4 weeks after the diet therapy and body weight was decreased at least over 2% by 4 weeks of the diet therapy.

In this study, 15 subjects were selected from 44 hospitalized patients for the control group and 20 of 60 patients for the IHD group, whereby age distribution was similar for both groups (53.9 $\pm$ 8.6 for control, 52.7 $\pm$ for IHD). I should like to mention that there was no significant difference in the level of lipids between the two groups because these subjects responded differently to diet fac-tors before the diet therapy.

First, these subjects were divided into two subgroups according to response of LDL-TCh to the diet. Table 1 shows the comparison of lipid composition of lipo-protein fraction in the subgroups with LDL-TCh increased by the diet between the control and IHD groups. The characteristics of this subgroup were a relatively

Table 1. Subjects with LDL cholesterol increased by calory restriction

	Control (N=7)		Ischemic heart disease (N=9)	
	Before	Difference	Before	Difference
Total cholesterol:				
LDL (mg/100 ml)	419 ± 112	+ 119 ± 91	413 ± 115	+ 79 ± 57
HDL (mg/100 ml)	99 ± 13	+ 34 ± 32	108 ± 38	+ 56 ± 38
LDL/HDL of TCh ratio	4.36 ± 1.13	-0.67 ± 1.88	3.97 ± 1.09	-0.05 ± 1.12
TCh/TG ratio in VLDL	0.39 ± 0.16	-0.10 ± 0.08	0.39 ± 0.07	+0.04 ± 0.16

VLDL: very low-density lipoprotein, LDL: low-density lipoprotein, HDL: high-density lipoprotein, TCh: total cholesterol, TG: triglyceride.

high content of TCh in VLDL decreased by the diet and a low level of TCh in high-density lipoprotein (HDL) which could be estimated more clearly if one calculated the ratio of LDL-TCh to HDL-TCh. Though the IHD group in this subgroup had the same characteristics as the control group, the response to the diet was not seen in the ratio of TCh to TG in VLDL. On the other hand, the characteristics of the subgroup in whom LDL-TCh decreased by the diet (Table 2) were no response of the ratio of TCh to TG in VLDL by the diet and high content of TCh in HDL accompanying a high TCh content in LDL. The IHD group of this subgroup HDL-TCh was significantly low if compared with this level in control ($P < 0.01$); this difference becomes especially clear when estimated by the ratio of LDL to HDL.

It is well-known that VLDL-TG is increased by dietary carbohydrate. The mechanism which enhanced output of VLDL-TG was reported by Quarfordt et al. in 1970. Moreover, we reported in 1975 that high VLDL-TG led to different movement of LDL-TCh in plasma lipoprotein metabolism (Kimura and Nanbu, 1975). So we tried to clarify the difference in response to the diet therapy between IHD and non-IHD, using the subjects with an initial VLDL-TG level over 180 mg/100 ml. It is clearly revealed that there are poor responses of VLDL-TG to the diet associated with no change of the ratio of TCh to TG in VLDL in the IHD group. One possible explanation of this difference is the high relative body weight in the control group. There are some interesting results in the IHD group after 50 g oral glucose tolerance (50 g OGTT). There is a marked decrease in plasma-free fatty acids (FFA) by 50 g OGTT in spite of a similar level of glucose rise and maximum increased level of plasma insulin after 50 g OGTT. Though we will need more experiments to explain this fact, excessive sensitivity to glucose on release of FFA into plasma might be related to an abnormal response of VLDL to calorie restriction seen in IHD (Tables 3 and 4).

It is obvious that dietary factors affect serum lipids in different ways. Patients with initially low HDL total cholesterol levels and with VLDL triglyceride over 180 mg/dl will respond to diet by reduction in VLDL total cholesterol. The ratio of total cholesterol to triglyceride in VLDL of IHD is not generally responsive to diet.

Table 2. Subjects with LDL cholesterol decreased by calory restriction

	Control (N=8)		Ischemic heart disease (N=11)	
	Before	Difference	Before	Difference
Total cholesterol:				
LDL (mg/100 ml)	501 ± 152	−142 ± 104	609 ± 132	−138 ± 85
HDL (mg/100 ml)	162 ± 32	−39 ± 49	120 ± 28	−20 ± 46
				$p < 0.01$
LDL/HDL of TCh ratio	2.99 ± 1.00	+0.53 ± 0.76	5.10 ± 2.02	+0.01 ± 0.07
				$p < 0.02$
TCh/TG ratio in VLDL	0.31 ± 0.09	+0.04 ± 0.11	0.32 ± 0.11	−0.52 ± 1.11

VLDL: very low-density lipoprotein, LDL: low-density lipoprotein, HDL: high-density lipoprotein, TCh: total cholesterol, TG: triglyceride.

Table 3. Subjects with initial VLDL-TG level over 180 mg/100 nl

	Control (N=9)		Ischemic heart disease (N=10)	
	Before	At 4 weeks	Before	At 4 weeks
VLDL-TG (mg/100 ml)	274 ± 31	135 ± 66	251 ± 57	170 ± 48
difference		−138 ± 78		−77 ± 52
TCh/TG ratio in VLDL	0.44 ± 0.15	0.28 ± 0.06	0.38 ± 0.11	0.38 ± 0.08
difference		−0.15 ± 0.13		−0.01 ± 0.11
Relative body weight (%)	125 ± 14	111 ± 8	112 ± 12 [a]	107 ± 10
% decrease of body weight		−8.3 ± 3.0		−2.8 ± 1.7

VLDL: very low-density lipoprotein, TG: triglyceride, TCh: total cholesterol.
[a] $p < 0.05$.

Table 4. Subjects with initial VLDL-TG level over 180 mg/100 ml

	Control (N=9)		IHD (N=10)
High-density lipoprotein	136 ± 46		121 ± 44
LDL/HDL (TCh) ratio	3.11 ± 0.81	— $p < 0.005$ —	4.54 ± 1.03
Free fatty acids	590 ± 70	— $p < 0.05$ —	505 ± 97
50 g OGTT:			
minimum level of FFA	420 ± 57	— $p < 0.001$ —	297 ± 47
maximum level of insulin	92 ± 15		76 ± 32
area of blood glucose	2.32 ± 0.50		2.39 ± 0.36

LDL: low-density lipoprotein, HDL: high-density lipoprotein, FFA: free fatty acids (μEq/l). TCh: total cholesterol.

PRACTICAL CONSIDERATIONS OF CHANGING DIETARY CHOLESTEROL AND FAT

P.J. Nestel

Changes in cholesterol intake are generally reflected in changes in plasma cholesterol levels. Equations that describe this relationship are based on studies
of populations and do not exclude marked variability among individuals. This
variability may be attributed to genetic heterogeneity and interaction of the
effects of dietary cholesterol with other components of the diet. The metabolic
responses to increased amounts of absorbed cholesterol include, in man, a reduction in the synthesis and an increase in the re-excretion of cholesterol.

Studies in our laboratory have examined the effectiveness of these compensating
mechanisms in two populations: a group of six New Guinea Highlanders (Whyte et
al., 1977) and in nine Australian whites (Nestel and Poyser, 1976). The New
Guineas were healthy males drawn from a population whose plasma cholesterol
levels are low by western standards and whose predominantly sweet potato diet
contains little fat, cholesterol or protein and about 90% of its calories as
carbohydrate. Faecal sterol excretion studies were carried out during their ha-
bitual very low-cholesterol intake and again after they had eaten, under close
supervision, an additional 1 g cholesterol as egg yolk powder. Table 1 shows: (a)
the failure of the plasma cholesterol to rise despite the "normal" absorption of
about 390 mg cholesterol per day, and (b) the excretion of 1245 mg of sterols
per day. Since the intake of cholesterol was 1000 mg, the synthesis of cholesterol was 1245 − 1000 = 245 mg per day. This compares with a synthesis rate of
750 mg per day on the control diet, i.e. synthesis was reduced by 505 mg per
day on average in response to an increase in absorption of 390 mg. Compensation,
brought about by reduced synthesis, was therefore adequate and prevented a rise
in the plasma cholesterol.

The findings in the Australians only partly resembled those in New Guineas, as
shown in Table 2. Some subjects showed a negligible increase in the plasma cholesterol with an additional intake of 500 mg while others showed a very large increase. The "theoretical" rise for the given increase in intake was calculated
to be 22 mg/100 ml. Two distinct compensating mechanisms were observed. Those
who showed a smaller than expected rise in the plasma cholesterol also showed a
substantial reduction in cholesterol synthesis. By contrast, the three subjects
whose plasma cholesterol concentrations rose greatly compensated for increased
absorption with increased re-excretion. Although this mechanism prevented accumulation of cholesterol in the body, it did not prevent the rise in the plasma.
Re-excretion, therefore, appears to be a secondary event and follows expansion
of the plasma cholesterol pool. This study clearly demonstrates the variability
in the response to cholesterol feeding and points to the need for a practical
screening test that will distinguish hyperresponders from hyporesponders.

A possible interaction between cholesterol intake and the amount and type of fat
eaten has practical implications since dietary advice to lower plasma cholesterol
levels includes reduction in cholesterol and total fat intake and a relative increase in the proportion of polyunsaturated fatty acids. We have re-examined
these three variables in studies in normal subjects (Table 3). In the first study,
we have compared the effect of increasing the P/S ratio during the course of
raising the cholesterol intake from 300 to 800 mg per day. At a P/S ratio of 0.3,
the additional 500 mg of egg yolk cholesterol raised the plasma cholesterol by
the expected 22 mg/100 ml. However, at a higher P/S ratio (1.5) the effect of the
dietary cholesterol was greatly modified, the increase in the plasma cholesterol
being limited to 12 mg/100 ml. This suggests that restriction of dietary cholesterol need not be as stringent in normal people provided the intake of polyunsaturated fatty acids is raised.

The second part of Table 3 shows the interaction of the amount of dietary fat
with the P/S ratio of the fat. The plasma cholesterol level was not affected by

Table 1. Cholesterol absorption and faecal sterol excretion during the last 8 days of a test period with 1 g daily of egg yolk cholesterol in the diet, and plasma lipid concentrations during the control (C), test (T) and control (C) periods of 28, 35 and 35 days respectively

Subject	Body weight kg	Plasma lipids cholesterol (nmol/l)			Triglyceride (nmol/l)			Cholesterol absorption %	Faecal sterol excretion (T) mg/day		
		C	T	C	C	T	C		Neutral	Acidic	Total
14	68	4.74	4.79	4.90	1.78	1.21	1.56	39	978	287	1265
15	62	5.80	6.48	5.75	2.58	1.78	2.00	48	924	294	1218
16	58	4.40	4.56	5.00	1.99	1.83	1.77	47	853	357	1210
17	53	4.61	4.84	4.51	2.11	1.72	2.01	39	961	284	1245
18	62	4.51	4.35	4.51	1.64	1.31	1.62	33	859	373	1232
19	71	3.81	3.88	4.35	1.40	1.31	1.30	29	996	307	1303
Mean	62	4.66	4.82	4.84	1.92	1.52	1.71	39	928	317	1245
SD	6.5	0.72	0.91	0.75	0.60	0.44	0.47	7.5	61	38	34

Cholesterol synthesis during control period was 750 mg per day on average.
Cholesterol synthesis during egg yolk diet was 1245 - 1000 = 245 g per day.
Reduction in synthesis therefore = 505 mg which exceeds increased absorption of 390 mg per day.

Table 2. Effectiveness of compensating mechanisms (sum of changes in cholesterol synthesis and re-excretion) in relation to amounts of cholesterol absorbed

Subject	Change in plasma cholesterol	Increase in absorbed cholesterol	Increase in re-excreted cholesterol	Decrease in synthesized cholesterol	Total Compensation
	mg/100 ml	mg/d	mg/d	mg/d	mg/d
1	+ 3	178	−119	227	108
2	+ 7	269	−89	420	331
3	+ 8	173	28	164	192
4	+ 11	250	−96	287	191
5	+ 12	261	84	242	326
6	+ 26	202	70	146	216
7	+ 64	250	268	40	308
8	+ 47	236	162	58	220
9[a] a	+142	240	137	11	148
b	−190	−238	−145	−74	−219
Mean ± S.D.		230 ± 34			226 ± 75

[a]9a: Changes following increase in dietary cholesterol.
9b: Changes following decrease in dietary cholesterol.

Table 3. Dietary fat and cholesterol: interdependent of independent

Percent fat in diet	P/S ratio	Cholesterol intake mg	Change in plasma cholesterol mg/100 ml
40	0.3	300	0
40	0.3	800	+ 22
40	1.5	300	0
40	1.5	800	+ 12
13	2S−P=0	1100	0
40	2S−P=0	1100	0

lowering the intake of fat from 40% to 13% of dietary calories, provided the P/S ratio in both diets was such that the equation $2S - P = 0$. These two studies demonstrate the interaction of dietary factors with respect to their overall effect on the plasma cholesterol level and suggest that the most useful advice in this regard is a reduction in saturated fat intake and an increase in the proportion of fat eaten as polyunsaturated fatty acid.

There is increasing interest in the effectiveness of dietary modification on the plasma cholesterol levels of infants and children. We have recently shown that increasing the linoleate content of breast milk by increasing the mother's intake of polyunsaturated fat will lower the plasma cholesterol in the suckling child (Potter and Nestel, 1976a). In artificially fed infants, the plasma cholesterol level can be lowered by substituting soy bean milk for cow's milk. This is associated with an increase in sterol excretion that is quantitatively greater than es seen in adults (Potter and Nestel, 1976b). It has been suggested that children may be more responsive than adults to diets that lower the plasma cholesterol. We have examined this by comparing the long-term response of hypercho-

Table 4. Effect of diet alone in familial hypercholesterolaemia

| | Mean plasma cholesterol (mg/100 ml) | | | |
	Year 0	Year 1	Year 2	Year 3
5 Parents	442	402	396	389
12 Children	367	322	279	243

Percent change in parents: 12%
Percent change in children: 34%

lesterolaemic adults and their affected children to a cholesterol-lowering diet. The results in Table 4, of the findings in five families comprising five parents and their 12 children, suggest that from a practical point of view, the children are either more responsive or compliant. The satisfactory 34% fall in the plasma cholesterol in this moderately affected group of children also cautions against the premature use of cholesterol-lowering drugs.

DIETARY PROTEIN, HYPERCHOLESTEROLEMIA, AND ATHEROSCLEROSIS*

Kenneth K. Caroll, Murray W. Huff, and David C.K. Roberts

It has been known for nearly 20 years that rabbits become hypercholesterolemic and develop atherosclerotic lesions when fed semipurified diets, even though the diets contain little or no cholesterol. The hypercholesterolenia and atherosclerosis have been observed with low-fat diets and with diets containing saturated fats, but can largely be prevented by incorporating polyunsaturated fats into the diet (Lambert et al., 1958; Malmros and Wigand, 1959).

These findings led to the suggestion that the observed effects were manifestations of essential fatty acid deficiency, but later studies by Kritchevsky and Tepper (1968) indicated that something more than dietary fat was involved. They noted that hypercholesterolemia and atherosclerosis do not develop in rabbits fed commercial chow, even when saturated fat is added to the diet. The Purina Chow used for their experiments contained 2-3% of polyunsaturated fat, but this did not seem to account for the protective effect. When this fat was extracted and added to a semisynthetic diet, it made little difference to the results obtained with either the commercial or semisynthetic diets.

Results of experiments in our laboratory, which were reported at the Third International Symposium on Atherosclerosis in Berlin (Hamilton and Carroll, 1974), showed that the elevation of plasma cholesterol levels in rabbits fed low-cholesterol, semipurified diets was primarily due to the casein commonly used as the protein component of such diets. The hypercholesterolemia was not observed when the casein was replaced by a plant protein such as isolated soy protein.

This findings has been confirmed and extended by further experiments in our laboratory over the past several years (Carroll and Hamilton, 1975; Hamilton and Carroll, 1976). Protein preparations from about a dozen different plant sources

*This work was supported by the Ontario Heart Foundation and the Medical Research Council of Canada. Soy protein isolate (Promine-R) was generously provided by Dr. E.W. Meyer, Central Soya, Chemurgy Division, Chicago, Illinois.

have been fed to rabbits in semipurified diets, and in no case has a significant hypercholesterolemia been observed. Conversely, protein preparations from milk, eggs, and meat have nearly all produced an elevation of plasma cholesterol levels in rabbits, when fed in a semipurified, cholesterol-free diet. Some feeding trials have also been carried out with diets containing a mixture of plant and animal protein. A significant hypercholesterolemia was obtained with a 3:1 mixture of casein and isolated soy protein, but no elevation of plasma cholesterol was observed when the diet contained a 1:1 mixture of these proteins.

In most of these experiments, the diets were fed for 4 weeks to groups of five or six young, male, New Zealand white rabbits. Over this period of time, the plasma cholesterol level normally increased from about 50 mg/dl to 200 mg/dl on a cholesterol-free, low-fat, semipurified, casein-containing diet. In a longer-term feeding trial carried out during the past year, the mean plasma cholesterol continued to increase to a maximum of about 300 mg/dl at 2-3 months, then decreased to about 200 mg/dl over the period of 4-7 months, and remained significantly elevated throughout the 10-month feeding period (Fig. 1). No signficant hypercholesterolemia was observed during this period of time in rabbits fed a similar diet containing soy protein isolate rather than casein. This illustrates the marked and continuing influence of dietary protein preparations on the level of plasma cholesterol in rabbits.

As part of this long-term experiment, analysis of plasma lipoproteins was carried out after 5 months on diet, with the results illustrated in Figure 2. It can be seen that the hypercholesterolemia produced by the casein diet was primarily due to an increase in LDL1 (d 1.006-1.019), with some increase in VLDL (d < 1.006) and in LDL2 (d 1.019-1.063).

Some of the rabbits on the long-term feeding experiments were killed after varying time intervals, and the aortas were stained with Sudan III. Few, if any, lesions were observed at time intervals of less than 6-8 months on diet, but from 8 months onward, sudanophilia was readily apparent and was sometimes quite widespread in rabbits fed the low-fat, cholesterol-free, casein, semipurified diet. However, no gross sudanophilia was observed in rabbits fed the corresponding diet containing soy protein isolate for periods of as long as 11 months.

It is obviously of interest to obtain more information on the exact nature of the dietary components responsible for the observed hypercholesterolemia and atherosclerosis. The differing effects of casein and soy protein isolate could be

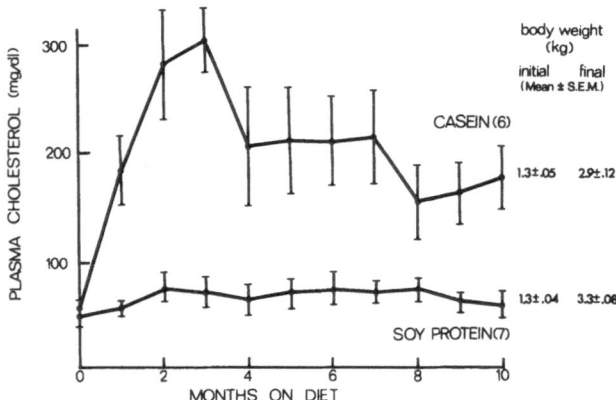

Figure 1. Plasma cholesterol levels of male New Zealand white rabbits fed cholesterol-free semipurified diets for 10 months. Numbers in brackets indicate the numbers of rabbits maintained on the casein and soy protein diets for the full 10-month period. The vertical bars indicate SEM

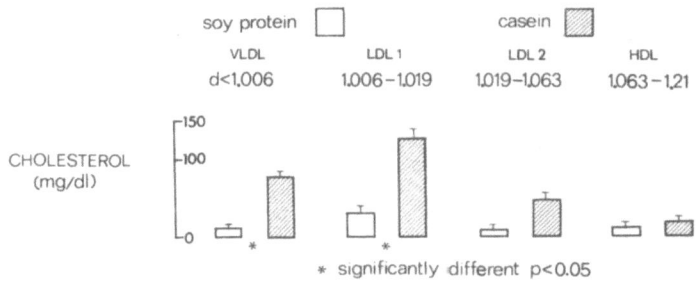

Figure 2. Analysis of plasma lipoproteins of rabbits after 5 months on semipurified diets containing either soy protein isolate or casein. Results are expressed
as mean ± SEM for groups of 4 rabbits

due to differences in their amino acid composition. It is also possible that other
substances associated with the protein preparations may be responsible, although
the casein preparation contains over 90% protein and the soy protein isolate better than 92% protein. In attempts to resolve this question, feeding trials have
been carried out with diets containing either ezymic digests of the proteins or
mixtures of amino acids corresponding to the amino acid composition of the proteins. Results of such experiments are shown in Figure 3. It can be seen that
the enzyme hydrolysates gave results very similar to those obtained with the intact proteins. The mixture of amino acids corresponding to casein also gave results similar to those obtained with the protein itself. Evidently, the hypercholesterolemia obtained by feeding the casein diet is not due to any extraneous
materials associated with the casein. However, the mixture of amino acids corresponding to soy protein isolate gave a somewhat higher level of plasma cholesterol than the intact protein. It is not certain at this time that the hypocholesterolemic effect of plant proteins is due entirely to their amino acid composition. Further experiments are being carried out with other combinations of amino
acids to examine in more detail the effects of individual amino acids or groups
of amino acids on plasma cholesterol levels.

The ultimate aim of experimental atherosclerosis research is to obtain information which can be used for prevention or treatment of the disease in humans. The
possible role of dietary protein in human atherosclerosis has so far attracted
relatively little attention, since it is generally considered that dietary protein has little or no influence. Epidemiological data from different countries of
the world show, however, that the positive correlation between animal protein intake and mortality from coronary heart disease is as strong as that with fat intake (Yudkin, 1957; Connor and Connor, 1972). A survey of the literature also
provided some evidence that dietary protein can influence serum cholesterol levels
in humans (Carroll and Hamilton, 1975).

In view of the evidence that dietary protein can have a marked influence on plasma cholesterol levels in rabbits, it seemed worthwhile to carry out further experiments to investigate its effects on plasma cholesterol levels in humans.
Dietary trials for this purpose are currently in progress in our laboratory. In
these trials, the aim is to have dietary protein as the only major variable, so
that effects of animal and vegetable protein can be compared. These experiments
should help to determine whether dietary protein does, in fact, play a role in
the etiology of atherosclerosis in human populations.

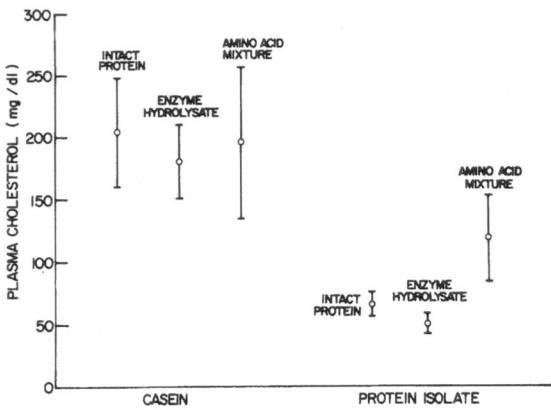

Figure 3. Effect on rabbit plasma total cholesterol of diets containing protein
hydrolysates or mixtures of amino acids equivalent to casein or soy protein isolate. Diets were fed for 4 weeks to groups of 6 male New Zealand white rabbits.
The vertical bars indicate SEM

SOYBEAN PROTEIN DIET IN THE TREATMENT OF HYPERCHOLESTEROLEMIA

Cesare R. Sirtori, Elisabetta Agradi, Franco Conti, Oreste Mantero,
and Ennio Gatti

Introduction

The availability of a soybean textured protein (Koury and Hodges, 1968), free of
cholesterol and saturated fat, suggested its use in therapeutic diets for hyperlipidemia. A dietary study with soybean protein totally replacing animal proteins
was carried out in patients with type II hyperlipidemia. Following a crossover
protocol, the soybean protein diet was compared, in the same subjects, with a
standard low-lipid, low-cholesterol diet. The results of this study have provided
evidence that soy protein exerts a hypocholesterolemic effect per se, independent
of the lipid content of the diet, and may be a valuable addition to therapeutic
diets for hyperlipidemia.

Materials and Methods

The study was carried out on 22 patients with stable type II hyperlipoproteinemia,
admitted to a metabolic ward. All had been following a low-lipid, low-cholesterol
diet for at least 3 months prior to admission and were not taking hypolipidemic
drugs. After 1 week of adaption to the hospital environment following the diet
customary to the patient, during which three blood samples for lipid analysis
were drawn, each was assigned to one or the other of two dietary sequences: *low-
lipid-soybean* and *soybean-low-lipid*. Each dietary period lasted 3 weeks.

Composition of the two diets is reported in Table 1. Soybean was available in the
form of granules of textured protein isolate (Temptein, Miles Laboratories,
Elkhart, Ind., USA). These were adjusted to prepare a variety of food items,
suitable to the Italian type of nutrition (Zoppi et al., 1976). Calories assigned
to each patient were calculated from the dietary record and reduced approximately
10-25% according the previous physical activity.

Plasma samples were drawn on Monday, Wednesday, and Friday of each experimental
week, after a 12-hour fast, and analyzed for cholesterol and triglycerides by

Table 1. Composition of the two diets

Low-lipid	Protein	20.98[a]	(62% animal 38% vegetable)
	Lipids	20.84	(46% polyunsaturated 33.1% monounsaturated 20.9% saturated) P/S 2.2
	Carbohydrates	58.81	
	Cholesterol 100 mg/1,000 kcal		
Soybean	Protein	20.60	(63% soybean protein 30% other vegetable protein 7% animal)
	Lipids	25.92	(44% polyunsaturated 49.6% monounsaturated 16.4% saturated) P/S 2.7
	Carbohydrates	53.48	
	Cholesterol:0 mg (max. 6 mg if skimmed milk was available)		

[a] % of total calories.

automated techniques. The Monday sample was also used for the electrophoretic and ultracentrifugal separation of plasma lipoproteins.

Two of the 22 patients started on this protocol did not finish. One, because of some gastric discomfort and constipation after a few days of soy protein, the other having refused to be switched to the low-lipid diet, after completing the soybean period, being satisfied with the results just achieved. The 20 patients with complete data are ten males and ten females (aged, respectively, 22-63 and 40-68), nine of which were classified at entrance as type IIa (LDL cholesterol levels above 190 mg/dl, VLDL cholesterol below 35 mg/dl; weak pre-β band in electrophoresis), 11 as type IIb (LDL cholesterol above 190 mg/dl; VLDL cholesterol above 35 mg/dl, prominent pre-β band in electrophoresis.

Results

The soybean diet, both when given first, or after the low-lipid diet, caused very significant decreases of total and LDL cholesterol levels. The mean decrease of total cholesterol was 14% after 2 weeks and 21% after 3 weeks (Fig. 1; Table 2). The low-lipid diet induced very modest variations of plasma total and LDL cholesterol. Switching from the soybean to the low-lipid diet was followed by a clear increase of plasma cholesterol. The response was not different in type IIa and IIb patients. The cholesterol decrease induced by the soybean diet was significantly correlated to the pretreatment cholesterolemias (Fig. 2). Triglycerides were slightly decreased by both diets during the first dietary period, and generally tended to stabilize during the second treatment. Body weights were stable throughout the study. All patients having completed the protocol felt generally well, and were satisfied with the appearance and flavor of the soybean entrees. Routine laboratory tests were not affected by the diets. In some patients, some improvement of clinical symptoms was also noted. In three, with familial type IIa disease, tendinous and buttock xanthomata were reduced after the soybean diet.

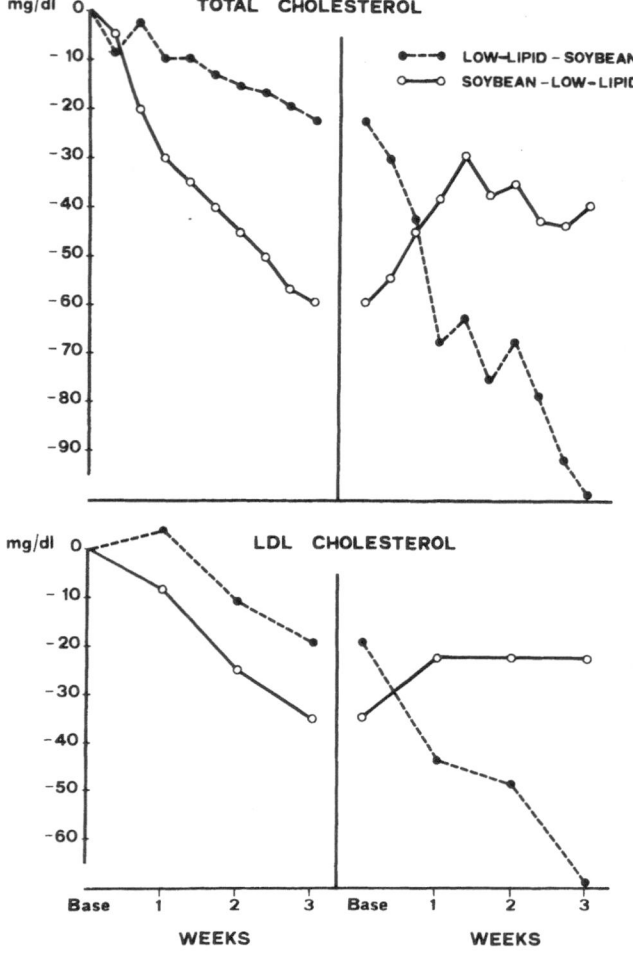

Figure 1. Mean total and LDL cholesterol changes following the two dietary sequences

Discussion

The results of this study indicate that the soy protein diet exerted a remarkable hypocholesterolemic effect, whereas a standard low-lipid, low-cholesterol diet, although responding to optimal criteria for diets of this type (Lewis et al., 1970), was ineffective. It may be noted that all patients had already been following a diet of this latter type at home.

A comparative analysis of two diets (Table 1) only indicates a slightly lower P/S ratio in the low-lipid diet, which also contains a small amount of cholesterol. By applying published formulas for calculating effects of dietary lipids on plasma cholesterol levels (Keys et al., 1965a, 1965b), these small differences of lipid composition fail to explain the decrease of cholesterolemia after the soybean diet. To further verify the effect of a cholesterol addition to soybean, a second experiment was carried out in eight type II patients, selected with the same criteria as in the first experiment, and divided into two groups of four. These patients followed two successive dietary periods, of 3 weeks each, both with textured soy replacing animal proteins (soy 2). During the soy 1 period, 500 mg of cholesterol daily (egg powder of known cholesterol concentration) were given to four of the patients to the other four during the soy 2 period. As shown

Table 2. Lipid levels in the two sequences ($\bar{x} \pm$ SEM)

	Low-lipid				Soybean			
	Base	1 wk	2	3	Base	1	2	3
Cholesterol	353.1	344.0	341.3	335.1	335.1	291.0b	292.9c	257.7c
(mg/dl) ±	22.9	23.3	27.1	29.0	29.0	18.7	24.8	20.3
LDL cholesterol	263.7	268.4	252.6	244.7	244.7	221.2	216.6a	188.7b
	18.7	18.2	19.6	23.1	23.1	16.7	20.8	20.7
Triglycerides	197.9	153.2	178.0	177.2	177.2	143.1	145.5	149.3
	23.9	20.4	35.8	32.2	32.2	16.2	19.2	27.7

	Soybean				Low-lipid			
	Base	1 wk	2	3	Base	1	2	3
Cholesterol	313.1	283.2a	268.8c	253.6c	253.6	275.9a	278.8b	276.5b
±	16.5	17.3	16.0	13.0	13.0	14.1	16.3	17.0
LDL cholesterol	220.5	213.2	194.4b	184.0c	184.0	196.8	197.5	196.6
	11.4	15.3	13.5	16.3	16.3	13.9	16.6	16.2
Trilgycerides	217.4	189.5	175.0	180.6	180.6	195.1	174.6	165.9
	21.1	18.5	20.8	23.9	23.9	20.7	15.5	13.1

P: a <0.05; b <0.01; c <0.0001 compared to baseline levels.

451

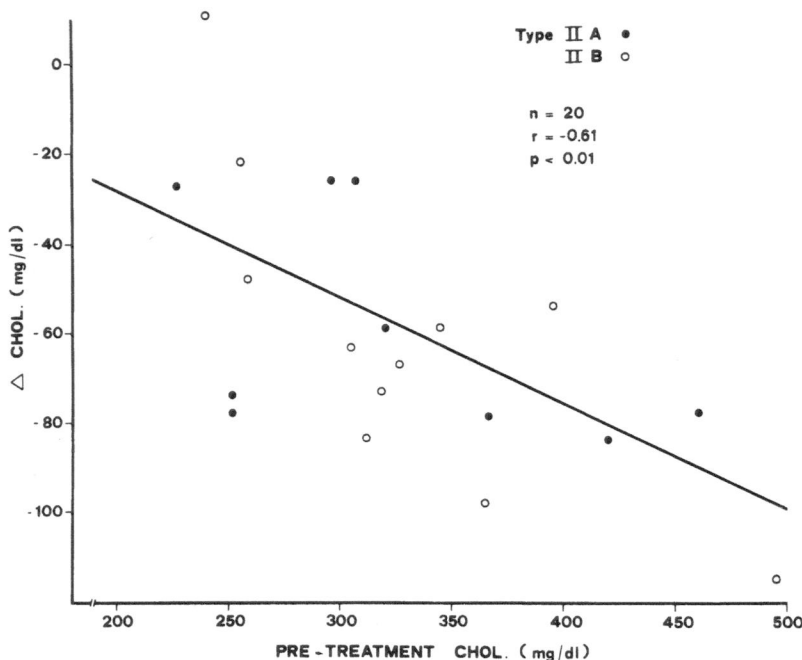

Figure 2. Correlation between the cholesterol changes induced by the soybean diet and the cholesterol levels immediately preceding this diet (i.e., data are from patients who took soybean first, or after the low-lipid diet)

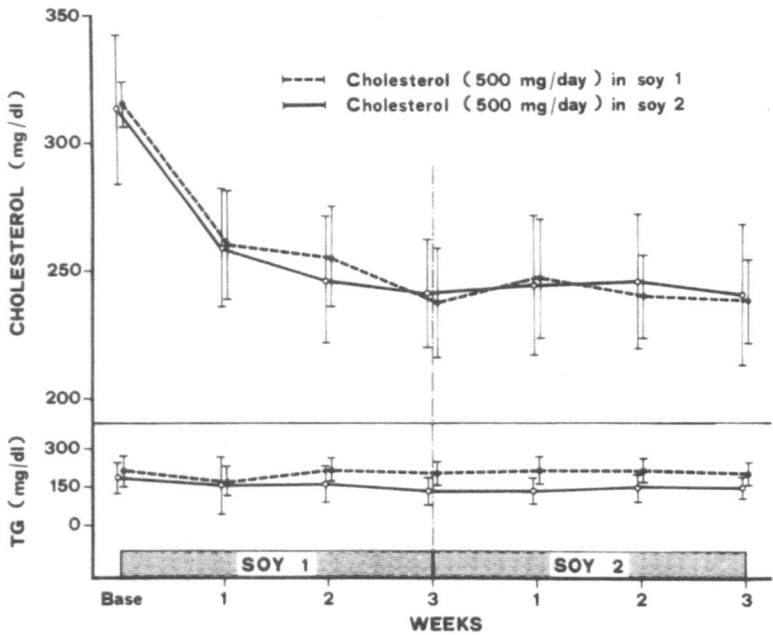

Figure 3. Effect on plasma lipids of the addition of cholesterol to the soybean diet. The group of four patients indicated with the dashed line received the cholesterol addition during the first 3 weeks of soybean diet; the other four patients during the second 3 weeks

in Figure 3, addition of cholesterol to soybean did not influence either the rate of decrease of cholesterolemia (when given during soy 1) or its stabilization (when given during soy 2).

These results suggest a hypocholesterolemic effect of soy proteins per se, independent of the lipid composition of the diet.

This tentative conclusion is supported by recent experimental studies (Carroll and Hamilton, 1975) as well as by epidemiological data on populations who consume large amounts of vegetable proteins (Sacks et al., 1975). It may be noted that vegetarians consume eggs and milk derivatives in addition to vegetable proteins. The hypocholesterolemic effect of the soybean protein diet in this study was remarkable and achieved within a few weeks of treatment. It was more diet even after many months of treatment. The exact mechanism of this effect remains to be elucidated.

METABOLISM OF RABBIT LIPOPROTEINS ALTERED BY DIETARY CHOLESTEROL, AND SATURATED AND POLYUNSATURATED FATS

E.F. Stange, M. Alavi, and J. Papenberg
Medizinische Universitätsklinik, Heidelberg/BRD

As was shown in a recent investigation, there is a marked change in the structural properties of rabbit lipoproteins by dietary cholesterol, and saturated
and polyunsaturated fats. Based on these electrophoretic, chemical and electron-
microscopic findings we now examined the metabolic behaviour of ^{125}I labelled
VLDL (d <1.006 g/ml) from normal rabbits (group I) as well as animals fed 1%
cholesterol (group II), 1% cholesterol + 5% coconut oil (group III) or 1% cholesterol + 5% corn oil (group IV). The activity decay curves were analysed for the
fractional catabolic rate per hour by the curve peeling technique. The F.C.R.
obtained for VLDL I was 0.082/h. All hypercholesteremic fractions were metabolized significantly (p <0.01) faster with respective F.C.R. values of 0.119,
0.157 and 0.173. The apoprotein decay curves of delipidated plasma resulted in
similar values: 0.083 (VLDL I), 0.145 (II), 0.224 (III) and 0.240 (IV). Already
10 min after injection most of the activity was recovered in the IDL class (d
1.006-1.019). The LDL of the normal group had the lowest decay rate, in all
other groups HDL was delayed. The metabolism of hypercholesteremic VLDL differs
from normal VLDL both quantitatively and qualitatively.

THE EFFECT OF A CHANGE FROM SATURATED TO POLYUNSATURATED FAT ONLY IN AN ORDINARY SWEDISH DIET ON SERUM LIPID AND LIPOPROTEIN CONCEN-TRATIONS IN PATIENTS WITH DIFFERENT TYPES OF HYPERLIPOPROTEINEMIA

Jonas Boberg, Merike Boberg, Inga-Britt Gustafsson, Brita Karlström, Hans
Lithell, Bengt Vessby, and Ivar Werner
Department of Geriatrics, University of Uppsala, Uppsala/Sweden

Seven patients with type II A, five with II B and eighteen with IV hyperlipoproteinemia habe been studied on a metabolic ward. Each patient had for two weeks
a control diet (very similar to an average Swedish diet with calories from protein 11, fat 43 and carbohydrates 46 per cent) followed by two weeks on a similar
diet except that the ratios polyunsaturated to saturated fatty acids was changed
from 0.2 to 2.0. Each patient received 126 KJ (30 Kcal) per kg body weight. Body
weight was unchanged during the studies. Average decrease of S-cholesterol concentration was 10.0 ± 2.6, 12.8 ± 2.4 and 12.1 ± 2.0 per cent in the three
groups of patients and corresponding decreases for S-triglycerides were 10.1
± 5.5, 13.8 ± 5.0 and 12.6 ± 4.0 per cent. Data of how the triglyceride and
cholesterol concentrations did change in the different lipoprotein fractions
will be presented as well as how the serum fatty acid patterns of S-triglycerides,
S-cholesterol esters and S-phospholipids were changes. No significant changes
occurred in adipose tissue lipoprotein lipase activities or in intravenous fat
tolerances. These decreases of S-cholesterol concentrations are about 50 per
cent and of S-triglyceride concentrations about 30 per cent of the greatest decrease that can be achieved by only diet treatment of these patients.

WEIGHT REDUCTION AND DIETARY MODIFICATION IN LOWERING SERUM LIPID LEVELS IN OBESE MEN

Boonseng Leelarthaepin, Joan Woodhill, Jean Palmer, Clyde McGilchrist, and Ralph Blacket
Department of Medicine, University of New South Wales, Prince Henry Hospital, Sydney/Australia

The relative contributions of weight reduction and modification of dietary fat in lowering serum lipids have been studied in eighty two moderately overweight subjects. Sixty one men had type 2 hyperlipidaemia and twenty one had "normal" lipid levels on entry. The subjects were divided according to weight loss after dietary intervention. In fifty four men relative body weight (RBW) at entry 117, serum cholesterol (SC) 289 mg/100 ml, serum triglyceride (ST) 193 mg/100 ml weight reduction to RBW 103 led to 18% fall in SC and 35% fall in ST. Twenty eight men RBW 118, SC 284 mg/100 ml, and ST 173 mg/100 ml did not lose weight on a similar fat modified diet. SC fell 6% and ST 5%. We conclude that weight reduction has a powerful lipid lowering effect. In obese subjects failure to lose weight greatly impairs the effectiveness of lipid lowering diets.

THE CHOLESTEROL INCREASING AND TRIGLYCERIDES LOWERING EFFECT OF A VERY HIGH CALORIC, HIGH FAT DIET

Daniel Brunner, Moshe Fischer, Kurt Loebl, and Sara Schwartz
Donolo Institute of Physiological Hygiene, Tel Aviv University, Tel Aviv/Israel

26 Yemenite Jewish smallfarmers volunteered in a 12-months dietary trial to consume in an especially established kitchen and dining room a very high caloric, high fat diet. The average daily intake was 4553 calories, which was 2.2 times higher than the original Yemenite diet. In the trial diet 35% of the calories were provided by carbohydrates and 50% by fats. The volunteers consumed the trial diet for 7 months, and after an interval of 3 months for 2 additional months. Serum cholesterol (CH) rose from a mean of 150 mg% at the start to a peak value of 199 mg%, dropped to 154 mg% at the 3-months interval, and rose steeply to 195 mg% during the last 2 months of the trial. Triglycerides (TG) were like a reflected image of the CH curves. From an initial value of 101 mg%, they dropped to 62 mg%, rose in the interval to the pre-trial level, and again decreased to 76 mg% during the last 2 month of the trial. Age-specific, pre-trial CH- or TG-specific subgroups showed similar curves.
It is suggested that the ratio between fats, carbohydrates and proteins in the total caloric intake, rather than their absolute weight, is of great importance in the determination of serum lipid values.

HYPOCHOLESTEROLEMIC EFFECT OF ALFALFA IN CHOLESTEROL-FED MONKEYS

M.R. Malinow, P. McLaughlin, L. Papworth, H.K. Naito, and L.A. Lewis
Oregon Regional Primate Research Center, Beaverton, OR/USA, University of Oregon Health Sciences Center, Portland, OR/USA, and Cleveland Clinic, Cleveland, OH/USA

Sixty-two adult female *Macaca fascicularis* were fed a semipurified diet containing 1.2 mg of cholesterol (C)/cal for 6 months. Plasma C was 833 ± (SE) 40 mg/dl; triglycerides (TG) were 71 ± 14 mg/dl; and phospholipids (PL) 518 ± 23 mg/dl. Each monkey was ranked and stratified according to plasma C, and randomly assigned to one of 3 dietary groups: (a) semipurified without additions (N=18), (b) semipurified with 50% alfalfa (N=18), or (c) stock chow (N=26). Diets (a) and (b) contained 0.34 mg C/cal and were isocaloric for protein and fat. Plasma C, TG, and PL were determined 4 and 6 months later. Similar body weights in the 3 groups were maintained throughout the experiment. Results shown in the table indicate that alfalfa reduced plasma C and PL levels but had no effect on TG, which were not elevated by the semipurified diet.

Plasma levels (mg/dl) (mean ± SE)

Group	C		TG		PL	
	4 mos.	6 mos.	4 mos.	6 mos.	4 mos.	6 mos.
(a)	371±28	350±20	67±12	59±6	318±23	254±12
(b)	238±16[c]	223±12[c]	67±9	60±8	266±22	211±9[c]
(c)	169±6[c]	161±4[c]	36±6[a]	52±4	215±9[c]	174±9[b]

p [Student's "t" test vs (a)] [a]<0.05. [b]<0.01. [c]<0.001.

EFFECTS OF ANTICALCEMIC DRUGS ON PROGRESSION AND REGRESSION OF
ATHEROSCLEROSIS IN RABBITS AND CYNOMOLGUS MONKEYS

Dieter M. Kramsch, and Catherine T. Chan.
B.U. Medical Center, Boston, MA/USA

Eight groups of 8 rabbits were studied for 8 weeks: 1 control group and 7 groups
on a fibrogenic atherogenic diet (FAD) including 1 group on FAD alone and 6
groups on FAD and ethane-hydroxy-diphosphonate (EHDP), Colcemid (Co), EHDP+Co,
thiophene carboxylic acid (ThCA), bromo-ThCA (B-ThCA) or methyl-ThCA (M-ThCA),
respectively. Seven more groups of 8 rabbits were fed FAD for 8 weeks followed
by 8 weeks on normal chow either alone or with the above drugs added separately
to 6 of there groups. In addition, 5 groups of 3 monkeys were studied for 18
months: 1 control group and 4 groups on FAD including 1 group on FAD alone and 3
groups on FAD and EHDP, Co or ThCA, respectively. In animals on FAD, serum elevations of calcium were suppressed by all drugs; serum cholesterol elevated only
in monkeys on EHDP and ThCA. The atherogenic rabbits without drugs showed marked
increases in aortic cholesterol (8-fold), collagen (55%), elastin (45%) and calcium (5-fold) with comparable aortic changes in monkeys on FAD alone. When drugs
were added to FAD, accumulations of these aortic constituents were greatly inhibited with the order of effectiveness being EHDP+Co=M-ThCA>B-ThCA>Co>ThCA>EHDP
for rabbits, and EHDP>Co for monkeys. Drug treatment of rabbits after cessation
of FAD resulted in regression of pre-established atherosclerosis with M-ThCA or
EHDP+Co being the most effective. Conclusion: The drugs tested appear to be useful agents for primary prevention and regression of atherosclerosis. (Supported
by USPHS NIH Grants HL 13262 and HL 15512).

STUDIES ON OCULAR FUNDUS AND SERUM LIPIDS IN VEGETARIANS

Jui-san Chen, Yen-Fei Yang, Ping-Kang Hou, and Kuei-Fang Tsai
Department of Clinical Pathology and Department of Ophthalmology, National Taiwan
University Hospital Taipei, Taiwan/Republic of China

Eye-ground changes and serum lipids were studied on 130 vegetarians with ages
over 35 with 3 to 40 years of vegetarian history. The eye-ground changes were
divided into three categories, viz: (1) abnormal eye-ground group showing abnormal findings of more than arteriosclerosis retinae grade I and retinopathia
hypertonica group I according to Scheie's classification, (2) normal eye-ground
group and (3) venous engorgement group. Serum cholesterol, triglyceride and phospholipid of them were determined. Significantly enough, all lipid fractions of
abnormal eye-ground, without a single exception, yielded values higher than the
other two groups. The finding of the third group as venous engorgement can be
due to systemic hypotension as they suffered neither from anemia nor from heart
failure, and their mean blood pressure was lower then normal group.

POLYUNSATURATED FAT AND CHOLESTEROL BALANCE IN MIDDLE AGED MEN

P. Hill, B. Reddy, and E. Wynder
American Health Foundation, Valhalle, New York, NY/USA

This study reports the effects of a prudent diet (PD) (2500 cals./day, 35% cals. from fat, P/S 1.2; 250 mg cholesterol/day) and a common diet (CD) (2500 cals./day, 40% cals. from fat, P/S 1.2, 600 mg cholesterol/day) composed of customary foods on the serum lipids, faecal neutral sterols (NS) and bile acids (BA) using either sunflower (II), corn (III) and soybean oil (IV) or margarine (I). On PD, serum cholesterol and phospholipids (PL) decreased except in I, while the percentage of (PL) polyunsaturated fatty acids (PUFA) increased in III and IV. These changes were maintained on CD in III, and IV. Reduction in total BA and NS occurred on PD except in IV. The total BA and degradation to secondary BA was decreased. Coprostanol (CL) and coprostanone (CE) decreased except in I. CD increased the excretion of CL and CE, while BA excretion was unaltered in II, III, and IV., Changes in the excretion of NS appeared to depend on the P/S ratio. Excretion of BA was maintained in IV in spite of the reduction in dietary cholesterol. As the serum lipids were unaltered on CD and as the BA and NS excretion were not increased on CD, evidence suggests that the cholesterol balance depends mainly on the cholesterol and calorie intake.

IV
Epidemiology

EPIDEMIOLOGICAL STUDIES OF ATHEROSCLEROTIC DISEASE IN JAPAN

Noboru Kimura

Of the three major causes of death in Japan, stroke ranks first, followed by cancer and heart disease. Accordingly, it can be said that the epidemiological studies of atherosclerotic diseases in Japan have been conducted centering on stroke.
This is the same reason why epidemiological studies in the USA and European countries have advanced, majoring in ischemic heart disease.

In Figure 1, the vital statistics for Japan and the United States are compared.
At the age of 55, the death rate ascribed to coronary heart disease in Japan is
less than one-tenth that in the United States in 1949.

In 1953, we undertook a study examining 1007 hearts that had been saved without
regard to whether or not heart disease was present. For each of the seven decades
of age, there were about 100 hearts from males and 50 from females.

A longitundinal cut to open the coronary arteries from the ostia to the terminal
pericardial branches was made and the degree of atherosclerosis found was classed
into grades 1, 2, and 3. Figure 2 shows that the incidence of grade 3, severe
coronary atherosclerosis in Japanese, is about one-tenth that in persons of the

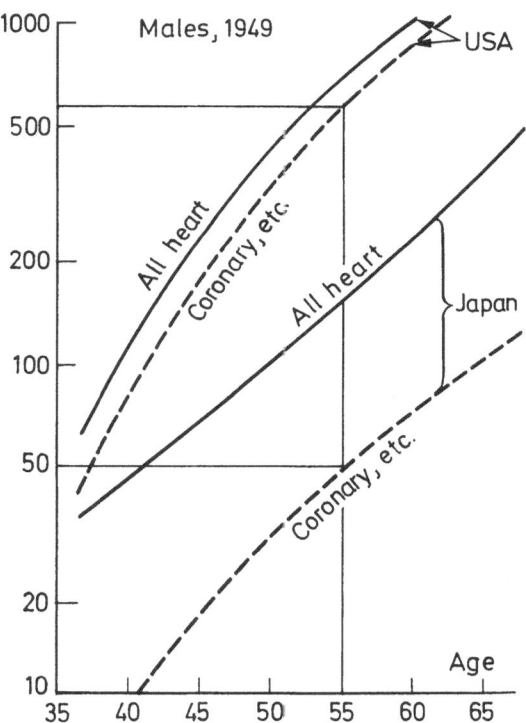

Figure 1. Analysis of 10,000 post-
mortem examinations in Japan. Data
from Kimura, 1956

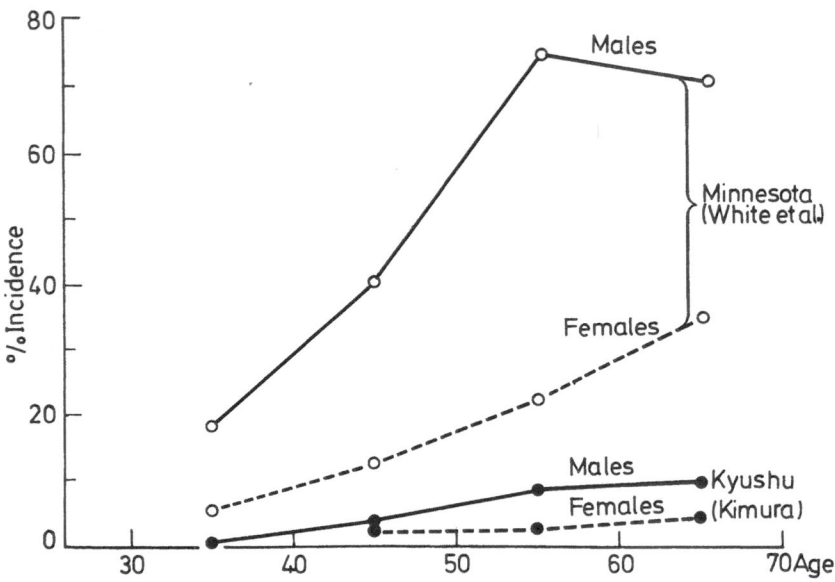

Figure 2. Data from Kimura, 1956

same age in the United States. This is about the same difference as is indicated
in the vital statistics. For any given age and sex the ratio of mortality, as
well as the incidence of severe coronary atherosclerosis is roughly ten to one
in the two countries (Kimura, 1965). This is the story of coronary atherosclerosis 20 years ago.

Since that time, the vital statistics in Japan have changed very much. Figure 3
shows the change of the death rate of stroke and ischemic heart disease during the last 20 years in Japan. The death rate of ischemic heart disease per
100,000 persons/year was 9.9 in 1950 and 25.9 in 1970. This is nearly a threefold
increase in the last 20 years.

The death rate of stroke per 100,000 persons/year was 128.4 in 1950 and 118.6 in
1970. There have been no significant differences in the death rate of stroke
during the last 20 years. But it might be said for sure that when it comes to
cerebral infarction only, the death rate has increased from 3.9 in 1950 to 37.1
in 1970. This is a tenfold increase in the last 20 years (Vital Statistics, 1975)

Figure 4 shows the change of nutritional intake per person in Japan according to
the national nutrition survey conducted by Japanese Goverment. The fat intake
represents a threefold increase in the last 20 years.

Before discussing the epidemiology of atherosclerotic disease in Japan, I would
like to explain something about the geography of Japan (Fig. 5) and also about
the life-style of the Japanese. The country of Japan, as you know, is made up of
Hokkaido, Honshu, Shikoku, and Kyushu islands, lying slender and long from north
to southwest. Its area is about the same size as the state of California. The
average temperature throughout the year is 5.9°C in the north and 21.1°C in the
south. The life-style can be generally divided into three types. One is the farm
land type, Japan's traditional life-style with a diet consisting mainly of rice.

Another is a fishing village type, where the people eat more fish. The third is
an urban type very similar to the Western world in terms of life situation after
World War II.

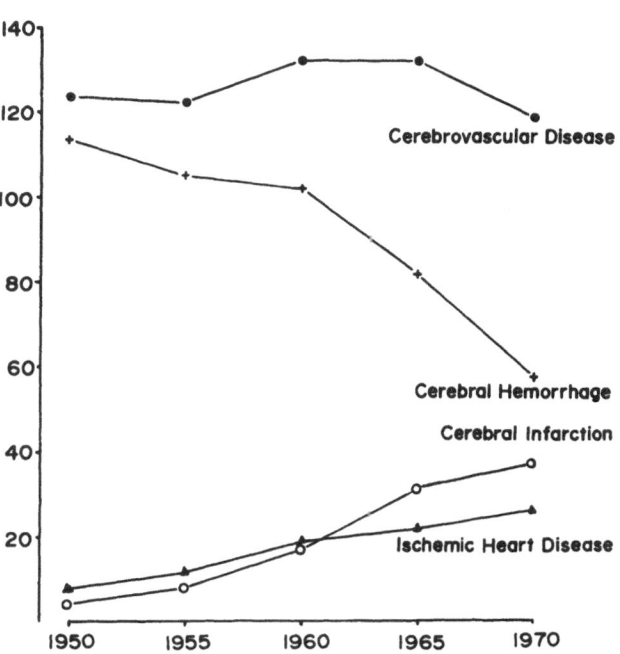

Figure 3. Cerebrovascular disease and ischemic heart disease in Japanese vital statistics, revised (1935) death rate, per 100,000

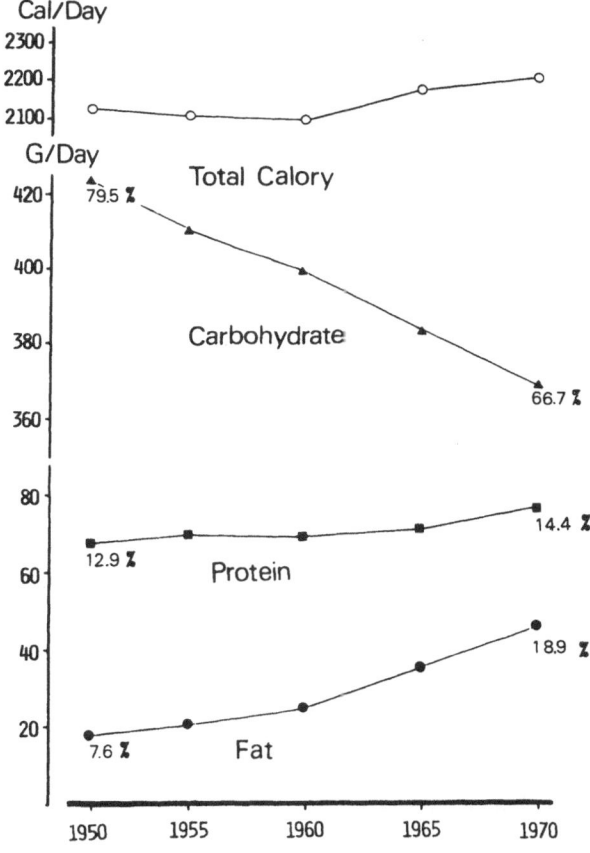

Figure 4. Daily food intake in Japan (data from National Nutritional Studies)

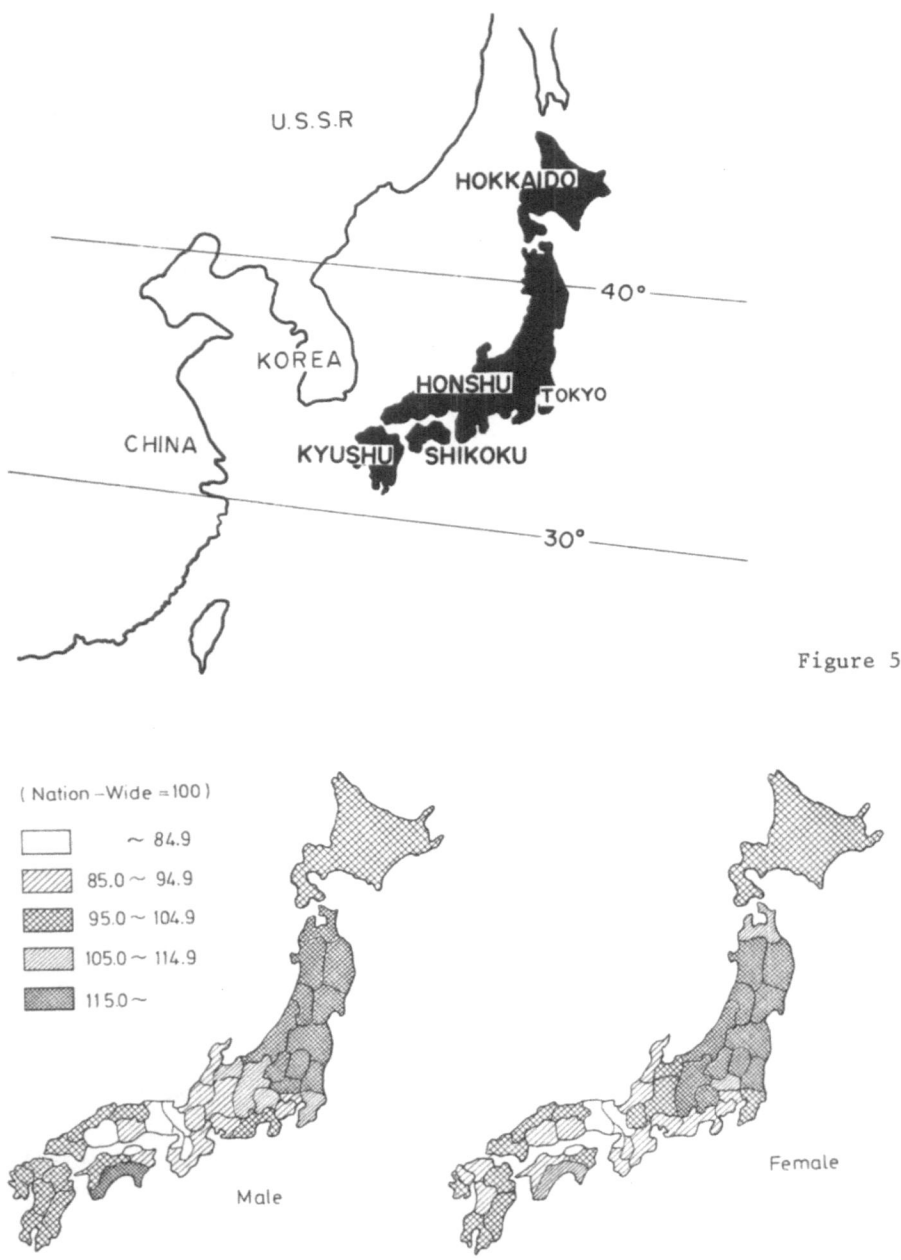

Figure 5

Figure 6. Cerebrovascular disease, revised death rate index

Figure 6 geographically illustrates the revised nationwide death rate indice of
stroke. The upper island on the map is Hokkaido, the coldest area in Japan. The
slender and long island beneath Hokkaido is called Honshu and the northern part
of Honshu has the highest incidence of stroke in Japan. In general terms, there
is a high incidence of stroke in agricultural areas, with a rice-centered diet.

A full-scale population survey in Japan was initiated by Kimura and his co-workers
in 1958 and also in 1961 by Katsuki and his associates. Ever since, in many parts
of Japan extensive surveys have been made.

464

At this time, I wish to bring you up-to-date on outstanding population surveys
in Japan. I feel my mission is completed if you can understand the characteristics involving stroke and ischemic heart disease in Japan.

Figure 7 shows the Hisayama study conducted by Katsuki. Diagnosis was made mainly
on the basis of autopsy findings. The study disclosed that of 1621 entrants,
143 developed stroke during a subsequent 10-year period with 98 of them dying.
Among these victims of stroke, cerebral infarction was four times more frequent
than cerebral hemorrhage. This is a population survey of an urban type. The
response rate is 90.1%, so we cannot discuss the incidence or death rate in this
survey. But we may get some information on risk factors. In this survey, the
risk factors of cerebral infarction and myocardial infarction are not equal. For
cerebral infarction, age, family history, hypertension, ECG abnormalities, and
glucose tolerance abnormality are considered risk factors, but for myocardial
infarction, ECG abnormality is only one risk factor (Omae and Takeshita, 1972).

A farming village (Tanushimaru) and a fishing village (Ushibuka) in Kyushu were
checked out by us (Keys et al., 1970; Kimura et al., 1959) (Fig. 8). The group
was all male, aged 40 – 64 from the general population. The examination coverage
was 100% at the farming area and 99.7% at the fishing village. The lost of follow up after 15 years, were one person from the farming group and two from the
fishing group.

Figure 9 shows the death rate in the 15-year follow-up. It was found that the
death rate of stroke was 4.3 persons per 1000 persons/year in the farming village
and 4.9 persons in the fishing village. The death rate of myocardial infarction,
on the other hand, was 0.6 persons in the farming village and 1.5 persons in the
fishing village.

Risk factors	No. of Subjects	Cerebral 88 (cases)	Infarction 32.5%	Myocardial 23 (cases)	Infarction 8.5%
Age (60 years or more)	206	83	40.3[a]	17	8.3
Family history (stroke, hypertension)	88	40	45.5[a]	8	9.1
Hypertension (WHO)	193	79	40.9[a]	18	9.3
ECG abnormalities (Minnesota codes 1·1,3·1,4·1~3)	85	40	47.1[a]	12	14.1[b]
Glucose tolerance (Minnesota codes 1·1,3·1,4·1~3)	40	20	50.0[b]	2	5.0
Heavy drinking habits	66	27	40.9	6	9.1
Fundus abnormalities (Kw II~IV)a	81	31	38.3	9	11.1
Serum cholesterol (200 mg/dl or more)	36	10	27.8	2	5.6

[a] $p < 0.01$. [b] $p < 0.05$.

Figure 7. Ten-year follow-up of Hisayama study. Roster: 1841 persons, examined:
1658, rate: 90,1%. Cerebrovascular disease free cohort: 1621. Unavailable for
10-year follow-up: rate 0.3%. Start: 1961, age: 40 years or more.
Risk factors of cerebral infarction, myocardial infarction — Studies on 271 autopsies. Follow-up period: Nov. 1961 - Oct. 1971

Area: Tanushimura (farmer), Ushibuka (fisherman)

Examination coverage: general population   age 40 – 64, male

Roster:

		No. of men	Examined	Rate
	Tanushimaru	639	639	100.0%
	Ushibuka	614	612	99.7%

Start: Tanushimaru   1958
         Ushibuka   1960

Unavailable for follow-up: Tanushimaru   0.2%
                           Ushibuka   0.3%

Figure 8. 15-year follow-up of Rural Kyushu, Japan

No. of subjects	Tanushimaru 639	Ushibuka 614
Stroke	41(4.3)	45(4.9)
Hemorrhage	19	18
Infarction	15	23
Hemorrhage or infarction	7	4
Myocardial infarction	6(0.6)	14(1.5)
Others	115	131
Total	162(16.9)	190(20.6)

( ): Rate per 1000/year

Figure 9. Deaths in 15 years

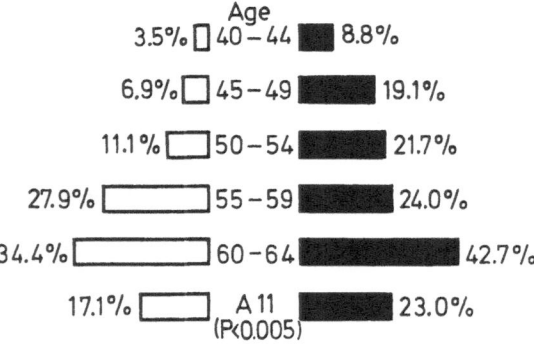

Age
3.5% 40 – 44 8.8%
6.9% 45 – 49 19.1%
11.1% 50 – 54 21.7%
27.9% 55 – 59 24.0%
34.4% 60 – 64 42.7%
17.1% All (P<0.005) 23.0%

Figure 10. Prevalence of hypertension at entry. ☐ Farmer (N = 639); ■ Fisherman
(N = 614)

Figure 10 shows the incidence of hypertension at entry. Hypertension is more
frequent at the fishing village than the farming village. Figure 11 shows the
relation between blood pressure and stroke obtained from our 10-year follow-up
studies in our farming village of Tanushimaru and also the fishing village of

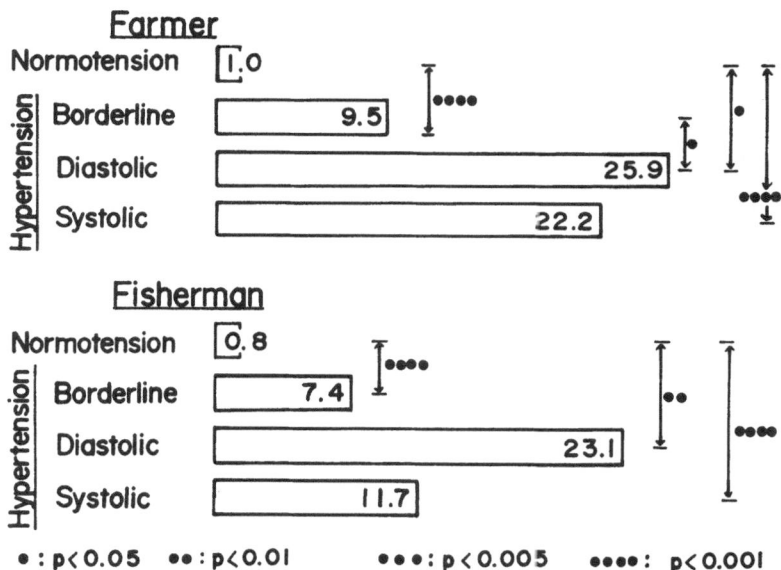

Figure 11. Blood pressure vs. stroke (10-year incidence/1000/year)

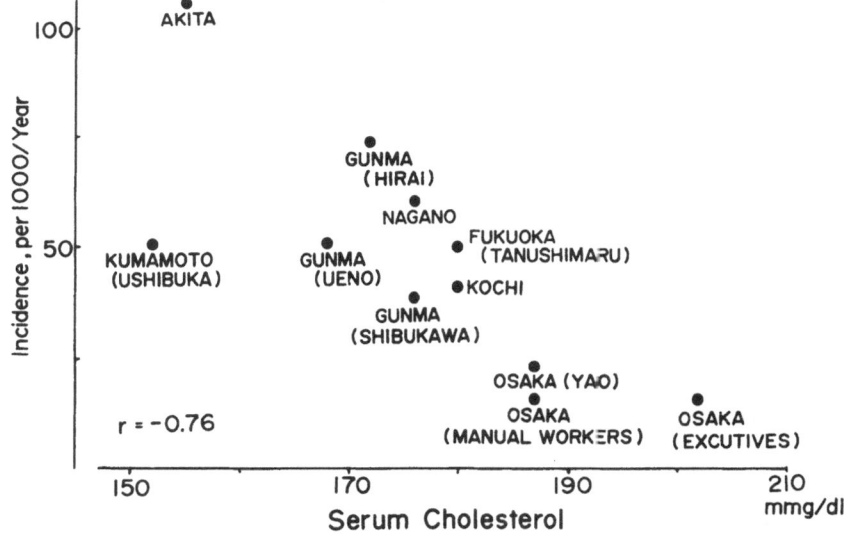

Figure 12. Mean serum cholesterol value vs. stroke (age: 40 - 64, male) (Shigiya et al., 1972)

Ushibuka. Among farmers, the incidence of stroke from hypertension is more than 20 times the incidence rate of the normotensive population. This holds true with fishermen. However, even though stroke has a very close connection with hypertension in Japan, it cannot be said that all hypertensive individuals will have a stroke.

As can be seen in Figure 12, serum cholesterol levels are low in inhabitants of Akita's agricultural areas where I said there is a predilection for stroke, whereas they are medium in those of Osaka's urban areas. There is a distinct negative correlation between serum cholesterol and incidence of stroke (Shigiya et al., 1972).

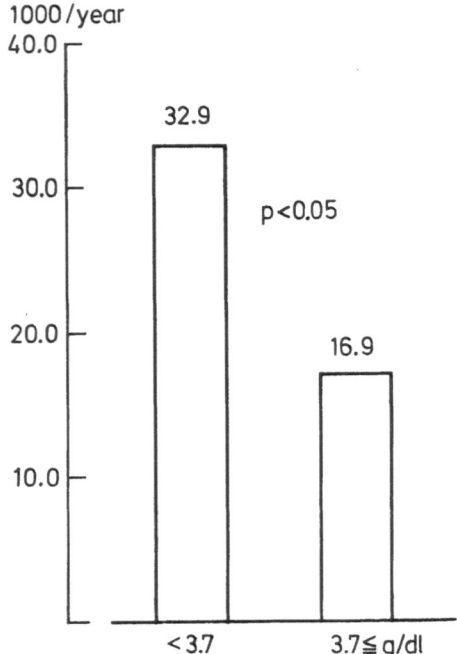

1000/year

Serum albumin levels

Figure 13. Serum albumin vs. stroke,
5-year follow-up, hypertensive group

Accordingly, at the time of the 10th year's systemic reexamination in the farming
and fishing villages, we measured serum protein in addition to serum lipids
(Kimura et al., 1972; Kimura, 1973).

Figure 13 shows the results of a follow-up for the subsequent 5 years. As you can
see, stroke occurred frequently among those persons with hypertension and low levels of serum albumin.

Finally I shoud like to discuss the influence of cigarette smoking. Figure 14
shows our results of the effect of cigarette smoking on the incidence rate of
stroke. In the hypertensive, smoking appears to decrease the incidence rate of
stroke.

But for the incidence rate of myocardial infarction (Fig. 15), smoking is a risk
factor in our survey.

Figure 16 shows that hypertension is a risk factor in myocardial infarction. But
Figure 17 shows that the serum cholesterol level is not high enough to influence
the incidence of myocardial infarction. The persons with a serum cholesterol level of over 230 mg/dl are only 3.2% of our roster.

Conclusion

I wish to say that what I have been talking about pertains to a population with
less than 200 mg/dl of serum cholesterol. Hypertension, among other factors,
most strongly links up with the development of stroke and ischemic heart disease
in Japan.

The low incidence of myocardial infarction is explained by extremely low serum
cholesterol levels.

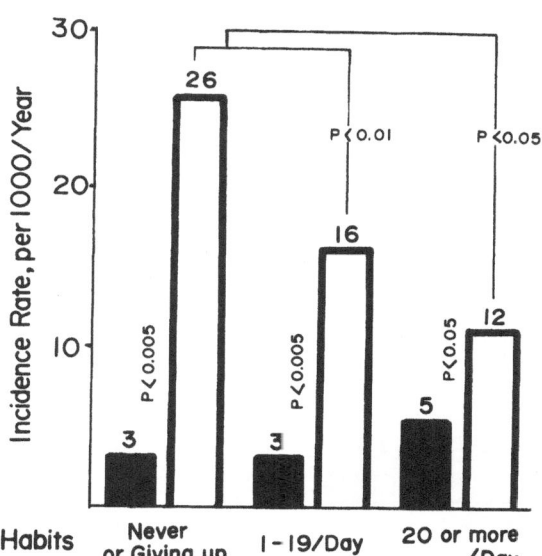

Figure 14. Smoking and blood pressure vs. stroke. 15-year follow-up of Rural Kyushu, Japan (Kimura et al.) ☐Hypertensive: 160-190 mm Hg or more; ■Nonhypertensive

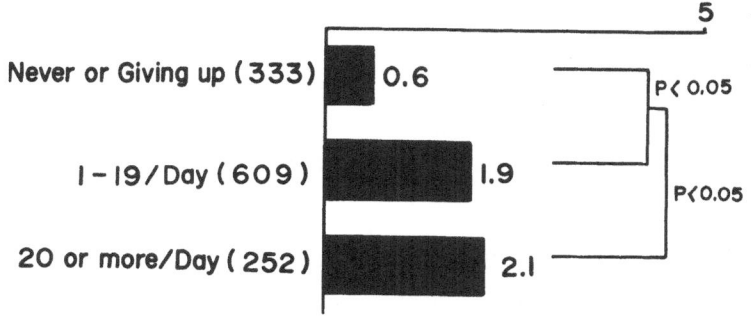

Figure 15. Smoking habits vs. myocardial infarction. 15-year follow-up of Rural Kyushu, Japan (Kimura et al.)

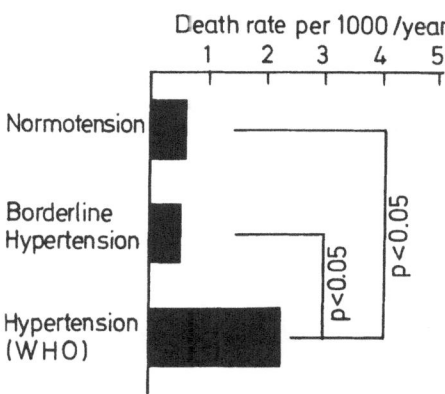

Figure 16. Blood pressure vs. 15-year myocardial infarction (Tanushimaru and Ushibuka)

469

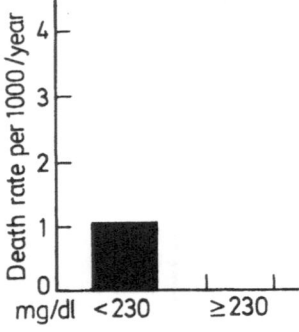

Figure 17. Serum cholesterol vs. 15-year myocardial infarction (Tanushimaru and Ushibuka)

	N	Obs	%
U.S. switchman	836	167	20.0
U.S. sedentary clark	858	201	23.4
East Finland	808	244	30.2
West Finland	859	93	10.8
Zutphen (Netherlands)	875	265	30.3
Slavolnia (Yugoslavia)	697	115	16.5
Verika Krusma (Yugoslavia)	511	57	11.2
Dalmatia (Yugoslavia)	670	107	16.0
Crevalcore (Italy)	984	229	23.3
Montegiorigio (Italy)	718	81	11.3
Crete (Greece)	678	82	12.1
Corfu (Greece)	529	63	11.9
Tanushimaru (Japan)	509	38	7.5
Uschibuka (Japan)	500	58	11.6

(N = total men; Obs = cases of observed)

Figure 18. Prevalence of hypertension (number of men with diastolic blood pressure of 95 mm Hg or more) (Keys et al., 1967)

All in all, we are inclined to think that the incidence of hypertension among
the Japanese population is not high enough to explain the frequency with which
Japanese are affected with stroke (Fig. 18). Although any general conclusion is
not warranted yet, it seems that low levels of serum albumin and cholesterol,
caused by mulnutrition of protein and fat, constitute risk factors for stroke
in the Japanese.

F.H. Epstein

A short review must necessarily be selective. To select objectively is difficult since some subjectivity must enter into the decision of what is most important. Here, the emphasis will be on two questions:
1. To what extent do currently known risk factors predict and, therefore, "explain" the occurrence of coronary heart disease and how much remains to be learned?
2. What can be expected from preventive measures taken to postpone the onset of clinical coronary heart disease?
These two questions touch the main purpose of epidemiological research: to contribute to the knowledge of causes and to suggest measures of disease prevention.

Risk Factors

The term "risk factor" seems to have come suddenly, like a nova, from nowhere. It has become a medical household word of great usefulness to describe the precursors of coronary heart disease, singly and in combination. Multivariate analysis of prospective data from epidemiological studies leaves no doubt that serum cholesterol and blood pressure levels and cigarette smoking are the most powerful predictors amongst the currently identified risk factors. By means of such analyses, it can be shown that as much as around 50% of the new events of first myocardial infarctions and sudden deaths occur amongst the 20% of men at the highest risk in terms of a risk score to which the three stated risk factors contribute most (Table 1 ; Truett et al., 1967; Keys et al., 1972; Wilhelmsen et al.,

Table 1. Predictive power of multiple risk factors by multivariate analysis

Study	Risk factors[a]	Endpoints	Age	Number of events	Events falling within the upper 20% of the risk function
Framingham, USA	a - g	Angina Myocardial infarct sudden death	30-62	258	49%
Railway workers USA	a - e	Myocardial infarct sudden death	40-59	78	49%
"Four-study-pool" USA	a - e	" "	"	223	49%
"European men"	a - e	" "	"	136	55%
Swedish men	b - d	" "	60	44	50%
Swedish men	b - d	" "	51-55	44	57%
Israeli men	a - d, h	" "	40+	205	48%

[a] (a) Age, (b) Serum Cholesterol, (c) Blood Pressure, (d) Cigarette Smoking, (e) Weight, (f) ECG, (g) Hemoglobin, (h) Diabetes.

Table 2. Predicting coronary heart disease (CHD) by means of the multiple logistic function. Positive test: men with a risk score in the upper fifth (20%) of the distribution

		Test +	Test −	Total
New events of CHD in 10 years	+	50	50	100
	−	150	750	900
Total		200	800	1000

$$\text{Sensitivity} = \frac{50}{100} \times 100 = 50\%; \text{Predictive power } (+) = \frac{50}{200} \times 100 = 25\%;$$

$$\text{Specificity} = \frac{750}{900} \times 100 = 83\%; \text{Predictive power } (-) = \frac{50}{800} \times 100 = 6.3\%;$$

$$\text{Risk ratio} = \frac{25}{6.3} = 4.$$

1973; Goldbourt et al., 1975). This reflects a remarkably high predictive power, indicating that as much as around half of the disease events can be explained, as it were, by these risk indicators. Even though the countries shown differ appreciably in incidence, i.e., absolute risk, the predictive value of the risk factors is very similar from place to place, suggesting similar etiological mechanisms. The Göteborg group in Sweden has developed a useful nomogram which permits determination of individual risk, as observed in that city, for any combination of the three major risk factors; the numbers indicate the percent chances of developing a heart attack within 10 years. These vary from 50% down to almost nothing (Wilhelmsen et al., 1976).

It is not necessary to have a computer to calculate multiple risk scores. Rose (1974) has developed a risk score point system and compared it with computer calculated scores based on the multiple logistic risk function developed by Cornfield; the two methods give comparable estimates of risk for a population of men in Belgium (Thilly et al., 1975).

In summary, let us take 1000 men (Table 2) and consider the 20% with the highest risk. With a 10-year incidence of 10%, 50 of the 200 men will develop a heart attack within 10 years - a chance of 25%. By contrast, only 6.3% of the men not at the highest risk will run the risk of clinical disease.

The question is sometimes asked how predictive power compares amongst the risk factors. A Table, published by the Framingham group, shows blood pressure as being the most powerful predictor, with serum cholesterol and cigarettes coming next. Blood glucose comes considerably lower down the scale (Kannel, 1976). However, a Table presented a year earlier places cholesterol much lower than glucose, with glucose about equal to cigarettes (Kannel and Sorlie, 1975). In view of such discrepancies, it is perhaps not surprising that a recent, well-publicized paper (Werkö, 1976) was entitled: "Risk factors and coronary heart disease-facts or fancy?" The fact is that risk factors are facts! The evidence which links risk factors to the disease is not based on epidemiological studies alone but much concurrent clinical, pathologic and experimental evidence. Furthermore, regardless of inconsistencies, it is very questionable whether statistical calculations based on multivariate regression coefficients lend themselves to the statement made that blood pressure is a more important risk factor than others. Apart from the matter of interactions between risk factors, the numerical values in which risk factors are measured and statistically evaluated do not necessarily reflect their quantitative effects on the arterial wall and the myocardium.

The belief in the importance of lipid metabolism, as expressed by serum cholesterol levels, should not in the least be influenced by such data.

Concerning serum triglycerides, there is still no unanimity whether they carry
predictive value independent of elevations of serum cholesterol. This controversy is important only from a practical point of view since it has bearing on the
question of whether serum triglycerides determinations should be part of a
screening examination. From the point of view of pathogenesis, triglycerides may
be important whether or not they have independent predictive value.

Recent studies have reopened the question whether high-density lipoproteins protect against coronary heart disease. In a study amongst Japanese men in Hawaii,
the prevalence of the disease was inversely related to HDL levels, independent
of β-cholesterol (Rhoads et al., 1976). In the epidemiological study in Evans
County, Georgia, black men had higher HDL levels than white men, independent of
serum cholesterol, possibly explaining in part their relative immunity toward
coronary heart disease (Tyroler et al., 1975). The British Medical Research Council, in collaboration with the Panamerican Health Organisation, is planning an
epidemiological investigation in Trinidad to explore these relationships further
(Miller, 1976). There is a sense of *déjà vu* in all this, going back to over 20
years, and it remains to be seen whether high-density lipoproteins will come into their own as useful disease predictors.

Earlier and more recent epidemiological observations have confirmed the long-
known association between clinical diabetes and coronary heart disease risk.
Whether, in addition, glucose intolerance behaves as a continuous, quantitative
predictor variable, like serum cholesterol or blood pressure, is still not established by prospective, epidemiological studies. As in the case of serum triglycerides, the evidence is not unequivocal, nor is it yet certain to what extent
blood glucose levels have a predictive value independent of other risk factors.
This is an important area for further research, which should take into account
not only blood glucose concentrations but the underlying changes in serum insulin and, perhaps, other hormones (Epstein, 1976). In assessing lipid-carbohy-
drate metabolic interrelationships, obesity probably provides an important link.
The importance of obesity as a risk factor, at least in some populations, has
long been underestimated because it is not so much a direct risk factor but acts
as a risk factor for others, in particular blood pressure, some lipoprotein
classes, and glucose intolerance. When considering any risk factors, the evolution of atherosclerosis over time must always be kept in mind, recognizing that
almost all prospective epidemiological studies to date have only started close
to middle-age or later when the optimal period for recognizing risk or starting
prevention may already have passed. The pediatric aspects of atherosclerosis
will be dealt with elsewhere in this symposium.

Psychosocial risk factors have been measured in a great variety of ways, but it
is not clear to what extent the various methods identify the same or different
characteristics, how strongly they are related to the disease, and how they
interact with other risk factors. Psychosocial influences, whether inherent in
the individual or in the pattern of culture, may not only be harmful through
neurohormonal mechanisms, but they determine as well detrimental ways of eating,
the smoking and drinking habits, and lack of exercise. The independent contribution of psychosocial attributes to risk is known in a quantitative way only for
the well-known behavior types A and B (Brand et al., 1976). When risk is determined by means of the multiple logistic risk function, being a type A man approximately doubles the risk at any level of the other major risk factors. Twin studies in Sweden have also suggested that psychological traits carry an independent
risk (Liljefors, quoted by Biörck, 1975).

The inclusion of factors involved in thrombosis amongst the risk factors measured in prospective epidemiological studies has always been hampered by methodological difficulties. However, such a study, to include about 3000 persons, is
now in progress in Britain under the egis of the Medical Research Council. The

results will not be available for some time since enrollment is continuing until 1978 (Meade, 1976). In this connection, ongoing prevention trials using aspirin to reduce platelet adhesiveness should be mentioned.

Hereditary factors were discussed at this symposium 3 years ago. Since then, a task force convened by the National Heart and Lung Institute in Bethesda has compiled a comprehensive review of the field (U.S. Dept. of HEW, 1975). The need is for more and more definitive studies. These include the study of families for aggregations of disease and predisposing factors. Amongst the latter, interest attaches to a recent report showing a correlation between the frequency of the histocompatibility antigen HLA-8 and mortality from ischemic heart disease in six European countries, Japan, and the USA (Matthews, 1975). A large study of twins in the United States has shown very surprisingly that there is no detectable hereditary contribution to the determination of serum cholesterol level, in contrast to blood pressure (Feinleib, 1975); these findings require recalculation and confirmation.

Amongst studies assessing the effect of physical inactivity, a recent report of a large study in Britain suggests that a relatively large amount of exercise is protective while lesser amounts carry no demonstrable benefit (Epstein et al., 1976). The relationship between physical activity and coronary heart disease risk has been critically reviewed by Blackburn (1976).

Finally, concerning risk factors, the presence of organic disease must be considered. Mortality from sudden cardiac death was much higher for men with such disease, especially when they carried any two or all three of the major risk factors (Stamler, 1975). Similar data were published this year by the World Health Organization (1976), based on the Myocardial Infarction Community Registers Study.

Incidence

Having discussed risk factors, the question arises whether changes in incidence over time and differences in incidence between populations are explained by changes or differences in the distribution of risk factors.

Table 3. Changes in mortality (%) from "arteriosclerotic and degenerative heart disease" (A 81) ——— 1961 to 1967

Region	Country	Mortality change, men age 45–54	age 55–64
Northern Europe	Finland	+36	+15
	Sweden	+10	+ 5
Western Europe	Ireland	- 5	+19
	Netherlands	+35	+19
	U.K.	+13	+ 7
	F.R. Germany	+ 6	+21
	Austria	+18	- 1
Eastern Europe[a]	Czechoslovakia	+36	+22
	Hungary	+27	+32
	Poland	+16	+17
	Romania	+26	+ 9

[a] No data for GDR, Lithouania, Bulgaria. Adapted from: Public Health in Europe, WHO 1973.

474

It is generally, though not entirely unanimously, agreed that coronary heart disease has become more common in the last decades. Data for men in Europe (Table 3) show this to be true for the 1960's. Unfortunately, there are no data which would permit a correlation between these trends and changes in risk factors. However, cigarette consumption has increased in most countries and increasing affluence has probably enabled a greater proportion of the population to eat more of the more expensive foods, resulting in an increased consumption of animal fats.

In the United States, death rates for coronary heart disease have decreased in recent years (Gordon and Thom, 1975). The trend is probably real and may be related to better treatment of hypertension, an increase in the proportion of ex-smokers and, conceivably, to some changes in eating habits since there are data to suggest a fall in mean cholesterol levels in the population. Therefore, both in Europe and the United States, there may be a relation between mortality trends, upward as well as downward, and changes in environmental conditions.

There has been a concern about rising rates of coronary heart disease in younger women, due to the use of oral contraceptives and an increase in the smoking habit. In the United States, such a general trend, as just shown, cannot be demonstrated. In England and Wales, however, there is such a trend, in contrast to Scotland and Northern Ireland where, however, the rates were initially higher (Shaper, 1976). Such data provide only pointers to keep on the watch.

In many ways, coronary heart disease epidemiology started with the observation of geographic differences and attempts to explain them. Within the last very few years, it has become possible to approach the question to what extent some of these differences relate to the major risk factors. Within Europe, there are striking differences in coronary heart disease mortality (Rose, 1973). Until now, it was difficult to counter convincingly the argument that such differences are largely artifactual. However, the WHO Moycardial Infarction Community Registers have provided reliable incidence data in a number of European cities which can be compared with the national mortality rates in the corresponding countries (Table 4). There is a remarkable correlation, indicating that many of the differences within Europe are largely real and providing a basis for selecting areas for field studies in order to explain the observed variations. Data available already from the WHO Myocardial Infarction Community Registers provide some intriguing findings (Table 5; World Health Organization, 1976). Why are the rates for acute myocardial infarction so much higher in Helsinki, Finland than in Gothenburg, Sweden, and why are the rates in Boden, Northern Sweden so much higher than those in Gothenburg further south? Similar questions arise from looking at the data from Western and Eastern Europe, or Perth in Australia and Tel-Aviv in Israel. From what relatively little there is known about the distribution of serum cholesterol and blood pressure levels and the frequency of smoking in these countries, it is unlikely that many of the differences shown are explained to a major extent by differences in the major risk factors. Indeed, a few years ago, it was already apparent from the Seven-Country Study (Keys et al., 1972) that men in Europe, at any combination of levels of serum cholesterol, blood pressure, and smoking, run only about half the risk of CHD than a comparable man in the United States. A similar trend is well-illustrated by the coordinated studies in Framingham, Puerto Rico, and Honolulu (Gordon et al., 1974). At any level of blood pressure, serum cholesterol, and smoking, the risk of developing CHD was much higher in Framingham, USA.

The Israeli Civil Servants Study provides additional evidence for the operation of as yet unspecified risk factors (Goldbourt et al., 1975). Jewish men born in Eastern and Central Europe had a higher than expected risk, calculated from the multiple logistic function for all the men in the study, while those from South-East Europe and the Middle East had a lower than expected risk. In the study in Evans County, Georgia in the United States, the risk of white men was higher than that of black men when major known risk factors were controlled (Kleinbaum et al., 1971).

Table 4. Incidence rates for acute myocardial infarction amongst men age 20-64 from who Myocardial Infarction Community Registers versus annual age-adjusted mortality from ischemic heart disease (A 83)

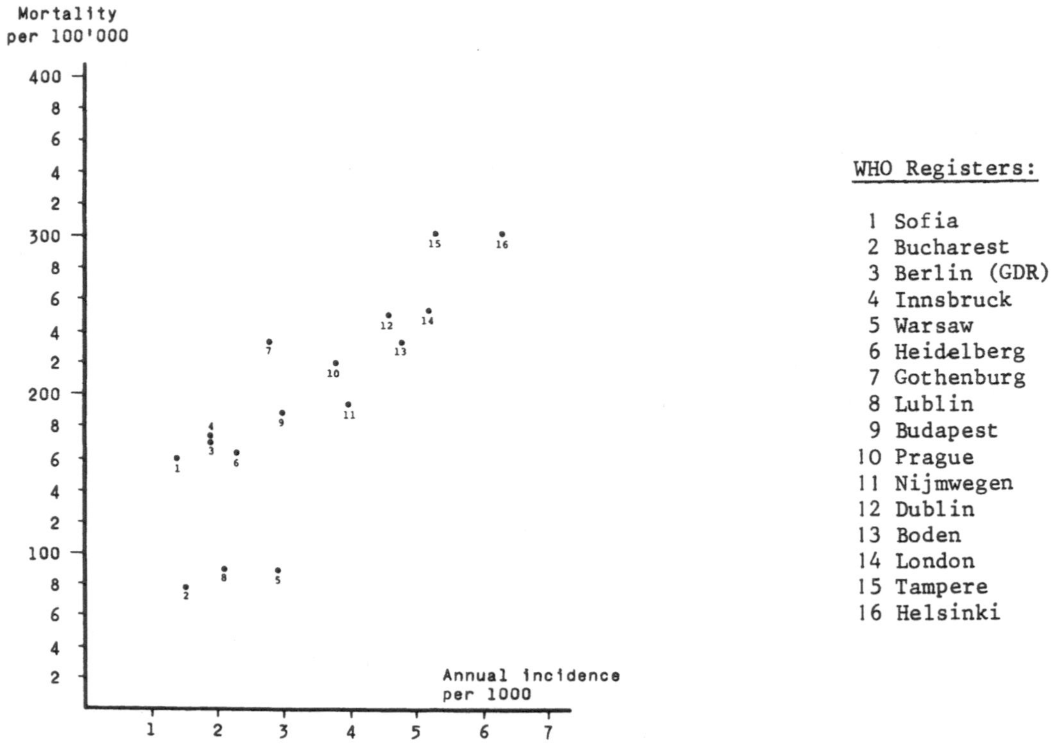

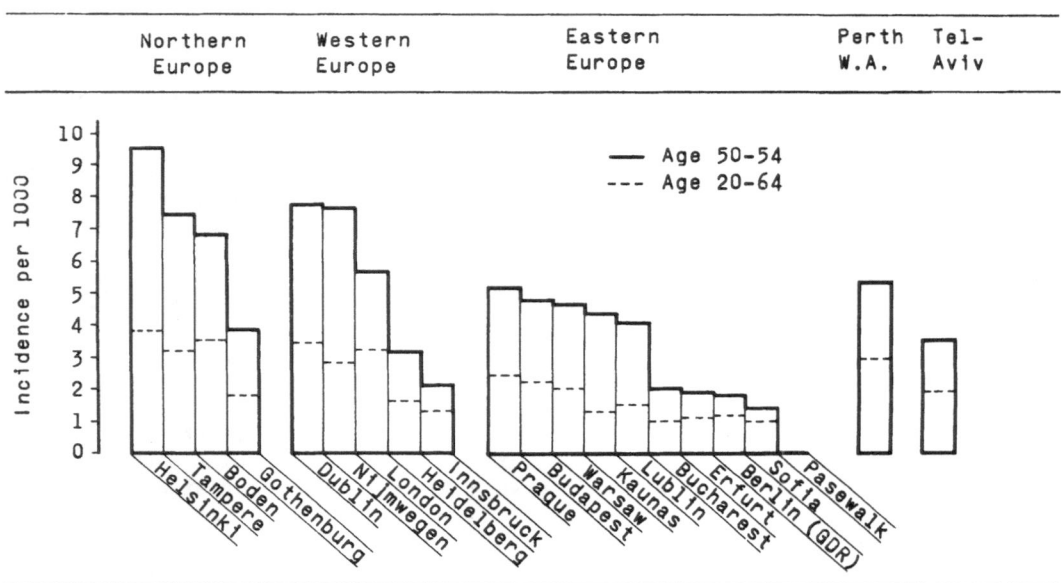

Mortality per 100'000
400
300
200
100
Annual incidence per 1000
1 2 3 4 5 6 7
WHO Registers:
1 Sofia
2 Bucharest
3 Berlin (GDR)
4 Innsbruck
5 Warsaw
6 Heidelberg
7 Gothenburg
8 Lublin
9 Budapest
10 Prague
11 Nijmwegen
12 Dublin
13 Boden
14 London
15 Tampere
16 Helsinki

Table 5. Annual incidence of acute myocardial infarction (first attack) — men. Adapted from "Myocard. Infarct. Community Registers", WHO 1976

Northern Europe	Western Europe	Eastern Europe	Perth W.A.	Tel-Aviv

Incidence per 1000
0 1 2 3 4 5 6 7 8 9 10
— Age 50-54
--- Age 20-64
Helsinki
Tampere
Boden
Gothenburg
Dublin
Nijmwegen
London
Heidelberg
Innsbruck
Prague
Budapest
Warsaw
Kaunas
Lublin
Bucharest
Erfurt
Berlin (GDR)
Sofia
Pasewalk

In a parallel study in Stockholm and Edinburgh, it was also noted that the higher frequency of coronary heart diseases in Edinburgh was not explained, except perhaps to a minor degree, by differences in the risk factors measured (Oliver et al., 1975). That social status does not necessarily reflect risk factor status is demonstrated in a study of relatively poor Mexican-Americans, as compared with the better-to-do white majority in three Californian communities: cardiovascular risk factor status was similar in the two groups (Stern et al., 1975).

Unpublished data from Norway (Bjartveit, 1976) indicate that serum cholesterol levels are higher in a northern community than in two communities further south; the trend for smoking was similar. Data on prevalence and incidence in these two Norwegian areas will be awaited with interest. Another ongoing investigation, the Norwegian-British migrant study will also provide information on the influence of ethnic and environmental factors on the frequency of coronary heart disease (Reid, 1975). It is thought that some of the regional differences in cardiovascular mortality in Britain at least, may be related, in part, to differences in water hardness (Shaper, 1976).

The data on regional differences just shown provide a great challenge. The associations, most likely largely causal, between a number of risk factors and coronary heart disease are firmly established. At the same time, it is now evident that there are additional factors as yet inadequately defined or perhaps even unsuspected, which contribute to causing the disease or protecting against it. In this particular review, it would seem idle to speculate on what they might be. Many of them were presumably included in the account on the risk factors mentioned earlier. From the all-important point of view of prevention, it is essential to recognize that these remaining grey areas of uncertainty call for further research but provide no excuse for inaction with regard to the firmly established risk factors.

Prevention

Current indirect evidence for a causal relationship between the major risk factors discussed is very strong. Nevertheless, evidence from preventive trials is desirable. Therefore, in the 1960's, a number of such trials especially in regard to dietary intervention, came into existence. Their results have been generally encouraging. While conclusive evidence for their effectiveness has not emerged, the results cannot and should not be discounted. The need for more definitive evidence led to the large field trials now in progress in a number of countries. None of the new trials intervene on diet only so that the diet-heart question, as originally posed, will presumably never be answered except within the context of simultaneous intervention on multiple risk factors. Therefore, even if these multifactor trials will yield positive results, it will not be possible to say with assurance that any single component of the total prevention package, such as change in eating habits, was responsible for the outcome. Consequently, anyone insisting today that a change in individual or national eating habits can only be justified if a cause-and-effect relationship between such changes, lowering of serum lipids, and reduction in coronary heart disease incidence can be demonstrated in terms of results from preventive trials would in effect condemn mankind forever to continue eating or start eating in a way which, from almost everything that is known on the basis of practically all other evidence, is responsible in large part for the premature threat of this disease.

Therefore, official and responsible agencies in several countries have now gone on record to advise even the general population that obesity be avoided, fat intake be reduced, regular exercise be encouraged, and smoking be curtailed. Such recommendations, while differing in detail, have been made in the Netherlands, the United Kingdom, Ireland, the Federal Republic of Germany, the Scandinavian countries, the German Democratic Republic, Czechoslovakia, Yugoslavia, as well as in the United States, Australia, and New Zealand (European Society of Cardiology, in preparation). These actions reflect a growing concern and the belief that there is now a scientific basis for preventive action.

What might be expected from preventive action in the population? Assuming a quantitatively causal relationship between risk factors and risk, the expected risk reduction from reducing risk factor averages in the population may be estimated, as done in an unpublished calculation by Menotti, using the European cohort data from the Seven-Country Study for men aged 40-59. Reducing serum cholesterol, blood pressure, or smoking alone, depending on degree, may reduce risk between a fifth and a third. Even modest reduction of all three risk factors simultaneously would result in a 30% reduction in risk; a 60% reduction might follow greater risk factor reductions. These calculations are not intended as an accurate forecast but merely as a guide to magnitudes of change within the range of expectation, if prevention were started only relatively late in life instead of early.

A number of community prevention studies are now in progress or being planned to discover the best ways to motivate people to change harmful living habits and to measure the effect of these health education methods on risk factor levels and risk. The earliest example is provided by the Stanford Study (Farquhar et al., 1975). Two different methods of intervention resulted in an almost 20% reduction of the multiple logistic risk score, comprising serum cholesterol, blood pressure, and smoking, in the population, in striking contrast to the control community. These trends are very encouraging.

Conclusion

Main aspects of coronary heart disease epidemiology, based on the state of current knowledge, were reviewed. Two principal directions for future research emerge: (1) investigations to identify the factors of susceptibility or resistance which are responsible for differences in disease frequency between individuals and populations but are not explained by associations with the firmly established risk factors, and (2) preventive programs to postpone disease onset in individuals and in the population at large.

SERUM TRIGLYCERIDES IN RELATION TO AGE, SEX, AND WEIGHT INDEX

Haruo Uzawa and Nobuhisa Nakamura
Department of Internal Medicine, Institute of Constitutional Medicine, Kumamoto
University, Kumamoto/Japan

As part of an ongoing health examination service in this area of Japan, serum
triglycerides concentration (TG) of 1807 males and 3534 females (both 20 - 69
yrs. of age) were determined. The changes of TG in relation to age, sex, and
weight index were investigated. When "normal" subject was selected by the criteria listed below, the TG was independent of age in male, while it increases
with age in female. The criteria of "normal": Weight index 1.09, systol. and/or
diastol. blood pressure mean+1SD, normal ECG, albuminuria and glucosuria negative,
GOT 45, Total Bil. 1.0, Alk-Pase 12, and CCLF negative. Total subjects were subdivided into six groups according to sex and weight index as follows: 1.09,
1.10 - 1.19, 1.20. In female the change of TG with age of the three groups were
almost same though TG in 1.20 group was higher than that of other groups.
Whereas in male the TG of 25 - 59 yrs. of age subjects of 1.20 group were
highest among all six groups.

TRIGLYCERIDES, CHOLESTEROL, FATTY ACID COMPOSITION OF LIPOPROTEINS IN IHD-PATIENTS AND IN HEALTHY PERSONS

Daniel Brunner, Shmuel Altman, Kurt Loebl, and Sara Schwartz
Donolo Institute of Physiological Hygiene, Tel Aviv University, Tel Aviv/Israel

Serum triglycerides (TG), cholesterol (CH) and fatty acids (FA) in CH-esters, TG
and phospholipids were determined. 130 male and 58 female patients 35 - 64 yrs
old, 3 months after myocardial infarction or suffering from angina pectoris, and
2219 male and 1469 female healthy, normotensive subjects were investigated.
In 10-years age-specific subgroups no significant differences in CH between coronary patients and healthy people (except males 35 - 44 yrs) were found, whereas
TG-values were significantly different in all age groups. In TG-specific subgroups no significant differences of CH were found. However, in CH-specific subgroups, ther were significant differences in TG.
The composition of myristic, palmitic, palmitoleic, stearic, oleic, linoleic and
arachidonic acids in CH-esters, TG and phospholipids were determined by gas-
liquidchromatography. Almost no differences were found between young sportsmen,
healthy subjects with high or low CH, and post-myocardial infarction patients.
The results indicate that in the examined population increased TG, not associated
with increased CH, are an independent marker for clinical coronary disease. FA
composition of lipoproteins are similar in healthy persons and in coronary patients.

CHOLESTEROL AND TRIGLYCERIDES AS FACTORS OF RISK FOR CORONARY HEART DISEASE IN MEN OF THE BASLE STUDY

Georges Hartmann, Hannes B. Stähelin, and Catherine Nissen
Department of Internal Medicine, University of Basel and Medical Clinic, Kantonsspital Chur, Chur/Switzerland

A population at risk of 1575 males aged = 25 years having determinations of
cholesterol and triglycerides (and other lipid fractions) could be followed for
10 years.

A total of 127 non-fatal coronary events were recorded (62 necrosis, 65 ischemia). Elevation of cholesterol proved to be a strong risk factor in the group of myocardial necrosis (4-fold increase of incidence from quartile I to quartile IV), but not so for ischemia. No correlation was found for triglycerides.
The incidence of fatal coronary events (n=31) increased in the presence of cholesterol as well as isolated triglyceride elevation. Mortality was highest with increase of both lipids. The frequency of other risk factors in the group of myocardial deaths is also shown.

SERUM CONCENTRATIONS OF α- AND β-LIPOPROTEIN CHOLESTEROL IN ATHEROSCLEROSIS, OBESITY AND BILIARY TRACT DISORDERS

Akira Yamamoto, Yuji Matsuzawa, and Hiroshi Sudo
The Second Department of Internal Medicine, Osaka University Medical School, Osaka/Japan

Distribution of serum cholesterol and phospholipids between lipoprotein classes was determined in normal male and female subjects of different ages and in some diseases in which lipid abnormalities are involved. An increase in ratio of β-lipoprotein (β-Ch) to α-lipoprotein cholesterol (α-Ch) took place along with an increase in total serum cholesterol in males, while there was no correlation between the total serum cholesterol and the ratio (β:α-Ch) in normal females.
In cases of coronary heart disease, cerebral vascular diseases, biliary tract disorders and obesity, there were significant decreases in α-Ch with increases in β-Ch, so that the ratio (β:α-Ch) was markedly increased in these diseases, even if the total cholesterol level was in normal range.
As an increase in total serum cholesterol was statistically significant only in coronary heart disease, the elevation of the ratio of β- to α-lipoprotein cholesterol seems to be of great value for prediction and prophylaxis of cerebral vascular diseases and gallstones. Effects of weight reduction in obese patients will also be presented.

CORRELATIONS OF SOME CORONARY RISK FACTORS WITH ALPHA-LIPOPROTEINS: THE ROMAN PROJECT OF CHD PREVENTION RESEARCH GROUP, ROME, ITALY

Alessandro Menotti, Giorgio Ricci, and Giancarlo Urbinati
Centro Malattie Cardiovascolari, Ospedale S. Camillo and Centro per la Lotta alle Malattie Dismetaboliche e all'Arteriosclerosi dell'Università Roma, Roma/Italy

The Roman Project of CHD Prevention is a controlled trial of CHD prevention as part of the WHO European Multifactor Preventive Trial of CHD, coordinate by the Regional Office for Europe of WHO, with the participation of centers in Great Britain, Belgium and Poland, beside Italy. The main characteristic of this trial relies in the allocation to either treatment of control of working units (factories) instead of single individuals. The entry screening performed in Rome on most men belonging to the treatment factories and on random samples of the control factories (over 3,000 men in 4 factories), has allowed to analyze up-date information on the distribution and interrelationships of risk factors in Rome, covering about 20 characteristics among which - for the first time in Italy, on large population scale - also electrophoresis of serum lipoproteins. The most striking result in terms of relationships among factors is the systematic negative correlation of alpha-lipoproteins with most other risk factors of biochemical and non-biochemical nature. Such data are in line with recent suggestions on the possible role of alpha-lipoproteins as a protective factors. Statistical and physio-pathological attempts are presented for explaining such findings.

HIGH DENSITY LIPOPROTEINS IN CORONARY PATIENTS WITH REFERENCE TO DIET AND BODY WEIGHT CHANGES

Horace Micheli, Bernard Grab, and Daniel Pometta
Division de Diabétologie, Département de Médecine, Université de Genève,
Genève/Switzerland

Male coronary patients (CAD, n = 143) have been examined 3 to 18 months after myocardial infarction. Lipid composition of serum lipoproteins was analyzed by preparative ultracentrifugation (VLDL d <1.006, LDL, HDL d >1.063) and compared to 212 age matched controls. CAD were divided into 4 groups according to diet (restriction vs no restriction of saturated fat) and to body weight changes (more vs less than 5% loss in weight). There were no differences in serum and LDL cholesterol (CH) between CAD and controls. Restriction of saturated fats was associated with slightly lower serum and LDL-CH. HDL-CH was lower in patients than in controls (0.43 vs 0.54 g/1, p <0.001). CAD had significantly higher serum triglycerides (TG, 1.68 vs 1.28 mMol/1) and VLDL-Tg (1.06 vs 0.73). Decreased body weight was associated with lower TG. The lower HDL-CH found in CAD cannot be only explained by the negative correlation existing between VLDL-TG and HDL-CH, and hence by their higher VLDL-TG. It was actually at the low and medium values of VLDL-TG that the difference of HDL-CH between controls and CAD was greatest, while it was not significant in the highest quartile of VLDL-TG values. Low HDL-CH appears to characterize coronary artery disease mostly when TG are in a normal range no matter what diet is followed.

CLINICAL AND EXPERIMENTAL STUDIES ON THE DELETERIOUS EFFECT OF POST-ALIMENTARY LIPEMIA IN ISCHEMIC HEART DISEASE

Hisashi Fukuzaki, Ryozo Okamoto, Yuichi Ishikawa, Takefumi Matsuo, and Tatsuya Tomomatsu
Internal Medicine Division I., Kobe University, School of Medicine, Kobe/Japan

In order to elucidate the pathophysiological significance of postalimentary lipemia in patients with ischemic heart disease (IHD), clinical and experimental studies were attempted. 1. In patients with IHD, high fat meal was given and 4 hours after that the physical stress was loaded. Serial observations were made on the changes in ECG and PaO_2. Ischemic changes in ECG were observed 4 hours after fat intake. These ischemic changes were augmented by physical stress. PaO_2 was lowered 4 hours after fat intake and then elevated by physical stress. 2. In dogs, intramyocardial oxygen tension (P_TO_2) and coronary sinus blood flow (CBF) were measured by Medspect and by direct measurement method, respectively, under the simultaneous treatments with atrial pacing (170/min) and infusion of Intralipid (TG). P_TO_2 was decreased significantly, and CBF was increased during TG infusion. From these results, it is concluded that myocardial hypoxia is induced by high fat loading and as its mechanism, the disturbance of tissue oxygen diffusion is highly probable.

CHARACTERISTICS OF ATHEROSCLEROSIS IN KOREANS

Esuk Sohn
Department of Internal Medicine, Paik Foundation Hospital, Seoul/South Korea

In recent years hypertensive cardiovascular disease became one of the greatest national health problems. The mean blood pressure of Koreans is compatible with those of white American and the prevalence was 17%. The admission rate among medical in patients in 1964 - 1967 was 4.4 - 9.1% and it showed marked increase to 13.7 - 18.4% in 1970 - 1973. The most common complication was cerebrovascular accident accounting 33.4%. It showed annual increase. In 1964 it was 9.7% and

33.4% in 1970 - 1973. In contrast ot the high incidence of cerebrovascular accident ischemic heart disease was extremely rare accounting only 0.6%. The serum cholesterol in hypertension was relatively low. However, the serum triglyceride was quite high. The most common phenotype of serum lipoprotein was Type IV and III. The high serum triglyceride seems to have intimate connection with carbohydrate rich Korean diet. Thus the hypertension in Korean appears to effect and accelerate the atherosclerosis of cerebral artery more than in coronary artery and the high serum triglyceride and low serum cholesterol seems to have intimate relationship in this point.

A FIVE YEAR EXPERIENCE IN THE BUCHAREST MULTIFACTORIAL INTERVENTION TRIAL FOR CORONARY HEART DISEASE

Marc Steinbach, Mihai Constantineanu, Petru Harnagea, Sanda Theodorini, Mircea Georgescu, Florin Cucu, Radu Voiosu, Stefăniţă Tănăseanu, Sebastian Mitu, Mihai Voiculescu, Coman Tănăsescu, Speranţa Teodorescu, Agata Suciu, Cornel Stănescu, and Mihai Cherciu
Institute of Internal Medicine, Bucharest/Rumania

The "at entry" examination in the 5000 males born 1911 - 1931 randomly selected by their home address was aimed to determine the risk factors prevalences: (F1.1)-serum cholesterol (Abell and Kendall) $\geq$220 md/dl = 34,1%; (F1.2)-serum cholesterol $\geq$250 mg/dl = 17,6%; (F2.1)-systolic blood pressure $\geq$160 mmHg and/or diastolic blood pressure $\geq$95 = 20,7%; (F2.2)-bordeline hypertension = 21,7%; (F3)-smoking of 15 or more cigarettes daily = 33,9%; (F4.1)-deviation from the ideal weight $\geq$20% = 32,6%; (F4.2)-deviation from the ideal weight $\geq$30% = 14,3%; (F5)-diabetes = 3%; (F6)-minor ecg abnormalities = 27,3%; (F7)-family history = 30,9%. After a 4 year of complex intervention with reexaminations every six months, the rates correction of risk factors detected at entry or subsequently which take into account a synthesis of the last 3 examinations, irrespective of the responsiveness to summons are the following: for (F1.1) = 43,2%; for (F1.2) = 50,2%; for (F2.1) = 35,6%; for (F2.2) = 61,6%; for (F3) = 35,1%; for (F4.1) = 19,6%; for (F4.2) = 33.8%.

FACTORS INFLUENCING CHOLESTEROL STUDIED BY MEANS OF MULTI- VARIATE ANALYSIS

Hugo Kesteloot and Omer Van Houte
Department of Pathophysiology, Section Cardiology, St. Raphael University Clinic, Leuven/Belgium

An epidemiological cross-sectional survey of the distribution of the serum cholesterol value has been performed in a male population group of 42,804 subjects, between the ages of 15 - 59 y. The following factors have been found by multivariate analysis to be independently associated with the cholesterol value: age, height, weight, arcus senilis, cigarette smoking, pathological Q-waves and ST-T-waves (classified according to Minnesota Code), blood pressure, blood group, geographical distribution, physical activity and social class (R - 0.420). The mean cholesterol value measured by the Pearson method at the age of 18 y. was 193 mg%, and it increased to a maximum of 256 mg at the age of 52 y. A higher prevalence of pathological O-waves and of early parental death was present in subjects of blood group A, in whom the serum cholesterol value was about 4 mg% higher than in subjects with blood group O. The cholesterol value was consistently higher in subgroups with ischemic heart disease compared to the "normal" population.

EPIDEMIOLOGY OF HYPERLIPOPROTEINEMIA IN JAPANESE

Fumio Kuzuya, Noboru Yoshimine, and Kunio Mori
The Third Department of Internal Medicine, Nagoya University School of Medicine,
Showa-Ku, Nagoya/Japan

The epidemiological study on hyperlipoproteinemia was investigated in a suburban
city near Nagoya in 1970. The subjects of the study were 858 male workers of the
automobile company whose ages were between 40 to 60 years. They were all healthy
by physical examination. The blood was sampled before meal in the morning. Serum
cholesterol, triglyceride, phospholipid and lipoprotein electrophoresis on cellulose acetate (Sepraphore III) were analysed. The tentative normal ranges of
serum lipid were defined from distribution curves of each lipid; cholesterol:
150 - 250 mg/dl, triglyceride: 45 - 120 mg/dl, phospholipid: 150 - 220 mg/dl.
The number of the subjects whose lipid values were higher than normal range was
as follows; cholesterol: 56 (6.5%), triglyceride: 88 (10.1%), phospholipid: 38
(4.4%). They were typed according to the W.H.O. hyperlipoproteinemia classification. The results were as follows; normal: 745 (86.8%), IIa: 41 (4.8%), IIb: 12
(1.4%), III: 3 (0.3%), IV: 48 (5.6%), not classified: 9 (1.1%). In 1973, 3 years
after the first examination, the subjects who were judged as hyperlipoproteinemia were investigated again. The changes of the type were as follows; IIa→ IIa:
2 of 10, IIa→ 0: 4 of 10, IIa→ IIb: 1 of 10, IIa→ IV: 3 of 10, IIb→ IIb: 4 of 8,
IIb→ 0: 1 of 8, IIb→ IIa: 1 of 8, IIb→ IV: 2 of 8, IV→ IV: 7 of 12, IV→ 0: 5 of
12, IV→ IIa: 0 of 12, IV→ IIb: 0 of 12.

RELATION OF BLOOD LIPIDS TO OBESITY AND MATURATION IN A BIRACIAL PEDIATRIC COMMUNITY STUDY — BOGALUSA HEART STUDY

Ralph R. Frerichs, Larry S. Webber, Sathanur R. Srinivasan, and Gerald S. Berenson

Specialized Center of Research-Arteriosclerosis (SCOR-A), Louisiana State University Medical Center, New Orleans, LA/USA

Serum lipids and anthropometric measurements including an assessment of maturation by the method of Tanner were obtained on 3,524 children, ages 5 - 14 years
(93% participation in the community). Four obesity indices, including the triceps skinfold (TSF) and three weight(W)-height(H) relationships (W/H^2; $W/H^{2.77}$;
W/H^3) showed in white boys a weak but significant positive correlation with
total cholesterol (TC), triglycerides (TG), β-lipoprotein (β-LP), pre-β-lipoprotein (pre-β-LP) and a slight negative correlation with α-lipoprotein (α-LP).
White girls showed similar correlations except for TC which exhibited no relationship. Only pre-β-LP and TG were correlated with obesity in black children. Using
multiple linear regression, knowledge of the children's age, race, TSF, maturation, and $W/H^{2.77}$ explained only 5% to 9% of the variation in the lipids in boys
and between 3% to 10% of the lipid variations in girls. In order to analyze the
extremes of body size for each of the race-sex categories, an obese and a lean
group were formulated based on W, H and TSF. In white boys, the obese group had
significantly higher levels of TC, TG, β-LP and pre-β-LP, lower levels of α-LP,
and no difference in TC when compared to lean girls. Within black children there
were no differences for boys while girls differed significantly but only for β-
LP and pre-β-LP. Obesity, commonly associated with hyperlipidemia in adulthood,
exhibits only a weak association in children.

THE NATURAL HISTORY AND PROGNOSTIC FACTORS IN ISCHEMIC HEART DISEASE IN JAPAN

Osamu Iumira, Mitsuo Miyahara, and Yuichi Hamagami
The Second Department of Internal Medicine, Sapporo Medical College, Sapporo/ Japan

In order to clarify the natural history of the ischemic heart disease (IHD) in Japan, follow-up studies were made on 764 patients with IHD examined during ten years from 1964 to 1974. The patients were divided into four groups; (I) effort angina, (II) old myocardial infarction, (III) rest angina, (IV) IHD without pain. The three, five, and ten year survival rate of the whole series was 89.3, 83.4, and 70.7 percent, respectively. The survival rate of the group I, II, III, and IV was 91.6, 69.2, 92.1, and 83.3 in five years, and 86.2, 44.5, 81.6, and 76.6 percent in ten years, respectively. The male patients in group I and II and total series, the older patients over sixty years old in total series, and the patients with diabetes mellitus in group I and total series showed significant lower survival rate and higher cardiac death rate. However, no significant difference was found between the patients with and without hypertension, hypercholesterolemia, cardiac enlargement, or arrhythmias. Although the continued medical treatment slightly improved the survival rate, it did not show significant effect on complete disappearance of anginal attack.

RISK FACTORS AND ARRHYTHMIA AT ACUTE MYOCARDIAL INFARCTION AND SUDDEN DEATH

Egbert Nüssel, Lutz Buchholz, and Christoph Hasslacher
Clinical Research Institute of Myocardial Infarction at University, Medicine School, Heidelberg/BRD

Criteria are to be deduced from the risk factors and cardiac arrhythmia to specifically predict acute myocardial infarction (MI) on the one hand and sudden death (SD) on the other. For this purpose the data of 3441 patients are being analysed. These patients constitute the Ischaemic Heart Disease Register established according to recommendations of the WHO and are controlled annually. Since 1973 the patients of the Register are being observed with respect to ventricular premature beats (VPB) also in the WHO follow-up "study on symptoms and signs predicting acute MI and SD". On the basis of these WHO-projects a retro- and prospective research program was possible. Considering the quantified chest pain and enzyme-diagnostic multi-variable statistical analyses are being carried out. The surviving patients with VPB were similar in the constellation of risk factors to the patients of the SD group. The patients of both groups differed from the surviving without VPB at and after MI. Leaving apart the constellations of the criteria and considering the individual risk factors, the close positive relation of diabetes mellitus to SD and to VPB is of special importance.

HISTOLOGICAL AND MORPHOMETRICAL EVALUATION OF CORONARY ARTERY SCLEROSIS IN INDONESIAN SUBJECTS

Soemiati Ahmad Muhammad
Department of Anatomy, Faculty of Medicine, Gadjah Mada University, Yogyakarta/ Indonesia

Coronary arteries of Indonesian subjects between 10 and 70 years have been studied for histological and morphometrical age-induced changes. Arteriosclerotic thickenings of the intima were found in all subjects, more pronounced in the central regions of the coronary artery, beginning as a thin diffuse fibrocellular

proliferation in the second decade and becoming increasingly prominent with an uneven distribution with advancing age. Medial alterations were seen as an increase of elastic tissue up to the end ot the third decade, followed by a decrease of elastic tissue and an increase of collagen.
Morphometric examinations show a positive correlation between intimal area, intima-medial index, lumen circumference and age.

FATTY ACID COMPOSITION OF PHOSPHOLIPIDS IN SERUM LIPOPROTEIN CLASSES IN NORMAL AND HYPERLIPEMIC SUBJECTS

Akira Yamamoto
The Second Department of Internal Medicine, Osaka University Medical School, Osaka/Japan

Fatty acid composition of lecithin and sphingomyelin in serum high-density (HDL) and low-density (LDL) lipoproteins was determined in normal subjects and in cases of hyperlipemia. The fatty acid composition of lecithin was essentially the same for HDL and LDL, except a minor difference in concentration of polyunsaturated fatty acids, which was slightly higher in HDL than in LDL. Major fatty acids of sphingomyelin were nervonic acid (24:1) and palmitic acid (16:0), but there was a marked difference in distribution of these fatty acids between HDL and LDL in normal subjects.
The concentration of 24:1 was much higher than that of 16:0 in HDL, while the concentration of 16:0 was almost at the same level as that of 24:1 in LDL, so that the average chain length of sphingomyelin fatty acids was about 1.0 shorter in LDL than in HDL. In hyperlipemia, the difference in fatty acid composition of sphingomyelin between HDL and LDL was not significant. But the difference markedly appeared by the treatment with a derivative of nicotinic acid. The formation of long chain fatty acids seems to be a factor which regulates the metabolism of lipoproteins in blood plasma.

V
Pediatric Aspects of Atherosclerosis

RISK FACTORS IN CHILDREN — THE EARLY NATURAL HISTORY OF ATHERO-SCLEROSIS *

Gerald S. Berenson

Introduction and Background

A concept of risk factors in adults as a tool for predicting morbid events related to coronary artery disease and hypertension has now been clearly established by the superb epidemiological studies conducted in Framingham, Tecumseh,
Albany, and other similar programs. Less clear, however, is a means of prevention, which is our ultimate goal. Heretofore, most studies have been directed at
understanding risk factors and their modification in adults, often already mani-
festing clinical evidence of coronary heart disease. Only recently has attention
been directed toward younger people, with efforts being made to treat those with
extremely high levels of risk factors and to develop guidelines for modification
of risk factors in children.

Epidemiological studies of another type, the study of vascular lesions, show that
atherosclerosis involves a population in the United States and other countries
that is much broader than indicated by defined risk factor levels (McGill, 1968).
It is apparent that the "silent" phase of the disease (Fig. 1) begins much earlier than the complications that attract so much interest. We must appreciate
and emphasize that the disease remains silent until significant lumen-occupying
lesions result in complications.

Several investigations 20-30 years ago began to point to the need of studying
young persons for the early development of atherosclerosis. Holman and his co-
workers (Holman et al., 1958), as well as other pathologists demonstrated morphologic evidence of the disease in childhood. Quite dramatic has been the evidence of extensive and significant coronary artery raised lesions observed in
necropsies of young soldiers killed in the military service (Enos et al., 1955).

Risk factors such as hypertension, obesity, elevated blood lipids, and cigarette
smoking have been extensively investigated; yet, much remains to be learned about
the role of these and other factors in the early pathogenesis of atherosclerosis.
The concept of risk factors is well-accepted, and epidemiological programs have
demonstrated the association of clinical manifestations, biochemical and physiologic parameters, with morbid events. However, all of the potential factors and
the early association of these factors with disease have not been elucidated.
For example, although genetic aspects obviously contribute to atherosclerosis,
they are not yet clearly formulated to account for the widespread occurrence of
this disease in the general population. Obviously, the same risk factors observed
for adults also need to be studied in children, but they are more difficult to
interpret in children because of a single limitation — inability to observe the
severity or progressiveness of the disease. This then poses a major question:
"How does one begin to describe the early natural history of atherosclerosis,
and we could equally include the early natural history of essential hypertension?" (To encompass the two diseases, the terms "arteriosclerosis" will be
used.) Observations have not been sufficient to answer this question, and certainly it requires critical attention. Clinical morbid endpoints are not yet
available, nor are there noninvasive methods for assessing severity of onset of

---

*Appreciation is expressed to the Louisiana SCOR-A staff and to the children of
  Bogalusa, Louisiana, without whom this program could not be possible.

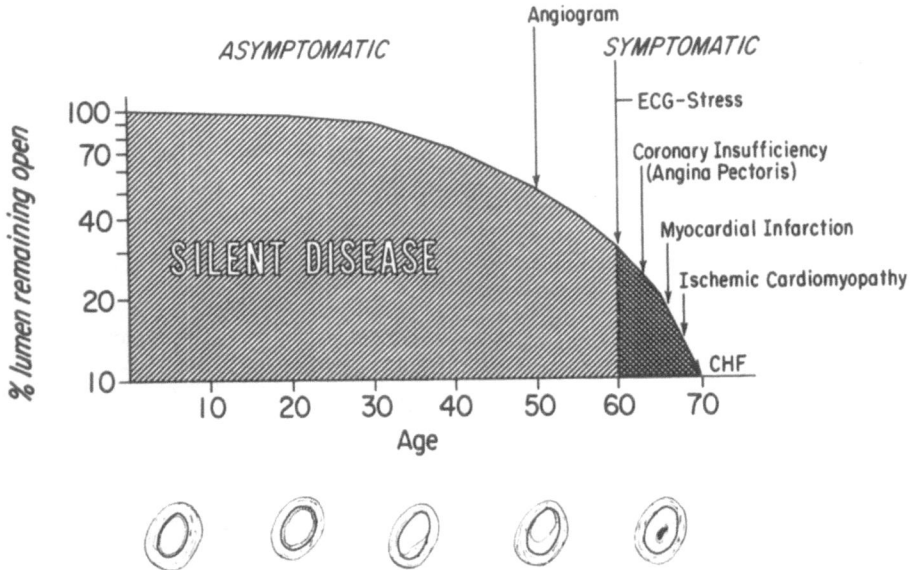

Figure 1. The early natural history of arteriosclerosis is silent. Currently, major cardiologic interest concerns end-stage disease and clinical manifestations. An understanding of the early natural history is needed for prevention of coronary heart disease

disease in an epidemiological study of children. Despite this limitation, risk factors associated with arteriosclerosis in adults are so important that a careful description of them in children is paramount.

Methodological Approach

Major Questions

In a discussion of risk factors in children, certain major questions become part of the description of the early natural history of arteriosclerosis. Shown in Table 1, these represent the major questions to be answered before we can begin to seriously consider broad-scale prevention to reduce arteriosclerosis in the general population. The distribution of some risk factor variables has been investigated earlier in children, specifically for blood pressure, serum cholesterol, and growth characteristics. Unfortunately, most studies have been cross-sectional in design, lacking extended observations and often conducted independently on variables without observing their interrelationships or studying them within the context of arteriosclerosis. It becomes obvious in a study of children that there are many areas of interest, each important and each with a certain degree of overlap (Fig. 2). This presentation will focus primarily on three areas — weight, blood pressure, and lipids.

Table 1. Risk factors in children

Major questions
1. What are the *distribution* and *prevalence* of risk factors in children?
2. What are the *interrelationships* of risk factors in children?
3. What is the *time-course* of risk factors in children?
4. What are the *determinants* of risk factors in children?
<div align="center">Genetic VS environmental</div>

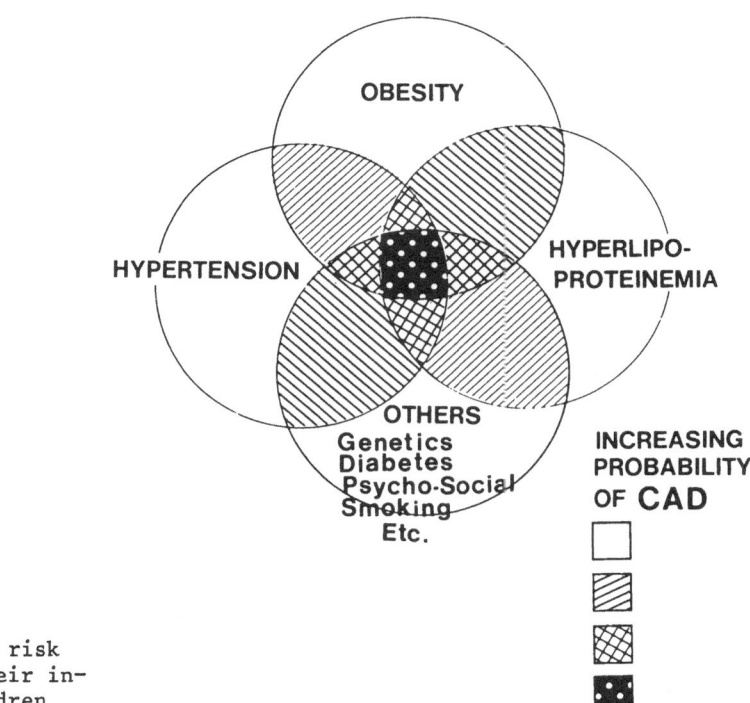

OBESITY

HYPERTENSION

HYPERLIPO-
PROTEINEMIA

OTHERS
Genetics
Diabetes
Psycho-Social
Smoking
Etc.

INCREASING
PROBABILITY
OF CAD

Figure 2. An overlap of risk
factor variables and their interrelationship in children

Population Sample

A research study designed as a model for examination of children for risk factors is being conducted in a biracial, rural community in southern Louisiana.
The Bogalusa Heart Study proposes to study the total population of approximately
5000 children in a geographic area of 22000 people, 63% of whom are white and
37% black. Observations on the school-aged children, 5-14 years, represent 91%
of the white children and 97% of the black in this targed population. Additional
observations have been conducted on 700 preschool children, ages 2 1/2 - 5 1/2
years, representing approximately 80% of this age group. The observations on the
children consist of a fasting blood sample for serum lipids, measurements of
height, weight, and triceps skinfold, a general physical examination, and a series of nine blood pressures recorded with the mercury sphygmomanometer and an
automatic recording device. The children are randomized through three stations,
two equipped with the mercury sphygmomanometer and one with the automatic instrument. At each station, three blood pressures are recorded by well-trained nurses.

Laboratory Studies

Serum samples are analyzed in a Core Lipid Laboratory that is designated as standardized for cholesterol and triglyceride by the Center for Disease Control in
Atlanta, Georgia. Both cholesterol and triglyceride determinations are done with
the Technicon Autoanalyzer II with cholesterol values converted by the Abel-Ken-
dall standard technique. The lipoprotein levels are measured using a heparin-
calcium precipitation and agar-agarose gel electrophoresis method developed in
our laboratory (Srinivasan et al., 1970). This method compares favorably with
blind analyses obtained with the analytic ultracentrifuge and shows good agreement with an ultracentrifuge method developed by Dr. Ralph Ellefson and used at
the Mayo Clinic.

Quality Controls

Each day of screening, an additional blood sample is collected in a random order on 10% of the children for assessment error. In addition, a random sample of children rotate back through the examinations, except for repeat blood sampling.

Results

Anthropometric Studies

Selected anthropometric studies included observations on height, body weight, and skinfold. Observations of the children within our described total population were quite similar to those of the National Health Examination Survey. Certain racial differences were noted, however, in that our black girls tend to be somewhat taller and heavier than the white girls, and perhaps an increase in weight of the black girls occurs in the older age group when compared to the national sample. When the distributions of weight over height were observed (Fig. 3) a slight kurtosis was found in the taller children, suggesting that based on height and weight, increases or excesses become more apparent in the older children. Many studies on growth characteristics have been conducted, but our studies give us an opportunity to relate them to the other risk factor parameters, as discussed below.

Skinfold studies indicated a thicker skinfold in white children than in black children, and significantly thicker skinfolds in girls than boys.

Blood Pressure Studies

The major findings in these cross-sectional observations on blood pressure were that blood pressure appears to increase with age and with insignificant differences related to race and sex. Progressive elevations were observed at about

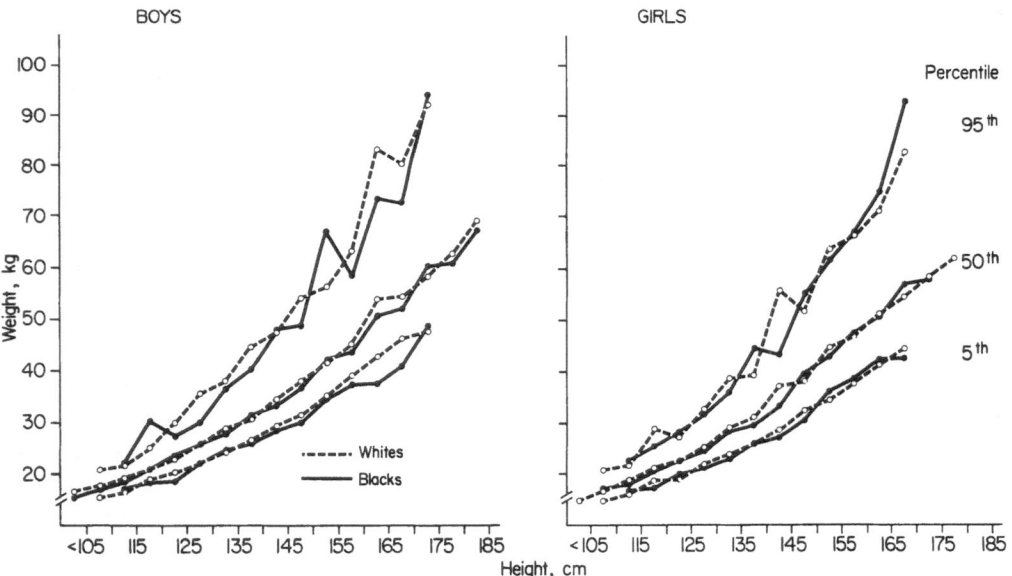

Figure 3. Distribution of weight at the 95th, 50th, and 5th percentiles for various heights. Note the relative increasing weight in the taller (and older) children (Bogalusa heart study, 1973-1974)

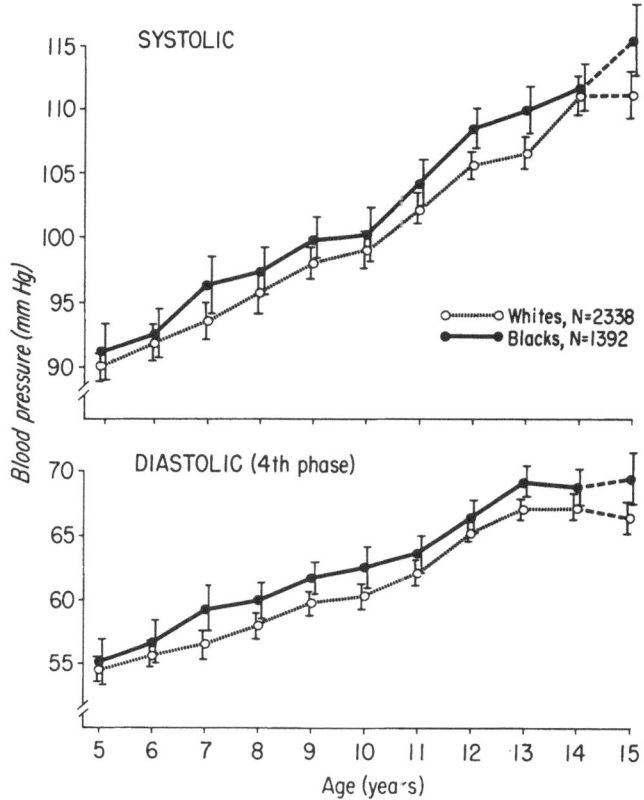

Figure 4. Blood pressures recorded by an automatic recorder indicating higher levels in black children. Physiometrics instrument blood pressure measurements of school children, by age and race (Bogalusa heart study, 1973-1974)

1.5 mm Hg per year for systolic and 0.7 mm Hg for diastolic or fourth-phase pressures. However, the measurements recorded with an automatic blood pressure recorder showed significantly higher levels in black children (Fig. 4). Of importance, these values were consistently lower than other cross-sectional observations on children, and are considered to approach basal blood pressures. We felt that the lower blood pressures were obtained because the children were relaxed, accepted the examination by a friendly staff, and could observe measurements being taken on other children. Achieving basal levels is important since reportedly these are more reliable for observing changes over time.

Although the current concept holds that essential hypertension does not occur in children (Dustan, 1976), we feel that tracking of hypertension can take place at a young age, as suggested by our data, by observations of Harlan and co-workers (Harlan et al., 1973) on young adults followed over two decades, and by the studies of Zinner and co-workers (Zinner et al., 1975) in children, which show aggregation of hypertension in families. The theoretical design of Figure 5 shows a concept of tracking. Although regression toward the mean occurs in epidemiological studies and marked variability of blood pressure, including momentary fluctuations, is known, we feel that children with consistently higher levels of blood pressure with regard to their body size may represent those children destined to become recognized as hypertensive in adulthood.

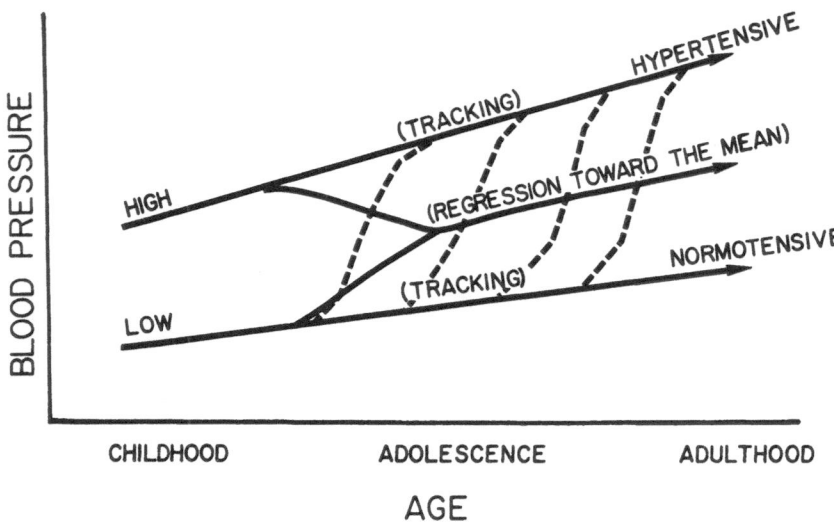

Figure 5. A concept of tracking of essential hypertension with an onset in children. Although marked variability of blood pressure occurs, it is suggested that children with consistently higher levels of blood pressure relative to height and weight become hypertensive adults. Regression toward the mean occurs in epidemiological studies; translocation from low to high levels also occurs as found in accelerated hypertension observed clinically. Projected trends of blood pressure over time

Lipid Studies

In the studies of lipids, the most interesting observations indicated somewhat higher serum total cholesterol levels in black children and higher triglyceride levels in whites. α-lipoproteins were higher in black children and pre-β-lipoproteins were higher in whites. The difference in the α- and pre-β-lipoproteins accounts for the racial differences observed in cholesterol and triglyceride levels. The cross-sectional values for β-lipoproteins related to age indicate the curve to be horizontal, with a slight decrease starting around age 11, especially in boys. In contrast, there appears to be an increase in pre-β-lipoproteins, more so in girls and especially in white girls. Since these studies occur over a relatively narrow age range, Figure 6 illustrates cholesterol over the age span of our target population compared to adults examined in the National Health Examination Survey. It is quite interesting to observe the rather dramatic change of serum cholesterol during the first year of life; adult levels are approached by 2 years of age.

For each of the studies of weight, blood pressure, and lipids it is not possible to define abnormal levels. Since the observations being reported are largely descriptive in nature and since risk factors are considered to occur essentially as a continuum, it now becomes necessary to define risk factor variables significantly elevated based on percentiles rather than previously published cutpoints.

Interrelationship of Variables

Significant interrelationships were observed among the anthropometric variables, blood pressure, and lipids. The analysis of blood pressure data revealed a remarkable relationship to height and weight which accounts for almost 40% of the variability of blood pressure observations. This relationship is so marked that when controlled for, age has no effect on blood pressure levels. From these data, it is recommended that normative blood pressure tables for this decade should

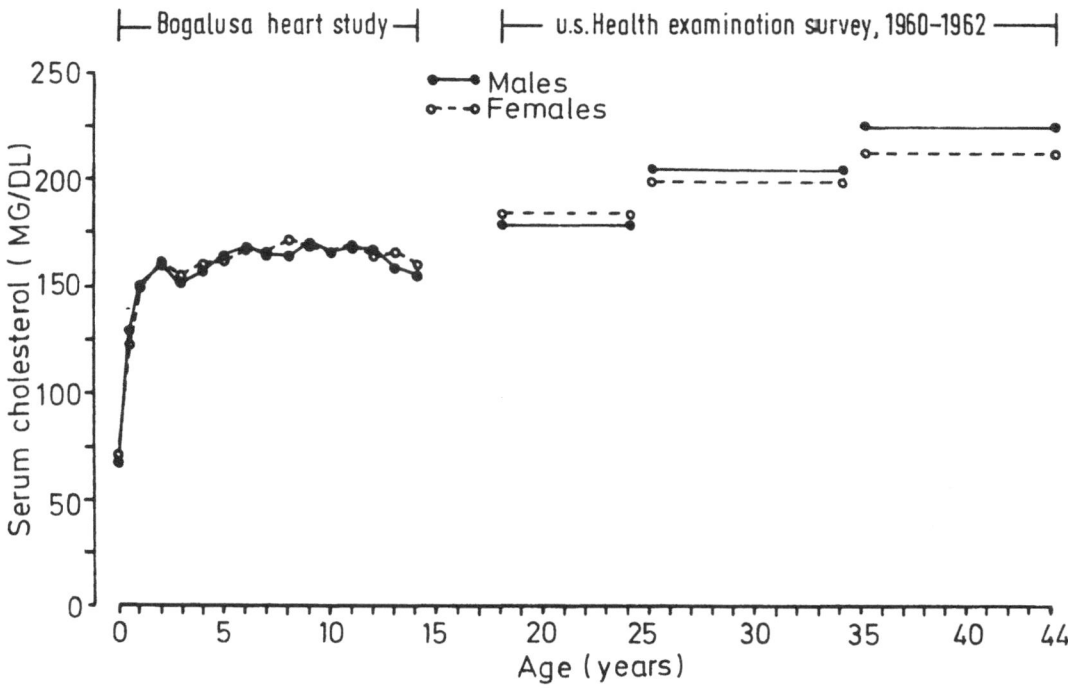

Figure 6. Total serum cholesterol levels in infancy, childhood and adulthood.
Data are from the Bogalusa Heart Study and the National Health Examination Survey

consider body mass of the child; that is, blood pressure in children should be
related to height, weight, or both instead of age.

Weight can also be related to lipid levels in children. Our studies show that
cholesterol levels at the 95th percentile cluster in the children at the higher
weight levels. This observation was noted for white boys and to some extent for
white girls, but was not observed in the black children (Fig. 7). Although there
is an interrelationship of obesity and lipid levels when analyzed by means of
correlation coefficients, these relationships account for as little as 13% of
the total variability.

Other Questions

What are the trends over time or the time-course of risk factors? We are unable
to show any longitudinal data at this time. Obviously, more information is
needed on this point but significant observations on young adults in the Navy
(Harlan et al., 1973) and from Evans County (Tyroler et al., 1976) suggest that
tracking does occur with blood pressure. Lastly, what are the determinants of
risk factor variables? It is obvious that genetics and environmental factors have
an interplay. Although certain specific genetic influences are understood, particularly with regards to type II A, little is known of their influence on the majority of the population. The variability of risk factors with regard to genetics is not entirely clear. Equally limited is our capability of understanding the
impact of environmental factors on risk factor variables.

We do have some information about dietary composition from a segment of 11-year-
old children, but as stated earlier by Kannel and co-workers from the Framingham

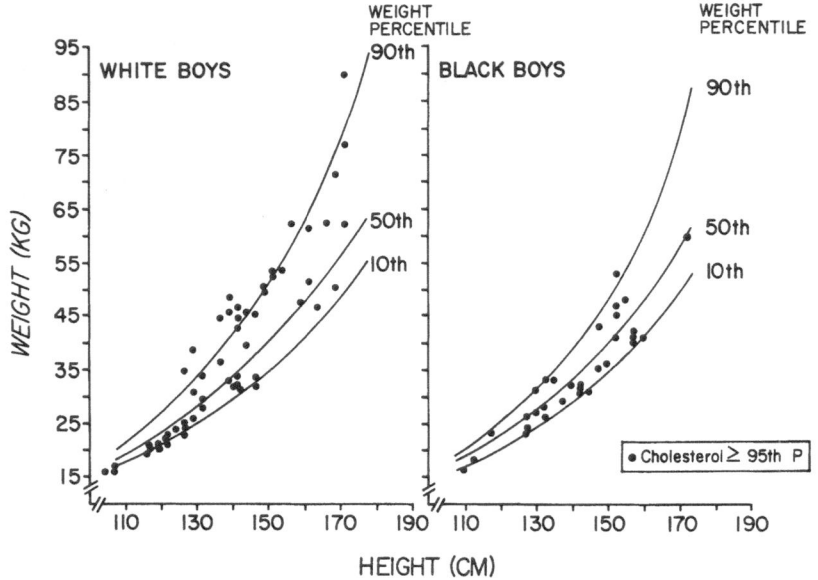

Figure 7. Clustering of white boys with serum cholesterol levels at the 95th percentile and of heavier weight. Similar observations were noted for white girls and for serum triglycerides in both girls and boys. These relationships were not found in the black children (Bogalusa heart study; ages 5-14 years)

Study (Kannel et al., 1971) and by Keys and co-workers (Keys et al., 1965), within a given population little correlation is observed between dietary fat or cholesterol and the serum lipid levels. Similar results were observed in our studies; only low and likely biologically insignificant correlations were observed. However, as shown in Table 2, we have found significant differences in correlations of cholesterol with specific dietary components between those children with the lowest level of cholesterol and those with median and high levels. These encouraging studies lead us to further areas of investigation.

Table 2. Mean intake of dietary components for children grouped according to serum cholesterol levels, Bogalusa Heart Study

Dietary components/ 1000 calories	Serum cholesterol levels percentile		
	<25th N = 49	25 ≤ X <75th N = 81	≥ 75th N = 49
Total fat	38.1	44.8[c]	44.3[c]
Animal fat	23.1	29.4[b]	28.5[b]
Saturated fatty acid	15.6	18.4[c]	18.5[c]
Unsaturated fatty acid	20.2	23.6[b]	22.9[b]
Carbohydrate	133.3[b]	119.5	120.2
Sucrose	53.1[a]	43.5	43.1

[a](p <.05). [b](p <.01). [c](p <.001).

Comment

The future will reveal how risk factors change with time. For the present, we must determine whether methods of measurement are sufficiently precise to observe biological variations over time. Ultimately, we must also determine when the risk factor variables we are describing become risk factors for coronary artery disease or hypertension and ascertain what levels are significant. With such observations, it will be possible to construct the evolution of risk factors from childhood through adulthood and to evaluate the role of these risk factor variables in the development of morbid events. We can then begin to develop means of preventing end-stage disease. The study of risk factor variables in children needs to be intensified and related to the silent anatomical changes occurring in the vascular system. Only with continued clinical and anatomical studies and efforts to correlate the two can be begin to appreciate and fully understand the early natural history of arteriosclerosis.

MORPHOLOGIC APSECTS OF CHILDHOOD ATHEROSCLEROSIS

Leonard C. Blieden and N. Neufeld

The treatment of atherosclerosis in adulthood does not get to the root of the problem, which is obviously prevention. The latter must of course start at an early age. In order to do this, we must understand the etiology and pathogenesis of atherosclerosis.

It is the purpose of this paper to discuss the morphologic features of childhood atherosclerosis. Hopefully, some of the features to be discusses will aid in the better understanding of this condition and thus in its prevention and treatment. We will briefly review the normal development of the coronary arteries and its influence on atherosclerosis. We will then consider the anatomical features in different ethnic groups and the possible effect of these differences on the prevalence of atherosclerosis.

The ultrastructural features of the coronary microcirculation will then be briefly described and we will attempt to relate these features to subsequent pathologic findings. We will then consider the effect of congenital heart lesions — especially those producing coronary hypertension — on the development of atherosclerosis. The coronary arterial changes in metabolic disorders will also be dealt with briefly. Finally, we will discuss the end result of coronary artery disease — namely myocardial infarction — in the childhood period.

Normal Coronary Arteries

The natural history of the development of coronary heart disease may be divided into three periods (Abramovici and Neufeld, 1965):

1. Incubation period (ab ova): fetal life, infants, children, young adults
2. Latent period: asymptomatic, but with pathologic changes present
3. Clinical period: signs and symptoms present

The last period is the one with which we all are familar. In the search for etiological factors, one must start in the infancy period and even back into fetal life. With this in mind, we developed our studies of the histology of coronary arteries. Two main aspects were considered: the normal child and the child with congenital heart disease. In the latter, we attempted to learn how the structural changes in the coronary arteries develop, particularly in those lesions where coronary artery hypertension exists because of its possible implications in the development of atherosclerosis. We have also placed special emphasis in our studies on the differences in structural changes of coronary arteries in different ethnic groups.

From the investigations performed up to the present, the histologic changes which appear in the coronary arteries during the different stages of development in fetal life as well as after birth have now been determined (Neufeld and Vlodauer, 1971).

In fetuses, the intima is not developed and consists of a very thin layer of endothelial cells. Immediately beneath it lies the internal elastic membrane (lamina elastica interna), which separates the intima from the media.

The first visible changes are seen a few days after birth and are localized in the internal elastic membrane, in the form of splitting or fragmentation. In the region of the splitting of the elastic membrane, fibroblasts proliferate (Fig. 1). In the first postnatal month, the splitting of the elastic membrane becomes more prominent and the adjacent smooth muscle cells of the media lose their shape and position and show degenerative changes.

Between the fibers of the split internal elastic membrane, smooth muscle cells begin to appear, tending to run in a longitudinal direction. In some instances, proliferation and thickening of the intimal layer are present with an increase of mucopolysaccharides under the endothelium.

The number of smooth muscle cells between the elements originating from the splitting of the internal elastic membrane increases and, in addition, fragmented elastic fibrils begin to appear among the ingrowing muscle fibers. As a result of these changes, a new layer, the musculoelastic layer, is formed between the obvious intima and media.

Differences in the quantity and intensity of the intimal changes between the sexes are found even in early life. These differences are apparent soon after birth, but are more obvious at the end of the first year of life. These alterations in the coronary arterial internal elastic membrane and intimal changes have been considered by some to be the basis for the development of coronary arteriosclerosis, but this theory has not been proven. It was therefore, decided to see whether the structural changes present in the population studied also occurred in other ethnic groups with low prevalence and incidence of coronary heart disease. Therefore, Yeminite Jews and Bedouins — both groups living in Israel — were also studied. It was assumed that if these changes appeared among them, this would then constitute strong evidence against an anatomical basis for development of atherosclerosis. On the other hand, it was felt that if the structural characteristics of these two groups were different from the original one studied, this would not prove, but would lend support to the theory of an anatomical basis underlying the development of coronary atherosclerosis. The histologic changes in the coronary arteries in full-term fetuses, infants, and children of three ethnic groups in Israel were studied. These were Ashkenazy Jews (European in origin), Yeminite Jews (from Yemen), and Bedouins.

Calculations of the ratio of intimal plus musculoelastic tissue area to total area per individual were based on weighted average of the ethnic groups at very early ages. The Ashkenazy males were found to have more intima and musculoelastic tissue than the Bedouin or Yemenite males and for the females of their group and

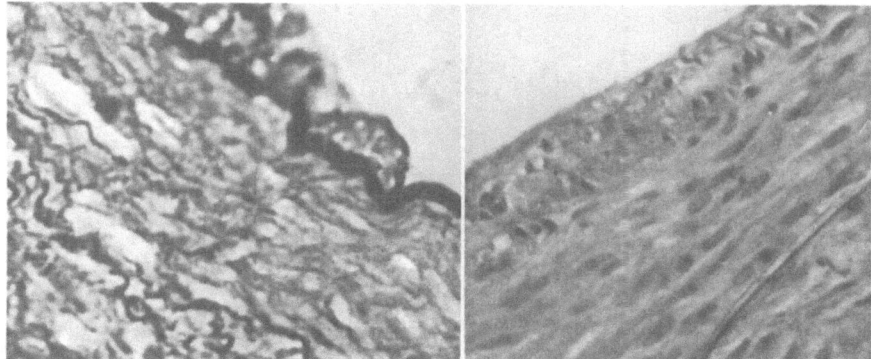

Figure 1. Right coronary artery of a 2-week-old male. Left: splitting and fragmentation of the internal elastic membrane. Elastic tissue stain (X 200). Right: proliferation of fibroblasts H and E (X 200)

in the others. No differences were found between the right and left coronary
arteries in any of the ethnic groups. In the Bedouins, the initial elastic changes
do not become more pronounced with age as they do in other ethnic groups. The
intima of the Ashkenazy males develops in an eccentrid form and has a richer
collagenous tissue component than that of the children of the Yeminite and Bedouin group (Fig. 2).

These differences in the findings between sexes and ethnic groups in children
up to 10 years of age are consistent with the known differences in the prevalence
of coronary arteriosclerosis and atherosclerosis, coronary heart disease, and
myocardial infarction in the corresponding adult populations (Neufeld, 1974).

Ultrastructure of the Microcirculation

A great deal of literature has appeared on the clinical, pathologic, and functional aspects of the main coronary arteries. To the best of our knowledge,
there have been no publications on the ultrastructural features of the coronary
microcirculation. Drs. Sherf and Neufeld of the Heart Institute of the Chaim
Sheba Medical Center, Tel Hashomer have recently studied this subject (Sherf and
Neufeld, 1976).

The features described apply to the findings in adult hearts. As they may play
a role in the morphogenesis of atherosclerosis, we feel it appropriate to discuss
these features in this presentation. In addition, in the near future a study of
the findings in children is to be undertaken.

The coronary arterial tree may be divided into three groups:
1. Main coronary arteries
2. Small coronary arteries
3. Terminal coronary vascular bed (microcirculation 100 – 8 – 100)
We are here concerned mainly with group "3". Table 1 shows the sizes of the various vessels. These measurements alone, however, are insufficient to characterize
the vessels, and specific features are necessary to aid in identification. In the

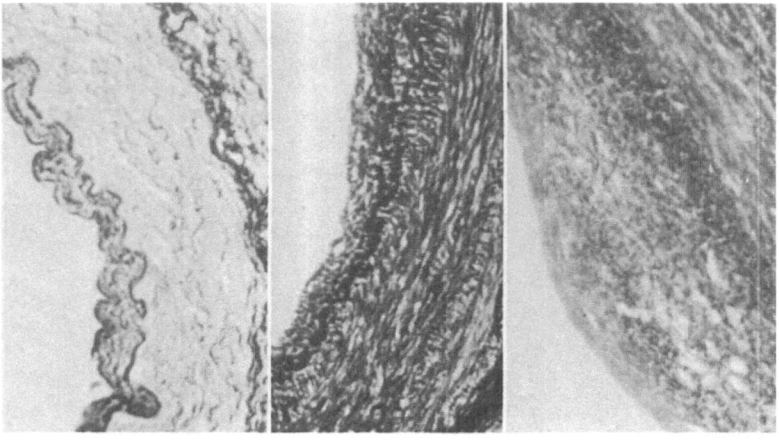

A   B   C

Figure 2. A. A right coronary artery of a 6-year-old Bedouin male. B. Left coronary artery of an 8-year-old Yemenite male. C. Right coronary artery of a 7-year-
old Ashkenazy male. Note the splitting of the elastic membrane in the Bedouin (A)
is now more pronounced than in the younger age groups; the Yemenite (B), localized area of musculoelastic layer; the Ashkenazy (C) marked changes in intima in
musculoelastic layer and media

Table 1. The microcirculation of the human coronary tree an electronmocroscopic study

Vessel	Lumen caliber
Arterioles and terminal arterioles	100 – 25 μ
Precapillary sphincters	25 – 10 μ
Metarterioles	10 – 8 μ
Capillaries	8 – 5 μ
Venules	20 – 45 μ
Small veins	45 –100 μ

arterioles, the cells of the endothelium are prolonged as are the nuclei which do not bulge into the lumen. In addition, there are two to three layers of smooth muscle. In the precapillary sphincters, the cells of the endothelium are shorter, the nuclei are larger, and bulge into the lumen of the vessel. There is a single layer of smooth muscle cells around the endothelium.

The details of other anatomical structures are outside the scope of this paper. In this study, however, of note is the fact that the precapillary sphincter was demonstrated "on end" as well as longitudinal sections.

Capillary hemodynamics may be regulated by one (or more) of three methods:
1. Periodicity of flow
2. Unequal duration of flow time
3. Lack of relation to systemic pressure
The capillaries do not control themselves; thus, the process which controls the blood flow must be upstream.

Rhodin was the first to correlate structure with function. He did this by observing the circulation — the smooth blood vessels — in muscle taken from the leg of a rabbit. Rhodin presented only longitudinal sections. In the "enface" sections from Dr. Sherf's material, open and closed sphincters may be seen. He showed that three or four sphincters are able to control the blood flow in a whole capillary network.

The exact significance of the sphincter mechanism remains to be seen. If, under certain conditions, the sphincters close and remain closed for a varying period of time, the blood supply to an area of the microcirculation may be impaired. Localized ischemia may be produced. Depending on the number of sphincters and the area involved, the effect on the myocardium will also vary.

Much work still remains to be done in this area. However, the changes outlined hint at a possible role that the microcirculation may play in the development of "coronary artery disease."

Histologic Changes of the Coronary Arteries in Congenital Heart Disease

Histologic changes occur in the coronary arteries in several congenital heart lesions; only those in which the coronary arteries are involved in a process resembling atherosclerosis will be discussed. These changes are usually "secondary" in nature. Secondary changes in the coronary arteries occur when there is hypertension associated with certain congenital cardiovascular anomalies (Neufeld et al., 1962). These changes consist of nonspecific intimal changes in the coronary arteries which are thickened; atherosclerosis is present in young adults.

The media of the coronary arteries is thickened and elastic changes are evident. Such changes are particularly well-developed in the following conditions.

Supravalvular Aortic Stenosis

The anomalies causing obstruction to aortic blood flow above the aortic valve are relatively rare and clinically difficult to distinguish from aortic valvular or subvalvular (subaortic) stenosis. The anomalies are of three types: 1) a localized zone of obstruction resembling a diaphragm in the ascending aorta, 2) localized narrowing of the ascending aorta, and 3) uniform narrowing of the entire ascending aorta. In a necropsy report of a 2-year-old, the last type was found. The media of the coronary arteries was thickened and deposition of elastic fibers was evident. The changes are attributed to systolic hypertension in the coronary vessels. The proximal segments of the coronary arteries dilate presumably because they fill during ventricular systole and are, therefore, subjected to the high lefel of systolic pressure proximal to the obstruction (Ogden, 1970).

Coarctation of the Aorta

In a histologic study of the coronary arteries in the hearts of patients in whom coarctation of the aorta was the sole anomaly, marked intimal changes and excess collagen tissue were present (Vlodaver and Neufeld, 1968). Atherosclerotic lesions were conspicuous. The media was markedly thickened with rich elastic fibers interspersed between muscle bundles. Studies in coarctation of the aorta have shown the left ventricular pressure to be elevated and equal to the pressure in the proximal aorta. Hypertension in the aorta proximal to the coarctation is due not only to the increased resistance, but also to the limited capacity and distensibility of the proximal aorta and the physiologic reactions of the left ventricle. Since the coronary arteries originate proximal to the aortic obstruction, elevated pressure in the aorta proximal to the coarctation increases the central coronary perfusing pressure.

Development of coronary hypertension in patients with coarctation of the aorta may well explain the severe changes in the intima in early life and the severe atheroma found in young adults. With coarctation of the aorta, the coronary capacity is larger than normal; this is confirmed by the measurements of the external lumen area, which are larger than those in a control group.

Inherited Disorders of Metabolism

Inherited disorders of metabolism are genetically determined abnormalities of enzymic function that result in either an absence or a low concentration of a specific enzyme. The enzymic deficiency leads to an accumulation of a specific metabolic product proximal to the enzymic block. The concentration of the product proximal to the enzymic block. The concentration of the product increases in tissues where the metabolic pathway exists, and its accumulation may lead to organ malfunction. Coronary artery involvement has been noted in several of these so-called storage diseases (Blieden and Moller, 1974). In some of these conditions, the findings are identical with those in typical atherosclerosis. In others, the findings are similar although not identical. In addition, however, the damage to the coronary arteries produced by the storage material may stimulate the production of atherosclerosis.

Mucopolysaccharidoses

The mucopolysaccharidoses are a group of inherited diseases characterized by the abnormal tissue deposition and/or urinary excretion of mycopolysaccharides. Cardiac involvement occurs in six syndromes of mucopolysaccharidosis. In two of these, Hurler's and Hunter's syndromes, the coronary arteries are involved.

Myocardial involvement occurs in areas adjacent to blood vessels. Large cells filled with storage material (gargoyle cells) move into these areas and, if extensive, interfere with myocardial contractility. In both these syndromes, the major branches of the coronary arteries may be narrowed by intimal plaques composed of deposits of mucopolysaccharide (Fig. 3).

Protein Metabolism

Primary hyperoxaluria describes two rare disorders of the metabolism of oxalic acid, each involving excessive synthesis of ocalic acid and following a pattern of autosomal recessive inheritance.

The clinical course is dominated by calcium oxalate accumulation in various tissues. The heart is one of the major sites and the coronary arteries may show calcium oxalate deposits.

Amino Acid Metabolism

Because homogentisic oxidase is absent in patients with alkaptonuria, homogentisic acid is not metabolized further. The major clinical features reflect the accumulation and urinary excretion of homogentisic acid: dark urine, pigmentation of cartilage and other tissues, and arthritis.

Myocardial infarction is a common cause of death and is related to atheromatous plaques, the blue-black pigmentation of these atheromata being a unique feature.

Homocystinuria

An enzymic defect in the formation of cystathionine from serine and homocystine results in this condition. The affected individuals show several features similar to Marfan's syndrome; however, osteoporosis, mental retardaticn, and thrombotic vascular disease are also present.

Extensive changes occur in the media of the coronary arteries and lead to dilation and thrombosis. Clinical manifestations include symptoms of coronary occlusion.

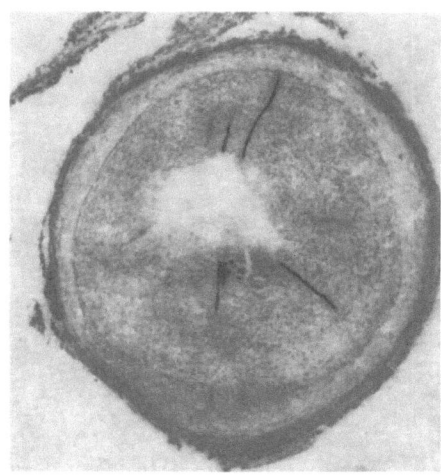

Figure 3. Hurler's syndrome. Coronary artery. Note marked accumulation of storage material

Lipid Metabolism

Fabry's disease is caused by a deficiency of ceramide trihexosidase. Ceramide trihexoside accumulates in most organs, primarly in relation to small blood vessels. The endothelial, perithelial, and smooth muscle cells of blood vessels are the vascular sites of accmulation. The disease is inherited as a sex-linked recessive trait.

Clinical manifestations of cardiac involvement include anginal chest pain, myocardial infarction, congestive heart failure, and cardiac anlargement.

Sandhoff's disease results from deficient activity of hexosaminidase A and B. Clinical features resemble those of Tay-Sachs disease. In two patients recently described (Blieden et al., 1974) the coronary arteries showed areas of luminal narrowing due to intimal proliferation of fibroblasts, although no areas of myocardial infarction were present.

G_{M1} gangliosidosis is a condition in which G_{M1} ganglioside accumulates mainly in the central nervous system and less prominently, in the viscera. In one patient, atheromatous plaques, present in the right coronary artery and descending aorta, contained balloon cells of foamy PAS-negative cytoplasm.

Hyperlipidemia plays a major role in the development of coronary artery disease. Elevation of serum cholesterol is associated with an increased risk of vascular disease. In the past few years the possible role of genetic factors is receiving increasing attention. Five main types of hyperlipidemia have been described in man. Type II is probably the most important as far as the pediatrician is concerned because it can be identified in childhood with a prevalence of about 1:200, and the disease in the homozygote state is definitely associated with an increased risk of premature coronary heart disease before the age of 20 years (Fig. 4). In the heterozygote state it also appears to be associated with premature coronary heart disease in the fourth and fifth decades.

Tangier disease is characterized by deficiency or absence of high-density lipoprotein in plasma, and by storage of cholesterol esters in many tissues. The enzymic defect has not been defined. Cardiovascular involvement is believed to be related to the deposition of cholesterol esters. Patients with coronary artery disease have been described.

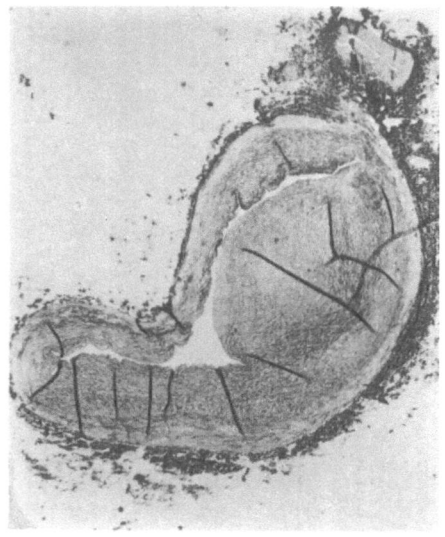

Figure 4. Hyperlipoproteinemia (type II). 18-year-old male. Note severe intimal changes with partial occlusion of lumen. H and E stain

Myocardial Infarction and Ischemia

The function of the coronary arteries is to serve as channels of delivery of oxygenated blood to the myocardium. Failure to perform this task adequately results in damage to the cardiac muscle and possible myocardial infarction. The latter entity is not often considered in a discussion of cardiac disease in the pediatric age range. However, since the incidence of myocardial infarction in children is higher than is usually appreciated, a consideration of this condition is appropriate.

Regarding etiology, failure of the coronary arterial system to supply oxygenated blood to the myocardium may be due to (1) intrinsic coronary artery disease, which in turn may be congenital or acquired (inflammatory, metabolic, traumatic, neoplastic, degenerative) or (2) normal coronary arterial tree with abnormal perfusant (due in some cases to congenital cardiac lesions). Only the first group of conditions will be discussed here. It should be emphasized that the conditions described in the first part of this paper including congenital cardiac lesions and the inherited disorders of metabolism may be associated with the development of myocardial infarction.

Intrinsic Coronary Artery Disease

Congenital Disease

Congenital malformations of the coronary arteries which may result in infarction include: anomalous left coronary artery from the pulmonary trunk, single coronary artery, coronary artery aneurysm, short coronary arteries, and coronary arteriovenous fistulae. In addition, anomalous coronary arteries may be compromised at the time of surgery, thus leading to infarction.

Acquired Conditions

The list of acquired conditions (diseases) of the coronary arteries is long and includes: rheumatic fever, lupus erythematosus, syphilis, polyarteritis nodosa, medial calcification of the coronary arteries, progeria, Friedreich's ataxia, hypertension, and miscellaneous other causes. A detailed discussion of these conditions is outside the scope of this paper.

In several of these conditions, the changes are very similar to those in atherosclerosis. Of note is one case of a young woman who suffered from Lupus erythematosus and died of myocardial infarction (Blieden et al., 1973). At necropsy, severe atherosclerotic changes were present. There was no evidence of arteritis; also no significant additional factors such as hypertension were present to explain the changes. The possibility exists that arteritis damaged the vessels and stimulated the development of atherosclerosis.

Conclusion

In this paper we have attempted to correlate the morphologic aspects of childhood atherosclerosis. Some of the features described are directly related to atherosclerosis. Some of the other conditions described may be related to the subsequent development of atherosclerosis by damaging the vessel wall and thus stimulating the production of atherosclerosis. In other instances, as in the description of the ultrastructural features of the coronary arteries, the exact role of the changes described still remains to be elucidated.

PREVALENCE OF FATAL CORONARY ARTERY DISEASE IN RELATIVES OF HYPER-TRIGLYCERIDEMIC SCHOOL CHILDREN

Peter H. Abrahams, Helmut G. Schrott, William R. Clarke, and Ronald M. Lauer
Cardiovascular Center and Department of Anatomy, University of Iowa, Iowa City, IA/USA

In each survey, 1973 and 1975, over 4,000 Muscatine school children had fasting lipid determinations. Index cases for family study were children with the following: triglyceride (TG) ≥90th% x 2 and cholesterol (C) >70th% (I), N = 39; TG ≥90th% x 2 and C <70th% (II), N = 33; TG ≤10th% x 2 (III), N = 31; a control group, C and TG between 5th and 95th% x 2 (IV), N = 44. Preliminary results indicate the total death rate of relatives ≥30 years of age was as follows: I, 13.3% (60/451); II, 11.1% (46/416); III, 15.1% (54/357); IV, 13.6% (60/441). The age specific coronary artery disease death rate is as follows:

Age Range	I	II	III	IV
30 - 55	2.1% (6/287)	0.7% (2/284)	1.9% (4/207	0.7% (2/288)
30 - 65	4.1% (15/364)	1.5% (5/337)	1.5% (4/266)	2.0% (7/355)
≥30	5.1% (23/451)	2.9% (12/416)	3.4% (12.357)	4.1% (18/441)

Hypertriglyceridemia, alone, in school children does not appear to identify coronary-prone families.
Supported by Lipid Research Clinics Program NIH-NHLI-NO1-HV-2-2913-L, SCOR: Atherosclerosis Thrombosis, Lipid HL14230-05S1 and Iowa Heart Association.

THE INHERITANCE OF BODY FAT IN CHILDREN AND ITS CONTRIBUTION IN THE RISKS OF CORONARY HEART DISEASE

Joan Slack
MRC Clinical Genetics Unit, Institute of Child Health, London C.G.D. Brook, Department of Paediatrics, Middlesex Hospital, London/England

Body fat is closely associated with the known risk factors for coronary heart disease (CHD) hypertension, hyperlipidaemia and physical inactivity. Lauer et al. (Journal of Pediatrics 86, 697 (1975)) have reported significant correlations of triceps skinfold thickness with blood pressure and serum triglycerides in schoolchildren. An understanding of the determination of body fatness in childhood would give an opportunity for preventive action designed to reduce the incidence of CHD.
The contribution of heredity and environment in the determination of body fat has been measured in 222 pairs of like sex twins aged 3 - 15 years (78 MZ and 144 DZ), by an analysis of triceps and subscapular skinfold thickness.
Genetic factors were estimated to contribute 74% ± 17 to the variation of total body fat in all twins, the contribution being greater in children over 10 years (98% ± 23) than in younger children (52% ± 26). Different methods of estimating heritability suggested that the contribution of common family environment was small, especially in the older age groups.
The high heritability of body fat in older children indicates that environmental measures must be vigorous if they are to be effective. The measures are likely to be most effective if they are taken during periods of rapid increase in body fat, that is in infancy and at adolescence.

EFFECTS OF FOOD STUFFS ON HUMAN SERUM CHOLESTEROL LEVEL AND ANIMAL CHOLESTEROL METABOLISM

Shinjiro Suzuki, Sumiko Oshima, Keisuke Tsuji, and Etsuko Tsuji
National Institute of Nutrition, Tokyo/Japan

Edible fats and oils, eggs, oligo- and poly-saccharides and mushrooms were given to several hundreds of human subjects to clarify their effects on serum cholesterol level. Animal experiments were also conducted to prove the mechanism of cholesterol metabolism.
Rice bran-, corn-, wheat germ-, safflower-, sunflower-oils, especially a brand oil of rice bran and safflower oils at a rate of 7:3 showed the most remarkable lowering effect on serum cholesterol level. Japanese mushroom Shiitake and Konjac mannan also lowered the human serum cholesterol. Eggs and sugars did not evidently increase the serum cholesterol level as generally told.
Animal experiments were carried out in order to make clear the influence of mucilaginous polysaccharides and plant pigments on their cholesterol metabolism.

A SIMPLE SCREENING PROCEDURE FOR HYPERLIPIDEMIA

Ingeborg R. Kupke
Pediatric Clinic, University of Düsseldorf, Düsseldorf/BRD

For the diagnosis of disorders in lipid metabolism, the determination of the lipid profiles in human plasma is widely used. For TLC analysis, usually the lipids have to be extracted prior to TLC. This is time consuming. In order to avoid lipid extraction, the plasma can be applied directly on self-prepated plates (Buckley and Little, 1969). HCL was used to denature the serum proteins on commercial plates (Kupke, 1975). In both procedures, the development of the neutral lipids was achieved only. *Micromethod*: 1 µl plasma from capillary blood is applied on commercial HPTLC plates (Merck) and it is overspotted with organic solvents. TLC results in a sharp separation of the neutral lipids and the main phospholipids. Rechromatography showed that no lipids remain at the origin. For quantitation, the absorbance of fluorescent derivatives is measured at 290 nm. Precision in the series (CV,%): CE = 2.1, C = 4.2, TG = 2.2, LFA = 2.4, PC = 3.2.- This procedure can be also carried out on macro-scale. - *Application*: 12 µl plasma are required for the determination of the lipid profiles by HPTLC, of the lipoprotein (LP) pattern by electrophoresis (E) and of the cholesterol (C) conc. in the LP fractions separated by E (Kupke, 1975, 1976). Thus a large data base can be obtained. 23 healthy children of Düsseldorf were examined. In 4 children Type II HL was observed. One child had a normal LP pattern and a low C level (116 mg/100 ml). However, an equal percentage of this C was found in the β- and pre-β fraction. This was only observed in adults with Type IV HL (Kupke, 1975, 1976).

CORD BLOOD CHOLESTEROL (TC), TRIGLYCERIDES (TG) AND LIPOPROTEIN AGAROSE GEL ELECTROPHORESIS IN 124 ITALIAN INFANTS

A. Pagnan, R. Cerutti, W. Donadon, and C. Dal Palù
Clinica medica II, Università di Padova, Padova/Italy

TC, TG and lipoprotein agarose-gel electrophoresis were determined in the Cord blood of 124 Italian infants (Verona country). Mean TC (69 $\pm$ 17 mg/dl) and TG (37 $\pm$ 19 mg/dl), in comparison with the data reported in other studies, turned out to be remarkably uniform; no sex differences were observed. The TG distribution curve resulted skewed superimposing the adults pattern. Cord blood TC and TG were not modified by the presence of perinatal factors. The total prevalence of hyperlipidemia was 8%:3.2 type IV, 2.4% type II and 2.4% mixed type. Both beta and alfa bands, were present all in the cases. Pre-beta band was clearly detectable in 90% of the cases; it was barely visible for TG values below 20 mg/dl. Sporadically a discrepancy between the intensity of the pre-beta band and TG was observed. In 4% of the cases a small band at the origin of the electrophoretic run was present, consisting with the cumulation of chylomicrons. In the serum of both a newborn and the mother a double band migrating in pre-beta position was detected, suggesting a familial transmission of the above abnormality.

VI
Treatment of Human Atherosclerosis

DIETARY MANAGEMENT OF ATHEROSCLEROSIS*

G. Schlierf, P. Oster, D. Seidel, H. Raetzer, B. Schellenberg, C.C. Heuck, and R.L. Wicklein

In spite of different opinions still existing with regard to the exact position of dietary factors within the multifactorial etiology of atherosclerosis, the prominent role played by the mode of life and particularly by nutritional habits is not seriously questioned. Diet should therefore be considered foremost in prophylaxis and management of atherosclerosis and its complications.

In *experimental animals* there is firm evidence that development, progression and even regression of atherosclerosis in various vascular areas is markedly affected by dietary measures. Dr. Armstrong has provided morphologic and biochemical evidence on this point during this symposium. To assess the effects of nutrition on *human atherosclerosis* is far more difficult since with methods generally available and applicable, the disease can only be detected late in its course when perfusion of organs is already markedly impaired and secondary changes have taken place. Although it is very tempting to equate complications such as myocardial infarction, stroke, or peripheral arterial occlusion with the process of atherosclerosis itself, one should proceed cautiously since it has been demonstrated that many factors other than degree and location of atherosclerosis may determine the appearance and extent of clinical complications. Nevertheless, in epidemiological studies designed to examine the diet-heart issue, such clinical complications and resultant mortality are usually counted rather than "atherosclerosis", which cannot accurately be measured during life. With these reservations in mind, the following questions should be discussed at this time:
1. The potential for regression in man
2. Correction of risk factors by diet
3. Epidemiological evidence that diet may prevent coronary heart disease

1. The Potential for Regression in Man

Regression of visible cholesterol deposits occurring as xanthomas of skin and tendons holds, for many investigators, the promise of regression occurring in other locations. Schettler (1961) described the case of a patient with severe xanthomatosis and evidence of coronary heart disease who had a mixed hyperlipidemia which was later characterized as type III hyperlipoproteinemia. Successful management of hyperlipidemia resulted in complete disappearance of xanthomatosis and, at the same time, reversal of ECG changes.

A more recent example of regression in a 12-year-old girl, homozygous for type II hyperlipoproteinemia, has been described by Starzl et al. (1974). This girl underwent end-to-side portocaval shunt in an attempt to lower cholesterol levels after she had a myocardial infarction and was almost completely immobilized owing to angina pectoris. Within a 6-month postoperative period, the cholesterol levels fell markedly and the chest pain disappeared. Follow-up at 17 months presented documentation of the disappearance of cardiovascular lesions in the human following the lowering of cholesterol and low-density lipoprotein levels. Raised yellow xanthomas over the heels, knees, knuckles, elbows, and eyelids continued to disappear and in some areas, they remained only as light discoloration of the

*Supported by Deutsche Forschungsgemeinschaft, SFB 90.

skin. The serum cholesterol level, preoperatively always above 600 mg/100 ml remained below 400 mg/100 ml. Cardiovascular findings were remarkable. The pressure gradient of aortic stenosis, preoperatively 56 mm Hg, decreased to 10 mm Hg and the decrease was, in the opinion of all examiners, associated with a diminished systolic murmur. The aortic valve, which was thickened and relatively immobile in previous studies, was normally mobile. Coronary arteriograms before the operation revealed diffuse narrowing of the coronary arteries, and the circumflex coronary artery was not displayed. The coronary studies 16 months after portocaval shunt revealed all three coronary arteries, none of which had diffuse narrowing. Although management in this patient was by surgery, it is of great interest that comparable lowering of the plasma cholesterol level was achieved prior to the operation by parenteral alimentation. Both procedures have in common that the liver is by-passed by nutrients and should be the subject of intensive research.

Complimentary evidence for regression comes from biochemical studies. Sodhi et al. (1973) performed experiments using labeled cholesterol in man. Their results indicate that tissue cholesterol was mobilized by lowering the plasma cholesterol level by diet or drugs. After incubating human arteriosclerotic arterial tissue in various media, Bjonders (1975) reported that cholesterol was removed from such tissues if the medium contained high-density lipoproteins.

Findings such as these have already been commented on by Drs. Stein and Stein and might explain data from epidemiological studies, which have been summarized by Miller and Miller (1975), indicating a negative correlation of HDL to various parameters of human atherosclerosis.

2. Correction of Risk Factors by Diet

The efficacy of dietary measures regarding several cardiovascular risk factors is well-known. Although the relationship between hyperlipidemia and diet will be focused upon below, we might recall the excellent responsiveness of other risk factors to rather simple dietary measures. Thus, *hypertension* is almost uniformly ameliorated with hypocaloric (low salt) nutrient and, in our own experience, was normalized in any case where total fasting was used for the treatment of gross obesity. We should mention the subject of *diabetes* and note that there is evidence, for instance from Japan, our host country, and from Israel, that diabetes as such, without associated risk factors may be less atherogenic than usually assumed (Heyden, 1975). With regard to *Hyperuricemia*, we have evidence from Germany (Ernährungsbericht, 1976) that the prevalence of hyperuricemia in adult male subjects approximates 5-10%. There was a rise of the plasma concentration of uric acid in adult males from 4.9 to 6.0 mg/100 ml between the years 1962 and 1971 which can be explained entirely by increased dietary purine intake, which occurred during this time due to increased consumption of meat and meat products (Griebsch and Zöllner, 1973).

Risk Factor Hyperlipidemia

The measures which affect *plasma cholesterol* levels in individual patients and in groups of the population are well-known and have been amply tested. They consist in *reduction of dietary saturated fat and cholesterol intake* and *partial substitution of saturated by polyunsaturated fatty acid sources, in that order.* There is a considerable range of dietary fat intake, compatible with low-plasma cholesterol levels if the relation of saturated and polyunsaturated fatty acids is maintained. An example is given in Figure 1 which shows a study in children with familial hypercholesterolemia using three low cholesterol diets with varying total fat content. Therefore, one could probably treat familial type II hyperlipoproteinemia in countries such as Japan and Germany without aggressive alteration of the total fat intake, provided the appropriate P/S ratios are maintained.

Effect of diet on plasma cholesterol levels
(inpatient studies)

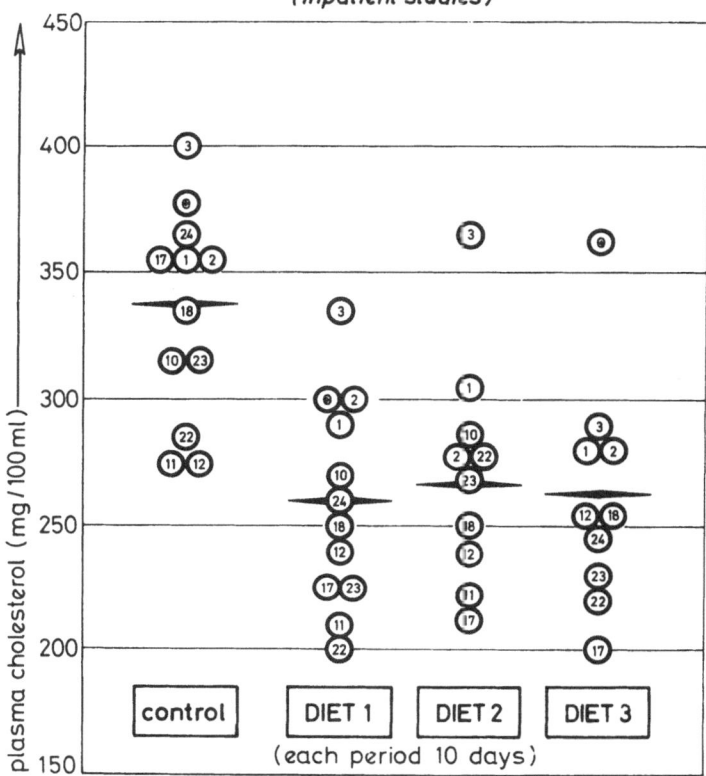

Figure 1. Dietary effects on plasma cholesterol levels in 12 children with familial hypercholesterolemia (inpatient study). Diet 1: isocaloric formula, 37% fat
as corn oil, P/S ratio 3.5. Diet 2: isocaloric formula, 8% fat as polyunsaturated margarine, P/S ratio 2.0. Diet 3: isocaloric mixed diet, P/S ratio 1.5 - 2.0
(from: Schlierf et al., Monatsschrift für Kinderheilkunde, in press, 1977)

With regard to *endogenous hypertriglyceridemia*, we have been continuously interested in acute plasma lipid and lipoprotein changes as affected by dietary measures. It has been acknowledged for many years that alimentary lipemia, the rise
of plasma triglycerides and very low-density lipoproteins/chylomicrons following
fat feeding, is dependent on the quantity and quality of the test meal, in particular the amount of dietary fat. Since we presented some data on this phenomenon at the 2nd International Symposium on Atherosclerosis 7 years ago, there
has been increasing evidence relating alimentary lipemia to atherogenesis. Dr.
Zilversmit's (1973) hypothesis has already been mentioned by Professor Schettler
in his keynote address. According to these most interesting considerations and
speculations, atherogenesis may result from the liberation of cholesterol-rich
fragments in proximity to the arterial endothelium when pre-β-lipoproteins or
chylomicrons are degraded by arterial lipoprotein lipase. High local concentrations of cholesterol-rich lipoproteins resulting from surface lipolysis and the
release of potentially injurious fatty acids would enhance the uptake of cholesterol by the arterial intima.

Accordingly, data from Bierman et al. (1973) show the avid uptake of chylomicron
"remnants" by vascular cells in tissue culture which far exceed uptake of other
lipoproteins. Similar findings have been presented by Bierman and Albers (1975)

with regard to the pre-β-lipoproteins. We have further studied the dietary factors which affect alimentary lipemia and postprandial lipoprotein changes. Partly confirming earlier studies with single test meals (Eggstein and Schettler, 1958), we found that even in normal subjects not only the amount of dietary fat but also it's kind, and not only the amount of dietary carbohydrates but also their kind and even the spacing of dietary constituents during the day markedly affects postprandial changes of plasma lipid concentrations (Schlierf et al., 1977). Let us now show a few data from a recent study on *patients with endogenous hypertriglyceridemia* using dietary fat at three caloric percent levels.

In this study, acute and chronic effects of three isocaloric diets on plasma lipids and plasma lipoproteins were studied in ten patients with primary endogenous hypertriglyceridemia (type IV hyperlipoproteinemia). The diets used contained 20% protein, 50, 37 and 1% fat and 30, 43 and 79% carbohydrates, respectively. Cholesterol levels were similar with all diets (Fig. 2). Fasting values of plasma triglycerides were lower with the fat-containing diets compared to the high-carbohydrate diet. Diurnal patterns, however, were significantly higher with the former diets in eight of the ten patients (Fig. 3). Postprandial lipoprotein patterns on fat-containing diets were characterized by chylomicronemia and marked changes of concentration and composition of other lipoprotein classes.

Ginsberg et al. (1976) have recently published evidence that even with 30 calorie percent fat, alimentary lipemia may be marked. Thus, if, analogous to diabetic therapy, control of hypertriglyceridemia is meant to imply low all-day levels rather than low fasting levels, a rather low-fat, high-carbohydrate diet seems to be superior in most patients with endogenous hypertriglyceridemia to diets containing more than 30 calorie percent of fat.

3. Epidemiological Evidence that Diet May Prevent Coronary Heart Disease

It is not necessary to remind this audience that the definite "Diet-heart study" has not been performed and, in the opinion of many, will never be performed. According to estimates of the Diet-Heart Review Panel (Ahrens, 1969) required sample size will vary inversely with the square of anticipated reduction of a coronary event by the experimental diet. If the reduction in the incidence of coronary heart disease associated with a reduction in serum cholesterol is estimated from the weight of the risk factor "hypercholesterolemia" in prospective studies, for a primary preventive study, reduction of serum cholesterol levels by about 10% could result in a reduction rate of coronary events by 25%. The Diet-Heart Review Panel estimates that in this case, for primary prevention studies, a minimum of 11,000 participants in a closed study population and a maximum of 219,000 participants in an open study would have to be recruited for 5 years. It should be stated that a study according to these criteria has not been performed up to now.

There were, however, a number of smaller studies involving a few hundred up to a few thousand persons, which were all started in the late 1950's or early 1960's (Heyden and Durham, 1972). All these studies aimed at primary prevention using dietary measures have shown a trend toward favorable results. The latest are data by Frantz and co-workers (1976) from the Minnesota Coronary Survey. In a total of 2298 person-years in < 50-year-old men participating in an institutional dietary trial of a cholesterol-lowering diet, the experimental group experienced considerably fewer atherosclerotic events (3/10) and deaths (2/12) than the control group. There was, however, no effect of diet in older men and in women (Frantz et al., 1975).

The results of multifactorial trials presently in progress in the United States are eagerly awaited but should not delay action in those countries where atherosclerosis and coronary heart disease is a major public health problem.

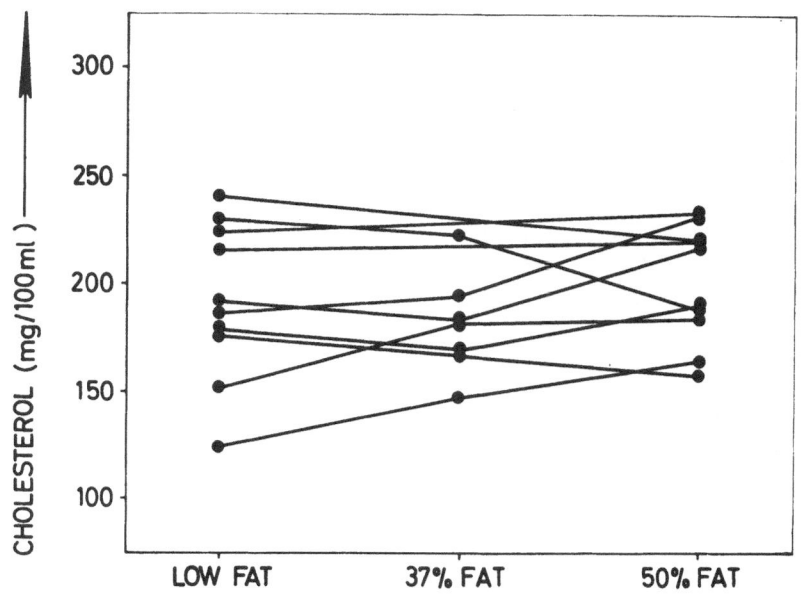

Figure 2. Plasma cholesterol levels in patients with endogenous hypertriglyceridemia (type IV hyperlipoproteinemia) with various diets differing in fat and carbohydrate content (P/S ratio 1.5 - 2.0)

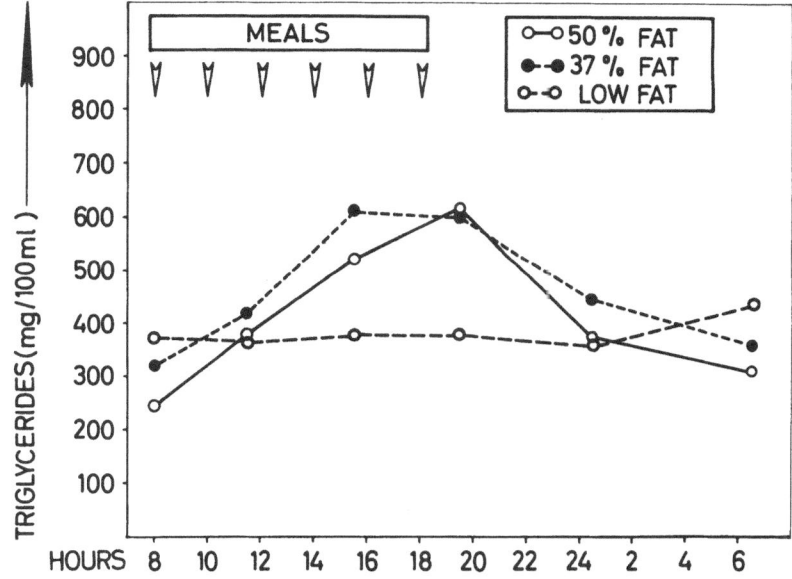

Figure 3. 24-h plasma triglycerides in 10 patients with primary endogenous hypertriglyceridemia (type IV hyperlipoproteinemia) with isocaloric diets of different
fat content (P/S > 1.5). The food was given during the day in 6 equal portions.
24-h studies were performed on each diet after 10 days on this particular regimen (from: Schlierf et al., Klinische Wochenschrift, in press, 1977)

The combined evidence, which comes from epidemiological studies on the relation between dietary fats, plasma lipid levels, and coronary heart disease, from case control studies, from clinical research and observations, in particular in hereditary disorders of lipid metabolism, from animal experiments, from pathologic investigations, and from primary and secondary prevention trials, points toward the high likelihood that dietary (saturated) fat and cholesterol cause atherosclerotic disease in a multifactorial frame. It would be indicated to reverse developments in dietary habits and other ways of life which have been brought into the industrialized societies only in very recent times and which most probably are detrimental. Prudent behavior does not carry any risk and is entirely feasible.

We believe that action is required now instead of waiting for "final" proof from a prospective unifactorial trial which will not be forthcoming. There are other examples in medicine that highly successful preventive programs are often begun before all the facts are known, e.g., the story of Edward Jenner, who in 1796 conducted the classical experiments leading to prevention and finally eradication of smallpox.

Accordingly, a number of governmental and voluntary health agencies have taken official positions on the diet and heart disease issue. The latest of these was issued by a Joint Working Party of the Royal College of Physicians of London and the British Cardiac Society in April, 1976. While differing in detail, these recommendations all include the advice that calories and total fat content of the diet be reduced, including reduction in the content of saturated fat. Most statements have advised, in addition, partial substitution of saturated by unsaturated fat. Generally, some dietary modification is recommended for the population at large, more stringent measures are recommended for particularly high-risk individuals, e.g., with hypercholesterolemia, which in these populations in adult men make up a proportion of 30% or more.

DRUGS AND ATHEROSCLEROSIS

R. Paoletti, A. Catapano, G.C. Ghiselli, and C.R. Sirtori

Introduction

Drug therapy of lipid disorders and atherosclerosis has changed scope in the
past few years. Attempts are made to induce regression of the arterial lesions,
instead of simply modifying plasma lipids levels. Drugs affecting lipoprotein
synthesis, structure, and turnover have been given increasing consideration. In
the preceding Atherosclerosis Meeting, Carlson et al. (1974) also noted that
drug and diet effects on lipoprotein composition are not identical for all lipoprotein classes, i.e., reciprocal changes between very low-density (VLDL) and
low-density lipoprotein (LDL) cholesterol may be observed when patients with
hypertriglyceridemia are treated with clofibrate, nicotinic acid, and/or a calorie restricted diet.

These observations, along with others, also dealing with altered lipoprotein composition following clofibrate (Wilson and Lees, 1972) had already cast some
doubts on the real significance of decreased plasma lipid levels as an index of
decreased atherogenicity. These doubts were further supported by the results of
the Coronary Drug Project (1975), a multicenter study of secondary prevention of
coronary heart disease (CHD), involving over 5000 patients, where clofibrate and
nicotinic acid were tested against a placebo in a double blind protocol. This
study provided, on the whole, negative findings, summarized in Tables 1 and 2.
The effects of the two drugs on cardiovascular morbidity and mortality were
negligible; there was also a significant incidence of side effects, particularly
with clofibrate, some of which may be explained on the basis of the drug's mechanisms of action, some others are of less clear origin, and possibly of doubtful
clinical significance (Sirtori et al., 1977a).

The results of the Coronary Drug Project should probably not be wholly ascribed
to a therapeutic inefficacy of the two hypolipidemic agents tested. The modest
reduction of plasma lipid levels in the treated groups may suggest an erratic
adherence to drug treatment. It should be noted that no plasma drug levels were
measured in the Coronary Drug Project. In addition to this, hyperlipidemia may
not be the most significant risk factor in the secondary prevention of CHD. Analysis of the placebo group in the Coronary Drug Project indicated that the first
six risk factors in secondary cardiovascular mortality cannot be corrected by
drugs of this type (Stamler, 1977). Among these risk factors are, in fact: ST segment depression, cardiomegaly on x-ray, and presence of Q waves on EKG. Plasma
cholesterol is only the seventh risk factor, lack of exercise the tenth, cigarette smoke the 13th; hypertriglyceridemia was not classified among the first 20
risk factors.

In spite of these considerations, and in spite of the positive results of a similar study with the anion exchange resin colestipol (Table 3), the Coronary Drug
Project was a strong incentive to revise the current beliefs in the pathogenesis
of atherosclerosis and in the role of plasma lipids in the development and reversal of the atherosclerotic lesions. It stimulated, in fact, further research
on the specific roles for some lipoprotein classes in the process of lipoprotein
deposition and removal from the arterial walls.

This review will, therefore, only marginally deal with strictly lipid-lowering
drugs. The main emphasis will be given to the present status of drugs affecting
lipoprotein composition, turnover, and uptake by the arterial walls.

Table 1. Clofibrate (CPIB), nicotinic acid (NA) and prevention of coronary heart disease (data from the Coronary Drug Project, 1975)

	Placebo	CPIB (1.8 g/day)	NA (3.0 g)
Total patients	2,789	1,103	1,110
% Mortality:			
Total	20.9	20.0	21.2
Cardiovascular	18.9	17.3	18.8
Lipid changes (% of pretreatment levels)			
Cholesterol	+0.3	−6.2	−9.6
Triglycerides	+6.7	−15.6	−19.4

Table 2. Clofibrate (CPIB, nicotinic acid (NA) and reventation of CHD (data from the Coronary Drug Project, 1975)

% Mortality Pretreatment cholesterol (mg/dl)	Placebo	CPIB	NA
< 250	19.7	20.4	21.5
> 250	22.3	19.6	20.8
Pretreatment triglycerides (mEq/L)[a]			
< 5	20.9	18.5	21.7
> 5	20.9	21.4	20.7

[a]5 mEq/L = 147.4 mg/dl.

Table 3. Colestipol and prevention of coronary heart disease[a]

	Placebo	Colestipol
Pretreatment mean plasma cholesterol (mg/dl)	313	308
Total myocardial infarctions	41	33
Deaths:		
Total	27	14[b]
Coronary	20	8[b]

[a]2100 patients with type II hyperlipoproteinemia were followed for 3 years. Reported data are from one-fourth of them, who had a history of prior myocardial infarction (Dorr et al., Adv. Exp. Med. Biol. *63*, 447, 1975).

[b]$P < 0.05$ vs. Placebo.

Drugs Modifying Lipoprotein Distribution

In addition fo lowering of plasma lipid fractions, a promising approach to the prevention of atherosclerosis is that of modifying lipid distribution in lipo-proteins. Different lipoproteins are in fact suspected of playing different, and at times opposite, roles in the atherosclerotic process.

Epidemiological and experimental evidence points out, in fact, that elevations of circulating low-density (LDL) and very low-density lipoproteins (VLDL) are a definite risk factor for the atherosclerotic disease (Goldstein et al., 1973). By immunological techniques (Hoff et al., 1976), the presence in the atheroscle-rotic lesions of apoproteins (B, C-III), which are major components of VLDL and LDL, has been clearly demonstrated. On the other hand, recent reports analyzing the lipoprotein profile of patients with and without CHD (Miller and Miller, 1975), have reported a negative correlation between high-density lipoprotein (HDL) levels and the incidence of CHD. Similar findings have been reported in different populations by comparing patients with similar cholesterol levels but differing incidence of CHD (Wiklund et al., 1975).

At present, two experimental interpretations may be offered for this likely "pro-tective" effect of HDL. The first interpretation suggests a role for HDL in the transport of free cholesterol from lipoproteins and tissues to the liver (Glom-set, 1976): in vitro studies on Landschütz ascites cells (Stein and Stein, 1973; Stein et al., 1975) and on cultured smooth muscle cells from rats (Stein et al., 1975; Jackson et al., 1976), have, in fact, shown that the exchange of choles-terol between cell membranes and HDL occurs in a nonenzymic way, concomitant with a transfer of phospholipids. Another protective mechanism is based on the inhibitory effect of HDL on the LDL uptake and cholesterol accumulation, both in cultured swine muscle cells (Carew et al., 1976) and in human endothelial cells (Stein and Stein, 1976) (Table 4). A possible explanation for these findings would consider competition between LDL and HDL for the same cellular binding sites (Goldstein and Brown, 1975). Although both of these hypothetic mechanisms remain speculative, they support the epidemiological and experimental evidence for a protective role of HDL in the atheromatous process and encourage pharmaco-logic studies toward the development of agents increasing the concentration of HDL or decreasing the cholesterol ratio between LDL and HDL.

Table 4. Effect of HDL on the binding, uptake, and degradation of ^{125}I labeled LDL[a]

Lipoprotein	Binding	Uptake	Degradation
LDL (10 ng/ml)[b]	1	1	1
LDL (10 ng/ml) + HDL (50 ng/ml)[b]	0.72	0.66	0.72
LDL (10 ng/ml) + HDL (100 ng/ml)[b]	0.51	0.57	0.41
LDL (40 ng/ml)[c]	1	1	1
LDL (40 ng/ml) + HDL (50 ng/ml)[c]	0.58	0.69	0.71
LDL (40 ng/ml) + HDL (100 ng/ml)[c]	0.47	0.53	0.53
LDL (40 ng/ml) + HDL (200 ng/ml)[c]	0.39	0.40	0.34

[a] Results from experiments with LDL alone are taken as 1.

[b] Data adapted from Stein et al. (1976). Human endothelial cells and human lipoproteins.

[c] Data adapted from Carew et al. (1976). Swine smooth muscle cells and swine lipoproteins.

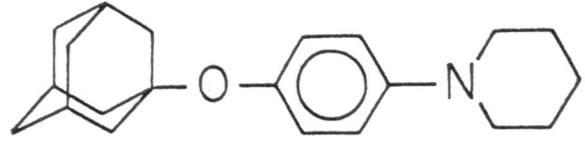

Figure 1. Chemical structure of U-41,792

Table 5. Effect of various hypolipidemic agents on plasma cholesterol and lipoprotein levels in male rats after fat feeding[a]

	Dose of drug mg/kg	Cholesterol	HPL[c]	HPL/TC[d]
Controls	--	1[b]	1[b]	1[b]
Clofibrate	200	0.61[e]	0.71	1.16
	100	0.77	0.76	0.98
Niacin	400	0.64[e]	0.74	1.15
Probucol	200	0.84	0.86	1.03
Lentysine	25	0.53[e]	0.54[e]	1.01
	3	0.63[e]	0.59[e]	0.94
D-thyroxine	3	0.28[e]	0.29[e]	1.04
Estrone	6	0.38[e]	0.47[e]	1.25[f]
	3	0.63[e]	0.59[e]	0.94
U-26,328	100	0.52[e]	0.42[e]	0.81[f]
	50	0.68[f]	0.66[f]	0.96
U-41,792	50	0.50[e]	0.34[e]	0.69[e]

[a] Data from Shurr et al. (1976).

[b] Values from control rats are taken as 1.

[c] Heparin precipitable lipoprotein cholesterol (d < 1.040).

[d] Ratio between heparin precipitable lipoprotein and total cholesterol.

[e] $P < 0.01$ vs. controls.

[f] $P < 0.05$ vs. controls.

A screening of compounds which may affect the cholesterol ratio between HDL and LDL was recently carried out by Shurr et al. (1976). The ratio of heparin-Ca^{++} precipitable lipoprotein cholesterol (d < 1.040) to total plasma cholesterol (HPL/TC) was tested in rats, receiving a lipid-rich diet for 4-5 days (Day et al., 1976). Among 3500 tested compounds, a bicyclooxyaniline (U-26,238) was found effective in lowering the HPL/TC ratio as well as plasma total cholesterol.

It was later shown that U-41,792 (Fig. 1), a derivative of U-26,238, was the most effective compound of this series (Table 5). In contrast to these agents, drugs presently used in the clinical management of hyperlipidemias (clofibrate, nicotinic acid, etc.) do decrease total cholesterol levels, but without influencing the HPL/TC ratio. By ultracentrifugal analysis of the two lipoprotein fractions (d < 1.040 and d 1.040-1.21), it was also noted that U-41,792 markedly decreases d < 1.040 lipoproteins while increasing those in the density range between 1.040-1.21 (Day et al., 1976). These effects are evident in rats, less so in mice and quails. In rats, at high doses, U-41,792 induces hepatomegaly and decreased food intake; for these reasons, it was not entered into clinical testing. To date, no agent of clinical interest affecting the HPL/TC ratio has been described with the possible exception of lipantyl, a clofibrate congener, which reportedly loweres the HPL/TC ratio in rats on a lipid-rich diet (Wülfert, personal communication).

Compounds specifically increasing HDL levels are also under investigation. A synthetic estrogen derivative with such properties, and devoid of hormonal activity, is currently under study (Day, personal communication). It may be noted that another estrogen derivative, DBCO (dibenzylcyclooctanone), which displays potent hypolipidemic properties, was instead recently found ineffective on the HPL/TC ratio (Cayen et al., 1976).

Drugs Modifying the Interaction of Lipoproteins With the Arterial Wall

Constituents of the arterial wall change during the course of the aging process, as well as in the various phases of atheromatosis. In particular, sulfated mucopolysaccharides (MPS) and glycoproteins increase with age and with the development of atherosclerosis (Smith, 1965; Gan et al., 1976). The presence of arterial MPS appears to be necessary for the interaction with lipoproteins (Srinivasan et al., 1972). Extraction of lipids and lipoproteins from the atheromatous arterial walls in humans and experimental animals has demonstrated the presence of both soluble and insoluble complexes of MPS with LDL, indicating that a similar interaction may occur in vivo (Berenson et al., 1971). It was recently shown that "free" MPS (i.e., sulfate-rich species) are more reactive with LDL in human serum than "bound" MPS (Nakashima et al., 1975).

In the case of *glycoproteins,* a significant advance in the understanding of the development of the atheromatous process has been the isolation of an aortic fraction which specifically binds VLDL and LDL in vitro (Camejo et al., 1975). Some human LDL fractions, more reactive with this arterial binding component, were recently analyzed (Camejo et al., 1976); "hyperreactive" LDL has a high cholesterol/phospholipid ratio and possibly specific apoprotein components. Atherosclerotic lesions in patients are strongly correlated to the presence of LDL of high reactivity (Camejo et al., 1976).

A pharmacologic approach to the MPS-lipoprotein interaction was suggested by Day et al. (1975). These authors demonstrated a significant inhibition of the in vitro binding of ^{125}I LDL to isolated arterial segments, by adding heparin, chondroitin sulfates, and different heparinoids to the system (Day et al., 1975; Day and Levy, 1975). The hypothesis that addition of hexogenous MPS may saturate the LDL binding sites, thus making the lipoprotein unavailable for arterial binding, was further supported by in vivo data (Sirtori et al., 1977b). By infusing intravenously a sulfated MPS of duodenal origin (3-GS) to rabbits injected with a ^{125}I HC-VLDL, which has a high affinity for the arterial wall, a significant inhibition of arterial uptake occurred (Fig. 2). 3-GS also inhibited in vitro the interaction between the same lipoprotein and the binding glycoprotein previously described.

The protection by sulfated MPS, in addition to the above-mentioned competitive mechanism, may also have other explanations. Lipoprotein lipase, released by sulfated MPS from the arterial surface (Zilversmit, 1973), may in fact inhibit lipoprotein uptake. MPS, as shown by Goldstein et al. (1976), release LDL from the cell surface receptors.

Heparin and parenteral heparinoids have several disadvantages when used in the prevention of atherosclerosis. They are expensive, require continued parenteral administration, and may have long-term side effects (Wessler, 1974).

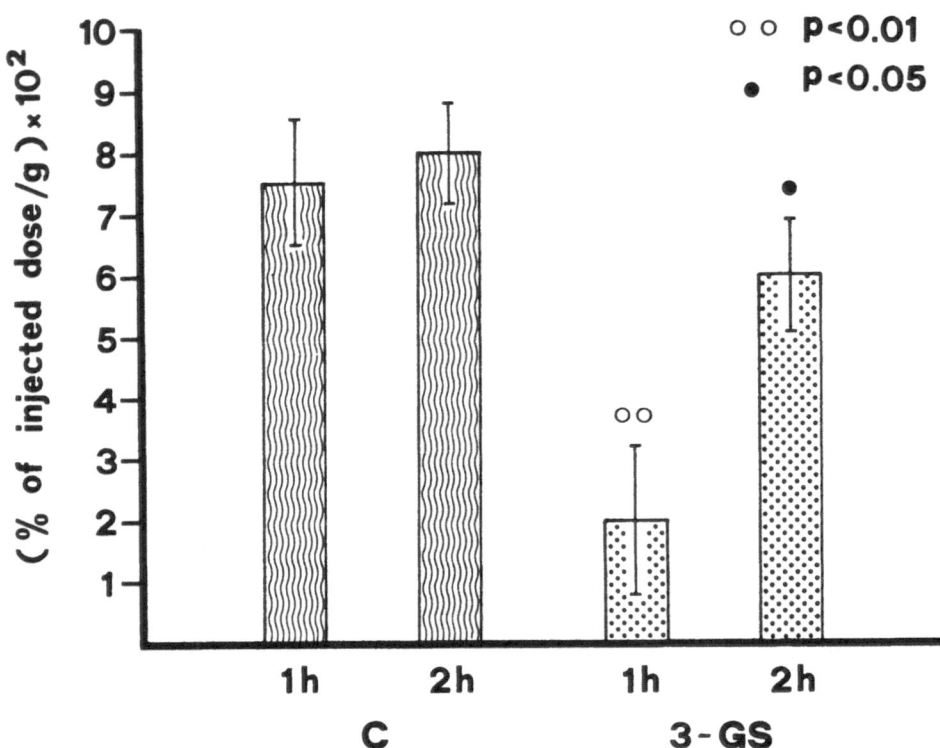

Figure 2. Effect of the infusion of a sulfated mucopolysaccharide (3-GS) on the aortic uptake of radioactivity in rabbits after i.v. injection of ^{125}I VLDL (d < 1.019) from cholesterol-fed rabbits (HC VLDL). C = rabbits infused with saline, 3-GS = rabbits infused with 3-GS

Phospholipids, which also represent a very effective preventive treatment of atherosclerosis in animals (Stafford and Day, 1975), also pose the same problem. Although there is no general agreement on the mechanism of the protective effect of phospholipids, both their surfactant properties (Adams and Morgan, 1967), as well as an inhibited interaction between lipoproteins and polyanions, such as arterial MPS, (Day and Levy, 1975) have been suggested. Recently, Blaton et al. (1976) noted decreased plasma cholesterol levels, as well as changes in lipoprotein composition after a course of intravenous and oral administration of "essential phospholipids" (i.e., linoleate-rich phospholipids) in type II and IV patients. In particular, linoleate concentration was markedly increased in HDL.

Drugs Modifying Lipoprotein Structure and Composition

The above considerations on the intrinsic atherogenicity of specific lipoprotein classes (namely, VLDL and LDL in humans), suggested the development of animal models with atherogenic lipoproteins. Pharmacologic treatments may be studied in these models, which may be natural or obtained after appropriate dietary or drug treatments.

This is the case of cholesterol-fed rabbits, which develop an abnormal lipoprotein in the density range d < 1.019, rich in cholesterol esters, and with an apoprotein composition similar to that of patients with type III hyperlipoproteinemia (Shore et al., 1974). Turnover studies with this lipoprotein indicated a delayed catabolism and an increased uptake in the aortic wall as compared to a control lipoprotein (Rodriguez et al., 1976a).

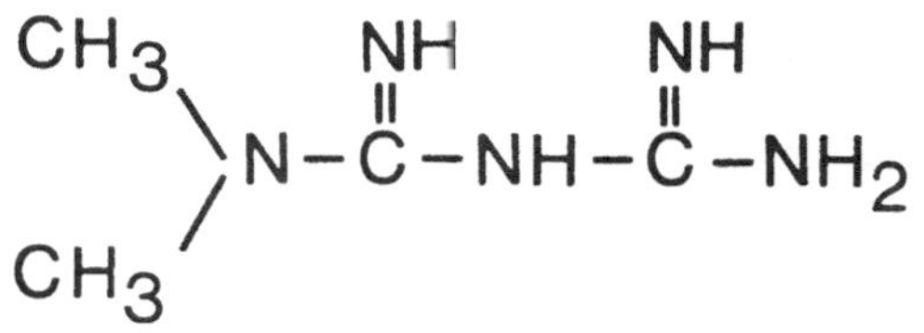

Figure 3. Chemical structure of metformin

Other atherogenic lipoproteins have been described in the cholesterol-fed pig
(Mahley et al., 1974). These animals carry the excess cholesterol in an HDL (HDL-
C), whose apoprotein composition is similar to that of the VLDL from patients
with type III hyperlipoproteinemia. HDL-C suppresses HMG-CoA reductase of pig
and human fibroblasts (Bersot et al., 1976), a property considered typical of
human LDL. HDL from cholesterol-fed rats also suppresses HMG-CoA reductase
(Breslow et al., 1975), an indication of potential atherogenicity.

Atherogenic lipoproteins, as pointed out, are often similar to the human VLDL observed in type III hyperlipoproteinemia. This lipoprotein is characterized by an
apoprotein rich in arginine (arginine-rich protein = ARP), whose presumable role
in atherogenesis is under investigation (Shore et al., 1974). It is suggested
that the ARP, similarly to apoB, may suppress HMG-CoA reductase. A lipoprotein
class with prominent ARP has been described in other animal models not necessarily developing atherosclerosis, such as sucrose-fed rats, where both HDL and VLDL
have increased ARP (Bar-On et al., 1976), or in cholesterol-fed guinea pigs
(Sardet et al., 1972). Mahley et al. (1974) described, on the other hand, hypo-
and hyperresponders among cholesterol-fed hypothyroid dogs. Hyporesponders show
a modest increase of VLDL cholesterol esters, the VLDL apoprotein does not show
a prominent ARP and there is no atherosclerosis. Hyperresponders have marked increase of cholesterol esters in VLDL, with a prominent ARP; they also develop
atherosclerosis.

Experience with drugs on these models has been limited. *Clofibrate*, whose antiatherosclerotic action in humans has been questioned due to unfavorable lipoprotein changes (increased LDL cholesterol in some patients after treatment) (Carlson et al., 1974), was tested by Roheim et al. (1974) in sucrose-fed rats. These
authors noted that C-proteins, as well as the ARP, increased by the diet, were
diminished by clofibrate. Clofibrate also reduced the A-proteins and the C II/
C III ratio in HDL, which had been increased by sucrose. It appeared also that
the B-apoprotein was moved from LDL to VLDL.

A more complete analysis of plasma lipoprotein changes in a model of experimental
atherosclerosis after pharmacologic treatment was recently provided by the administration of *metformin* to cholesterol-fed rabbits (Marquié and Agid, 1968).
Metformin (Fig. 3), a biguanide drug used in the clinical treatment of maturity
onset diabetes (Sterne, 1964), showed a promising antiatherosclerotic effect,
when administered to cholesterol-fed rabbits. This effect is independent from
the reduction of plasma cholesterol (Sirtori et al., 1977c). When given to cholesterol-fed rabbits, in fact, metformin only slightly reduces plasma total cholesterol, but a dramatic reduction of the aortic concentration of cholesterol
esters takes place (Table 6). The compositions of plasma VLDL (d < 1.019) (which
show the most marked modifications after cholesterol feeding) from rabbits fed
cholesterol (HC) and cholesterol + metformin (HC+Met) differed, on the whole,
only for a significant increase of phospholipids in HC+Met. The relative concentration of cholesterol esters and their fatty acid composition were not modified
by metformin (Sirtori et al., 1977c).

Interesting differences were, however, observed in the phospholipid distribution
and in the apoproteins of drug-treated animals. The phosphatidylcholine/sphingo-
myelin ratio (PC/Sph) is increased from 2.5 (HC VLDL) to 3.8 (HC+Met VLDL) (Table 7). HC+Met VLDL also show an elevation of phosphatidylinositol (PI), which
is about three times higher than in control and HC VLDL. This finding is of par-

ticular interest, because PI has been associated with an inhibited LDL-polyanion precipitation, an in vitro model of atherosclerosis (Day and Levy, 1975); it may also be related to the different ultrastructure of HC and HC+Met VLDL (Fig. 4).

Table 6. Plasma and tissue cholesterol from control (C) cholesterol-fed (HC)[a] and cholesterol+metformin fed (HC-Met)[b] rabbits ($\bar{x} \pm$ SD of six animals, after 60 days of treatment)

	C	HC	HC + Met
Plasma cholesterol (mg/dl)	80 ± 14	1409 ± 297[c]	1085 ± 212[c]
Aortic cholesterol esters (mg/g of tissue)	0.11 ± 0.03	1.39 ± 0.19[c]	0.38 ± 0.07[cd]
Liver cholesterol (mg/g of tissue)	1.97 ± 0.24	24.56 ± 3.02[c]	23.71 ± 2.4[c]

[a] 2 g/day of cholesterol.

[b] 2 g/day of cholesterol + 135 mg/kg/day of Metformin.

[c] $P < 0.01$ vs. C.

[d] $P < 0.01$ vs. HC.

Table 7. Distribution of phospholipids of VLDL from control (C), hypercholester-emic (HC) and hypercholesteremic treated with metformin (HC+Met) rabbits ($\bar{x} \pm$ SD of six animals)

	C	HC	HC + Met
Origin	1.89 ± 0.61	1.80 ± 0.60	2.26 ± 1.10
Phosphatidylcholine	73.06 ± 2.54	61.90 ± 1.09[a]	65.05 ± 2.00[a]
Lysophosphatidylcholine	3.96 ± 1.52	5.98 ± 1.40	6.49 ± 1.20
Phosphatidylinositol	3.23 ± 0.31	2.44 ± 0.42	4.84 ± 0.90[ab]
Sphingomyelin	6.94 ± 0.89	22.09 ± 1.01	17.23 ± 1.20[ab]
Phosphatidylethanolamine	11.94 ± 0.94	3.76 ± 0.70[a]	4.82 ± 0.80[a]

[a] $P < 0.01$ vs. C.

[b] $P < 0.01$ vs. HC.

Table 8. Aortic uptake of radioactivity (2 hours) after the injection of differ-ent VLDL (d < 1.019) into control (C) and treated rabbits ($\bar{x} \pm$ SD)

C VLDL into C	HC VLDL into C	HC+Met VLDL into C	HC VLDL into HC	HC+Met into HC+Met
4.00 ± 1.05[a]	6.79 ± 1.36	1.15 ± 0.58	6.00 ± 0.81	2.00 ± 0.80

[a] Values as (% of injected dose/g of tissue) x 10^2.

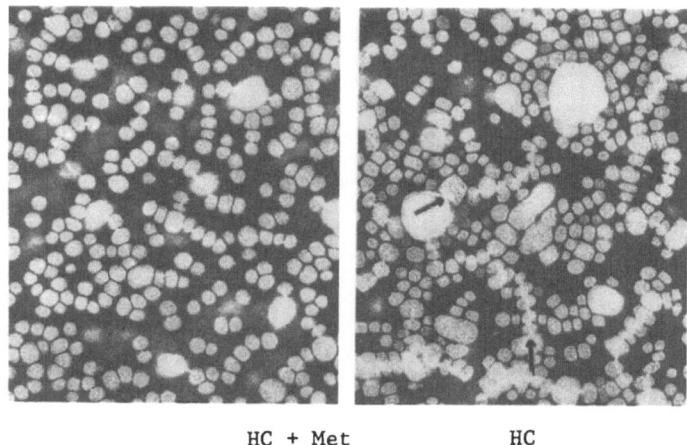

HC + Met   HC

Figure 4. Electron microscopy of VLDL (d < 1.019) from cholesterol-fed (HC) and cholesterol + metformin-fed (HC+Met) rabbits. The arrows indicate the presence of fusions and stickiness between particles (X 60,000)

In the latter, in fact, lipoprotein particles are more homogenous in size and show a markedly decreased stickiness.

The apoprotein composition of HC+Met VLDL shows a reduced content of the ARP, as compared to HC VLDL. Moreover, preliminary studies on the apoprotein components, after amino acid analysis of apoproteins, show the presence of protein constituents which are not found in HC VLDL. A major component is albumin, which moves in polyacrylamide gels containing urea with a similar mobility as the ARP, and which increases constantly with treatment. Albumin increases in the chylomicrons, VLDL and HDL of drug-treated animals (Shore et al., in preparation).

The presence of a significant amount of albumin probably explains the faster catabolic rate of HC+Met VLDL as compared to the HC lipoprotein (Rodriguez et al., 1976b). In steady state, in fact, ^{125}I labeled HC+Met VLDL has the same half-life of a control lipoprotein (whereas the half-life of HC VLDL is 40% longer). The distribution of radioactivity in the different lipoproteins at various intervals after injection is similar to that found after injection of similarly labeled control lipoproteins, whereas radioactivity from HC VLDL is not transferred to lipoproteins of higher density at an equivalent rate (Rodriguez et al., 1976b). These results are obtained both when lipoproteins are reinjected into the donor animals or into control rabbits.

The difference in the physicochemical properties of lipoproteins, after the various treatments, possibly explains also the different affinity for the arterial wall. Aortic uptake of radioactivity, measured at different intervals after the injection of control, HC and HC+Met VLDL clearly shows that HC+Met VLDL has the lowest uptake (Table 8). VLDL and LDL from HC+Met rabbits also have a reduced affinity for the isolated arterial binding component (Camejo et al., 1975) as compared to HC VLDL.

The mode of action of metformin on rabbit lipoprotein biosynthesis is debatable. A direct effect of metformin is supported by its preferential accumulation in the intestinal wall even after parenteral administration (Cohen and Costerousse, 1961); this observation is of particular interest, following recent data which suggest an important role for the intestine in lipoprotein biosynthesis (Eisenberg, 1976).

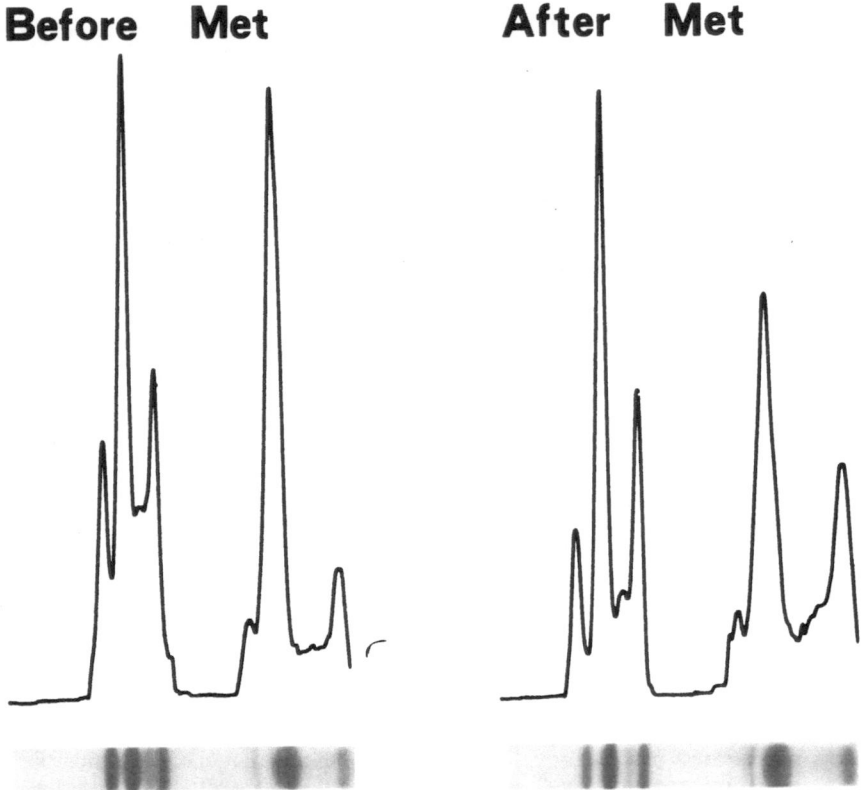

Before Met   **After Met**

Figure 5. Polyacrylamide gel electrophoresis of d < 1.019 apoproteins from a type III patient before and after 12 weeks of treatment with metformin (2,550 mg/day). 10% acrylamide gels containing 8M urea. The densitometric scans show a clear reduction of the area corresponding to the ARP band

Treatment with metformin of patients with hyperlipidemia has resulted in a significant lowering of plasma triglycerides, without reciprocal elevation of LDL cholesterol, and independent from the patients' glucose tolerance and insulin secretion (Sirtori et al., 1977d). Preliminary findings in patients with peripheral vascular disease treated with metformin have indicated some improvement of symptoms, as well as promising plethysmographic changes (Conti et al., 1976). Lipoprotein patterns were analyzed by us in four patients with type III hyperlipoproteinemia, where, as pointed out, lipoprotein changes similar to those of cholesterol-fed rabbits may be observed. In these patients, analysis of the composition of d < 1.019 lipoproteins consistently showed a decreased relative concentration of the ARP (Fig. 5), associated with a decrease of the cholesterol/triglyceride ratio and of sphingomyelin. These results indicate a good correlation with the data obtained in cholesterol fed rabbits.

The present status of drug therapy of atherosclerosis is one of great challenge: on the one hand, the basic knowledge of lipoprotein structure, metabolism, and arterial uptake provide new sites of action for specific drugs; on the other hand, the availability and recognition of drugs affecting specific pathways in lipoprotein metabolism may provide new powerful tools for the dynamic analysis and control of atherogenic lipoproteins.

Summary

Drug treatment of atherosclerosis through lipid lowering should be extremely selective. Indeed, lipid lowering per se may be accompanied by lipoprotein changes, i.e., increased LDL levels, which are considered unfavorable for the control of the atherosclerotic process.

1. Inhibited lipoprotein deposition in the arterial wall may be achieved by changing the ratio between atherogenic (VLDL and LDL) and antiatherogenic lipoprotein (HDL) fractions. This ratio, optimal in women and in populations with a lower incidence of CHD, may be reduced by pharmacologic treatments still under investigation.

2. Agents, such as mucopolysaccharides or phospholipids, inhibit lipoprotein deposition in the arterial wall. The affinity of lipoproteins for the artery may be reduced by inhibiting the uptake or by inducing specific physicochemical changes.

3. Another approach may be that of drugs modifying lipoprotein composition. This is exemplified by metformin, which, in cholesterol-fed rabbits, significantly reduces atheromatosis without markedly modifying plasma cholesterol levels. Analysis of lipoproteins from treated animals show striking changes, as compared to animals fed a high-cholesterol diet. These changes indicate the feasibility of reducing atherogenicity of lipoproteins without markedly decreasing plasma lipid levels.

SURGICAL MANAGEMENT OF HYPERLIPIDEMIA*

Henry Buchwald, Ignacio J. Guzman, Richard B. Moore, and Richard L. Varco

At the present time, there are three clinical surgical procedures that have been demonstrated to lower the circulating lipids: jejunoileal by-pass for management of morbid obesity, end-to-side portacaval shunt, and partial ileal by-pass. The primary purpose of jejunoileal by-pass is to achieve a caloric absorptive defect and subsequent weight reduction; an accompanying effect is plasma cholesterol and triglyceride lowering. Systemic diversion of the portal blood stream, long employed in the treatment of portal hypertension and esophageal varices, has been suggested as a therapeutic approach in the treatment of type IIa homozygous hyperlipoproteinemia in children. The partial ileal by-pass was designed specifically as a means to achieve cholesterol lowering.

Jejuno-Ileal By-Pass

Morbid obesity, which can be described as a maintained body weight 100 pounds over "ideal" insurance table weights for age and sex, is a serious medical problem in many parts of the world today, especially in the industrialized Western countries. There is essentially no organ system not afflicted by the complications of obesity. Indeed, actuarial tables clearly document a reduction in life expectancy as a near exponential function of excess body weight (Dublin and Marks, 1951). Wadd as early as 1819 was correct when be stated, "Corpulency is not only a disease itself but an harbinger of others."

The balance sheet on jejunoileal by-pass must yet be tallied. We have yet to judge a mean 100 poind weight loss, reduction in blood pressure, improved cardiac function, improved respiratory function, reversal or mitigation of diabetes mellitus, improvement of osteoarthritic problems, some relief of peripheral venous insufficiency, improved exercise capacity, improved quality of life, and a probable prolongation of life for the majority *against* operative mortality and morbidity, diarrhea, vitamin B_{12} malabsorption, transient electrolyte malabsorption, and, in about 5 - 10%, transient alopecia, episodic polyarthralgia, oxalate nephrolithiasis, and liver failure. Critical analysis of the operative results, over the past 15 years, by surgeons, internists, and psychiatrists, is shifting from condemnation of the procedure to strong affirmation (Buchwald et al., 1975b; The Kroc Foundation, 1977)

We have completed a study of the frequency and distribution of lipid levels among 274 morbidly obese patients. These patients were not hypercholesterolemic. The distribution of cholesterol levels was identical to that found in a normal weight population, corrected for age and sex. Triglyceride data revealed that 26% had fasting triglyceride values greater then 200 mg%.

All patients in our jejunoileal by-pass series (now numbering about 600) have had a marked reduction in their serum lipids. The cholesterol lowering has averaged 41% and seems to be independent of the preoperative cholesterol concentration. A significant number of our patients have a postoperative cholesterol value

*Supported by National Heart and Lung Institute Grants HL 11901 and HL 15265 and a Special Legislative Appropriation of the State of Minnesota. Direct reprint requests to Dr. Henry Buchwald, Box 290, University of Minnesota Hospitals, Minneapolis, Minnesota 55455.

below 100 mg%. In distinction, the serum triglyceride response appears to be directly relalated to the initial triglyceride level. The average triglyceride reduction has been 35%; however, for those individuals with preoperatively low triglyceride concentrations, the postoperative reduction was relatively small, whereas the triglyceride lowering in the hypertriglyceridemic subjects was marked.

Portacaval Shunt

Patients with type II homozygous hyperlipoproteinemia usually will die of cardio-vascular complications before reaching 30 years of age. Furthermore, these individuals rarely have a normal childhood, since they are often afflicted with symptomatic xanthomata and coronary artery disease very early in life, frequently prior to puberty. Medical treatment for this disease has been disappointing, both biochemically and clinically. The role of partial ileal by-pass in the management of this genetic defect has not, as yet, been clearly defined (see the following Section). Starzl et al. suggested in 1973 that the end-to-side portacaval shunt might play a positive role in the treatment of these children.

Winter et al. demonstrated in 1941 that portacaval shunt would reduce the serum cholesterol in dogs. The opposite result was reported by McAllister et al. (1961) in cholesterol-fed, hypothyroid dogs. Waddell and Hurley (1964) showed a de-creased serum cholesterol after portacaval transposition in diabetic dogs. In 1971, Kader et al. confirmed cholesterol lowering after portacaval shunt in the dog and, in 1973, this group (Kader et al., 1973) reported nine patients who had undergone portacaval shunt for portal hypertension, all had lower postoperative serum cholesterol values.

Starzl and associates (1973) have observed a decrease in the serum cholesterol concentration after portacaval shunt in their patients with glycogen storage disease. They performed the first portacaval shunt in a homzygous type II hyper-lipoproteinemic patient. This 12-year-old girl had severe angina pectoris and a previous myocardial infarction. The patient had a satisfactory response in the serum cholesterol level and symptomatic improvement; unfortunately, she died 18 months after operation of a probable cardiac arrhythmia.

By personal communications, we surmise that about 20 patients have been treated with portacaval shunt for homozygotic hypercholesterolemia. Published data are available for only eight for them; two have been operated upon by Starzl (Starzl et al., 1973) (lipid dynamics performed on the latter by Bilheimer and asso-ciates, 1975), four by the Johannesburg group of Stein et al. (1975), and two by Cywes' group (1976) in Capetown (Table 1). The first patient operated upon by Cywes showed a cholesterol lowering for months, followed by a rise to baseline levels secondary to thrombosis of the shunt. Three patients have been alluded to by Fischer in a published discussion on portacaval shunt mechanisms (Coyle et al., 1976).

It should be noted that most of these patients were preoperatively treated by intravenous hyperalimentation, which has a demonstrated potential for marked cholesterol lowering as long as the intravenous infusion is maintained. The largest cholesterol reductions in the eight patients listed on Table 1 occurred while they were on intravenous hyperalimentation. The subsequent portacaval shunt improved but little on this earlier cholesterol lowering. Indeed, for one of the patients reported by Stein and associates (1975), the postportacaval shunt-induced cholesterol reduction was not as marked as that of the postintravenous hyperalimentation cholesterol lowering. Fischer (Coyle et al., 1976) has stated that the portacaval shunt was not as effective in lowering the plasma cholesterol as hyperalimentation. An implication of these data is that a preoperative trial of hyperalimentation might be useful in predicting the magnitude of the potential response after portacaval shunt.

Table 1. Published portacaval shunt (PCS) results

Reference	Pt.age years	Prehyperali- mentation cholesterol (mg%)	Posthyperali- mentation cholesterol (mg%)	Post-PCS choles- terol (mg%)	Total · follow-up (mos.)
Starzl et al. (1973)	12	769	390	239[b]	18
Starzl et al. (1973)	6	997	-	578	5
Stein et al. (1975	7	1000[a]	880[a]	600[a]	5
Stein et al. (1975	27	1100[a]	650[a]	600[a]	2
Stein et al. (1975)	16	1350[a]	800[a]	750[a]	1 1/2
Stein et al. (1975)	10	800[a]	550[a]	650[a]	1 1/2
Cywes et al. (1976)	2 1/2	950[a]	-	700[a] [c]	13
Cywes et al. (1976)	4	681	-	435	9
Mean values		956	654	569	
Mean %↓			32%	40%	

[a]Values as best determined from published graphs; actual numbers not published.

[b]Six months after PCS.

[c]Just prior to thrombosis of the PCS, 8 months, postop.

The mechanism of action of the portacaval shunt in reducing circulating cholesterol remains to be ascertained. This brief clinical review does not permit discussion of the controversial data that have been published from several different
laboratories (Bilheimer et al., 1975; Coyle et al., 1976; Starzl and Lee, 1975;
Carew et al., 1974). The full potential of the portacaval shunt may only be realized when it is combined with other means of cholesterol reduction. For that
reason the elucidation of the mechanism(s) of action of the portacaval shunt is
imperative and not merely academic.

Few conclusions can currently be drawn regarding portacaval shunt in the treatment of the hyperlipidemias. We believe the operation should only be performed
by investigational groups in type II homozygous individuals. Only time and more
data will ascertain the cost-benefit ratio, taking into consideration the incidence of encephalopathy, the operative risk, and the fact that the cholesterol
level achieved has fallen short of the recommended "safe" upper limit. In the
published cases, the cholesterol reduction has been 40% from the prehyperalimen-
tation baseline with a mean postportacaval shunt cholesterol of 570 mg%.

Partial Ileal By-Pass

In a review of 1,305,805 patient-months experience, type specific diet therapy
for hyperlipidemia, initiated in adulthood, has been shown to cause a net mean
cholesterol lowering of 6-7% (Buchwald et al., 1974a). Members of a free-living
population, as a rule, do not adhere to a prudent dietary program, if it is contrary to their national and customary food preferences (Brown and Green, 1962;
Lewis et al., 1970). Evaluation of the effect of cholestyramine in a large well-
controlled clinical trial will need to await completion of the Lipid Research
Clinics study. The comparably large Coronary Drug Project (1975) showed only a
6.5% cholesterol reduction for clofibrate and 9.9% for nicotinic acid. Furthermore, the Coronary Drug Project (1975) documented numerous and significant complications associated with the use of clofibrate and nicotinic acid. It should be

remembered, when new drugs are being considered for future clinical use, that the ethics group of the Coronary Drug Project was forced by the number and life-threatening nature of the complications to break the code of the study program twice and remove estrogens and dextrothyroxine from use in this trial (Coronary Drug Project, 1970, 1972). On the basis of these results after years of diet and drug therapy, as well as the undeniable implication of the Cornfield (1962) exponential risk equation, we concluded in the early 1960's that there was a great need for more effective, safe, lasting, and obligatory hyperlipidemia management.

In this brief survey, we will review only the clinical partial ileal by-pass data. The animal experimental literature for partial ileal by-pass through 1974 has been complied and analyzed (Buchwald et al., 1974a). Knowledge of certain of these metabolic studies in cholesterol dynamics is, we believe, essential to an understanding of this field.

The partial ileal by-pass operation is relatively simple and can be done by the experienced surgeon, in about 1 1/2 hours. After measuring the entire length of the small intestine, and end-to-side anastomosis is established between the proximal small intestine and the cecum, 200 cm or one-third the length of the small bowel (whichever is longer) from the ileocecal valve. We have published details of this procedure elsewhere (Buchwald et al., 1975a).

In our experience, the circulating cholesterol concentration is reduced an average of 41% from the preoperative and postdietary baseline after partial ileal by-pass (Buchwald et al., 1974a, 1974b). In combination with type-specific dietary management, a 53% cholesterol level lowering, on the average, has been achieved in type IIa individuals (Fig. 1) (Buchwald et al., 1968). Partial ileal

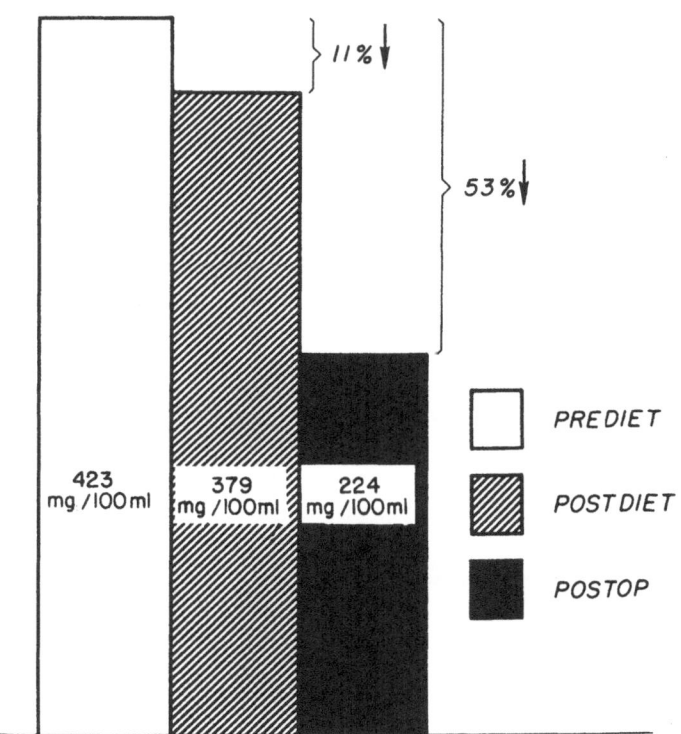

Figure 1. Effect of cholesterol-lowering diet and partial ileal by-pass on serum cholesterol levels in a cohort of 24 type II patients (reprinted by permission from Buchwald et al., 1974a)

by-pass, in addition to its effectiveness in the type IIa patient, lowers the cholesterol concentration in all of the hyperlipidemia types. These results have not been compromised by effect escape in our 13 years of experience.

The cholesterol lowering effect of the operation is neither uniform nor is it precisely predictable for each person. The lowering of cholesterol from the pre-operative, postdietary baseline has varied from 5% to 79%. In the series reported by investigative groups elsewhere in the United States and Europe, the mean additional cholesterol concentration reduction after that caused by dietary therapy has been virtually identical to our findings; namely, another 40% (Fritz and Walker, 1966; Lewis et al., 1968; Strisower et al., 1968; Swan and McGowan, 1968; Helsinger and Rootwelt, 1969; Rowe et al., 1969; Miettinen, 1970; Sodal et al., 1970; Clot et al., 1971; Streuter, personal communication; Morgan and Moore, personal communication)

To date, the least impressive responders have been the type IIa homozygous young people. Yet, Balfour and Kim (1974) reported two homozygous children followed for 3 years, with sustained cholesterol reductions of 42% and 33%.

Let us examine more closely the cholesterol responses as a function of lipopro-tein typing carried out prior to operation. We will employ "mixed type" to de-scribe those individuals with electrophoretic staining patterns characteristic for both type II and IV, and IIx for those imprecisely classifiable because they were operated upon prior to the general use of plasma triglyceride determinations. One year postoperatively, the plasma cholesterol reductions from the postdietary, preoperative baseline were: type IIa – 34.8%, type IIb – 41.3%, type IIx – 32.0%, type III – 47.5%, type IV – 45.6%, and mixed type – 41.1% (Fig. 2).

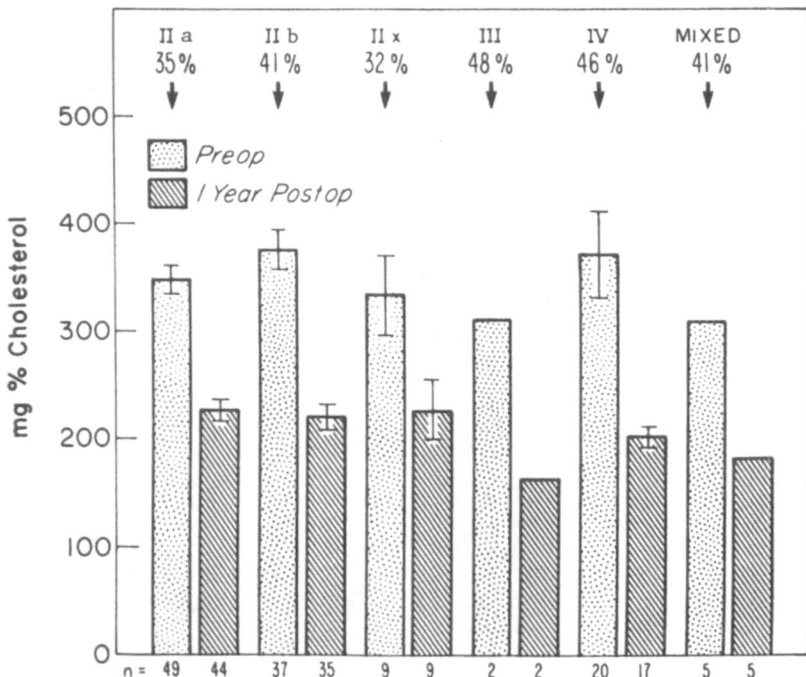

Figure 2. Average 1-year postoperative plasma cholesterol level response by lipo-protein type (± SE); type IIx = no triglyceride values before operation (re-printed by permission from Buchwald et al., 1974b)

The average cholesterol concentration of middle-aged men in the United States is about 250 mg%; the average preoperative cholesterol concentration reported for individuals who have undergone partial ileal by-pass has been over 330 mg%. Following partial ileal by-pass, better than 80% of these subjects have circulating cholesterol levels below 250 mg% and better than 50% have levels below 200 mg%.

Partial ileal by-pass has also demonstrated its effectiveness in lowering triglyceride levels following maximum type-specific dietary therapy (Buchwald et al., 1974a, 1974b). The largest reductions have been achieved in the type IV individuals with an average lowering of 53% from the postdietary baseline. A small paradoxical increase in triglyceride levels has been noted in the type IIa patients; nevertheless, despite this increase, the average triglyceride level has remained within the accepted normal range.

The partial ileal by-pass procedure has a documented operative mortality well under 1%, the presence of coexisting coronary artery disease in many of these patients notwithstanding (Buchwald et al., 1975b, 1974a). Wound infections, pulmonary emboli, or other serious postoperative complications have occurred in 2% of these patients (Buchwald et al., 1975b, 1974a).

Diarrhea is the one annoying side effect experienced by the majority of individuals after partial ileal by-pass (Buchwald et al., 1974a, 1974b; Strisower et al., 1968; Swan and McGowan, 1968; Helsinger and Rootwelt, 1969; Brown, personal communication; Miettinen, personal communication; Streuter, personal communication). Commonly, it is not persistent. Within a year or so, approximately 90% of patients have less than five bowel movements daily, without bowel control medications. The patients generally also report an increase in the firmness and consistency of stools with time.

Following partial ileal by-pass, vitamin B_{12} absorption is either severely impaired or totally lost (Buchwald, 1964). After several years, however, absorptive adaptation for vitamin B_{12} occurs in about one-half of these patients (Nygaard et al., 1970; Coyle et al., 1977). Nevertheless, we indefinitely prescribe parenteral vitamin B_{12} supplementation.

Contrary to jejunoileal by-pass, there are no electrolyte abnormalities, nutrient malabsorption, long-term weight loss, arthritic phenomena, nephrolithiasis, or hepatic dysfunction after the partial ileal by-pass operation.

Various investigators have reported a postoperative decrease in size, or even disappearance, of periorbital xanthelasma, subcutaneous xanthomata and tendon xanthomata, especillay of the plantar extensor tendons (Buchwald et al., 1974a; Helsinger and Rootwelt, 1969; Buchwald, 1970). By analogy, a reduction in size of xanthomatous lesions might indicate that other tissues' stores of lipid have been mobilized and excreted from the body.

Many individuals afflicted with angina pectoris have testified to a reduction in the frequency of their attacks, or to the complete disappearance of these symptoms during comparable effort after partial ileal by-pass (Buchwald et al., 1974a; Fritz and Walker, 1966; Swan and McGowan, 1968; Sodal et al., 1970. Sixty-nine percent of our patients with angina pectoris present prior to partial ileal by-pass experienced significant improvement postoperatively (Fig. 3). We have no proven explanation for this finding; however, in in vitro experiments utilizing rabbit blood, oxygen extraction from blood with a high-cholesterol content was significantly less than from blood with a low-cholesterol content (Steinbach et al., 1974).

Serial evaluation of coronary atherosclerotic plaque changes by arteriography yields data which are inconclusive (Rowe et al., 1969; Baltaxe et al., 1969; Knight et al., 1972). A randomized control population for objective statistical comparison has not been available. An appraisal of our patients indicates an apparent nonprogression rate of coronary artery disease in 55% of patients followed

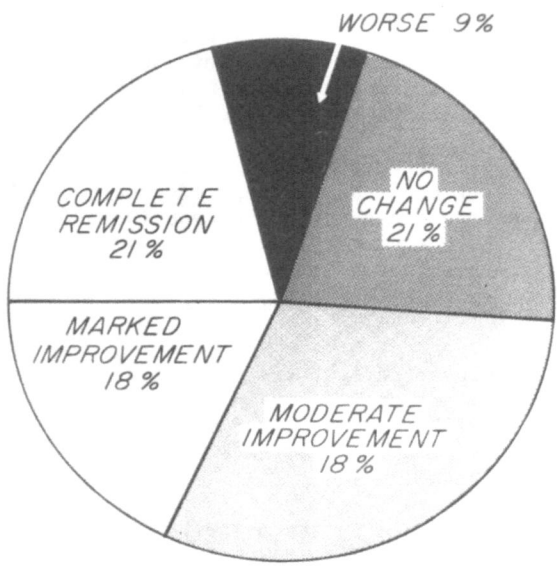

WORSE 9%

COMPLETE
REMISSION
21%

NO
CHANGE
21%

MARKED
IMPROVEMENT
18%

MODERATE
IMPROVEMENT
18%

Total Improvement: 69%

Figure 3. Relative change in angina pectoris symptomatology following partial ileal by-pass (reprinted with permission from
Buchwald et al., 1975b)

for up to 3 years (Knight et al., 1972). Also, coronary arteriographic evidence
of plaque regression has been noted in three partial ileal by-pass patients at
1 - 2 years (Fig. 4).

In conclusion, partial ileal by-pass is not proposed as the treatment of choice
for hyperlipidemia. We do believe, however, that it is the treatment of choice
for certain patients with hyperlipidemia.

Prospectus

If current intervention trials, one of which utilizes the partial ileal by-pass
operation, affirm the lipid-atherosclerosis hypothesis and clearly demonstrate
a reduction in cardiovascular risk by cholesterol lowering, then it will be imperative in clinical therapeutics to be able to reduce the plasma cholesterol
concentration. Not only reduce it by a modest degree for a transient period of
time but reduce it markedly, permanently, and without voluntary or involuntary
response escape. We suggest that optimal posttherapy cholesterol levels be 40%
or more below pretreatment values and below 200 mg%. Surgical methods of cholesterol lowering have the documented capacity to achieve optimal results. Singly,
in combination, and together with diet and drug therapy, the current lipid-lowering operations are part of the clinical lipodologist's armamentarium. Inventive
minds will, undoubtedly, suggest yet other surgical approaches to the hyperlipidemias.

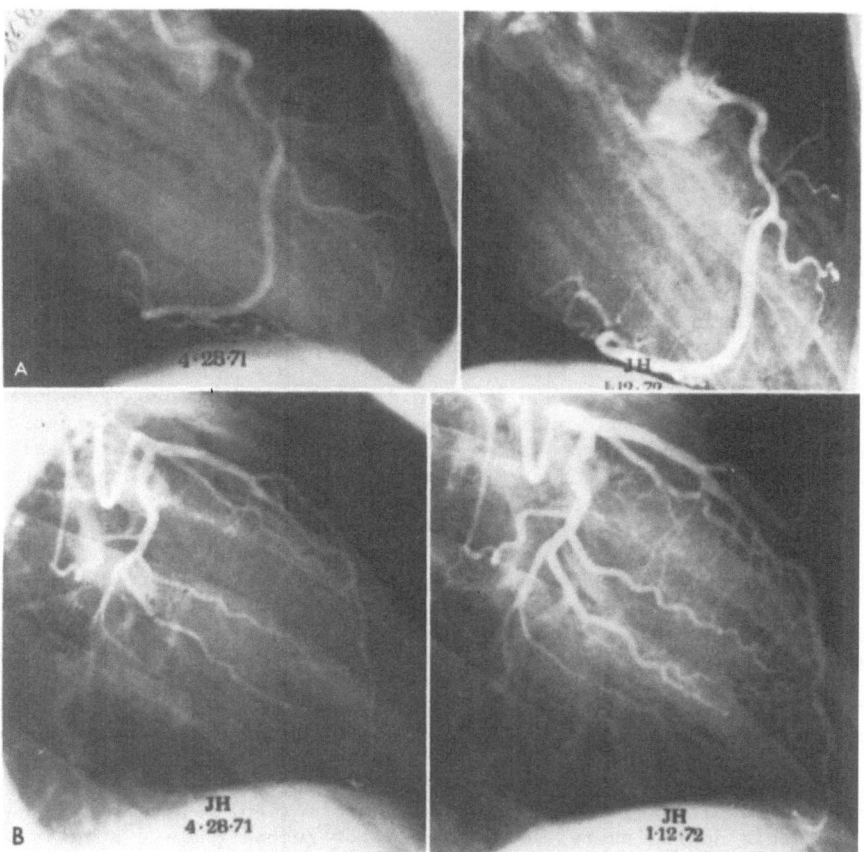

Figure 4. (A) Right coronary arteriograms showing plaque regression following partial ileal by-pass (preoperative x-ray on the left, 1-year postoperative on the right). (B) Preoperative (left) and 1-year postoperative (right) left coronary arteriograms of the same patient (reprinted by permission from Buchwald et al., 1975a)

METABOLIC ASPECTS OF THE MANAGEMENT OF OBLITERATIVE ATHEROSCLEROSIS*

Bengt Pernow

An obliterative atherosclerotic process reduces the inflow capacity to the affected tissue. Numerous studies in animals have yielded a detailed picture of the cellular and subcellular effects of a decrease in blood flow below a critical level. The consequences of ischemia have been studied most extensively in the myocardium (Bergström, 1962) and brain (Carlson and Ericsson, 1975). It is thus well-documented that tissue hypoxia due to a decreased oxygen delivery in relation to oxygen demand causes metabolic disturbances in the affected area, notably a decreased oxidative phosphorylation, increased glycolysis, decreased total rate of ATP regeneration and decreased tissue content of high energy phosphate compounds. In the heart, the ischemia produced by coronary obliteration impairs myocardial contractility and ventricular performance.

Similar studies have been presented concerning the effect of an impaired blood flow and ischemia on the metabolism of human tissues. It is thus clear than in man, too, myocardial ischemia reduces cardiac performance, and studies on the underlying metabolic changes in the myocardium are now in progress (Kaijser et al., 1976). In skeletal muscle, arterial obstructions lead to pain and fatigue during physical exercise, and it can be presumed that these symptoms are induced primarily be metabolic changes based on an inadequate supply of blood and oxygen.

This presentation illustrates how impairment of the blood flow capacity due to arterial obliteration will cause profound metabolic disturbances in human skeletal muscle during exercise. The effect of reconstructive surgery on physical performance as well as on blood flow and metabolism of skeletal muscle in patients with occlusive arterial disease of the leg is also described.

Subjects and Procedures

Thirty male patients with angiographically verified complete or almost complete occlusions of the iliac and/or femoral artery were studied. Their ages ranged from 43 to 65 years. Walking distance on an even level did not exceed 100 m and was limited by pain in the thigh and calf. No patient showed signs of congestive heart failure or diabetes and none was obese. All patients had normal intravenous glucose tolerance. Total serum cholesterol and total serum triglycerides were both above the 90th percentile of the Swedish population in every patient (Carlson and Ericsson, 1975). None took any drug regularly. The results were compared with data obtained under similar conditions in 12 healthy men of comparable age (40-49 years).

Leg blood flow was analyzed with a dye dilution technique (Wahren and Torfeldt, 1973). Samples were drawn from arterial and femoral venous blood via percutaneously inserted catheters for analyses of individual free fatty acids (FFA) and FFA radioactivity, $^{14}CO_2$, O_2, lactate, and glucose (Hagenfeldt et al., 1972). Lipid metabolism of the leg muscles was analyzed by a radioactive technique using ^{14}C-labeled oleic acid as tracer (Hagenfeldt et al., 1972). Muscle content of energy phosphate compounds and metabolites was studied on needle biopsy material

*This study was supported by grants from the Swedish Medical Research Council (04X-4554) and Petrus and Augusta Hedlunds Foundation.

(Bergström, 1962; Karlsson et al., 1970). Physical exercise was performed on a bicycle ergometer.

The values are given as mean ± SE.

Preoperative Results

Leg blood flow during exercise was considerably lower in the patient group than in the normals at comparable work intensities. Furthermore, as the work load gradually increased, there was a leveling of the leg blood flow instead of the linear relation observed in the control subjects. The arterial-femoral venous (a-v) oxygen difference was very high during exercise due to the considerable decrease in oxygen saturation of the femoral venous blood (Fig. 1). In spite of this, leg oxygen uptake (calculated as the product of leg blood flow and a-v oxygen difference) was in all patients significantly lower during heavier work than in the controls (Pernow et al., 1975).

The arterial concentration at rest and the changes during exercise of four main FFA (palmitic, stearic, oleic, and linoleic acid) were similar in the patients and the controls. At rest the turnover of oleic acid (calculated as the amount of radioactivity infused per unit time divided by the oleic acid specific activ-

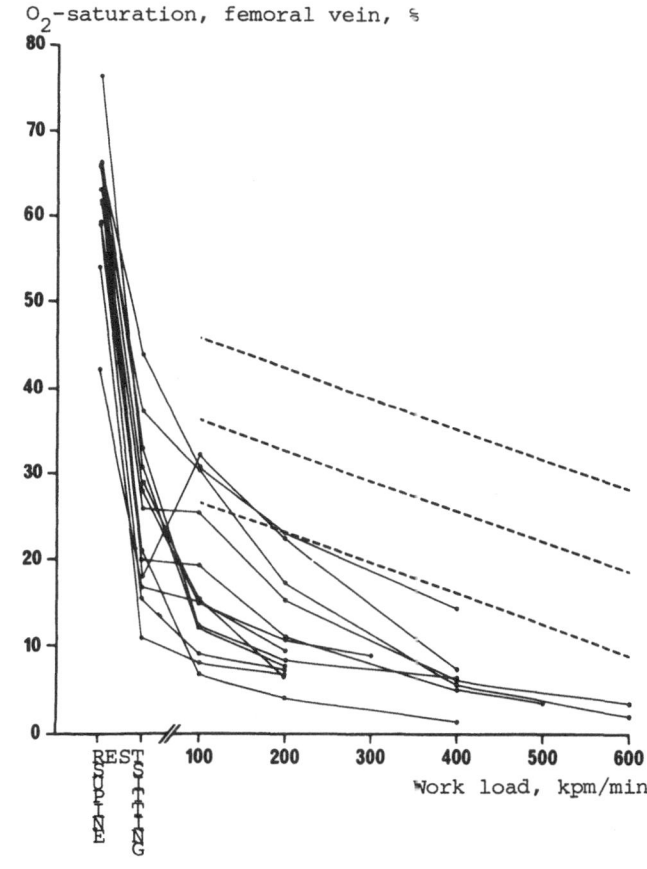

Figure 1. Oxygen saturation of the femoral venous blood at rest and during exercise in patients with occlusive arterial disease of the leg. Broken lines indicate mean ± 2 SD of the controls

ity) was the same in controls and patients, but during exercise the increase in turnover was significantly smaller in the patients. Neither the uptake of FFA (μmol/l plasma) nor the fractional uptake of FFA (the a–v difference of the radioactivity as a fraction of the arterial radioactivity) differed significantly, either at rest or during exercise, between patients and controls. Due to the significantly lower plasma flow, the rate or uptake of FFA (μmg/min) during exercise was much lower in the patients. Furthermore, the fractional oxidation of FFA (calculated as the v–a difference in $^{14}CO_2$ radioactivity divided by the a–v difference in ^{14}C oleate radioactivity) during exercise was significantly lower in the patients ($53 \pm 6\%$) than in the controls ($84 \pm 2\%$) and showed a negative regression on the simultaneous release of lactate (Fig. 2) and the lactate/pyruvate ratio measured in femoral venous blood (Hagenfeldt et al., 1972).

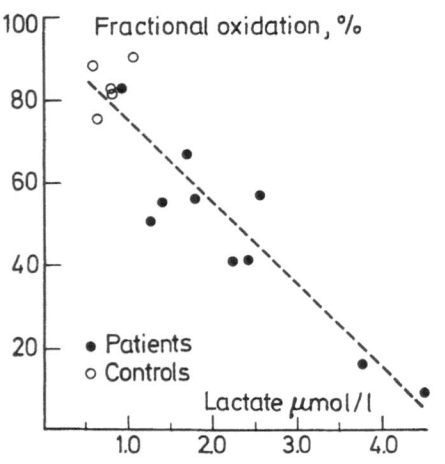

Figure 2. Fractional oxidation of FFA during exercise in relation to release of lactate

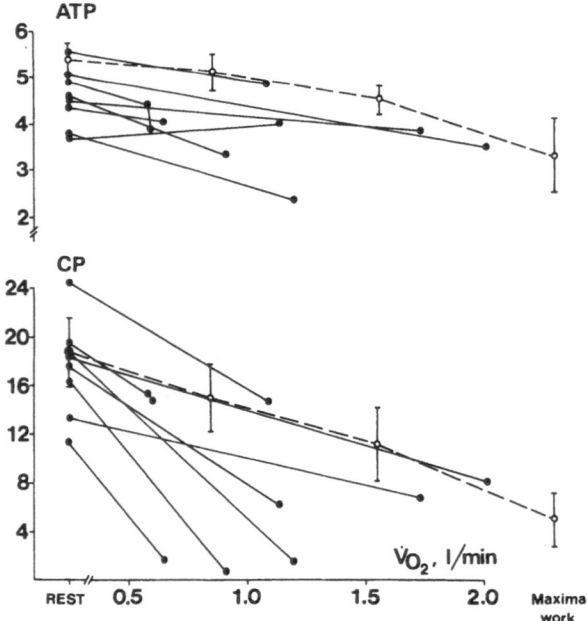

Figure 3. Muscle concentration of ATP and creatine phosphate at rest and immediatel after maximal work in patients with occlusive arterial disease of the leg (filled circles). Open circles and vertical bars indicate mean values $\pm$ 2 SD in the controls after submaximal and maximal work. The work intensity is indicated as oxygen uptake in the lungs ($\dot{V}_{O_2}$)

The arterial level of glucose did not differ at rest and rose approximately equally in both groups during exercise. The a-v glucose difference during exercise was, however, somewhat greater in the patients than in the controls ($p < 0.02$).

Muscle ATP concentration was significantly lower in the patients than in the controls both at rest and immediately after an identical exercise. Creatine phosphate was normal at rest, but the decrease in connection with exercise was considerably greater in the patients. Thus, some patients displayed an almost total exhaustion of creatine phosphate at work intensitites at which no decrease was observed in the controls (Fig. 3). Muscle glycogen was normal at rest and the decrease during exercise was of the same order of magnitude in patients and controls, although the exercise was experienced as very light by the controls but as completely exhaustive by the patients. Muscle lactate concentration increased rapidly in the patients during exercise, in contrast to the very slow rise in the controls. Thus, the mean lactate level for the patients was $12.1 \pm 2.3 \, \mu mol/kg$ wet tissue, compared with 2.7 ± 0.5 for the controls at an identical work load (Pernow et al., 1975). Similarly, the release of lactate from the exercising muscles was considerably increased (Fig. 4).

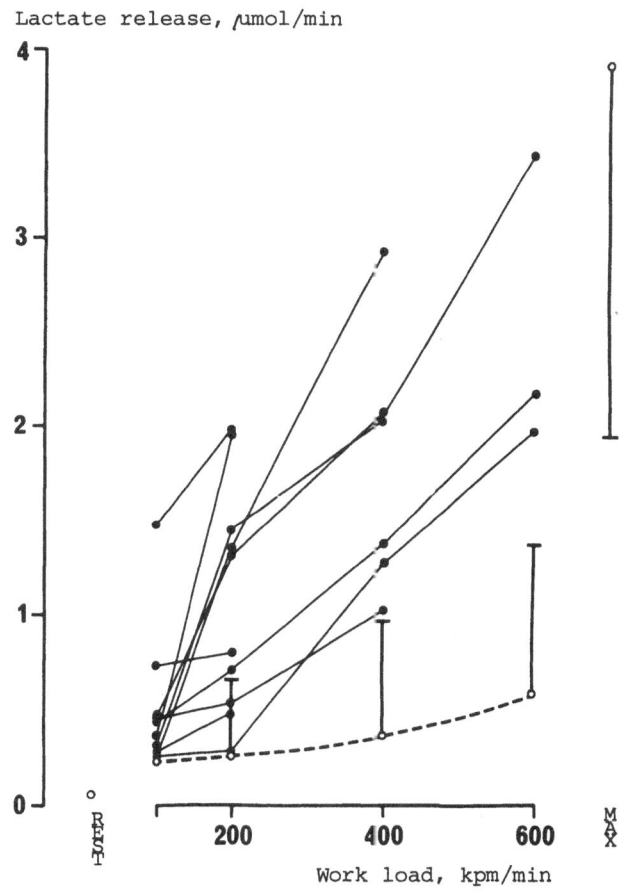

Figure 4. Release of lactate from the exercising muscles in patients with occlusive arterial disease of the leg. Broken line and vertical bars indicate mean ± 2 SD of the controls. The open circle and solid bar to the right indicate mean ± 2 SD of the controls performing exhaustive work

Postoperative Results

(Table 1). Repeated exercise test 3-6 months after reconstructive surgery (thrombendarterectomy + femoro-popliteal by-pass) showed a considerable improvement in physical working capacity. The postoperative metabolic study was performed at the same work loads as in the preoperative study and with the same experimental procedure. No symptoms of fatigue or pains occurred during the exercise period, in contrast to the severe pains experienced by the patients in the preoperative study. At comparable work intensities, leg blood flow (Fig. 5) and oxygen uptake were significantly higher than before surgery and increased linearly in relation to work intensity. A-v oxygen difference was much lower at comparable work loads. The arterial FFA level as well as the leg uptake of FFA per liter plasma had not changed significantly, while the fractional oxidation of oleic acid in the leg during exercise increased from a preoperative mean of $47 \pm 8\%$ to $90 \pm 10\%$ in the postoperative study ($p < 0.001$). The a-v glucose difference and the calculated glucose uptake by the leg muscles were unchanged. Release of lactate from the exercising muscles was significantly less than before surgery (Fig. 6).

There were no consistent pre- and postoperative differences with regard to the basal muscle concentration of ATP, creatine phosphate, glycogen, or lactate. During exercise, the decrease in creatine phosphate was considerably less postoperatively, while no significant change was seen in ATP. The breakdown of muscle glycogen was more pronounced postoperatively while production of lactate was considerably less.

Table 1. Effect of reconstructive surgery on the circulatory and metabolic adaptation during exercise in 11 patients with occlusive arterial disease

Variable	Significance of difference (p) pre- vs. postop
Heart rate	< 0.01
Pulmonary oxygen uptake	ns
Leg blood flow	< 0.01
Leg a-v O_2 difference	< 0.01
O_2-saturation, femoral vein	< 0.001
Leg O_2-uptake	< 0.05
Arterial lactate concentration	< 0.001
Leg a-v lactate difference	< 0.001
Leg lactate release	< 0.001
Arterial glucose concentration	ns
Leg a-v glucose difference	ns
Leg glucose uptake	ns
Muscle ATP	ns
Creatine phosphate	< 0.01
Glycogen	< 0.01
Lactate	< 0.01
Glucose	ns
Glucose-6-phosphate	ns

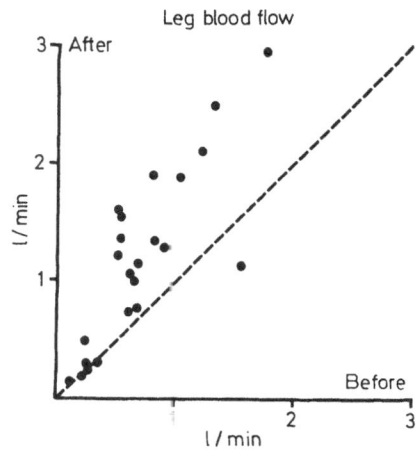

Figure 5. Leg blood flow analyzed at identical work loads before and after reconstructive surgery in patients with occlusive arterial disease of the leg. Broken line indicates line of identity

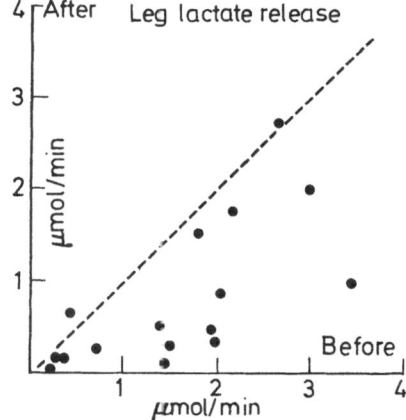

Figure 6. Release of lactate from the exercising muscles before and after reconstructive surgery in patient with occlusive disease of the leg. Broken line indicates line of identity

Discussion

The highest work load chosen in the present study, identical in controls and patients as well as pre- and postoperatively, provoked severe leg pains and cramps in the preoperative study but no symptoms postoperatively or in the controls. The leg blood flow reaction to exercise differed in two respects between the pre- and postoperative studies. Thus, the blood flow level on each load was significantly lower preoperatively and the flow pattern was different, with an early leveling off to a plateau which obviously represented the maximal blood flow permitted by the mechanical obstruction of the leg arteries. After surgical treatment, a linear relation was obtained between flow and work load in all patients and the flow pattern was now very similar to that of the controls at comparable work loads.

The limitation of blood flow through the untreated diseased legs was compensated to some extent by an more efficient extraction of oxygen from the blood during exercise, as evident from the larger a-v oxygen difference. The considerably lower oxygen uptake indicates, however, that this increased oxygen extraction did not entirely make up for the reduction in blood flow.

The reduction of blood flow capacity elicits profound changes in the metabolism of the exercising muscles. The lower turnover of oleic acid was probably a consequence of a reduced inflow of FFA to the exercising muscles. The most important finding with regard to FFA metabolism is obviously the severely impaired fractional oxidation of FFA in the preoperative patients compared with the postoperative state and the controls. Evidently, this is due to a lack of oxygen in the muscle cells, restricting the oxidative phosphorylation. The correlation between the decrease in fractional FFA oxidation and the increased accumulation of lactate in the muscle cell or the venous outflow speaks in favor of this hypothesis. It is interesting to note that in contrast to this finding, an increase in the fractional oxidation of oleate is found in heart muscle when anginal pain is induced by atrial pacing in patients with ischemic heart disease (Kaijser et al., 1976).

Surgical treatment resulted in a significant increase in the turnover of oleic acid and, above all, a normalization of the fractional oxidation of FFA, evidently due to an increased availability of oxygen, since the production of lactate was simultaneously decreased and the lactate/pyruvate ratio normalized.

The fate of the ^{14}C-labeled FFA not appearing as $^{14}CO_2$ is still somewhat obscure. However, in a few patients receiving high rates of oleic acid — ^{14}C infusions it was possible to demonstrate that the FFA label not recovered as $^{14}CO_2$ left the leg muscles quantitatively in the form of perchloric acid extractable, water-soluble metabolites, preferentially as radioactive acetate (Hagenfeldt et al., 1972). These findings support the theory that the restriction of fatty acid oxidation occurs at the level of acetyl-CoA utilization (Hagenfeldt and Wahren. 1972).

As for oxygen, the a-v difference for glucose was significantly larger in the preoperative patients than in the controls. However, as a consequence of the lower leg blood flow, the calculated uptake of glucose in the exercising muscles was not significantly greater in the patients. In addition, the decrease in muscle glycogen in relation to work intensity was of the same order of magnitude in the two groups, suggesting that the rate of carbohydrate utilization by muscle during exercise was similar in the patients and the controls. Furthermore, the marked increases in muscle and blood lactate concentrations in the patients, even at very low work intensities, indicate that a larger fraction of the pyruvate produced in the muscle during glycolysis was reduced to lactate instead of being oxidized in the tricarboxylic acid cycle. After reconstructive surgery, calculated glucose uptake and glucogen depletion during exercise were found to be the same as preoperatively while the breakdown of muscle glycogen was accelerated. In addition, the utilization of carbohydrates was more efficient as is indicated by the much lower production of lactate and evidently due to an improved delivery of oxygen to the muscles.

The profound preoperative impairment of both FFA and carbohydrate metabolism of the exercising muscles results in a critical reduction of the energy required for the regeneration of muscle phosphagens. Thus, the almost total depletion of creatine phosphate at the end of work in some of the patients has never been observed in normal subjects, even after exhaustive exercise (Karlsson et al., 1970). The ATP concentration also decreased substantially and a further depletion would, for several reasons, be unlikely to occur. One is tempted to speculate that the onset of the severe muscle symptoms during exercise in patients with occlusive arterial disease is related to the profound reduction observed in muscle phosphagens.

CLINICAL INVESTIGATION ON THE EFFECTS OF A NEW HYPOLIPIDEMIC AGENT, S-8527

Iwao Fukuki and Koichi Ogino
Cent. Lab. for Clinical Investigation, Kyoto Pref., University of Medicine and
The Third Department of Internal Medicine, Kyoto University, Medical School,
Kyoto/Japan

A new hypolipidemic agent, S-8527 with the chemical structure of 2,2'-(4,4'-cyclohexylidenediphenoxy)-2,2'-dimethyldibutyric acid, is one of the derivatives of clofibrate. S-8527 has an equivalent serum lipid lowering effect to that of clofibrate at one-tenth dose of clofibrate in normal rats.
We have studied clinically the effects and adverse effects of this compound in 56 patients of high cholesterol or of high triglicerides level by administring each 100 mg of S-8527 three times a day for 12 weeks. Serum lipids decreased in two weeks after initiation of S-8527 administration. Decrease per cents of cholesterol and triglyceride are approximately 5.0% and 20.0%, respectively. No adverse effects were so far observed. We have been continuing the study at higher dosage of S-8527.

"LT-178", A POTENT HYPOLIPIDEMIC DRUG. FIRST RESULTS FROM A 12 MONTHS CONTROL TRIAL ON 5O PATIENTS WITH HYPERLIPOPROTEINEMIA TYPE II

P. Drouin, J.P. Sauvannet, B. Martin, and G. Debry
Service de Médecine Générale "G" orienté vers les Maladies Métaboliques et les
Maladies de la Nutrition; C.H.U. Hôpital Jeanne-d'Arc, Nancy Cédex/France

The authors have studied the hypolipidemic effect of LF-178 in a group of 50 patients affected by type II. H.L.P. (IIa, IIb, W.H.O.) for a period of 12 months. This dietary controlled trial was divided into two parts: during the first period the patients were only given an individually and specifically adapted hypolipidemic dietary regimen. During the second period (3rd to 12th month) diet therapy was maintained and LF-178 given concomitantly at a daily average dose of 300 mg. The specific hypolipidemic action of the drug has been assessed by comparing blood lipid levels during the first period (dietary regimen only, mean value on the basis of a min. of 3 indiv. determinations) with those obtained during the second period (diet plus drug therapy). Lipid values were as follows: First period, type IIa, chol.: 390 mg/dl $\pm$ 0,28, type IIb, chol.: 371 mg/dl $\pm$ 0,32, T.G.: 193 mg/dl $\pm$ 0,25.
Drug induced lipid lowering effect was: IIa, Chol. 24-26% (6th - 12th month), IIb, Chol. 24-25% (6th - 12th month), T.G. 45-48% (6th - 12th).
The results are discussed according to the different types of H.L.P. by comparing these data to those obtained from a statistically significant control group located in the same geographic area and having the same food habits. Drug tolerance was assessed according to standard clinical and biochemical methods and drug efficiency discussed in the light of circulating plasma levels of the active drug principle.

TREATMENT OF HYPERLIPOPROTEINEMIC SUBJECTS WITH SELECTIVE ACUPUNCTURE

Chun-Chung Wu
Department of Medicine, Taiwan University Hospital, Taipei/Taiwan

The author reported the effectiveness of selective acupuncture (S.A.) on lowering hyperlipidemia in 1974. To confirm the similar effects in hyperlipoproteinemic patients observations of one month to 12 months were carried out in the S.A. group ov 79 cases and in control group of 23 cases. Those patients were kept in the ordinary diet without diet restriction and kept the same body weight. S.A. was carried out at specific points depend on their phenotype of lipid once every day or other day about 12 times in one month. Serum cholesterol decreased significantly after one week. S.A. treatment and kept the effect by 12 months in 20 type IIa cases (mean cholesterol 286 mg%) 13 and 24 percent respectively, in 9 type IIb cases (cholesterol 329 mg%) 17 and 29 percent, and in 3 type V cases 47 and 36 percent. Serum triglyceride (T.G.) decreased significantly after one week S.A. treatment until 12 months in 47 type IV (mean T.G. 279 mg%) 30 and 44 percent respectively, in type IIb (T.G. 287 mg%) 46 and 65 percent and in type V (T.G. 1358 mg%) 56 and 86 percent. Eye ground examination showed disappearance of arteriosclerotic retinopathy grade 1 (A-V cross phenomenon) five in 15 cases, 33 percent, one year after normalization of serum lipid. Serum free fatty acid, uric acid and lactic dehydrogenase decreased significantly after one to two weeks S.A. treatment.

A STUDY OF HYPOLIPIDEMIC EFFECT OF ACETIROMATE (TBF-43) — COMPARATIVE STUDY WITH CLOFIBRATE BY DOUBLE BLIND METHOD

Iowa Fukui and Yutaka Nakano

Cent. Lab. for Clinical Investigation, Kyoto Pred. University of Medicine and The Second Department of Internal Medicine, Kyoto University, Medical School, Kyoto/Japan

The several clinical studies are being tried with 3,5-diiodo-4-(3'-iodo-4'-acetoxyphenoxy) berzoic acid (Acetiromate, TBF-43), a derivative of Triiodothyronin which is said to exert the serum lipid lowering effect and is less calorigenic.

109 subjects with over 220 mg/dl of serum cholesterol or over 120 mg/dl of triglyceride were selected in order to carry out the clinical study by the double blind cross-over method on this compound with a reference drug of Clofibrate. The subjects received 15 mg of TBF-43 a day for the first 4 weeks and 30 mg a day for the consecutive 4 weeks. Clofibrate group received 1000 mg a day. All subjects were assessed on the last day of the initial treatment of 4 weeks for determination of the lowering effects of both drugs on the serum lipid. TBF-43 group responded significantly in lowering the serum levels of TC, TG, PL and β-L (P <0.01) and the lowered rates were 12.0%, 12.2%, 7.4% and 10.8%, respectively. Clofibrate group responded also significantly in lowering the serum levels of TC, TG and β-L (P <0.0a) and the lowered rates were 5.3%, 25.0% and 13.1%, respectively.

In comparing the lowering rate of both drugs, it can be concluded that TBF-43 exceeded Clofibrate in TC and PL, and Clofibrate excelled TBF-43 in TG, both significantly (P <0.05).

PRELIMINARY REPORT OF MECHANISM OF HYPOLIPIDEMIC EFFECTS OF SELEC-
TIVE ACUPUNCTURE IN CHOLESTEROL-FED RABBITS

Chun-Chung Wu

Department of Medicine, Taiwan University Hospital, Taipei/Taiwan

The author reported hypolipidemic effects of acupuncture in experimental hyperlipidemic rabbits and hyperlipidemic patients in 1974 and 1975 respectively. To
clear up the mechanism and the real effective hypolipoproteinemic points 28
cholesterol-fed rabbits were divided into control and selective acupuncture
groups (S.A.) 1 and 2. The latter S.A. received each selective on point once
every day for six weeks when their serum cholesterol (T.C.) reached 400 mg%. In
another experiment both control and S.A. groups received 14C cholesterol intra-
muscular injection followed by needling. Serum beta-lipoprotein (LP.) free-fatty
acid (F.F.A.) radioimmuno assay of corticosterone , insulin, radioactivity of
14C cholesterol and 24 hour stool deoxycholic acid, neutral sterol, total lipid
and neutral fat were measured. Serum T.C. and F.F.A. decreased 40 percent after
3 days and 2 weeks in SA 2 and SA 1. Serum LP. decreased after 3 day S.A., T.C.
content and fatty streak of aorta and LP. content of liver signigicantly decreased only in S.A. 2. T.C. content of liver decreased in S.A. 1. Enhanced excretion of deoxycholic acid and neutral fat in 24 hour feces were found in S.A.
groups and of total lipid in S.A. 1. Increased insulin and corticosterone were
found in S.A. 2. Different ways of hypolipidemic effects were found in S.A.
groups.

LIPOPROTEIN METABOLISM ON A MOLECULAR LEVEL DURING ATROMID-S
THERAPY

Robert C. Bahler and Jan J. Opplt
Cleveland Metropolitan General Hospital, Case Western Reserve University, Cleveland, OH/USA

Lipoprotein metabolism, on a molecular level, was studied in thirteen patients
with proven coronary disease before and during therapy with Atromid-S.
Preseparated serum lipoproteins were isolated in eight standard subfractions
by molecular filtration. Every subfraction was characterized by the elution volume, electrophoretic mobility, chemical and immunochemical properties, ultracentrifugation, estimation of the particle size and analysis of the apolipoproteins. These parameters were compared with traditional measurements of cholesterol, triglycerides and with the conventional measurements of electrophoretic
and ultracentrifugal types. Nine patients, all with hypertriglyceridemia, significantly improved their lipoprotein metabolism by decreasing both the fractions containing particulate fat and very low density particles as well as
those composed of intermediary metabolites (remnants). The high density lipoproteins generally increased. These changes in molecular distribution of serum
lipoproteins were not as evident by standard methods, although normalization of
the dyslipoproteinemia, according to the usual typing, was achieved.
This complex study of isolated lipoprotein associations has helped define
clofibrate's locus of action in the metabolic sequence of pathologically changed
lipoproteins.

MANAGEMENT OF HYPERLIPIDAEMIA BY A NOVEL 1,3-DIARYLOXYPROPANOL-(2) DERIVATIVE

R. Zschocke, H. Grill, G. Hofrichter, and H. Enomoto
Research Laboratories of Klinge Pharma, Munich/BRD, and Nippon Shinyaku Co.Ltd., Kyoto/Japan

A new 1,3-diaryloxypropanol-(2) derivative (G267) was compared with known hypo-lipaemics — clofibrate (CPIB), nicotinic acid (NiAc), and L-thyroxine (L-Th) — in five models to differentiate modes of action, using δ Wistar rats, 180-220 g b.wt. unless otherwise stated. Given comparable acute toxicities (LD50, rat p.o.: G267/CPIB/NiAc: 2440/2300/ca.3000), hypolipaemic activities are expressed as ED50% (mg/kg/day) for serum total cholesterol (TC) or triglycerides (TG). Oral treatment time (days) is given in parentheses. A. Normal rats (3.5), TC: G267/CPIB/NiAc: 100/220/$\geq$2000; B. Fructose hypertriglyceridaemia (3), TG: G267/CPIB/NiAc: 19/40/inactive; C. Triton hypercholesterolaemia (1), TC: G267/CPIB/NiAc: 75/inactive/$\gg$500; D. Thiouracil hypercholesterolaemia (4), TC: G267/CPIB/L-Th: 18/27/0.3; E. Cholesterol feeding (1% in diet) in weaned rats (50-60 g b.wt.) (3), TC: G267/CPIB: 33/158. LP electrophoresis and prep. UC in normal rats indicated reduction of total lipoproteins, unchanged α/β, and reduced β-TC by G267. CPIB produced a fall of the α/β ratio and reduced pre-β-TC and α-TC. The main feature differentiating G267 is its much greater effect on TC in all models. This hypocholesterolaemic activity was substantiated in youg δ baboons. It is suggested that the compound acts at a key step of lipoprotein assembly or release and thus appears particularly promising for treatment of human type II hyperlipidaemias.

LONG TERM EVALUATION OF THE HYPOLIPIDEMIC ACTIVITY OF LF-178 IN 340 PATIENTS AFFECTED BY ATHEROGENIC ENDOGENOUS HYPERLIPOPROTEINEMIA (IIa, IIb, IV)

J. Rouffy, C. Dreux, Y. Goussault, and R. Dakkak
Centra de Recherche et d'Etude des Facteurs Métaboliques de l'Athérosclérose, Université Paris VII, C.H.U. Hôpital Lariboisière Saint Louis, Paris/France

The authors report their experience of the treatment of the atherogenic type of pure hyperlipoproteinemia with the hypolipidemic drug, LF-178: 340 patients affected by hyperlipoproteinemia, types IIa, IIb and IV (W.H.O.) (associated with tendinous xanthomatosis) so far unresponsive to any diet-therapy, were selected for the study.
The daily dose administered to these patients varied from 200 to 400 mg during a 3 year-long drug treatment period. Under these conditions, cholesterol values were significantly depressed proportionally to the selected dose. The mean reduction of blood cholesterol observed varied from 20% to 36% in types IIa and IIb. Triglyceride levels were substantially depressed with mean reductions from 2o% to 50% in types IIb and IV. No "escape phenomenon" during the drug trial. In some patients, extravascular lipid deposits have sometimes been almost reduced (cutaneous, tuberous and tendinous xanthoma) which confirms our conclusion that LF-178 is far superior to Clofibrate in depressing blood lipid levels.
The clinical and biological tolerance was excellent and no adverse reaction could be recorded throughout the 3 year-long trial.

PRIMARY PREVENTION OF ATHEROSCLEROTIC VASCULAR DISEASES BY CONTROLLING THE RISK FACTORS. RESULTS OF 6 YEAR TRIAL

Motoo Tsushima, Tetsuya Tsuchida, Eiichiro Asano, Yoshiya Hata, and Yuichiro Goto
Department of Medicine, Keio University, School of Medicine, Tokyo/Japan

Out of 3 free-living populations in the northern and middle part of Japan, 320 subjects over 40 years of age were randomly selected, and divided into two groups: one group treated daily with 0.75 mg of an anabolic steroid, and the control group on placebo. Serum lipids, blood pressure, ECG and physical states were examined once or twice a year from 1969 to the present. The mean serum cholesterol and triglyceride levels of the treated group were significantly lower than those of the control group throughout the observation period. Hypertension being treated by local physicians decreased in prevalence without significant difference between the groups. The mean euglobulin lysis time was 342 ± 45 min. for the treatment group and 373 ± 50 min. for the control group ($p < 0.05$), while no significant difference was seen in platelet adhesiveness between the two groups. No correlation was seen between serum lipids and platelet adhesiveness. The ischemic cerebral and coronary diseases occurred, though not statistically significant, less in the treatment group than in the control group: 6 vs 8 in cerebral thrombosis, 1 vs 2 in myocardial infarction and 4 vs 2 in intracranial bleeding, respectively.

ACTION OF BM 15075 {2-[4(CHLORO-BENZOYL-AMINO-ETHYL)-PHENOXY]2-METHYL-PROPIONIC-ACID} ON RAT LIPID AND LIPOPROTEIN CONCENTRATION

Harald Stork, Giovannella Baggio, and Dietrich Seidel
Boehringer Mannheim, Medical Research Department, Mannheim/BRD, and Medical University Clinic, Heidelberg/BRD

The effect of 75 mg/kg/day BM 15075 and of 150 mg/kg/day Clofibrat on plasma lipid and lipoprotein concentrations was studied in male Sprague-Dawley rats (180 - 220 g) after 7 days of drug treatment under a standardized diet and compared to controls. Serum total Cholesterol (tot.CH), Tryglycerides (TG) and Phospholipids (PL) as well as HDL and lipoproteins d <1.063 (LP <1.063) were measured.
Results are expressed in % of the values found in the control group (n=10)

	tot.CH	TG	PL	LP<1.063	HDL
BM 15075 (n=17)	81	40	77	78	56
Clofibrat (n=12)	69	47	77	77	41

and inicate that both drugs similarly lower TG and HDL concentration. Comparison of our results with previous reports on the effect of these drugs in other species suggests that the marked and uniformly described reduction of plasma TG is independent of the properties of the lipoprotein particles which transport TG in plasma.

HYPOLIPIDEMIC EFFECTS OF 4-O-METHYLASCOCHLORIN (MAC)

A. Akcasu, and B. Berkarda
Department of Pharmacology and Therapeutics, Cerrahpasa Faculty of Medicine, Istanbul/Turkey

Hypolipidemic effects of MAC were evaluated in 16 hypercholesterolemic subjects (9 males, 7 females) aged 40 - 82 (mean 55). The drug was administered orally on a daily basis: 1 mg/kg Week 1, 2 mg/kg Week 2, 6 mg/kg Week 3, 17 mg/kg Weeks 4-8, followed by 4 Weeks of placebo treatment. Hematopoietic, renal, and hepatic functions remained normal throughout the course of treatment, as did prothrombin time and all physical parameters. Slight, transient diarrhea occurred in 2 subjects, and mild vertigo and an acneform eruption in each of 2 other subjects; all symptoms subsided without reduction of MAC dosage. Total serum cholesterol (TC), serum triglycerides (TG) and serum free fatty acids (FFA) were determined before treatment and at weekly intervals thereafter. MAC induced a mean reduction of 33.9% in cases where TC/TG<1.50, but TG reduction was not statistically significant when TC/TG<1.50. FFA reduction averaged 33% when TC/TG<1.50, but was statistically insignificant when TC/TG<1.50.

Analysis of variance of hypolipidemic response showed that MAC was effective in a dosage as low as 2 mg/kg.

THE PHARMACOKINETICS OF THE ANTIATHEROSCLEROTIC AGENT PHOSPHATIDYL-CHOLINE

R.A. Chaplain
Nattermann Pharmaceutical Company, Cologne/BRD

Regression of experimental atherosclerosis, together with a normalization of lipid metabolism, can be induced in baboons, miniature pigs, Japanese quails, cockerels, rabbits and rats by administering 28-400 mg/kg of polyunsaturated phosphatidylcholine (PU-PC, Lipostabil®) over a period of 8 - 24 weeks. To study the metabolic fate of the PU-PC 1,2-dilenolenyl phosphatidylcholine labelled both in the choline and fatty acid moieties has been used. Most of the PU-PC is hydrolyzed and absorbed as 1-acyl-lyso-phosphatidylcholine by the intestine. While 50 - 60% is reacylated and stored as an intermediary pool in the intestinal wall, the remainder is further hydrolyzed to glycerophosphorylcholine and free gatty acids. Of the absorbed PU-PC virtually all appeared in the lymph, the time course of the total dosage being 5% after 3.5 hrs, 17% after 6.5 hrs, 26% after 2.5 hes and around 50% after 19 hrs. Whole-body autoradiography revealed radiolabel mainly in the liver and intestinal mucosa at 12 hrs after dosing. After 24 hrs 24% of the dose was contained in the liver, declining to 4% at 8 days. In the striated muscle radioactivity increased from 6% at 6 hrs to 25% after 8 days. When expressed in terms of gram tissue weight, the 6-hr-dosage concentration was as follows: liver (2.4%), lungs (0.4%), kidneys (0.8%), adrenals (o.4%), spleen (0.3%).

EXPERIMENTAL AND CLINICAL EVALUATION OF TIBRIC ACID, A NEW HIPO-LIPIDEMIC AGENT

E. Marmo, F.G. Caramia, C. Vacca, G. Brita, A. Imperatore, C. De Bac, G. Ceccarelli, R. Spadaro, and R. Di Nola
Second Chair of Pharmacology (Head: Prof. E. Marmo), First Faculty of Medicine, University Naples, Second Chair of General Pathology (Head: Prof. F.G. Caramia) and Chair of Infant Diseases (Head: Prof. G. Ricci), Faculty of Medicine, University Rome, Rome/Italy

In rats the tibric acid presented significative hypolipidemic effects in various forms of hyperdislipidemias (hyperdislipidemia by Triton and by a diet rich in cholesterol; hypertriglyceridemia by margarine). The activity of tibric acid has been greated than that of clofibrate and clofinol. *In vitro* the tibric acid presented at high conc. antiaggregant effects on the platelets. In rats tibric acid does not show choleretic activity and does not effect liver function. In rats tibric acid contrarely to clofibrate, clofinol and tetralinic acid does not increase the mortality induced by thromexan. In patients suffering from hepatomegalic steatosis, together with hyperlipemia, a three weeks treatment with tibric acid produced in the liver a slight proliferation of the endoplasmatic plain reticulum and a slight dilatation of the biliar canaliculi. No decrease of the glycogen, nor variations of the mitochondria number was found.

EFFECT OF METFORMIN ON LIPID LEVELS AND LIPOPROTEIN STRUCTURE IN PATIENTS WITH HYPERTRIGLYCERIDEMIA

Cesare Sirtori, Marina Bertoli, Enzo Cocuzza, and Franco Conti
Center E. Grossi Paoletti for the Study of Metabolic Diseases and Hyperlipidemias, University of Milano, Milano/Italy

Patients with different types of hypertriglyceridemia (types II B, III, IV, V) were treated with metformin (N,N-dimethylbiguanide) with the objectives of defining patients with a positive response, as well as of identifying lipoprotein alterations induced by treatment. A total of 32 patients underwent an oral and i.v. glucose tolerance test before and after 16 weeks of drug treatment (2,500 - 3,000 mg/day). 5 patients had clinical diabetes, while 11 showed varying degrees of glucose intolerance. Metformin induced significant decreases of cholesterol and triglycerides in all types of hyperlipoproteinemia considered. Response to treatment was not related to weight loss of to previous diabetic abnormalities. Decrease of serum cholesterol (26%) in hypercholesterolemic patients exceeded that expected from triglyceride fall (-47%). Preliminary data on VLDL structure indicated changes in type II B and III patients.

NEW GROUP OF EFFECTIVE ANTIATHEROSCLEROTIC AGENTS: PYRIDO(1,2-a)-PYRIMIDINES

István Hermecz, Zoltán Mészáros, Lelle Debreczy, Ágnes Horváth, and Sándor Virág
Research Centre, CHINOIN Pharmaceuticals Ltd., Budapest/Hungary

In the course of our past years pharmaceutical research work concerning pyrido-(1,2-a)pyrimidine derivatives, we have found a group of compounds displaying significant antiatherosclerotic activity. Beside a lipolytic effect, they were also found to posses central nervous system actions. With systematic study of the structure-activity relationship, we have succeeded in eliminating the central nervous system effects while increasing the lipolytic activity of the compounds. When tested in normolipaemic rats, the compounds were found to reduce the serum cholesterol level to a greater extent than Clofibrate without producing a change in the liver size. Further screening of the compounds in rabbits rendered hypercholesterolaemic by cholesterol feeding, CHINOIN-123 was found to produce the strongest reduction in the amount of lipids deposited in the aorta. The present work is a description of our activities leading to the selection of CHINOIN-123.

EFFECT OF A PYRIDO-1.2.-A-PYRIMIDINE DERIVATIVE ON DEPOSITION AND SYNTHESIS OF LIPOPROTEINS AND GLYCOPROTEINS

Antal Ferencz, Sándor Virág, Judit Kovács, Lászlo Varga, Zoltán Mészáros, and Egon J. Hidvégi
Frédéric Joliot-Curie National Research Institute for Radiobiology and Radiohygiene, Budapest/Hungary

There are evidences that anti-atherosclerotic effect of the CHINOIN-123, a pyrido-1.2-a-pyrimidine derivative is exerted by affecting the mechanism resulting in lipid deposition in aortic tissue. The effect of CHINOIN-123 was studied on deposition and synthesis of lipoproteins and glycoproteins. The Golgi complex of hepatocytes was choosen first as a model for glycoprotein synthesis and was studied in detail. It was found that the administration of CHINOIN-123 at a dose of 5o mg/kg/day per os for 7 to 10 days led to a significant increase of 3H-glucosamine incorporation into the Golgi complex, as compared with untreated controls. At the same time there was no change in the incorporation of 3H-glucosamine into the smooth membrane fraction. Further on the deposition and synthesis of lipoproteins and glycoproteins in liver and aorta subcellular fractions of atherosclerotic rats was studied after treatment with CHINOIN-123 and clofibrate, respectively, and was compared with the atherosclerotic and untreated controls.

EFFECT OF A SYNTHETIC PYRIDO-(1,2a)-PYRIMIDINE DERIVATIVE (CHINOIN-123) ON THE COLESTEROL INDUCED CHANGES IN THE COMPOSITION OF THE HEART AORTA

Magdolna Bihari-Varga, Amalia Kardos, S. Virág, and S. Gerő
Arteriosclerosis Research Group of the Ministry of Health, Budapest/Hungary

1. In the aorta of cholesterol-fed rabbits a slight increase of glycosamine-glycan (GAG) concentration and of structural hydration, and an intensive lipid deposition was found by biochemical and histochemical methods. By thermal analysis the presence of aortic GAG - serum beta-lipoprotein complexes and the accumulation of "pathological" cross-links within the fibrillar tissue proteins could be demonstrated.
2. Chinoin-123 treatment resulted in a further increase of the structural water-, and GAG-content on the aortas of the cholesterol-fed rabbits. At the same time a significant de crease could be established in the amount of accumulated lipids and of GAG-beta-lipoprotein complexes.

NOCTURNAL INHIBITION OF LIPOLYSIS BY NICOTINIC ACID (NA) DERIVATES IN MAN

H. Raetzer, W. Kruse, W. Eggert, C.C. Heuck, P. Oster, B. Schellenberg, and G. Schlierf
Department of Medicine, University of Heidelberg, Heidelberg/BRD

Hepatic (endogenous) triglyceride production rates under most circumstances are highly correlated with plasma free fatty acid (FFA) levels. The "carbohydrate-induced" rise of plasma triglycerides which occurs at night when FFA levels are high can be inhibited by suppression of nocturnal lipolysis using nicotinic acid infusions. A comparative study was undertaken with oral administration of long-acting nicotine acid derivatives in order to suppress FFA levels at night. The study was performed in 12 normal subjects in a controlled, randomized fashion.
Significant lowering of nocturnal FFA levels was obtained with beta-pyridyl-carbinol and xanthinol nicotinate although both oral preparations were inferior to prolonged infusion of NA. It appeared that the time course rather than the absolute concentrations of plasma NA determined the behaviour of FFA levels. Side effects, in contrast, were directly related to NA levels.

A NEW METHOD FOR PRODUCING EXPERIMENTAL ATHEROSCLEROSIS IN RATS
AND THE INFLUENCE OF CHINOIN-123. A NEW PYRIDO-(1.2a)-PYRIMIDINE
DERIVATE ON THE DEVELOPMENT OF VASCULAR CHANGES

Sándor Virág, Csaba Vértesi, Zoltán Mészáros, and István Hermecz
Research Centre, Chinoin Pharmaceuticals Ltd., Budapest/Hungary

The adjuvant arthritic type of experimentally induced inflammatory reaction in
rats is very often accompanied by the development of "fibrinoid" and "hyalinoid"
types of vascular lesions. Considering the polyethiologic character of atherosclerosis both in human and laboratory animals a successful attempt was made to
provoke atherosclerotic type of vascular lesion in rats by combining the method
of adjuvant arthritis with cholesterol feeding.
Indomethacin and sodium salicylate were effective only in suppressing inflammatory reactions, while Clofibrate proved to be effective in decreasing the
severity of vascular lesions with lipid depositions. Chinoin-123, a new pyrido-
(1,2a)-pyrimidine derivate was effective in diminishing the inflammatory reactions and decreasing the severity of lipid depositions in different vascular
areas as well.

THE INFLUENCES OF NICOTINIC ACID THERAPY ON THE CHOLESTEROL BAL-
ANCE IN PATIENTS WITH HYPERLIPIDAEMIA TYPE IIa AND IV

Barbro Leijd, Kurt Einarsson, and Kjell Hellström
Department of Medicine, Karolinska Institute at Serafimerlasarettet, Stockholm/
Sweden

The kinetics of ^{14}C-cholic acid and ^{14}C-chenodeoxycholic acid and fecal excretion
of neutral steroids were studied in 10 patients with the IIa and in 5 patients
with the type IV lipoprotein pattern before and during treatment with nicotinic
acid for 3 to 12 months.
The serum lipid levels decreased in all patients. This change in type IIa was
not associated with any significant effects on the total bile acid formation and
the net steroid balance (defined as total bile acid formation plus neutral fecal
steroid excretion minus cholesterol intake). In all the type IV patients total
bile acid formation decreased by 25 to 30%. The fecal excretion of neutral
steroids increased and the net steroid balance was unchanged. Thus the effect of
nicotinic acid in patients with hyperlipoproteinaemia type II and IV were essentially the same as those previously recorded for clofibrate.

ACTION OF NICOTINIC ACID, NICERITROL AND β-PYRIDYLCARBINOL ON EX-
PERIMENTAL HYPERCHOLESTEROLEMIA AND ATHEROSCLEROSIS IN MINI-PIGS

L. Lundholm, L. Jacobsson, R. Brattsand, and O. Magnusson
Department of Pharmacology, Linköping University, Linköping/Sweden

In 50 female mini-pigs of Göttingen strain hypercholesterolemia was produced by
adding 12% dried egg yolk + 0.5% cholesterol to basal pig food for 40 - 90
weeks. In the 15 untreated animals the mean plasma cholesterol levels during
the experimental period varied between 400 - 700 mg/100 ml. Most of the cholesterol was located to LD-lipoproteins. Marked atheromatosis developed in the abdominal aorta and coronary arteries. Matched groups of animals were after 2
months of hypercholesterolemia treated with nicotinic acid compounds corresponding to 0.5% nicotinic acid in the diet. In the matched groups (n=20) with mean
cholesterol levels ~ 500 mg/100 ml niceritrol and β-pyridylcarbinol was most
effective during 90 weeks of treatment to reduce (~150 mg/10C ml; p <0.01) the
mean plasma cholesterol level and inhibit (p <0.01 - 0.001) the accumulation of
free and esterbound cholesterol in the coronary arteries and abdominal aorta.

Nicotinic acid was less effective in these respects despite that the plasma levels of free nicotinic acid were highest in these animals. Several metabolic parameters were compared in atheromatotic and normal pieces of intima + media from the same vessel (abdominal aorta) of untreated animals. O_2-consumption, lactate production, C^{14}-leucine incorporation in protein, C^{14} acetate-incorporation in lipids and the cyclic GMP level were increased whereas the ATP and cyclic AMP levels were reduced in atherosclerotic samples in comparison to normal pieces. In animals treated with nicotinic acid compounds these differences were less or not present.

SITOSTEROL TREATMENT OF FAMILIAL TYPE II HYPERLIPOPROTEINEMIA IN CHILDREN AND ADULTS

P. Oster, G. Schlierf, C. Heuck, H. Greten, U. Gundert-Remy, W. Haase, G. Klose, A. Nothelfer, H. Raetzer, and B. Schellenberg
Department of Internal Medicine, University Heidelberg, Heidelberg/BRD

Sitosterol was given in a controlled, randomized double blind study to 25 adults (24 gm) and 12 children (12 gm) for 4 resp. 6 months. Plasma lipids, lipoproteins, bromide and sitosterol levels were determined every 2 (4) weeks. Sodium bromide was used for control of drug intake.
Of the 25 adults 10 had to be excluded from further evaluation because of changes in body weight exceeding 3 kg or unreliable drug intake. In the remaining 15 patients total plasma cholesterol fell from 368 to 322 mg/dl (p <0.01, range + 5 to - 25%), LDL cholesterol from 231 to 186 mg/dl (p <0.05). Plasma sitosterol levels were always below 0,3% of cholesterol levels.
In the 12 children plasma cholesterol was slightly reduced from 311 to 292 mg/dl (n.s.). In 4 children plasma cholesterol actually increased. Drug intake was good in all children as estimated from bromide and sitosterol levels. Side effects were not observed.
In 11 adult type II patients sitosterol administration was continued for periods up to one year.

PROBUCOL IN THE LONG TERM MANAGEMENT OF HYPERCHOLESTEROLEMIA

Donald McCaughan
Department of Cardiology, West Roxbury, Veterans Administration Hospital, MA/USA

Probucol was administered to 57 patients for a period of 60 months for the control of hypercholesterolemia. Initiation of therapy was based on pretreatment levels of cholesterol greater than 250 mg% (average of 3 values). Cholesterol values were determines at 2 monthly intervals. The average of the final 3 values was compared with the pretreatment average. All cases showed a decline, mean of -29% (S.D.9). The range of declines was -45% to -8%. No significant differences were observed in the different lipid types. Red and white cell counts, hemoglobin, hematocrit, urinanalysis, serum SGPT, BUN, bilirubin and physical examination were carried out at 2 monthly intervals. No significant deviation from control values were observed. Slit lamp examinations at yearly intervals did not reveal any adverse effect in the ocular media. Electrocardiograms performed at baseline and yearly intervals showed no change in P-R intervals; the QT and QRS durations were not affected. The number of ventricular extra systoles observed was similar to that found in an untreated population. No ventricular tachycardias were observed. Two patients with previous histories of arrhythmias, developed atrial fibrillation, which converted easily with digitalis, and dit not recur.
Probucol appears to be an effective and safe agent for the long term treatment of hypercholesterolemia.

EFFECT OF A NEW HYPOLIPIDEMIC DRUG (LL 1558) ON PRIMARY HYPERLIPO-PROTEINEMIA

G. Briani, P. Balestrieri, G. Baggio, H.R. Baiocchi, R. Fellin, and G. Crepaldi
Department of Internal Medicine, Division of Gerontology and Metabolic Diseases, Policlinico, Padua/Italy

24 patients with primary hyperlipoproteinemia (8 type IIa, 11 type IIb, 5 type IV) of both sexes (age 20 - 65 years) have undergone 6 months treatment with 2.400 mg/die bis-(idrossietil-tio)-1,10 decane (LL 1558, Tiadenol). Mean serum total cholesterol (TC) and triglyceride (TG) levels were:

Month		0	2	4	6
IIa	TC	302 ± 22	265 ± 14	235 ± 14	261 ± 16
	TG	106 ± 11	104 ± 10	123 ± 16	107 ± 13
IIb	TC	283 ± 18	263 ± 19	245 ± 16	262 ± 20
	TG	284 ± 41	262 ± 39	309 ± 54	209 ± 41
IV	TC	307 ± 12	243 ± 22	242 ± 26	251 ± 29
	TG	751 ± 190	472 ± 97	515 ± 153	354 ± 80

In type IIa TC decrease was significant at 4th ($p < 0.02$) and 5th ($p < 0.05$) months. In type IIb IC decrease was significant at the 1st ($p < 0.01$) and 4th ($p < 0.05$) months, while variations in TG levels were not significant. In type IV TG decrease was significant at 4th ($p < 0.05$), 5th ($p < 0.025$) and 6th ($p < 0.05$) months; TC decrease was always significant. The drug was well tolerated and no side effects nor biochemical variations were noted.

EFFECT OF CHOLESTYRAMINE TREATMENT ON ENDOGENOUS SERUM TRIGLYCERIDE TRANSPORT IN HYPERCHOLESTEROLAEMIC SUBJECTS

Bo Angelin, Kurt Einarsson, Kjell Hellström, and Barbro Leijd
Department of Medicine, Karolinsky Institute at Serafimerlasarettet, Stockholm/Sweden

In order to study the effect of increased cholesterol and bile acid synthesis on triglyceride dynamics, ^{3}H-labelled glycerol was administered intravenously to 10 patients with hyperlipoproteinaemia type IIa or IIb before and after the institution of cholestyramine treatment. By means of consecutive blood sampling and plasma triglyceride radioactivity determination, endogenous triglyceride synthesis and fractional turnover rate were determined, averaging 9.2 mg $kg^{-1}h^{-1}$ and 0.18 h^{-1} in the basal state. After minimum 1 month of therapy, leading to lowered cholesterol and unchanged triglyceride levels, both parameters showed an increase in all subjects with means of 12.6 mg $kg^{-1}h^{-1}$ and 0.24 h^{-1}, respectively. The results indicate that the metabolism of cholesterol/bile acids and triglycerides is integrated, and they also suggest a regulatory role of cholesterol in very low-density lipoprotein triglyceride metabolism.

INHIBITION OF HUMAN FAT CELL ADENYLATE CYCLASE BY CLOFIBRATE

Horst Kather, Gabriela Simon-Crisan, and Bernd Simon
Klinisches Institut für Herzinfarktforschung an der Medizinischen Universitätsklinik, Heidelberg/BRD

The lipid lowering effect of clofibrate has been supposed to be mediated by inhibition of the fat cell adenylate cyclase system either directly or via biotransformation to a derivative. We studied the effects of this drug on adenylate cyclase of human fat cell.

Enzyme activity was assayed in fat cell ghosts by the method of Salomon et al. (Anal. Biochem. 58, 541 (1974)). Increasing concentrations of clofibrate (0.01 to 1 mg) caused a dose-dependent inhibition of all expressions of enzyme activity (basal, noradrenaline as well as NaF-stimulated enzyme activity) up to 45% of controls. The inhibitory action was found to be non-competitive with respect to substrate (ATP) and Mg^{2+}-ions and was detectable after s.5 min. Our results show that clofibrate by itself can inhibit the adenylate cyclase system in human fat cells. They support the hypothesis that inhibition of adenylate cyclase may represent one of the mechanism contributory to the lipid lowering action of clofibrate.

ANALYSIS OF THERAPEUTIC RESISTANCE TO CLOFIBRATE IN MIXED HYPER-LIPIDEMIA WITH SLOW MIGRATED PREBETA LIPOPROTEIN (prebeta 1). ANALYSIS OF 50 CASES

J.L. de Gennes, J. Truffert, and G. Turpin
Department of Endocrinology-Metabolism, Hospital La Pitié, University Paris VI, Paris/France

An unusual resistance to regular treatment of mixed hyperlipidemia by diet low in carbohydrate low in cholesterol with replacement of saturated fat by polyunsaturated fat was been met in 50 cases followed over several months and years.- This resistance was therefore submitted to a careful analysis. No striking difference in the age of patients in adhesion to diet was found by comparison to apparied patients classified in the same hyperlipidemic group, and easily corrected by the same treatment for their blood lipid disorders. Glucose tolerance disturbances with excessive insulin were frequently, though not constantly observed. But electrophoretic studies on agarose gel by Noble technic showed a significant increase of slow migrating préblipoprotein of $préb_1$ lipoprotein in the group of resistant patients. Additional studies have shown an unusual binding of a large part of Clofibrate with VLDL binding of $préB_1$LP and Clofibrate is suspected in this group as a major factor of resistance.

COMPARISON OF THE EFFECT OF CLOFIBRATE AND BM 15.075 ON SERUM LIPID AND LIPOPROTEIN LEVELS IN HYPERLIPIDAEMIA

Anders G. Olsson, P. Dieter Lang, Stephan Rössner, Göran Walldius, and Lars A. Carlson
King Gustaf V Research Institute, Stockholm/Sweden

The hypolipidaemic effect of BM 15.075 ((2-(4-(Chloro-benzoyl-amino-ethyl)-phenoxy)-2-methyl propionic acid) has been described in animals and man[*]. In a single blind cross over study the effect of clofibrate, 500 mg x 3 daily, and BM 15.075, 200 mg x 3 daily, was followed during four consecutive 4 week periods in 29 patients with different types of hyperlipoproteinemia. The fasting concentration of cholesterol and triglycerides was determined in whole serum and in very low (VLDL), low (LDL) and high (HDL) density lipoproteins. Over all there was a reduction in total triglycerides of 26 and 37 and total cholesterol of 8 and 14% with clofibrate and BM 15.075 respectively. The corresponding figures for VLDL were 39 and 54 for triglycerides and 39 and 45 for cholesterol. The treatment effect was analyzed in relation to the pretreatment levels of the various lipoprotein classes. The changes in LDL cholesterol and VLDL triglycerides were significantly related to the pretreatment levels. The activities of the two compounds were evaluated against these regression lines. No subjective side effects were noted on BM 15.075. No differences were observed in safety laboratory parameters between both drugs.

---

[*] Stork H. and Lang P.D., Adv. Exp. Med. Biol. 63, 485 (1975)

DETERMINATION OF BLOOD LEVELS OF NICOTINIC ACID AND CLOFIBRATE BY GLASS CAPILLARY GAS-LIQUID CHROMATOGRAPHY

H. Jaeger, J. Wechsler, H.U. Klör, J. Schönborn, and H. Ditschuneit
Department of Medicine, Division of Metabolism and Nutrition, University of Ulm, Ulm/BRD

One of the major problems in the evaluation of lipid lowering drugs is the correlation of drug levels in the body to their pharmacological effects. We have therefore developed a micromethod for the determination of nicotinic acid and clofibrate in serum, whole blood and tissues. After extraction of the sample with acetone and chloroform nicotinic acid was recovered from the aqueous and clofibrate from the organic phase. Both substances were methylated. Total recovery was 85%. Detection limit was about 200 pg for nicotinic acid and 1 pg for clofibrate. The samples were chromatographed on a Carlo Erba Fractovap equipped with a nitrogen-specific detector and a micro-electron capture detector and a 15 m glass capillary column. The levels of inositol-nicotinate, xantinol-nicotinate, β-pyridyl-carbinole, free nicotinate, and clofibrate given separately and in combination were analysed after oral administration in normal volunteers and in patients with hyperlipidemia type IIa, IIb, and IV. The determination of drug levels in adipose tissue seems to be a reliable parameter for the adherence to medication.

SERIAL LIVER BIOPSIES DURING CLOFIBRATE TREATMENT: EFFECT ON ULTRA-STRUCTURE, GLYCOGEN AND TRIGLYCERIDE CONTENT

Markolf Hanefeld, Christa Kemmer, Wolfgang Leonhardt, Werner Jaroß, and Hans Haller
Medical Academy "Carl Gustav Carus", Dresden/DDR

In about 40 patients with primary hyperlipoproteinemia liver specimens were obtained by needle biopsy before and during Clofibrate treatment. At the first controll after 3 months we found a distinct increase of number and size of mitochrondria and microbodies, desorientations of mitochondrial cristae and proliferations of the smooth endoplasmic reticulum (SER). Liver glycogen decreased from 4.17% wet weight to 2.69% (p <0.02). TG content did not change significantly (27.4% and 25.5% dry weight, respectively) whereas FFA, TG, Cholesterol and VLDL levels of the serum decreased highly significant. At a third biopsy 2 to 5 years later the most impressive ultrastructural change of the organelles was the proliferation of SER as well as of rough ER. At this time mitochondrial alterations were less pronounced. The relation between liver findings and different blood parameters are analysed.

CHANGES IN PLASMA LIPIDS AND IN LIPOPROTEIN CONCENTRATION AND COMPOSITION IN HYPERLIPIDEMIAS TYPE IIa, IIb and IV UPON TREATMENT WITH COMBINATIONS OF CLOFIBRATE AND NICOTINIC ACID

J. Wechsler, V. Hutt, H.U. Klör, J. Jäger, and H. Ditschuneit
Department of Medicine, Division of Metabolism and Nutrition, University of Ulm, Ulm/BRD

30 patients with hyperlipidemias type IIa, IIb and IV were treated first with a diet rich in polyunsaturated fatty acids until stable lipid levels were reached. 10 patients with type IIa were given 1.5 g clofibrate (Cl) and 2.4 g inositol-nicotinate (IN) daily (group 1), 10 patients with IIb and type IV received 0.75 g clofibrate and 0.45 g IN daily (group 2) and another 10 patients with type IIb and IV were administered 1.5 g Cl and 0.9 g IN (group 3). Plasma total cholesterol was lowered by 25% in group 1, by 12% in group 2 and 11% in group 3.

Plasma triglycerides decreased by 30% in group 1, and by 40% in both group 2 and 3. The concentration of triglycerides, esterified cholesterol, free cholesterol, phospholipids and protein were determined in VLDL, LDL and HDL before therapy, on therapy and on placebo in all patients. In all groups, the composition of the lipoprotein classes was identical in the pretreatment and posttreatment placebo phase. All VLDL constituents decreased upon treatment by about one third. The same rate of reduction of the different components was obtained in the LDL, while the HDL constituents did not change very much.

EFFECT OF COLESTIPOL PLUS CLOFIBRATE ON SERUM LIPIDS IN FAMILIAL TYPE II HYPERLIPOPROTEINEMIA

R. Fellin, G. Baggio, G. Briani, P. Balestrieri, M.R. Baiocchi, and G. Crepaldi
Department of Internal Medicine, Division of Gerontology and Metabolic Diseases, Policlinico, Padua/Italy

Colestipol (15 g/die) and Clofibrate (2 g/die) were administered to 20 subjects with familial hyperlipoproteinemia (12 type IIa and 8 type IIb) for 15 months. These patients had been previously treated with Colestipol, 12 months with 15 g/die and 4 months 30 g/die. The figure obtaines after the 16th month Colestipol treatment was taken as basal value. Mean serum total cholesterol (TC) and triglyceride (TG) levels during treatment were:

Month		0	4	9	15
IIa	TC	389±35	334±25	345±26	310±23
	TG	121±15	88±7	93±13	87±11
IIb	TC	346±19	360±16	381±30	328±28
	TG	293±36	163±17	105±35	208±31

In type IIa TC decrease was significant at the 3rd ($p < 0.05$), 4th ($p < 0.001$), 7th ($p < 0.05$) and 15th ($p < 0.05$) months; TG decrease was always significant. The hypotriglyceridemic effect of the combined therapy was particularly evident in type IIb; TG decrease was significant at evera month while TC showed a moderate increase. These results show that Colestipol + Clofibrate treatment is effective in lowering both serum TC and TG levels in type IIa and TG levels in type IIb.

4-O-METHYLASCOCHLORIN, A NEW HYPOLIPIDEMIC AGENT FROM FUNGAL ORIGIN

M. Sawada, T. Okutomi, H. Hosokawa, K. Ando, and G. Tamura*
Research Laboratories, Chugai Pharmaceutical Co.,Ltd., and *Department of Agricultural Chemistry, University of Tokyo, Tokyo/Japan

Hypolipidemic property and mode of action of 4-O-methylascochlorin (MAC) was studied using experimental animals. MAC at a daily dose of 10 mg/kg for one month effectively lowered serum cholesterol and triglyceride together with preventing lipid deposit in liver, heart and aorta in the rat fed on lipid-rich diet. The agent also reduced serum cholesterol and triglyceride of beagle dog at doses of 5 and 20 mg/kg for 4 weeks. Protection from degeneration of cardiac muscle and prolongation of life span in addition to prevention of cholesterol deposit in liver, heart and aorta were observed in MAC treated rabbit fed on atherogenic regimen for 14 weeks. In the quail fed on cholesterol-rich diet for 9 months, MAC at daily doses of 1 - 64 mg/kg was capable of inhibiting atheroma and retarding elevation of serum and organ lipid levels.
Fecal excretion of acidic steroid was much increased by MAC, although that of neutral steroid was unchanged. Increas in secretion of cholic acid was observed by MAC with bile-duct cannulized rat. MAC inhibits active transport of bile acid through everted gut sac. Thus, two mechanisms participate in its hypolipidemic activity.

EFFECT OF PHOSPHATIDYLCHOLINE (EPL) i.v. ON RED BLOOD CELL MOR-
PHOLOGY AND LIPOPROTEIN (LP) COMPOSITION IN CHOLESTASIS

Gianfranco Salvioli, and Roberto Salati
Istituto Clinica Medica, Università di Modena, Modena/Italy

We have studied the morphology of red blood cell (RBC) in 30 cirrhotics with
cholestasis (CC); the following parameters were also evaluated: RBC osmotic
fragility (OF), cholesterol (C) and phospholipids (PL) contents, the serum bile
acids (SBA), LCAT activity and fatty acid composition of RBC lecithin (PC), and
LP composition. In 12 (40%) patients with CC, spur cell (SC), acantocyte-like
with slight alteration of OF were present; the ratio C/PL is 1.3 (vn 0.7); SBA
2100 µg dl (vn 300), with ratio CA/CDCA 0.5 (vn 1.3); linoleic acid content of
RBC PC in SC is 14.2 (vn 21.6). The great molar ratio C/PL and the less content
in polyunsaturated fatty acids increase viscosity and surface area of RBC. The
irregular folds of the membrane regress after EPL administration (2 gi.v. for
5 days) in 8 patients with SC; the treatment decrease the molar ratio RBC C/PL
from 1.22 to 0.88 and the ratio CL/PL in HDL of cirrhotics with SC (from 0.32
to 0.21); the content of linoleic acid of RBC PC (from 14.2 to 20.5%) and LCAT
activity (from 31.2 to 54.4 µmole/L/h) both increase after EPL infusion.

SERUM LIPIDS AND LIPOPROTEINS, BLOOD COAGULATION AND PLATELETS DUR-
ING A DOUBLE-BLIND TRIAL OF CLOFIBRATE/CLOFIBRATE-EPL IN HYPERLIPO-
PROTEINEMIA

J. Schneider, G. Fuchs, H. Kaffarnik, R. Schubotz, L. Hausmann, G. Mühlfellner,
O. Mühlfellner, and P. Zöfel
Medical Policlinic University, Marburg/Lahn/BRD

80 patients with hyperlipoproteinemias type IIa, IIb, IV and V according to
Fredrickson were treated with clofibrate and Clofibrate-EPL in a double-blind
study for 4 months. Total cholesterol, phospholipids and triglycerides were determined in the HDL, LDL, VLDL fractions and in the whole serum. The decrease of
the triglycerides exceeded that of cholesterol and phospholipids in both experimental periods, LDL-cholesterol was lower after clofibrate-EPL than after
clofibrate alone. An extensive study of hämostasis was performed. The following
parameters were determined: thromboplastin time, partial thromboplastin time,
thrombin time, thrombelastography, factor V, euglobin lysis time, number of
platelets, platelet-spreading and platelet-aggregation by PAT I and PAT III
tests.

PREVENTION OF ATHEROMATOUS LESIONS IN RABBITS AND RATS BY A NEW
Δ^8-DIHYDROABIETAMIDE

Hiroshi Enomoto, Yoshiaki Yoshikuni, Katsuhide Saito, and Gernot Hofrichter
Research Laboratories, Nippon Shinyaku Co., Ltd., Kyoto/Japan and Klinge Pharma,
Munich/BRD

This study was to investigate the effect of a new non-toxic Δ^8-dihydroabietamide
(THD-341) on aortic atheroma formation in male albino rabbits induced by cholesterol (C) feeding and on the coronary arterial or aortic lesions induced in male
rats by C and vitamin D_2 treatment. The compound is a very active hypolipaemic
since in C fed (1% in diet) weaned rats less than 1 mg/kg reduce serum total C
by 50%. Rabbits were fed a 1% C containing diet for 7 weeks. Addition of THD-341
(0.01% in diet) after the 3rd week caused a dramatic drop serum total C levels
and significantly prevented aortic athermoa formation. Using arbitrary scores
the extent of atheroma formation in the arch, thoracic, and abdominal parts, was
respectively: C-fed control: 2.1, 0.9, and 0.5, THD-341 treated: 1.1, 0.2, and

0.0. Rat arterial lesions were induced by 40,000 I.U. vitamin D_2/rat/day for an initial period of 5 days and 1% C feeding for 3 weeks. Addition of THD-341 (0.03% in diet) almost completely prevented aortic and coronary arterial damage even when compared with C-free, vitamin D_2 treated control group. It is concluded that THD-341 prevents atheromatous lesions mainly by virtue of its profound hypocholesterolaemic properties, but may also have a direct protective action on the arterial wall.

EFFECT OF A PYRIDO-1.2.-A-PYRIMIDINE DERIVATIVE ON DEPOSITION AND SYNTHESIS OF LIPOPROTEINS AND GLYCOPROTEINS

Antal Ferencz, Sándor Virág, Judit Kovács, László Varga, Zoltán Mészáros, and Egon J. Hidvégi
"Frédéric Joliot-Curie", National Research Institute for Radiobiology and Radiohygiene, Budapest/Hungary

There are evidences that anti-atherosclerotic effect of the CHINOIN-123, a pyrido-1.2.-a-pyrimidine derivative is exerted by affecting the mechanism resulting in lipid deposition in aortic tissue. The effect of CHINOIN-123 was studied on deposition and synthesis of lipoproteins and glycoproteins. The Golgi complex of hepatocytes was choosen first as a model for glycoprotein synthesis and was studied in detail. It was found that the administration of CHINOIN-123 at a dose of 50 mg/kg/day per os for 7 to 10 days led to a significant increase of 3H-glucosamine incorporation into the Golgi complex, as compared with untreated controls. At the same time there was no change in the incorporation of 3H-glucosamine into the smooth membrane fraction. Further on the deposition and synthesis of lipoproteins and glycoproteins in liver and aorta subcellular fractions of atherosclerotic rats was studied after treatment with CHINOIN-123 and clofibrate, respectively, and was compared with the atherosclerotic and untreated controls.

MANAGEMENT OF HYPERLIPIDAEMIA BY A NOVEL 1-ARYLOXY-3-ARYLAMINO-PROPANOL-(2) DERIVATIVE

H. Enomoto, Y. Yoshikuni, T. Ozaki, and R. Zschocke
Research Laboratories, Nippon Shinyaku Co., Kyoto/Japan and Klinge Pharma, Munich/BRD

Differentiation of the mode of action at an early stage appears essential for the development of new, nore effective hypolipaemic agents. In this study the effect of a new 1-aryloxy-3-arylamino-propanol-(2) derivative (OCO-508, LD50, rat p.o.: >12000 mg/kg), was investigated mainly in comparison with clofibrate (CPIB) in various types of hyperlipidaemic and normal male rats. 50% inhibitory doses (ID 50%, mg/kg/day), unless otherwise stated, were evaluated after oral treatment over the number of days given in parentheses. Data are presented in the order: OCO-508/CPIB. A. Fructose hypertriglyceridaemia (3): 13/50 (nicotinic acid: >500). B. Cholesterol feeding (1% in diet) (3): 290/300 (nicotinic acid: >1000). C. Thiouracil hypercholesterolaemia (4): 26/32 (L-thyroxine: 0.6). D. Normal rats (aged 8 weeks) (3.5): 50% serum triglyceride (TG) reducing dose: 5/50, 40% serum total cholesterol (TC) reducing dose: 60/100. There was consicerable variation in control TG and TC levels, possibly age-related. The effect of OCO-508 was the greater the higher the lipid levels. Prep. UC analysis of LP indicated that both OCO-508 and CPIB primarily decrease VLDL and HDL corresponding with TG and TC reductions. LP-electrophoresis gave reduced α/β and unchanged or slightly increased $\alpha/pre\beta$ ratios with both drugs. These results indicate that OCO-508 is promising for the treatment of human type 2b and 4 hyperlipidaemia.

Chairmen: J. Davignon, Canada
          S. Yamazaki, Japan

Participants: P.J. Nestel, Australia
              A.G. Olsson, Sweden
              J.A. Little, Canada
              S. Sailer, Austria
              J. Davignon, Canada
              A.N. Howard, England
              S. Yamazaki, Japan
              I. Fukui

MECHANISMS OF HYPERLIPOPROTEINAEMIA DERIVED FROM MULTICOMPARTMENTAL ANALYSIS OF VERY LOW-DENSITY APOLIPOPROTEIN B-KINETICS

P.J. Nestel

Three forms of hyperlipoproteinaemia are commonly encountered in clinical practice:
1. Hypercholesterolaemia
2. Hypertriglyceridaemia
3. Combined hyerplipidaemia.
Genetic and environmental factors are implicated in the causation of all three.
A better understanding of the underlying mechanisms has been derived from measurements of the turnover of the lipid and the protein constituents. With an increase in the knowledge of the functions of the various apoproteins, kinetic
studies of the individual proteins will clarify the relative importance of overproduction and reduced catabolism as the cause of specific hyperlipoproteinaemias.
Unique apoproteins are associated with the assembling, degradation and reconstitution of lipoproteins; it is likely that the final classification of hyperlipoproteinaemias will be based on the functional adequacy of these apoproteins. Furthermore, the modes of action of foods and drugs on plasma lipoprotein levels will
be better understood when their effect on apolipoprotein metabolism is clarified.

Although studies with the peptides of very low-density and high-density lipoproteins are in their infancy, the measurement of low-density lipoprotein protein
has established the importance of diminished protein degradation as a major cause
of one form of hyperlipoproteinaemia. Measurements of cholesterol and bile acid
kinetics had earlier failed to define the metabolic defect.

In this discussion, we shall compare data derived from measurements of the turnover of the B-apolipoprotein and the triglyceride components of very low-density
lipoproteins. The kinetics of both protein and lipid are described more accurately in terms of multicompartmental rather than one-pool models (Fig. 1). VLDL B-
apolipoprotein turnover was measured by injecting autologous 125I and 131I labelled lipoproteins of various densities (Reardon et al., 1976) and VLDL triglyceride turnover was measured after injecting radioglycerol (Grundy et al., 1975).
Multicompartmental analysis of protein and of lipid showed that overproduction
of lipoprotein was a major cause of VLDL accumulation in plasma, though the data
from apolipoprotein kinetics suggest that at higher concentrations, removal mechanisms become saturated (Fig. 2; Table 1).

VLDL B-protein kinetics conformed to a two-pool model during the first 48 h of
catabolism. The turnover within pool A accounted for most of the turnover within
both pools. The mass of pool A exceeded the intravascular content of VLDL B by

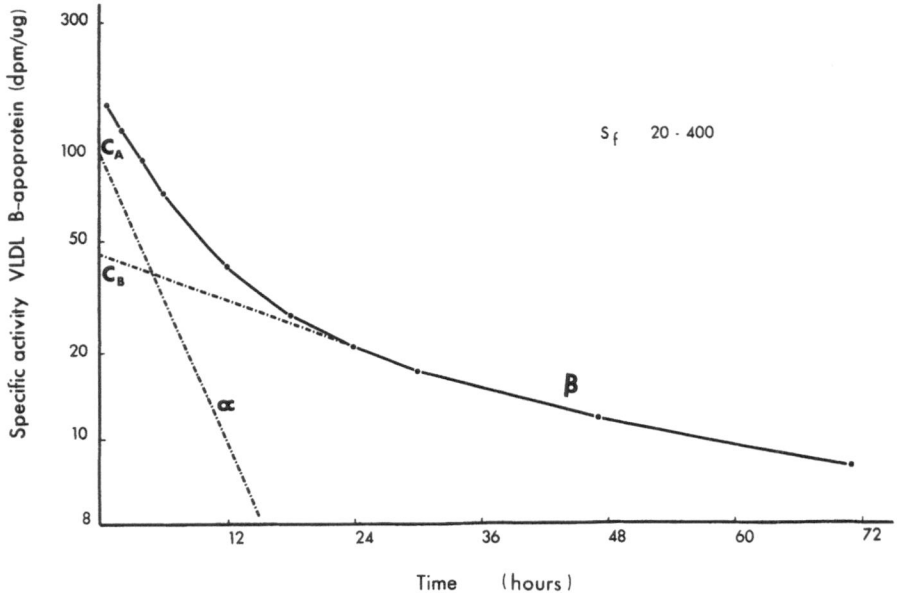

Figure 1. Two-pool nature of Sf 20–400 VLDL B-apolipoprotein turnover

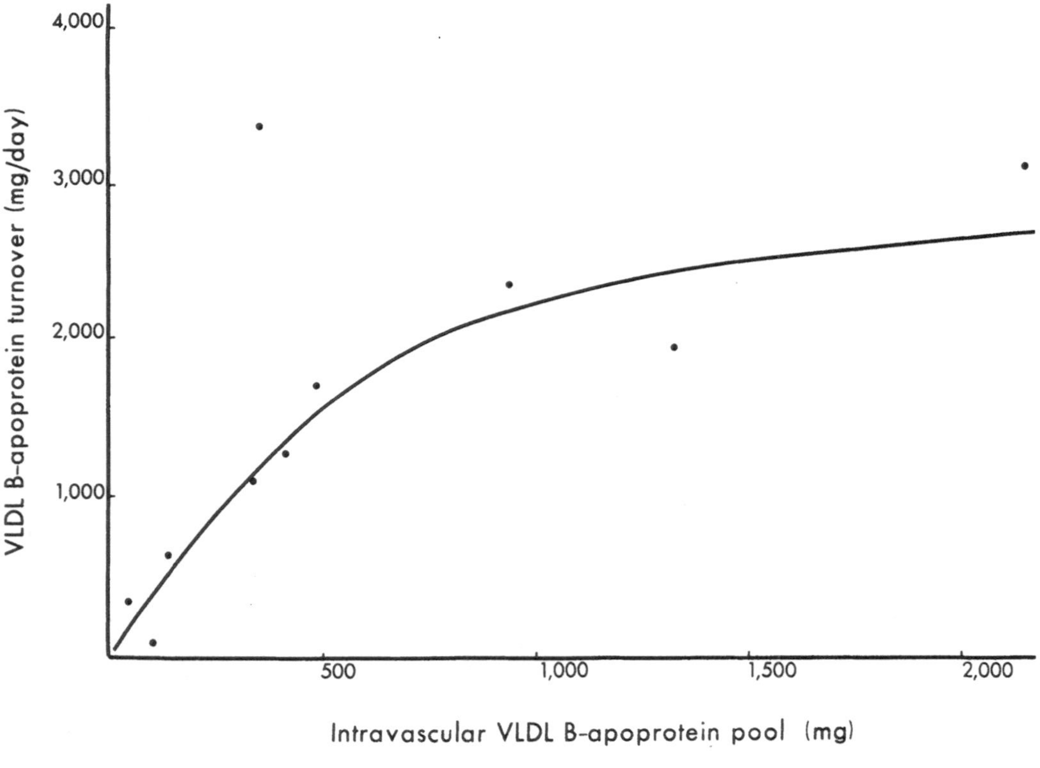

VLDL B-apoprotein turnover (mg/day) vs Intravascular VLDL B-apoprotein pool (mg)

Figure 2. Relation between plasma concentration and turnover of Sf 20–400 VLDL B-apolipoprotein

Table 1. Turnover of Sf 20-400 VLDL B by two-pool analysis

Lipoportein phenotype	Plasma VLDL B (mg)	Turnover VLDL B (mg/day)
N	44	359
N	131	637
2a	334	1092
2b	415	1238
2b	485	1671
4	355	3345
4	942	2323
4	1326	1928
5	2147	3060

24% on the average, indicating extravascular metabolism of VLDL. The two-pool model might reflect the input of several populations of particles or heterogeneity of catabolic processes. This was tested by injecting subclasses of VLDL (Sf 100-400, 60-400, 12-60 and 12-20) either alone or two at a time labelled with ^{125}I or [131]I. The findings revealed the following:

1. In hypertriglyceridaemic subjects, more than one population of VLDL may be secreted into plasma.
2. Catabolism of VLDL may proceed by more than one route.
3. The probable intermediate lipoprotein of VLDL catabolism was in the S_f 12-60 rather than S_f 12-20 range (Table 2).
4. The complexity of both influx and efflux of VLDL contribute to the multiexponential nature of VLDL B-apolipoprotein turnover.

The turnover of low-density lipoprotein B-apolipoprotein (LDL B) which is believed to be dereived from VLDL catabolism was calculated from the area between the specific activity-time curves of VLDL B and LDL B. In subjects with normal plasma triglyceride concentration, LDL B turnover was from 80-107% of that of VLDL B,

Table 2. Major intermediate lipoproteins of VLDL catabolism

Lipoprotein phenotype	Lipoproteins studied	Turnover B-apoprotein (mg/day)
4	S_f 60-400	605
	S_f 12-60	544
2b	S_f 60-400	512
	S_f 12-60	462
4	S_f 20-400	2323
	S_f 12-20	462
N	S_f 20-400	637
	S_f 12-20	200

Lipoprotein fractions labelled with ^{125}I or [131]I.

turnover, LDL B turnover was only one-third that of VLDL B (Table 3). This suggests that when VLDL B turnover is high, VLDL is substantially catabolized by a route other than through LDL (Fig. 3).

The increased turnover of VLDL B-protein and triglyceride in hypertriglyceridaemia is, therefore, consistent with previous reports of increased plasma cholesteryl ester and bile acid turnover (Nestel, 1974).

Table 3. Comparison of turnover of VLDL B (S_f 20-400) & LDL B (S_f 0-12)

Lipoprotein phenotype	VLDL B turnover (mg/day)	LDL B turnover (mg/day)
N	359	315
N	637	579
2a	1092	1177
2b	1238	990
2b	1671	1542
4	3345	1144
4	2323	772
4	1928	1368
5	3060	1074

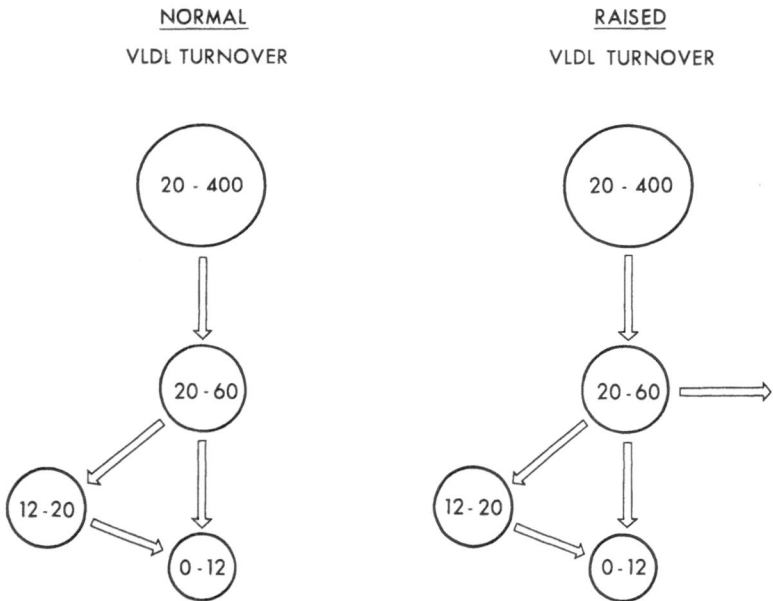

Figure 3. Possible pathways of VLDL catabolism, showing S_f 20-60 lipoprotein as the major intermediate lipoprotein and an alternate pathway of catabolism in hypertriglyceridaemia

ON THE SIGNIFICANCE OF TYPING OF HYPERLIPOPROTEINEMIA IN PRIMARY ASYMPTOMATIC HYPERLIPIDEMIA*

Anders G. Olsson

Introduction

In recent years typing of HLP according to Fredrickson et al. (1967) or according to its modification by Beaumont et al. (1970) has become the most common way of defining these conditions. This typing system was a great advance as it facilitates communication and stimulates thinking in terms of LP instead of in total lipid levels. The typing system of HLP was originally applied to patients with familial HLP with often extreme elevations of one LP class (Fredrickson and Levy, 1972). In those subjects, typing of HLP bears no problem. Therefore, the problems that arise when dealing with moderate elevations of one or more LP were not fully apparent. Another lack of the initial system was that combined HLP, later introduced as type IIb HLP (Beaumont et al., 1970) was not recognized.

This paper describes the applicability of the modified typing system to a free-living, asymptomatic population who were found to have elevated serum cholesterol and/or triglyceride (TG) concentrations at a routinely performed health check.

Material and Methods

Serum cholesterol and TG concentrations were determined in about 20,000 subjects attending a health control center linked to their employment (Olsson and Carlson, 1975). Three hundred and fourteen asymptomatic subjects with serum cholesterol >350 mg/100 ml and/or TG >3.5 mmol/l in the screening test but without secondary hyperlipidemia or history of cardiovascular disease were examined further. LP analyses with preparative ultracentrifugation separating very low-(VLDL), low-(LDL) and high-(HDL) density LP classes and the determination of cholesterol (Block et al., 1965) and TG (Kessler and Lederer, 1965) concentrations in each fraction was performed (Carlson, 1973). LP paper electrophoresis (Lees and Hatch, 1963) was run on whole serum and on top and bottom fractions after separation in the ultracentrifuge at d=1.006. Typing of HLP was performed according to WHO (Beaumont et al., 1970).

Results

Type of HLP

The following proportions of types of HLP were found (males/females, %): IIa 16/37, IIb 7/10, III 6/5, IV 50/24, V 2/1, and normal type 19/25 (Fig. 1). Thus, of all HLPs, type IIa was most abundant in women while type IV was so in men.

The Effect on Typing of Changing Cutoff Points for LP

The effect of moderate changes of the cutoff points in defining elevated concentrations of VLDL TG and LDL cholesterol is demonstrated in Table 1. As expected, the higher the cutoff point, the more sera was classified as normal. However, the most dramatic effect of going from low to high cutoff points was in both sexes a pronounced reduction of the number of type IIb. Thus, minor changes in the cutoff points not only changed the number of HLP subjects but also the relative frequencies of different types of HLP.

---

*Supported by grants from King Gustaf V 80-years foundation.

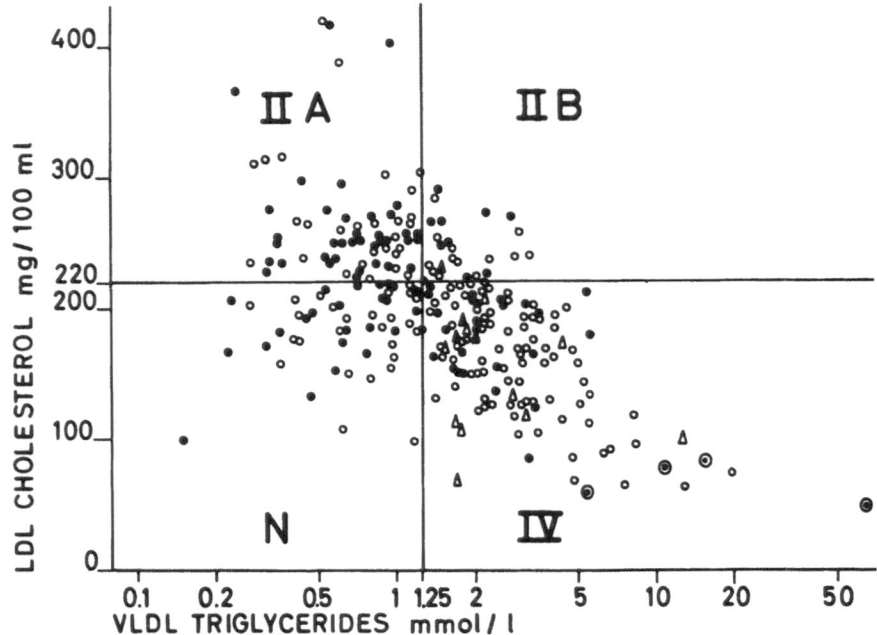

Figure 1. VLDL TG and LDL cholesterol concentrations in males (open symbols) and females (closed symbols). The lines indicate the cutoff points in the typing of HLP. Δ and $\blacktriangle$: type III HLP, ⊚ and ◉ : type V HLP

Table 1. The effect of the use of different cutoff points for defining elevated VLDL TG and LDL cholesterol on the distribution of the HLP men on different types

VLDL TG mmol/1	1.10	1.25[a]	1.40
LDL cholesterol mg/100 ml	200	220	240
N[b]	22	35	49
IIa	31	31	26
IIb	40	14	3
IV	81	94	96
V	3	3	3

[a]Cutoff points used for classification in this study.

[b]N = normal LP type despite hyperlipidemia at screening

Continuous Relation for Single LP in HLP

As seen in Figure 1, when VLDL TG is "elevated" this HLP is further subdivided into type IV with "normal" LDL cholesterol and type IIb with "elevated" LDL cholesterol. When the LDL cholesterol of type IIb and IV were pooled, however, the distribution curve of LDL cholesterol did not indicate the presence of two LDL populations (Fig. 2). On the contrary, the LDL cholesterol distribution curve was continuous and fairly normal. A similar picture evolves if we consider instead HLPs with elevated LDL cholesterol. VLDL TG in these types (type IIa and IIb) did not show any significant signs of bimodality but was fairly continuous (Fig. 2). From these fairly continuous distribution curves, the cutoff points used for both LDL and VLDL seem artificial.

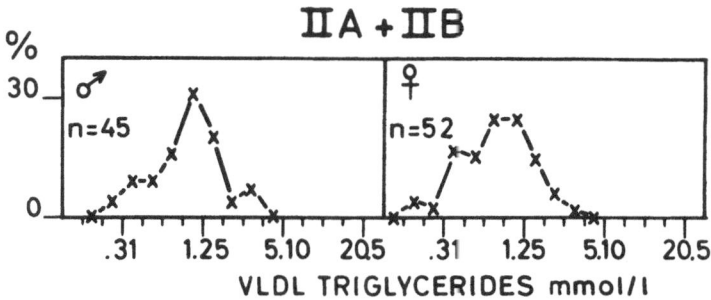

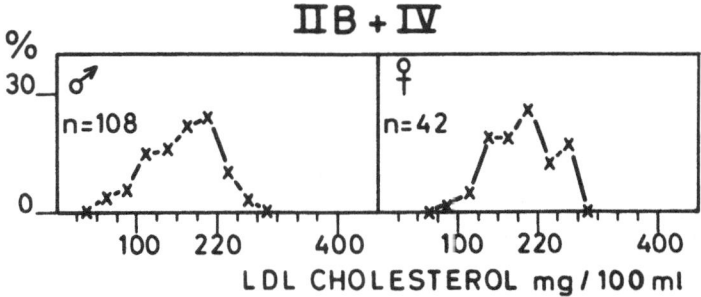

Figure 2. Distribution of VLDL TG in males and females with elevated LDL cholesterol concentration (above) and of LDL cholesterol when VLDL TG were elevated
(below)

Continuous Relation Between LP in HLP

It is also clear from Figure 1 that a continuous relation existed between VLDL
TG and LDL cholesterol. Except at the highest levels of VLDL TG, LDL cholesterol
could vary within rather wide limits. However, at every level of VLDL TG, the
maximal cholesterol concentration seemed to be very definitely determined. Therefore, only low and never high LDL cholesterol concentrations were seen with high
VLDL TG levels. All types of HLP appeared to fit into this regression.

Discussion

The present study shows that in a free-living, asymptomatic population types IIa,
IIb, III, IV, and V HLP could be diagnosed. The lack of specific pattern for total
serum cholesterol and TG concentrations in all types, except IIa, demonstrated
the necessity for lipoprotein determination and the inadequacy of only total
lipid determinations for correct typing of HLP.

Obvious advantages of the typing system for HLP are that it facilitates communication and it stimulates thinking in LP terms instead of total cholesterol and TG
levels.

However, the typing system also has several drawbacks. It has been argued that
individuals often oscillate between several types of HLP within a short time.
Also, one may easily become inclined to look erroneously at the types of HLP as
separate disease entities. It has to be born in mind that the typing system has
nothing to do with etiology and pathogenesis and that the typing is done on the
plasma sample and not on the patient (four-P problem, see Carlson, 1970). In the
present study, some other disadvantages of the typing system were evident:

1. By necessity, cutoff points must be arbitrarily defined as the distribution curves of the LPs are unimodal and continuous.

2. The allocation of subjects into different types of HLP was highly dependent on the cutoff points chosen, not only in the sense that the increasing or decreasing cutoff points altered the number of subjects having HLP but also in that the relative frequencies of the various types changed. From Figure 2 it is evident that looking at all subjects with elevation of LDL cholesterol or VLDL TG, an approximate normal distribution is achieved with other diagnostic LP, e.g., VLDL TG in type IIa and type IIb formed together a normal continuous relation.

3. The continuous relation between LDL cholesterol and VLDL TG in the HLP population (Fig. 1) is completely interrupted by the use of cutoff points for these LP lipids and misleadingly transforms a continuous relation into discrete populations. These findings make the typing system appear highly arbitrary, even artificial, and sometimes misleading.

This study demonstrates that the different types of HLP indeed are no discrete entities with regard to LP characteristics. Nevertheless, the current typing system for HLP is of great use to facilitate communication and to stimulate thinking in lipoprotein terms instead of total lipid levels. Today, no better way of defining hyperlipidemia is available. In the future, it is hoped that the system based on etiology will replace the current typing system.

SECONDARY CAUSES AND AGGRAVATING FACTORS FOR HYPERLIPOPROTEINEMIA

J.A. Little

Serum cholesterol (C) and triglyceride (TG) levels in a population are continuous variables and the risk from complicating diseases increases continuously with the levels. Thus, there is no sharp distinction between normal and abnormal. In Canada, where lipid levels and the prevalence of atherosclerotic disease (Statistics Canada, 1970) are high as compared to some other countries, it seems logical to choose relatively low upper "normal limits." Therefore, arbitrarily we consider that a person with a C and/or TG greater than the 90th percentile for their age and sex group has borderline hyperlipoproteinemia (HLP) and greater than the 95th percentile has definite HLP.

When a physician investigates a patient with HLP he must always consider the secondary causes and aggravating factors since this influences treatment. The ones of major clinical importance are obesity, alcohol ingestion, hypothyroidism, diabetes mellitus, estrogen therapy, and pancreatitis.

If one of these conditions is present, the physician should not forget that there may also be an underlying, genetically determined, primary HLP. Evidence for this will be found in the laboratory data, the family history of disease, screening the relatives for HLP, and in following the patient while on treatment. Examples of such evidence will be given in the following case reports. From our experience, the majority of patients with HLP have a combination of primary and secondary disease.

Family Screening

Table 1 shows the division of 25 type IV HLP probands into the group of five patients who could be said to have "primary" HLP without any recognizable aggravating factors and a group of 20 patients having either obesity, mild chemical dia-

Table 1. Hyperlipoproteinemia in first degree relatives of 25 type IV probands

Probands		First degree relatives			
Type	No.	Total	Normal	Borderline[b]	Definitely abnormal[c]
"Primary" IV	5	10	0	7	3
"Secondary" IV[a]	20	65	36	13	16

[a]"Secondary" to obesity, mild chemical diabetes or ingestion of alcohol.

[b]Serum C and/or TG levels >84th and <97.5 percentile.

[c]Serum C and:or TG levels >97.5 percentile.

betes, or excessive ingestion of alcohol, who could be considered to have "sec-ondary" HLP. A high percentage of the relatives of both proband groups had border-line or definite HLP. The finding of HLP in the family members of patients with so-called "secondary" HLP is evidence in favor of some genetic basis for their disease.

Obesity

In our population, there is a strong correlation between the ponderal index, $3\frac{ht}{\sqrt{wt}}$, and serum TG levels (LRC Program, unpublished data). From practical experi-ence with patients, there can be no doubt that obesity aggravates HLP and weight reduction is essential in the treatment of HLP. The first treatment of the gross-ly obese HLP patient is a reducing diet without regard to the type of fat, as shown by the patient in Table 2. Mr. G.W., age 30, was 128% of his ideal weight and had an elevated serum C and borderline elevation of TG. On a simple reducing diet of 1800 calories and increasing the amount of exercise, the serum lipids fell to normal as his weight decreased. Longer follow-up of such patients usually shows that any return to a positive caloric balance produces a quick reoccurrence of HLP.

Alcohol

Alcohol ingestion by humans having a tendency to hypertriglyceridemia often raises the serum levels significantly (Amatuzio and Hay, 1958; Wilson et al., 1970; Little, 1971; Little et al., 1970). The patient most susceptible to alcohol in our experience had type I HLP. Only 16 ml of ethanol before supper for 3 days consistently doubled the fasting serum TG level. Another patient, J.F. with type IV HLP, had an increase in TG from 1000 to 2000 mg/dl within a few hours of in-gesting 42 ml of ethanol. Healthy subjects show no increase in serum TG under these conditions. Treating patients with controlled fat diets usually will not lower serum lipids to normal if they continue to use alcohol.

Alcohol produces a number of metabolic changes during its oxidation including an increase in hepatic lipid content and release of VLDL from the liver and intes-tine (Freinkel et al., 1963; Kalant and Khanna, 1969; Lieber et al., 1965; Gordon, 1972; Mistilis and Ockner, 1972). In Canada, the per capita consumption of alcohol is equivalent to 5% of calories (the same as for potatoes). However, most of the alcohol is drunk by a fraction of the population. Thus, among our clinic patients, 10 - 40% of calories as alcohol in their customary diet is common. Sometimes mere-ly stopping the use of alcohol may quickly restore serum lipids to normal.

Table 2. The effects of a reducing diet on serum lipids in Mr. G.W., age 30 years, type II HLP and obesity (chart 1582)

| Date | Diet | Wt., kg. | Serum, mg/dl | |
			Cholesterol	Triglyceride
14.10.75	Customary 3200 cal	103	271	245
23.10.75	"	103	288	185
15. 1.76	Reducing 1800 cal	-	-	-
3. 2.76	"	101	205	165
24. 2.76	"	99	221	120
16. 3.76	"	95	210	170
29. 6.76	"	91	208	127

Hypothyroidism

Every patient with HLP should be screened for hypothyroidism because it can be associated with any of the usual lipoprotein patterns from I through V (Fredrickson and Levy, 1972). In the past, we screened our patients by measuring serum l-thyroxine. More recently, in patients with borderline low levels of l-thyroxine, we have also measured serum TSH looking for so-called "subclinical" hypothyroidism (Hall, 1972; Evered et al., 1973; Gordin et al., 1974). Indeed, there is a hypothesis, as yet unproved, that subclinical hypothyroidism may be one cause of secondary HLP. It is characterized by normal thyroid indices, except for an elevated basal serum TSH level. Although our experience is still limited in this regard, we have not yet found this as a cause of HLP. So far, thyroid medication in such patients has been unimpressive, as compared to the effect of diet and lipid-lowering drugs on serum lipid levels. However, definitely myxedematous patients, with low serum l-thyroxine levels and HLP, may have their serum lipid levels reduced to normal with thyroid replacement therapy alone. One should be careful to avoid cardiotoxic doses of thyroxine in these high risk patients.

An unusual example of HLP secondary to frank hypothyroidism is a 56-year-old lady, V.L., who presented with a serum C of 513 and TG of 400 mg/dl, serum l-thyroxine <1.0 μg/dl, T3 resin uptake 19% and TSH <80 μU/ml. There was a type III lipoprotein electrophoretic pattern, a floating β-fraction and a negative Wieland-Seidel test (1973), and a VLDL C/total TG ratio of .26. On 0.1 mg of l-thyroxine daily, the signs of myxedema disappeared, the C fell to 154 and TG to 94 mg/dl, and the lipoprotein pattern became normal within 4 weeks.

Diabetes Mellitus

Patients with insulin-dependent diabetes mellitus as a group have slight but significantly increased serum lipid levels (Nikkila, 1974; Kaufmann et al., 1975; New et al., 1963). However, frank HLP may be aggravated by poorly controlled insulin-dependent diabetes, but is certainly not caused only by the diabetes. Two cases illustrate the varied association between diabetes and HLP.

Mr. A.Sq., an obese man of 37, developed thirst and severe widespread eruptive skin xanthomata. The fasting blood sugar was 276, C 483, TG 980 mg/dl, and the electrolytes were normal. On a 1500 calorie diabetic diet and 500 mg of tolbutamide twice daily, the blood lipids fell to normal within 3 weeks (C 219, TG

222 mg/dl), he lost only 1.5 kg and the fasting blood sugar was still elevated at 148 mg/dl. The skin xanthomata disappeared. As discussed by Reaven et al. (1975), the balance between this patient's VLDL synthesis and utilization must have been very sensitive to dietary restriction and the insulin released by tolbutamide.

Another diabetic male, A.Se., age 52 with HLP, responded differently to treatment. He was not obese and had been on traditional diabetic diet and insulin for years. The fasting blood sugar was 357, C 567, TG 777 mg/dl, and the lipoprotein electrophoresis showed increased β and pre-β fractions with normal separation by ultracentrifugation. Increasing the insulin dose and replacing some of the animal and dairy fat and simple sugars in the diet with polyunsaturated vegetable fats and starch lowered the fasting blood sugar to the range of 50 - 250 mg/dl. However, the HLP persisted with a type IIb lipoprotein pattern and a C of 320, LDL C of 242, and a TG varying from 120 to 260 mg/dl. A family screen revealed numerous members with HLP. Therefore, this patient has both diabetes and familial type IIb HLP.

Patients having both HLP and diabetes, if followed carefully, usually continue to have some elevation of serum lipids inspite of good diabetic control. In contrast, the majority of well-controlled diabetics do not have HLP.

Estrogens

Oral estrogens definitely elevate the serum C and TG levels of younger and middle-aged women. This is evident from the population survey by the Lipid Research Clinic Program (Hoover et al., 1976) and the clinical observations by Rossner et al. (1971) and others.

Hyperlipoproteinemia and the use of oral estrogens are commonly associated in women referred to the Lipid Clinic. One striking example was B.V., a 25-year-old female, who developed eruptive skin xanthomata soon after staring .05 mg of ethinyl estradiol daily. The blood serum had a chylomicron layer, a C of 320, and TG of 2400 mg/dl, a type V lipoprotein pattern and a normal post heparin lipolytic activity (PHLA) of .294 µEq/ml/min (Fredrickson et al., 1963). The medication was stopped. After 1 month, the serum TG remained elevated at 1800 mg/dl and the C was 265 mg/dl.

Then a diet was prescribed having 20% of calories as fat and limitation of simple sugars and alcohol. The C fell to 170 and TG to 420 mg/dl, and the lipoprotein pattern changed to type IV. While not on estrogens, her Apo CII polypeptide in the VLDL fraction was decreased in proportion to Apo CIII, as described previously by Carlson et al. (1976) in type IV and V patients. Her father was found to have type V HLP and two other relatives have diabetes. Therefore, this patient probably has primary familial type V HLP and the estrogen was only an aggravating factor. On no estrogens and a strict diet, she still has some residual triglyceridemia.

Pancreatitis

Pancreatitis may precede or be a consequence of the triglyceridemic forms of HLP. Often it is difficult, if not impossible, to decide whether the HLP is primary or secondary to the pancreatitis. Exacerbations of recurrent pancreatitis may occur, especially when the serum TG levels become greatly elevated above 3000 mg/dl. Such patients must abstain from alcoholic or dietary excesses which produce triglyceridemia and attacks of potentially fatal pancreatitis. Obviously, treatment for one condition is beneficial for the other in a preventive sense.

In three patients, we were able to find evidence that the HLP was primary, inspite of the long history of chronic recurrent pancreatitis prior to our investigation. One had no PHLA in her plasma and is the type I HLP who, as mentioned above, was so sensitive to alcohol. Another is a man with a 40-year history of abdominal pain, a type V lipoprotein pattern, and no Apo CII polypeptide on poly-acrylamide gel electrophoresis (Breckenridge et al., 1976). A third is a man with a type V pattern and two close relatives with type IV HLP. All of the several other patients with the syndrome of pancreatitis and HLP have no detectable lipid metabolic defects or relatives with HLP to indicate that there is a genetic basis for their disease.

Conclusion

HLP which appears to be secondary to other conditions or drugs or diet may, after careful investigation and follow-up, prove to have a genetic basis. It is the interaction of environmental factors or drugs or acquired diseases with certain genetic traits which produces their HLP.

DIAGNOSIS OF TYPE III HYPERLIPOPROTEINEMIA BY MEANS OF RATE ZONAL ULTRACENTRIFUGATION

S. Sailer, J. Patsch, and W. Patsch

The partial conflicting reports regarding the definition and diagnosis of type III hyperlipoproteinemia gave rise to our investigation of the main lipoprotein density classes in the plasma of type III patients. Since not only the VLDL frac-tion is altered in these patients, we separated the lipoprotein fractions d <1.063 by means of zonal ultracentrifugation. This technique allows a good separation of the main density classes within a short period of time (Patsch et al., 1974) and seems therefore suitable for diagnosis of type III patients as well as for the study of changes in the concentration of the different lipopro-tein density classes as a result of an altered metabolic situation, for example, during fasting.

Using a linear density gradient from 1.00 - 1.30, in the postabsorptive state in type III subjects three distinct lipoprotein fractions, namely chylomicrons VLDL, an intermediate density class and the "normal" LDL were found (Fig. 1). In normal subjects and in hyperlipoproteinemic patients other than type III, only two lipo-protein peaks, namely chylomicrons VLDL and LDL were found in the postabsorptive state. The concentration of this "intermediate" lipoprotein (or as we call it "LP III") was 286 ± 81 mg/dl, it contains about 40% (wt/wt) total cholesterol, 20% triglycerides, 20% phospholipids, and 20% protein (Patsch et al., 1975). On agarose gel electrophoresis, LP III exhibited a migration rate which was faster than that of LDL and slower than that of VLDL. Using the double immunodiffusion technique or immunoelectrophoresis, B-apolipoprotein and C-apolipoprotein could be detected, but no A-apolipoprotein albumin.

In order to find optimal conditions for the preparation of LP III in angle head rotors, ultracentrifugation was carried out in an angle head rotor at 1.4×10^8 g min at different densities. The appropriate density for the separation of LP III from LDL proved to be d 1.025. At this nonprotein solvent density, LP III floats, whereas LDL remains quantitatively in the bottom fraction (Fig. 2).

It is of further interest that for quantitative separation of VLDL from the slower migrating LP III at least 1.4×10^8 g min is required, because after ultra-centrifugation at 1.01×10^8 g min, d 1.006, LP III did not sediment completely, as was shown by slicing the tube at different levels and recentrifugation of the supernate in the zonal rotor. Therefore, the "floating β-lipoprotein" or the "β-VLDL" could in some instances at least partly be due to contamination with LP-III.

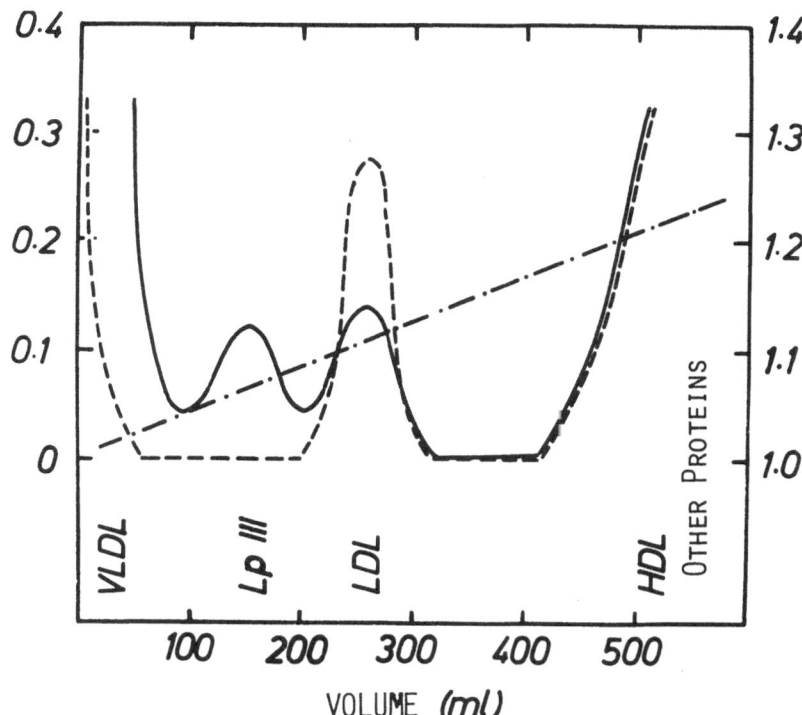

Figure 1. ——— — — — — Absorption (280 nm)
-.-.-.-.-.-.-. Specific gravity

The changing ratio of LP III/LDL observed in one person (0.73 – 1.84) over a period of 15 months suggests that the plasma concentration of LP III and LDL is
closely related to the actual metabolic state of the individual. Therefore, the
effect of starvation for 6 days and a subsequent isocaloric carbohydrate-rich,
fat-free diet was studied. During fasting, in normals and in patients with type
IV hyperlipoproteinemia, the VLDL concentration decreased rapidly and the LDL
concentration increased. In contrast, in type III patients, the VLDL concentration decreased much lower and the LP III ("intermediate") increased, while the
LDL fraction remained unchanged. The opposite effect was obtained by a carbohydrate-rich diet (Fig. 3).

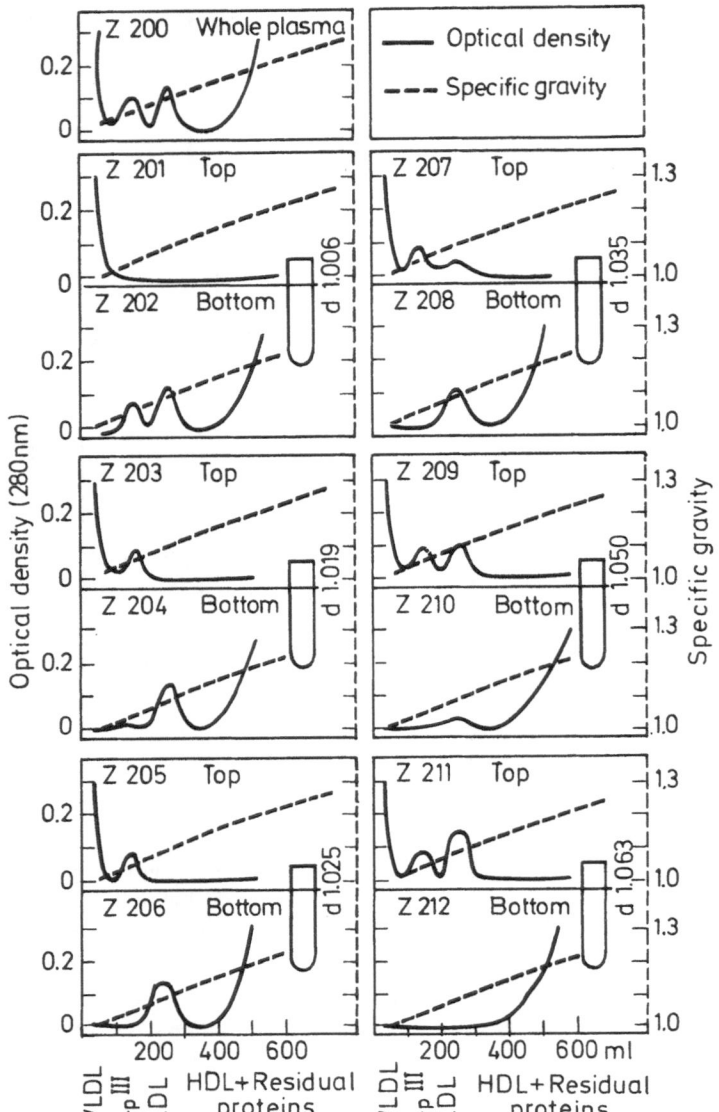

Figure 2

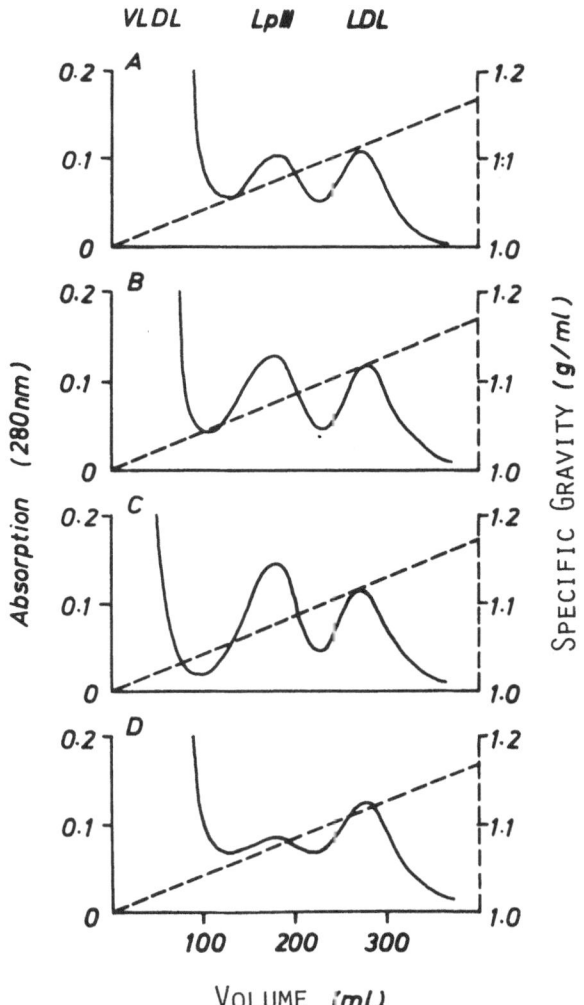

Figure 3

SOME ASPECTS OF SENSITIVITY AND RESISTANCE TO THE CHOLESTEROL LOWER-ING EFFECT OF CLOFIBRATE*

R. Pichardo and J. Davignon

Clofibrate (CPIB) is not generally considered the drug of choice in the treatment of familial type II hypercholesterolemia (Levy et al., 1972). This is unfortunate because in our experience (Davignon et al., 1971), and in that of others (Crepaldi et al., 1974), it has been found to be a potent cholesterol and β-lipoprotein cholesterol-lowering agent in a good proportion of patients affected with this disease. The problem, however, is to identify the potential responders among these patients. A few years ago, we were able to demonstrate a negative correlation between the average plasma triglyceride/cholesterol (TG/TC) ratio of a control period and the cholesterol-lowering effect of clofibrate in familial type II (Davignon et al., 1971). Thus, type IIa patients with low plasma triglycerides

*Supported by grants from the Quebec Heart Foundation and the Macdonald-Stewart Foundation.

were more likely to have their plasma cholesterol concentration lowered by this drug than type IIb patients with higher plasma triglycerides. Since a line arbitrarily drawn at a TG/TC ratio of 0.40 separated the majority of the responders from the majority of the nonresponders, we have been using this ratio in our laboratory as a cutoff point for separating type IIa from type IIb. At one extreme, the responsive type II patient may show a 30% decrease in plasma cholesterol while at the other extreme a 10% increase may be observed. These findings allowed us to account for some of the discrepancies in the literature on the effectiveness of clofibrate in familial hypercholesterolemia as a function of the relative proportion of types IIa and IIb (or of responders and nonresponders). In addition, the TG/TC ratio turned out to be helpful in recognizing potential responders. Since β-cholesterol is probably the most atherogenic of plasma lipoproteins, it is important to identify the nonresponders and stop clofibrate administration especially in those patients who show an increase in β-cholesterol on the drug. In the Coronary Drug Project (1975) greater reductions in plasma cholesterol concentrations were achieved by clofibrate treatment in patients with low baseline levels of triglycerides than in those with high triglyceride levels. It is thus possible that a relatively large proportion of type IIb patients or nonresponders might have been responsible for the rather modest overall fall in cholesterol concentration observed (6.5%) and perhaps for the adverse effects reported in this study.

In an attempt to find an explanation for the striking difference in response to the cholesterol-lowering effect of clofibrate in familial type II hypercholesterolemia, we have selected patients at the two extremes of response and measured their plasma clofibrate concentrations. The CPIB-responsive patients were defined as those showing at least a 20% fall in plasma cholesterol and/or at least a 15% fall in plasma β-lipoprotein cholesterol. The CPIB-resistant patients were those who had a increase or less than a 10% fall in cholesterol concentration and/or an increase or less than a 5% fall in β-cholesterol. Assessment of responsiveness on 2 g per day of clofibrate, and measurement of plasma lipids and lipoprotein cholesterol were done according to standard techniques used in our laboratory (Davignon et al., 1971, Davignon and Langelier, 1975). Plasma CPIB concentration was determined by gas-liquid chromatography (Bruderlein et al., 1975) on blood samples obtained from patients who had been receiving 1 g of clofibrate twice a day for at least 2 months. Blood was drawn after an overnight fast and 10 hours after the last evening dose taken exactly at 22:30 h.

Thirty-three patients were studied, 18 responders and 15 nonresponders. Details on each patient group and the results obtained are given in Table 1. Both groups had the same proportion of patients with tendon xanthomas and were comparable for age. The body weight, however, was slightly higher in the CPIB-resistant group. The mean plasma cholesterol and β-cholesterol levels were comparable in both groups. The selection of patients in each group accounted for the greater than 20% fall in plasma cholesterol and β-cholesterol in the CPIB-sensitive patients, and for the modest lowering of cholesterol and the increase in β-cholesterol in the CPIB-resistant group. As expected, triglycerides were higher in the resistant group which included more type IIb patients, but the degree of triglyceride lowering was the same in both experimental groups.

Plasma clofibrate levels (measured as nonesterified clofibric acid) were significantly higher (p <0.001) in the CPIB-responsive patients whether all patients in each group were considered or only those with tendon xanthomas. Plasma clofibrate levels were found to be inversely correlated with body weight in the responsive group but not in the resistant one. Expressed differently, plasma CPIB was directly correlated with the dose of clofibrate (mg/kg) in the responders (r = 0.77, p <0.001) but no such correlation existed in the resistant group (r = 0.17, NS). When the changes in plasma β-cholesterol were plotted against plasma clofibrate levels, a marked difference between the two groups were observed. In the CPIB-resistant patients, the β-cholesterol tended to be higher with increasing levels of plasma clofibrate (r = 0.64, p <0.05). In contrast, the opposite was true in the responders, the greater the plasma CPIB, the greater the fall in β-cholesterol (r = 0.84, p <0.001).

Table 1. Clinical data. Plasma lipid changes, and plasma CPIB levels

	CPIB-responsive	CPIB-resistant	p [b]
Number (females)	18(12F)	15(7F)	
Number of types IIa	14	7	
Number with tendon xanthomas	10	8	
Age ($\bar{x} \pm$ SD)	48.2 ± 15.8	41.9 ± 10.5	N.S.
Weight (kg ± SD)	59.9 ± 8.9	67.3 ± 13.0	<0.05
Fasting blood sugar[a]	92.6 ± 6.2	95.0 ± 7.0	N.S.
Basal plasma cholesterol[a]	327 ± 71	334 ± 44	N.S.
Cholesterol on CPIB[a]	247 ± 46	321 ± 50	<0.001
Percent change ($\bar{x} \Delta\%$)	-24.2 ± 5.3	-3.4 ± 5.1	<0.001
Basal β-cholesterol[a]	264 ± 66	258 ± 57	N.S.
β-cholesterol on CPIB[a]	185 ± 39	259 ± 60	<0.001
Percent change ($\bar{x} \Delta\%$)	-28.1 ± 9.8	+1.3 ± 8.2	<0.001
Basal plasma triglycerides[a]	113 ± 56	206 ± 128	<0.01
Triglycerides on CPIB[a]	78 ± 31	142 ± 76	<0.01
Percent change ($\bar{x} \Delta\%$)	-22.0 ± 36	-25 ± 23	N.S.
Plasma CPIB (μg/dl ± SD)	131.4 ± 24.8	94.7 ± 26.0	<0.001
Plasma CPIB in patients with tendon xanthomas only	141.8 ± 22.7 (n = 10)	98.6 ± 24.6 (n = 8)	<0.001

[a] mg/dl ± SD.

[b] Student t test comparing CPIB-responsive and CPIB-resistant patients.

Increasing the dose of clofibrate in resistant type II from 2 to 3 g per day always resulted in an increase in plasma CPIB levels. However, this was followed in some patients by a decrease in β-cholesterol and in other subjects by an increase in this parameter so that the net result was not significantly different between the two groups (Table 2).

Table 2. Effect of increasing the dose of CPIB in resistant type II

Plasma levels of	Control period (A)	CPIB 2 g/d (B)	p [b]	CPIB 3 g/d (C)	p [c]
Cholesterol[a] (n=8)	318 ± 29	304 ± 34	NS	285 ± 33	<0.02
β-cholesterol[a] (n=8)	239 ± 28	256 ± 20	NS	221 ± 21	N.S.
CPIB (μg/ml SD) (n=7)	-	108 ± 27	-	135 ± 25	0.05

[a] mg/dl, $\bar{x} \pm$ SD.

[b] Paired t test comparing A and B.

[c] Paired t test comparing B and C.

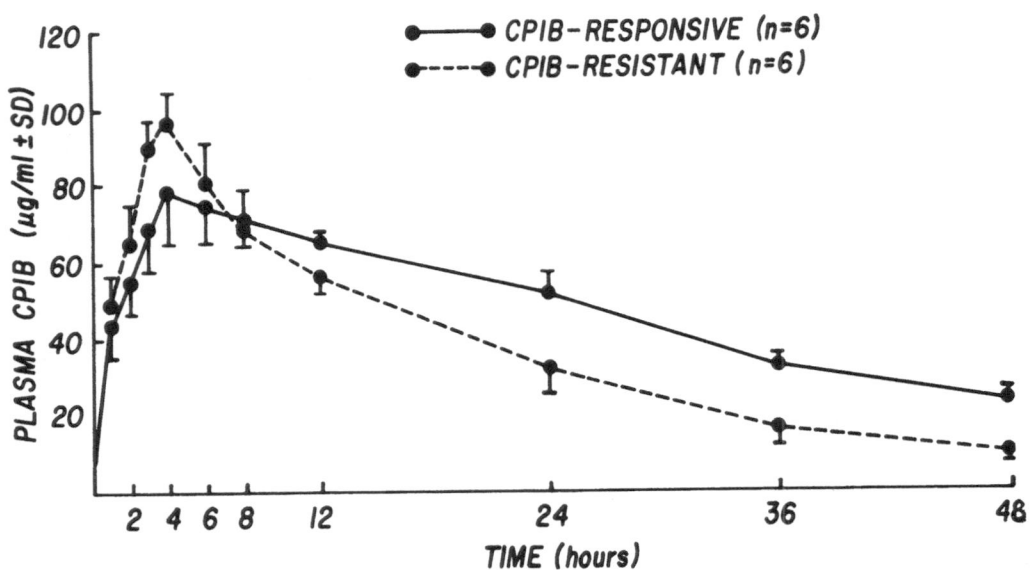

Figure 1. Plasma levels of CPIB after the oral administration of 1 g of clofibrate in patients who are responsive or resistant to the cholesterol-lowering effect of this drug and who have been off clofibrate for at least 3 weeks

To further investigate the difference observed between the two groups, the plasma levels of CPIB were measured over a 48-hour period after a single oral dose of 1 g of clofibrate. This was carried out on six patients of each group after they had stopped receiving the drug for at least 3 weeks. The half-life calculated by computer on the log-linear part of the disappearance curve was found to be higher on the average in the responsive group (22.6 ± 1.52 h) than in the resistant patients (15.3 ± 0.83 h). The degree of significance for the difference in this small sample was p <0.01, the curves obtained for the two groups are plotted in Figure 1. The plasma levels are slightly higher (although nit significantly so) at 4 hours in the resistant group, but because of the more rapid clearing of CPIB in this group, the plasma concentrations are lower from the 8th hour on.

In conclusion, it appears that the metabolic handling of clofibrate differs if a patient affected with familial hypercholesterolemia is "responsive" or "resistant" to the cholesterol-(or β-cholesterol-) lowering effect of this drug. This difference does not seem to be due to an absorption defect for CPIB or a lesser sensitivity to its cholesterol-lowering action in the resistant patients; it may reflect basic differences in β-lipoprotein-cholesterol metabolism between the two groups which should be explored further.

NEWER METHODS OF TREATMENT OF THE HYPERLIPOPROTEINEMIAS

A.N. Howard

The drugs commonly used for the treatment of type IIa hyperlipoproteinaemia are the anion exchange resins, neomycin and D-thyroxine. However, none of these drugs alone is capable of lowering serum cholesterol by more than about 20%. For this reason, various combinations of drugs have been tried. Of these, the most successful have been the combination of any of the above-mentioned drugs with clofibrate (Howard, 1975). Clofibrate inhibits liver biosynthesis and increases biliary cholesterol and bile acids in animals. All of these properties could enhance the action of anion exchange resins.

One of the most potent combinations with clofibrate is polydexide, Secholex®, (Howard and Hyams, 1971) which appears superior to cholestyramine or colestipol. This difference is surprising since cholestyramine is a stronger base than poly-dexide, and causes a much greater increase in faecal bile acids (Simons and Myant, 1976).

Neomycin, which is also a weaker base than cholestyramine, has the same order of activity as polydexide, when combined with clofibrate. This would suggest that the mechanism of action of polydexide and neomycin is related to their weaker basicity. Although neomycin is a bile acid sequestrant, it also inhibits the formation of fat micelles in the intestine, leading to malabsorption of fat and increased excretion of neutral and acidic sterols (Thompson et al., 1971). In this respect, the removal of long chain fatty acids seems to be of more importance than the removal of bile acids. Thus, a new explanation of the synergistic effects of the two classes of drugs can be proposed. Clofibrate causes an increase in biliary cholesterol, much of which would normally be reabsorbed in the entero-hepatic circulation. Neomycin and polydexide, being weak bases, preferentially combine with fatty acids rather than bile acids, interfering with the micellar formation and hence the absorption of cholesterol (Fig. 1).

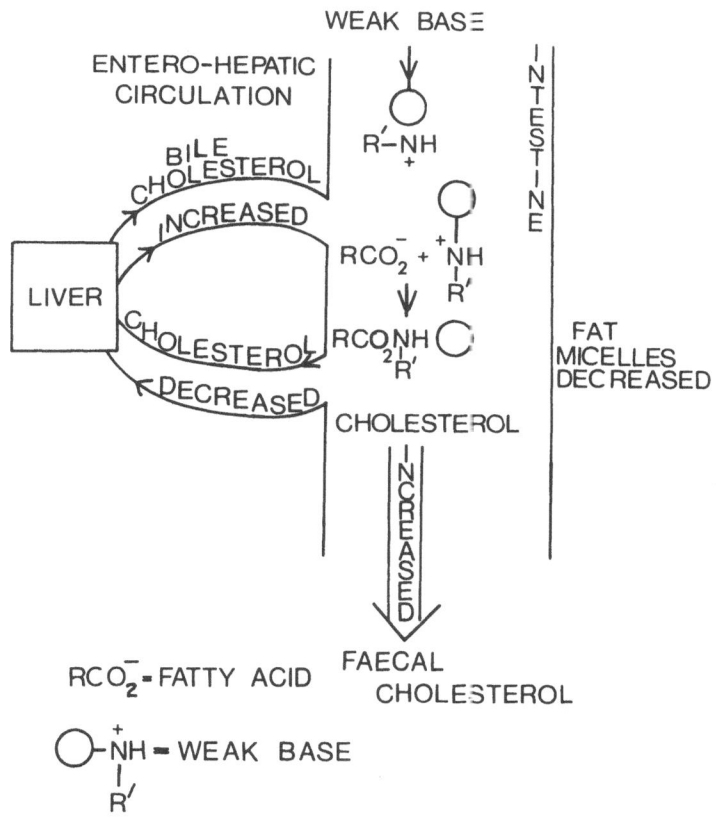

Figure 1. Alternative mechanism of action of weak basic drugs in combination with clofibrate

This explanation seems preferable to that previously proposed, namely, that it is the combination of bile acid sequestration, the inhibition of cholesterol biosynthesis, and increase in biliary bile acids, which is responsible. The defect of the latter hypothesis was that it was difficult to explain why cholestyramine and clofibrate should have such a weak combined activity. Also, clofibrate does not cause an increase in biliary bile acid in man (Pertsemlidis et al., 1974) as it does in animals.

Calcium salts will also decrease blood lipids (Bierenbaum et al., 1972) and act as bile acid sequestrants. Calcium salts of glycine but not taurine conjugated bile acids are insoluble and can be excreted in the faeces. Calcium also forms insoluble soaps with long-chain fatty acids and would be expected to interfere with fat micellar formation.

A combination of calcium salts and clofibrate might be expected to show the same effect as that described above (Howard et al., 1977). Patients were asked to continue their normal diet, and blood was taken after an overnight fast. After 4 weeks treatment they were given clofibrate (Atromid-S, 500 mg thrice daily), calcium carbonate (0.65 g thrice daily) or a combination of both. As shown in Table 1, treatment with clofibrate gave a mean reduction of 11% in serum cholesterol. With calcium carbonate, a 4% decrease was seen. When both clofibrate and calcium carbonate was used in combination, a 23% reduction occurred. Thus, the average reduction was over 50% greater than the sum of the individual effects. Clofibrate caused a 35% decrease in serum triglycerides when given alone. Calcium carbonate had no influence on serum triglycerides alone or in combination.

Other metallic cations which form insoluble salts with bile acids are also effective in combination with clofibrate (Fig. 2). Thus, magnesium, aluminium and bismuth salts also demonstrate a synergistic effect with clofibrate (Howard et al., 1977). Since all these anions form insoluble soaps with fatty acids, the mechanism of action of the combination may be the inhibition of micellar formation as already described above.

Attempts are currently being made to develop alternative drugs with the same activity as clofibrate. One such drug currently under international investigation is Gemfibrozil (2,2-dimethyl 5-(2,5-xylyloxy) valeric acid, Parke-Davis) which has a structure somewhat related to clofibrate. Gemfibrozil has a pronounced ability to decrease serum triglycerides in rats, mice and monkeys, after oral administration but has no effect on serum cholesterol. If it is possible to extrapolate these data to man, the hyperlipoproteinaemias most likely to be affected are types IIb, III, IV and V.

In our studies, Gemfibrozil proved an effective drug for the reduction of serum triglycerides (Howard and Ghosh, 1976). As shown in Figure 3, serum cholesterol

Table 1. Effect of clofibrate and calcium carbonate alone and in combination. Serum cholesterol (mg/100 ml)

Type	Nil	A	% Change	Nil	Ca	% Change	Nil	A + Ca	% Change
IIa	255	230	10	260	255	2	250	180	28
IIa	255	235	8	250	240	4	255	195	24
IIb	265	215	19	270	260	4	265	190	28
IIb	290	250	14	295	280	5	290	225	22
V	310	300	3	305	295	4	300	260	13
Mean			11			4			23

CaCO₃ 2g/day; A = Clofibrate 1.5 g/day; treatment: 4 weeks.

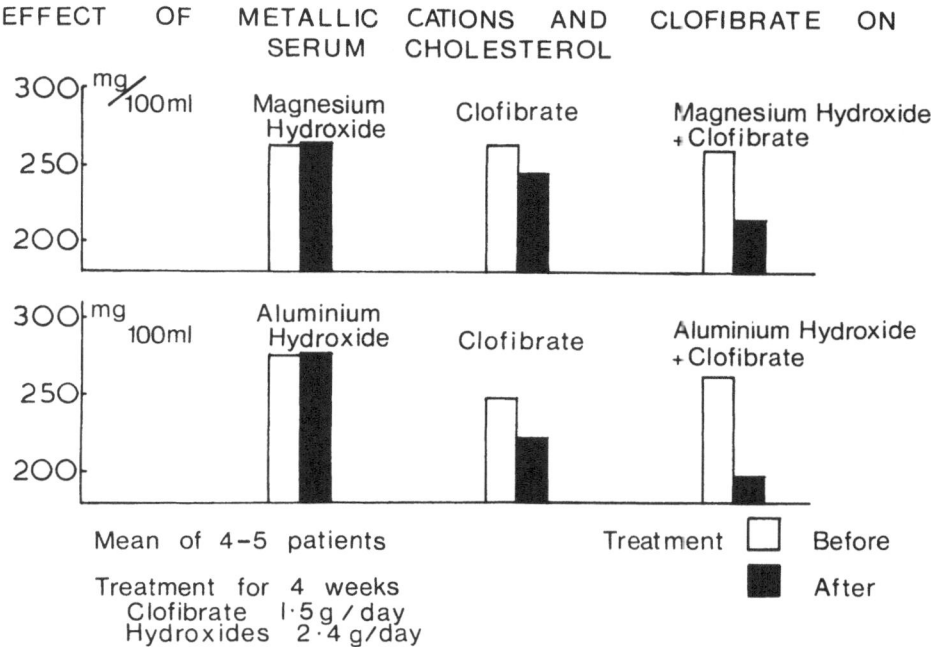

Figure 2. Combination therapy with metallic anions

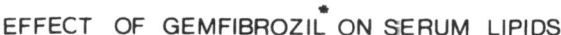

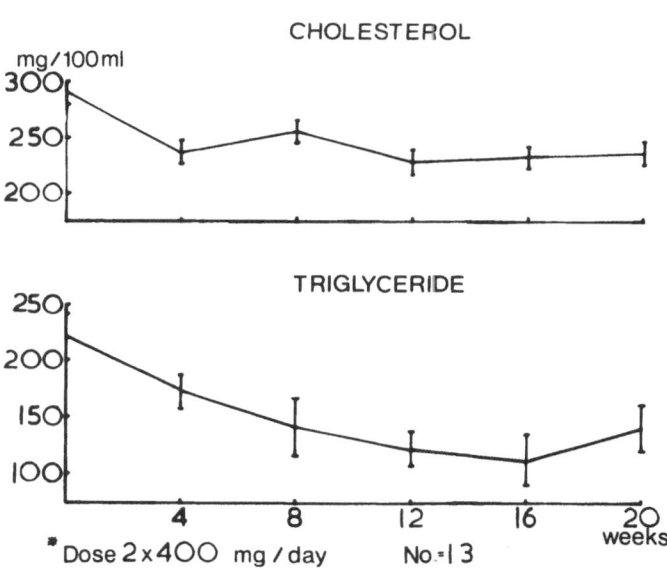

Figure 3. Effect of Gemfibrozil on serum lipids (mean ± SEM)

and triglycerides were decreased to a minimum after 3 months treatment, to values of 21% and 45% respectively, below the normal baseline values. Likewise, VLDL and LDL were decreased 32.5% and 21%. In addition, one type V subject was investigated. An initial serum triglyceride value of 1295 mg/100 ml was reduced to 230 mg/100 ml after 12 weeks treatment. Both chylomicrons and VLDL were effectively reduced accordingly.

Clofibrate, the most widely used drug for the treatment of hypertriglyceridaemia (Howard, 1975), has one major side effect, namely, it increases the incidence of gallstones (Coronary Drug Project, 1975). A study of the effect of Gemfibrozil on the lithogenicity of bile would appear to be of high priority since there is a need for a safer hypotriglyceridaemic drug.

ANALYSIS OF THE CHARACTERISTICS OF β-K BAND IN THE FRACTION OF LIPOPROTEIN BY POLYACRYLAMIDE GEL-DISC ELECTROPHORESIS AND THE FREQUENCY OF ITS APPEARANCE IN IHD

S. Yamasaki

The β-lipoprotein band was separated into a few subunits (midbands) by polyacrylamide gel-disc electrophoresis. Of these midbands, one which migrates nearest the pre-β band had been described as a β-k band in our previous reports (Yano et al., 1974; Nanbu et al., 1973, 1975). This paper presents additional evidence in respect to the β-k band, especially its characteristics on the composition of lipids and protein in each lipoprotein fraction. The frequency of its appearance in the patients with ischemic heart disease (IHD) was also examined.

Methods

The subjects were 150 patients that were hospitalized in the Kurume University Hospital and divided into two groups, control group and IHD group. The control group consisted of 102 patients. Forty-eight patients with IHD were diagnosed by physical examination, laboratory findings, and clinical symptoms. Blood samples were collected in ethylene diaminotetra-acetic acid before and after the diet therapy for 4 weeks. This diet was characterized by 1000 calories, consisting of 140 g of carbohydrate and 80 g of protein. Each lipoprotein fraction, very low-density lipoprotein (VLDL), and low-density lipoportein (LDL) were separated using ultracentrifugation as described by Havel et al. (1955) 25 μl of whole plasma or each lipoprotein fraction were inserted into the tubule of polyacrylamide gel-disc electrophoresis (Canarco, QDL). Electrophoresis was carried out for 28 min at a constant current of 5 mA. After the disc electrophoresis, its densitograph was traced by densitometry (Tokyo, DMU-33C). Concentration of total cholesterol (TC), triglyceride (TG) and protein in plasma and each lipoprotein fraction were measured by the method of Abell et al. (1952), STG 5 (Nishimoto and Nishimoto, 1965), and Lowry et al. (1951), respectively.

Results

A β-k band was clearly separated by polyacrylamide gel-disc electrophoresis and its densitograph (Fig. 1). Pre-β band was observed in the fraction of VLDL, whereas the β-k band was found in the fraction of LDL. This band was completely separated from pre-β band. In the densitograph, the solid line represented the blood sample having β-k band and the dotted line represented the sample without β-k band in the same patients. While the sample with this band showed a lower β-band and a higher pre-β band, the sample without this band showed a higher β-band and a lower pre-β band. It showed the characteristic phenomenon that ordinary β-band decreased with the appearance of β-k band in the same patients.

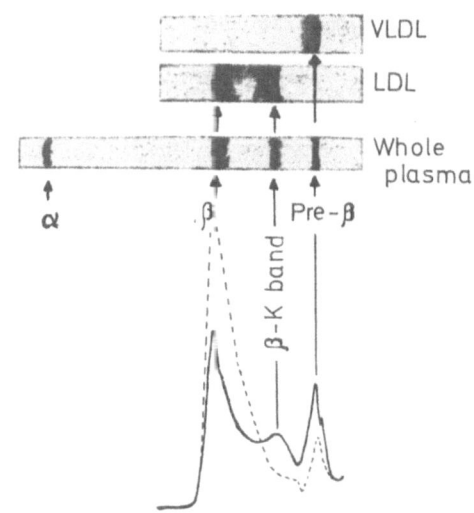

Figure 1. Demonstration of β-k band. Top: a β-k band was observed in the fraction of LDL by polyacrylamide gel-disc electrophoresis. Bottom: simultaneous tracings of densitograph. Solid line = sample with β-k band. Dotted line = sample without this band. Two samples were collected at separate stages from the same patient

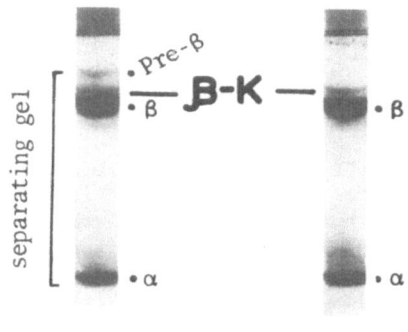

Figure 2. Effect of heparin infusion (polyacrylamide gel-disc electrophoresis). S.T. 49-year-old female

Lipoprotein fraction with β-k band was shown to have the characteristics of low TC containing LDL. After the activation of LPL by the heparin injection, pre-β band was disappeared from its densitography by hydrolysis of TG in pre-β band, whereas the β-k band was still found in β-band (Fig. 2). It is possible, therefore, that the appearance of β-k band is not dependent on hydrolysis of TG in VLDL and is associated with cholesterol metabolism. And so it can be estimated that β-k band after the heparin infusion is derived from suppression of an exchange between free cholesterol and cholesterol ester. In consequence, the remnant type was observed by an incomplete catabolysis of VLDL. From these findings, the β-k band seems to be a remnant lipoprotein.

Plasma TC levels when the β-k band was present ranged from 140 to 294 mg/100 ml (mean, 221) and 66 to 246 mg/100 ml (mean, 146) for TG, respectively. When the β-k band was absent, these levels ranged from 118 to 343 mg/100 ml (mean, 233) for TC and 44 to 142 mg/100 ml (mean, 96) for TG. The β-k band appeared in two (subject O.R. and S.H.) of six patients after 4 weeks of the diet therapy even though plasma TG in all cases were decreased by the diet. This fact indicated

Table 1. Comparison of lipid compositions in plasma lipoprotein with or without β-k band

	Very low-density lipoprotein						Low-density lipoprotein			
	Triglyceride mg/100 ml		Total cholesterol mg/100 ml		Ratio of TC/TG		Triglyceride mg/100 ml		Total cholesterol mg/100 ml	
β-k band	(+)	(−)	(+)	(−)	(+)	(−)	(+)	(−)	(+)	(−)
Subjects:										
S.T.	330	193	262	60	0.79	0.31	232	126	534	811
M.T.	311	204	198	98	0.64	0.48	182	166	409	568
N.O.	120	76	49	29	0.41	0.38	79	60	240	270
K.A.	120	81	41	22	0.34	0.27	126	121	708	824
O.R. [a]	324	232	155	79	0.48	0.34	188	140	281	521
S.H. [a]	253	218	97	70	0.38	0.32	163	131	897	1130
Mean	243	167	134	60	0.51	0.35	162	124	512	687
Mean difference	−76		−74		−0.16 0.74 [b] (0.39−0.93)		−38		+176	

[a]The β-k band of these subjects appeared 4 weeks after the diet therapy.

[b]This value was determined by the TC/TG ratio when β-k band was absent over its ratio when β-k band was present.

that the β-k band might be metabolically unstable and was not affected by diet factors. The lipid levels in each LP fraction are shown in Table 1. Although the differences in the concentrations recorded were not significant, TG and TC levels in very low-density lipoprotein (VLDL) were relatively high when the β-k band was present as compared with levels recorded in the absence of β-k band. Mean difference of these levels was 76 mg/100 ml (range, 35-137) high for TG and 74 mg/100 ml (range, 19-202) high for TC. Moreover, there was a relatively high content of TC against TG in VLDL of the group with the β-k band. As shown in Table 1, the TC/TG ratio of VLDL in the absence of the β-k band was 0.74 of that found in the presence of the β-k band. These results suggested that the β-k band might be occasioned by a disturbance of cholesterol catabolism in VLDL rather than by a disturbance of hydrolysis of TG in VLDL. However, our recent reports (Kimura et al., 1974, 1975) have suggested that VLDL catabolism was controlled by the balance of both hydrolysis of TG and removal and/or esterification of free cholesterol.

The concentrations of lipids recorded in LDL were also variable. However, the composition of LDL lipids, especially as shown by a comparison between patients with and without β-k band, was characterized by the reciprocal change between TG and TC. The relatively low level of LDL cholesterol might be due to inhibition low level of LDL cholesterol might be due to inhibition of conversion of VLDL to LDL.

The β-k band in PAG-disc electrophoresis was characterized by the relatively high content of VLDL TC with a relatively low LDL TC, and the composition was originally unafffected by the diet factor for hyperlipidemia. The impaired catabolism of VLDL cholesterol rather than that of VLDL TG might play an important role in the genesis of the β-k band.

Table 2. Frequency of the appearance of β-k band in the patients with and without IHD

| | Total | | In the presence of β-k band | |
	No.		No.	Frequency
IHD group	48		15	31.2%[a]
Control group	102		18	17.6%[a]

[a] P <0.01.

Finally, we attempted to examine the frequency of the appearance of the β-k band in the patients with IHD (Table 2). The frequency of the β-k band was not different before and after the diet therapy. This frequency was also not observed in the singularity of the various types from WHO's classification for hyperlipoproteinemia. While the frequency of the appearance of the β-k band in the control group was found to have a value of 17.6%, in the IHD group the value was 31.2%. This difference was statistically significant (p <0.01).

The present study indicated that the appearance of β-k band was produced by an incomplete hydrolysis of TG in the fraction of VLDL, and the characteristics of this mechanism was a TC-rich VLDL. Additionally, measurement of this frequency may serve in researching a risk factor for ischemic heart disease or atheroclerosis.

NUTRITIONAL FACTORS AND ATHEROSCLEROSIS
A study on Cholesterol Concentration in Foods - Shellfish

Iwao Fukui, Hideto Kushiro, Kazutaka Arisue, Yoshihisa Yamaguchi, Zensuke Ogawa, Chozo Hayashi, and Yuichi Yamamura

It is said that the use of foods low in cholesterol content is essential to dietary treatment, because of the close relationship between the serum cholesterol level and the onset or progress of atherosclerosis.

It has been warned that patients with serum hypercholesterolemia should refrain from intake of foods with high-cholesterol content such as eggs, shellfish, or Cephalopoda. However, it must be pointed out and stressed at this time that such analytic findings of high contents of cholesterol were obtained by incomplete pretreatment and colorimetric reaction of low specificity for cholesterol.

In order to find the accurate cholesterol contents in foods, analytic measurement methods, colorimetric, enzymic, thin layer chromatography, gas-liquid chromatography, and gas chromatography-mass spectrometry, were applied to the shellfish.

Materials and Methods

1. Materials

Five kinds of shellfish, corb shells, bloody clams, shortneck clams, clams, and oysters, were used as samples for this experiment.

2. *Extraction of Lipids*

The lipids used for the analyses were extracted from 100 g samples of shucked shellfish.

3. *Analyses*

a) Colorimetric Method
The Liebermann-Burchardt, Killian, and orthophthal-aldehyde (OPA) reactions were employed.
b) Enzymic Method
The principle of this method is to first produce the free cholesterol and fatty acids by the action of cholesterol ester hydrolase on the esterified cholesterol and to produce Δ4-cholestenone and hydrogen peroxide by the action of cholesteroloxidase on free cholesterol. The hydrogen peroxide thus quantitatively produced was assayed by the colorimetric determination of the red quinone produced by the oxidative condensation of 4-aminoantipyrine and phenol in the presence of peroxidase. This method, which is said to have high specificity, was employed for cholesterol determination in this study.
c) Thin Layer Chromatography
Thin layer chromatography was applied to the extracts previously obtained for separation of the lipids. Two methods were employed for detecting the spots: The UV lamp and spraying the mixture of sulfuric acid-acetic acid (1:1). Cholesterol was detected by heating at 90°C for 15 minutes.
d) Gas-Liquid Chromatography
Shimadzu GC-5A was used for determination.
e) Gas Chromatography-Mass Spectrometry
Shimadzu LKB 9000 GC-MS was used for identification of the sterols.

Results and Discussion

1. *Quantitative Findings Obtained by Colorimetry*

As is shown in Table 1, the cholesterol contents obtained per 100 g of each shellfish by the Liebermann-Burchardt reaction were 216 mg in corb shells, 160 mg in bloody clams, 115 mg in shortneck clams, 113 mg in clams, and 153 mg in oysters. By the Killian reaction, the cholesterol contents were 174 mg in corb shells, 124 mg in bloody clams, 100 mg in shortneck clams, 93 mg in clams, and 154 mg in oysters. By the OPA reaction, the cholesterol contents were 191 mg in corb shells, 114 mg in bloody clams, 112 mg in shortneck clams, 99 mg in clams, and 169 mg in oysters. As is shown in Table 1, the average values of these three reactions are given in order of the content of cholesterol per 100 g of each shellfish, i.e., corb shells with 194 mg, oysters with 159 mg, bloody clams with 136 mg, shortneck clams with 109 mg, and clams with 102 mg.

Table 1. Cholesterol content in shellfish by colorimetric methods

Shellfish	Cholesterol content			
	Liebermann-Burchardt reaction (mg/100 g)	Killian reaction (mg/100 g)	OPA reaction (mg/100 g)	Colorimetric method (mg/100 g)
1. Corb shell	216	174	191	194
2. Bloody clam	160	124	114	136
3. Shortneck clam	115	100	112	109
4. Clam	113	93	99	102
5. Oyster	153	154	169	159

Average of triple determination.

Table 2. Comparison of cholesterol values between reference and our data

Shellfish	Cholesterol content			
	Reference data[a]		Our data	
	Colorimetric method (mg/100 g	Colorimetric method (mg/100 g)	Enzymic method (mg/100 g)	Enzymic and GC method (mg/100 g)
1. Corb shell	497[a]	194	147	136
2. Bloody clam	65[a]	136	100	76
3. Shortneck clam	192[a]	109	95	67
4. Clam	118[a] 121[b]	102	89	56
5. Oyster	115[b]	159	107	71

[a] Y. Goto. [b] Joslin's diabetes mellitus.

2. Assay Values Obtained by Enzymic Method

As shown in Table 2, the cholesterol contents obtained per 100 g of each shell-fish by the enzymic method were 147 mg in corb shells, 100 mg in bloody clams, 95 mg in shortneck clams, 89 mg in clams, and 107 mg in oysters. Table 2 compares the average values of cholesterol content obtained by enzymic and colorimetric methods. Comparing the corresponding values, the colorimetric method showed generally higher values: 32% in corb shells, 36% in bloody clams, 15% in shortneck clams, 15% in clams, and 49% in oysters. Further investigation was, therefore, carried out to find the cause.

3. Investigation by Thin Layer Chromatography (TLC)

a) Detection by UV Method
When the UV method was employed to the plate, four spots in corb shells and three spots each in bloody clams, shortneck clams, clams, and oysters, caused by the double bond, were observed in addition to the cholesterol fraction.
b) Detection by Colorimetry
The plate was colored with the detecting reagent composed of sulfuric acid and acetic acid by the so-called Liebermann-Burchardt reaction. In addition to the cholesterol fraction, five spots in corb shells, three spots each in bloody clams and shortneck clams, and two spots in clams were detected. Of these spots, the corb shells and oysters displayed those with the larger dimension. It can be concluded that the difference between the colorimetric and enzymic methods is due to the existence of coloring substances other than cholesterol in the extracts of the shellfish, as is obviously shown by the Liebermann-Burchardt reaction in TLC. Therefore, the assay values by the colorimetric method do not show the real cholesterol content of the shellfish.

4. Separation by Gas-Liquid Chromatography and Calculation

In order to obtain the real cholesterol contents in the shellfish, the cholesterol fractions of each shellfish were collected from the plate for gas-liquid chromatographic determination. The results are shown in Figure 1. As is evident from Figure 1, in addition to cholesterol, five more sterols, C26-sterol, 22-dehydrocholesterol, brassicasterol, 24-methylencholesterol, and C29-sterol, were detected. Campesterol and C29-sterol were detected in oysters as β-sitosterol in the position of 24-methylencholesterol. The proportion and the basic chemical structures of these sterols are shown in Table 3. The proportions of cholesterol in sterols were found to be 70% in corb shells, 56% in bloody clams, 61% in short-

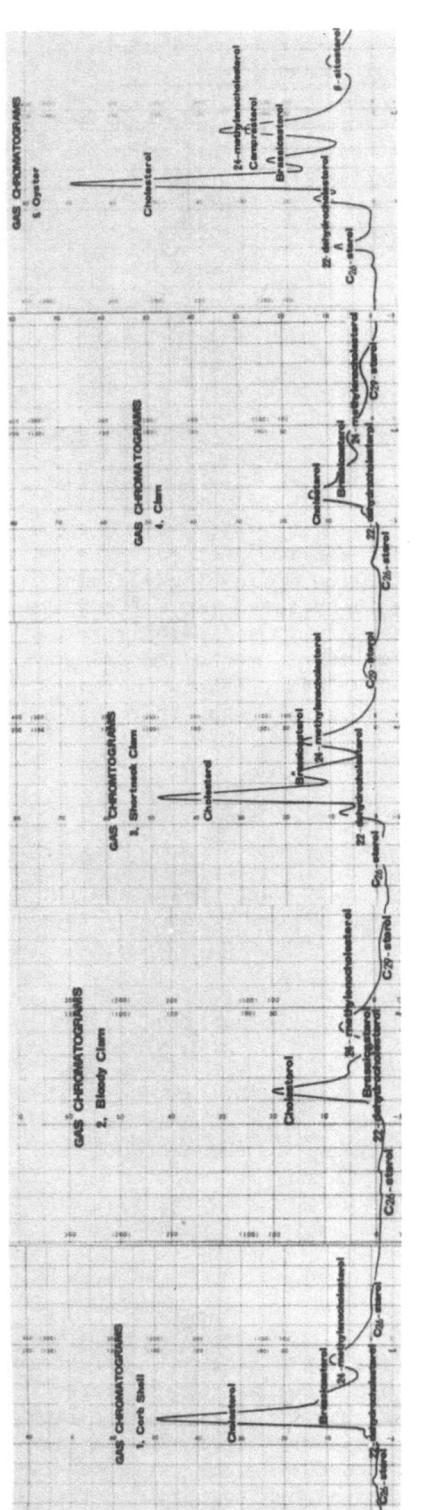

Figure 1. Gas chromatograms of cholesterol fraction of each shellfish

Table 3. Composition of sterols in shellfish

Shellfish	C26-sterol %	22-dehydrocho-lesterol %	Cholesterol %	Brassicasterol %	24-methylene-cholesterol %	C29-sterol %
1. Corb shell	1.0	4.0	70.0	10.0	15.0	1.0
2. Bloody clam	1.8	3.5	56.0	11.0	25.0	3.0
3. Shortneck clam	2.0	9.6	61.0	16.0	26.0	5.1
4. Clam	5.0	10.0	55.0	6.6	12.0	12.0
5. Oyster	4.0	7.0	44.5	10.0	26.0	8.0
						(β-sitosterol)

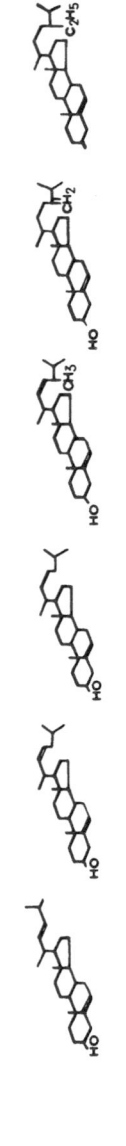

neck clams, 55% in clams, and 44.5% in oysters. Among the sterols, except for cholesterol, 24-methylencholesterol and brassicasterol were most frequently detected.

5. *Identification by Gas Chromatography-Mass Spectrometry*

Each peak of sterol separated by gas chromatography of shellfish was identified by mass spectrometry. The important peaks in mass spectra of the sterols are shown in Table 4.

The values of the cholesterol contents in the foods published in the paper by Goto are currently prevailing as a dietetic standard. As shown in Table 2, according to Goto, the cholesterol contents obtained in 100 g of each shellfish were found to be 497 mg in corb shells, 65 mg in bloody clams, 192 mg in shortneck clams, and 118 mg in clams.

However, as previously reported, we have obtained divergent values by both the colorimetric and enzymic methods, particularly the remarkably low cholesterol content in corb shells, originally considered problematic because of the high cholesterol content.

On the assumption that the six kinds of sterols in the so-called cholesterol fraction separated by TLC will give the same level of the molecular extinction coefficient at the color reaction, the cholesterol contents were calculated on the basis of concentration in percentage obtained by gas chromatography. The results per 100 g of each shellfish were even lower: 136 mg in corb shells, 76 mg in bloody clams, 67 mg in shortneck clams, 56 mg in clams, and 71 mg in oysters. These sterols analogous to cholesterol are thus additionally determined by the colorimetric method, as previously mentioned. From the results obtained, it can conclusively be stated that the real cholesterol contents in the shellfish are lower than have been reported. However, since these sterols are contained in the shellfish in considerable amounts, it is considered necessary to study in more detail the possible antilipemic effect of these sterols, with the possible expectation that these sterols will physiologically prevent the absorption of cholesterol. Further study will, therefore, be undertaken for corroboration. In addition extensive studies are being performed on other foods, and the new findings will be reported on the next occasion.

Table 4. The important peaks in the mass spectra of sterols

Peak	GC retention time	MS						Sterols
		Parent	Base	2nd		4th	5th	
	min							
1	18.7	442 (9.7)	97	129 (41.6)	255 (23.9)	313 (20.4)	352 (19.5)	C26-sterol
2	22.0	456 (20.0)	121	129 (56.8)	255 (49.1)	327 (40.3)	366 (34.7)	22-dehydro-cholesterol
3	23.0	458 (18.3)	129	329 (84.6)	368 (52.3)	353 (28.1)	458 (18.3)	Cholesterol
4	24.1	470 (18.2)	125	129 (77.2)	255 (50.7)	380 (31.9)	470 (18.2)	Brassicasterol
5	25.5	472 470	129 129	343 341	382 380	367 365	472 470	Campesterol 24-methylene-cholesterol
6	28.0	486 (10.4)	129	357 (43.5)	396 (32.1)	381 (16.1)	486 (10.4)	β-sitosterol

X GC-MS ( ): Percent of relative intensity.

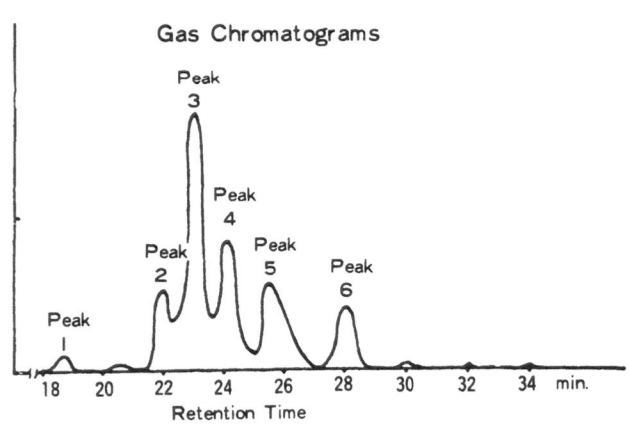

Gas Chromatograms

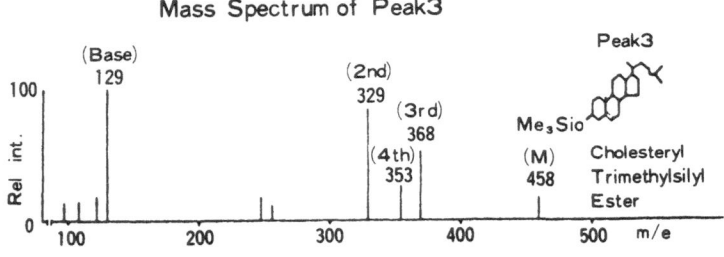

Mass Spectrum of Peak3

ABSTRACTS

PREVALENCE OF ATHEROSCLEROSIS IN DIFFERENT TYPES OF FAMILIAL HYPER-LIPOPROTEINEMIA

G. Crepaldi, R. Fellin, G. Briani, G. Baggio, E. Manzato, P. Balestrieri, and M.R. Baiocchi
Department of Internal Medicine, Division of Gerontology and Metabolic Diseases, Policlinic, Padua/Italy

308 patients of both sexes (age 10 - 60 years) with different types of hyperlipoproteinemia were studied. Prevalence of coronary artery disease (CAD) and peripheral artery disease (PAD) in 280 patients (age 19 - 60 years) was studied; other risk factors (hypertension, cigarette smoking, diabetes, overweight) were also evaluated. In the 3 type I patients either CAD and PAD were not observed; CAD was present in 3 of 8 type III patients. Prevalence of CAD and PAD in the other Fredrickson's types was:

Type	n.	CAD	PAD
IIa	93	42 (45%)	8 (9%)
IIb	70	33 (47%)	15 (21%)
IV	71	27 (38%)	8 (11%)
V	35	6 (17%)	7 (20%)

CAD was more frequent than PAD in all types except type V. Serum cholesterol levels were directly correlated with CAD prevalence in type IIa. Statistical evaluation of additional risk factors was carried out and their influence in CAD and PAD prevalence in comparison to hyperlipidemia is discussed.

STUDY ON TWIN WITH ISCHEMIC HEART DISEASE

Goro Mimura, Tomio Jinnouchi, Shoji Kido, Shojiro Ishimoto, Keizo Kajihara, Shunsaku Miyagawa, Kenichi Hirabaru, Shoji Fukumitsu, Yoshikuni Haraguchi, Kazumitsu Koganemaru, Yasuhiro Sakamoto, and Michimasa Kono
Department of Geriatrics, Institute of Constitutional Medicine, Kumamoto University, Kumamoto/Japan

80 pairs of monozygotic (MZ) twins and 18 pairs of dizygotic (DZ) twins were studied. The average difference of electrical axis, depth of S_{V1} and height of R_{V5} in electrocardiogram was smaller in MZ than in that of DZ twins. The average difference of cardiothoracic ratio in MZ was also smaller than in that of DZ twins. The concordance of onset of ischemic heart disease in MZ twins was found to be 75%, while in DZ twins it was found to be 25%. A significant differense was obtained between them. The number of paris with concordarce of ischemic heart disease among 9 pairs of MZ twins, was found to be 3 pairs in the same environment and 6 pairs in different environment. This results suggests that MZ twins tend to be concordant, even if environment is different.

EVIDENCE FOR GENETIC HETEROGENEITY IN FAMILIAL HYPERCHOLESTEROL-AEMIA (FH)

Arvid Heiberg, and Joan Slack
Institute of Medical Genetics, University of Oslo, Oslo/Norway and MRC Clinical
Genetics Unit, London/England

2 family studies of F.H. have been conbined to examine the evidence for genetic
heterogeneity. All index patients were identified by the presence of hypercholesterolaemia and tendenous xanthomata and correlations between the age at
coronary death between 1st degree relatives have been calculated.
Among heterozygotes for F.H. there was a sib/sib correlation for age at coronary
death of 0.69 (p <0.001) in 42 pairs. Among sib pairs in families of unselected
patients with myocardial infarction there was a sib/sib correlation of 0.31 in
14 pairs. The sib/sib correlation for total serum cholesterol concentration
among heterozygotes for F.H. was 0.30 in 37 pairs and the heterozygote parent/
child correlation was 0.44 (p <0.05) in 20 pairs. No correlation was found between the total serum cholesterol concentration and the age of coronary death in
8 heterozygotes for F.H.
The findings suggest that at least 2 genetic forms of F.H. exist, each having
its own expected age at death, but that the age at coronary death is modified
by other polygenic or environmental influences.

HLA-ANTIGENES IN A FAMILY WITH TYPE II HYPERLIPOPROTEINEMIA

H.B. Stähelin, P. Buchmann, P. Strub, H. Göschke, G. Thiel, and F. Koller
Department of Internal Medicine, Kantonsspital, University of Basle, Basle/
Switzerland

Coronary heart disease (CHD) is particularly prevalent in subjects with hereditary hyperlipidemias. Recently, it was suggested that HLA 8, espc. type 1-8
and ev. W15 are genetic markers for CHD being linked to genes responsible for
hypercholesterolemia. In order to elucidate further the relation between the
HLA and the inheritance of lipid disorders a family (7 females, 12 males aged
15 - 72, belonging to two generations) with combined hyperlipidemia (CHL) was
investigated.
Analysis of the data suggested a bimodal distribution for triglycerides (TGL) as
well as cholesterol (CH. The CHL appeared to be transmitted in an autosomal
dominant mode. Phenotype IIb was observed 7-, IIa 5 times, IV once. No correlation was found between the HLA-type and the inheritance of the lipid disorder.
Furthermore, only the younger generation, normolipidemics and hyperlipidemics
had HLA 1-8 or W15. However, subjects of this generation with CHL and HLA 1-8 or
W15 had higher CH-concentrations (304 ± 33 vs 260 ± 25 mg/dl; ns) and higher
TGL-concentrations (166 ± 13 vs 120 ± 7 mg/dl; p <0.01). Genes linked to certain
HLA types seem not to be responsible for the transmission of the lipid disorder.
They may, however, aggravate the manifestation of an otherwise determined lipid
disorder.

ON THE INHERITANCE OF TYPE III HYPERLIPOPROTEINAEMIA. LIPOPROTEIN PATTERNS IN FIRST DEGREE RELATIVES

Bengt Vessby, Hand Hedstrand, and Lars-Gustav Lundin
Department of Geriatrics, University of Uppsala, Uppsala/Sweden

The lipoprotein (LP) patterns were studied in 20 families affected with hyperlipoproteinaemia (HLP) type III. 70 adult first degree relatives (92% ascertain-
ment) were reached for analysis. There was a marked overrepresentation of HLP
type III among the relatives (27%) compared to the normal population of Uppsala.

There was also an increased frequency of hypertriglyceridaemia (29% against expected 15%) mainly because of a high prevalence of HLP type IV (24%). A "late pre-β band" in the very low density (VLDL) fraction on agarose electrophoresis, probably indicative of an increased amount of intermediary LP particles, was frequently present (42%) among relatives not classified as HLP type III.
A genetic analysis of the LP patterns within the families showed several examples of vertical transmission of HLP type III. There was no sex linkage. Six of 13 analysed parents showed LP patterns classified as HLP type III. 23% of the siblings to the probands showed a type III pattern, another 4 siblings (7%) showing patterns very similar to HLP type III. The data support the concept that HLP type III is inherited as an autosomal dominant gene. It was indicated that HLP type IV with a "late pre-β band" in VLDL may represent an other expression of the gene for HLP type III.

VERY LOW DENSITY LIPOPROTEIN (VLDL) COMPOSITION IN FAMILIAL HYPER-LIPOPROTEINAEMIA

I.C. Ononogbu, and B. Lewis
Royal Postgraduate Medical School, England

VLDL concentration varies substantially in the different hyperlipoproteinaemic states. In the rare entity type III hyperlipoproteinaemia, VLDL composition is known to be abnormal, but in most forms of human hyperlipidaemia this has not been extensively studied. The cholesterol and triglyceride contents of VLDL, isolated by precipitation with sodium dodecyl sulphate was measured in 19 controls and 26 patients with familial hyperlipoproteinaemia. In the controls, cholesterol to triglyceride ratio was 0.32 ± 0.01 (S.E.M.). The VLDL lipid ratio was not significantly different in patients with raised low density lipoprotein (LDL) levels (0.29 ± 0.03, n = 6). In type III the ratio was confirmed to be high (0.51 ± 0.03, n = 4) (p <0.001). In 8 patients with raised levels of LDL and VLDL (type IIb), VLDL composition was also abnormal (0.38 ± 0.02) (p <0.05). Those with high VLDL levels (tape IV) had a significantly (p <0.01) low ratio (0.24 ± 0.02, n = 8). In this condition, enhanced endogenous triglyceride transport may be mediated by increased triglyceride content of VLDL as well as increased number of circulating VLDL molecules.

FOUR CASES OF TYPE III HYPERLIPOPROTEINEMIA ASSOCIATED OR SECONDARY TO EITHER NEPHROTIC SYNDROME, DIABETES OR HYPOTHYROIDISM

Horace Micheli, and Daniel Pometta
Division de Diabétologie, Département de Médecine, Université de Genève,
Genève/Switzerland

Type III hyperlipemia has recently been redefined as an increased ratio of cholesterol to triglycerides content in very-low-density lipoproteins (VLDL) reflecting the presence of particles of intermediary density between VLDL and LDL. We describe four cases associated with a nephrotic syndrome, 2 diabetes and one hypothyroidism. Repeated ultracentrifugations of lipoproteins showed initially or later during treatment of the primary illness a cholesterol (g/l) to triglycerides (mmol/l) ratio in VLDL between 0.42 and 0.64 at time when serum triglycerides were above 3 mmol/l. The patients with nephrotic syndrom had been known for ten years as having a type IIa hyperlipemia and the type III pattern coexisted transitorily and disappeared while on treatment with prednisone and clofibrate for 4 months. The renal disease completely recovered. Both diabetic patients initially had a type IV pattern and the VLDL lipid composition characteristic of type III was present for a short time only. One patient normalized his lipemia under insulin treatment and weight loss. The other was on diet only but did not loose weight and turned again to be a type IV. The hypothyroid patient normalized his lipemia at the same time as betafloating pattern and palmar xanthomata disappeared under thyroid treatment.

THE SERUM CHOLESTEROL VALUE DURING THE FIRST 5 WEEKS AFTER BIRTH

Hugo Kesteloot, Jos Claes, and Josephine Dodion-Fransen
Department Pathophysiology, Section Cardiology, St. Raphael University Clinic, Leuven/Belgium

The serum cholesterol value has been measured in the cord blood of 303 newborns by means of the method of Abell. The mean value was 72 mg% for the newborns. By multiple regression analysis it has been shown that a significant independent correlation exists between cord blood cholesterol and the cholesterol of the mothers, birth weight, sex and the blood group of the ABO system of both, the newborn and their mother. This demonstrates that several factors known to influence cholesterol in adult life are already operating at birth. In a group of 39 newborns it has been shown that the cholesterol value increases rapidly from 71 mg% at birth to 91 mg% the first day, 106 mg% the second day and 115 mg% the third day of life and they slowly decrease to 112 mg% the twelfth day of life. The behaviour of cholesterol value, the first two weeks of life, is largely independent from birth weight and from the cholesterol content of the diet. In an independent sample of 45 newborns the mean cholesterol value increased from 77 mg% at birth to 131 mg% at the age of 5 weeks.

EFFECTS ON LIPOPROTEIN LIPID CONCENTRATIONS AND FAT TOLERANCE OF COLESTIPOL WHEN ADDED TO DIET + CLOFIBRATE THERAPY

Hans Lithell, Jonas Boberg, Bengt Vessly, and Ivar Werner
Department of Geriatrics, University of Uppsala, Uppsala/Sweden

Colestipol (Upjohn) reduces low density lipoprotein (LDL) cholesterol concentrations by 25% when given to patients with type II A or II B hyperlipoproteinemia, who are on diet treatment. However, a disfavourable increase of very low density lipoprotein (VLDL) triglyceride concentrations of about 1.5 times the pretreatment value occurs in earlier reports.
In this double-blind cross-over study including 22 patients the effects of adding Colestipol to an ongoing treatment with diet + clofibrate was studied. Average S-cholesterol concentration was 292 (range 209 - 432) mg/100 ml and average S-triglyceride concentration was 2.17 (range 1.20 - 4.66) mmol/l before treatment. Earlier reported increase of VLDL concentration did not take place and the removal rate of fat as Intralipid (i.v. fat tolerance test) was not changed during Colestipol treatment. LDL-cholesterol concentration decreased by 23% and a small but significant increase of HDL-cholesterol occurred. These results will be discussed and related to other parameters studied, e.g. P-fibrinogen and fasting S-insulin concentrations.

GLUCOSE KINETICS IN TYPE IV HYPERLIPEMIA

George Steiner, Soichiro Morita, and Mladen Vranic
Department of Medicine, University of Toronto, Toronto/Canada

To determine why carbohydrate tolerance is often impaired in type IV hyperlipemics (HLP) glucose-^{14}C kinetics during, and pancreatic β cell response to, physiologic glucagon infusions were examined. Normal (N) and lean HLP humans were tested. Both groups were selected to have normal glucose tolerance tests (GTT) and had the same basal plasma levels of insulin (IRI in N 14 ± 2; HLP

16 ± 3 μU/ml) and glucagon (IRG in N 120 ± 11; HLP 141 ± 33 pg/ml). In both groups during the GTT the IRI rose equally (7x) but the IRG fell more in HLP (52%) than in N (27%). Basal glucose turnover was the same in both (74-78 mg/m^2-min). During glucagon infusion both glucose production and IRI:glucose ratio rose in direct relation to IRG. The IRI:glucose at all IRGs was the same in both groups. Although the effect of IRG to increase glucose production was the same in both groups, the restraining effect of insulin on hepatic glucose production in HLP was less than in N. Also, at the same glucose concentration, changes in IRI had a much smaller effect on glucose utilization in HLP than N. The interaction of insulin and glucagon on glucose turnover in HLP resembled that we observed in normolipemic obese.

Conclusions: In lean type IV HLPs (1) the pancreatic β cell response is normal; (2) there is a peripheral and hepatic resistance to insulin similar to that of normolipemic obese humans; (3) insulin resistance may account for the glucose intolerance.

Chairmen: R.H. More, Canada
          T. Takeuchi, Japan

Participants: R.H. More, Canada
              T. Takeuchi, Japan
              I. Sakurai, Japan
              S. Moore, Canada
              H.R. Baumgartner, Switzerland
              S. Renaud, France
              K. Tanaka, Japan

INTRODUCTION

Robert H. More

Almost everyone will accept the importance of thrombosis to atherosclerosis in
the context of clinical disease. At the extreme distal end of events, it is often
the precipitating factor in occlusion of an artery. There is, however, less evidence of its role in the initiation of events, but a good deal of evidence has
been put forward indicating that thrombosis may be an important factor in the
progression of the lesion. Today, evidence of the role of thrombosis in the
pathogenesis of the different stages of atherosclerosis will be discussed. The
importance of studying risk factors in relation to atherosclerosis has received
much attention in the past year. In their consideration of the role of thrombosis
in atherosclerosis, it is important to study the relation of these same risk factors as possible causal agents in thrombosis, and the panelists will discuss
these in relation to their particular subject. None will deny that if we could
control thrombosis, many of the problems of atherosclerosis would disappear or
be delayed. The observations and conclusions of the symposium this afternoon are,
therefore, of relevance to the problem of the morbidity and mortality of atherosclerosis and hopefully to its etiology and pathogenesis.

STRUCTURE OF THE RENAL ARTERY AND ITS VASOCONSTRICTION
(Orientation to Sclerotic Change and Hypertension)

T. Takeuchi

The structure of the renal arteries within the kidney is characterized by well-
developed smooth muscle in the media. The smooth muscle cells are connected with
each other by intercalating pattern; protrusion of cytoplasma of one smooth muscle cell invaginating into the cytoplasma of neighboring cells (Burnstock, 1970;
Somlyo and Somlyo, 1968). With the aid of high magnification of the electron
microscope, there are seen a considerable number of nexus where two cytomembranes
are merged inperseptively. The fluorescent method according to Falck (1962)
reveals that monoamines involving noradrenaline and adrenaline are located at the
outer most layer of medial smooth muscle cells. No site of monoamine deposition
within the media is discernible. This indicates that sympathetic innervation ter-
minates subjacent to the adventitia. And the stimulus leading to vasoconstriction
is conducted by action potential running on the surface of cytomembrane of the
medial cells from the outer most cell to the inner most one, when the sympathetic
nerve is excited.

Vascular constriction requires two steps to proceed:
1. Conduction of stimulus to initiate smooth muscle constriction
2. Shortening of myofilament in the medial smooth muscle cytoplasma resulting in vasoconstriction.

For understanding the mechanism of vasoconstriction it is inevitable to know how the stimulus is conducted throughout the entire thickness of the arterial media (Prosser et al., 1960). In case of intensive vasoconstriction as in shock, one can note (Takeuchi et al., 1974; Takeuchi, 1974) that perinuclear vacuoles of the arterial media increase markedly, whereas the number of perinuclear vacuoles decrease at the relaxation. Electron microscopic study of this particular vacuole discloses that the vacuolic structure is indentical with the protrusion of smooth muscle cytoplasma where electron density becomes even less watery and is lacking deposition of large molecular substances such as glucose, lipid material, and protein. Electron chemical study (Mizuhira, 1971) exhibits that there is a linear accumulation of potassium ion subjacent to the inner cytomembrane which is attenuated at the normal part of the cytomembrane. There seems to be little increase of deposition of sodium inside the cytoplasma. No particular evidence of calcium ion is discernible. Conclusively, it can be stated that intracellular potassium ion is mobilized to shift toward the protrusion and deposit itself in linear fashion in the zone subjacent to the cytomembrane (Takeuchi et al., 1974; Takeuchi, 1974). At relaxation, the potassium accumulation is disintegrated by movement of potassium ion out of the protrusion to the main body of cytoplasma. Though much remains obscure and undetermined, it is most likely that the perinuclear medial vacuole possesses a close relationship with conduction of stimulus toward vasoconstriction because the potassium accumulation (Takeuchi et al., 1974; Takeuchi, 1974) in the protrusion can certainly alter the concentration of ion against a biomembrane generating electric potential which differs from that at relaxation. It is still uncertain, however, whether or not the change of membrane potential at vasoconstriction would be a cause of electric generation or the sequelae of altered potential.

On the basis of the knowledge above in conjunction with vasoconstriction, it could be promising to explore the initiation of vascular sclerosis of the renal artery. The clue for exploration is as follows: 1. It could be assumed that potassium ions accumulated subjacent to the cytomembrane of smooth muscle could spill out into the interstitial space where there is a considerable amount of acid mucopolysaccharide of the chondroitin sulfate types. 2. Sulfate radical has been proven to penetrate rather easily into the intermuscular space, as well as glycin by employing radioisotopes. 3. This could happen rather rapidly when the vasoconstriction takes place intensively. 4. The vascular sclerotic change is seen where the vasoconstriction occurs repeatedly and persists for a fairly long time. 5. There exists a possibility that the formation of fibrous components, either elastin or collagen, is accelerated in the presence of higher concentrations of potassium and comparatively larger amounts of mucopolysaccharides. Due to the increase in fibrosis in the very narrow intercellular space, the nexus could be demolished resulting in the paralysis of transmission of membrane potential. This provides some evidence about the initiation of sclerotic changes and hypertension as well. The research is continuing in order to determine more exactly the relation between vasoconstriction and sclerosis of the renal arteries.

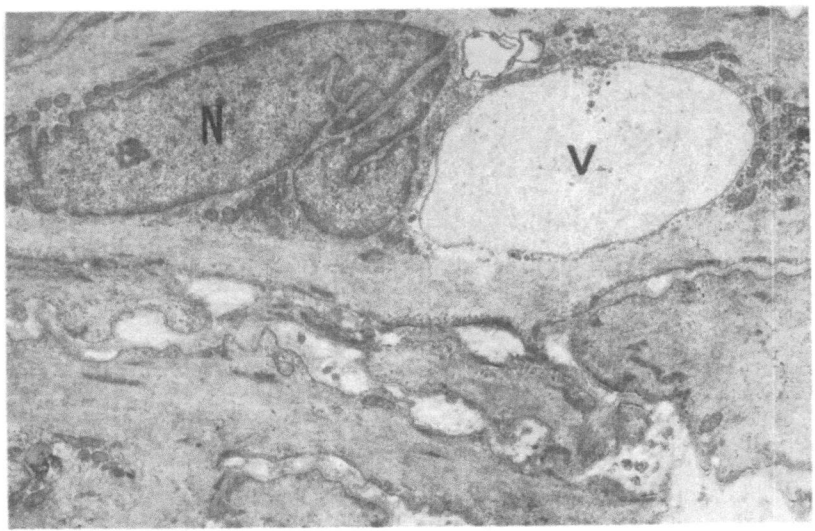

Figure 1. Perinuclear vacuole, as interpreted to be a parameter of vasoconstriction, is usually seen in the arterial medial smooth muscle

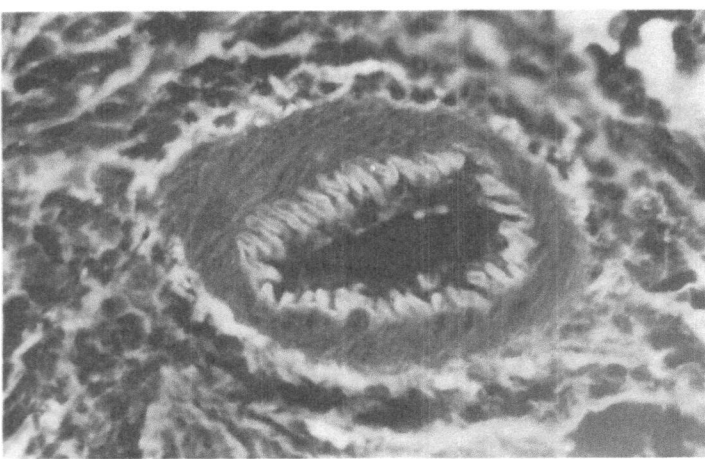

Figure 2. Fluorescence picture indicating the presence of monoamine at the outer most part of the media

CORONARY ARTERIAL CHANGES IN CHILDHOOD AND YOUNG ADULTS WITH RE-
SPECT TO PROGRESSION OF CORONARY SCLEROSIS AND A BRIEF COMMENT ON
THROMBOSIS AS A COMPLICATION

I. Sakurai

Is a Microthrombus a Factor in the Initiating of or in the Progression of
Atherosclerosis?

Mural thrombosis on the arterial intima may play some role in the progression of
atherosclerosis in its early period. By a careful study of human material, microthrombi can be found in young people (Duguid, 1946, 1955; Haust et al., 1959;
More and Haust, 1961). By various experimental methods including injection of
fibrin or blood clots, traumatizing the arterial wall with plastic tubes, or by
various irritants, mural thrombi can be formed, entrapped, and organized into
the arterial intima (Harrison, 1948; Heard, 1952; Barnard, 1953; Heptinstall,
1959). However, many of the experimental studies have been carried out on pulmonary arteries, which are not suitable for correlation with human arterial atherosclerosis. Recently Sumiyoshi et al. (1973) and Sumiyoshi (1976) reported that
fully developed atheroma similar to that in man could be produced in aortas of
even normolipidemic rabbits, following mural thrombi formed by intubation of the
aorta from the femoral arteries. But the interpretation remains still controversial, because it is not clear whether the atheromas can be produced purely secondary to mural thrombi and their organization, or whether they are influenced
by other factors. For instance, thrombosis or minor trauma of the intima may accelerate vascular permeability which allows much infiltration of plasma constituents into the vascular walls.

A total of 60 autopsy cases under 20 years of age were employed in the study. For
56 of 60 cases, serial sections of the left main and anterior descending coronary
arteries were made. The arteries were examined histologically from the orifices
of the left coronary artery to the point of the apex of the heart. Microthrombi
were found in four cases, two cases out of nine from 1 to 4 years of age, one
case out of eight from 5 to 10 years of age (Fig. 1), and one case out of nine
from 11 to 20 years of age, from a total of 56 cases.

None of the cases below 1 year of age among 30 cases had any mural thrombi. Two-
thirds of the newborn babies below 1 month of age, however, show some degree of
intimal thickening, diffuse or localized, where fibrocellular proliferation and
acid mucopolysaccharide deposits with splitting of the internal elastic lamina
were observed, but no fat was observed using oil red-O stain. The degree of
severity in intimal thickening increases with age even in young people from the
newborn period to 20 years of age. Groups of 5 - 10 years and of 11 - 20 years of
age presented some fatty streaks or dots in thickened intimas. These were present
sent in seven out of 17 cases above 5 years of age. Localized eccentric elevation
of the intima tends to begin at the points of branching even in the baby group
(Fig. 2).

Eight cases, aged 1 day - 17 years were selected for immunohistochemical study.
Antifibrinogen fluorescent antibody was positive in one case aged 9 years, and
β-lipoprotein was positive in two cases, aged 7 and 17 years. Albumin was negative in all cases. Both fibrinogen and β-lipoprotein infiltrations were observed
in the superficial intima beneath the endothelial lining.

Results of comparative biochemical analysis of lipids in platelets, whole fatty
streaks of coronary arteries, and inner walls of coronary arteries at different
age groups are shown in Table 1. Platelets have a high percentage of phospholipid and free cholesterol, and only a trace of triglyceride and esterified cholesterol, whilst fatty streaks have much more esterified cholesterol. From the point
of view of lipid chemistry, the lipid composition of platelets and fatty streaks
are significantly different. Also from the morphologic point of view, comparing

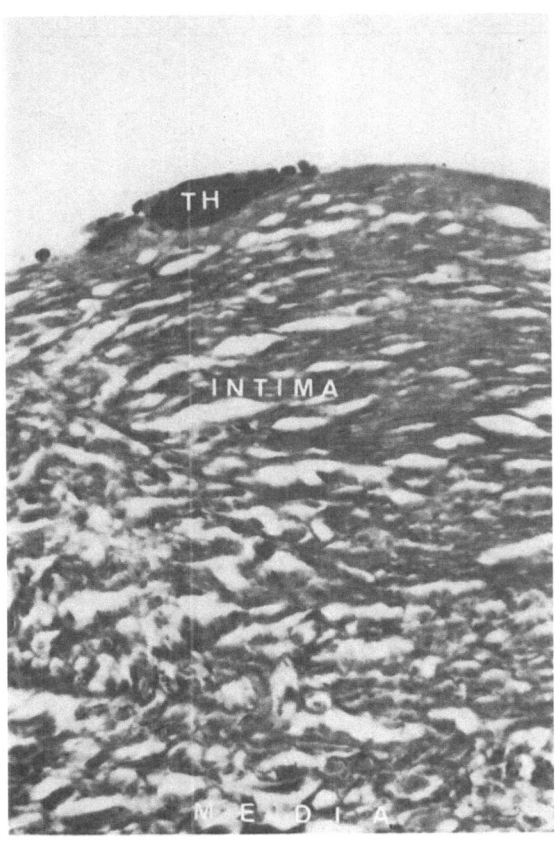

Figure 1. A microthrombus at the tip of localized intimal elevation. Phosphotan-
gustic acidhematoxylin stain. 10-year-old girl (AN-4960)

the size and numbers of fatty steaks and dots to those of microthrombi, the former is significantly greater than the latter.

Therefore, it seems reasonable to think that most of the fatty streaks and dots
may not develop secondary to microthrombi entrapped within the intima. Microthrombi, however, once developed and organized, may be responsible for intimal
fibrotic thickening, and lead to a more ischemic state resulting in damage of
intimal or medial cells, with an increased permeability which allows more plasma
constituents to pass into the vascular walls.

Thrombosis and Intramural Hemorrhage as a Complication of Coronary Athero-
sclerosis

Twenty-three coronary arteries obtained from 22 cases with myocardial infarction
were investigated morphologically with serial sections for some cases with an
intramural hemorrhage or a thrombus.

The incidence of coronary thrombosis in cases with myocardial infarction is quite
varied from one report to another (Genton et al., 1973). In this study thrombi
were found in 12 arteries (52.5%). Six out of 12 are associated with intra-ath-
eromatous hematoma, and one associated with microhemorrhage in the arterial wall.

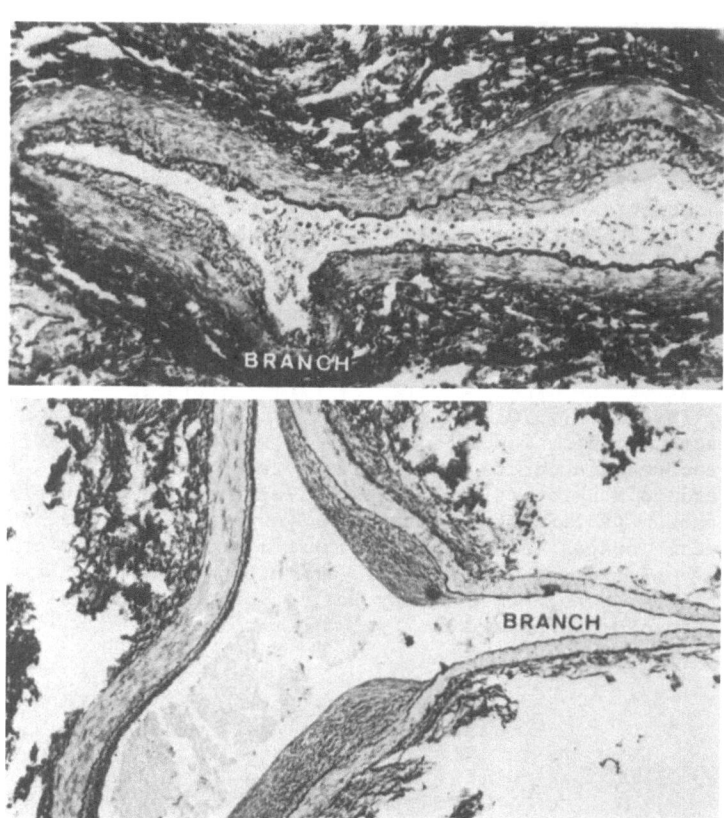

Figure 2. Localized eccentric intimal thickening at brachning points. One-day-old baby boy (upper, AN-5164), and 20-year-old female (lower, AN-5030)

Table 1. Comparison of lipids in "normal" inner walls of coronary arteries at different age groups, in whole fatty streaks of coronary arteries, and in platelets in Japanese

		PL	FCH	FFA	TG	MEFA	ECH
N o r m a l	Child	25.3%	12.4%	8.8%	43.1%	−	10.2%
	Young adult	13.3	13.7	9.3	24.5	−	39.0
	Elder	19.6	17.9	20.1	10.1	−	31.4
	Fatty streak	23.1	23.7	5.2	6.5	−	41.6
	Platelet	36.9	37.4	14.8	Trace	−	Trace

PL   = Phospholipid;
FCH = Free cholesterol;
FFA = Free fatty acid;
TG   = Triglyceride;
MEFA = Methyl ester of fatty acid;
ECH = Esterified cholesterol.

The remaining five arteries have thrombosis only. Thrombi were formed at the location where atheromas had been ruptured in about half of the cases with thrombi.

Sixteen arteries (69.6%) reveal intramural hemorrhages, consisting of eight with massive hematoma and eight with microhemorrhages or hemosiderosis within atheromas. Histologic analysis of cases with intramural hemorrhages showed that micorhemorrhages usually occur around the vas vasora entering from the adventitia into the atheromas, while two cases among eight with massive intramural hematoma showed direct continuation from the ruptured vas vasora adjacent to the hematomas.

Among six arteries with both thrombosis and hematoma, where both processes communicated with each other through the site at a ruptured atheroma, only one coronary artery is considered to have developed an intramural hematoma by blood entering the atheroma directly from a ruptured site of the atheroma as reported by Friedman (1970). Among the other five arteries, two disclose evidence of direct communication of a vas vasore with the hematomas, and many others have vasa vasorum adjacent to the hematomas, as mentioned above (Fig. 3). These results may lead to a hypothesis that in the later period of development of atheroma, vasa vasorum proliferate in the atheroma mainly from the adventitial side, and these become congested and finally cause microhemorrhages or hematomas. After the massive hematoma develops within the atheroma, it may break out of the atheroma into the lumen where thrombi may easily form by a release of tissue factors and hemodynamic disturbances that promote thrombosis.

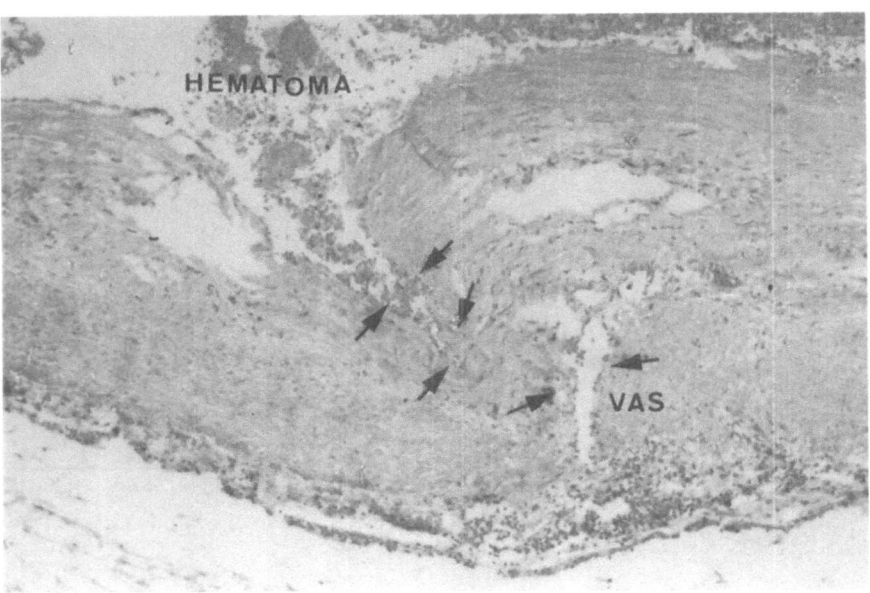

Figure 3. Intramural hematoma communicating with a vas vasora (myocardial infarction, AN-5256)

THROMBOSIS AND ENDOTHELIAL INJURY IN ATHEROGENESIS

S. Moore, J. Mustard, M.A. Packham, and R.L. Kinlough-Rathbone

In considering the relationships among thrombosis, endothelial injury, and atherogenesis, several aspects of this topic seem to be particularly relevant. These are the effects produced by a single injury and by repeated injury to the vessel wall, the types of lesions produced, changes in these when the injury stimulus is removed, the role of platelets and thrombi in the development of lesions, factors which may injure the vessel wall, and the effect on all these of environmental or therapeutic influences.

A single injury to the vessel wall such as that which can be produced by removing the endothelium with a balloon catheter leads to the accumulation of platelets on the surface of the denuded vessel (Baumgartner, 1974). There is no proliferation of the smooth muscle cells or thickening of the intima, but platelets can be seen adherent to the subendothelial surface.

The examination of such lesions several weeks after the balloon catheter injury shows that the smooth muscle cells have proliferated and the intima has thickened. Studies which have been carried out by many investigators (Haust et al., 1960; Stemerman and Ross, 1972; Ross and Glomsett, 1973) indicate that the smooth muscle cells from the media migrate into the intima and proliferate to produce this thickening. Following a single injury which involves extensive removal of the endothelium, it takes a long time for the endothelium to recover the lesions. These lesions gradually reendothelialize and regress and seldom if ever show gross evidence of lipid accumulation within them.

However, if the animals are fed a hypercholesterolemic diet in association with the balloon catheter injury, lipid accumulates in the lesions. Ross and Harker (1976) have shown in monkeys that balloon catheter injury coupled with hypercholesterolemia leads to extensive lipid accumulation in these lesions. Lipid accumulation and smooth muscle cell proliferation were localized to the sites of injury. Thus, proliferation of smooth muscle cells in the wall of an artery occurs after vessel injury, but the lipid content of the lesions that develops is dependent on the dietary lipid supplement.

In our own studies, we found that if polyethylene catheters were left in the aortas of rabbits so that the catheters caused repeated injury of the vessel wall, not only did smooth muscle cells proliferate at the sites of injury but a variety of atherosclerotic lesions developed (Moore, 1973). These included fatty streaks or edematous plaques, fibrous lipid-free plaques, and raised lesions, generally covered or partly covered by thrombus. The raised lesions contained abundant lipid material both intracellularly and extracellularly and frequently a central lipid pool was observed. Refractile lipid and cholesterol clefts were seen in these lesions, as early as 2 weeks following catheter placement, but were more prominent up to 8 months of continuous or repeated catheter injury (Moore, 1971). Accumulation of cholesterol ester in these lesions resulted in part from synthesis in the arterial wall (Day et al., 1974).

Repeated arterial injury produced by other methods such as exposing the inner surface of the vessel to an endothelial antibody leads to the development of similar lesions (Friedman et al., 1975).

Thus, with a single injury, a fibromusculo-elastic plaque, free of histologic lipid is produced (Fig. 1). With continued or repeated injury, either mechanical or immunologic, lipid-rich lesions similar to complicated lesions in man are produced (Fig. 2).

Although the animals are not fed a diet rich in fat to induce hypercholesterolemia, in the experiments where repeated injury is induced either by the catheter

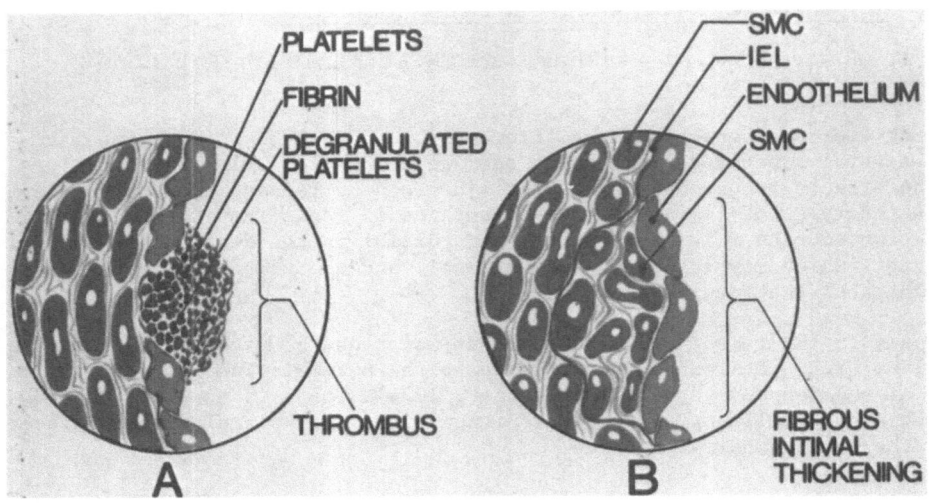

Figure 1. Response to a single injury

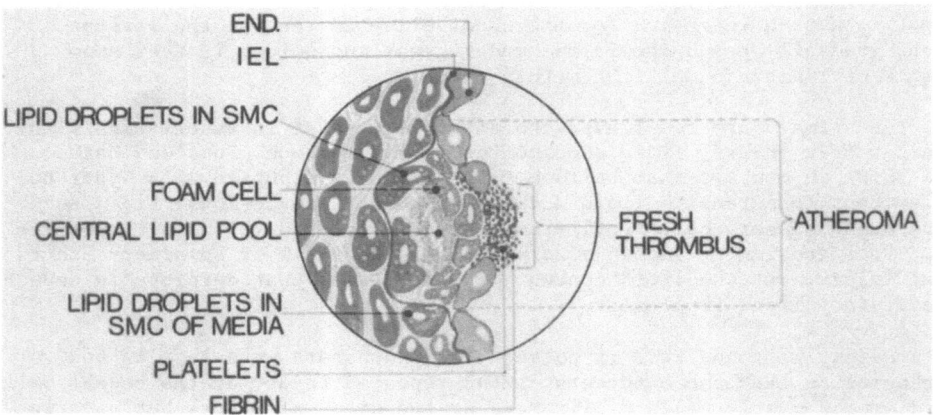

Figure 2. Response to repeated injury

or by the antibody, we find that the serum cholesterol level in the experimental animal increases to about twice the normal level (Moore, 1971; Friedman et al., 1976a). At the present time, we do not know the explanation for this or whether it has any significance in relation to the lipid accumulation that occurs in these lesions.

We have examined the pattern of change of the lesions in these animals following withdrawal of the injury stimulus in repeated injury experiments (Friedman et al., 1976a). The atheromatous lesions decrease in size and number, and as they decrease the number of fibrous plaques increases. Although a definite conclusion cannot be drawn at present, there is some indication that the fatty streaks may be an intermediate state in the transition from the atheromatous lesions to the fibrous, lipid-free plaques. This has some very interesting implications in light of the generally accepted theory that fibrous plaques develop into atheromatous lesions. In the repeated injury experiments, the observations indicate that fibrous plaques may develop after the atheromatous lesions and represent a healing stage in the process.

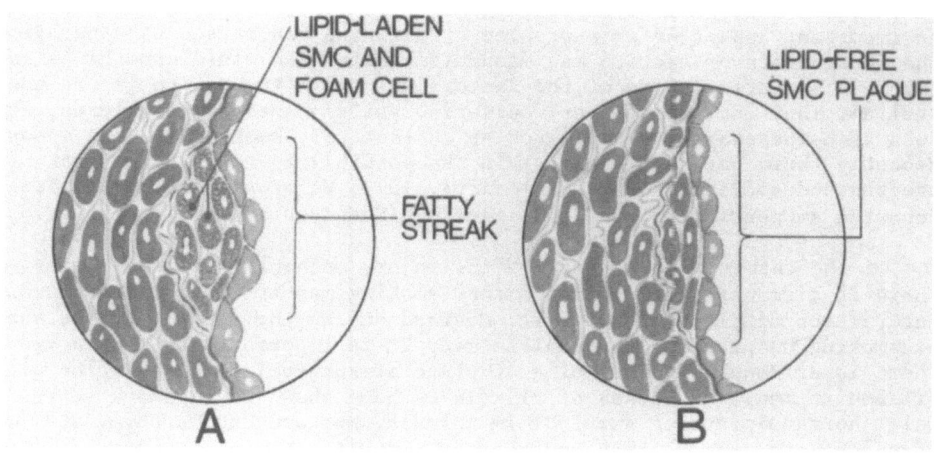

Figure 3. Response when injury stimulus is removed

When the injury stimulus is removed, in the setting of repeated injury, lipid-containing lesions regress to fibrointimal thickenings, in which stainable lipid is not seen (Fig. 3).

Of course, in all these animal experiments, the objection can be raised that artificial means of causing vessel wall injury are being used. The key question is whether injury occurs normally in the intact human being or other animals. Jørgensen et al. (1972) have found in both pigs and humans that in and around vessel orifices the endothelium often appears to be injured or lost and intimal thickening can be observed. These findings have subsequently been confirmed by Gutstein et al. (1973). Jørgensen's work in humans has shown the relationship between intimal thickening and the accumulation of white cells and platelets on the surface of the thoracic aorta adjacent to vessel orifices. When the endothelium is injured, it is not uncommon for thrombi and white cells to accumulate on the surface. The relationship, therefore, between these sites and formed element accumulation indicates that spontaneous injury probably does occur at these sites in intact human beings and may be a major factor in the localization of the proliferative lesions which occur in man. The explanation for this relationship may reside in the findings of Ross and his co-workers (1974). The observation that platelets release a factor which is mitogenic for smooth muscle cells seems to be of very major importance in establishing the relationship among endothelial injury or loss, smooth muscle cell proliferation, smooth muscle cell proliferation, and thrombosis.

To examine the question of whether platelets are crucial to the development of proliferative lesions with repeated vessel wall injury, we prepared an antibody against rabbit platelets. Then rabbits were treated with the antibody to make them thrombocytopenic during the period of the study. When we induce vessel wall injury with an indwelling catheter in the abdominal aorta, we found that in the thrombocytopenic animals there was a marked inhibition of atheromatous lesions and fibrous plaques (Moore et al., 1971).

When very low platelet counts of the order of $1000/mm^3$ were observed, lesions were completely inhibited. Thus, thrombocytopenia prevented or markedly inhibited the development of proliferative lesions in these animals.

In subsequent studies, we have shown that thrombocytopenia prevents the development of proliferative lesions in animals subjected to a single balloon catheter injury of the aorta (Friedman et al., 1976b).

An important aspect of this problem of defining the causes of atherogenesis is the recognition of factors and mechanisms which can cause endothlial injury. Figure 4 summarizes some of the factors which are thought to injure the endothelium. They include viruses, bacteria, antigen-antibody complexes, chemicals such as homocysteine, lipids such as cholesterol, smoking, carbon monoxide, etc. Recently there has been interest in the possibility that cholesterol might damage the endothelium (Ross and Glomsett, 1973; Wu et al., 1975) and Jørgensen has reported supporting data at this meeting (Svendsen and Jørgensen, 1976).

One of the interesting aspects of the injury mechanisms is the effect of smoking. There is circumstantial evidence that smoking may affect the vessel wall and the interaction of platelets with it. Mustard and Murphy (1963) studied the effect of smoking on platelet survival in man. It is important to bear in mind that there is evidence of shortening of platelet survival in association with vascular disease in man, and Harker et al. (1974) have shown that damage to the vessel wall shortens platelet survival in animals. Mustard and Murphy (1963) found that when subjects smoked, they had shorter platelet survival times than when they were not smoking. This effect on platelet survival was a great or greater than that produced in animals by damaging the endothelium. Astrup (1973) considers that the damaging effects of cigarette smoking are due to carbon monoxide and he has shown subendothelial edema in the aorta of rabbits exposed to this gas. Thomsen (1974) has made similar observations in monkeys. These observations, together with the epidemiological data linking smoking and atherosclerosis, provide evidence for the hypothesis that the mechanism by which smoking leads to enhanced risk of vascular disease is its damaging effect on the vessel wall, which enhances platelet interaction with the wall, and thus causes proliferative atherosclerotic lesions to form. If this should be established to be a mechanism in the development of atherosclerosis, then one of the key strategies in prevention will be to produce a cigarette that satisfies the smoker but does not damage the vessel wall.

We now know that there are a number of drugs which inhibit platelet function (Mustard and Packham, 1975). Among these are some, such as sulphinpyrazone, which appear to inhibit the interaction of platelets with the subendothelial surface of a damaged vessel wall. It is possible that as a temporary measure to minimize the development of atherosclerosis associated with injury, therapy with such drugs could be useful. However, it seems long-term therapy with such compounds will not prove to be a practical way to prevent the development of atherosclerosis because of the problem of drug toxicity and the difficulties of achieving long-term patient compliance.

1. Bacteria-endotoxin
2. Viruses
3. AG/AB complexes
4. Hemodynamic
5. Blood platelets white cells
6. Hormones
7. Homocystine
8. Carbon monoxide-smoking
9. Hypercholesterolemia

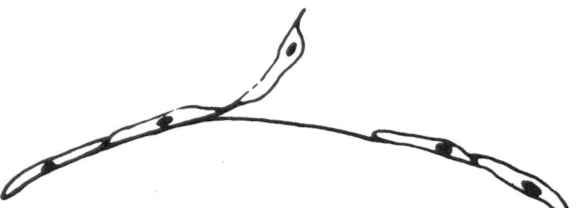

Figure 4. Endothelial injury

Summary

The evidence which I have reviewed from an experimental point of view indicates
that damage to the vessel wall leads to the interaction of the formed elements
of the blood with the vessel wall and that the platelets which adhere to the vessel wall release their constituents, particularly a mitogenic factor which causes
the smooth muscle cells to proliferate. The proliferating smooth muscle cells
migrate into the intima and produce an atheromatous lesion. With a single injury,
the lesion tends to be essentially a fibrous plaque. With repeated injury, lipid-
rich lesions develop, which include atheromatous plaques with extensive cholesterol deposits. Although vessel wall injury leads to the development of atherosclerotic lesions, lipid accumulation in the lesions is not dependent upon hypercholesterolemia and occurs in experimental animals on normal diets, provided the
vessel wall is repeatedly injured. Hypercholesterolemia, however, may enhance the
accumulation of lipid in lesions caused by injury to the vessel wall.

PLATELET FACTORS AND THE PROLIFERATION OF VASCULAR SMOOTH MUSCLE CELLS

Hans R. Baumgartner and Alfred Studer

Blood platelets play a predominant role in arterial thrombosis. This has long
been recognized by pathologists. However, only recently the pathophysiologic
prerequisites which lead to increased platelet participation in arterial thrombosis were more fully understood. These prerequisites include the exposure of
subendothelial tissue to the blood stream and high blood shear rates. Unaltered
platelets do not adhere to vascular endothelium; however, they rapidly react with
subendothelium (French et al., 1964; Baumgartner et al., 1967). The rate of this
reaction, i.e., the rate of platelet deposition on subendothelium, was found to
be proportional to the blood shear rate (Turitto and Baumgartner, 1975). In the
absence of blood flow, virtually no platelets reach the vessel wall. With increasing flow and by concomitant oscillation of red blood cells, increasing numbers of platelets per unit time arrive at the vessel wall (Goldsmith, 1972;
Turitto and Baumgartner, 1975) and can interact with reactive substrates. Thus,
the extent of platelet vessel wall interaction increases with the area of subendothelium exposed and the blood shear rate.

Loss of Endothelium: Short and Long-Term Consequences

The pathophysiologic conditions which may lead to desquamation of vascular endothelium have been summarized by Moore et al. (1976). We have studied the subsequent events at the cellular level in an experimental model in vivo.

Rabbit iliac artery and abdominal aorta were denuded of endothelium by balloon
catheter injury (Baumgartner and Studer, 1966; Baumgartner, 1973). At time intervals following denudation, the arteries were fixed by perfusion of 2.5% glutaraldehyde in phosphate buffer at 110 mm Hg. Interaction of blood cells with subendothelium and subsequent intimal thickening were measured morphometrically in
0.8 μm thick and stained Epon sections.

Platelets rapidly covered the subendothelial surface (Fig. 1). Up to 3 days after
removal of the endothelium, most platelets adhered to the subendothelial surface
itself, later they were also observed in association with amorphous material
produced by neointimal cells. As revealed by electron microscopy, some platelets
were overgrown by neointimal cells, most of them were probably lysed and/or phagocytosed by leukocytes which adhere to the platelet layer in large numbers; neu-
trophiles with a peak after 3 hours, monocytes with a peak after 2 - 3 days.

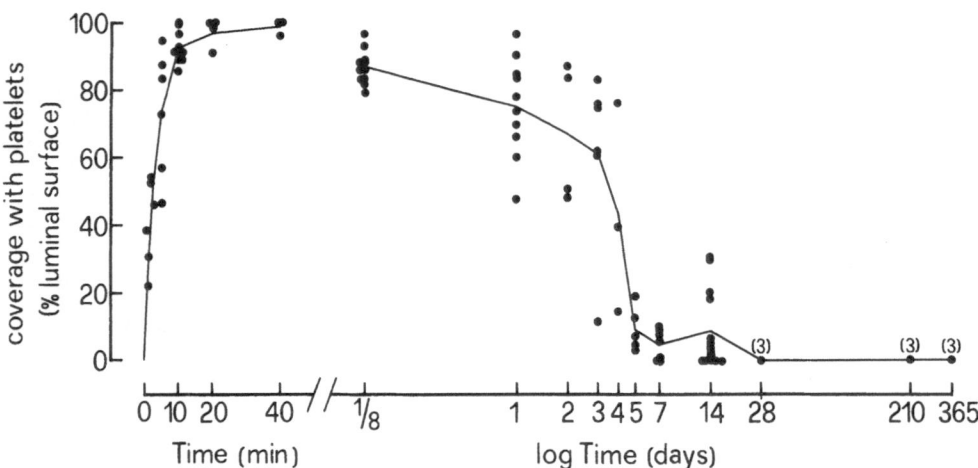

Figure 1. Platelet interaction with the luminal surface of iliac artery at different time intervals after the removal of the endothelium by balloon catheter. Initially, platelets adhere to the subendothelial surface, from day 4 on, platelets mainly adhere to connective tissue newly formed by neointimal cells. In this and the following Figures, each point represents the average of morphometric measurements in a rabbit, numbers in brackets indicate the numbers of rabbits investigated

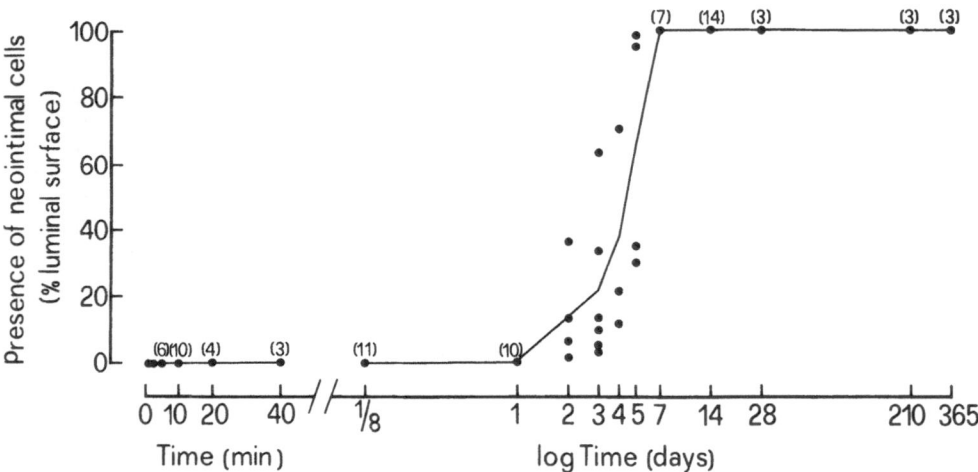

Figure 2. Presence of neointimal cells on the luminal side of the internal elastic lamina. Sequence after removal of endothelium from iliac artery in rabbits. At day 2 mainly processes of smooth muscle cells migrating from the media through fenestrations of the internal elastic lamina are seen on the luminal side, at day 4 numerous complete smooth muscle cells are already present. Early after desendothelialization, new endothelial cells were found near branches only. For further explanation see Figure 1

Within 7 days, the subendothelial surface was fully covered with neointimal cells (Fig. 1). These are mostly smooth muscle cells which are observed to migrate from the media, through the fenestration of the lamina elastica interna to its luminal side and proliferate (see below). Proliferation of smooth muscle cells and accu-

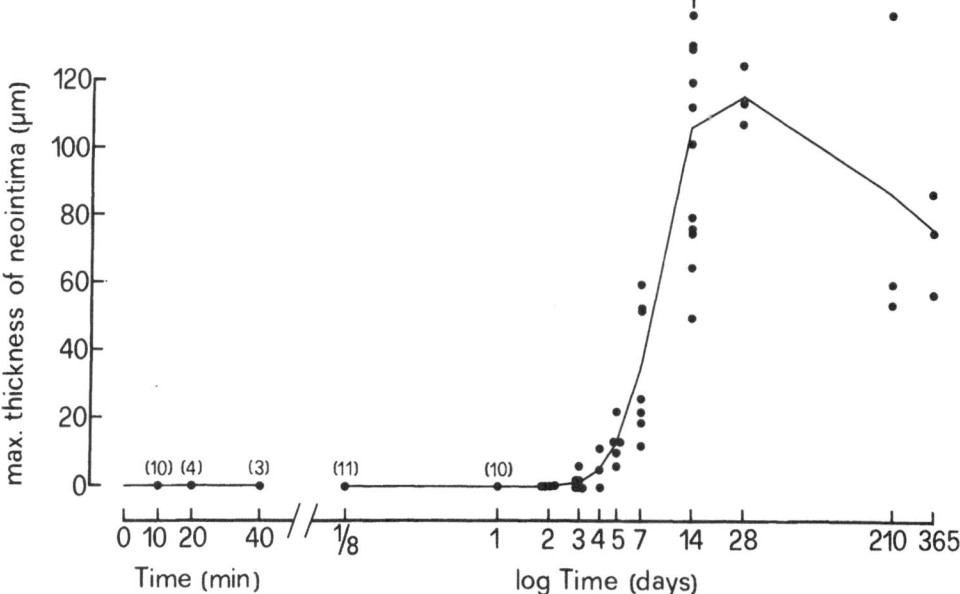

Figure 3. Formation and regression of neointima in rabbit iliac arteries after desendothelialization. In most specimens, intimal thickening was excentric. However, when minimal intimal thickening was plotted instead of maximal (shown), a similar curve was obtained. In more recent experiments the volume of the neointima is measured morphometrically instead of maximal and minimal thickness of the hyperplastic intima. For further explanation see Figure 1

mulation of connective tissue produced by them resulted in a markedly thickened neotinima. Maximal thickness of the neointima (about twice the thickness of the media) was observed 4 weeks after removal of the endothelium, then very slow regression took place (Fig. 3).

In order to determine the site of proliferative activity, rabbits were injected with tritiated thymidin 2 1/2 hours prior to perfusion fixation. 3H-thymidin incorporation into the media started at day 2, was maximal at day 4, and at control level again after 2 weeks. In the neointima, the largest number of labeled cells was found after 2 weeks, and even after 4 and 6 weeks thymidin incorporation was still above control level (Baumgartner et al., 1971; Baumgartner and Studer, 1976). These data indicate that proliferative activity takes place in the media only initially after removal of endothelium, but then goes on at a high rate for at least 2 weeks in the neointima. The mechanism which stops proliferation is unknown. It may be related to the coverage of the neotintima with new and fully functional endothelium.

Factors Released from Platelets

Platelets which adhere to basement membrane, collagen fibrils, or other collagenous material selectively release many of their components (Holmsen et al., 1969 and many others). The biological activities (their chemical nature) released include: platelet aggregation-promoting agents (adenosine diphosphate, endoperoxides, thromboxanes, serotonin), vasoactive substances (serotonin and other amines, intermediates of prostaglandin synthesis), a proliferation-stimulating factor (Ross et al., 1974; probably a polypeptide), and a number of other activities (lysosomal enzymes, collagenase, elastase, PF4, β-thromboglobuline, protoglycan). It is conceivable that all these factors or at least some of them are released not only toward the vessel lumen but also or even selectively toward the vessel wall. At present, no direct evidence is available for the latter possibility which certainly deserves more attention in the near future.

Platelets and Atherosclerosis

In the introduction to the symposium, Dr. Moore has discussed the role of mural platelet thrombi in the progression of atherosclerosis: platelet thrombi which develop (on ruptures plaques, for example) are organized and incorporated into the vessel wall. This is a physical, a visible contribution of platelets. However, our studies show that platelet adhesion to subendothelium and subsequent aggregation are also transient events. Platelets are not always organized and incorporated, mural thrombi are often washed away by the blood stream and platelets may be lysed and phagocytosed by leukocytes. Nevertheless, the close relationship between platelet adhesion to subendothelium and the subsequent migration and proliferation of medial smooth muscle cells suggested a working hypothesis: factors released from adhering platelets trigger the migration and proliferation of smooth muscle cells and thus initiate the proliferative response to endothelial injury. Ross et al. (1974) and Moore et al. (1976) provided the first indirect evidence that a platelet factor might indeed play a very significant role in atherogenesis. Ross et al. (1974) have shown that platelets contain a factor(s) which is essential for smooth muscle cell proliferation. This factor is present in serum (released from platelets during blood clotting) but absent in plasma. The proliferation-stimulating factor is a heat stable, nondialysable, basic protein which is currently purified by several laboratories Rutherford and Ross, 1976; Busch et al. (1976). Moore et al. (1976) have shown that the formation of raised lesions and fibrous plaques induced by chronic injury in rabbits is inhibited in animals made thrombocytopenic by an antiplatelet serum.

Effect of Antiplatelet Agents on Intimal Thickening

The platelet factor hypothesis nourishes hopes that antiplatelet agents might inhibit not only platelet aggregation but also influence the proliferative response after endothelial injury. Some recent findings obtained in rabbits after

Table 1. Effect of treatment with antiplatelet agents on the volume of the neointima which developed after balloon catheter injury in rabbit iliac artery within 2 weeks

	Number of rabbits	Volume of neointima (% of media)
All controls	18	68.0 ± 5.6
Control I	6	64.0 ± 7.9
Dipyridamole (50 mg/kg twice daily)	7	65.7 ± 7.6
Control II	5	76.9 ± 12.9
Aspirin (30 mg/kg)	3	97.1 ± 39.0
Control III	7	65.2 ± 9.5
Sulfinpyrazone (67 mg/kg)	9	40.6 ± 9.5[a]

Drugs were fed aily by stomach tube, starting the day before balloon injury. Means ± SEM are given.

[a] Signficantly different from corresponding control III (p 0.05) and from all controls (p 0.01; Student t test).

balloon injury are shown in Table 1. Sulfinpyrazone seems to have an effect on intimal thickening; dipyridamole and aspirin not. Additional experiments are necessary and definite results will be presented elsewhere.

THROMBOGENIC AND ATHEROGENIC EFFECTS OF DIETARY FATS*

S. Renaud

Since 1930, numerous epidemiological studies have shown that coronary heart disease (CHD) was closely associated with the saturated fat intake. So far, much of the energy in this field has been concentrated on elucidating the role of cholesterol and fat in inducing atherosclerosis. However, coronary death appears to be, most of the time, the result of a thrombotic occluding event superimposed on an atherosclerotic plaque. In recent years, indications are accumulating that dietary fats, in addition to inducing atherosclerosis, might predispose to thrombosis, directly through certain blood components.

During World War II, in Norway and also in other European countries, a decrease in the incidence of CHD as well as of venous thrombosis was observed in relation to a marked decrease in the consumption of saturated fats (Stormoken, 1973, 1974).

It has also been shown that a high incidence of thromboembolisms could be observed solely in countries where the incidence of CHD was high as in the U.S.A. as compared to Japan (Gore et al., 1964) or to Uganda (Thomas et al., 1960). Those studies indicate that some environmental factor, most probably the saturated fat intake, might directly predispose to thrombosis (both arterial and venous).

The intial event of a thrombus, arterial or venous, appears to be the formation of platelet aggregates consolidated by fibrin threads. Several in vitro experiments have shown that some components of saturated fats, the long-chain saturated fatty acids, mainly stearic acid, are effective in inducing platelet aggregation (Hahadevan et al., 1966) and promoting coagulation (Didisheim and Mabashan, 1963).

Numerous experimental studies in animals have indicated that among the lipids only saturated fats, in the diet, appear to predispose to thrombosis. Those results were confirmed and extended recently by the aorta technique in rats fed various fats (Hornstra, 1937, 1974). With this technique, it was found that the severity of thrombosis was mostly related to the content of the fat in long-chain saturated fatty acids, which in practice means palmitic (16:0) and stearic acid (18:0).

In our studies on venous thrombosis, we found that the thrombogenicity of a dietary fat was mostly dependent on the ratio stearic acid/linoleic acid (Renaud and Lecomte, 1970), since linoleic acid appears to be the most antithrombogenic fatty acid.

Our studies in rat and rabbit (Renaud and Lecomte, 1970; Renaud et al., 1970) have shown that the thrombogenic fats predispose the animals to thrombosis essentially by:
1. Increasing the susceptiblity of platelets to aggregation (mostly to thrombin)
2. Accelerating fibrin formation, chiefly by increasing the clotting activity of pletelets (PF$_3$) (Gautheron and Renaud, 1972).

*Part of the work reported here has been supported by grants from the USDA (Contract N°12-14-100-599), the INSERM (ATP N°12-74-33), the "Fondation pour la Recherche Médicale", and the University of Montreal.

This PF$_3$, the only clotting factor of lipidic origin (phospholipids), appears to be the limiting factor of coagulation. Thus, from an increase in its activity which appears to depend on its content in stearic and oleic acids results a comparable acceleration of clotting (Renaud and Gautheron, 1974).

In a study, still in progress, on farmers from two French regions (Moselle and Var) differing in the incidende of CHD and in the type of fat consumed, identical results to those of the experimental studies reported above were obtained.

As shown in Figure 1, the PCT of the subjects in Moselle was markedly shorter than of the subjects in Var. This clotting acceleration could be completely reproduced by platelets alone (F$_3$-CT).

By contrast, the CEP-CT did show a slight prolongation in the subjects from Moselle. Those three tests demonstrate that the hypercoagulability observed in the subjects from Moselle by the PCT is entirely due to an increase in the clotting activity of platelets.

In addition, the Moselle subjects presented a tremendous increase in the primary aggregation induced by thrombin and ADP, but not by collagen or epinephrine. Of interest is that there was no difference in plasma cholesterol between the two regions. In animals also, the studies of Hornstra (1973, 1974), as well as ours, indicate no close relationship between serum cholesterol and the susceptibility to thrombosis or platelet functions. Still, the incidence of death from CHD in men 35 – 44 years old in those two regions, as determined by the death certificates

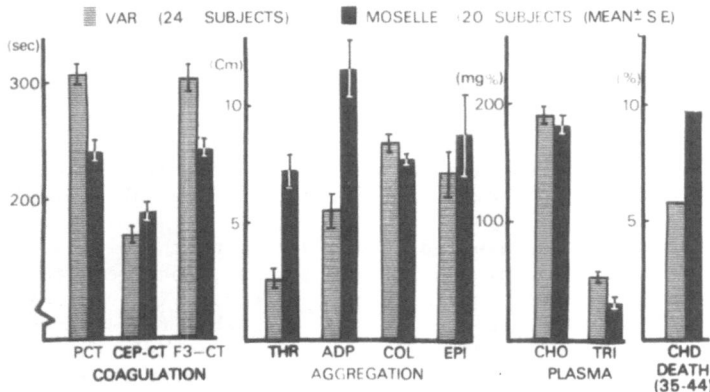

Figure 1. Blood parameters in healthy male farmers (40 – 45 years) from two French regions differing in the incidence of CHD and the fat intake
PCT recalcification plasma clotting time of platelet-rich plasma (evalueates the clotting activity of the whole blood)
CEP-CT cephalin clotting time of platelet-poor plasma (evaluates the clotting activity of the plasmatic clotting factors)
F$_3$-CT clotting of washed platelets, resuspended in a standard platelet-poor plasma (400,000 platelets/mm^3) (evaluates the clotting activity of platelets)
All the clotting tests have been performed in a recording turbidimetric coagulometer.
The platelet aggregation in platelet-rich plasma (300,000 platelets/mm^3) was evaluated by turbidimetry as the maximum height of the curve (Thr: thrombin, ADP, Epi: epinephrine) with agents inducing a reversible aggregation. The susceptibility to collagen (COL) was evaluated as the distance from origin for the curve to be 5 cm above the initial level.
CHO cholesterol; TRI triglycerides in plasma

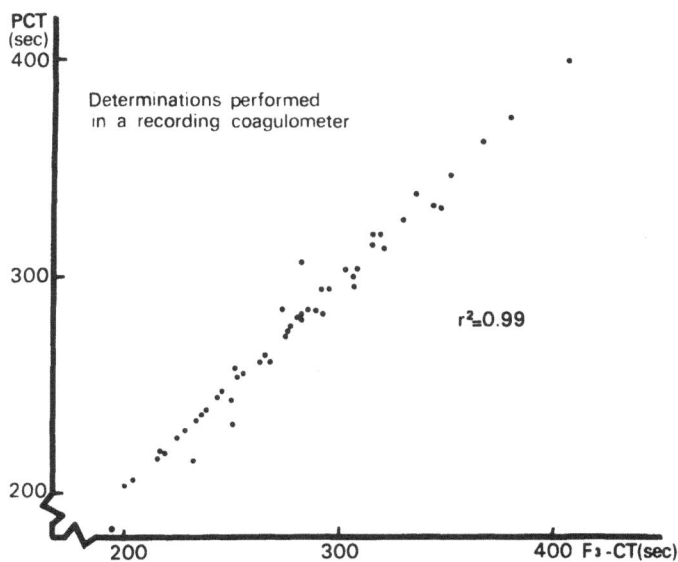

Figure 2. Correlation between the PCT and the F_3-CT in the totality of subjects studied in the two French regions

from the French Official Statistics, is 9.8% in Moselle as compared to 5.7% in Var. The saturated fat intake, and particularly stearic acid, appears to be much higher in Moselle than in Var.

Figure 2 illustrates the marked correlation between the PCT and the F_3-CT tests in subjects studied in those two regions.

We had previously shown that in CHD patients submitted to coronarography as compared to normal subjects an increase in the clotting activity of platelets, apparently due to changes in the fatty acid composition of their phospholipids, could also be observed. The platelets of the CHD patients were also more susceptible to aggregation, mostly to thrombin.

Contrary to thrombosis and to platelet functions, atherosclerosis, as noted in human populations or in rabbits fed various fats (Fig. 3), appears to be related to blood cholesterol. Consequently, cholesterol might be of importance solely for one of the two components of CHD, namely atherosclerosis. Studies in man and in animals have shown that myristic and palmitic acids might be the fatty acids responsible for the hypercholesterolemic effects of saturated fats and most probably of their atherogenic effects. Stearic acid does not seem to be hypercholesterolemic at all, both in man and in animals. Consequently, the main contributions of the saturated fatty acids to CHD might be illustrated as in Figure 4.

Conclusions

1. Epidemiological studies have shown that CHD (arterial thrombosis) and venous thrombosis were closely associated with the dietary saturated fat intake.
2. In vitro and in vivo studies are unanimous in that long-chain saturated fatty acids, mostly stearic acid, are thrombogenic, while linoleic acid has protective effects.
3. Stearic acid appears to modify the fatty acid composition of platelet phospholipids resulting in an increase in the aggregating and clotting capacities of platelets.

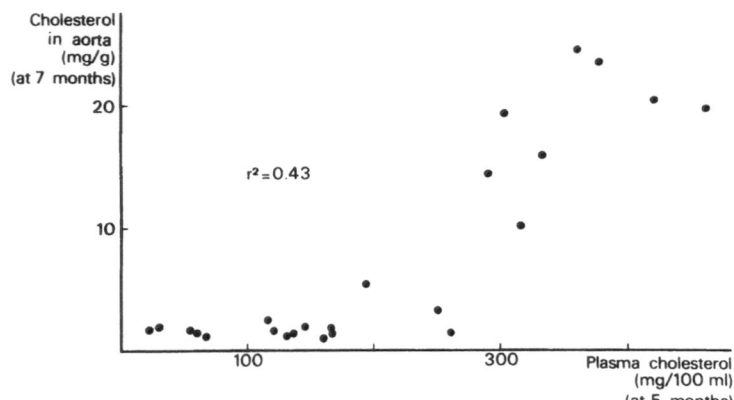

Figure 3. Correlation between the plasma cholesterol 5 months after the beginning of diet feeding and the aortic cholesterol at 7 months, in rabbits fed various dietary fats (12% + 0.1% cholesterol)

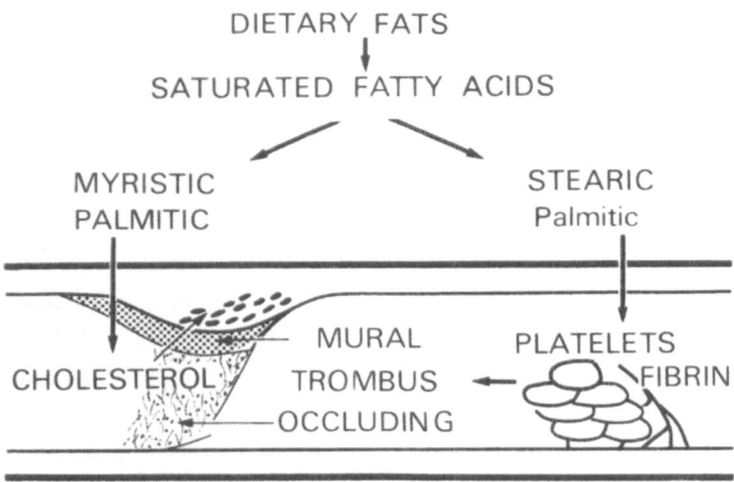

Figure 4. In a schematic way, mechanisms involved in the effects of saturated dietary fats on both atherosclerosis and thrombosis through the long-chain saturated fatty acids

4. In coronary patients or in subjects eating saturated fats, similar modifications in platelet behavior can be observed related to changes in platelet phospholipids.
5. Those results appear to confirm the hypothesis that certain dietary saturated fats, in addition to inducing hyperlipemia and atherosclerosis, predispose to thrombosis mostly through blood platelets.

SCANNING AND TRANSMISSION ELECTRON MICROSCOPIC STUDIES ON EXPERIMENTAL THROMBOSIS IN RABBITS

K. Tanaka

Platelet adhesion on the surface exposed to blood is considered to be the earliest event in the formation of mural thrombus in vivo, and much attention has been given recently to the interaction of platelets with subendothelial materials (Baumgartner, 1974; Sumiyoshi and Tanaka, 1976). In the present study, the effect of a minute injury on the intima was studied by transmission and scanning electron microscopy as well as immunohistochemically.

Materials and Methods

Intimal injury was induced in the aorta and inferior vena cava of rabbits by inserting polyethylene tube (external diameter 0.038 in) into the aorta and inferior vena cava via the femoral artery and vein, respectively. Rabbits were allowed to survive for experimental periods ranging from immediately after to 7 days after tube insertion. Specimens were obtained from various parts of the injured areas and were examined with scanning and transmission electron microscopy. Ruthenium red stained was carried out in some of the specimens. In all rabbits, 40 mg per kg body weight of Evans blue was injected intravenously at the tubing or before sacrifice. The injured areas were also observed under a fluorescence microscope and studied by immunofluorescent technique with antirabbit fibrinogen antibody.

Results

Immediately after tube insertion into the aorta, by scanning electron microscopy, platelets with pseudopods adhered in a scattered manner on the exposed subendothelial materials which were composed of finely fibrillar components. Adhesion of platelets was not found on the normal appearing or disintegrated endothelial cells located at the margins of the denuded area. By transmission electron microscopy, platelets adhered on the exposed surface of the subendothelial material, containing microfibrils. Adhered platelets showed pseudopod formation and degranulation. Fibrin threads were not found. By fluorescence microscopy, specific yellowish-green fluorescence of fibrinogen was found in the superficial layer of the denuded intima, and red fluorescence of Evans blue-albumin complex was found in the intima and inner most layer of the media where denudation of the endothelium was induced.

Five minutes after tubing, localization of fibrinogen and Evans blue-albumin complex was almost similar to that described above. By ruthenium red staining, the denuded area was covered by a thick, electron-dense layer of glycosaminoglycans containing cellular debris, possibly degranulated platelets (Fig. 1).

Fifteen minutes after tubing, by scanning and transmission microscopy, the findings were almost similar to those found immediately after tubing (Fig. 2). Occasionally, dense aggregates of degranulated platelets with pseudopods were found on the denuded area.

One hour after tube insertion, the findings of the denuded area were almost similar to those found in the earlier stage, but larger platelet aggregates were occasionally found.

Twenty-four hours after tube insertion, fibrin nets covered the platelet aggregates. Several erythrocytes and a few leukocytes were trapped in the fibrin network (Fig. 3).

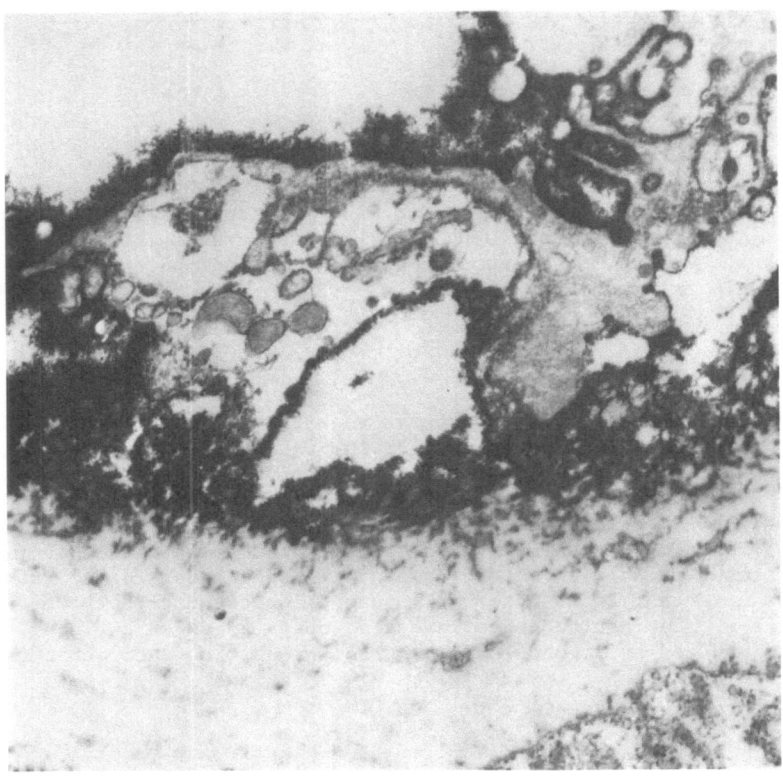

Figure 1. A transmission electron micrograph of a denuded area of the aorta immediately after tube insertion (ruthenium red staining). Denuded area is covered by thick, electron-dense layer of glycosaminoglycans containing cellular debris, possibly degranulated platelets

Fourty-eight hours after tubing, aggregates of deformed platelets and granular materials probably derived from disintegrated platelets, intermingled with a small amount of fibrin nets, covered most parts of the injured surface, and leukocytes were occasionally found. Transmission electron microscopic observation of these areas revealed that degranulated and/or nondegranulated platelets covered some parts of the injured areas with exposure of the microfibrills. Mononuclear cells attached occasionally on the platelets. Fibrin formation was mainly found in the larger thrombi.

Seven days after tubing, newly formed endothelial cells covered the injured areas showing more or less fibrous thickening. Larger thrombi in various stages of organization were also covered by newly formed endothelial cells.

These cells were continuous with the endothelium lining of the adjacent undamaged area. They were irregular in shape showing cytoplasmic processes, and their attachment appeared incomplete. Platelets adhered on the incomplete intercellular junctions of these cells. By transmission electron microscopy, intercellular junction of these cells was incomplete. Proliferation of the modified smooth muscle cells was noted.

These serial changes occurred on the injured surface of the inferior vena cava where the tube was inserted, but aggregation of the platelets and adhesion of leukocytes were more prominent. The size of thrombi tended to be larger than that formed in the aorta 48 hours after tubing. The findings 7 days after tubing

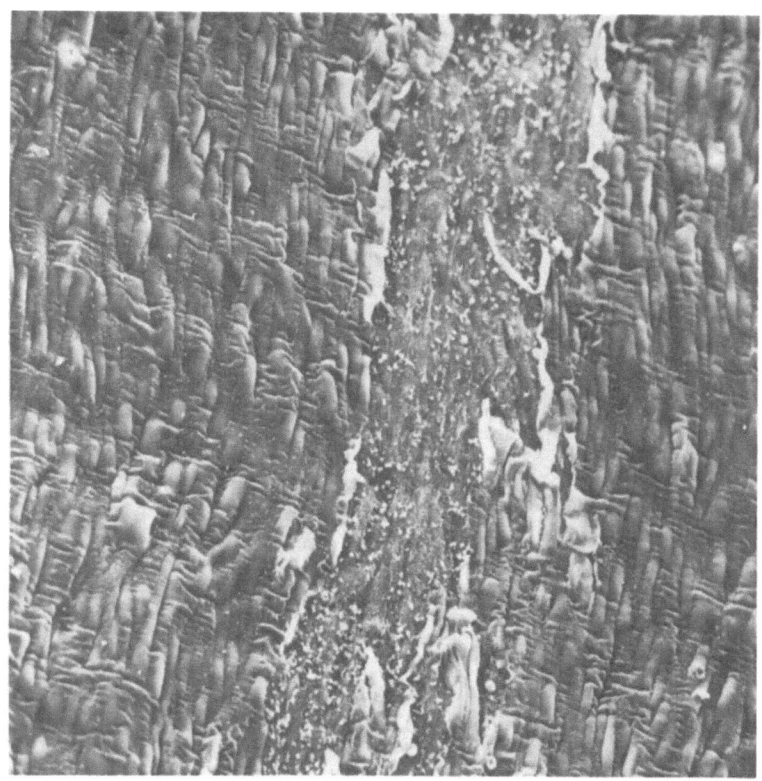

Figure 2. A scanning electron micrograph of a denuded area of the aorta 15 minutes after tube insertion. Platelets with pseudopods adhere on the deendothelialized surface composed of subendothelial fibrillar components

were almost similar to those of the aorta, though the localized intimal fibrous thickening was more prominent than that found in the aorta.

Discussion

Denudation of endothelial cells and direct exposure of the subendothelial materials, containing microfibrills, was apparently necessary for the initiation of the in vivo mural thrombosis in the aorta as well as in the inferior vena cava, but platelets did not adhere over the entire surface of the denuded areas, and adhesion, aggregation, and dissociation of the platelets on the injured area appeared to take place repeatedly.

Thrombus was further developed by formation of fibrin networks surrounding the platelet aggregates and appeared to be settled as a mural 24 hours after tubing.

Cellular components of blood other than platelets might play little role in the primary event of thrombogenesis.

Injured areas showed slight fibrous thickening covered by newly formed endothelial cells 7 days after tube insertion. Some platelets adhered on the immature intercellular junctions of these cells.

Finally, immediately after the denudation of the endothelial cells, blood constituents containing fibrinogen insudated into the denuded intima and innermost layer of the media.

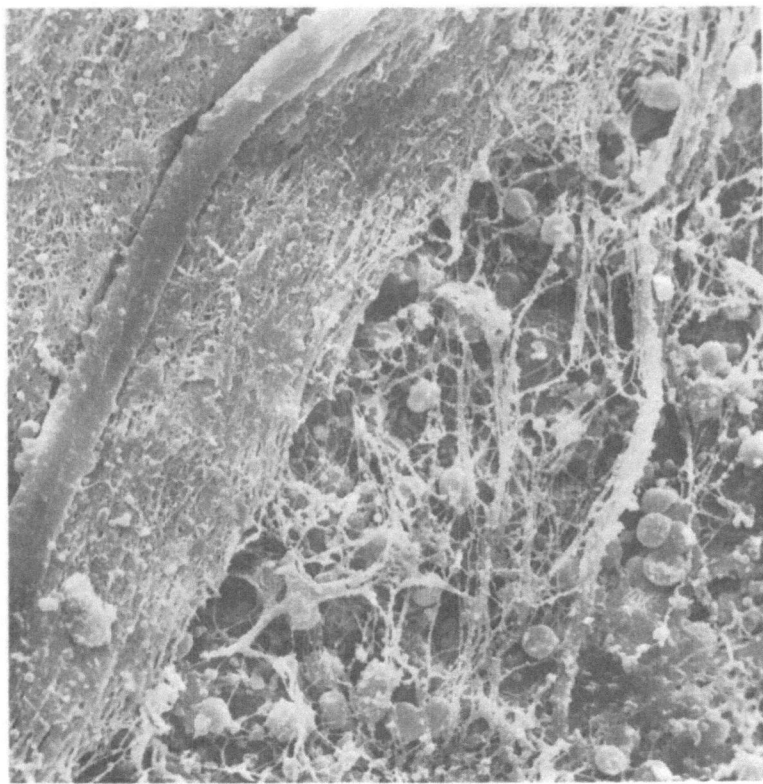

Figure 3. A scanning electron micrograph of a thrombus of the aorta 24 hours after tube insertion. Fibrin nets covering the platelets aggregate

A complex of glycosaminoglycans and fibrinogen formed in some cases and may play a role in the platelet adhesion. Insudated blood constituents containing fibrinogen may have some relation to the proliferation of smooth muscle cells, because vascular wall, especially intima, contained tissue thromboplastin (Onoyama and Tanaka, 1969) and proliferative reaction induced by plasma was more severe than that induced by serum (Tanaka, 1973).

Summary

The initial event of thrombus formation was platelet adhesion and subsequent aggregation on the denuded intima of the aorta and inferior vena cava and fibrinogen and its derivatives might have some relation to the platelet adhesion. Not only the organization of thrombi, but also the intimal fibrous thickening following platelet adhesion on the denuded intima and insudation of blood constituents containing fibrinogen into the vascular wall seem to be important in the development of atherosclerosis.

ATHEROMATOSIS OF THE RABBIT CAROTID ARTERY: II. THE PREVENTATIVE EFFECT OF ANTICOAGULANTS AND PERMEABILITY AFFECTING AGENTS

C.Th. Smit Sibinga, H.O. Nieweg, and H.B. Lamberts
Loagulation Laboratory, Department of Radiopathology, University Hospital,
Groningen/Netherlands

The prevantative activity of drugs with an effect on fibrin formation or vessel wall permeability, was tested on irradiation induced vessel wall damage. An experimental irradiation model was used: rabbits were fed on a 0.5% chol. diet, irradiated one week later on one carotid artery (single dose 2000 R, dose rate 12o R/min) and killed 4 weeks after the irradiation-procedure. The carotid art. (the non-irradiated one being the control to the irradiated one) were excised for histological examination. Fibrin formation, platelet function, serum chol. were measured throughout the whole experiment. As a control 11 rabbits were fed on a 0.5% chol.diet without addition of any drug. Durgs used: I. *anti-coagulants*-calcium heparin, warfarin sodium. II. *permeability affecting agents*- etamsylate, prednisone, H.R., benzarone. *Results*: It is shown that heparin protected the vessel wall from being infiltrated with lipid from the serum. In the prednisone treated group there was a limited infiltration (intima) of lipid. The other drugs did not show any preventative effect as compared to the hypercholesterolaemic control. The effect of heparin and moderate effect of prednisone seems to be related to permeability support, and to an effect on lipid metabolism.

THE PROTECTIVE EFFECT OF ACETYLSALICYLIC ACID AND HEPARIN IN EXPERIMENTAL ARTERIAL THROMBOSIS AND ATHEROSCLEROSIS

R. Zimmermann, W.W. Höpker, P. Barth, D. Lange, and C. Zeltsch
Medizinische Universitätsklinik Heidelberg, Heidelberg/BRD

Antiplatelet drugs may inhibit arterial thrombosis and possibly development of atherosclerosis. In a *first series* of experiments the antithrombotic effect of acetylsalicylic acid (ASA) was studied in 620 experiments using 320 rabbits in which thrombus formation by vessel injury, hypercoagulability or stasis was standardized. The effect of ASA and anticoagulants were examined in the arterial and venous system. In addition, in 12o rabbits, thrombus composition was investigated by measurement of platelets (labelled with Cr^{51}), fibrinogen (J^{125}) and red cells (Fe^{59}). In the arterial system ASA reduced thrombus size by 61% and was as effective as heparin. The composition of thrombi was altered by antithrombotic therapy. In the venous system heparin was superior to ASA. In the *second series* the direct action of ASA on the development of atherosclerosis was tested in 40 rabbits. Atherosclerosis was induced by atherogenic diet and by extreme restriction of physical action. No preventive effect of ASA could be demonstrated. *Comment*: Treatment with ASA reduces the formation of arterial thrombi. The antithrombotic action of ASA is as effective as heparin. The evolution of the atherogenic process cannot be inhibited by ASA.

DECREASED PLATELET SENSITIVITY IN SPONTANEOUS HYPERTENSIVE RATS MAY
BE RELATED TO REDUCED PLASMA FREE FATTY ACID LEVELS

R.N. Saunders, E.R. Waskawic, D.J. Fretland, T.S. Burns, and L.F. Rozek
Searle Laboratories, Skokie, IL/USA

Platelets from spontaneous hypertensive (SH) rats were shown to require twice as
much collagen or adenosine diphosphate (ADP) to achieve a comparable *in vitro*
aggregation response when compared to platelets from normotensive Sprague-Dawley
(SD) rats. Similar finding were reported by Nagaoka et al. (Jap. Circul. J. $\underline{35}$,
1379 (1971)). No difference in plasma glucose, calcium or uric acid was noted,
but a significant ($P < 0.05$) difference was found in plasmy free fatty acid (FFA)
levels (SH, 188 ± 21 μ Eq/L vs. SD, 289 ± 33 μ Eq/L). Fasting the rats for 24
hours eliminated the difference in plasma FFA (SH, 348 ± 36 μ Eq/L vs. SD, 378
± 49 μ Eq/L) and resulted in the platelets having similar ADP-induced aggregation response profiles. Decreased 24 hour urinary prostaglandin (PG) E metabolites were also observed with SH rats (123 ± 40 ng) compared to the SD (1091
± 209 ng) or normotensive Kyoto-Wistar (338 ± 72 ng) rats. This data suggests
that decreased aggregation sensitivity of the SH rat platelet may be related to
lower FFA levels and a reduced prostaglandin synthesis rate.

ATHEROMATOSIS OF THE RABBIT CAROTID ARTERY: III - THE PREVENTATIVE
EFFECT OF ANTIAGGREGATIVE AGENTS AND TRANEXAMIC ACID

C.Th. Smit Sibinga, H.O. Nieweg, and H.B. Lamberts
Coagulation Laboratory, Department Radiopathology, University Hospital, Gronin-
gen/Netherlands

The preventative effect of anti-aggregating agents and tranexamic acid on irradiation induced vessel wall damage was tested. An experimental irradiation model was
used: rabbits were fed on a 0.5% cholesterol diet, irradiated one week later on
one carotid artery (2000 R single dose, 120 R/min dose rate) and killed 4 weeks
after the irradiation procedure. The carotid arteries (the non-irradiated one
being the control to the irradiated one) were excised for histological examination. Platelet function, serum cholesterol were measured throughout the whole
experiment. A a control 11 rabbits were fed on a 0.5% chol. diet without addition
of any drug. Drugs used: 1. *anti-aggregating agents-* acetylsalicylic acid (ASA),
indomethacin, phenylbutazon and the pyrimido-pyrimidin derivatives: VK 744 and
RA 233. 2. *anti-fibrinolytic agent-* tranexamid acid (TA). *Results*: a striking
protective effect on irradiation induced vessel wall damage is seen in the rabbits treated with ASA and TA. Of the other drugs used, indomethacin, phenylbutazon and VK 744 showed even more severe vessel wall damage in comparison to the
hypercholesterolaemic control. It is concluded that the favourable effect of ASA
and TA predominantly is the result of an inhibitory activity on irradiation induced local inflammatory reaction and therefore secondary on vessel wall permeability.

EFFECT OF SUSTAINED ISOMETRIC HANDGRIP EXERCISE ON PLATELET AGGREG-
ABILITY AND LEFT VENTRICULAR FUNCTION IN AHTEROSCLEROTIC PATIENTS
AND CYCLIC AMP PHOSPHODIESTERASE INHIBITOR PRETREATMENT

Takeshi Motomiya, Tadahiro Sano, Hiroh Yamazaki, and Takio Shimamoto
Department of Medicine, Aoyama Tokyo Metropolitan Hospital, Tokyo Metropolitan
Institute of Medical Science and Japan Atherosclerosis Research Foundation,
Tokyo/Japan

A striking enhancing effect of EG626, a potent cyclic AMP phosphodiesterase inhibitor, on regression of atherosclerotic plaque of rabbits and a potent anti-

thrombotic effect of this compound on experimental thrombosis (Furlow and Bass, 1974) have been reported by Shimamoto and Numano 1975. In this paper the preventive effect of EG626 on the increase in platelet aggregability as well as the deterioration of cardiac function induced by exercise test in man has been reported. Thirty healthy adults, 29 patients suffering from coronary sclerosis and 20 patients with cerebral arteriosclerosis were subjected to the 50% maximal voluntary handgrip exercise test. During the rest and the exercise, the platelet aggregability (TDH 25,524 (1971)) and systolic time intervals were measured. A statistically significant increase in platelet-aggregability and a statistically significant deterioration of the left ventricular performance were found in the patients, but not in healthy controls. The pretreatment of the patients with single dose of 100-300 mg (p.o.) of EG626 prevented the above mentioned changes in platelet-aggregability and in the systolic time intervals.

THROMBOSIS IN VIVO WITH SPECIAL REFERENCE TO SCANNING ELECTRON MICROSCOPIC STUDY ON ENDOTHELIAL DAMAGE

Akinobu Sumiyoshi and Kenzo Tanaka
Department of Pathology, Medical College of Miyazaki, Miyazaki/Japan and Department of Pathology, Faculty of Medicine, Kyushu University, Fukuoka/Japan

Thrombosis is an important pathological process but initial changes of thrombogenesis in vivo are not fully understood. In the present study, significance of endothelial damage and effects of hemodynamics on thrombogenesis in vivo and fate of organized thrombus of the aorta were studied by light microscopy, and scanning and transmission electron microscopy. Direct exposure of the subendothelial structures, mainly of microfibrils and collagen, was apparently necessary for initiation of in vivo mural thrombosis in the aorta as well as in the inferior vena cava. Thrombus formation was initiated by platelets adhesion to the areas where the endothelium was completely absent. Some platelets aggregates were followed by formation of fibrin nets around them and developed into the thrombi. Platelet adhesion was more prominent and thrombus tended to be larger in the inferior vena cava where blood flow was slow than in the aorta where the blood flow was fast.

THE RELATIONSHIP BETWEEN PLASMA FACTOR VII, AND SERUM CHOLESTEROL AND TRIGLYCERIDES IN MEN AND WOMEN

W.R.S. North, T.W. Meade, R. Chakrabarti, Y. Stirling, and M. Brozovic, N. Noble, and J. Slack
MRC-DHSS Epidemiology and Medical Care Unit, and MRC Clinical Genetics Unit, London/England

Levels of blood lipids and several haemostatic variables including factor VII have been measured in a prospective study of ischaemic heart disease in an industrial population in N.W. London. Results are currently available for 507 white men and 192 white women aged 20 - 49; of the women, 46 were on oral contraceptives (OC). As previously reported, cholesterol, triglycerides and factor VII levels all increase with age in men, and in women not on OC, and at younger ages all 3 variables are lower in women than in men. Two original observations are: (1) In women on OC there is presently no significant regression with age in any of the 3 variables, the younger women on OC having values similar to those of older women not on OC. (2) There are presently significant correlations, after age adjustment, and log. transformation, between factor VII on one hand and cholesterol and triglycerides on the other:

	Men	Women not on OC
Cholesterol	+0.23[a]	+0.10
Triglycerides	+0.25[a]	+0.16

[a] $p = <0.0001$.   [b] $p = <0.05$.

The findings suggest that in considering liability to ischaemic heart disease, the relationship between factor VII, cholesterol and triglycerides should be considered.

CONCENTRATION OF PLASMA ANTITHROMBIN III IN ATHEROSCLEROTIC DISEASES

Tamotsu Matsuda, and Mototaka Murakami
Tokyo Metropolitan Institute of Gerontology, Department of Physiology, Division of Clinical Physiology (II), Tokyo/Japan

Concentration of plasma antithrombin III was measured in 39 cases of acute myocardial infarction, 58 cases of acute cerebral infarction and 16 cases of acute cerebral hemorrhage, using single radial immunodiffusion method.
Plasma antithrombin III content was significantly decreased before and after the development of myocardial infarction. In ten autopsied cases of acute myocardial infarction, three cases with extremely low levels of plasma antithrombin III were complicated with disseminated intravascular coagulation, acute cerebral infarction and/or thromboembolism of lower extremities, while the other seven cases in whom plasma antithrombin III concentration was more than 20 mg/dl exhibited no thromboembolic episodes following the attack of myocardial infarction.
Plasma antithrombin III levels were not decreased before and after the onset of stroke.
These data suggest that there may be a relation between development of myocardial infarction and the low levels of plasma antithrombin III.

RELATIONSHIP BETWEEN HYPERLIPAEMIA AND FIBRINOLYTIC SYSTEM

Hiromichi Okuda, Toshiharu Muraoka, Yasushi Saito, Nobuo Matsuoka, Akira Kumagai, and Hideo Shio-
Department of Medical Biochemistry, Ehime University Medical School, Department of Internal Medicine, Chiba University, Medical School, and Department of Geriatrics, Kyoto University, Medical School, Kyoto/Japan

Lipoprotein lipase (LPL) was found to be located at endothelial cells of arterial walls and evidence was obtained suggesting that serum non-specific esterase might become a precursor of LPL. It was demonstrated that free fatty acids (FFA) produced by action of LPL induced agglutination of blood platelets and release of coagulative factors. Furthermore, FFA was found to inhibit plasmin activity. The inhibitory effect of FFA was demonstrated only with fibrin as substrate. No inhibition was observed with casein or tosylarginine methylester as substrate. Based on these results, relationship between hyperlipaemia and fibrinolytic activity was discussed.

TIME, TEMPERATURE, pH AND THE PRIMARY SHAPE CHANGE OF PLATELETS IN VITRO; ITS INFLUENCE ON DIFFERENT PLATELET FUNCTION TESTS

K. Breddin, M. Ziemen, O. Bauer, U. Pietsch, H. Grun, and R. Wiedemann
Center of Internal Medicine, Department of Angiology, University, Frankfurt/BRD

In citrate blood and PRP platelets show characteristic morphologic changes. They are loosing their original disc like form and develop tentacles. This process is enhanced by low temperatures (4^oC, 10^oC) and slowed at 37^oC; it is also enhanced by rising pH and by heparin and heparinoids. ASA ($10^{-4}M$) delays this primary shape change in vitro. Morphologic platelet changes are also slowed in blood taken from patients who have ingested aspirin. The speed of this primary shape change is closely correlated with the pattern of spontaneous and induced platelet aggregation. A close correlation between different function tests is found in clinical investigations, of the time dependent variations of these tests are being considered. Examples showing the correlation between ADP-, collagen-, and epinephrine induced and spontaneous aggregation (PAT III) are presented. Considering these findings we are able to explain why several investigators came to differing results in studies of similar patient groups. Our studies stress the need for a better standardisation of platelet function tests in clinical use.

PHOTOMETRIC PLATELET AGGREGATION TEST III. A NEW TOOL FOR THE DETECTION OF ENHANCED PLATELET AGGREGATION. FIRST RESULTS IN DIABETICS, PATIENTS WITH RECENT MYOCARDIAL INFARCTION AND VASCULAR DISEASE

H.J. Krzywanek and K. Breddin
Center of Internal Medicine, Department of Angiology, University, Frankfurt/BRD

PAT III was developed for the study of "spontaneous" platelet aggregation. PRP is rotated in a disk shaped polystyrol cuvette at 37^oC and 20 rpm. Changes of optical density which are induced by the formation of platelets aggregates are continuously recorded. The tendency of platelets to aggregate increases in the 60 - 300 min following blood sampling. Test results are further influenced by temperature, changes of pH, platelet count and plasma turbidity. The time dependent changes of platelet aggregability are with all probability caused by the primary shape change of thrombocytes which occurs after blood drawing. Like in previous studies enhanced platelet aggregating activity was observed more frequently in patients with diabetes mellitus, vascular disease and recent myocardial infarction as compared with age matched healthy controls. Prospective studies will have to prove whether PAT III is a useful tool for the early detection of vascular disease in the individual patient and whether enhanced platelet aggregation indicates the risk of thromboembolic complications.

EFFECT OF TOBACCO SMOKE AND CARBON MONOXIDE ON PLATELET AGGREGATION AND ADHESION TO THE ARTERIAL WALL IN THE MINIPIG

Markward Marshall, Hans Hess, and José Fdez. B. de Quiros
Medical Polyclinic of the University of Munich, Munich/BRD

26 minipigs were exposed to tobacco smoke or a carbon monoxide-air mixture with 150, 200 or 500 ppm CO. Duration of exposure varied between 1 x 4 and 16 x 4 hours. COHb saturation reached values between 5 and 35% according to the supplied CO concentration. Scanning electron microscopy of the arteries reproducibly showed platelets adherent to the superficially intact appearing endothelium after cigarette smoke and CO exposition. The tendency of platelets to aggregate (PAT I according to Breddin) increased significantly. The blood viscosity showed a marked rise with cigarette smoke and high CO concentrations, but no changes at moderate CO concentrations.

We conclude that the initial mechanism of atherosclerosis include a disturbed interaction between platelets and the arterial wall. In this interaction platelets have a key role. In the risk of tobacco smoke inhalation in inducing angiopathy carbon monoxide appears to be a significant factor.

PLATELET AGGREGATION IN ATHEROSCLEROSIS

Toshio Ozawa, Yuzo Nagakawa, and Masaki Yoshikawa
Department of Geriatrics, University of Tokyo, Tokyo/Japan

The aim of this report is to clarify the significance of platelet aggregation in atheriosclerosis compared to healthy subject as well as the effect of exercise and smoking on the platelet aggregation. One hundred arteriosclerotic patients including ischemic heart disease and cerebral infarction in chronic state and 60 controls were examined. Serum cholesterol, triglyceride, free fatty acid, plasma fibrinogen and euglobin lysis time were also measured at the same time. The responses of platelet rich plasma to 2×10^{-6} M of ADP, collagen solution using bovine tendon, and 1×10^{-6} M of adrenaline were observed by the optical density method of Evans (EEL-169). All of these three types of aggregation were increased in arteriosclerosis compared to control (P <0.001). The index of maximal optical density showed the most significant difference.
The effect of submaximal exercise using bicycle ergometer on platelet aggregation was studied in normal and ischemic heart disease. In both groups platelet aggregation was increased following exercise. The effects of smoking was also examined in the heavy smokers after 12 hours of breaking off with smoking. The control showed an increase of platelet aggregation to ADP, collagen and adrenaline, but there was no definite change in arteriosclerosis.

THROMBOSIS AND FIBRINOLYTIC SYSTEM IN THE RAT EXPERIMENTAL ATHEROSCLEROSIS

C.A.-Villaverde, L. Badimón, and F.G.-Valdecasas
Department of Pharmacology, P. "Juan de la Cierva", C.S.I.C. Barcelona/Spain

Atherosclerosis (At) was produced by Altman's technique, in 5 days treatment, in Sprague Dawley rats of approx. 250 g. The mesenteric circulation was observed, inducing thrombosis by lactic acid perfusion "in situ", by our personal technique already described. We studied the thrombosis time in normal and (At) rats, on a group of 30 rats, and we found a value of 11.05 ∨ 2.5 m. in the normal rats and of 3.4 ∨ 2.3 in the (At) rats, significant reduction for p 0.0005. Euglobulins level in (At) rats was 0.016 Ploug U/ml blood, against a value of normal rats of 0.042 Pl U/ml. Blood activation with 100 Pl U/ml Urokinase gave the following results in (At) rats: Whole blood 4.9, whole plasma 3.2, diluted plasma 40.4 Pl U/ml blood; and in untreated rats the values were: 4.2, 2.5, 28.5, respectively. Conclusions: It was shown the highest sensibility of (At) rats to the acidotic thrombi induction, that there is a derease in the euglobulins activity and similar or slightly increase response to the urokinase activation; these results suggest that the thrombogenic state is caused by a decrease of the fibrinolytic activators.

PLATELET FUNCTION AND SERUM LEVELS OF CHOLESTEROL, TRIGLYCERIDES, URIC ACID AND BLOOD SUGAR IN POSTMYOCARDIAL INFARCTION PATIENTS DURING A TWO YEAR STUDY

Ellen Weber, Erhard Walter, and Theo Pfleiderer
Unit of Clinical Pharmacology, Department of Medicine, University of Heidelberg, Heidelberg/BRD

The Department of Medicine of the University of Heidelberg takes part in a two year trial for secondary prevention of myocardial infarction. This is a multi-center, prospective, randomized, double-blind study. Males and females between 45 and 70 years, who have suffered at least one myocardial infarction are allocated to one of three groups. They receive either phenprocoumon or 1,5 g aspirin a day or placebo. The two last groups are running double blind. The observation period and the special medication are started 6 – 8 weeks after the acut event and last for two years. Controlled are the arterial pressure, pulse rate, ECG, serum cholesterol, triglycerides, uric acid, blood sugar and platelet function. Although the starting point of the cholesterol and triglyceride levels was indentical, we found a higher increase of both levels in the anti-coagulant group in comparison to the combined ASA-placebo group. There was no difference in the uric acid levels. Elevated platelet stickiness, controlled with the Wright-test and the PAT was normalized under ASA-treatment, whereas with the Hellem-method we determined higher values in the ASA-placebo group and lower in the anticoagulant group.

Chairmen: A.S. Daoud, USA
         K. Murata, Japan

Participants: K. Fischer-Dzoga, USA
             G.H. Rothblat, USA
             K. Murata, Japan
             T. Zemplenyi, USA
             S.N. Jagannathan, USA
             A.S. Daoud, USA

PROLIFERATIVE RESPONSE OF ARTERIAL SMOOTH MUSCLE CELLS TO HYPER-LIPEMIA

K. Fischer-Dzoga and R.W. Wissler

We have long been interested in the smooth muscle cell as one cell type actively involved in the process of atherogenesis. Our main focus has been its response to hyperlipemia as compared to its behavior in normal serum. To this effect we developed a tissue culture system of primary or subculture of aortic medial cells. Rhesus monkeys and rabbits were used as donors for the explants, as well as the hyperlipemic serum.

The technique and morphology of these cells have been described previously (Fischer-Dzoga et al., 1973). Briefly, we use the outgrowths from 2 mm round explants of aortic media, stripped free of intima and adventitia. These primary cultures grow to 15-20 mm in diameter in about 6-8 weeks, after which time they become stationary, with little mitotic activity and little increase in size.

These cells show morphologic characteristics of smooth muscle cells when examined by electron microscopy. They grow in a characteristic pattern of mono- and multilayers of rather large, elongated cells, often arranged in a parallel fashion. The presence of collagen, elastin, and mucopolysaccharides can be demonstrated using special staining techniques.

Our main findings so far have been that such arterial smooth muscle cells in vitro react to the presence of hyperlipemic serum, and in particular its LDL fraction with increased uptake of lipids, accumulation of cholesterol esters and increased esterification of cholesterol. However, there is also an increased hydrolysis of cholesterol ester, increased lipid efflux, and a suppression of cholesterol synthesis.*

While the former are atherogenic in nature, the latter may be looked upon as defense mechanisms, always assuming that these cells show a similar reaction pattern in vivo.

At the same time, and maybe related to these changes in lipid metabolism, there is also a remarkable increase in cellular proliferation, often accompanied by accelerated cell necrosis. We will now focus on this phenomena, namely, increased cell proliferation, another important factor in atherogenesis.

---

*Work done by Drs. R. Chen and S. Bates in our laboratory.

Table 1. Proliferation studies using arterial smooth muscle cells in vitro

Type of culture	Measurement of growth	Results
Primary cultures	**Monkey:** Culture size: direct measurement of diameter or measurement of surface by point counting techniques, incorporation of ^{3}H-thymidine visualized by autoradiography	Proliferative effect of hyperlipemic serum, within 24 hours LDL$_2$ (1.02 – 1.05) most active fraction Normal LDL has no effect No linear dose-response relationship No relationship to food fats Proliferative effect not due to platelet factor(s) Serum from hypertensive, normolipemic donors also stimulatory

	Rabbit:	Proliferative effect of hyperlipemic serum
		  blocked by estrogen
		  decreased by insulin
		Stimulatory effect of diabetic, normolipemic serum

Rabbit subcultures	Cell count protein determination ^{3}H-thymidine incorporation and release	Increased proliferation and increased cell detachment due to hyperlipemic serum or its LDL

These results are summarized in Table 1. Proliferation was evaluated by either measuring the increase in culture size and by computing the percentage of labeled nuclei after a ^{3}H-thymidine pulse. The main finding and also the basis for all future work is the fact that these cells can be restimulated to another phase of growth by the addition of hyperlipemic serum to the culture medium.

This restimulation occurs in cultures which are stationary despite optimal culture conditions (Fig. 1), that is, the presence of 10% normal serum in the medium, which indicates that we are not dealing with a growth factor, generally necessary for optimal growth of these cells.

By autoradiographic assessment, we found this proliferative response to start after a relatively short lag phase (Fischer-Dzoga et al., 1974). The active fraction in the hyperlipemic serum has been identified as the LDL, density 1.019–1.063 g/ml. When this fraction is further narrowed down to density 1.019-1.05 g/ml — which yields a fraction with apoprotein B only — it is still proliferative. The results of two experiments are illustrated in Table 2. Although the percentage of labeled nuclei — after an 8-hour ^{3}H-thymidine pulse — was not as high as in the whole hyperlipemic serum group, it still was double the value for normal serum. Normal LDL of the same density had no effect, despite the fact that it was given in higher concentration, in order to achieve comparable cholesterol levels. This brings up another fact, namely, that this effect is not dose related, that is, we have not been able to establish a linear-dose-response relationship. Likewise, the food fat fed to the donor animals in order to produce hyperlipemia does not have any bearing on this proliferative effect in vitro. They are all proliferative in this system despite different total lipids and cholesterol levels (Fischer-Dzoga and Wissler, 1976).

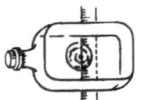
a)

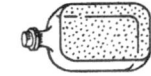
b)

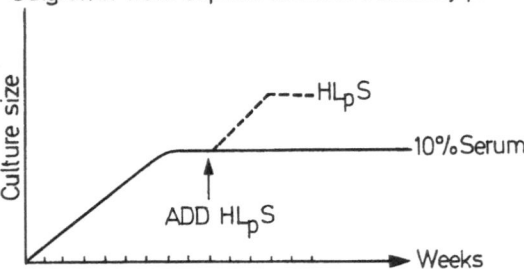

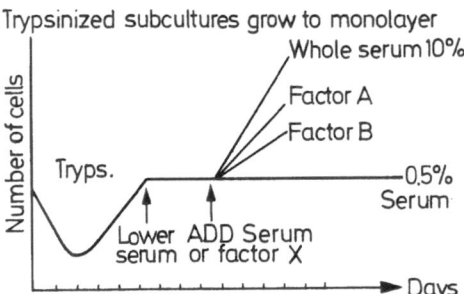

Figure 1. Primary vs. subculture in assay of growth promoting factors.
a) Primary cultures reach a stationary phase despite optimal culture conditions
(10% serum). They are stimulated to a second phase of proliferation by addition
of homologous hyperlipidemic serum.
b) Trypsinized subcultures artificially arrested in G_1 phase by lowering serum
to near zero level in order to study growth factors in general

Table 2. Mitogenic effect of hyperlipemic serum and its LDL (density 1.02-1.05)
on primary cultures of arterial smooth muscle cells

Addition to culture medium	% of nuclei labeled by H^3-thymidine	
	Experiment A	Experiment B
5% Normal monkey serum	2.56 ± 1.9	2.41 ± 1.7
5% Hyperlipemic monkey serum	17.99 ± 7.1	11.10 ± 5.2
Bottom fraction equivalent to 5% hyperlipemic serum	1.78 ± 2.6	0.50 ± 0.4
"Narrow cut"[a] from hyperlipemic serum	5.09 ± 4.4	4.20 ± 2.9
"Narrow cut"[b] from normal serum	0.68 ± 0.5	0.46 ± 0.6

[a]Equivalent to 5% serum

[b]10x concentrated.

Platelets have recently been implicated very strongly as carriers of a proliferative factor in vascular repair and also in atherogenesis (Ross et al., 1974).
Testing out this possibility, namely, that a platelet factor might be responsible for the proliferative effect, we compared platelet-poor and platelet-rich
serum from the same hyperlipemic donors as to their proliferative effect on
these cultures. We found the platelet-poor serum to be as effective in stimulating proliferation as the platelet-rich serum (Fig. 2), concluding that the platelet factor does not play any decisive role in this system.

In the course of these studies, we also explored additional substances which
were of interest to us, e.g., estrogen (Ledet et al., 1976), which we found to
block the stimulatory effect of the hyperlipemic serum on rabbit primary cultures. It also largely suppresses the production of collagen and elastin in

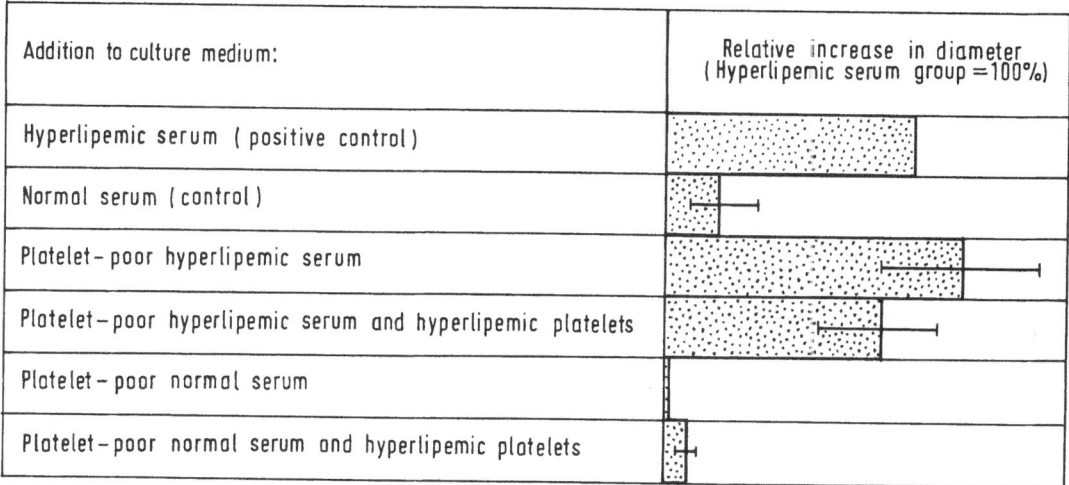

Addition to culture medium:	Relative increase in diameter (Hyperlipemic serum group = 100%)
Hyperlipemic serum (positive control)	
Normal serum (control)	
Platelet-poor hyperlipemic serum	
Platelet-poor hyperlipemic serum and hyperlipemic platelets	
Platelet-poor normal serum	
Platelet-poor normal serum and hyperlipemic platelets	

Figure 2. Increase in culture diameter during 10-day treatment period (summary of three experiments)

these cultures. A similar blocking effect was obtained with insulin. On the other hand, serum from diabetic rabbits (Vesselinovitch et al., 1974) had a stimulatory effect, despite the fact that it was normolipemic. The same is true for serum from hypertensive, normolipemic monkeys.

Thus, the direction for further research is three-fold, namely to further analyze the hyperlipemic LDL molecule as compared to the same fraction from normolipemic serum, or to modify the normal LDL in the search for the active component; to find a common pathway — if any — for the proliferative activity of hyperlipemic, diabetic, and hypertensive serum, and the search for further substances which might be able to block this proliferative effect.

CHOLESTEROL ESTER SYNTHESIS BY MICROSOMAL FRACTIONS FROM Fu5AH RAT HEPATOMA CELLS: STIMULATION BY LIPOPROTEINS FROM HYPERLIPEMIC SERA

G.H. Rothblat, M. Naftulin, and L.Y. Arbogast

Summary

Cholesterol ester synthesis by the microsomal fraction from rat hepatoma cells was stimulated by preincubation with lipoproteins obtained from hyperlipemic rabbit sera. Lipoproteins from normolipemic sera had no stimulatory effect. Growth of cells in hyperlipemic rabbit sera also increased microsomal cholesterol ester synthesis. Increased cholesterol ester synthesis appears to be correlated with increased microsomal-free cholesterol content.

Introduction

Our previous studies (Rothblat, 1974) on the metabolism of cholesterol ester (EC) in hepatoma cell cultures demonstrated that growth of these cells in the presence of hyperlipemic rabbit serum (HRS) lipoproteins resulted in a marked accumulation of EC, not seen during culture in equivalent free cholesterol (FC) concentrations of normolipemic sera (NRS) lipoproteins. Quantitation of the source of the accumulated EC demonstrated a contribution of both exogenous EC and FC to cellular EC (Rothblat et al., 1975). Increased cellular incorporation of FC was closely correlated with increased FC esterification. The present study was conducted to investigate the influence of HRS lipoproteins on the synthesis of EC by the acyl-CoA-cholesterol acyltransferase (ACAT) (EC 2.3.1.26) from hepatoma cells. This enzyme has been found in various tissues with marked elevation of activity in atherosclerotic aorta (Goodman et al., 1963; St. Clair et al., 1970; Hashimoto and Dayton, 1975; Brecher and Chobanian, 1974; Hashimoto et al., 1974).

Methods

The Fu5 rat hepatoma cell lines were grown in Eagle's minimal essential medium supplemented with 10% fetal bovine serum (Flow Labs) and exposed to 2.5% HRS or NRS for 24 h prior to harvest. Procedures for obtaining lipoproteins have been previously described (Rothblat, 1974), the density <1.019 g/ml being such as to include the "intermediate" or "remnant" particles present in HRS (Camejo et al., 1973; Shore et al., 1974) in the very low-density lipoprotein (VLDL) fraction.

Washed cell pellets were resuspended in 10^{-3} M phosphate buffer (pH 7.4), disrupted by sonication, and diluted with equal volumes of 0.5 M sucrose prior to centrifugation at 12,000 x g for 15 min. The $S_{12,000}$ fraction was preincubated with isolated NRS or HRS lipoprotein, 1 mg FC/4 mg $S_{12,000}$ protein, for 2 h at 37°C. A microsomal fraction was then pelleted at 100,000 x g for 45 min, suspended in 0.1 M phosphate buffer (pH 7.1), and adjusted to 100 µg microsomal protein/0.45 ml buffer. In designated experiments, isolated microsomes (1 mg protein) were preincubated with VLDL (1 mg FC), reisolated, and washed. Untreated $S_{12,000}$ or isolated microsomal controls were preincubated in the absence of added lipoprotein.

The assay mixture for cellular ACAT activity consisted of 0.5 ml 0.1 M phosphate buffer (pH 7.1) containing 100 µg microsomal protein, 2.5 µm $MgCl_2$, 0.5 µm dithiothreitol, and 0.6 mg fatty acid free bovine albumin (Sigma). 1-[^{14}C]palmityl-CoA (New England Nuclear, 57.8 mCi/mM), adjusted to a specific activity of 1.16 µCi/µm was added at 0.5 nmol to 30 nmol as indicated. Incubations were at 37°C for 30 min unless otherwise stated. Values presented are the average of at least two replicate assays. The reaction was stopped by the addition of chloroform methanol and lipids were extracted by the method of Bligh and Dyer (1959). Total lipid extracts were spotted on silica gel G thin-layer chromatographic (TLC) plates and developed with petroleum ether/ethyl ether/acetic acid (85/15/1). The lipid bands on the TLC plate were counted by liquid scintillation techniques. The efficiency of recovery of radio-labeled lipids was >95%. PalmitylCoA was assayed using the method described by Barnes and Wakil (1968). All other analytic procedures have been previously described (Rothblat, 1974; Rothblat et al., 1975).

Results

Microsomal ACAT activity reached a broad maximum between pH 7.1 and pH 8.1 with no activity below pH 6.3. No activity could be detected at any pH in the 100,000 x g supernatant fraction. Maximum levels of [^{14}C]palmitate were incorporated into EC at substrate concentrations between 10 and 20 nmol palmityl-CoA/100 µg microsomal protein.

Because of the known stimulation of FC esterification in whole cells by H VLDL, the time-course of [^{14}C]palmityl-CoA utilization was quantitated. Figure 1 shows the utilization of 100 and 200 nmol of [^{14}C]palmityl-CoA mg microsomal protein. Preincubation with H VLDL stimulated [^{14}C]palmitate incorporation into EC (Fig. 1a) at all time points over that seen in untreated microsomal fractions. Esterification in H VLDL-treated microsomal fractions was similar at both substrate concentrations during the first 15 min of incubation, with a greater increase occurring between 15-30 min with 200 nmol palmityl-CoA/mg protein. Exposure to

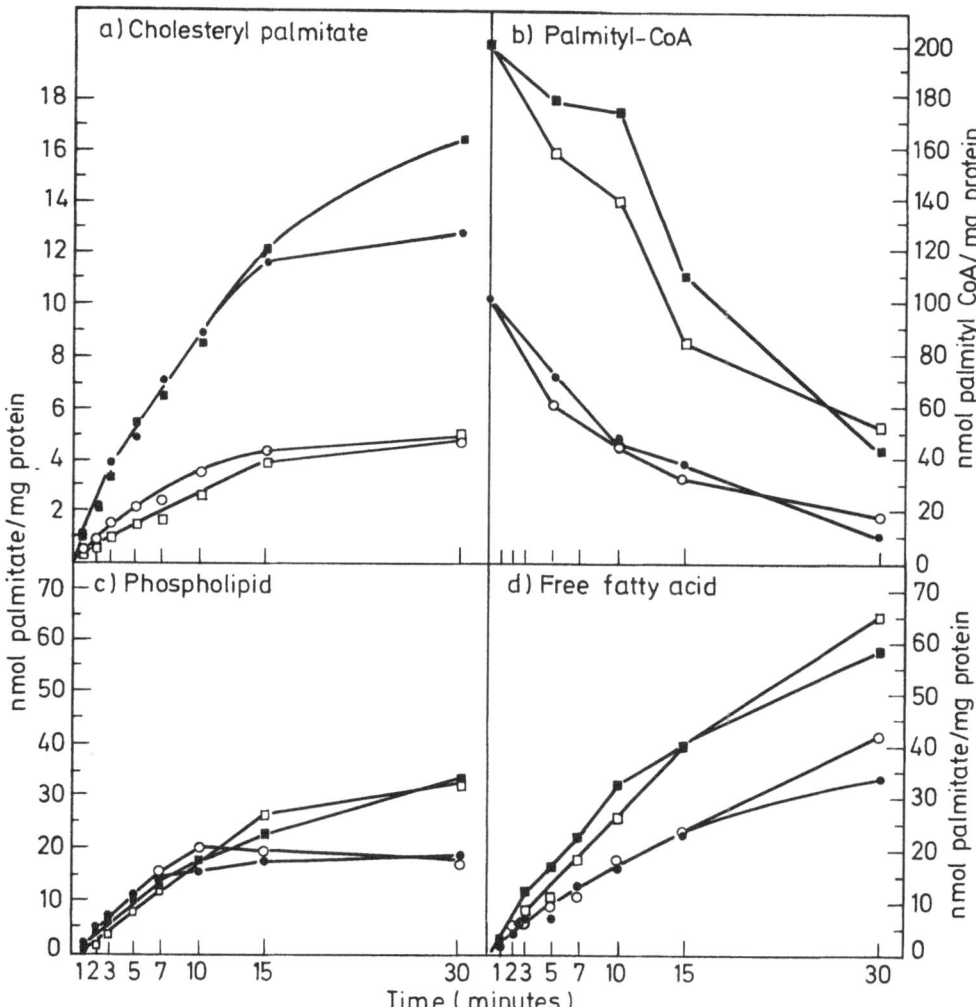

Figure 1. Utilization of palmityl-CoA by microsomal preparations from Fu5AH cells: ● —— ● 100 nmol palmityl-CoA, preincubated with H VLDL, ■ —— ■ 200 nmol palmityl-CoA, preincubated with H VLDL, ○ —— ○ 100 nmol palmityl-CoA, no VLDL treatment, □ —— □ 200 nmol palmityl-CoA, no VLDL treatment. Values presented for 1 mg microsomal protein

H VLDL had no significant effect on palmitate incorporation into phospholipid (PL) (Fig. 1b), deacylation of palmityl-CoA to free fatty acids (FFA) (Fig. 1c), or the overall utilization of labeled substrate as measured by the amount of un-reacted palmityl-CoA (Fig. 1d). Increased substrate concentration resulted in in-creased palmitate recovery as PL and FFA at the later time points. The stimula-tory effect of H VLDL was dependent on the amount of H VLDL added to the $S_{12,000}$ fraction, with maximum stimulation at 1 mg lipoprotein FC/4 mg $S_{12,000}$ protein.

Increased ACAT activity could also be elicited by adding H VLDL directly to iso-lated microsomal fractions (Table 1, No. 1 and 2), indicating that no factor in the $S_{12,000}$ was essential for stimulation. Washing the treated microsomal prepa-rations after incubation with VLDL had no significant effect on ACAT activity. Table 1 also shows the results from a series of experiments in which normal mi-crosomes from Fu5AH cells (as $S_{12,000}$) were preincubated at 37°C in the absence

Table 1. Microsomal cholesterol palmitate synthesis in Fu5 cells

No.	Material	Preincubation conditions	Cholesterol palmitate (nmol/mg microsomal protein)	
			Fu5AG cells	Fu5-5cells
1.	Microsomal fraction	− VLDL	$5.31 \pm .48$ (9)	
2.	Microsomal fraction	+ H VLDL	11.76 ± 1.11 (10)	
3.	$S_{12,000}$	− VLDL	$5.01 \pm .25$ (20)	$0.96 \pm .06$ (6)
4.	$S_{12,000}$	+ N VLDL	$5.83 \pm .40$ (7)	
5.	$S_{12,000}$	+ H VLDL	$11.36 \pm .72$ (20)	$2.12 \pm .19$ (6)

[a] Preincubation at 37°C for 2 h N and H VLDL added at 1 mg lipoprotein FC/4 mg $S_{12,000}$ protein. 30-minute assay with 10 nmol [^{14}C]-palmityl-CoA/100 µg microsomal protein. Values given as nmol $\pm$ SE (No. of determination).

or presence of VLDL. The addition of N VLDL (St. Clair et al., 1970) to the pre-incubation mixture had no significant effect on EC synthesis, whereas H VLDL (Hashimoto and Dayton, 1975), added at similar FC concentrations elicited a 2.8-fold increase over the control microsomal fraction (Goodman et al., 1963). Although H VLDL was the most stimulatory density fraction, other lipoproteins isolated from HRS also resulted in increased incorporation of palmitate into EC.

In a previous study, it was observed that the Fu5-5 rat hepatoma, a cell line closely related to Fu5AH, exhibited elevated EC content and FC esterification when grown in HRS (Rothblat et al., 1975). Table 1 (No. 3 and 5) demonstrates increased EC synthesis in Fu5-5 microsomes pretreated with H VLDL. Growth of both Fu5AH and Fu5-5 cells in HRS also stimulated EC synthesis more than two times that seen in control NRS grown cells. The amount of cholesterol palmitate synthesized was less than that seen with equivalent material obtained from Fu5AH cells. The stimulation of EC synthesis was directly related to the concentration of HRS in the growth medium, with maximum stimulation at concentrations between 1.25% and 2.5%.

Table 2. Unesterified cholesterol content of microsomal fractions from Fu5AH

Microsomal fraction (preincubation)[a]	Lipoprotein concentration[b]	Microsomal FC content[c] (µg/mg microsomal protein)
Control	0	42.2
H VLDL	0.2	55.6
	0.5	58.6
	0.8	63.0
	1.0	75.9
N VLDL	0.2	41.3
	0.8	41.6

[a] Lipoproteins preincubated for 2 h with $S_{12,000}$.

[b] mg lipoprotein FC/4 mg $S_{12,000}$ proteins.

[c] Average of at least two determinations.

Table 2 shows the FC content of the microsomal fraction of FBS-grown cells after preincubation in the presence of either N VLDL or H VLDL. Exposure of the microsomal preparation to normal lipoprotein had no effect on unesterified cholesterol content whereas incubation in the presence of H VLDL produced a dose-dependent net increase in microsomal FC content.

Discussion

The data clearly indicate that both microsomal fractions isolated from Fu5AH rat hepatoma cells grown on HRS and microsomal fractions preincubated in vitro with hyperlipemic lipoproteins synthesize more cholesterol palmitate than do untreated controls. The results obtained with isolated microsomal preparations closely parallel the increased incorporation and esterification of serum lipoprotein FC shown by cells cultured in HRS (Rothblat et al., 1975). The higher ACAT activity of treated and untreated microsomes from Fu5AH cells as compared to those from the closely related Fu5-5 hepatoma was of the same order of magnitude as was previously observed with whole cells (Rothblat et al., 1975).

Although an increase in cholesterol esterification has been demonstrated in atherosclerotic aortas (St. Clair et al., 1970; Hashimoto and Dayton, 1975; Brecher and Chobanian, 1974; Hashimoto et al., 1974; Kritchevsky et al., 1974), and in cultures of fibroblasts exposed to LDL and oxygenated sterols (Goldstein et al., 1974; Brown et al., 1975b), the mechanism responsible for increased EC synthesis has not been elucidated. A number of mechanisms could be proposed to explain the apparent increase in ACAT activity in hepatoma cells grown in HRS. The ability of HRS to stimulate EC accumulation and FC esterification in cells treated with cycloheximide (Rothblat, 1974; Rothblat et al., 1975) together with the stimulation of EC synthesis in isolated microsomal fractions incubated with H VLDL indicates that increased enzyme levels are not responsible for increased synthesis. The data suggest that increased EC synthesis in both whole cells and isolated microsomes is linked to greater substrate availability. The present experiments use endogenous FC as the acyl acceptor and Table 3 indicates that preincubation with H VLDL, but not N VLDL, can increase the microsomal FC content. The reduced synthesis of EC in untreated microsomes, where acyl donor is not limiting, could be due to reduced availability of FC. This interpretation is consistent with the recent observation of Nilsson (1975) that stimulated synthesis of cholesterol in hepatocytes is correlated with increased esterification.

Cells in culture are able to incorporate exogenous lipoprotein (Brown et al., 1975a; Bierman et al., 1974). Further experiments are needed to determine whether hyperlipemic serum lipoproteins exert their effect on microsomal ACAT:
1. Directly as the native lipoprotein
2. As a partially metabolized lipoprotein fragment, or
3. Through a cellular sterol carrier
These studies on hepatomas demonstrate that there are cell-recognizable differences between the lipoproteins of NRS and HRS and, further, illustrate a high degree of specificity of serum lipoproteins in regulating cellular cholesterol metabolism.

Acknowledgements

This investigation was supported by Public Health Service Grant ROI-HE-09103 from the National Heart and Lung Institute and by funds from the Department of Health, Commonwealth of Pennsylvania. This investigation was performed during the tenure of an Established Investigatorship from the American Heart Association (G.H.R.).

INHIBITION OF LIPID SYNTHESIS BY SULFATED GLYCANS IN CULTURED AORTIC CELLS

K. Murata

Introduction

The preventative effects of certain sulfated glycans on experimental lipemia and atherosclerosis have been reported in cholesterol-fed rabbits (Murata, 1962a, 1962b; Murata et al., 1969). These sulfated glycans possess not only potential anticoagulant properties but also antilipemic functions, having a similar mechanism as shown by heparin (Murata, 1962b). The present paper reports an effect of sulfated glycans on lipid synthesis in cultured aortic cells under various conditions. The application of the sulfated glycans such as charonin sulfate and chondroitin polysulfate resulted in the reduction of ^{14}C-acetate incorporation into lipid fractions in the aortic monolayer culture system.

Materials and Methods

Aortic monolayer sheets were cultured from the single cell suspensions which were prepared by trypsinization from stripped aortic intimal layers of 3-week-old chicks, as reported previously (Murata et al., 1965, 1967). When the cells made monolayers after a 1-week culture period, the cells were daily treated with sulfated glycans, ranging 1 μg - 50 μg/ml Eagle's minimum essential media (MEM) with 5% calf serum for 24, 48, or 72 hours. Two sulfated glycans used here were prepared as follows. Charonin sulfate, which was prepared from the mucin of *Charonia lampas*, consisted of sulfated polyglucose with about 15% sulfur content. Chondroitin polysulfate, which was obtained synthetically by sulfation of chondroitin sulfate, consisted of the repeating units of glucuronic acid, galactosamine, and sulfate with 15.7% sulfur.

Sodium ^{14}C-1-acetate (specific activity, 3.0 mC/mmol, Volk Radiochemicals, Calif.) was then added to the treated cells at the rate of 0.4 μC/ml in MEM for 6 hours. After exposuring, the cells were washed with MEM until the washing media was not counted radioactive. After trypsinization, lipids in the cells were extracted with methanol-chloroform (1:2, v/v) and purified (Murata et al., 1967; Murata, 1969). Further separation of lipids was performed by the method reported previously (Murata, 1969); the cold acetone-insoluble fraction was designated as phospholipid and the acetone-soluble fraction was designated as neutral fat. Free sterol was precipitated as digitonide from the acetone-soluble fraction. Radioactivity in each fraction was measured by a liquid scintillation spectrometer.

Results

The preliminary experiment indicated a linear relation between exposure time and the synthesized lipids during 6 hours except the first lag time. In the present study, the incubation with ^{14}C-acetate was performed for 6 hours.

The suppression of total lipid synthesis by two sulfated glycans in the chick aortic cells under various conditions is shown in Table 1. The suppression by both sulfated glycans was different between the primary and succeeding cultured aortic cells at the rate of 10 μg/ml MEM, 36% in the primary culture cells, and 23-25% in the secondary culture cells. When the aortic cells were pretreated with 10% human lipemic serum (HLS, 940 mg% total lipids and 387 mg% total cholesterol) for 72 hours, the suppressing effect of charonin sulfate was more pronounced in MEM plus HLS than in MEM only, in both generations; 66% in the primary cells and 37% in the secondary cells. The difference of the inhibition by charonin sulfate was statistically significant between the HLS-treated and untreated groups.

Table 1. Suppression of total lipid synthesis by sulfated glycans in aortic cells

Generation	Media used	Number of samples	Control	Sulfated glycans	Suppression rate
			Specific activity of total lipid synthesized (dpm/µg)		
			Charonin sulfate		
Primary	MEM	8	244 ± 7[a]	181 ± 4	36%
Primary	MEM plus HLS	6	283 ± 14	125 ± 4	66%
Secondary	MEM	8	212 ± 7	163 ± 8	23%
Secondary	MEM plus HLS	7	149 ± 13	94 ± 5	37%
			Chondroitin polysulfate		
Primary	MEM	7	240 ± 12	154 ± 12	36%
Secondary	MEM	7	192 ± 6	143 ± 7	25%

Aortic cells were treated with or without sulfated glycans (10 µg/ml) in minimum essential media (MEM) for 72 h in each experiment. After the media was removed, the cells were exposed for 6 h with media containing ^{14}C-acetate (0.4 µg/ml).

[a]Mean and standard error. The values between the treated and the control groups were all significant at the p value of 0.001.

The effect of the concentration of charonin sulfate on the lipid synthesis was studied during the treatment for 72 hours. The reduction of lipid synthesis by sulfated glycans was related to the concentration both in total lipids and free sterol at 72-hour treatment; the higher concentrations of sulfated glycans produced a greater reduction of lipid synthesis in both generations (Fig. 1).

The inhibitory effect of the lipid synthesis was also dependent upon the incubation time with sulfated glycans. Figure 2 shows the time-dependent effect of charonin sulfate at the concentration of 10 µg/ml MEM. The significant reduction of lipid synthesis was obtained in both generations after the cells were treated with charonin sulfate for 48 or 72 hours.

The suppression of ^{14}C-acetate incorporation into the lipid fractions by sulfated glycans was studied using primary cells. When the cells were treated with two substances (10 µg/ml MEM) for 72 hours, the inhibitory effect was observed in total lipids, phospholipid, neutral fat and free sterol fractions (Table 2). As can be seen from Table 2, the predominant reduction was constantly observed at the neutral fat and free sterol fractions.

Discussion

The present study clearly indicated that two sulfated glycans namely charonin sulfate and chondroitin polysulfate show a pronounced suppressing activity of lipid synthesis in cultured aortic cells. It is of interest to note that the pretreatment with HLS resulted in a greater inhibition of lipid synthesis by sulfated glycans. This may be interpreted that sulfated glycans were more effective on reducing the lipid synthesis in the lipid-loaded cells which may be analogous to lipid-deposited aortic cells in the atherogenic process in vivo. The similar behavior of the primary and secondary aortic cells in the inhibitory effect of lipid synthesis by the sulfated glycans would favor an understanding of lipid

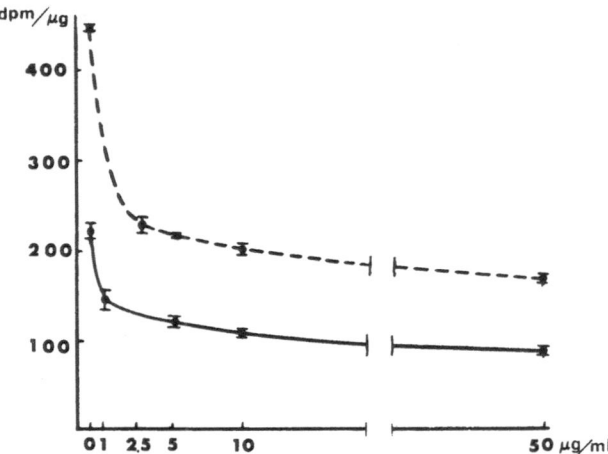

Figure 1. Concentration effect of charonin sulfate on lipid synthesis in aortic cells. Aortic cells were incubated with the media containing various concentrations of charonin sulfate as shown in the figure. After the removal of the media, the cells were exposed with the media containing C^{14}-acetate for 6 h
The points indicate averages of 4-9 samples and the vertical lines indicate the standard deviations. The solid line indicates total lipids and the broken line indicates free sterol

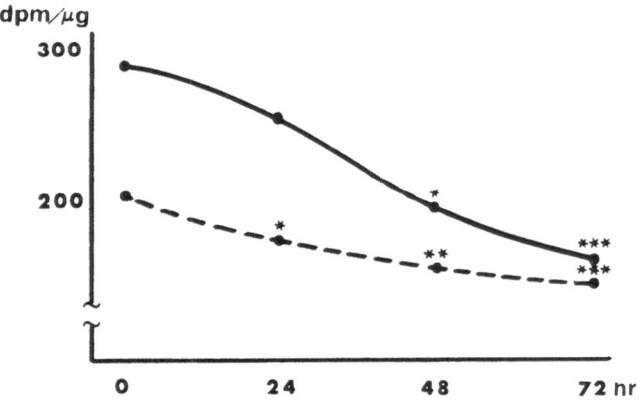

Figure 2. Effect of exposure time of charonin sulfate on total lipid synthesis in aortic cells. After treatment with charonin sulfate (10 µg/ml MEM) for the indicated hours, aortic cells were incubated with new media containing C^{14}-acetate for 6 h
The points indicate averages of 4-6 samples and the vertical lines indicate the standard deviations. The solid line indicates primary cells and the broken line indicates secondary cells. Statistical differences were shown as follows: * = $p < 0.05$, ** = $p < 0.01$, *** = $p < 0.001$

synthesis on an equilibrium basis. The fact that the suppressing rates of sulfated glycans on lipid synthesis depended upon the concentration and incubation time of the substance would be an adequate proof of the inhibition effects by the sulfated glycans.

In the course of the experiments, the cell numbers and lipid weights in aliquots as well as the morphologic changes in the cells were carefully tested in order

Table 2. Suppression of ^{14}C-acetate incorporation into lipid fractions by sulfated glycans in aortic cells

Specific activity of synthesized lipids (dpm/μg)	Control	Charonin sulfate	Control	Chondroitin polysulfate
Total lipids	365 ± 23[a]	229 ± 23[c]	387 ± 15	273 ± 6[d]
Phospholipid	101 ± 4	60 ± 8[c]	151 ± 4	138 ± 6
Neutral fat	375 ± 10	274 ± 16[d]	393 ± 35	267 ± 16[b]
Free sterol	721 ± 37	406 ± 63[c]	510 ± 22	312 ± 38[b]

Primary cells were used. After pretreatment with 10% human lipemic serum for 72 h, the monolayer cells were exposed with ^{14}C-acetate containing media for 6 h. Each determination consisted of 6 samples.

[a] Mean and standard error.

[b] $p < 0.05$.

[c] $p < 0.01$.

[d] $p < 0.001$.

to define the possible toxicity of the substance. The suppressing effect of sulfated glycans on lipid synthesis, however, was not associated with any discernible effects on the above-mentioned subjects of the treated cells. Accordingly, the present data support the inhibitory effect of sulfated glycans on lipemia and atherosclerosis experimentally induced in vivo, by illustrating at least in part the suppression of lipid synthesis by the substance in aortic cells.

The relation of the inhibitory effects of lipid synthesis and anticoagulant activity of sulfated glycans is uncertain. Since the other sulfated glycosaminoglycans in the aortic tissue possessing anticoagulant properties showed antilipemic and antiatherogenic activities (Murata et al., 1975; Nakazawa and Murata, 1975), further studies are required to clarify the mechanism based on this line.

Summary

1. Suppressing effects of two sulfated glycans, charonin sulfate and chondroitin polysulfate on lipid synthesis in the chick aortic cells were studied with ^{14}C-acetate as a precursor in the dynamic cellular level.
2. The suppression of lipid synthesis by sulfated glycans depended not only on the concentration but also on the incubation time.
3. The inhibitory effect of lipid synthesis by sulfated glycans was found in, in order of the effect, free sterol, neutral fat, and phospholipid fractions.
4. Pretreatment with human lipemic serum resulted in more pronounced lipid suppression by the sulfated glycans.

THE EFFECT OF HYPOXIA AND CARBON MONOXIDE ON ARTERIAL SMOOTH MUSCLE CELL CULTURES

T. Zemplenyi, W.J. Paule, D.E. Rounds, V.K. Kalra, and D.H. Blankenhorn

Experimental and clinical studies indicate that carbon monoxide and tissue hypoxia may play an essential role in accelerating atherogenesis. The mechanism of their action until now is not clear.

In the present studies, we worked with piglet aortic smooth muscle cell cultures grown in flasks containing Eagle's MEM or diploid media supplemented with 10% fetal calf serum. The medium was usually changed every 3rd day and cells were subcultured about twice a month (May et al., 1975).

After a minimum of 6 weeks in culture, multiple T-60 flasks were seeded with an equal number of cells and when almost confluent, separated into control and experimental groups. The experimental groups were subjected to either 4-5% O_2, 5% CO_2, and N_2, or 0.02% CO, 5% CO_2 and 94.08% N_2 over a period of 4-7 days.

For morphologic studies, common histologic, histochemical, and electron microscopic techniques were used. For biochemical studies, the cells were washed at least twice with 5 ml of basic salt solution. Afterwards, the cells were scraped into ice-cold 0.85% neutral saline, centrifuged, and homogenized using a Polytron homogenizer. For measurement of metabolic intermediates, the cells were handled the same way but scraped into 8% $HClO_4$ instead of saline and neutralized with K_2CO_3.

Enzyme activities were assayed as described before (Zemplenyi and Rosenstein, 1975); metabolic intermediates were measured by modifications of the fluorometric methods described by Lowry and Passoneau (1964). The activity of the lysosomal hydrolases N-acetyl-ß-glucosaminidase and ß-glucuronidase was measured using 4-methyl umbelliferyl derivatives.

A. Light and Electron Microscopic Findings

The morphology of arterial smooth muscle cells grown in a normal atmosphere is well-known. Suffice it to mention that after the cells have proliferated for a period of at least 2 weeks, groups of cells begin to make contact with one another and become polarized and spindle-shaped. Later they form characteristic "hills and valleys." A few lipid droplets can be detected in some of these cells.

After 4-5 days exposure to an atmosphere of 4-5% O_2, the organizational pattern of the cells becomes disrupted. Many cells show an increase in large granules, most of which are positive to oil red-O. In some focal areas, the cells aggregate and they form mound-like protuberances which are very different from the hills and valleys commonly seen throughout the culture. They measure 0.1 - 0.5 mm in height and always have a cap of viable cells and a core of debris (Fig. 1). In the core of these mounds, birefringent material can be observed, as well as accumulations of lipid material with an affinity for osmium tetroxide. Furthermore, fibrillar material and various amounts of PAS-positive accumulations are also components of the core of the mound (Paule et al., 1977).

At the electron microscope level, the cells acquire an appearance resembling the cells usually seen in younger cultures. Thus, there is a loss of myofilaments, the Golgi increase in amount, and a rise in other cell organelles can be observed. There is a large increase in the number of pinocytotic vesicles beneath the cell surface and myelin figures of various complexities increase in number. Many of the granules observed at the light microscopic level are identified as secondary lysosomes (Fig. 2). Under the light microscope, cells grown in the car-

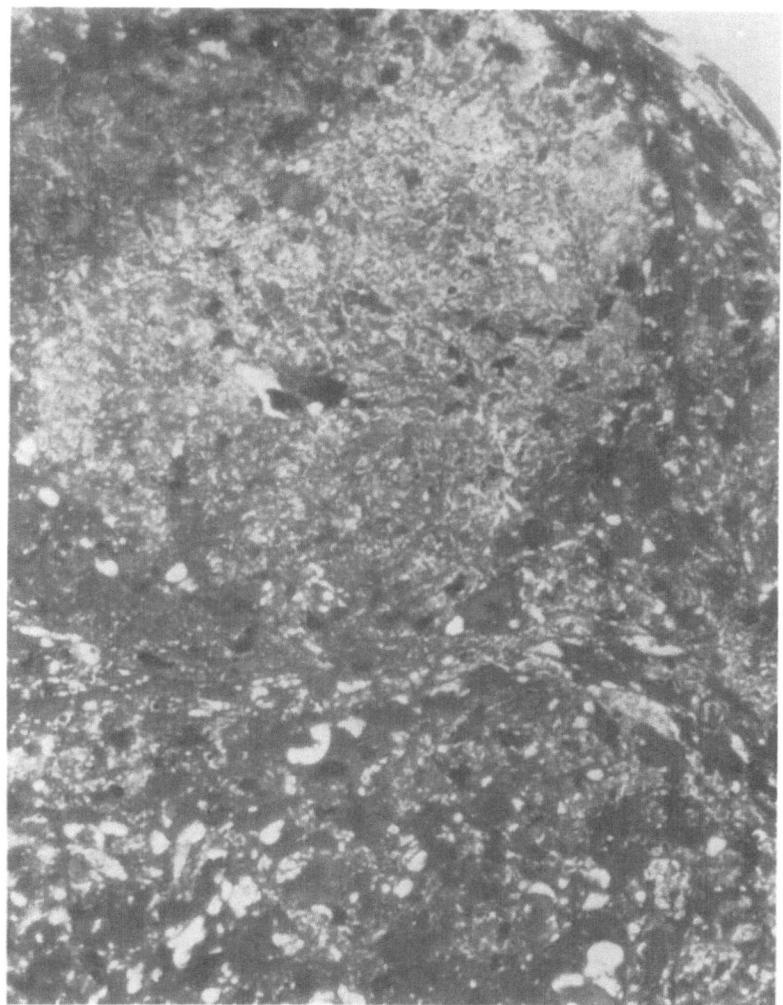

Figure 1. Light microphotograph of a culture of smooth muscle cells subjected to hypoxia. The large light area is the core of a mound. It contains fibrillar material, occasional cells, and necrotic debris. The cup of viable cells merges with the surrounding cells. Toluidine blue (X 700)

bon monoxide-enriched atmosphere look usually as healthy as the control cells. However, the lysosomes are usually quite dense and their number is clearly higher than in either the hypoxic cells or control cells.

Time-lapse cinematography revealed that the smooth muscle cells undergo isometric contraction. Spontaneously synchronized contractile activity continued in well-formed mounds, indicating that these contain active muscular cells.

B. Biochemical Findings

Enzyme activity studies showed that hypoxia of 3 or 4 days duration caused a very high increase of activity of glycolytic enzymes and also an unequivocal elevation in the activity of Krebs cycle enzymes studied. Hypoxia of longer duration had a more moderate effect on most glycolytic enzymes and the activity of

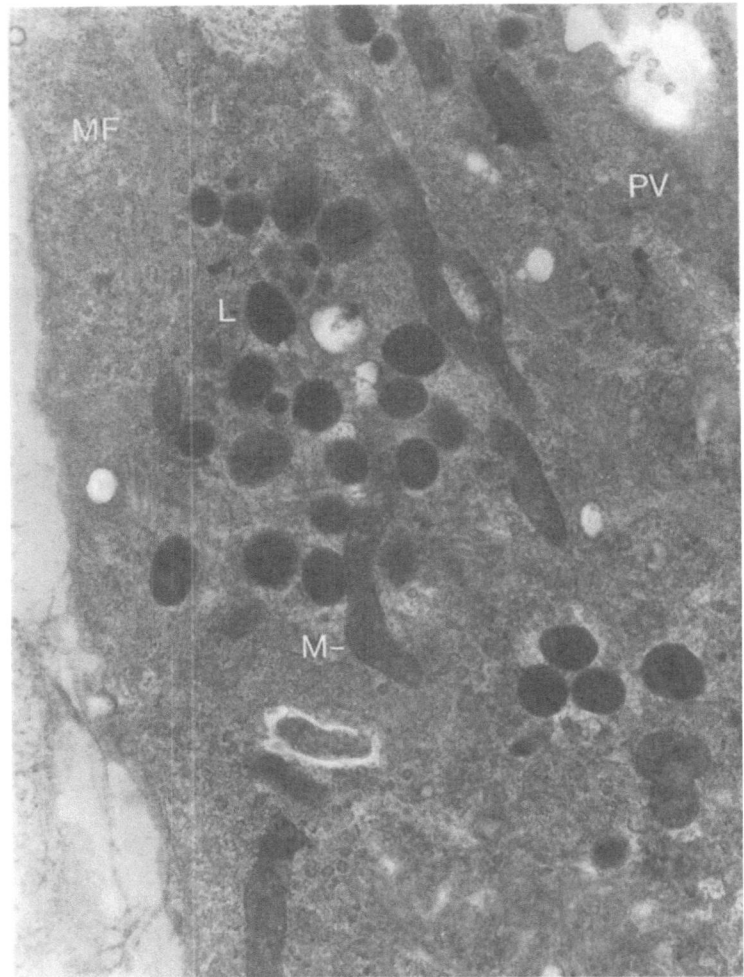

Figure 2. Electron microphotograph of a smooth muscle cell subjected to hypoxia. There is an increase in number of lysosomes (L) and pinocytotic vesicles (PV). Myofilaments (MF) decrease in number, while the number of mitochondria (M) remain the same. Lead citrate and uranyl acetate (X 26, 750)

Krebs cycle enzymes became lower than in the control cells. However, with increasing cell age the results became gradually less consistent. In the few experiments in which N-ß-acetylglucosaminidase and ß-glucuronidase activity was measured, both enzymes exhibited increased activity compared with control cells.

As far as intracellular metabolites were concerned, the hypoxic or carbon monoxide-treated cells were producing in most experiments more lactate than the control cells and the concentrations of direct intermediates of glycolysis such as G-6-P, F-6-P, and PEP were also increased.

An interesting and perhaps important finding is the rise of the α-glycerophosphate level in the majority of hypoxic experiments. This compound is well-known to be a precursor for the synthesis of some phospholipids and triglycerides. Nevertheless, the question whether hypoxia or carbon monoxide stimulates lipid synthesis could not be unequivocally answered from our studies. The extent of incorporation of 2-^{14}C acetate into different lipid fractions was usually, but not always, lower when cells were grown under hypoxic conditions. It appears that differing conditions such as cell age, duration of hypoxia, use of normal versus heat-inactivated calf serum, etc., may be causing the varying results in this regard.

In *summary*, the data show that hypoxic or carbon monoxide-treated smooth muscle cells *first* develop changes characteristic of young primitive cells. *Second*, they undergo alterations indicating increased permeability and/or uptake of extracellular material, especially lipids, and subsequent formation of mound-like protrusions. The significance of local lipid synthesis in this chain of events is questionable, if any. A *third* feature is a defense reaction characterized by increased lysosomal activity.

STEROL METABOLISM IN CULTURED HUMAN ENDOTHELIAL CELLS*

S.N. Jagannathan

The endothelium constitutes the interface between the circulating plasma lipoproteins and the arterial intima. A study of the lipoprotein and lipid metabolism in endothelial cells is, therefore, particularly relevant to understanding the evolution of atherosclerosis.

Material and Methods

For the studies reviewed here (Jagannathan et al., 1974b, 1976a, 1976b), morphologically and immunologically identifiable human endothelial cells, originally isolated from umbilical cord veins and maintained in monolayer culture (Lewis et al., 1973; Jaffe et al., 1973), were used during the second to the sixth serial passage.

Whole human plasma and ultracentrifugally isolated lipoproteins from normolipidemic and hyperlipoproteinemic subjects were labeled in vitro with $4-C^{14}$ cholesterol (Avidan, 1959) and included in the culture medium.

For sterol uptake and accumulation studies, the medium of a 70-80% confluent monolayer culture was replaced by media containing whole human plasma at 10% level or one or the other of isolated lipoprotein fractions (VLDL, LDL, and HDL) in amounts provided by 10% plasma. The cells were allowed to replicate for an additional 72 hours at which time there was a confluent monolayer. Fetal calf serum (FCS) included at 10% level served as a control for each experiment.

For sterol synthesis studies, monolayer cultures were incubated for 4 hours in the presence of tritiated acetate $(-2-^3H)$ in a medium containing intact human plasma or isolated low-density lipoproteins (LDL).

Six to eight flasks (75 cm^2) of monolayer cultures were needed to be pooled for each observation. The endothelial cell pellet was analyzed for free and esterified cholesterol (FC and EC) by gas chromatography (Jagannathan et al., 1974a), protein by Lowry's method (Lowry et al., 1951), and radioactivity by liquid scintillation counting.

*Supported in part by U.S. Public Health Service Research Grant HE-14,230 to the Specialized Center for Research in Arteriosclerosis at the University of Iowa and an Institutional Research Grant at West Virginia University.

Results and Discussion

Cultured human endothelial cells accumulated varying amounts of cholesterol, particularly esterified cholesterol (EC) depending upon the source of plasma- or lipoprotein-cholesterol in the culture medium (Fig. 1). Grown in a medium containing FCS, the cells had a total cholesterol content of 30 μg/mg protein, only 5 μg of which was EC. With normolipidemic human plasma (cholesterol 155 and triglycerides 40 mg/100 ml), cellular EC was a little higher at 7 μg (out of a total of 35 μg) per mg protein, whereas with hyperlipoproteinemic plasma included in the growth medium, the endothelial cells had nearly three-fold accumulation of EC as compared to that with FCS. The chylomicron positive type V hyperlipoproteinemic plasma evoked an EC accumulation of as much as 44 μg/mg protein.

Isolated high-density lipoproteins (HDL) included in the culture medium elicited a response similar to FCS (Table 1). Very low-density lipoproteins (VLDL) and low-density lipoproteins (LDL) evoked higher cellular accumulations of total and esterified cholesterol than did intact hyperlipoproteinemic plasma. VLDL caused a two-fold accumulation of EC as compared to whole plasma. The isolated LDL which evoked free cholesterol accumulations similar to that ofVLDL, elicited EC accumulations that were twice that of VLDL and four times that of intact plasma. Thus, LDL produced the highest accumulation of cholesterol (104 μg/mg protein), nearly 59% of which was esterified cholesterol.

Data from experiments with isolated LDL from six different subjects showed a significant correlation (r=0.93) between the EC content of the LDL-containing media and the EC content of the endothelial cell pellet (Fig. 2). Such a correlation was obtained only for LDL and not for intact plasma or the other lipoproteins. This observation provided the first clue that the predominant source of esterified cholesterol in the cell pellet is the esterified cholesterol of LDL in the media. Studies discussed below using labeled preformed cholesterol ($-4-^{14}C$) and labeled precursor of cholesterol (acetate-$2-^{3}H$), helped further confirm this hypothesis.

Uptake of labeled free cholesterol ($-4-^{14}C$) was least from intact plasma, viz., 2.7%, and was four or five-fold higher for isolated lipoproteins including LDL. However, the ^{14}C label was found predominantly (95%) in the free cholesterol fraction of the cell pellet despite considerable accumulation of esterified cholesterol in mass, especially in LDL-grown cells. Likewise, labeled acetate was incorporated predominantly into FC fraction of cells incubated with LDL, with no significant labeling of esterified cholesterol occurring in the cholesterol and/or fatty acid moieties, despite large accumulation of EC. These observations provided specific evidence that in cultured endothelial cells, the process of intra-

Table 1. Accumulation of cholesterol in cultured endothelial cells grown with whole plasma and isolated plasma lipoproteins[a]

| | Cholesterol (μg/mg protein) | | |
	Total	Free	Ester
Fetal calf serum	29.3 ± 1.97	23.5 ± 3.01	5.8 ± 1.70
Whole plasma	42.5 ± 3.52[b]	26.3 ± 4.15	16.3 ± 2.14[b]
HDL	28.8 ± 3.94	21.8 ± 3.75	7.0 ± 2.61
VLDL	75.0 ± 20.85	41.5 ± 11.21	33.5 ± 12.09
LDL	103.5 ± 16.55[b]	43.3 ± 10.50	60.3 ± 6.91[b]

[a]The data give mean ± SE of four experiments with plasma and isolated lipoproteins from four hyperlipoproteinemic subjects (one type IIa, one IIb, and two III).

[b]P <0.01

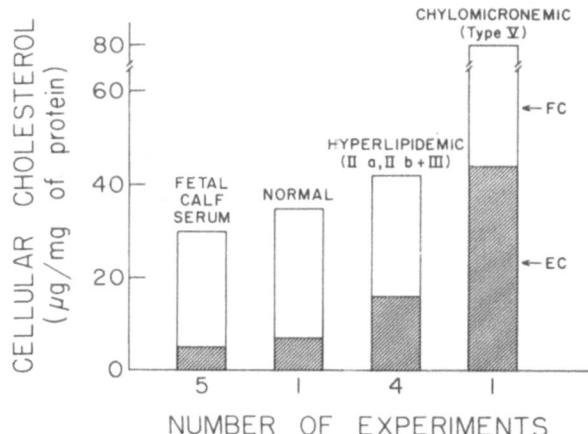

Figure 1. Cholesterol content of cultured human endothelial cells when grown in the presence of normolipidemic and hyperlipoproteinemic human plasma

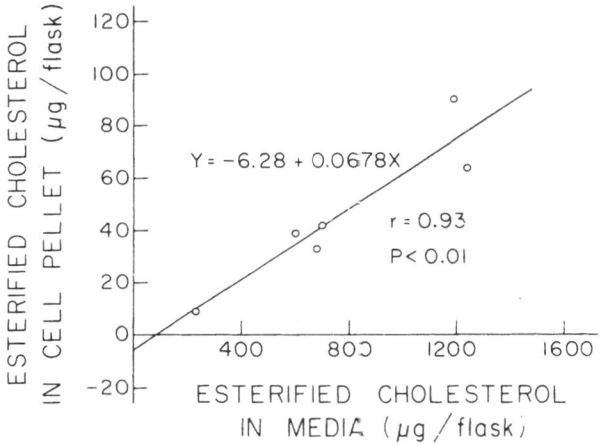

Figure 2. Correlation between esterified cholesterol content of the LDL in the culture media and esterified cholesterol content of the endothelial cell pellet

cellular esterification of free cholesterol was not the major contributory mechanism by which esterified cholesterol accumulated.

The extent of cholesterol synthesis in cultured endothelial cells depended upon whether the medium was free of cholesterol or contained plasma or LDL (Fig. 3). The cells readily incorporated labeled acetate into free cholesterol when the incubation medium was devoid of a cholesterol source. Inclusion in the incubation medium of a hyperlipoproteinemic (type II) plasma, caused a 51% inhibition of this cholesterol synthesis. Isolated LDL (type II) caused an almost complete (96%) suppression of biosynthesis. Normolipidemic plasma and its isolated LDL, likewise, caused significant suppression of cholesterol synthesis.

In Fig. 3, adjacent to the wide bars indicating cholesterol synthesis, there are slim bars which indicate the corresponding cellular accumulation of cholesterol. Comparing the data for plasma and LDL, one finds that the more esterified cholesterol was stored within the cell (the shaded part of the slim bar), the greater the suppression of cholesterol synthesis was.

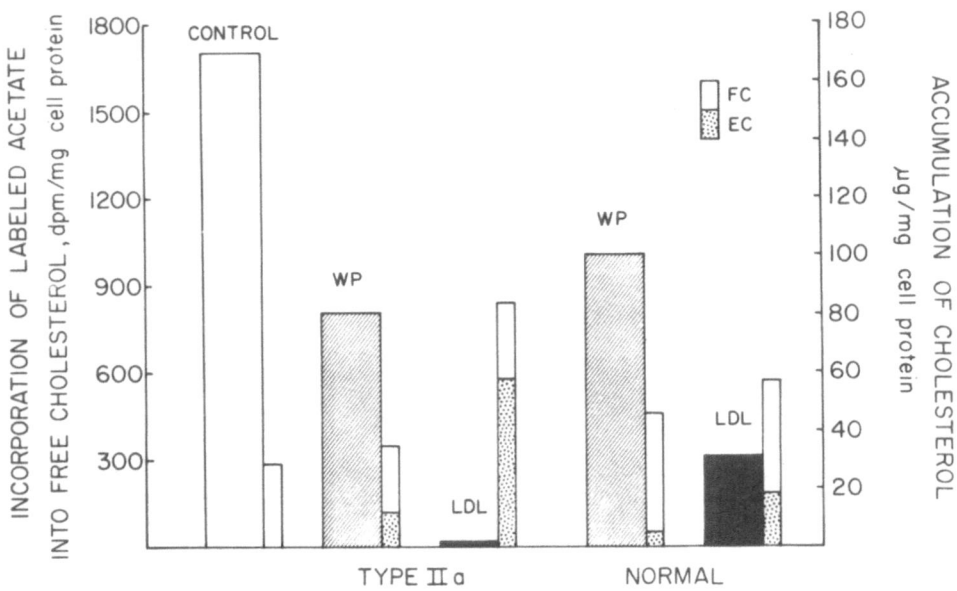

Figure 3. Cholesterol synthesis in cultured endothelial cells and its inhibition by human whole plasma (WP) and isolated low-density lipoproteins (LDL)

The above studies lead to the conclusion that the massive accumulation of esterified cholesterol in cultured human endothelial cells evoked by the presence of LDL in the medium is mediated through uptake of esterified cholesterol most likely by a process of pinocytic vesicular transport of the LDL macromolecule. This internalization of the LDL molecule, or part thereof, particularly esterified cholesterol, is suggested as a factor responsible for effective inhibition of cholesterol synthesis in cultured endothelial cells.

EFFECT OF HUMAN SERA ON DNA SYNTHESIS IN AORTIC EXPLANTS

Assaad Daoud, Katherine Fritz, Joan Augustyn, John Jarmolych, and Julio Sosa

In a previous study presented at the Third International Symposium on Atherosclerosis, we reported that the growth of swine aortic medial explants in the presence of human serum appeared analogous to that resulting from medium containing swine serum. The peripheral growth formed in cultures in the presence of human serum was qualitatively indistinguishable by light and electron microscopy from that resulting from cultures with swine serum in the medium (Daoud et al., 1973; Daoud, 1974). In addition, the peripheral growth resulting from either type of serum had many of the characteristics of the early atherosclerotic lesions, among them cell proliferation and cell necrosis, which are two important components of the lesion. In both types of culture, the cellular component of the peripheral growth was smooth muscle cells which secreted collagen, elastic tissue, and glycosaminoglycans. While qualitatively similar, quantitative differences between the two types of cultures were observed. These are:
1. Human sera resulted in more copious peripheral growth in most instances than the normal swine serum.

Table 1. DNA synthesis-stimulating activity of human sera[a]

Type	Number of sera	Mean activity	SEM[b]
Cardiac patients with angiographically detectable disease	329	229[c]	3.0
Cardiac patients with no angiographically detectable disease	77	200[c]	3.8
Healthy volunteers	56	149[c]	12.7

[a]Expressed as % of control normal swine serum activity.

[b]SEM = standard error of the mean.

[c]Significantly different from each other by analysis of variance.

2. Comparison of all human sera tested with control normal swine sera resulted in a significantly greater terminal rate of synthesis of DNA with the human sera.
3. The range of DNA synthesis-stimulating activities among the human sera was much greater than that among normal swine sera, as much as 15-fold within a single experiment.

In the current study, we compared the effect of sera from patients with angiographically defined amounts of coronary artery disease on one major parameter of atherogenesis, cell proliferation as measured by DNA synthesis, with that of sera from patients without angiographically detectable coronary artery disease and of sera from healthy volunteers.

Before catheterization, 40 ml of blood was drawn sterilely from each patient and total cholesterol and triglyceride levels measured. The presence of a defined type of hyperlipidemia was also determined according to the method of Fredrickson et al. (1967). Historical and clinical data were recorded for all patients and volunteers relative to age, sex, occupation, and to the presence or absence of the following risk factors: hypertension, diabetes, family history of atherosclerosis, and cigarette smoking. All patients received the same precatheterization medication, and information as to type and duration of periods of other medication was recorded.

Patients were identified only by number, and the assessment of amount of occlusive disease was not completed until some time after completion of the culture experiments, and again, with no knowledge of the laboratory results. In this study, a linear correlation between the amount of disease and the resultant DNA synthesis was not attempted because angiography measures only luminal narrowing and not wall thickness. Validation of luminal narrowing as an index of the amount of disease is now under consideration.

Of the total of 406 patients studied, 77 were free of angiographically detectable occlusive disease. In addition, sera from 56 healthy volunteers, with age and sex distribution fairly close to that of the patients, were also tested. The mean DNA synthesis activity was calculated for all patients with no detectable disease, for all patients with disease, and for all volunteers. Results are presented in Table 1.

The patients with detectable disease showed significantly greater DNA synthesis-stimulating capacity in their sera than either the patients with no disease or the volunteers. In addition, the rate of DNA synthesis resulting from sera from patients with no detectable disease was also significantly greater than that from volunteers.

The significance of these findings lies in their confirmation that at least one of the parameters we measure in our in vitro assay system, and for which a determining factor is demonstrable in sera, human or swine, is related to disease development, at least as measured by the most reliable in vivo method of assessment available. Thus, continued study of the serum factor(s) which govern DNA synthesis should be most pertinent to the ultimate understanding of the disease.

ABSTRACTS

BIOSYNTHESIS OF THE INTERCELLULAR MATRIX IN AORTA ORGAN CULTURES.
EFFECT OF AGE AND OF HYPERLIPEMIC SERA

D. Brechemier
Laboratoire Biochimie du Tissu Conjonctif, Faculté Médecine, Université Paris -
Val de Marne, Créteil/France

Rabbit aorta media organ cultures were used for the study of the regulation of
the relative rates of biosyntheseis of the intercellular matrix macromolecules
(IMM): collagen, elastin and glycoproteins. The effect of age, cholesterol-rich
regime and of hyperlipemic human sera was studied through their effect on the
incorporation of labelled precursors (14C-proline, 14C-lysine, 3H-glucosamine)
in the IMM-s. The rate of incorporation (dpm/mg DNA) decreased strongly with age
in all IMM-s. Some elastin biosynthesis could be demonstrated however (by 14C-
desmosine isolation) even in adult, non growing rabbit aortas. Hyperlipemic human
sera decreased the overall rate of incorporation except in collagen. A two week
2%-cholesterol diet had a profound effect on the incorporation pattern. The
modifications observed depended on the age of the animals and resulted in a
modification of the relative rates of synthesis of IMM-s. The observed effects
may explain the modification of the composition of the arterial wall in arteriosclerosis.

AN ACCELERATED METHOD FOR CULTURING RABBIT AORTIC SMOOTH MUSCLE
CELLS

C.Y. Rhee, F. Herz, and T.H. Spaet
Division of Hematology, Department of Medicine, Montefiore Hospital, Bronx, NY/
USA

A technique has been developed for accelerating the availability of smooth
muscle cells in culture. The basic principle is to start with a blood vessel in
which proliferative activity is already well under way and at a high level.
Other studies from this lab. show this time to be about one week after de-endothelialization. Experimental animals were rabbits. Their abdominal aortas were
de-endothelialized by passage of a balloon catheter, and after designated intervals, explants were prepared from dissected inner halves of these vessels. Explants from the outer halves of these vessels and inner half segments of the
non-ballooned thoracic aorta from the same animals served as controls. Similar
explants from non-ballooned rabbits were also included. The explants were placed
into culture bottles containing media. The parameter measured was the time of
appearance of cellular growth from each explant. Accelerated outgrowth of smooth
muscle cells was noted within 2 of 3 days with explants of inner halves of de-
endothelialized abdominal aortas when the animals were sacrificed 4 or 7 days
post-ballooning. By contrast, control specimens showed cellular outgrowth no
earlier than day 7 and more often about 2 weeks after implantation. Generally,
outgrowth from adventitial explants appeared earlier than that of intimal controls. Cells of explants from the medial inner half lost the accelerated proliferating properties by 3 weeks after balloon injury. In general, this time
relationship corresponds to that of mitotic activity seen in ballooned vessels
left in situ.

SYNTHESIS AND REMOVAL OF FREE CHOLESTEROL AND OF CHOLESTEROL ESTERS BY SMOOTH MUSCLE CELLS IN TISSUE CULTURE

Allan J. Day, Marion Sheers, and Sudipta Kar
Department of Physiology, University of Melbourne, Melbourne/Australia

Smooth muscle cells obtained from aortas of normal fed rabbits and maintained in tissue culture were used to investigate the synthesis and removal of free and ester cholesterol. Incorporation of ^{14}C-labelled acetate into cholesterol by the cells is inhibited in the presence of hyperlipemic serum. Partial esterification of the endogenously synthesised cholesterol takes place in the cells with increased formation of cholesterol ester in the presence of hyperlipemic serum. Cholesterol labelled lipoprotein is taken up by the smooth muscle cells and its conversion to cholesterol ester is increased by the presence of hyperlipemic serum. The removal rate of free cholesterol and of ester cholesterol was investigated in experiments in which the cells were pulse labelled for 24 hours with either labelled acetate or labelled lipoprotein and then followed for periods of 5 days ehereafter. Both endogenous and exogenous free cholesterol is removed from the smooth muscle cells in culture with a half life of less than 3 days. Most of the free cholesterol removed from the cells appears in the incubation medium. Relatively slow removal of the ester cholesterol takes place with little cholesterol ester appearing in the incubation medium. It is concluded that accumulation of cholesterol during atherogenesis results from its conversion to cholesterol ester in the smooth muscle cells.

ARTERIAL SMOOTH MUSCLE CELL CULTURE AND THEIR LIPID UPTAKE. A TRANSMISSION AND SCANNING ELECTRON MICROSCOPIC STUDY

Anna Kádár, and Éva Csonka
The Second Department of Pathology and Central Electron Microscop Laboratory, Semmelweis Medical University, Budapest/Hungary

The arterial smooth muscle cells play an important role in the pathogenesis of arteriosclerosis. The injury of endothelial cells is followed by the repair process, the growth of smooth muscle cells too. Smooth muscle cells were cultured from mini-pig aorta. The characteristics of smooth muscle cells become increasingly pronounced with the time of incubation. The appearence of lipid in the cultured cells suggests the possibility that not only the lipoproteins and cholesterols of the culture medium(serum)penetrate into the cells bus also the lipoprotein-cholesterol complexes or the phospholipids of the degraded cell membranes are accumulated in the smooth muscle cells. This phenomenon may throw some light on the metabolism and utilization of lipoproteins in atherosclerosis. The appearence of lipid like material in the cells grown in vitro depends on the lipid composition of the serum too. The incidence and shape of the intracellular lipid inclusion were investigated in cells cultured in serum with different (quanti- and qualitatively measured) lipid compositions.

GROWTH EFFECT OF HUMAN DIABETIC SERUM, INSULIN AND HUMAN GROWTH HORMONE ON PRIMARY AORTIC MEDIAL CELL CULTURES

Thomas Ledet
Department of Pathology and the Second University Clinic of Internal Medicine, Kommunehospitalet, Aarhus/Denmark

The report deals with the growth effect on primary aortic medial cell cultures of: -1) human diabetic and non-diabetic serum (dialysed and non-dialysed), -2) non-diabetic human serum with and without addition of insulin and human growth hormone (HGH). Serum was culled from young male diabetics and non-diabetics with equal lipid values. Growth was estimated by measuring the area of the cultures with a point count technique, by counting of mitotic cells and of H^3-thymidine labeled cells on autoradiograms. Both non-dialysed and dialysed diabetic serum enhanced the growth of cultures (2p <0.01). Also the fraction of labeled and mitotic cells was increased in diabetic medium (2p <0.005). Non-diabetic serum with addition of 50 µU, 100 µU, 200 µU and 2000 µU insulin/ml did not enhance the growth. However, growth was increased in normal medium with 1 ng and 5 ng HGH/ml (2p <0.001) but not with 0.5 ng HGH/ml. Medium with 1 ng HGH/ml increased the fraction of mitotic and labeled cells (2p <0.025 - 0.005).

The growth factor(s) in human diabetic serum cannot be glucose, fructose, amino-acids or ketones (all dialysable). It is not lipids or insulin. The molecular weight must be higher than 3000 - 4000. However, it may well be growth hormone.

LIPID REMOVAL FROM NORMAL AND ATHEROSCLEROTIC ARTERIAL EXPLANTS IN TISSUE CULTURE

A.K. Horsch, K. Hudson, and A.J. Day
Medizinische Universitätsklinik, Heidelberg/BRD and Department of Physiology, University of Melbourne, Melbourne/Australia

An organ culture system was used to maintain segments of normal or atherosclerotic rabbit aorta in a metabolically active state for periods up to six days *in vitro*. Using this system, the uptake and metabolism of ^{3}H-fatty acid labeled lecithin, ^{3}H-labeled oleic acid and ^{14}C-labeled linoleic acid were investigated. After a pulse label of 24 or 48 hours the uptake was measured in some of the explants and the removal of the endogenously labeled lipid fractions was then followed for a period of up to five days in the remaining explants. Labelled lecithin was taken up and incorporated into phospholipids, triglycerides and cholesterol esters in the explants. Uptake was higher in the atherosclerotic arterial wall with significantly increased incorporation into this cholesterol esters. The labeled phospholipid was removed rapidly from both normal and atherosclerotic arterial wall with a half life of 3.7 days. Synthesised triglyceride and cholesterol ester were more slowly removed from the arterial wall. Both labeled oleic and linoleic acids were incorporated into phospholipid, triglyceride and cholesterol ester in the atherosclerotic aortic explants was slower than phospholipid and triglyceride. No significant difference between the removal of cholesterol oleate and cholesterol linoleate was apparent.

LIPID METABOLISM OF CULTURED HUMAN ARTERIAL TISSUE FIBROBLASTS AS INFLUENCED BY p-CHLOROPHENOXYISOBUTYRATE (CPIB)

Ivan Flipovic and Eckhart Buddecke
Institute of Physiological Chemistry, University of Münster, Münster/BRD

Human aortic fibroblasty specifically bind and take up both the lipid and protein component of homologous ^{125}I-VLDL and ^{125}I-LDL in a ratio as present in these lipoproteins. 65 - 80% of the internalized lipids are distributed to the cellular lipid subfractions preferably to phospholipids, while the noncatabolized lipids and the total lipoprotein-protein are eliminated from the cells by regurgitation into the medium. Half of the regurgitated protein label is recovered as TCA soluble products.

5 mM CPIB elevated the intracellular lipid bound radioactivity of VLDL and LDL by about 30% and 40% via a reduced regurgitation. The lipoprotein-protein steady state and lipoprotein binding to the cell surface are not influenced by 5 mM CPIB.

CPIB lowers the uptake of ^{14}C-acetate, ^{14}C-pyruvate and ^{32}phosphate by aortic fibroblasts and the incorporation of their radioactivity into fatty acids and phospholipids, respectively. Under the influence of 5 mM CPIB the palmitic acid synthesis is reduced and a shift from de novo synthesis of palmitic acid to the mechanism of chain elongation is observed, but further elongation of palmitic acid to saturated C18 – C24 fatty acids is depressed.

The CPIB enhanced retention of lipoprotein lipid radioactivity is interpreted as a compensatory mechanism which provides essential cellular fatty acids deficient as a result of the CPIB inhibited synthetic process.

RAT LIPOPROTEIN UPTAKE AND CATABOLISM OF ISOLATED RAT LIVER PARENCHYMAL CELLS

Tsuguhiko Nakai and Thomas F. Whayne, Jr.
Oklahoma Medical Research Foundation, Oklahoma City, OK/USA

The catabolic site(s) and mechanisms of binding (B), uptake (U) and proteolytic degradation (P) of plasma lipoproteins are not established. Our previous studies indicate liver parenchymal cells (LC) and lysosomes are important cellular and subcellular catabolic site(s) for apolipoprotein (Apo) A-I in dogs. We investigated B, U and P, by rat LC, of rat ^{125}I-HDL$_3$ in which Apo A-I is the major polypeptide. After collagenase liver perfusion, structural and metabolic integrity of LC were verified by >95% trypan blue exclusion, low LDH leakage, EM morphology and constant gluconeogenesis from lactate including glucagon stimulation. ^{125}I-HDL$_3$ was incubated with LC at 37°C and 4°C in albumin and Krebs-Henseleit medium, pH 7.4. B and U were determined by radioactivity in washed LC and P by TCA soluble radioactivity in the medium. At 37°C, maximum B and U occurred at 30 min and plateaued to 2 hr; P showed a 15 min lag and then constant P to 2 hr with 5.2% of ^{125}I-HDL$_3$ protein degraded and released to the medium. 60% of cell radioactivity at 37°C was trypsin releasable. At 37°C, ^{125}I-HDL$_3$ B, U and P were inhibited markedly by unlabeled HDL$_3$ and minimally by VLDL and LDL. B, U and P, by Lc, of ^{125}I-HDL$_3$ were abolished by prior trypsin and by 4°C. Chloroquine, a lysosomotropic agent, enhanced ^{125}I-HDL$_3$ P at 1 mM and inhibited at 10 mM. Our data suggest binding, uptake and proteolytic degradation of HDL$_3$ by liver cells are effective and linked. There may be a specific HDL$_3$ (lipoprotein A) recognition site on the plasma membrane. Our data further confirm the important role of lysosomes in proteolytic degradation.

BIOSYNTHESIS OF COLLAGEN BY CULTURED SMOOTH MUSCLE CELLS FROM FETAL AND ADULT HUMAN AORTAS

J. Rauterberg, S.S. Allam, and U. Brehmer
Medizinische Klinik und Poliklinik der Universität Münster, Münster/BRD

Cells from the media of fetal and aortic specimens from adult persons were grown to confluency and incubated with (C-14)-glycine-containing medium. The newly synthesized collagen was treated with pepsin in order to degrade the nonhelical regions of the collagen preforms, and was then characterized by ionexchange and molecular sieve chromatography. Furthermore cyanogen bromide clearage was applied, and the occurrence of certain peptides being specific for different genetic types of collagen was determined.

Fetal aortic SMC were found to synthesize mainly type I collagen, and only a small amount of type III collagen. The proportion of type III collagen, however, is significantly enhanced in the newly synthesized collagen by SMC from adult aortas. On the other hand the proportion of type III collagen synthesized by aortic SMC is still lower than that found in the collagen of the original tissues.

TRANSPORT AND ACCUMULATION OF CHOLESTEROL IN MONKEY AORTIC MEDIAL CELLS GROWN IN HYPERLIPEMIC MONKEY SERUM

Sandra R. Bates, and Robert W. Wissler
Department of Pathology, University of Chicago, Chicago, IL/USA (USPHS HL00202 and HL15062)

The movement of cholesterol between hyperlipemic monkey serum (HMS) and monkey aortic medial cells was studied in a tissue culture system. The cellular sterol content of aortic medial cells was analyzed after 40 hrs of growth in 10% of either normal (NMS) or hyperlipemic monkey serum. Cells grown in NMS contained 26 μg free cholesterol (FC) and 2 μg esterified cholesterol (EC)/mg cell protein. The cholesterol content of HMS-grown cells showed a 15% increase in FC over that found for NMS-grown cells, with a 4-fold elevation in their EC content. In order to assess the contribution of the esterification process to the build up of EC, experiments using a double label were conducted where the fate of the FC in the cells at zero time (endogenous FC) and the FC of the 10% HMS in the media (exogenous FC) were followed. After 40 hrs of incubation, 1/3 of the endogenous FC remained in the cell, 1/2 of the cellular FC was derived from the exogenous FC of the HMS, and 1/2 of the cellular esterified cholesterol content was formed from the esterification of both endogenous and exogenous FC. The remainder of the free and ester cholesterol found in the cell were presumably derived from the unlabeled cholesterol esters of the HMS, which may have been taken up intact, or hydrolyzed and reesterified. Thus uptake of cholesterol esters and esterification of FC both contributed to the accumulation of cholesterol esters in aortic medial cells.

INFLUENCE OF LYSOSOMAL ENZYME STABILITY IN HYPERLIPEMIC SERUM-INDUCED METABOLIC CHANGES OF MONKEY AORTIC MEDIAL CELLS

Robert M. Chen, Katti Fischer-Dzoga, and Robert W. Wissler
Department of Pathology, University of Chicago, Chicago, IL/USA

Chloroquine was used as a lysosomal enzyme stabilizer to evaluate the possible role of this enzyme system in hyperlipemic serum-induced metabolic changes. Subcultured monkey aortic medial cells at stationary phase of growth were exposed to 10% normal or hyperlipemic monkey serum, with or without 50 microm. of chloroquine for up to 48 hours. These cells showed no change in their lysosomal enzyme (acid phosphatase) content during this period. However, some of the hyperlipemic serum-induced changes, namely suppression of cholesterol synthesis and enhanced cholesterol esterification, were blocked by chloroquine. Yet cells exposed to chloroquine, either with or without hyperlipemic serum, showed remarkable accumulation of cholesterol esters. This cholesterol ester accumulation is probably due to decreased hydrolysis or increased uptake. The hyperlipemic serum-stimulated cell proliferation was enhanced by chloroquine in the initial 24 hours and suppressed the second day. Cell damage, provoked by hyperlipemic serum as monitored by release of cytoplasmic enzyme, was enhanced by chloroquine. Some of the hyperlipemic serum-induced changes were unaffected by chloroquine. These included decreased consumption of glucose, and increased production of lactate, which exceeded the amount of glucose consumed and was presumably contributed by increased catabolism of amino acid. This study indicates that hyperlipemic serum-induced metabolic changes are partly attributable to the lysosomal enzyme system.

WORKSHOP 15. Atherosclerosis Without Major Risk Factors

Chairmen: A.L. Robertson, USA
            M. Murakami, Japan

Participants: A.L. Robertson, USA
               H. Sekimoto, Japan
               T. Fujinami, Japan
               P. Avogaro, Italy
               A.L. Robertson, USA
               J.P. Strong, USA

INTRODUCTION

Abel Lazzarini Robertson, Jr.

There is extensive, well-documented clinical evidence in many developed countries
that several major risk factors can be identified as accelerating and/or aggravating human atherosclerosis. Three of them have received well-deserved attention;
hyperlipoproteinemias in all forms, chronic hypertension, and diabetes mellitus.

The practicing physician if often confronted, however, with patients with symptomatic atherosclerotic disease in which such overt metabolic and functional abnormalities are not found. Many of these cases show striking regional variations
in both progression and severity of vascular lesions.

Individual differences in risk factors between cerebral vascular disease anc coronary atherosclerosis are well-known. The high male/premenopausal female ratio for
myocardial infarction and sudden cardiac death is not found in cerebral ischemia,
while the latter closely parallels overt hypertension and hypertensive heart disease.

Such clinical discrepancies may in part be due to the fact that atherosclerosis
is a multifactorial disease in which a variety of risk factors, both known and unknown, play independent but often synergistic roles in the accelerated development of overt vascular disease.

For example, environmental factors such as cigarette smoking, alcohol, caffeine,
and emotional stress are being increasingly considered important but as yet poorly defined contributors to the higher incidence of symptomatic vascular pathology
noted in younger age groups in recent years.

It is the purpose of this workshop to briefly review our current knowledge of
some of these less understood risk factors and their interplay with other environmental, metabolic, and genetic influences in atherogenesis.

STUDIES ON THE ATHEROGENESIS AND SUCROSE INTAKE IN CRAB-EATING MONKEYS

Hiroshi Sekimoto, Isao Nakada, Kunio Nakamura, Masaaki Takaori,
Satoru Takabatake, Hiroshi Hirai, and Mototaka Murakami

Judkin et al. have shown that the mortality from atherosclerotic heart disease
was more closely related to sugar consumption than fat consumption. Some people

claim that Judkin's data are not supported by experimental evidence. It has been reported by our group and Dalderup et al. that high sucrose feeding can induce vascular lesions in aorta, heart, and kidney in rabbits, rats, and beagle dogs. We reported precise pathologic findings of sucrose-induced vascular lesions in those animals. The purpose of the present study was to investigate the vascular lesions and metabolic changes in male crab-eating monkeys fed a high-sucrose diet for 42 months. Since the crab-eating monkey is more closely related to human phylogenetically, it is reasonable to postulate some aspects of human atherosclerosis by investigating the correlation between metabolic changes and pathologic findings observed in monkeys fed a high-sucrose diet.

Method

Eleven male crab-eating monkeys were fed a semisynthetic diet (Oriental A) containing approximately 53.5% of weight as carbohydrate, 27.4% as protein, 6.2% as fat with salt and vitamins A, B, D, and C for 42 months. Their body weight ranged from 1.7 to 3.4 kg at the start of the experiment. In sucrose-fed monkeys, 40% of calories were replaced by sucrose. Body weight and blood lipid levels were measured once a year. A glucose tolerance test including immunoreactive insulin levels, assays of enzyme activity such as alkaline phosphatase, GOT, GPT, LDH, CPK, aldolase, prothrombin time, partial thromboplastin time, and a platelet aggregation test were done on the last day of the experiment. The monkeys fed with a high-sucrose diet for 42 months were anesthetized with sodium pentobarbital (30 mg per kg body weight), and 3 g of glucose per kg of body weight was administered orally after fasting for 18 hours. Arterial blood was drawn for measurement of blood glucose and plasma immunoreactive insulin immediately before glucose ingestion and 30, 60, 120, and 180 minutes after glucose administration.

Results and Discussion

Figure 1 shows changes in body weight of monkeys during the experimental period. Increment of body weight of sucrose-fed monkeys was greater than that of control monkeys up to 36 months. The total serum cholesterol levels of sucrose-fed monkeys were higher than those of control monkeys for the initial 24 months and thereafter were almost the same in both groups, as shown in Figure 2. Blood triglyceride levels of sucrose-fed monkeys were significantly elevated compared to those of control monkeys after 36 months, as shown in Figure 2. Figure 3 shows the results of the glucose tolerance test. Sucrose-fed monkeys showed a higher glucose intolerance and higher blood immunoreactive insulin levels measured by radioimmunoassay than in control monkeys, shown in Figure 4. As shown in Figure 5, there was a significant rise in the enzyme levels of alkaline phosphatase, GOT, GPT, LDH, CPK, and aldolase in sucrose-fed monkeys. Although no significant differences were observed in prothrombin time between the two groups, shorter partial prothrombin time and increment of platelet aggregation were observed in sucrose-fed monkeys. Histologic examinations showed atherosclerotic lesions in

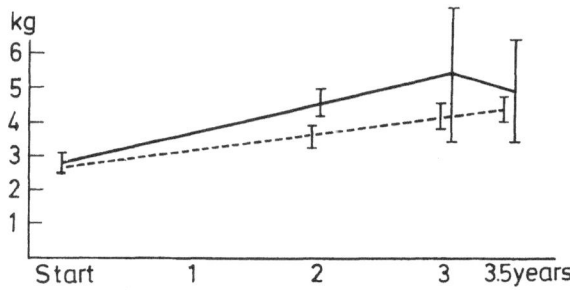

Figure 1. Body weight. ——— = sucrose group, — — — = control group

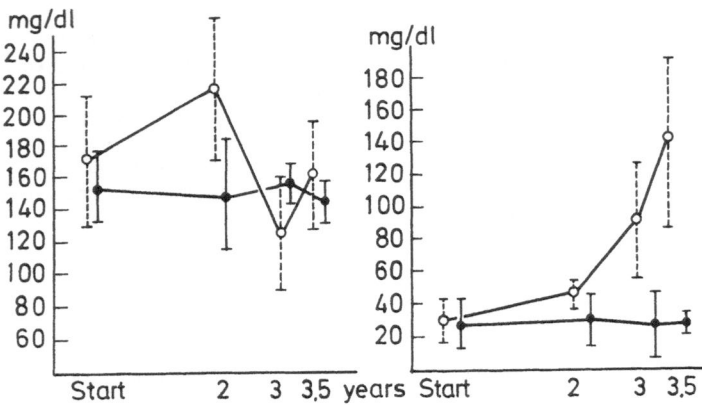

Figure 2. *Right*: cholesterol; *left*: triglycerides. o = sucrose group, • = control group

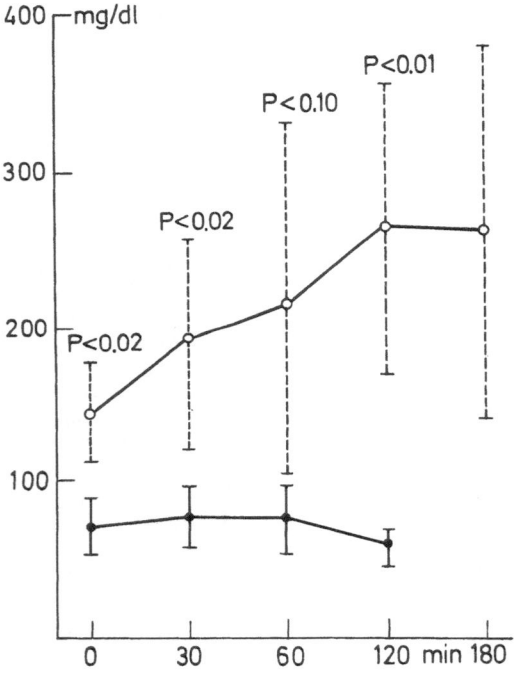

Figure 3. Blood sugar. —•— = control group, —o— = sucrose group

the aorta, coronary artery, and femoral artery. Nodular lesions of renal glomeruli compatible with human diabetic glomerulosclerosis were observed. A few monkeys developed myocardial infarction. Since 1966, we have demonstrated sucrose-induced atherosclerosis in rabbits, rats, and beagle dogs. However, no one hase reported such lesions in nonhuman primates fed a high-sucrose diet. In the present study, we could demonstrate vascular lesions in monkeys comparable to the lesions in other animals already reported. We may postulate that sucrose might play a role in the initiation and progression of human arterial lesions.

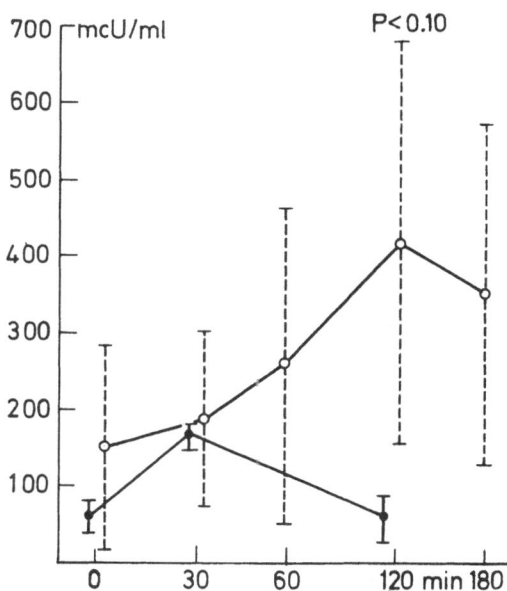

P< 0.10

Figure 4. Immunoreactive insulin. ——•—— = control group, ——o—— = sucrose group

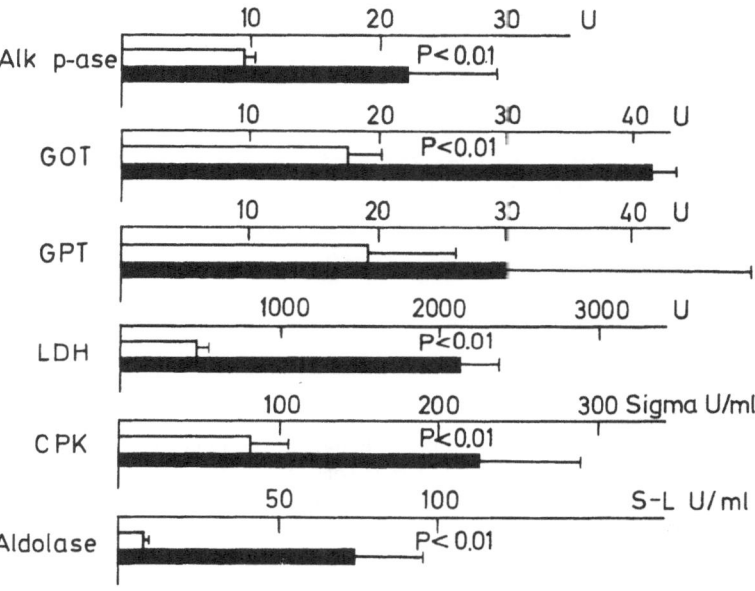

Figure 5. ▭ = control group, ▰ = sucrose group

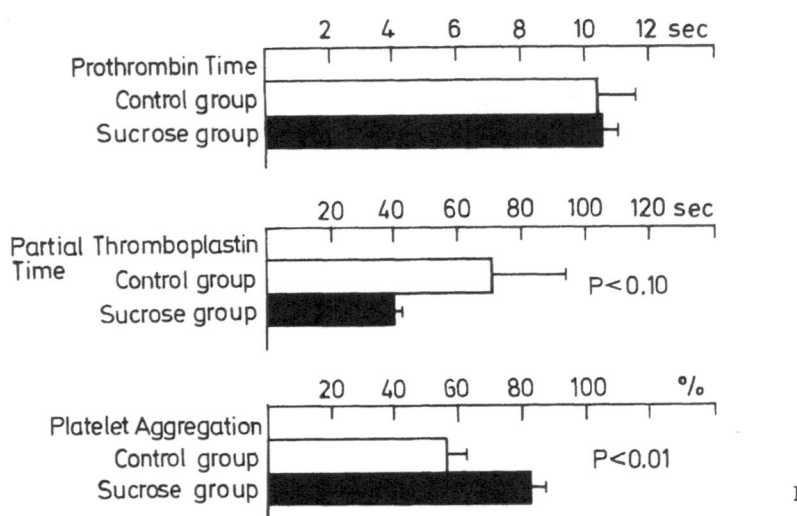

Figure 6

Summary

In crab-eating monkeys, a sucrose diet could induce atheromatous lesions in the aorta, coronary artery, and femoral artery. Sucrose-fed monkeys showed glucose intolerance and nodular lesions of renal glomeruli.

ASCORBIC ACID AND ATHEROSCLEROSIS: EFFECTS OF CHRONIC HYPOVITAMIN C ON AORTIC GROUND SUBSTANCE AND LIPID METABOLISM

Takao Fujinami, Reiji Higuchi, Sagami Nakano, Nagahiko Sakuma, Katsuhiko Hayashi, and Junichi Yokoi

Because ascorbic acid deficiency is a disease of the ground substance of the blood vessels and also induces an increase in serum lipids, hypovitamin C is considered to be an ideal model for atherosclerosis investigation. The use of an experimental model of ascorbic acid deficiency, obtained by restricting the ascorbic acid intake in guinea pigs allowed us to demonstrate alteration of the aortic endothelium and atherosclerotic lesions, as previously reported.

In the present studies, the influence of hypovitamin C on the ground substance of the aorta, the adrenal function, and lipid metabolism were investigated. Male guinea pigs weighing about 300 g were divided into two groups, i.e., chronic hypovitamin C and the control. Animals of both groups were fed a scorbutogenic diet supplemented in the hypovitamin group by 5 mg of vitamin C twice a week to prevent overt deficiency and 25 mg of the vitamin daily in the control group for 8 weeks.

In chronic hypovitamin C guinea pigs, atherosclerotic lesions were found in 16% of them at the 4th week and in 66% at the 8th week feeding. Histologic observations revealed thickening of the intima with subendothelial lipid deposition and lesions in the middle of the media accompanied by an accumulation of lipid, mucopolysaccharides, and calcium. Acid mucopolysaccharide in the aorta was analyzed using a cetylpyridinium chloride column according to the method of Seethanathan and the uronic acid content determined by the method of Bitter und Muir. An increase in the total acid mucopolysaccharides was observed in a grossly normal aorta of the hypovitamin C group at 4 weeks and a prominent increase in the aorta with atherosclerotic lesion of the hypovitamin C group at 8 weeks. In the constituents of mucopolysaccharides, and increase of hyaluronic acid, heparan sulfate, and chondroitin sulfate A and C, whereas a decrease of dermatan sulfate was a distinctive pattern of the chronic hypovitamin C group. Hydroxyproline content in the aorta was determined by the method of Woessner. In acute scurvy, the content of hydroxyproline in the aorta was significantly decreased as previously reported, but there was no apparent difference in the content between the chronic hypovitamin C and the control groups (Fig. 1).

Serum lipids estimated by the conventional methods revealed significantly higher serum triglyceride levels in hypovitamin C animals than in control animals at the 4th and 8th weeks and a high serum cholesterol level at the 4th week. Two μCi per 100 g of body weight of $4C^{14}$-cholesterol was injected intraperitoneally and radioactivity was measured in the serum, homogenate of the aorta, and liver at 3 and 7 days after the injection. Significantly higher activity in the serum and a relatively high activity in the aorta was observed in the deficient group as compared to the control group.

Analytic ultracentrifuge of lipoprotein revealed an apparent increase of HDL and VLDL in the deficient group, whereas only a trace of these lipoproteins was found in the control group. The amount of LDL was also significantly elevated in the deficient group. Subfraction of LDL and HDL obtained by filtration through a column of 2% agarose gel showed an abnormal absorbance at 280 μm which might indicate the existence of abnormal lipoproteins or polypeptides in HDL and LDL of chronic hypovitamin C animals (Fig. 2).

When the animals of both the hypovitamin C and the control groups were fed a scorbutogenic diet with 1% cholesterol added for 4 weeks, total serum cholesterol and triglyceride levels were significantly elevated in the hypovitamin C group.

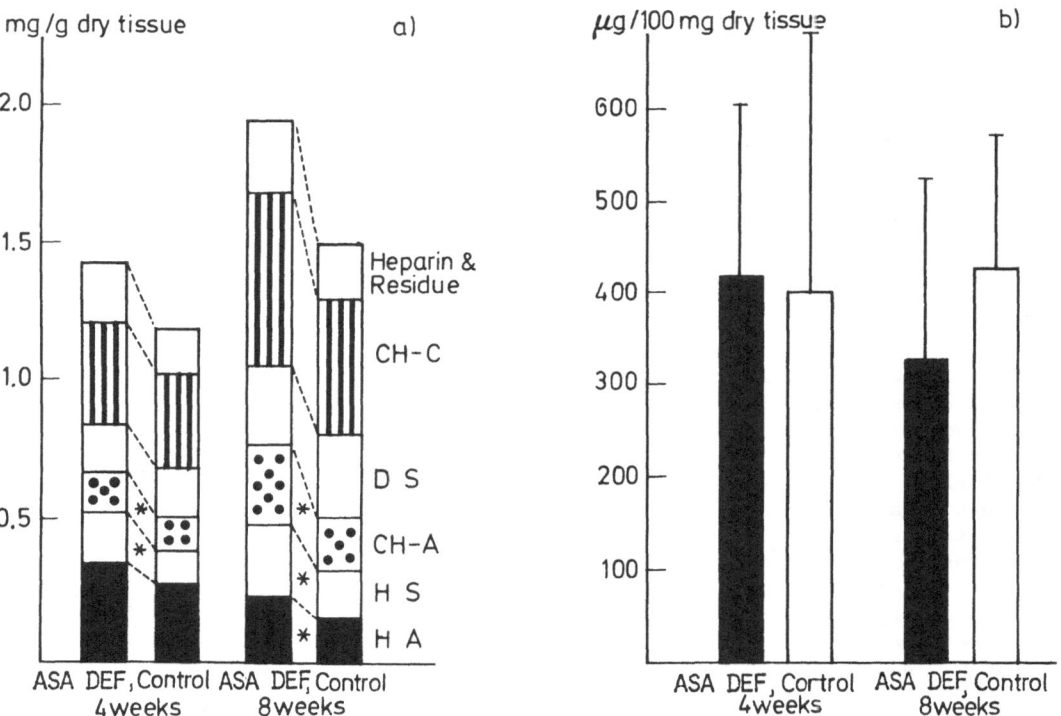

Figure 1. Acid mucopolysaccharide content (a) and hydroxyproline (b) in the aorta of chronic hypovitamin C and control animals shows a significant difference (P <0.05)

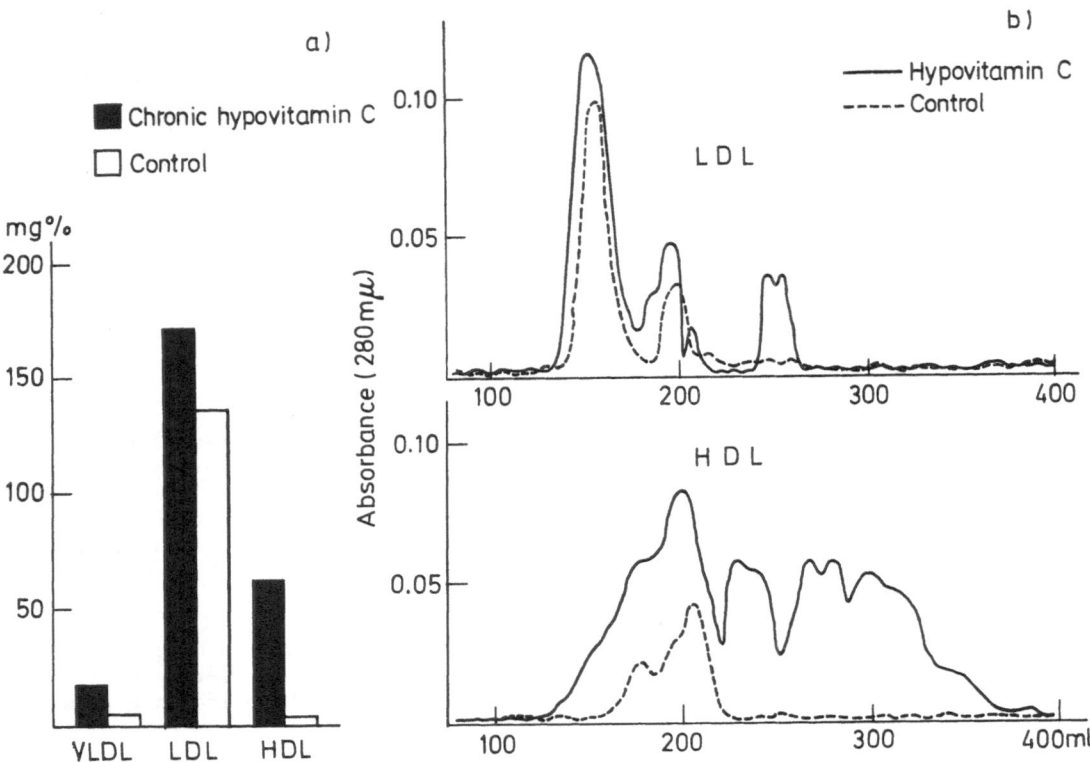

Figure 2. Serum lipoprotein content in the animals of the chronic hypovitamin C and control groups. Agarose gel filtration of HDL and LDL revealed abnormal absorbance at 280 μm suggesting an existence of variant lipoproteins or polypeptides in the HDL and LDL lipoprotein fraction of chronic hypovitamin C

Conversely, this finding means that dietary cholesterol-induced hypercholesterolemia is reduced by a supplement of vitamin C. The blood ascorbic acid level was low in the control group even though they received 25 mg of the vitamin daily. This suggests that cholesterol feeding increases the vitamin C requirement in guinea pigs.

A high concentration of ascorbic acid is present in the adrenal gland, and it is generally believed that the vitamin influences the biosynthesis of adrenocortical hormones. There was a marked enlargement of the adrenal gland in the hypovitamin C animal after 8 weeks feeding. With a urinary output of 17 KS and 17 OHCS, plasma cortisol was elevated at the 4th week and inversely depleted at the 8th week. Contrary to the decrease in plasma cortisol, the cholesterol content in the adrenal gland was elevated at the 8th week. Catecholamin content in the urine and the adrenal gland was not affected by chronic hypovitamin C. Since high plasma cortisol and serum lipids were observed at the time of earliest manifestation of atherosclerotic lesions in hypovitamin C animals, the influence of corticosteroid on blood ascorbic acid, serum lipids, and aortic ground substance was studied. Guinea pigs of both groups received 20 mg/kg of hydrocortison for 4 weeks. An increase in serum cholesterol and triglyceride levels by administration of the steroid was observed in both groups. Composition of the aortic acid mucopolysaccharide was not significantly influenced, whereas aortic hydroxyproline was markedly decreased by steroid administration in both groups. No atherosclerosis lesions were found in the animals of either group.

Table 1. Results of blood analysis and plasma cortisol and urinary output, catecholamine and cholesterol content in the adrenal gland of chronic hypovitamin C and the control. Significant difference between hypovitamin C and the control by probability less than 0.05 was shown with*

	Four weeks		Eight weeks	
	Control	Hypovitamin C	Control	Hypovitamin C
Blood ascorbic acid mg%	1.03±0.26 *	0.32±0.16	0.74±0.20 *	0.49±0.12
Serum cholesterol mg%	22.0±7.08 *	79.8±17.9	64.0±18.0	99.7±34.9
Serum triglyceride mg%	40.9±15.5 *	80.1±35.6	75.2±3.1 *	99.2±17.4
Plasma cortisol μg%	74.3±30.6 *	96.0±27.5	76.3±30.9	52.4±18.3
Urine 17-K S μg/day	7.2±2.2 *	10.6±2.0	6.9±1.7	9.4±4.0
Urine 17-OHCS μg/day	2.7±0.9 *	4.0±1.1	2.3±0.8	2.8±1.1
Urine catecholamine μg/day	1.54±0.34	1.16±0.41	1.69±0.38	1.51±0.32
Urine V M A μg/day	55.5±19.8	55.4±10.0	65.9±17.3	64.2±12.9
Weight of adrenal gland mg	243±38	249±85	358±85 *	453±93
Cholesterol in ADR, GL mg/g	54.4±9.6	61.3±11.7	48.3±3.7 *	79.2±15.9
Incidence of athero-sclerosis	0	16%	0	66.6%

Studies on how chronic hypovitamin C affects serum lipids and atherosclerosis in humans have not been definitive. In the present studies, the relationship of hyperlipoproteinemia and blood ascorbic acid and cortisol levels was investigated. One hundred twenty-six patients who had hypercholesterolemia above 250 mg% and/or hypertriglycemia above 150 mg% were divided into lipoprotein phenotypes according to the WHO classification. The plasma cortisol level was determined by the radio-immunoassay method. A low blood ascorbic acid level below 0,9 mg was observed in more than half of the patients with type IIa and IV. Thirty-nine percent of the type IIa and 15.6% of the type IV had a high plasma cortisol level above 20 μg% accompanied simultaneously by low ascorbic acid. This high cortisol level accompanied by low blood ascorbic acid in types IIa and IV was a similar feature of the ascorbic acid-cholesterol-cortisol relation in chronic hypovitamin C guinea pigs at the 4th week. These results may suggest that chronic hypovitamin C might be a pathogenic factor in some hyperlipidemia in human. It is apparent that vitamin C as concerned with the maintenance of normal vascular functions, and deficiency or hypovitamin of it may cause vascular disease. Some investigators have proclaimed that a characteristic biochemical lesion of ascorbic acid deficiency seems to be an alteration of the sulfated mucopolysaccharide in connective tissue. It has also been proposed that acid mucopolysaccharides bind with lipoprotein and fibrinogen and precipitate in the arterial wall. Altered aortic endothelium such as widened endothelial junction may provide an increase of plasma lipid infusion into the arterial wall. Thus, relative or localized hypovitamin C induces the altered ground substance and forms a mucopolysaccharide-lipid complex. The mechanism responsible for the elevation of serum lipids in chronic hypovitamin C is supposed to be: (1) reduced postheparin lipoprotein lipase activity

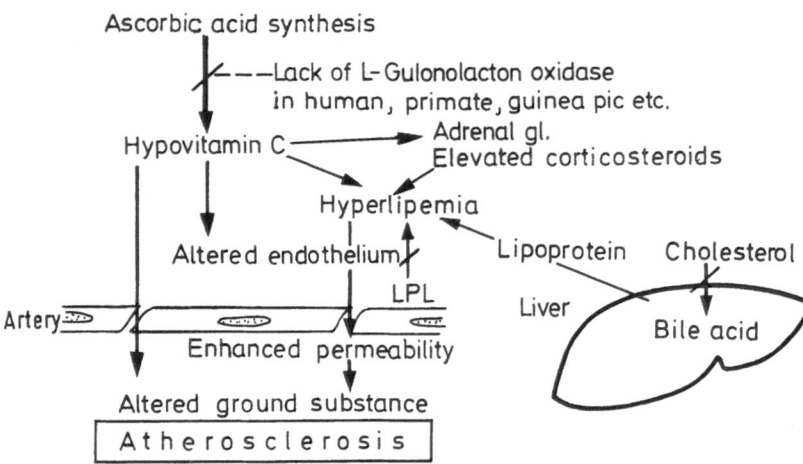

Figure 3. Hypothetic mechanism of chronic hypovitamin C in atherogenesis

as previously reported, (2) impaired 7 α-hydroxylation of the cholesterol cyclo-
hexan ring during conversion of cholesterol to bile acid, (3) enhanced cholesterol synthesis, and (4) abnormal lipoprotein formation. Accelerated release of
corticosteroids at the 4th week of hypovitamin C might be a contributing factor
to hypercholesterolemia.

Thus, vitamin C seems to occupy a position of importance by virtue of its involvement in the maintenance of vascular integrity, adrenocortical function, and lipid metabolism. Since the primate and guinea pig cannot synthesize vitamin C due
to lack of L-glunolacton oxidase, chronic covert ascorbic acid deficiency might
be an important factor of atherogenicity in humans, as observed in guinea pigs
(Fig. 3).

ETHANOL-LIPEMIA — A DOUBTFUL RISK FACTOR

P. Avogaro, G. Cazzolato, G. Bittolo-Bon, and F. Belussi

Introduction

Despite a recognized property of inducing hyperlipemia in both animals and humans
(Lieber et al., 1962; Jones et al., 1963; Losowsky et al., 1963; Schapiro et al.,
1965; Nestel and Hirsch, 1965; Baraona and Lieber, 1970; Baraona et al., 1973;
Wilson et al., 1970; Avogaro and Cazzolato, 1975), ethanol (EOH) is thought to
be a poor atherogenetic factor (Hirst et al., 1965; Viel et al., 1966; Spain and
Bradess, 1957). It is not known insofar whether the poor atherogenetic property
of EOH is due to any special feature of induced lipemia.

This paper gives further information about chemical variations induced by ethanol
in the lipoprotein classes, Information is also given about ethanol-induced variations of apolipoproteins.

Material and Methods

Four males, aged 40 - 60, were included in this study. Criteria for selection are
the same as employed in a previous study (Avogaro and Cazzolato, 1975).

At 7:30 a.m., each subject received 1.5 g/kg of ethanol p.o. in a 30% water solution after 12 hours fasting. Blood samples were collected on EDTA (1 mg/1 ml) before the test and 4 hours after the load.

Ultracentrifugal separation. The procedure for separation of the five major lipoprotein density classes was carried out on Beckman model L2-65 B ultracentrifuge equipped to accept the Ti-14 zonal rotor.

A Ultrograd LKB was used for programming the density gradient and a Bio-rad fiber pump module for filling the rotor.

For separation of VLDL, IDL, LDL, HDL_2, and HDL_3, the two-step procedure outlined by Kostner et al. (1974) was followed.

Methods

Estimations of the following components were carried out in all ultracentrifugally collected fractions: protein (Lowvry et al., 1951), phospholipids (Fiske and Subarrow, 1925), cholesterol (Liebermann and Buchardt, 1967), triglyceride (Eggstein, 1966), electrophoresis in agarose (Seidel, 1973), and in polyacrylamide gel (Mead and Dangerfield, 1974). Values of chemical constituents are given as percentage of total lipoprotein.

The content of individual polypeptide species was determined in 10% polyacrylamide gels using tetramethyl urea (TMU) according to Kane (1973).

Due to the semiquantitative nature of the polypeptides analysis in polyacrylamide gel, no effort have been made to give quantitative data. The corresponding patterns of the various polypeptides, both before and after the ethanol load, are shown in Figures 1-3.

B-apoprotein cotent of VLDL was determined as the difference between the content of total proteins and proteins soluble in TMU (Kane, 1973).

Results

Following ethanol, an increase of "areas" corresponding to VLDL, IDL, LDL, HDL_2, and HDL_3 has been recorded in all the studied subjects (Fig. 1).

Cholesterol percentage decreased significantly in LDL, HDL_2, and HDL_3 with minor meaningless variations in the other classes. Triglyceride concentration increased in all the fractions; however, the increase in HDL_2 was not significant (Table 1).

Phospholipids decreased significantly in all classes.

Protein percentage increased in HDL_2 and HDL_3 and decreased in VLDL, IDL, and LDL.

The cholesterol/triglyceride ratio decreased in all classes with the single exception of IDL. The major decrease was recorded in LDL.

The triglyceride/protein ratio increased in VLDL, IDL, LDL, HDL_3 and underwent no variations in HDL_2.

Polar components of VLDL (free cholesterol plus protein plus phospholipids) underwent a reduction (Table 2).

The triglyceride/cholesterol esterified ratio showed an increase.

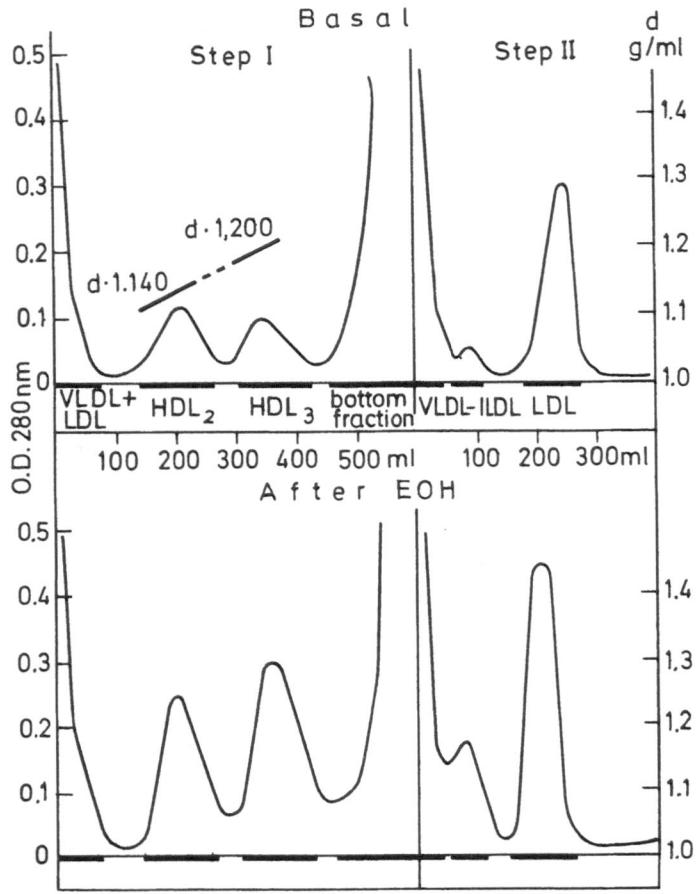

Figure 1. Densitometric areas of lipoprotein classes collected through a zonal rotor Ti-14-Beckman. The densitometric readings are obtained with an Uvicor-III LKB equipment at wave length 280 nm and checked with Shimatzu QV 50 spectrophotometer at the same wave length. At the left of the Figure, fractions obtained in step 1: *top* before EOH; *bottom* after EOH. At the rigt of the Figure, fractions obtained in step II

Apolipoproteins which are soluble in TMU (apoC, apoA, arginin-rich) increased while apolipoprotein B decreased.

The determination of soluble polypeptide recorded increased bands corresponding to CII, $CIII_1$, $CIII_2$ in VLDL, IDL and LDL (Fig. 2). Minor unrelevant variations have been recorded in HDL_2 and HDL_3.

Bidirectional, meaningless variations have been observed in the C_1, band in all the classes considered.

When a fraction with d <1006 was submitted to electrophoresis on agarose, a non-migrating band at origin was recorded in two out of the four subjects following ethanol (Fig. 3). In two out of four subjects in the fraction with d <1006 a pre-β band appeared which was not present in the fasting sample before ethanol (Fig. 3).

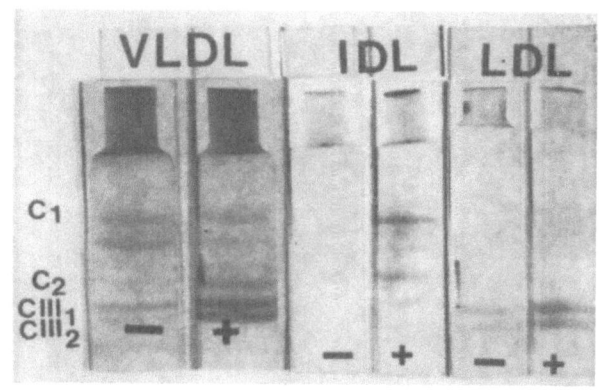

Figure 2. 10% polyacrylamide gel electrophoresis in urea 8 m variations in TMU soluble apolipoprotein bands before (-) and after (+) EOH (see text)

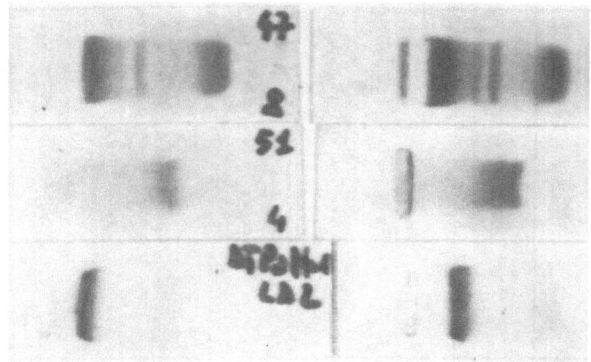

Figure 3. Electrophoretic patterns of total serum (top), VLDL (middle), LDL (bottom), before (left) and after ethanol load (right). The appearance of chylomicra and a pre-B_1 band in total serum and VLDL is evident

Discussion

The data referred to in the present paper confirm that ethanol exerts a deep effect on all blood lipoproteins. Its main effect, however, seems to be an enrichment in triglyceride content of all the lipoprotein classes and a decrease in LDL cholesterol.

The surcharge in the triglyceride content of lipoproteins with a density greater than 1.063 explains the increased electrophoretic α-lipoproteins recorded during intoxication by ethanol (Johansson and Laurell, 1969) and the increased areas of HDL recorded in our experiment (Fig. 1). Moreover, the unchanged percentage of cholesterol in HDL does not support the hypothesis that the poor atherogenetic property of ethanol may be related to increased levels of α-(HDL)-cholesterol.

It seems therefore likely that the enrichment in triglyceride content and percentage, associated with a decreased cholesterol level, may reduce the ability of the LDL to permeate the vascular wall.

In our experience, ethanol appeared to be particularly effective in promoting an increase of the "intermediate" area. This finding stresses the hypothesis that

Table 1.

	VLDL B	VLDL A	IDL B	IDL A	LDL B	LDL A	HDL2 B	HDL2 A	HDL3 B	HDL3 A
Total Lipo-P M	106.25	208.75	39.0	88.75	235	277.5	109.5	164.75	225.25	294
S.D.	±12.86	±55.77	±6.83	±36.59	±28.86	±41.12	±13.32	±18.73	±32.98	±38.78
Chol M̄	14.6	17.9	27.1	29.6	38.6	34.7	16.7	13.2	13.7	10.7
S.E.	±4.2 N	±0.1 S	±0.4 N	±0.3 S	±0.4	±0.9 **	±0.2	±0.6 **	±0.4	±0.2 **
Est. Chol. M̄	11.5	12.3								
S.E.	±0.4 N	±0.3 S								
TG M̄	50.9	60.6	31.8	35.2	14.2	28.5	7.9	9.7	5.0	7.1
S.E.	±0.7	±0.1 **	±1.2	±0.6 **	±0.4	±1.1 **	±0.5 N S	±0.6	±0.1	±0.4 **
PL M̄	18.0	13.3	21.7	19.8	24.3	22.3	34.1	30.1	31.2	24.3
S.E.	±1.7	±0.3 *	±0.7	±0.8 **	±0.7	±0.5 *	±1.0	±1.1 **	±0.5	±1.7 **
P M̄	11.9	8.0	19.5	15.6	22.9	14.8	42.3	47.9	50.8	59.5
S.E.	±0.2	±0.2 **	±0.6	±0.2 **	±0.6	±0.9 **	±0.5	±0.5 **	±0.9	±1.0 **
Chol. TG	0.36	0.29	0.87	0.83	2.73	1.23	2.16	1.37	2.74	1.61
	±0.016	±0.003 *	±0.027	±0.010 N S	±0.085	±0.074 **	±0.16	±0.032 *	±0.053	±0.080 **

	4.28 ±0.095	7.55 ±0.22	1.63 ±0.106	2.26 ±0.063 **	0.62 ±0.024	1.94 ±0.0127 ** N	0.18 ±0.093 S	0.20 ±0.102	0.10 ±0.003	0.12 ±0.007 *
TG P										

	Mean	S.E.
Soluble apo-Lp	55.7 ±1.1	61.4 ±1.1 **
Apo-B M	44.3 ±1.1	38.6 ±1.1 **

*P <0.05. **P <0.01. Values are given as mg/dl. B = before ethanol. A = after ethanol.

Table 2. Percentage composition of VLDL before and after EOH (1.5 g/kg p.o.)

Polar constituents % volume	37.7	27.9
TG/CE	4.2	5.2
Protein (weight %)	11.8	8.1
B-apolipoprotein (%)	44.7	39.5
TMU-soluble apolipoprotein	55.3	60.4

a Mean values for 4 subjects.

ethanol may be a trigger of type III hyperlipemia. The same finding may explain the high prevalence of peripheral atherosclerosis similar to type III recorded in alcoholic patients (Sirtori et al., 1974).

Conclusion

The main effect of ethanol in man is its property of inducing an enrichment of triglycerides in all the major lipoprotein classes even of greater density. At the same time, there is an increase of apo-C in VLDL and an appearance of these polypeptides in LDL and IDL. Cholesterol decreases not only in LDL but also in HDL. The effectiveness of ethanol in inducing a chylomicronemia and the appearance of an intermediate class is confirmed. One may speculate that the increased quantity and percentage of triglyceride in LDL lowers the ability of these lipoproteins to permeate the intima of vessels. This speculation might provide an explanation for the poor atherogenicity of ethanol-induced lipemia (Hirst et al., 1965; Viel et al., 1966; Spain and Bradess. 1957).

VASOACTIVE AGENTS AND POSTPRANDIAL CHYLOMICRONS AS RISK FACTORS IN ATHEROGENESIS*

Abel Lazzarini Robertson, Jr.

Epidemiological and experimental data suggests that atherosclerosis is a poly-etiologic and polypathogenetic disease (McMillan, 1973). Although at first asymptomatic, the disorder may progress at variable speeds to overt clinical manifestations under the influence of synergistic and often poorly understood risk factors. The great variability in geographic distribution, anatomical severity and rate of progression of individual arterial lesions (Strong et al., 1972; McGill, 1974) are indicators that local metabolic and functional alterations of the vascular wall may influence the rate of atherogenesis (Glagov, 1971).

Some early experimental observations (Gutstein, 1963) suggested to us that localized experimental trauma of the arterial wall may induce secondary vasomotor responses that significantly alter the rate and character of vascular repair. This "irritability" of the blood vessel wall resulted in the development of accelerated atherosclerosis in hypercholesterolemic animals at sites of limited injury.

More recently, studies with the octapeptide angiotensin II in rabbits and rats showed that this powerful vasoactive agent has multiple sites of action related not only to control of systemic blood pressure but to the permeability and function of the vascular wall as a whole (Robertson and Khairallah, 1972; Khairallah et al., 1972). Based on these findings, experiments were carried out with acute intravascular injections of several other vasoactive agents including norepinephrine, 5-hydroxytryptamine, prostaglandin E_1, bradykinin, and histamine at concen-

*These studies were partially supported by a Research Grant from Sanzod, Inc., U.S.A. Preliminary investigations were carried out while a Visiting Fellow at the John Curtin School of Medical Research, Australian National University under Prof. F.C. Courtice. The cooperation of Drs. G.I. Schoefl and A.D. Shannon, Canberra, is gratefully acknowledged.
The valuable assistance of L.S. Staikoff, Technical Associate in Macromolecular Sciences and K. Gruen, Senior Research Associate in Pathology at Case Western Reserve University allowed completion of the study.

trations below those able to produce significant increases in mean systolic blood pressures. The results obtained suggested that sudden and short-lived ("trap door" effect) increases on arterial permeability to circulating macromolecules occurred with entrapment of serum lipoproteins in the vascular wall (Robertson and Khairallah, 1973). It is important to emphasize that under focal stimulation by such vasoactive agents, the mechanism of "in bulk" transport of circulating lipoproteins across the so-called arterial endothelial "barrier" may differ and be considerably faster than that observed in the normal aorta both in vivo (Stein et al., 1973) and in vitro (Jensen, 1967). In nonstimulated arteries, endocytotic plasmalemmal vesicles (Jacques, 1969) seem to be the main route involved in the transport of labeled lipoproteins across the endothelium (Robertson and Rosen, 1977).

For the present study, preliminary observations were made with anesthesized "Canberra" Wistar rats in which retrograde aortic infusions of either angiotensin II (0.1 - 10 ng) or 5-hydroxytriptamine sulfate (10 - 100 ng) were carried out with or without simultaneous injection of 0.5 ml homologous whole lymph obtained by thoracic duct cannulation 30 min after administration by gastric tube of 1 ml of heavy cream. Following in vivo fixation with 1% glutaraldehyde solution in phosphate buffer injected at mean systolic pressures immediately thereafter, the specimens were processed for light and scanning electron microscopy as recently reported (Robertson and McKalen, 1975).

As shown in Figure 1, angiotensin II induced acute attachment of blood cells, particularly platelets and erythrocytes, at sites of aortic branching, specifically at regions corresponding to the distal or caudal tip of the branch opening. When lymph was simultaneously injected, these arterial sites also showed attachment of chylomicrons. To evaluate these phenomena further, lymph samples were pooled and separated by ultracentrifugation in samples containing "large" chylomicrons (2500 - 10,000 Å in diameter) (fraction A) and "small" chylomicrons (less

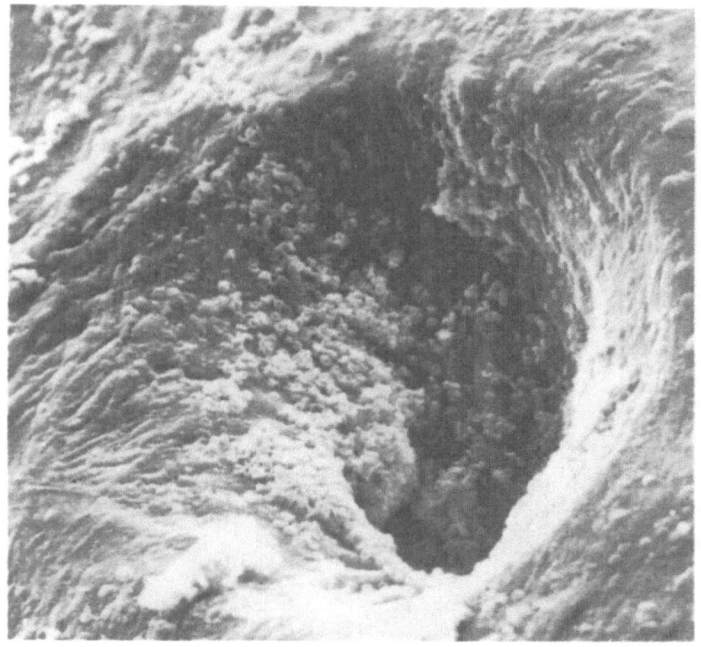

Figure 1. Scanning electron micrograph of the periostial region of an intercostal branch of the rat aorta showing localization of adherent blood cells to the lower edge or lip of the vessel (bottom) following intra-aortic injection of 0.1 ng of angiotensin II. Gold palladium coating (60X)

than 2500 Å) (fraction B). When injected with the vasoactive agent, fraction A chylomicrons were found 1 h after injection loosely attached to the aortic endothelial surface at sites of arterial branching (Fig. 2), while those from fraction B appeared by scanning electron microscopy tightly adherent to the vascular surface between leukocytes and red blood cells (Fig. 3). Control aortic injections of chylomicron fractions in saline alone failed to show any luminal changes.

Due to the relative higher cholesterol concentration of "small" chylomicrons (fraction B), a series of experiments were desinged in adult female Sprague-Dawley rats using cholesterol-1,2 ^{3}H to label the cholesteryl esters fraction as proposed by Redgrave (1970). Under anesthesia, an indwelling catheter was introduced through the left carotid artery to the descending thoracic aorta and a 0.3 ml injection of the chylomicron preparation made with or without the vasoactive agents at same concentrations as described above followed by sufficient Ringer's solution to rinse the catheter. During injection, mean systolic pressures were continuously monitored.

As shown in Table 1, animals were compared for plasma and aortic radioactivity determined by thin layer chromatography and liquid scintillation spectrometry at different intervals between injections. The results obtained indicated statistically significant differences in arterial cholesterol radioactivity for both angiotensin II and 5-hydroxytriptamine that were related to the length of time between administration of the vasoactive agents and the chylomicron preparations. Highest tritiated cholesterol uptake occurred in intimal-medial samples when chylomicrons and drugs were injected simultaneously.

Figure 4 shows results obtained 24 – 48 h after simultaneous injection of angiotensin II and fraction B chylomicrons by scanning electron microscopy. At sites of aortic branching, large numbers of "remnants" were found partially incorporated to the luminal arterial surface.

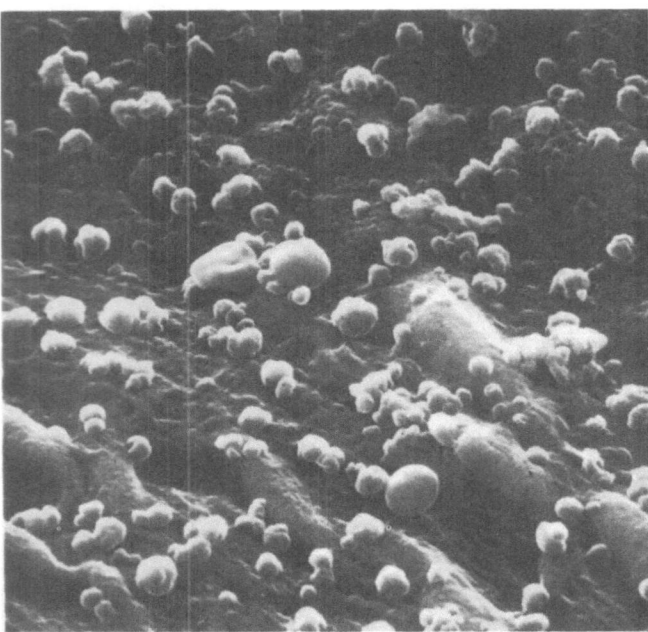

Figure 2. Scanning electron micrograph of "large" chylomicrons (fraction A) loosely attached to endothelial surface between scattered rounded platelets 1 h after simultaneous injection with 10 mg of 5-hydroxytriptamine. Gold palladium coating (20,000X)

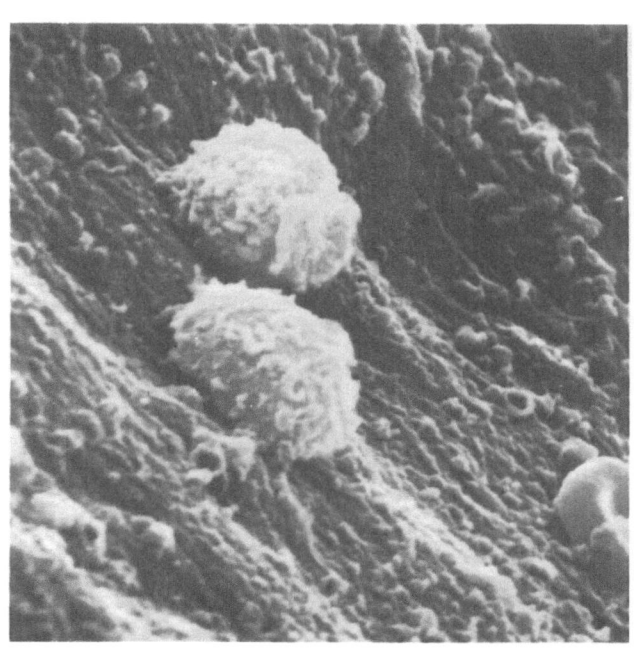

Figure 3. Scanning electron micrograph of "small" chylomicrons (fraction B) tightly adherent and partially incorporated to the aortic luminal surface, 1 h after simultaneous intra-aortic injection with 0.1 ng of angiotensin II. Two leukocytes and part of an erythrocyte with an adherent platelet can be seen on the lower right corresponding to the edge of the intercostal orifice. Gold palladium coating (34,000X)

Table 1. ^{3}H-cholesterol labeled fraction B postprandial chylomicrons

Rat aortic intima-media recovery/% radioactivity from plasma				
Injection of chylomicrons	0	60"	360"	900"
After injection with 0.10 ng angiotensin II:				
	12.6	8.3	1.6	–
Without:	1.64	2.72	1.04	–
After injection with 10 ng 5-hydroxytriptamine sulfate:				
	9.7	7.3	5.6	3.2
Without:	1.28	1.84	1.37	1.27

Some of the vasoactive agents were also shown to affect the behavior of fraction B postprandial chylomicrons in vitro. Short-term endothelial monolayer cultures of newborn aorta, carotid, and vena cava were tested and compared with those from umbilical veins in the presence of angiotensin II, 5-hydroxytriptamine, or prostaglandin E_1. As shown in Table 2, attachment or "stickiness" of small ^{3}H-labeled chylomicrons to endothelial cells as shown by autoradiography was significantly higher in arterial endothelial cells than in those from veins. Considerable variation in response to the three vasoactive agents tested was also noted.

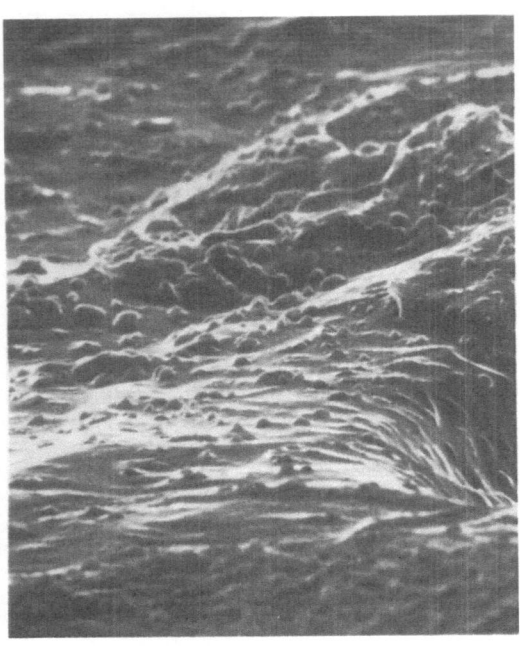

Figure 4. Scanning electron micrograph of an intercostal ostial region 48 h after simultaneous injection of chylomicron fraction B and 0.1 ng of angiotensin II. Compare with Figure 3. Note disappearance of adherent blood cells from the vascular luminal surface and widespread incorporation of chylomicron remnants. Gold palladium coating (34,000X)

Table 2. Variations on "stickiness" of homologous "small" ^{3}H-labeled chylomicrons[a] to confluent human endothelial monolayer cultures following in vitro stimulation

Cell origin	A	B	C
Thoracic aorta	82.4	69.3	42.8
Carotid arteries	62.1	52.6	39.7
Vena cava	15.0	16.4	1.2
Umbilical vein (fetal)	8.9	2.3	2.8

A = angiotensin II 1×10^{-9}G.
B = 5-hydroxytriptamine sulfate 1×10^{-8}G.
C = prostaglandin E_1 1×10^{-7}G.

[a]Average % of labeled cells from 20 matched cultures each.

In order to evaluate if these effects of angiotensin II on the uptake of post-prandial chylomicrons by the aortic wall also occurred with other blood lipid moieties, a study was conducted with pooled ^{125}I human-labeled lipoproteins obtained from another laboratory.

As shown in Table 3 and as described before for chylomicrons, simultaneous injections of the lipoprotein fractions and angiotensin II produced highest uptake rates. An interesting difference was noted, however, labeled low-density lipoprotein (LDL) as incorporated at a higher rate and for longer periods than very low-

Table 3. Incorporation of iodinated lipoprotein fractions[a] by rat aortic intima[b] after endothelial stimulation with angiotensin II[c]

% Radioactivity from plasma	Simultaneous injection with angio II	Injected 60 S after angio II	Injected 480 S after angio II
VLDL	7.8	5.4	–
S	1.24	1.82	–
LDL	16.2	8.4	0.4
S	4.64	1.49	–
HDL	4.8	0.4	–
S	1.47	0.12	–

[a] ^{125}I labeling by iodine monochloride method of Mac Farlene modified by Bilheimer et al. (1972).

[b] Intima and inner medial layers.

[c] Intra-aortic injection of 0.1 ng angiotensin II in 0.2 ml Ringer's solution by indwelling carotid catheter in a 200–210 g Sprague-Dawley female rat.

density (VLDL) or high-density (HDL) lipoproteins. Future studies will determine if these findings represent differences on transport or selective binding of these lipoproteins on the vascular surface of stimulated endothelial cells.

Single weekly simultaneous intra-arterial injections of the LDL fraction and angiotensin II or 5-hydroxytriptamine at subpressor doses induced lasting morphologic changes in the aortic wall. As shown in Figure 5, aortic intimal thickening and "foam cell" formation occurred, in the absence of sustained hyperlipemia.

The results of both these in vivo and in vitro studies strongly suggest that low concentrations of vasoactive agents such as angiotensin II, 5-hydroxytriptamine, prostaglandin E_1, and one or more platelet factors may not only affect permeability and function of the vascular wall as previously suggested (Robertson and Khairallah, 1972, 1973) but may have direct effects on the interaction of circulating chylomicrons and lipoproteins with the arterial lining. If as first suggested by Zilversmit (1975) lypolytic degradation of triglyceride-rich particles, chylomicrons, and VLDL in association with vascular endothelium requires binding of the lipids to surface mucopolysaccharides, vasoactive agents studies herewith may play an important role in the regulation of lipid uptake by the arterial wall. Sudden and short-lived increases in blood concentrations of these agents under stressful conditions may alter the balance and allow "undigestable" remnants (Zilversmit, 1975) rich in cholesteryl ester and apolipoprotein B to be incorporated into the vessel wall.

If, as shown, vasoactive agents and platelets are able to alter the permeability of the arterial wall at specific sites, they may not only accelerate the entrapment of lipid remnants but allow rapid incorporation of platelet factors able to stimulate propagation of primate smooth muscle cells and fibroblasts in vitro (Rutherford and Ross, 1976). Both phenomena could in turn greatly facilitate induction of intimal and medial cell proliferation, a key process in the intimal stages of atherogenesis (Robertson, 1974).

The noted preference for these experimental vascular lesions induced by vasoactive stimuli to localize at the distal lip of aortic branches is of particular

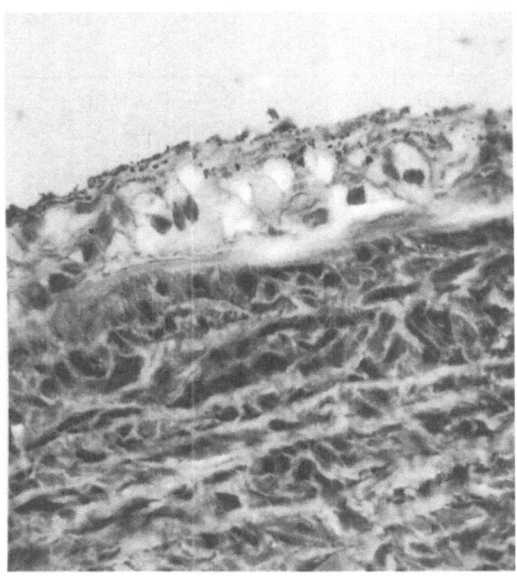

Figure 5. Photomicrograph of cross section of aortic wall 3 weeks after 1 single weekly injection of 1 ml (0.50 mg) of human LDL fraction simultaneously with 0.1 ng of angiotensin II. Note intimal thickening and abundant foam cells over irregular medial layers. Light microscopy, modified trichrome staining (250X)

interest. It is well-known that human atheromatous lesions as well as those produced in a variety of experimental models characteristically appear first in periostial areas. Giacomelli and Wiener (1974) have reported significant increases in the permeability of the rat thoracic aorta to electron markers at sites of intercostal orifices in the absence of appreciably ultrastructural differences in endothelial junctions compared with those of interostial regions. We have recently found accelerated lipoprotein uptake and increased turnover rates for human endothelial cells harvested from pooled distal lips of intercostal ostia compared with those from other areas of the same thoracic aorta (Robertson, 1976). These results were interpreted as indicating that at sites prone to accelerated atherosclerosis the endothelial lining of large human arteries may be genetically preprogrammed for rapid cell replacement and entrapment of circulating macromolecules.

While sustained hypertension has long been recognized both clinically and experimentally as a major risk factor in atherogenesis, little information is available, in the absence of increased blood pressure, as to the physiopathologic role of vasoactive agents in the autoregulation of the metabolic and functional characteristics of the arterial wall. The observations reported heretofore suggest that these agents may act as less conspicuous but important atherogenic risk factors that deserve closer scrutiny.

UNEXPLAINED VARIABILITY IN EXTENT OF ATHEROSCLEROSIS IN HOMOGENEOUS HUMAN POPULATIONS*

Jack P. Strong

The workshop topic, atherosclerosis without major risk factors, suggests concern for environmental or genetically determined variables other than the accepted major risk factors that might cause or accelerate the development of atherosclerosis and its sequelae. At a workshop on the epidemiology of atherosclerosis (Strong, 1976) earlier in this Fourth International Symposium, the relationship of atherosclerotic lesions and risk factors was discussed in detail. Most of that workshop's reports confirmed the associations between the major risk factors (elevated serum cholesterol levels, elevated blood pressure levels, and cigarette smoking) and the extent of mural atherosclerotic lesions in the coronary arteries and/or aorta. Significant associations were also reported for several other suspected risk factors for coronary heart disease. Even after these putative risk factors are considered, much of the variation in atherosclerosis in human subjects undergoing autopsy will undoubtedly remain unexplained. Strong and Eggen (1970) closed their report on risk factors and atherosclerotic lesions at the Second International Symposium with this paragraph:

"Unexplained Variability. One intriguing finding in all studies of human atherosclerosis is the wide variation among individuals in extent of lesions which persists in the most homogeneous subgroups. This variability is illustrated in... scatterplots of coronary raised lesions in 25–64-year-old New Orleans Negro men dying from accidental causes and other causes not known to be associated with cigarette smoking or atherosclerosis and classified according to smoking habits. Even after selecting cases according to race, sex, age, disease, and level of cigarette consumption, there is still much variability to be explained. For the 25–34 year age group the surface involvement with raised atherosclerotic lesions ranges from zero to 32% in the nonsmoker or light smoker and from zero to 63% in the heavy smoker. Great variability is also present in subgroups of subsequent decades. Even if other risk factors had been considered, there would still have been much variability remaining. This variability should be investigated intensively by epidemiologic, pathologic, genetic, and other methods. This unexplained variability could be the result of genetic influences which regulate susceptibility to other etiologic agents."

Figures 1 and 2, taken from a recently published report by Strong and Richards (1976), show the variability in coronary and aortic atherosclerosis among heavy smokers and among nonsmokers. These scatterplots of extent of raised atherosclerotic lesions in deceased white and black New Orleans men include only those persons dying of accidental causes and other causes not known to be associated with atherosclerosis, hypertension, or cigarette smoking. Known cases of such conditions as coronary heart disease, stroke, hypertension, diabetes, and lung cancer were excluded from these scatterplots. All the major known risk factors, however, were not excluded by this technique because cholesterol levels were not known for each case in this residual group. Nevertheless, the extent of lesions varies greatly for homogeneous groups of the same age, race, and smoking habits in basal cases where known hypertension and other associated diseases have been excluded.

Figure 3 shows another example of the large individual variability that exists within homogeneous subgroups of several human populations. Each point in the scatterplots represents the extent of raised lesions in the anterior descending branch, left coronary artery, of 45–54-year-old men undergoing autopsy as the basal cases from the International Atherosclerosis Project (Tejada et al., 1968).

*Supported in part by grants HL–08974 and HL–14496 from the National Heart, Lung and Blood Institute, National Institutes of Health, Bethesda, Maryland

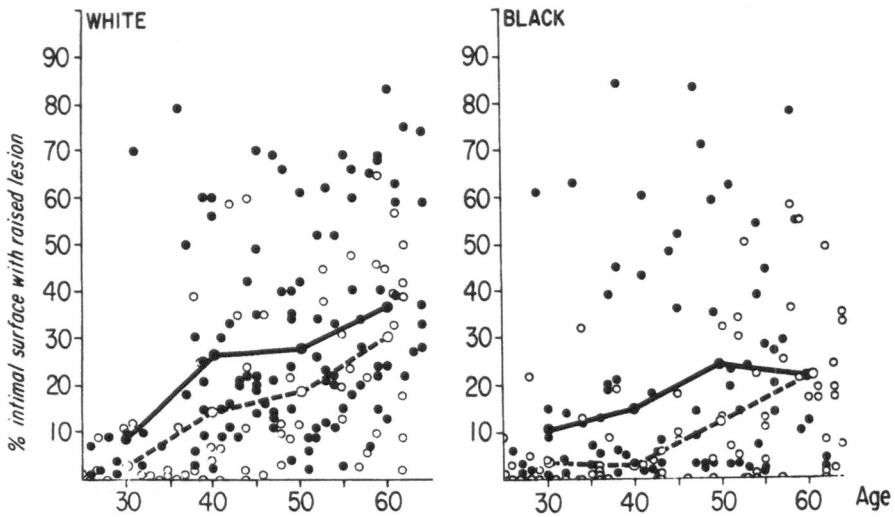

Figure 1. Percentage* of intimal surface of coronary arteries involved with raised lesions by age and average rate of smoking last 10 years of life, basal groups of white nonsmokers and heavy smokers and black nonsmoker and heavy smokers.
*Note: The lines connecting the mean percentages are used solely for the purpose of visual aid for the reader. (From Strong and Richards (1976), reprinted with the permission of Elsevier Scientific Publishing Company, Amsterdam)

●——— 25 or more } avg. No. cigarettes smoked/day last 10 years of life
o- - - none

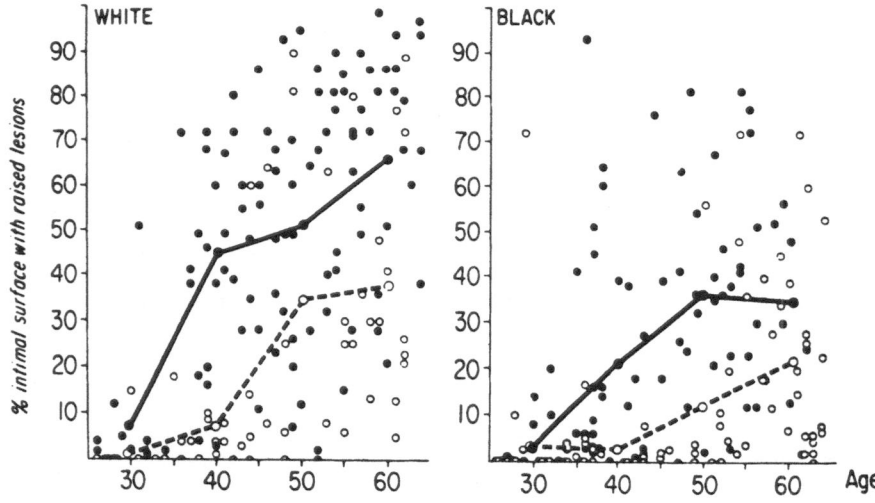

Figure 2. Percentage* of intimal surface of abdominal aortas involved with raised lesions by age and average rate of smoking during last 10 years of life, basal groups of white nonsmokers and heavy smokers and black nonsmokers and heavy smokers.
*Note: The lines connecting the mean percentages are used solely as a visual aid for the reader. (From Strong and Richards (1976), reprinted with the permission of Elsevier Scientific Publishing Company, Amsterdam)

●——— 25 ore more } avg. No. cigarettes smoked/day last 10 years of life
o- - - none

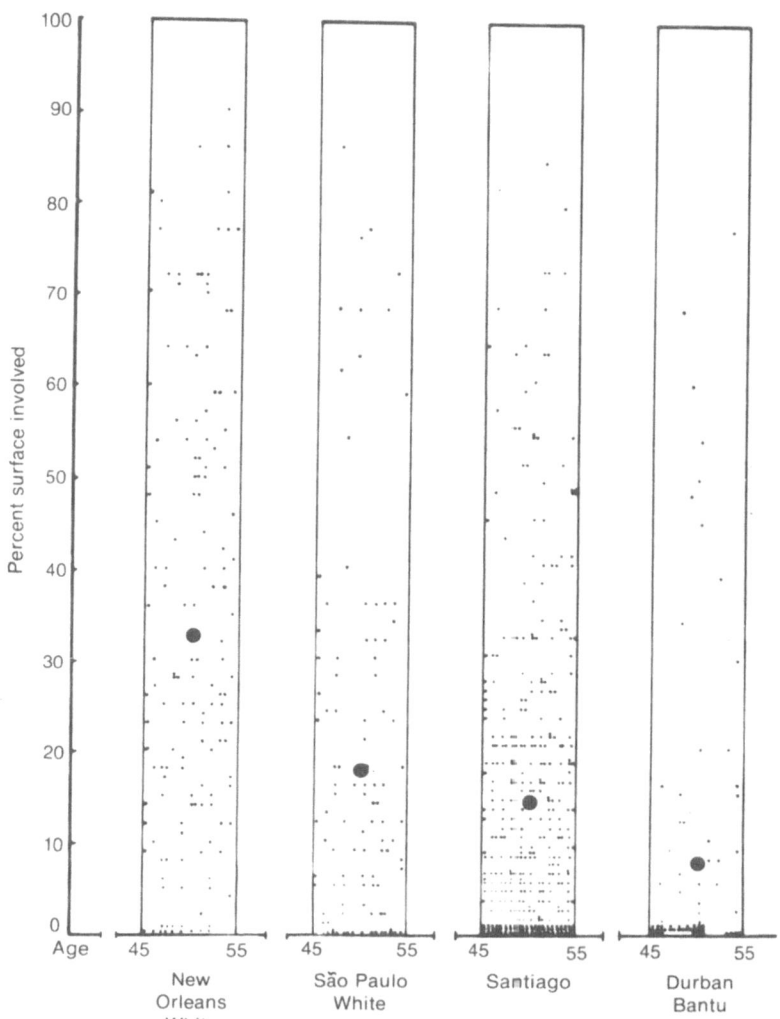

● Mean percent
    surface involved

Figure 3. Variability of raised atherosclerotic lesions in left descending coronary artery of mean, aged 45 – 54 years, who died of accidents, cancer, infection, and miscellaneous causes. Subjects were from the New Orleans white, São Paulo white, Santiago, and Durban Bantu location race groups. (From Tejada et al. (1968), reprinted with the permission of Williams and Wilkins Company, U.S. Canadian Division of the International Academy of Pathology)

Although the mean extent of lesions was clearly different among the four populations represented in this Figure, much variability in extent of lesions among subjects was present in each population. Large variability in extent of atherosclerotic lesions has now been documented both among persons of such "homogeneous" human populations and among experimental animals on identical atherogenic regiments (Eggen, 1976).

The major questions remaining are:
1. What fraction of the variability in the extent of atherosclerosis in humans can be explained by knowledge of known risk factors such as age, sex, race, serum lipid levels, blood pressure levels, cigarette smoking habits, and measure of obesity, glucose tolerance, and physical activity?

2. What is the cause or what are the causes of the remaining variability?
3. Are there other risk factors, as yet unknown, for atherosclerosis?
Clearly, the studies that have shown significant relationship of risk factors
to atherosclerosis have not "explained" all of the variability observed. After
all, the measures of some risk factors, such as serum lipids or blood pressure,
have usually been limited to one or a few points in time. With better information
on the cumulative exposure to known factors, with more appropriate measures of,
say, lipoprotein components and the noxious element in cigarette smoke, or with
the best "atherogenic" expression of elevated blood pressure, much more of the
variability in lesions would probably be explained. Although new risk factors
will likely "explain" another fraction of the variability in lesions, a residual
variability attributable to arterial "susceptibility" will certainly remain an
area of investigation.

ABSTRACT

STUDIES ON THE CHARACTERISTICS OF SERUM LIPID AND LIPOPROTEIN PATTERNS IN "NORMOLIPIDEMIC" ISCHEMIC HEART DISEASES

Takeshi Yamanaka, Chikayuki Naito, Tamio Teramoto, Hirokazu Kato, and Rihei Sato
First Department of Internal Medicine, Faculty of Medicine, University of Tokyo,
Tokyo/Japan

We studied on the lipid and lipoprotein fractions in sera of myocardial infarction (MI), angina pectoris (AP) and control groups, using routine chemical
methods, agarose gel (AGE) and polyacrylamide (PGE) electrophoresis and ultracentrifugation. While serum total cholesterol were almost equal among these three
groups, the concentration of free cholesterol, triglycerides, total phospholipids, total lipids and free fatty acids were higher in the AP and MI groups
than in control one. The percent concentration of pre-β, β and the ratio of β/α,
pre-$\beta+\beta/\alpha$ increased in the AP and MI groups significantly.
So-called extra pre-β lipoprotein (Elp) were seen in 18% cases of atherosclerotic
diseases (AS) by AGE, and 52% in AS, 38% in hypertension and 25% in controls by
PGE. Elp appeared and disappeared in the same individuals, but more consistently
appeared in persons with AS.
Lipid moiety in relation to protein moiety of VLDL and the ratio of total cholesterol in VLDL to serum triglycerides were higher in Elp(+) sera than Elp(-) ones.
These results suggested that even slight changes in serum lipid and lipoprotein
patterns might be related to atherogenesity.

Chairmen: W.L. Holmes, USA
          Y. Hata, Japan

Participants: S. Dayton, USA
              P. Leren, Norway
              J.L. de Gennes, France
              W.L. Holmes, USA

DIET AND CORONARY HEART DISEASE — PRIMARY PREVENTION TRIALS

Seymour Dayton

At least five trials of primary prevention of coronary heart disease by diet
have been reported, and all have been informative. This brief review will be limited to the three trials commonly considered to have been well controlled.

Let me first review the rationale for these difficult and costly studies. Particularly impressive are data from six prospective studies in the United States,
showing the now well-known increase in risk of ischemic heart disease as serum
cholesterol rises. This increase is evident even within the serum cholesterol
range 200-280 mg/dl, which is typical for most middle-aged Americans (Dayton,
1975). The international studies of Ancel Keys and his many collaborators not
only confirmed the relationship just cited, but also showed that intake of saturated fatty acid also is strongly correlated with incidence of ischemic heart
disease (Keys, 1970). In fact, this was the strongest single correlation encountered in those studies.

Although this information was not yet fully developed when prevention trials began in the late 1950s, many of the basic facts had begun to emerge. It seemed to
many investigators that the time for clinical tests was already at hand.

Let me first review our own trial, conducted in Los Angeles with the help of
many colleagues (Dayton et al., 1969). The subjects were middle-aged and elderly
men living in a home for military veterans. Those who volunteered were assigned
at random to experimental and control groups. In both groups, about 70% were
free of overt atherosclerotic complications. They were followed on a double
blind basis for periods averaging 6 years. Some men were followed for over 8
years.

We elected to use an experimental diet in which the type of fat was modified,
but the amount of fat was similar to that in the traditional American diet which
the control subjects received. Cholesterol content of the experimental diet was
reduced moderately.

The experimental group achieved and sustained a serum cholesterol level 13% lower than that of the control group.

Figure 1 summarizes the results in terms of atherosclerotic events. In each individual category, there were fewer events in the experimental group than in the
control group, but for no individual category was the difference statistically
significant. When these results were pooled, there were 96 men affected in the
control group and 66 in the experimental group. This difference was significant.

Most of the favorable effect was observed in the younger half of the population,
aged 54 - 65 when they entered the study. In analyses of results for fatal ath-

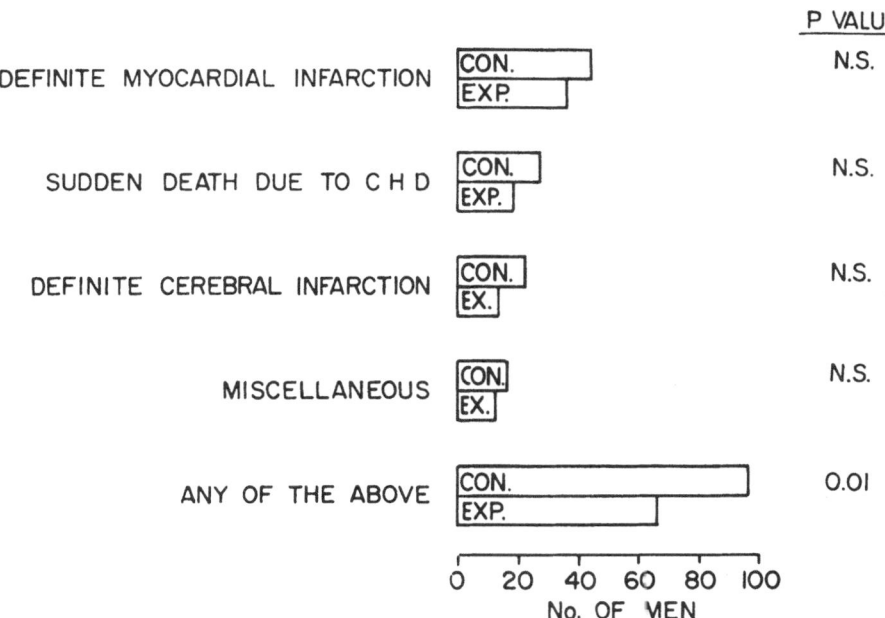

Figure 1. Main clinical end points in the Los Angeles trial

erosclerotic events, the difference in the younger stratum was particularly impressive (Dayton et al., 1969).

Some colleagues were surprised that we observed apparently favorable results at an age when coronary atherosclerosis is known to be quite advanced in many American men. But a year or two after the study was completed, the Framingham group reported age-specific data on many risk factors. This analysis showed that cholesterol still functions as a risk factor at age 65, although the gradient is less impressive than in younger men (Gordon and Verter).

Concurrently with our clinical trial, Turpeinen, Miettinen, and their colleagues conducted a trial in two mental hospitals in the Helsinki area. The diets were similar to those which our subjects received. Initially, one hospital's entire population received the control diet, while at the other hospital the experimental diet was served. Because the hospital populations differed in many ways, after years the diets were interchanged and the subjects were observed for additional years.

Table 1 summarizes the Helsinki trial's results in regard to death rates due to ischemic heart disease (Miettinen et al., 1972). Note that experimental rates were consistently lower than control rates. This is true if one compares the two hospitals or if one compares the two periods. The results in women appear less impressive than those in men. Not shown here are the data for electrocardiographic evidence of myocardial infarction. Those data produce a similar table — that is, a table with more favorable experience on the experimental diet (Miettinen et al., 1972).

These two trials had been reported at the time of the last International Symposium on Atherosclerosis in Berlin. Therefore, the most important news in this field is the completion of Frantz's study in seven mental hospitals in the state of Minnesota, USA. Like our own trial, Frantz's study randomized the participants and employed double blind follow-up technique. His experimental diet was more rigorous than those used in Los Angeles and Helsinki, and the experimental details were exceptionally meticulous. The resultant difference between experi-

Table 1. CHD death rates in the Helsinki study

| | | Age-adjusted CHD death rates per 1000 person-years | |
		Period 1 (6 years)	Period 2 (6 years)
		Experimental	Control
	Hospital N	5.7	13.0
Men		Control	Experimental
	Hospital K	15.8	7.5
		Experimental	Control
	Hospital N	4.0	7.7
Women		Control	Experimental
	Hospital K	8.1	6.5

Table 2. Major end points in the Minnesoty study of Frantz et al. (1975)

| | Age < 50 | | | | All ages | | | | | |
| | Men | | Women | | Men | | Women | | Combined | |
	Exp.	Con.	Exp.	Con.	Exp.	Con.	Exp.	Con.	Exp.	Con.
Number of subjects (person-years)	1192	1106	1124	1068	2505	2428	2417	2425	4922	4853
Myocardial infarct, sudden death, or stroke	3	10	6	6	67	78	67	51	134	129
All deaths	2	12	11	7	157	159	111	97	268	256

Table 3. Comparison of Los Angeles and Minnesota results stratified by age

Minnesota (trial duration = 4+ years)	Los Angeles (trial duration = 8+ years)
Age < 50: effective (in men only)	
Age > 50: ineffective	Age 54–65: effective
	Age > 65: ineffective

mental and control groups, in regard to serum cholesterol, was 14%. The study lasted 4 ½ years for some of the subjects.

Table 2 summarizes Frantz's results (Frantz et al., 1975). Let me first call your attention to the combined results for all ages and both sexes. Clearly, they show no evidence of benefit from the cholesterol-lowering diet. On the other hand, one subgroup appeared to experience a striking benefit: men under age 50.

Interpretation of these results certainly present a dilemma. Frantz has concluded that the experimental diet was ineffective.* Others may conclude that it is effective if started at an early enough age, but if so, that it will be difficult to explain the negative results in younger women.

The difference in results at different ages is superficially reminiscent of the Los Angeles results, but this point bears further examination. Table 3 compares the Los Angeles and Minnesota results. It is intended to emphasize that the young stratum in Minnesota was a good deal younger than the young stratum in Los Angeles. It is of interest to select from Frantz's data an age group close to our so-called young stratum. With Frantz's cooperation in making unpublished data available, I was able to establish that for ages 50-60 (roughly comparable to our younger stratum), his subjects showed little benefit, certainly none of statistical significance.

Duration of the Los Angeles trial was almost twice that of the Minnesoty study. This fact may help to account for some of the differences in outcome, that is, perhaps the longer study duration in Los Angeles explains the apparent effect in men 54-65 years old, whereas there was no effect in Minnesota among persons of comparable age.

Another problem in the outcome of all three trials is that, in the main, they fail to show significant effects on the most useful and convincing end point of all. I refer, of course, to death due to any cause. The main exception, you will recall, was among Frantz's subgroup of men under 50.

It is somewhat difficult to summarize, and certainly difficult to draw crisp and definitive conclusions. But the gloom which sometimes enters these discussions should be mitigated by several considerations. All three studies were too small, from a statistical viewpoint, to be sure that they would lead to definite conclusions. Possibly some or all of the trials were too brief; the appropriate duration for such a trial has always been an impenetrable issue. Remember that a man who is destined to have a myocardial infarct 3 years from today probably has advanced coronary atherosclerosis right now, regardless of his age. Perhaps, then, the candidates for meaningful dietary prevention are those with only mild atheromatosis at present. If this is the case, studies of 6 years or even much longer might be needed to show a convincing clinical effect. I don't seriously expect that anyone will ever undertake such a study. We may ultimately have to depend on end points other than clinical events. Meanwhile, we can only continue trying to give prudent advice based on inconclusive information.

---

*Presentation at the annual meeting of the Council on Arteriosclerosis, American Heart Association, Anaheim, California, November, 1975.

ATTEMPTS AT PRIMARY AND SECONDARY PREVENTION OF CORONARY HEART DISEASE

Paul Leren and Ingvar Hjermann

Secondary Prevention: A Monofactorial Diet Study

This trial includes 412 men, aged 30-64, discharged from medical departments in Oslo with a first diagnosis of myocardial infarction. The men were randomly allocated to the experimental, diet group and to the control group 1-2 years, an average of 20 months, after the infarction. Factors of age and clinical severity were successfully randomized.
Detailed reports have previously been published (Leren, 1966, 1970).

Diet

The diet was low in animal fats and dietary cholesterol and rich in vegetable oil (Table 1).

Cholesterol Reduction

The average serum cholesterol reduction during 5 years was 17.6% in the diet group (Fig. 1).

5-Year Results

There was a statistically significant lower incidence of myocardial reinfarction and of new angina pectoris in the diet group. The incidence of sudden death was the same in the two groups.
Table 2 presents the major events, showing a statistically reduced incidence of major CHD relapses. However, the differences in total cardiovascular deaths and in total deaths did not reach the 5% level of significance, although the same positive trends are present.

A 11-year follow-up showed that at age 60 and below, the serum cholesterol level was significantly lower in the survivors as compared with those who died of CHD (Table 3).

Table 1. Daily food intake of experimental group as measured during initial 5-year study

	Grams	% of calories
Carbohydrates (total)	269	45.5
Sugar	51	
Protein	92	15.0
Fat (total)	104	39.0
Saturated fat	22	8.5
Monounsaturated fat	27	10.1
Polyunsaturated fat	55	20.7
Dietary cholesterol	0.264	20.7
P/S ratio		2.4

P/S = ratio of polyunsaturated fat to saturated fat.

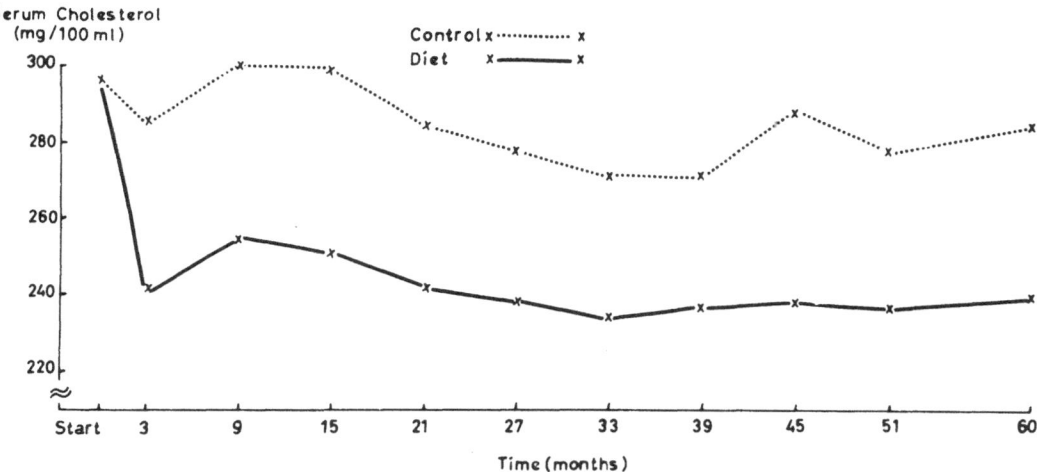

Figure 1. Mean serum cholesterol levels during the first 5 years of observation time

	N (at entry)	Value at entry (mg/100 ml)	Mean reduction (mg)	(%)
Control	206	296	11	3.7
Diet	206	296	52	17.6

Table 2. 5-year results

	Diet	Control
No. of men at risk	206	206
Fatal myocardial reinfarction	10	23
Sudden death	27	27
Nonfatal myocardial reinfarction	24	31
Major CHD relapses[a]	61	81
Total cardiovascular mortality[b]	38	52
Total mortality[c]	41	55

[a] p 0.05.   [b] p 0.09.   [c] p 0.13.

Table 3. 11-year report: mean serum cholesterol value in survivors and patients dead of CHD in relation to age

	Diet group at age		Control group at age		Both groups at age	
	<60	>60	<60	>60	<60	>60
Died of CHD	261[a]	248	301	276	281	265
Survivors	248	246	285	282	265	265

[a] Values in mg/100 ml.

Primary Prevention: An On-going Bifactorial, Diet-Anticigarette Study

In the Oslo study, 1972-73, 18,000 men, aged 20-49, were screened for CHD risk factors (Leren et al., 1975).
The age curve for serum cholesterol shows a steep increase from about 200 at age 20 to about 270 at age 50. When this age cholesterol curve is drawn separately for cigarette smokers, ex-cigarette smokers and noncigarette smokers (Fig. 2), three separate cholesterol age curves emerge, smokers at the top, nonsmokers at the bottom, and ex-smokers in between. Thus, a significant intercorrelation between the serum cholesterol level and cigarette smoking exists.

Among 16,000 men, aged 40-49, 1232 healthy men with a calculated CHD risk in the upper decile, as judged from serum cholesterol and number of cigarettes smoked, were randomly allocated to an experimental group and a control group, to see whether a change in eating and smoking habits would influence future incidence of CHD.

Table 4 presents some data of the two groups. The mean cholesterol level at onset was 330 mg/dl and 80% were daily cigarette smokers. All men were normotensive (syst. B.P. <150 mm Hg) and had a negative exercise ECG test.

Figures 3 and 4 present cholesterol values in the treatment and control groups. A 15% reduction has been maintained for 3 years in the treatment group.
Figure 5 presents the triglyceride values. In the treatment group, fasting triglycerides have been reduced by 14.5% and the nonfasting by 24.7%. In the control group, no reduction of fasting and nonfasting triglycerides has occurred.
Daily cigarette smoking has been reduced to one third, from an average of 13.5 to 4.6 cigarettes a day, while the controls have reduced daily cigarettes from 12.8 to 11.4 (Fig. 6).
Figure 7 shows that body weights have decreased by 3 kg in the treatment group in spite of the smoking reduction. In those who have stopped smoking, body weight

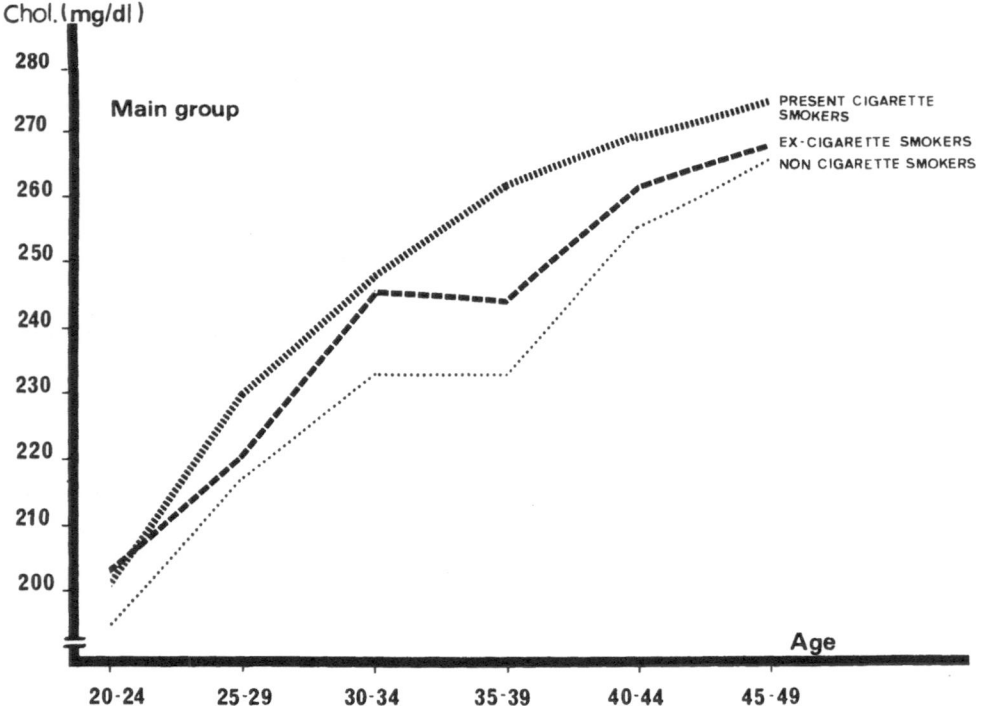

Figure 2. Serum cholesterol by age in different groups of smokers (Oslo study)

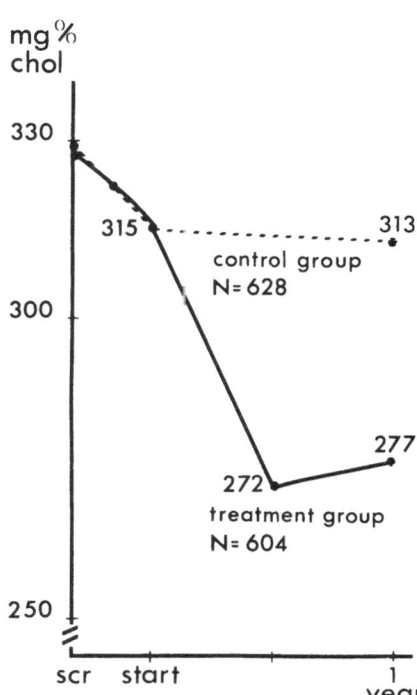

Figure 3. Dietetic lowering of serum
cholesterol (Oslo study)

shows a slight increase early in the study. However, this increase tends to be
overcome after some 2–3 years (Fig. 8).
Whether these changes in lipids and in smoking will influence future CHD rate
will be reported when the study has lasted for 5 years.

Table 4. Oslo study: smoking-lipid primary
prevention trial.
Age: 40–49; n: 1232; men

Treatment group	Control group
n = 604	n = 628
Chol. mean 330	Chol. mean 330
80% cig. smokers	80% cig. smokers

Randomized controlled trial. Duration 5
years.

Statisticians have calculated that the chances for obtaining statistical significance in this trial is 85%, provided that the 5-year CHD incidence is reduced by
50% in the treatment group as compared with the controls.

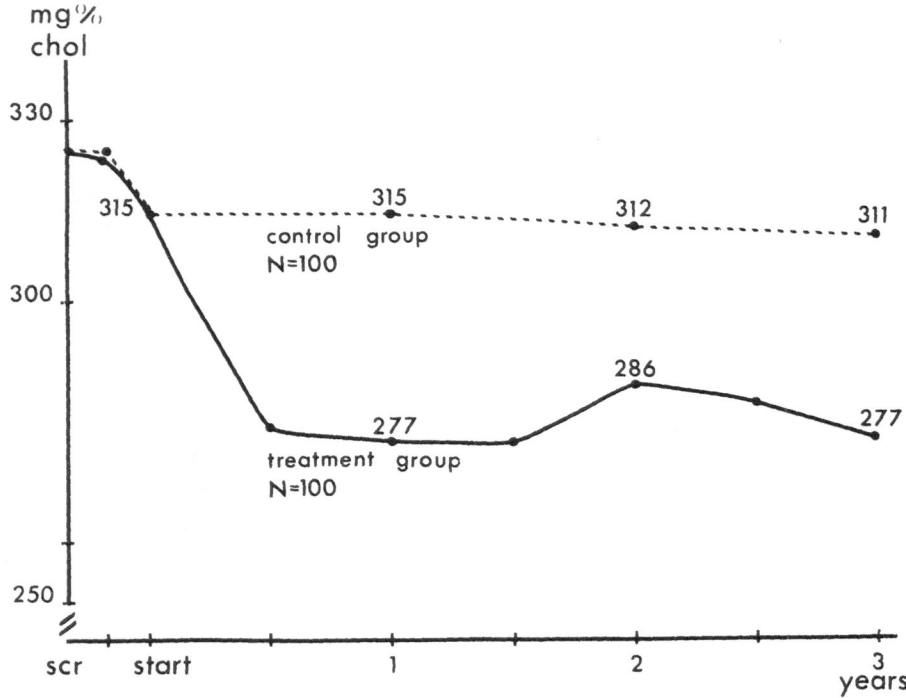

Figure 4. Dietetic lowering of serum cholesterol (Oslo study)

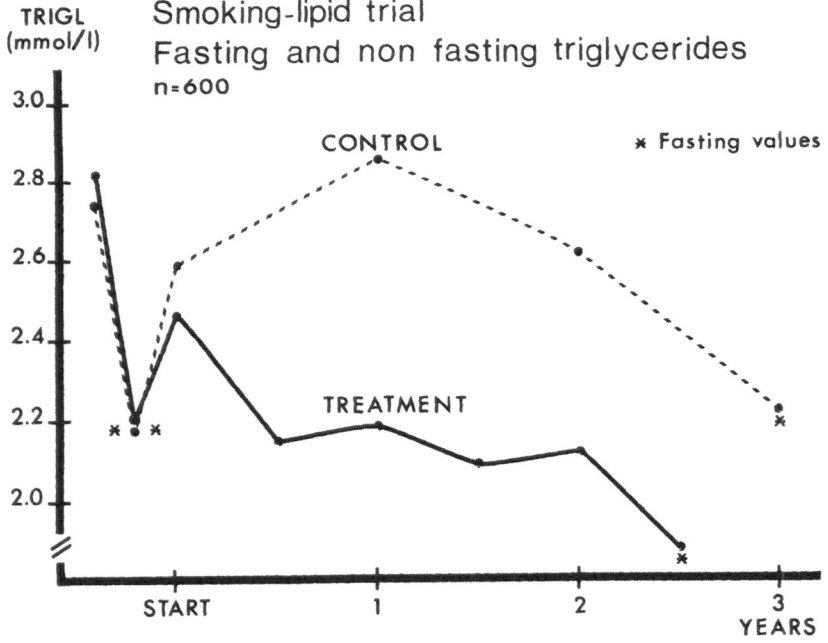

Figure 5. Dietetic lowering of serum triglycerides (Oslo study)

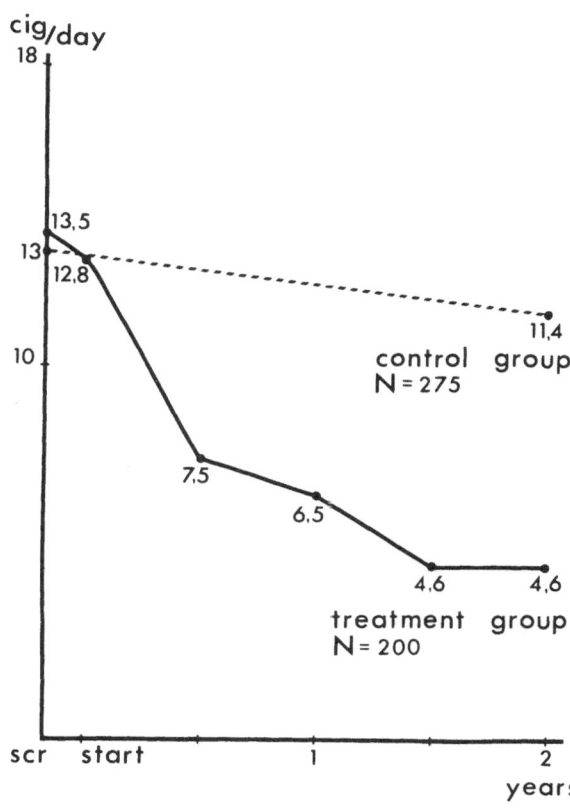

Figure 6. Effect on cigarette consumption by anticigarette counseling (Oslo study)

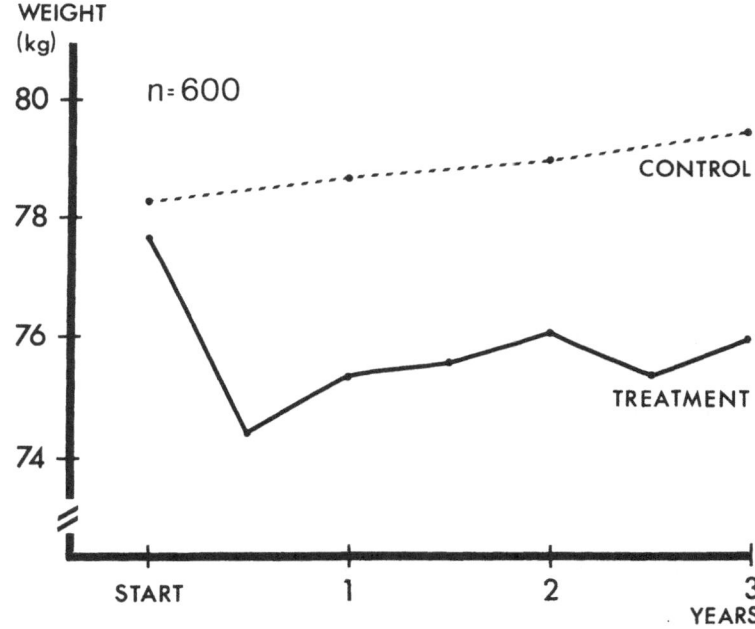

Figure 7. Body weight in smoking-lipid trial (Oslo study)

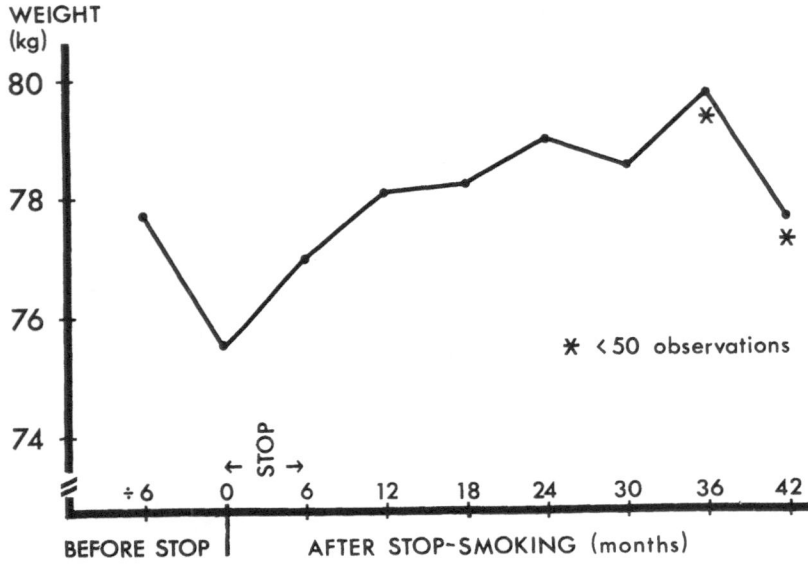

Figure 8. Effect on body weight before and after cessation of smoking (Oslo study)

INTERVENTION TRIAL FOR SECONDARY CV PREVENTION IN PRIMARY ATHERO-GENOUS HYPERLIPIDEMIAS

J.L. de Gennes

The positive benefit of correcting blood lipid or lipoprotein disorders in secondary CV prevention is still controversial because of lack of convincing evidence. Negative results, primarily those of the Coronary Drug Project, have
caused many people not only to accept that the correction of blood lipid disorders plays only a minor role in secondary CV prevention, but even to promote
this viewpoint.

It is difficult to understand this new view of denying the role of blood lipid
disorders in progressive and even accelerated atherosclerosis, and one must be
anxious about the potential hazards, even risks, of such a negative attitude.
One is obliged to recognize first that the substance of the problem is not easy
to elucidate because of the approximate and poorly defined clinical criteria of
defining atherosclerosis.
The situation has been further confused by recent statistical studies, such as
the Coronary Drug Project (Stamler, 1975) which, in considering the role of correcting lipids, took into account decreases of blood lipids as minor as 8%. So,
to check the CV benefit, even in secondary prevention, of correction of blood
lipid disorders in well-defined and well-identified atherogenic primary hyperlipidemias, it is highly desirable to include an elective evaluation and correction of other environmental and endogenous risk factors and to compare the results with very strict biological correction of lipids only.

We are only able to present, in this field, some preliminary results or approaches which do not suggest the undesirability of the specific treatment of
blood lipid disorders and which certainly do not allow us to give up any method-
ic and effective trials along these lines.

686

Although we are perfectly conscious of the eventual complexity of discriminating and evaluating all the important factors in such studies of secondary CV prevention, we have chosen, as a first approach to the problem, the use of simple methodology in a retrospective study that we are only now ready to present.

1. Selection of patients first, according not only to a precise definition of their lipid metabolic disease using classical typing and genetic information but also successive exclusions as follows:

    a. Of sex, (including only males).

    b. Of major additional risk factors such as: overt diabetes, severe hypertension, heavy tobacco smoking (≥20 cigarettes/day), and major irreducible overweight.

    c. As far as the first CV clinical criterion is concerned, we have selected only coronary ischemic disease (CID), either as angina or as myocardial infarction, in order to avoid a too controversial heterogeneity of cardiovascular damage. All the patients were entered into the study at least 3 months after their myocardial infarction (MI) or first symptoms of angina.

2. Selection of standardized therapeutic measures, including:

    a. Two standardized model diets set up by us: one model hypocaloric diet utilized first in cases of needed weight reduction (total calories 1000: 39% as fat, 36% as carbohydrate, and 25% as protein) and one alternative (or consecutive) model of long-term normocaloric hypolipidemic diet (2500 cal: 40% as fat, 40% as carbohydrate, 20% as protein, 17% as polyunsaturated fat, and cholesterol ≤300 mg).

    b. Standardized choice and posology of drug therapy including: clofibrate at a dosage of 1500 - 2000 mg per day in every case of mixed hyperlipidemia (MH) and in a large number of essential familial hypercholesterolenias (EFH) and cholestyramine at a daily dosage of 16 - 24 g in association with clofibrate, only in EFH tendinosum xanthomas (TX).

Of course, the majority of these patients have received, because of their ischemic heart disease, other therapeutic prescriptions, such as anticoagulants, vasodilators, ß-blockers, and neuroleptics, but the common use of all these drugs made no important or significant difference between subgroups of subjects with or without CV recurrence or new events.

3. In order to avoid the immediate objections to nonrandomization and noncomparative study of patients not treated for their blood lipid disorders in this program, the objective of this trial was simply limited to an *internal comparison of the follow-up during 3-5 years of their CV evolution, according to their long-term blood lipid response and the quality of the biological correction during the same period of time.*

4. The statistical analysis of these findings was conducted in several different ways. First we tested a large-scale and simple computer (IBM) program on analysis of contingence tables, with evaluation of CHI square test.
We studied 121 MH and 52 EFH of type IIa.

Thus, 173 patients were reviewed according to qualitative criteria or gradations of CV evolution and blood lipid correction. The grades of correction were estimated as percentage of correction of excess of starting levels of total cholesterol and triglycerides versus ideal age-adjusted levels, derived from personal studies and calculations for the French male population (Turpin et al., 1973). Four grades of blood lipid lowering correction have been set up: (1) <25%, (2) ≥25%, (3) ≥50%, and (4) ≥75%. Comparative gradation of CV evolution included three gradations: (1) improvement, (2) status quo, and (3) recurrent or new CV events.

The total cholesterol (TC) decrease index, which is defined as:

$$\frac{\text{mean TC before treatment } - \text{mean TC after treatment}}{\text{mean TC before treatment}}$$

was measured in 39 carefully selected type IIa with TX and the statistical difference between the group of patients with CV recurrence and the group without
CV recurrence was determined by the t test. In a special group of 41 MG cases
resistant to the usual and previously described treatment, the absence of a significant reduction of blood lipid abnormalities allows a direct estimation of
their CV prognosis when there is no effective treatment of blood lipid disorders.

Results

The results shown in Table 1 reflect, in the first large-scale computer study of
contingence analysis, a significant correlation between CV-favorable evolution
and quality of biological correction, but only in the series of 121 MH while a
statistical significance was not observed in the first series of 52 cases of EFH,
perhaps because of the small number of CV relapses or new events.

Therefore, we decided to recheck this last group of hyperlipidemics (type IIa) by
analyzing the results on a more severe form of EFH with TX in 39 consecutive
cases. In this study (Table 2), the results were more clear-cut than in the previous one (Table 1) probably because of the usually more severe CV evolution in
this gradation of EFH. Also, the blood lipid correction was significantly better
in the group without CV recurrence than in the group with.

In the selected final series of 41 MH resistant to treatment, the complete absence of decrease in abnormal blood lipid values permits a direct comparison
with the previous group of 121 MH as shown in Table 4, and clearly reflects the
excessively high prevalence of CV recurrence in this particular subgroup giving
strong support to the role of uncorrected blood lipid abnormalities in accelerated CV evolution of these cases.

Incidentally, it is worthwhile to notice in Table 4 that our figures for CV recurrence are rather better than the ordinary figures given for coronary evolution; we personally think that the help of anticoagulant therapy which has been
pursued in almost every case cannot be excluded for different reasons in this
special type of hyperlipidemia (MH).

In summary, this preliminary analysis of our therapeutic trial in CV secondary
prevention for idiopathic hyperlipidemias indicates a substantial and signifi-

Table 1. First results of IBM computer program

		χ^2	Probability of occurrence[a]	Hypothesis of interaction accepted[b]
EHC n = 51		5.8081	0.2410	/ (No)
(24 + XT)		(7.3385)	(0.3981)	
MH n = 121	↘ CT ↘ TG	3.0219	0.0366	+ (Yes)
	↘ CT	1.6724	0.0043	++ (Yes)
	↘ TG	8.1423	0.4801	/ (No)

[a] Probability of occurrence of such χ^2 if is no correlation.

[b] Interaction between improvement of lipid levels and
cardiovascular improvement.

cant benefit for correcting blood lipid disorders in reducing the frequency of
CV recurrence or new events as compared to results previously reported. These
findings provide a strong incentive for continuing and expanding this work.

Table 2. Follow-up study of 39 XTHF on a standardized secondary prevention trial
(diet and drug)

CV recurrence or new events	With	Without	Statistical significance
Number of patients	43 Mean survey: 3 years (1.6 - 5 years)	26 Mean survey: 4.5 years (3 - 9 years)	NS
Mean age (range)	42.8 years (18 - 56 years)	43.7 years (18 - 67 years)	NS
Initial TC (mg/100 ml) level	466	477 mg	NS
Therapeutic TC stabilized level	407 (- 12.6%)	375 mg (- 21.4%)	p <0.05[a]
Other risk factors	Tobacco HTA 31% Overweight 23% Patent diabetes 8%	28% 44%	NS NS NS
Other treatments	Anticoagulants 11/13	17/26	NS

[a]TC decrease index : $\dfrac{\overline{TC}\text{ before treatment} - \overline{TC}\text{ under treatment}}{\overline{TC}\text{ before treatment}}$.

Table 3. Further analysis of correlation in 39 XTHF (IIa+TX) between TC decrease
index and CV evolution on a secondary prevention trial

With recurrence		Without recurrence	Level cf statistical significance
New CV events in any territory	n = 13 patients index[a] = 12.6%	n = 26 index = 21.4%	p <0.05
New CV events from only one arterial involvement	n = 12 index = 12.0%	n = 23 index = 21.5%	p <0.05
New CV events from only coronary involvement	n = 10 index = 13.0%	n = 18 index = 23.3%	p <0.02
New CV events outside coronary areas	n = 6 index = 2.7%	n = 26 index = 21.4%	p <0.01

[a]TC decrease index: $\dfrac{TC\text{ before treatment} - TC\text{ under treatment}}{TC\text{ before treatment}}$.

Table 4. CV evolution ($\bar{m}$ 4 years) in MH compared with biological (lipid) evolution

CV grades grades lipid correction	Amelioration		Status quo		Aggregation or new CV events	
	n	%	n	%	n	%
Without consistent correction n = 9	3	33%	4	44%	2	22%
Partial or dissociated correction n = 25	9	36%	9	36%	7	28%
Perfect correction[a] n = 86	40	37%	40	47%	6	8%
MH resistant n = 41	4	9.8%	26	63.4%	11	26.8%

[a]Perfect correction means return to normal blood CT and TG values, adjusted for age and sex.

THE MULTIPLE RISK FACTOR INTERVENTION TRIAL (MRFIT)

William L. Holmes

The Multiple Risk Factor Intervention Trial was initiated by the National Heart, Lung and Blood Institute in 1971, in accordance with recommendations made earlier that year by a task force on atherosclerosis (Hew, 1971). It is a randomized, nondouble blind clinical trial of the efficacy of modifying multiple risk factors (elevated blood lipid levels, hypertension, and cigarette smoking) for the reduction of coronary heart disease mortality. The first eight participating clinical centers were selected in June of 1972, followed by the addition of 12 others during the next 18 months. Also established in 1972 were a coordinating center at the University of Minnesota, a central laboratory at the Pacific Medical Center in San Francisco, and electrocardiography centers at the University of Minnesoty and Dalhousie University in Halifax, Nova Scotia.

During the first year and a half the steering committee, comprised of the principal investigators of the clinical and ancillary centers and NHLBI staff, developed a protocol and manual of operations. The original proposal for a 6-year trial involving 11,000 male participants 40-59 years of age was modified to increase the population size selected to 12,000 and to broaden the age range from 35 to 57 years. The primary end point selected was death ascribed to coronary heart disease. The participants selected were to be in the upper 15% of the population distribution for risk of coronary heart disease as determined by serum cholesterol level, blood pressure, and degree of smoking by the Framingham Study predictions of risk. As the trial progressed (28% of participants screened), a number of considerations encouraged the steering committee to make the eligibility criterion somewhat more rigorous, hence only the upper 10% of the population distribution were selected from the final 72% of the population screened. Participants selected through a process of three screening visits (S_1, S_2 and S_3) would be randomized at S_3. Half of the group would be referred to their usual source of medical care and half would be entered into a 6-year intensive intervention program aimed at modifying their particular risk factors.

Screening

At S_1, the participants are introduced to the purposes and methods of the trial and are administered a brief questionnaire concerning cigarette consumption, geographic mobility, current treatment for diabetes, and extended hospitalization for heart attack. Systolic and diastolic blood pressures are determined three times and a nonfasting blood sample is obtained for determination of serum cholesterol.

Eligible participants from S_1 are invited to S_2 which consists of the following: a review of medical history and physical examination, measurement of height, weight, and blood pressure, urinalysis, resting ECG, PA chest x-ray, pulmonary function test, 1-hour glucose tolerance, and a battery of clinical chemistry tests including lipoprotein phenotyping.

Participants returning to S_3 complete a social-behavioral physical activity questionnaire at home. At the third visit, blood pressure is taken again, a baseline and exercise ECG are obtained, a smoking questionnaire is administered, and a 24-hour food recall is done by a nutritionist. After the participant has again had the trial explained to him and he signs a consent form to participate, he is randomized by the coordinating center into either the special intervention group or the usual care group.

The results of the screening phase of the trial completed in February, 1976 are summarized in Table 1. Seven percent of the participants seen at S_1 were eligible to return for S_2. In addition to ineligibility on the basis of a low risk factor score, participants were excluded if a history of myocardial infarction, a presence of diabetes mellitus, a serum cholesterol ≥ 350 mg%, a diastolic blood pressure of 115 mm Hg, or a suggestion of geographic mobility were determined. The overall exclusion rate at S_2 was 28%. About half of these were excluded because of evidence (Rose questionnaire and ECG) of coronary heart disease and the other half for reasons of dietary habit, other disease or specific medications, general unwillingness to participate, specific refusal to stop smoking, and obesity. A further 9% were excluded at S_3, mostly because of unwillingness to participate and a few because of chest x-ray findings or changes in the resting ECG between S_2 and S_3. The number of participants finally randomized, 12,854, represents approximately half of those meeting eligibility requirements at S_1.

A comparison of the average risk factor levels for men attending S_1, the "risk eligible group" for S_2, and the final randomized population is given in Table 2. The risk eligible group had a serum cholesterol level and diastolic blood pressure considerably greater than the mean value for all men attending S_1. The level of both variables decreased appreciably between S_1 and randomization, primarily because of regression toward the mean; however, the serum cholesterol is still 25.2 mg% and the diastolic blood pressure 6.7 mm Hg greater than the average for all men screened. The risk eligible and final randomized groups smoked an average of two to two and one-half times as many cigarettes per day as the entire group. Of the men attending S_1, 63% professed to be nonsmokers whereas only 40% of the randomized group fell into this category.

Intervention

The special care group attended ten integrated intervention sessions of approximately 2 hours each at weekly intervals. Each group was comprised of 10-12 participants and their spouses. The steering committee devoted an intensive effort to the selection and preparation of appropriate educational materials including films, slides, booklets, and pamphlets, all especially designed for the trial. The strategies of these sessions combined factual education, selected principles from the disciplines of behavior modification and group dynamics, and the use of group process to facilitate change in a supportive atmosphere.

Table 1. Yield summary - MRFIT screening

Visit	No. of men seen	% of those eligible	Eligible for next visit Number	Percent
S_1	366,287	–	25,350	7
S_2	22,400	87	15,800	72
S_3	14,200	90	12,854	90

Table 2. Comparison of risk factor levels at S_1 and baseline (S_2 or S_3)

	Men attending S_1 (N = 366,287)		Risk eligible for S_2 (N = 25,357)		Randomized men (N = 12,064)	
	Mean	SD	Mean	SD	Mean	SD
Age (years	45.9	–	46.6	–	–	–
Serum cholesterol (mg/dl)	219.0	40.5	255.1	37.5	244.2	37.3
Diastolic B.P. (mm Hg)	83.9	10.7	99.3	7.8	90.6	9.8
Number cigarettes/day	9.5	14.9	23.4	20.4	20.0	20.1

Emphasis in nutrition was on the use of an overall balanced diet low in saturated fat and cholesterol. The basic diet was planned to provide 30% of calories in the form of fat, less than 10% from saturated fatty acids and 10-13% from polyunsaturated fatty acids, approximately 300 mg of cholesterol per day, and modification of carbohydrate as required. A step-care program of weight reduction followed by appropriate drugs, if necessary, was selected for the management of hypertension. The smoking modality emphasized complete cessation using a variety of techniques, special supporting materials, and audiovisual aids.

Upon completion of intervention, all special care participants are seen regularly at intervals of 4 months. The usual care participants return annually for a medical history, physical examination, and laboratory studies. Those special care participants who attained risk factor modification goals are entered into a maintenance program. Those not attaining goals are placed in an extended intervention program. This includes frequent visits for management of hypertension, monthly or bimonthly visits for nutrition counseling, and determination of serum cholesterol for those individuals having difficulty in reducing their cholesterol level, and other special counseling sessions either individually or in small focal groups.

Summary

The successful completion of the planning, recruiting, and intervention phases of MRFIT have clearly demonstrated the feasibility and practicality of undertaking such a large, expensive, complex, multicenter, and multidisciplinary clinical trial. The accomplishments to date are a tribute to the many dedicated staff members, participants, and others who have contributed so freely and generously to the conduct of the trial. Although the final results will not be available for another 6 years, it might be anticipated that important knowledge will be gained with respect to prevention of coronary heart disease which will be of benefit not only to the MRFIT participants but to countless thousands of persons throughout the world.

PRACTICAL APPROACH BY HISTOCHEMICAL, ENZYMOLOGICAL AND IMMUNOLOG-
ICAL STUDIES OF THE CELLULAR AND INTERCELLULAR LESIONS IN MYOCAR-
DIAL ISCHEMIA AND INFARCTION

J. Roland, F. Chatelet, P. Chiche, S. Witchitz, and C. Seban
Laboratoire Central d'Anatomie-Pathologie et Service de Cardiologie de l'Hôpital
Tenon, Faculté de Médecine Saint-Antoine, Paris/France

Studies were carried out on the heart of patients prematurely deceased from myocardial infarction during intensive care treatment and also in cases of sudden
death in relation to coronary disease.
Macro enzymological (succinate dehydrogenase and β OH butyrate dehydrogenase),
standard histochemical, histoenzymological and histoimmunological (albumin, fibrin, and various types of immunoglobulins) techniques were used.
Thus the increased vascular permeability at the level of the terminal vascular
bed, the cell membrane damage permeability of the myocardial cells were estimated. Also the relation between clinical course and accurate topography of
interstitial and cellular damage was assessed; and a study of a natural history
of myocardial damage during the course of coronary disease with rapid evolution
to death was performed.

HISTOLOGICAL EFFECT OF CHINOIN-123 ON EXPERIMENTAL ATHEROSCLEROSIS

Ferenc Schneider, Árpád Hesz, Gábor Lusztig, and Sándor Virág
Pathology Institut and Research Laboratory of County Hospital, Kecskemét/Hungary

The effect of "Chinoin 123" on atherogenic-diet fed rabbits was investigated.
Plaque-planimetry of the aorta was carried out. Histologically the aortic wall
was investigated by normal light, and polarizing microscope.
Authors concluded, "Chinoin 123" having influence in development of aortic lesions.

THE PIGMENTATION OF HUMAN ATHEROMATOUS PLAQUES BY BILE PIGMENTS IN
THE CASES OF OBSTRUCTIVE JAUNDICE

Kyoh Adachi, and Teruyuki Nakashima
The Second Department of Pathology, Kurume University, School of Medicine,
Kurume/Japan

The aortic atherosclerotic plaques of the patients with obstructive jaundice
frequently look distinctly green after formalin fixation due to conversion of
infiltrated serum bilirubin into biliverdin. The intensity of staining of plaques
is often much more prominent than that of neighboring non-atherosclerotic intima.
The infiltration of bile pigment into the plaques was traced by making 50 100
serial cryostat sections. It was revealed that the entrance of bile pigment was
situated very often at the peripheral ridge of atheroma, and sometimes the pigment came through vasa vasorum originated from aortic branches. It was also recognized that bilirubin precipitation showed close relationship between lipid-
or fibrin depositions.

CONSULTATION BUREAU (CB) HEART PROJECT IN THE NETHERLANDS. IMPLE-
MENTATION OF A CORONARY PREVENTION PROGRAMM IN CHEST CLINICS

A.C. Arntzenius, J.H. de Haas, H.A. van Geuns, T.L. Mellema, J. Meijer, D.P. Sluyter, and K. Styblo
Royal Netherlands Tuberculosis Association (KNCV), Riouwstraat 7, Den Haag/ The Netherlands

The CB-Heart Project, a community project on coronary risk factor modification is financed by the Ministry of Health. The present study refers to the period March 1973 - March 1974, when 5560 persons were examined; 3674 of which belonged to the general populations of Doetinchem (ages 35-49)and of Tilburg (40-42 yrs), whereas 1886 were school employees in Rotterdam (20-40 yrs). Cholesterol levels rank The Netherlands under countries with high levels: 1243 (22%) had "border-line" values (240-280 mg%) and 538 (9%) "elevated" ones ($\geq$280 mg%). Bloodpressure (BP) results: 290 (5%) proved to have "elevated" BP's ($\geq$160 and/or $\geq$105 mmHg), and 717 (13%) "borderline" BP values (140/95 - 159/104). Of the 290 persons with "elevated" BP, 166 (57%) were newly detected and only 36 (14%) were being treated with drugs at the time of examination. Of the 2625 men, 832 (32%) smoked at least 15 cigarettes/day and 533 (20%) 5-14.
The CB-network can be used to recruit persons for coronary risk screening, it can devise a program and train a staff to provide reliable characterization of risk factors in those screened and high risk individuals will return in reasonable numbers (90%) for continued advice.

PATHOGENETIC ASPECTS OF INTERRELATIONS OF ARTERIAL HYPERTENSION AND
ATHEROSCLEROSIS IN AN EXPERIMENT

Igor K. Shkhvatsabaya, and A.L. Myasnikov
Institute of Cardiology AMS USSR, Moscow/USSR

Possible participation of emotional stress in the origin of arterial hypertension (AH) and atherosclerosis (A) is illustrated by experimental data obtained on rabbits with repeated 4-months irritation of hypothalamus, which led to stable increase of serum cholesterol and triglycerides (on an average by 43% and 75%, respectively) and to slight (on an average by 10%) but stable rise of arterial pressure (AP). More significant rise of AP (on an average by 50%) was obtained in repeated and long-term irritation of different regions of hypothalamus of cholesterol-fed rabbits. In rabbits with cerebro-ischemic hypertension induced by successive occlusion of extracerebral arteries we found by the 60th day of the experiment rise in AP, hypercholesterinemia and increase of renin-plasma activity of blood as well as thickening of arterial walls. In the aortas of cholesterol-fed rabbits (group I) and in normal rabbits (group II) 1 day later after 4-hour irritation of the anterior and posterior hypothalamus causing increase of AP we revealed predominance of processes of synthesis over catabolism of collagen in group I and retardation of synthesis in simultaneous potentiation of collagen catabolism in group II. Differences in the markedness of A in various forms of AH might be due to diverse changes of blood kinin system in animals with cerebro-ischemic and renovascular hypertension.

EFFECTS OF HYPOXIA, HYPERTENSION AND VESSEL WALL NECROSIS ON THE INTIMA AS STUDIED BY SCANNING ELECTRON MICROSCOPY. INFLUENCE OF MEDICATION ON THE HYPOXIC DAMAGE

H. Jellinek, Gabriella Elemér, and S. Virág
The Second Department of Pathology, Semmelweis Medical University, Budapest/
Hungary

Authors have studied the changes of the intima in hypoxia, hypertension or after acid treatment induced necrosis. The endothelial cells were destroyed the regeneration of the endothelial layer started already after 2 hours. More extensive damage resulted in the complete denudation of large areas. The subendothelial mucopolysaccharide layer was set free together with some collagen fibres. Not infrequently even the elastic fibres were denuded. In these very severe damages the regeneration process started from the endothelial cells along the adges. These cells exhibit characteristic features in scanning electron microscopy. At the end of the regeneration phase the surfaces of the endothelial cells appear normal. Occasional macrophages and leukocytes were detected by both methods. The changes described were identical in three independent experiments. The application of medication to animals with hypoxic vessel damage had two effects. First the damage was less pronounced as compared to the controlls, secondly the incidence of mitotic cells was higher and the regeneration speedier.

THE EFFECTS OF CARBON MONOXIDE EXPOSURE ON ATHEROSCLEROSIS IN THE WHITE CARNEAU PIGEON

R.F. Davies and D.M. Turner
Hazleton Laboratories Europe Ltd., Harrogate/England

We have exposed female white carneau pigeons to 150 ppm carbon monoxide (CO) for six hours a day and five days a week for periods of up to 84 weeks. The level of CO exposure was sufficient to produce a mean level of 10% COHb. CO exposure for 52 weeks caused a significant increase in the degree of coronary atherosclerosis in birds fed a standard diet containing 1% additional cholesterol. Differences between this group and the controls disappeared however during a further 32 weeks of exposure essentially because of an increased incidence of disease in the controls. The level of cholesterol in the diet is critical since 0.5% or 1% addition to the diet over a 52 week period gives rise to increased coronary artery disease in CO exposed birds whereas after 2% cholesterol feeding the incidence of disease is identical in both CO and control groups. Reduced triglyceride (TG) and phospholipid (PL) levels have been observed in the aortae of some birds exposed to CO for 52 weeks. By analogy with the observed inhibitory effects of CO on triglyceride metabolism in hepatic tissue it is suggested that CO inhibits the arterial synthesis of TG and PL.

ARTERIAL LESIONS BY OXIDATION PRODUCTS OF CHOLESTEROL

Hideshige Imai, V. Subramanyam, Nicholas T. Werthessen, and Albert H. Soloway
Pathology, Albany Medical College, Albany, NY; Northeastern University, Boston,
MA; Brown University, Providence, RI/USA

Short-term effects of specific oxidative derivatives of cholesterol on the arterial wall were examined in the rabbit. Physiological saline suspension of 25-hydroxycholesterol or cholestane-3beta,5alpha,6beta-triol was injected through the ear vein for 3 days. The doses were 5 and 10 mg/ml/kg. Controls were given cholesterol purified via dibromination or the vehicle alone. The pulmonary vasculature and aorta were pressure perfusion-fixed with buffered 3% glutaraldehyde at 20 to 25 mmHg on the 4th day under anesthesia with pentobarbital sodium. These cholesterol derivatives induced grossly visible, segmental thickening of the pulmonary arteries, but not of the aorta. These oxidative products were synergistic: the 1/2 dose of each combined induced a greater pulmonary arterial response than either agent alone at the full dose. Purified cholesterol or saline alone induced minimal changes that were grossly not visible. Pulmonary arterial changes induced by these cholesterol derivatives included those of acute necrotizing arteritis with exudation of true eosinophiles, relatively uninjured endothelium and adventitia, and those of intimal diffuse fibrous thickening. Supported by USPHS NIH Grant HL-14177.

ULTRASTRUCTURAL AND HISTOENZYMATIC BEHAVIOR OF AORTIC MYOCYTES DURING CALCIFEROL-INDUCED MEDIAL CALCINOSIS

P. Hadjiisky, J. Renais, and L. Scebat
Centre de Recherches Cardiologiques, Hôpital Boucicaut, Paris/France

Ultrastructural, histoenzymatic (28 enzymes activities-EA) and histochemical studies were performed at various stages of rat aortic medial calcification induced by hypervitaminosis D2 (4-8000 UI during 15, 30, 45, 90 and 120 days). The results indicate that some histoenzymatic changes precede the calcifying process. Later, during the medial calcinosis some round shaped, RNA enriched cells persisted in and around the calcified foci. They had the ultrastructural aspect of modified and morphogenetically activated myocytes. Furthermore these cells presented an enzyme hyperactivity (phosphatases; E.A. linked to Krebs cycle, pentoses pathway, glycolysis, lipogenesis, GAG and glycogen metabolism; lysosomial E.A.). Similarly these foci of medial calcinosis accumulated glycoproteins, GAG and acidic lipids. The present findings suggest that the modified and activated myocytes could favorably influence and accelerate the metastatic aortic calcification.

DEGENERATION OF AORTIC SMOOTH MUSCLE CELLS IN SWINE FED EXCESS VITAMIN D3

Akinori Kamio, Fred A. Kummerow, and Hideshige Imai
The Harlan E. Moore Heart Research Foundation, Champaign, IL/USA

Twenty-eight weanling swine were divided into 2 groups and fed a basal ration of corn and soybean meal or the basal ration containing a high fat and cholesterol supplement. One of the subgroups of each received 220,000 IU of vitamin D_3/kg. Distal abdominal aortas were used for quantitative comparison by electron microscopy of degenerated smooth muscle cells. Degeneration was classified into rarefaction and condensation and the frequency expressed per 100 nucleated cells. Statistical significance in the frequency of dead cells was demonstrable between the swine fed excess vitamin D_3 with or without high fat and cholesterol and those fed basal ration alone, or 7.9, 7.4 and 5.6 at 3 months of age ($P < 0.5$) and 7.3, 6.2 and 5.1 at 6 months of age ($P < 0.5$), respectively. No significant difference was observed between the swine fed high fat and cholesterol without excess vitamin D_3 and those fed the basal diet alone, or 5.7 and 5.6 at 3 months of age, and 5.5 and 5.1 at 6 months.

ON OPTIMAL EXPERIMENTAL CONDITIONS FOR TESTING THE ANTIATHERO-
SCLEROTIC PROPERTIES OF HYPOLIPEMIC DRUGS IN FAT-FED RABBITS

Ralph Brattsand
AB Draco, Fack, Lund/Sweden

The connection between the mean levels of cholesterol (chol.) in plasma (pl.),
the distribution of lipids between VLDL, LDL, and HDL in pl. and the extent of
aortic lipid accumulation (aort. lip. acc.) was studied in rabbits fed chol.
supplemented or chol. free semisynthetic diets for at least 5 months. On all
diets aort. lip. acc. started at 200 mg/100 ml of pl. chol. A close correlation
between mean pl. chol. and aort. lip. acc. existed especially between 200 and
400, but not above 600 mg/100 ml of pl. chol. The most human-like distribution
of lipoprotein lipids was obtained on semisynth. diets with pl. chol. 250-400
mg/100 ml. With respect both to pl. and aortic lipids the most relevant exp.
conditions for testing prophylactic effects of hypolipemic drugs would be to
use semisynth. diets inducing pl. chol. of 300-400 mg/100 ml and experimental
periods of at least 5 months.- Antiatherosclerotic action located to the arterial
wall can be studied by giving extra dietary fat to omit the hypochol. action.
Proposed conditions will be examplified by results with pentaerathritoltetra-
nicotinate and clofibrate.

THE ATHEROGENIC EFFECT OF DIFFERENT CHOLESTERYL ESTERS

Jack J. Gottenbos
Unilever Research, Vlaardingen/The Netherlands

Atherosclerosis is characterized by an accumulation of lipids, mainly cholesteryl
esters in the intima of the arterial wall. It has been concluded that the major
part of the cholesteryl esters in the advanced atherosclerotis lesion originates
directly from plasma-lipoprotein. The nature of the dietary fat influences the
degree of atherosclerosis as well as the amount and composition of the cholesteryl esters in plasma. A dietary fat-induced low plasma cholesterol level normally means a high lineleic:oleic acid ratio in the plasma cholesteryl esters
and conversely. Such experiments do not answer the question whether the individual cholesteryl esters differ in atherogenicity. However, other experimental
data point to such differences and suggest that cholesteryl oleate is the main
atherogenic factor. A model using rabbits is described which makes it possible
to determine the atherogenic effect of individual cholesteryl esters. The significance of the difference in atherogenic properties of cholesteryl esters for the
dietary management of coronary heart disease will be discussed.

ATHEROSCLEROSIS AND SKIN CHOLESTEROL CONCENTRATION IN MAN

Tom Björnheden, Sören Björkerud, and Göran Bondjers
Department of Medicine, University of Göteborg, Göteborg/Sweden

Lipid abnormalities involved in the formation of atherosclerotic lesions might
not only be reflected in serum, but also in disturbances at a cellular level. It
is possible that local disturbances in the exchange of different substances between blood and tissue may be primary and serum changes secondary to these. Is
there a value of skin biopsies in testing relevant variables cf lipid metabolism?
Skin biopsies were obtained peroperatively from two age-matched patient-groups
undergoing (T) thrombendarterectomia due to atherosclerosis in the femoral artery
and (V) varicectomia. Cholesterol- (c) and DNA-content (d) were analyzed.
In epidermis both c and d were significantly lower in T than in V. Both c and d
decreased with age in T, but only c in V. In dermis d was significantly lower in
T than in V.

Conclusions: Atherosclerotic changes are parallelled by changes in lipids of other tissues also. In skin such changes may be observed in apparently normal tissue. In atherosclerotic patients the cholesterol concentration was changed in different ways in different compartments, suggesting abnormalities in lipid transfer. The DNA-changes noted in atherosclerotic patients suggest abnormalities in cellularity. It is proposed that serum lipoprotein analyses should be complemented by tissue analyses, e.g. skin biopsies, in patients at risk for atherosclerotic, vascular disease.

MICRORHEOLOGICAL EFFECTS OF THE VASOACTIVE COMPOUND 3,7-DIMETHYL-1-(5-OXO-HEXYL)-XANTHINE (BL 191)

Hans-Günther Grigoleit, and Gabriele Jacobi
Pharmaceutical Department, Hoechst AG Werk Albert, Wiesbaden/BRD

BL 191 decreases whole blood viscosity in patients with peripheral arterial occlusive disease and increases red blood cell (RBC) ATP content. RBC-ATP content is a decisive factor in controlling RBC deformability. We measured in ageing banked blood the influence of BL 191 on RBC with a new device. Stored RBC deplete from ATP over time. Deformability was measured daily over 5 days from 4 banked ABC bloods. Daily 3 portions (A,B,C) were measured 6-fold at $37^{o}C$. A = control, B = 20 µg BL 191, immediate measurement, C = 20 µg BL 191, measured after 2,5 h incubation at $37^{o}C$. Measurements were done in a filter system allowing filtration of whole blood within 1,5 min for each filtration. The system consists of a membrane with pores of 5 µm diameter and works with a suction of 20 cm H_2O. The filtrability of A decreases from day 1 (100%) to approximately 6% at day 5. The difference between the days is statistically significant. Up from day 3 when filtrability of A in average is 14% the filtrability of B and C is higher compared to A. The difference is statistically significant. The highest filtration rate is achieved with portion C. It is suggested that this methodological approach is an advantage in microtheological studies. The results with BL 191 might be of a therapeutic relevance in the treatment of microcirculatory disturbances, since less deformable RBC with an average diameter of 8 µm can obstruct capillaries with pores less in diameter than RBC.

INTIMAL THICKENINGS AT BRANCHING SITES OF COLLATERAL OUTGROWTHS OF AN ARTERY

Soemiati Ahmad M., A.M. Djoyosugito, and Djoko Prakosa
Department of Anatomy, Faculty of Medicine, Gadjah Mada University, Yogyakarta/ Indonesia

Light microscopic studies on the early stage of developing collateral vessels produced by ligation of the femoral arteries were carried out in rats and rabbits. Special attention was given to the site of branching of a new collateral outgrowth from the main artery proximal to the ligature, in order to investigate the arterial wall structure at a newly developed branching.
In both animals intimal thickenings were found at the branching sites as early as 3 weeks after the ligation, located circumferentially around the collateral ostium, consisting of a cellular and fibro-elastic proliferation. In rats an increase of elastic lamellae was also found in the media around the collateral ostium. These wall changes were presumably caused by the changes in hemodynamic forces produced by the new flow of blood into the newly formed collateral vessel. The circumferentially located intimal thickening indicates that the entire margin of the ostium is subjected to accentuated hemodynamic forces.

HISTOLOGIC FEATURES OF ADVANCED ATHEROSCLEROSIS IN AORTOCORONARY VEIN GRAFTS

Joseph J. Barboriak, George E. Batayias, Michael E. Korns, Karl Pintar, and Diane L. Van Horn
Research Service, Wood VA Center and Department of Pharmacology, Medical College of Wisconsin, Milwaukee, WI/USA

The early lesions in aortocoronary vein grafts mainly consist of thrombosis and lumen narrowing or occlusion due to intimal proliferation. More recent findings indicate that some of the vein grafts removed several years after the bypass operation also developed atherosclerosis. Examination of vein graft athero-sclerosis by light and transmission electron microscopy has shown that the lesions were focal, penetrated into the media and occasionally were covered with nearly normal endothelium. Hyperlipidemia seemed to be the risk factor most frequently associated with the development of these late graft lesions. (Supported by NIH Grant #14378)

HISTOPATHOLOGIC STUDY ON ATHEROSCLEROTIC LESIONS OF HYPERLIPEMIC AND NORMOLIPEMIC PATIENTS

Minoru Suzuki, Roberto J. Bayardo, Alexander Braun, Han-Seob Kim, J.T. Lie, and Jack L. Titus
Department of Pathology, Baylor College of Medicine, Houston, TX/USA

In an attempt to establish a relationship of hyperlipemia with the disstribu-tion and severity of atherosclerosis, intimal lesions were evaluated on post-mortem arterial segments which were taken from specified sites. Arterial sam-ples of 10 hyperlipemic and 15 normolipemic patients were obtained at autopsy from: common carotid, ascending aorta, abdominal aorta right main coronary, left anterior descending coronary, left circumflex coronary, middle cerebral, basilar. Histologic slides were read independently by two pathologists. Fairly concordant relationships were observed between foam cell accumulation (intracellular lipids) and cholesterol cleft deposition, and between smooth muscle cell increase and acid mucopolysaccharide accumulation. Calcification, hemorrhage and thrombus formation were seen only in advanced lesions. Between the hyperlipemic and nor-molipemic groups, atherosclerotic changes were more severe in the former, but the severity of lesions varied greatly within each group and even between dif-ferent arterial segments of the same individuals. The results suggest that atherosclerotic changes of the hyperlipemic patients were more severe than those of the normolipemic, but none of the histopathologic characteristics of athero-sclerosis was useful in differentiating lesions of the hyperlipemic patients from those of the controls. (Supported by a grant HL-17269 from N.I.H., Bethesda, Maryland)

THE EFFECT OF ETHANOL ON THE ONSET OF EXPERIMENTAL ATHEROSCLEROSIS

Yoshio Goto, Hiroaki Kikuchi, Kanji Abe, Yuji Nagahashi, Sei-ichi Ohira, and Hajime Kudo
The Third Department of Internal Medicine, Hirosaki University School of Medi-cine, Hirosaki/Japan

Experiments were designed to ascertain whether hyperlipemia produced by chronic alcohol intake would accelerate cholesterol-fed experimental atherosclerosis. Young male rabbits (134-139 days after birth) were kept on a diet containing cholesterol)0.5%) and lard (5%) and some of them were kept on 5% or 10% ethanol in drinking water for thirteen weeks. There was no significant difference in the increase of body weight and in diet intake. Plasma lipids levels were significantly higher in the ethanol-fed groups than in the control group kept on plain water. The atherosclerotic changes of the aorta, however, were significantly less in the ethanol-fed rabbits than in the controls and even less in the rabbits kept on 10% ethanol than in those on 5% ethanol. The results suggest that ethanol has an inhibitory effect on cholesterol-induced experimental atherosclerosis despite its hyperlipemic action.

THE FAT TOLERANCE TEST AS A MEASURE FOR LIPID METABOLISM IN NORMAL AND PATIENS WITH PORTOCAVAL SHUNT

W. Schwartzkopff, M. Zschiedrich, G. Gründler, and I. Schlicht
Medical Clinic, Free University, Berlin/BRD

After performing a portocaval shunt there was observed improvements of glycogenosis and of homocygous hypercholesterolemia (Starzl et al. (1973); Riddel et al. (1966)). In patients with portocaval shunt (n=6) the kinetics of the lipomicrons and of the TG-elimination (k%/min) was determined by means of the intravenous tolerance test by Boberg (1 ml Intralipid 10%/kg body weight). The conversion of the exogenic into endogenic TC and the behaviour of the free fatty acids were measured furing 90 min. The results were compared with those of a normal collective (NC=20). In shunt patients the CH and the β- or LDL were decreased. The TG and the pre-β or VLDL were missed in part completely in the fasting serum. The disappearance rate of the lipomicrons was 4.4% min, in the NC=2.67%/min. The disappearance rates for the TG were 3.97%/min; NC=2.0%/min. In opposite to the NC the conversion rate of exogenic into endogenic TG and into pre-β or VLDL was decreased near the factor 5 in comparison with the NC. As a measure for that the planes for the Δ-TG, and the Δ pre-β or Δ-VLDL (0.16 cm^2/min); NC: 0.85 cm^2/min were taken. In spite of the missing or a very much reduced TG-conversion of the exogenic into endogenic fat there is nevertheless a more quickly hydrolysis in shunted patients than the NC. The concentration and the quantity of the free fatty acids were until to the 90th minute approximatively double so high as in the NC after the intravenous application of fat.
Results: Patients with portocaval shunt have a more increased hydrolysis of parenteral applied fat. The resynthesis to endogenic fat that means to TG and pre-β or VLDL was decreased in comparison to the NC. This may be one factor for lower incidence of atherosclerosis in patients with liver cirrhosis.

FAT TOLERANCE TEST AND ATHEROSCLEROSIS

Soichiro Takahashi, Fumiko Nagano, Takashi Tsuchida, and Hideaki Saito
The Second Department of Internal Medicine, Niigata University School of Medicine.
The College of Biomedical Technics of Niigata University, Niigata/Japan

The fat diet containing two eggs, the yolk of three eggs and fifty gram butter was ingested in the fasting state of the normal and atherosclerotic subjects in order to detect the variability in responses to the loading based on the analysis of serum lipids. Although all our subjects showed a rise in serum triglyceride levels by the diet, large absolute increments were confined to the atherosclerotic subjects in whom the gradual increments persisted until 6 hours after the loading. The normal subjects did not readily develop hypertriglyceridemia and the maximum levels were found in 4 or 6 hours after the loading. Increments of serum cholesterol after the loading were not correlated with the initial cholesterol levels. The atherosclerotic subjects revealed larger increments of serum cholesterol than the normal subjects. This test would be available to detect not only abnormal dietary hyperlipidemia but also predisposition to atherosclerosis.

INCREASED PULMONARY CLOSING CAPACITY AND RESIDUAL VOLUME IN PATIENTS WITH HYPERLIPOPROTEINEMIA

Franco Conti, Bruno Amaducci, Cesare Sirtori, Oreste Mantero, and Mario Morpurgo
Center E. Grossi Paoletti and Pulmonary Laboratory, Maggiore Hospital and University of Milano, Milano/Italy

14 patients with stable hyperlipoproteinemia (9 type IV, 4 type II and 1 type IIB), non smokers and not professionally exposed to noxious gases, underwent spirometry with determination of static and dynamic volumes. Total body plethysmography, Raw and SGaw were determinated; MMEF was calculated from the spirometry data, MEF 25 and 50 from the flow-volume curves. DLCO SS2, blood gas analysis and CC were measured at rest.
VR and VR/TLC ratio were increased significantly above C.E.C.A. standards, respectively by 23 ± 2.1% and 24.2 ± 5.9% CC exceeded values of our control population by 21.4 ± 4.0%. Occasional patients also exhibited alterations SGaw, MMEF and MEF 25-50. DLCL SS2, contrary to previous reports, was altered in only one patient. In three patients, marked decrease of lipid levels was followed by improvement of CC (pt.A: +40 to +5; pt.B: +35 to +8; pt.C: +33 to +7), RV (A: +86 to +31; B: +70 to +37; C: +65 to +38) and RV/TLD (A: +66 to +32; B: +38 to + 25; C: +70 to +45).

HYPOBETALIPOPROTEINEMIC ACTIVITY IN HYPERCHOLESTEROLEMIC ANIMALS

C.E. Day, P.E. Schurr, D. Lednicer, and W.E. Heyd
The Upjohn Company, Kalamazoo, MI/USA

Either a genetic increase in high density lipoprotein (HDL) or a decrease in lower density lipoproteins (LDL) appears to be beneficial in decreasing morbidity from atherosclerosis. Therefore, we randomly screened for pharmacologic agents that possess one or both of these activities. In hypercholesterolemic rats and mice 1-[p-(1'-adamantyloxy)phenyl]-piperidine (U-41,792) caused both a marked reduction in LDL and an increase in HDL. We have designated this activity hypobetalipoproteinemia. In addition to U-41,792 we have discovered numerous other compounds such as p-(bicyclo[2.2.2]oct-1-yloxy)-aniline and p-(1-adamantyloxy)-aniline that possess hypobetalipoproteinemic activity. These agents are active in hypercholesterolemic rats, mice, quail, pigeons, and gerbils. They are not active in normocholesterolemic animals. U-41,792 is active both intravenously and orally in hypercholesterolemic rats and causes qualitative changes in composition as well as quantitative changes in both LDL and HDL. After a single dose activity is evident at 8 hrs and persists for 96 hours. No other common hypocholesterolemic agent, such as clofibrate, exhibits hypobetalipoproteinemia in our test system. Hypobetalipoproteinemic agents will be quite useful for elucidating new aspects of atherogenic lipoprotein metabolism.

CHANGES OF CYCLIC AMP & CYCLIC AMP PHOSPHODIESTERASE IN AORTIC WALL OF RABBITS IN THE COURSE OF CHOLESTEROL FEEDING

Fujio Numano, Yoshinori Watanabe, Kyoko Takeno, Terukazu Takano, Tomoe Kuroiwa, Hidenori Maezawa, Kinya Moriya, and Takio Shimamoto
Tokyo Ika-Shika National University, Japan Atherosclerosis Research Foundation, Tokyo/Japan

Cyclic AMP has been recently highlighted as an intracellular second messenger of various hormones to regulate the function of cells. Changes of cAMP & its degradating enzyme, phosphodiesterase (PDE) activity in aortic wall of rabbits were pursued in the progression of atherosclerosis. Twenty four healthy rabbits were fed with 1% cholesterol-diet and cAMP & PDE activity in atheromatous lesion

and media of aortic wall of rabbits before 3, 6, 9, 12 and 15 weeks after cholesterol feeding, using Lowry's microbiochemical analysis modified by us. Cyclic
AMP in both media and atheromatous lesion exhibited a gradual decrease and especially remarkable decrease in atheromatous lesions in rabbits fed with cholesterol for more than 6 weeks.
Contrary PDE activity increased gradually and a statistically significant high
activity was obtained in both atheromatous lesion (P <0.01) and media (P <0.05)
of rabbits' aorta fed with cholesterol for 15 weeks. These changes make us sup-
pose the important role of cyclic nucleotide in the formation of the atheromatous
lesion.

GLUCOSE METABOLISM, ATP AND cAMP LEVELS IN AORTAS FROM RABBITS FED A STANDARD OR ATHEROGENIC DIET

Laura Caparrotta, Paola Dorigo, Rosita Gaion, Alberta Leon, and Marco Prosdocimi
Chair of Pharmacology and Pharmacognosy, Padua University, Padua/Italy

In an attempt to investigate the metabolic disorders occurring in the aortic
wall during atherogenesis, attention was given to energy metabolism. This was
suggested by the following data. (i) Anaerobic glycolysis prevails in the arterial wall. Oxidative processes and oxygen supply are scanty. (ii) Atheromal
mitochondria have a depressed capacity in oxiding long chain fatty acids: this
could result in increased cholesterol ester synthesis. Albino ♂ rabbits were
fed 45 days on a commercial or atherogenic diet according to Kritchevsky. Changes
in atherosclerotic aortas when compared with the normal ones were: glycogen/
glucose ratio increase, decrease of lactate and pyruvate, increase of DNA and
decrease of ATP. A question now arises: is glucose metabolism oriented towards
a different direction in the atherosclerotic lesions? (promoting biosynthetic
processes?).

METABOLIC DIFFERENCES BETWEEN ARCH AND THORACIC SEGMENT IN RABBIT AORTAS

Giuliana Fassina, Marco Prosdocimi, Laura Caparrotta, Paola Dorigo, and Gino
Toffano
Chair of Pharmacology and Pharmacognosy, Padua University, Padua/Italy

Anaerobic glycolysis prevails in the arterial wall. Oxidative phosphorylation is
very low but just sufficient to fulfill the energy request of this particular
tissue. Some parameters related to energy metabolism were investigated in two
different areas of rabbit aortic tissue. Each aorta was removed from the aortic
valve to the abdominal part, stripped of periadventitial debris and divided into
arch and thoracic segment. ATP, glycogen, glucose, lactate and pyruvate were determined in each aortic fraction of 8 animals. Differendes observed between the
two segments were: (i) a higher content of ATP and glucose in the arch, (ii) a
lower lactate/glucose and pyruvate/glucose ratio in the thoracic segment. These
variations could be of interest in view of the different sensitivity to atherosclerosis of the two districts.

LIPID TRANSPORT ACROSS THE INTESTINAL EPITHELIAL CELL: EFFECT OF COLCHICINE

Carlos Arreaza-Plaza, Virgilio Bosch, and Michel Otayek
Cátedra de Fisiopatologia, Facultad de Medicina, Universidad Central, Caracas/
Venezuela

Rats injected with colchicine (C), (0.5 mg/100 g body weight) one hour before
the ingestion of a margarine emulsion, do not show the postprandial rise in total
plasma triglycerides (TG) or in plasma chylomicrons TG concentration as compared
to controls. The effect of C has been observed, even in rats previously injected
with Triton WR-1339, a substance known to inhibit chylomicrons and very low density lipoproteins catabolism. In C treated rats, a seven fold increase in TG content of the proximal jejunal mucosa was also observed. D-(+)-xylose absorption
and pancreatic lipase secretion were not altered. When the margarine emulsion was
given at 6 and 10 hours after the C administration, the rise in plasma TG did not
differ from control, however the fatty intestine remains unchanged. These results
are consistent with the idea that C interfers with the intracellular phase of fat
absorption, suggesting that the microtubular-microfilament system could be involved in the absorptive process of fat by the jejunum.

The excellent help of Mrs. Marta Rodriguez is acknowledged. This study was supported by grants from CONICIT No. 31.26.SI-0696 and C.D.C.H. (1974) Universidad
Central, Caracas/Venezuela.

ESSENTIAL FATTY ACID DEFICIENCY IN OBESE KOLETSKY STRAIN OF RAT

Antanas Butkus, Eugene Tan, and Simon Koletsky
Research Division, Cleveland Clinic and Department of Pathology, Case Western
Reserve University, Medical School, Cleveland, OH/USA

In the Koletsky strain of spontaneously hypertensive rats, obesity, hyperlipemia
and premature atherosclerosis develop at an early age without dietary manipulation in association with an as yet unidentified mutant recessive trait. The hyper-
lipemiy in the obese rats was due mainly to a much larger increase in cholesteryl ester and triglyceride concentrations as compared to free cholesterol and/
or phospholipids. Concentration of neutral esterified lipids in liver and aortic
intima-media were also greatly elevated without corresponding increase in phospholipids. Tissues and blood from obese rats contained high levels of eicosatrie-
noic acid relative to arachidonic, ratios of these two being in excess of that
which is generally viewed as a chemical hallmark of essential fatty acid deficiency. These abnormalities were absent in the non-obese littermates. Studies *in
vitro* on obese and non-obese rats suggest that the enzymatic activity of choles-
terogenesis in the liver of obese rat was elevated, but the enzymatic activities
of cholesterol esterification and cholesteryl ester hydrolysis as well as choles-
terol-7α-hydroxylation as a function of substrate concentration were greatly reduced suggesting that the catabolic pathway of cholesterol is impaired in the
obese Koletsky rat. It is suggested that the impaired cholesterol metabolism is
related to the essential fatty acid deficiency. Supported by NIHL Grant HL-6835
and AHA-NEO Grant 8542.

NEPHELOMETRIC MEASUREMENT OF HEPARIN PRECIPITATED LIPOPROTEINS — A VALID SCREENING PROCEDURE FOR POPULATION STUDIES

Maurice Stone, Jeffrey Thorp, and John Wain
Clinical Research Unit, Leigh, Lancashire/England

The precipitation of lipoproteins by heparin in the presence of Ca^{++} is a useful
procedure for the detection of hyperlipoproteinaemia. The original papers de-

scribed turbidity measurements by spectrophotometer, but the results vary with
the optical characteristics of different instruments.
We have adapted the technique for use in the Thorp-Stone nephelometer which has
a standardized response to light scattering intensity (LSI), so that LSI values
can be interpreted by any nephelometer user. The nephelometric technique requires only 0.02 ml of serum instead of the original 0.2 ml, and costs only 0.5 p
(U.K.), i.e., less than 1 cent (U.S.) per analysis.
There is a high correlation (r = 0.94) between the LSI of heparin precipitated
LDL + VLDL (LSI_H), and the concentration of LDL + VLDL obtained by more detailed
analyses (Stone et al., Clin. Chim. Acta 30, 809 (1970)).
In 497 consecutive serum samples from a research clinic the range of LSI_H was
35 - 240 units. Of the 138 samples with LSI_H <90 units only 5 (3.6%) were classified as "abnormal" by more detailed analysis. Examination of the distribution
of LDL + VLDL in a population random sample suggests that measurement of LSI_H
as a screening procedure would eliminate the need for more detailed analysis in
almost 70% of serum samples in population studies.

A STUDY ON CHOLESTEROL CONTENTS IN FOODS (1) — SHELLFISH —

Iwao Fukui, Hideto Kushiro, Kazutaka Arisue, Yoshihisa Yamaguchi, Zensuke Ogawa,
Chozo Hayashi, and Yuichi Yamamura
Kyoto Pref., University of Medicine, Kyoto/Japan; Kinki University, Hospital;
Osaka University, Hospital, and Osaka University, Medical Scholl, Osaka/Japan

It is important to know the exact content of cholesterol in foods for prevention
of onset or progress of atherosclerosis. Such shellfish as corb shell (shijimi),
bloody clam (akagai), shortneck clam (asari), clam (hamaguri), and oyster (kaki)
were treated with organic solvent. The L-B reaction, Kiliani reaction, OPA reaction, and enzymatic method were applied to each extract for determination of
cholesterol. The findings obtained by enzymatic method showed 20 to 30% lower
in cholesterol content than those obtained by the colorimetric method.
Furthermore, these extracts were analysed by TLC, and UV method and L-B method
were applied to the plates. By these reactions, the several spots were observed.
The spot corresponding to cholesterol was collected and GCL analysis was carried
out for further separation. C_{26}-sterol, 22-dehydrocholesterol, brassicasterol,
24-methylenecholesterol, campesterol, and β-sitosterol were found in addition to
cholesterol. The ratio of cholesterol contents to the total amounts of sterols
were found from 44.5% to 70.0% in these shellfish. Of these sterols other than
cholesterol, much of 24-methylenecholesterol and brassicasterol were existing.-
As a result of these studies, it became known that the cholesterol contents in
these shellfish were far less than has been reported. The extensive studies are
continued on the other foods.

BOVINE XANTHINE OXIDASE, RISK FACTORS AND CARDIOVASCULAR DISEASE; AN INTEGRATED APPROACH

Kurt A. Oster
Department of Biology, Fairfield University, Fairfield, CT/USA

Xanthine oxidase from bovine milk can be absorbed in active form from the small
intestines and distributed through the entire organism by two possible mechanisms;
(a) pinocytosis of macromolecules, and (b) persorption of starch granules coated
with micronized enzyme particles. The chemistry involved constitutes a basis for
some of the established risk factors. Xanthine oxidase is activated by male sex
hormones and inhibited by female sex hormones. The possibility of its also being
activated by certain cholesterol-related substances and vitamin D is being investigated in our laboratories. The process of persorption is stimulated by particle size, coffee drinking, and cigarette smoking. For the first time, an inte-

grated causal and risk factor approach to the problem of the dietary initiation of the atherosclerotic process is provided. The statistical difference in incidence of myocardial infarction in various geographic locations described by Keys et al. could be reduced to the bioavailability of bovine xanthine oxidase and raw starch particles in the affected population groups.

A MORPHOLOGICAL STUDY ON MUTUAL RELATIONSHIP AMONG MYOCARDIAL INFARCTION, CORONARY SCLEROSIS AND THROMBOSIS IN JAPAN

Ryozo Okada, Tatsuji Kanoh, and Kazuo Kitamura
Department of Internal Medicine, School of Medicine, Juntendo University, Tokyo/ Japan

To clarify interrelationship among myocardial infarction, coronary sclerosis and thrombosis, 215 Japanese autopsy cases with myocardial infarction were morphologically studied. The overall incidence of coronary thrombosis in the infarcted cases was 53% and the incidence was higher in the massive necrosis (M) infarction, to 70% in male and 63% in female. In the M type infarction, the highest incidence of thrombosis was recorded in 60-69 years old male (84%) and 70-79 years old female (69%). The thrombosis is appeared only 43% in the M type infarction during initial 24 hours from the attack, and it was increasing thereafter up to 80%. The anterior infarction fairly matched thrombosis in the anterior descending (Ad) branch, but the posterior one which was increasing after 70 years old, did not show so intimate relation to thrombosis in the right coronary artery. The thrombosis was correlated to coronary stenosis up to 75%, but not so to the extent of atherosclerosis which was increasing with age. Thrombosis on moderate stenosis in the left coronary main trunk and proximal Ad branch was noted in 40-59 years old male. The site of thrombosis in the Ad branch was shifted distalwards and thrombosis just distal to the severe atheromatous stenosis became marked with advancing age. Thrombosis was predisposed at the median portion of the right coronary artery and circumflex branch with a shift both proximal- and distalwards with age.

CHANGES OF IMMUNOGLOBULINS AND OTHER GLYCOPROTEINS IN ACUTE MYOCARDIAL INFARCTION

Lajos Jakab, János Fehér, and István Siró
The Third Department of Medicine, Semmelweis University of Medicine, Budapest/ Hungary

The serum IgG, IgA, TgM, coeruloplasmin, alpha-2-macroglobulin and transferrin levels were estimated by the radial immunodiffusion technique and followed up over a period of 40 days in patients with acute myocardial infarction. IgG and IgA levels were elevated between the 16th and 21st days. The coeruloplasmin level showed the most marked elevation, and had not completely normalized by the 40th day. The alpha-2-macroglobulin level revealed a similar, though less marked, tendency. The transferrin level decreased.

RELATIONSHIP BETWEEN CORONARY THROMBOSIS AND ATHEROSCLEROSIS IN THE PATHOGENESIS OF ACUTE MYOCARDIAL INFARCTION. A HISTOPATHOLOGICAL STUDY OF CORONARY ARTERIES OF 108 AUTOPSIED CASES EMPLOYING SERIAL SECTION

Toshinobu Horie, Morie Sekiguchi, Koshichiro Hirosawa, and Akira Kajita
Heart Institute Japan and Department of Pathology, Tokyo Womens's College, Tokyo/Japan

An extensive histological study of acute myocardial infarction cases who died after having been admitted to our coronary care unit was done. Thrombosed segments of coronary arteries were studied at intervals of 100 microns, employing serial histological sections. A high incidence (80.3%) of thrombus formation, corresponding to the site of infarction, was observed. Such occluding thrombi were usually formed at the proximal portion of coronary arteries and at the portion of ruptured atheromatous abscess (incidence rate: 90.8%). We feel that such serial section is needed because pathology of the lumen is extremely variable within a 2 to 3 mm-wide segment. Increase of intra-plaque pressure resulting from a stone-wall-like accumulation of foam cells, cholesterin clefts, and blood infiltration from lumen to plaque through injured endothelial cells is, we feel, causing rupture of the atheromatous plaque. This fracture between the lumen and the plaque might precede and be responsible for formation of the thrombus and onset of acute myocardial infarction.

EVIDENCE AGAINST THE HYPOTHESIS THAT POLYUNSATURATED FATTY ACIDS ARE CO-CARCINOGENS

Seymour Dayton, and Sam Hashimoto
VA Wadsworth Hospital Center, and School of Medicine, Los Angeles, CA/USA

Past experiments in humans and animals have suggested that unsaturated vagetable oils may stimulate cancer growth. Availability of a mutant safflower, producing an oil rich in oleic acid, provided an opportunity for a critical test of the hypothesis that polyunsaturated fats act as co-carcinogens. Weanling female Sprague-Dawley rats were each given 5 mg of 7,12-dimethylbenz(α)anthracene intragastrically. They were then placed on diets containing 20%, by weight, of conventional high-linoleic safflower oil; high-oleic safflower oil; or coconut oil. Half of each group received supplementary α-tocopherol. Rats were pair-fed. Tumors were identified weekly and independently by two observers, by palpation. The high-oleic safflower group had more tumor-bearing animals than did the coconut oil group (p <0.01). High-linoleic safflower was intermediate, but not significantly different from either of the other groups. Numbers of tumors per tumor-bearing animal were significantly higher with both safflower oils than with coconut oil. Addition of tocopherol had no effect, and there were no differences between groups in time of first appearance of tumors. Conclusion: both safflower oils stimulated DMBA-induced tumors, but this was not attributable to polyunsaturated fatty acid. (Supported in part by Arthur Dodd Fuller Foundation.)

EARLY DETECTION OF CORONARY ATHEROSCLEROTIC LESIONS BY NON-INVASIVE, "TOTAL" ELECTROCARDIOGRAPHY

Fred Kornreich, Jo Snoek, Melvyn Fishel, and Judith Kornreich
Unit for Cardiovascular Research, School of Medicine, Free University Brussels (V.U.B.), Brussels/Belgium

A new electrocardiographic lead system has been described in the literature (Circulation 48 (1973) and 49 (1974)): 9 QRS waveforms, recorded at anatomically fixed location, were found capable of resynthesizing any ECG recorded on the tho-

racic surface; thus 9 ECGs could account for the total available surface wave-
form information.

This above described lead system is used in this study in order to investigate
wether early, asymptomatic lesions of the coronary arteries — as evidenced by
coronary angiography or by autopsy — could be detected in early stages (≤70%
obstruction in one mayor coronary artery). Two series were studied: series 1
(192 patients with coronary lesions with a ≤70% obstruction in one or more vessels), and series 2 (no coronary lesions in 155 patients). The concordance between our non-invasive system and the coronary arteriography was respectively of
94% for series 1 and of 91% for series 2.

FATTY ACID COMPOSITION OF ADIPOSE TISSUE IN PATIENTS WITH CORONARY HEART DISEASE

P. Dieter Lang, Michael Degott, and Joachim Vollmar
Klinisches Institut für Herzinfarktforschung, Department of Medicine, Heidelberg
University, Heidelberg/BRD

To study the relationship between the fatty acid composition of adipose tissue
and CHD two studies on male subjects on "normal" diets have been performed:
1. 34 patients with acute MI and 33 controls free of clinical CHD were selected.
Subcutaneous fat was obtained by needle biopsy and the fatty acids determined by
GLC. The only statistically significant difference in fatty acids between the
two groups was a lower proportion of stearic acid in patients with MI compared
with controls (3.25% vs. 4.13%). Using multivariate linear discriminant analysis,
age discriminated best between the two groups, followed by stearic acid. Age did
not correlate with the proportion of stearic acid. 2. 48 subjects undergoing
coronary angiography were studied. The proportions of the various adipose fatty
acids were compared in 4 groups with different ranges of a score indicating the
overall degree of coronary arteriosclerosis. Stearic acid tended to be lower in
subjects with coronary narrowing, but multivariate discriminant analysis showed
glucose tolerance to be the best discriminator between patients with and without
coronary arteriosclerosis.

The metabolic basis for a possible relationship between CHD and stearic acid is
not clear at present.

FACTORS INFLUENCING THE PROGNOSIS OF ESTABLISHED CORONARY HEART DISEASE (CHD), WITH REFERENCE TO THE VALUE OF THEIR TREATMENT

Carlo Caruzzo, Anna Salto, and Gualtiero Pozzallo
Istituto Unificato di Medicina Interna, Cattedra di Clinica Medica Generale,
Università di Torino, Torino/Italy

In order to evaluate which factors influence the prognosis of CHD, 200 patients
with myocardial infarction or angina pectoris were followed for at least 3 years
and subjected to the control of main Coronary Risk Factors (CRF) (including their
pharmacological treatment), to symptomatic therapy of angina and heart failure
(when necessary) and to randomized treatment with drugs acting on blood clotting.
Fatal or non-fatal Cardio-Vascular Events (CVE) in the first 3 years of follow-
up were related to the various CRF at entry and at the end of the observation,
and to the pharmacological treatments already mentioned. The results were evaluated both with dichotomic crosstabulation method and with factor analysis.
Results: The correlations between CVE and main CRF at entry and at the end of
the observation are either lacking or unexpected. Only hyperglycemia at entry
significantly increases the CVE, as well as hypertension at entry, to a lesser
extent. Overweight at the end unexpectedly decreases the CVE. The highly significant correlations between the use of diuretics and digitalis and the incidence
of CVE is explained by the severity of the disease in these patients. The lack of

correlations of CVE with other CRF and their drug treatments (antihypertensive, antidiabetic, different antihyperlipidemic drugs) suggest some comments: 1) the employed drugs have no therapeutic values, or the dosage and the adherence of the patients were inadequate; 2) the drugs were given in a too late stage of the disease; 3) other CRF were present, such as an hypercoagulable state. Our study confirms the last hypothesis. Fibrinolytic, platelet antiaggregating and heparinoid drugs showed in the crosstabulation analysis a preventive effect on CVE; this was not significant likely because of the small number of patients. Furthermore, the only drugs clearly related in the factor analysis to a reduction of CVE (clofibrate, biguanides, fibrinolytic drugs and nicotinic acid) have a fibrinolytic effect. On the contrary, the anticoagulants and the antianginal therapy did not influence the CVE.

LIGATION OF THE INTESTINAL LYMPHATICS IN THE TREATMENT OF ARTERIO-SCLEROSIS

M. Servelle
Paris/France

In patients presenting a substantiel loss of chyle (chyloperitoneum, exsudative arteriopethy, chylothorax) we observe a reduction of protifs and calcium, but also lipids and cholesterol.
So we think that the ligation of the intestinal lymphatics present the absorption of lipids and cholesterol. To make sure of the harmlessness of the procedure we carried out in 1966 numerous animal operations. During the last 9 years we did the ligature of the intestinal lymphatics in front of the renal vein on 600 arteriosclerotic patients. Lymphographies clearly demonstrate the blockage of the lacteals.
The biological and clinical results are very goods. We also ligate the lacteals in 12 coronary patients who had no infarction and no stenosis of the main coronary vessels: the results have been also very encouraging.

IN VITRO AND IN VIVO OBSERVATIONS ON THE PRIMARY SHAPE CHANGE OF THROMBOCYTES

R. Wiedemann, K. Breddin, H. Grun, and H.J. Krzywanek
University Center of Internal Medicine, Department of Angiology, Frankfurt/BRD

In vitro thrombocytes can be studied in their native shape by immediate fixation of blood at venepuncture. Under these conditions platelets appear as flat discs, less than 25% show pseudopodes. In citrate blood and PRP as well a progressing shape change occurs. Platelets tend to swell and tentacle formation continues. At room temperature 90% of thrombocytes have undergone these changes within 60 min. In contrast to this "primary shape change" the addition of ADP (10^{-6} M) to PRP induces the formation of large vesicles, the rupture of which is followed by the formation of platelet aggregates. Bencyclan (2×10^{-4} M) affects platelet morphology by inducing a spherical transformation, which is paralleled by changes of platelet adhesiveness, spreading and aggregability. In an animal model changes very similar to those of "primary shape change" can be observed at the site of a laser induced injury of the vessel wall.
The stimuli which initiate the "primary shape change" of thrombocytes are unknown. The morphologic platelet changes demonstrated in the film seem to present a basic process in hemostasis and thrombus formation.

THROMBOSIS - ATHEROSCLEROSIS

Georg Munck
Leonaris-Film, Böblingen/BRD

For 25 years the death-rate, caused by atherosclerosis has been rapidly growing so that R. Ross states: Atherosclerosis is the principal killer of western man. We know the risk factors, which alone are potentiating when in combination accelerate atherosclerosis and cause thrombo-embolic complications. Thus far we were not very successful in fighting against these risk factors. Modern man, living in a world of plenty often tries to overcome his psychosocial conflicts by indulging in all sorts of pleasure. Only too seldom we can convince him of the necessity to change his may of life. What other plans have we to offer our overstressed 45 to 60 years old patients than the all to often repeated Om Mani Padme Hum of the eternal prayer-wheel of risk factors. But even though the increasing death-rate shows that our efforts are in vain, we should not resign. On the contrary we should clutch at any straw. There is perhaps a possibility by using the long-known drugs, the antiplatelet effects of which have been discovered and are now discussed. This may be the way we should go as soon as possible.

ATHEROSCLEROSIS FROM A DIFFERENT POINT OF VIEW

Hans Hess, Holger Schmid-Schönbein and Coworkers
Medizinische Poliklinik and Physiologisches Institut, Universität München, München/BRD

The film presents a uniform theory of the pathogenesis of obliterating angiopathies of all sorts and localisations. In this theory the platelet function and blood flow are the main etiological factors. In experiments with minipigs and rabbits it was demonstrated, that various factors similar to the risk factors of the obliterating arteriopathies of man first lead to platelet adhesions on the inner surface of the vessel wall. Longterm experiments show then the development of such adhesions to mixed microparietal thrombi and to the atherosclerotic plaque.
In view of these results prophylaxis and therapy of the obliterating arteriosclerosis and their prognosis too have to be reassessed from a different point of view.
(Scientific coworkers: U. Gottstein, H. Poliwoda, D. Sinapius, H.M. Becker, H. Frost, H. Hartmann, R. Landgraf, M. Mallasch, M. Marshall, H. Müller-Faßbender, K. Oversohl, H. Rieger.)

REFERENCES

ABDULLA, Y.H., ORTON, C.C., ADAMS, C.W.M.: Cholesterol esterification by trans-acylation in human and experimental atheromatous lesions. J. Atheroscler. Res. 8, 967 (1968).

ABELL, L.L., LEVY, B.B., BRODIE, B.B., KENDALL, F.E.: A simplified method for the estimation of total cholesterol in serum and demonstration of its specificity. J. Biol. Chem. 195, 357 – 366 (1952).

ABRAMOVICI, A., NEUFELD, H.N.: Estimation of areas of histological sections. "A visopan-planimetric method." Israel J. Med. Sci. 1, 569 (1965).

ACHESON, R.M., JESSOP, W.J.E.: Tobacco smoking and serum lipids in old men. Br. Med. J. 2, 1108 – 1111 (1961).

ACKERKNECHT, E.H.: Rudolf Virchow – Doctor, Statesman, Anthropologist. University of Wisconsin: Madison, 1953.

ADACHI, K., NUMANO, F.: Phosphodiesterase inhibitors, their comparative effectiveness in vitro and in various organs. Jap. J. Pharm. 127, 97 (1977).

ADAMS, C.W.M., MORGAN, R.S.: The effect of saturated and polyunsaturated lecithins on the resorption of $4-^{14}C$-cholesterol from subcutaneous implants. J. Pathol. 94, 73 (1967).

ADAMS, C.W.M., MORGAN, R.S., BAYLISS, O.B.: No regression of atheroma over one year in rabbits previously fed a cholesterol enriched diet. Athero. 18, 429 (1973).

ADDISON, P., GULL, W.: On certain affection of the skin, vitiligoidea A. Plana, B. Tuberosa, with remarks. Guy's Hospital Report 7, 265 (1851).

AGGERBECK, L.P., KEDZY, F.J., SCANU, A.M.: Enzymatic probes of lipoprotein structure. Hydrolysis of human serum low density lipoprotein-2 by phospholipase A_2. J. Biol. Chem. 251, 3823 – 3830 (1976).

AHRENS, E.H., Jr.: Mass Field Trials of the Diet Heart Question. American Heart Association Monograph Number 28, (1969).

AHRENS, W., HIRSCH, J., OETTE, K., FARQUHAR, J.W., STEIN, Y.: Carbohydrate-induced and fat-induced lipemia. Trans. Assoc. Am. Physicians 74, 134 – 136 (1961).

AKANUMA, Y., KUZUYA, T., MAYASHI, M., IDE, T., KUZUYA, N.: Positive correlation of serum lecithin: cholesterol acyltransferase activity with relative body weight. Europ. J. Clin. Invest. 3, 136 – 141 (1973).

ALAUPOVIC, P.: Apolipoproteins and lipoproteins. Atherosclerosis 13, 141 – 146 (1971).

ALAUPOVIC, P., LEE, D.M., McCONATHY, W.J.: Studies on the composition and structure of plasma lipoproteins. Distribution of lipoprotein families in major density classes of normal human plasma lipoproteins. Biochim. Biophys. Acta 260, 689 (1972).

ALBERS, J.J., CABANA, V.G., HAZZARD, W.R.: Immunoassay of human plasma apolipoprotein B. Metabolism 24, 1339 – 1351 (1975).

ALBERS, J.J., SCANU, A.M.: Isoelectric fractionation and characterization of polypeptides from human serum very low density lipoproteins. Biochim. Biophys. Acta 236, 29 (1971).

ALBERS, J.J., WAHL, P.W., CABANA, V.G., HAZZARD, W.R., HOOVER, J.J.: Quantitation of apolipoprotein A-I of human plasma high density lipoprotein. Metabolism 25, 633 (1976).

ALBERS, J.J., WAHL, P., HAZZARD, W.R.: Quantitative genetic studies of the human plasma Lp(a) lipoproteinemia. Biochem. Genet. 11, 475 – 486 (1974).

ALBRINK, W.S., ALBRINK, M.J.: The hyperlipidemia of lymphoma-bearing hamsters. Yale J. Biol. Med. 43, 288 (1971).

ALEXANDER, C.A., Hamilton, R.L., HAVEL, R.J.: Subcellular localization of B apoprotein of plasma lipoproteins in rat liver. J. Cell Biol. 69, 241 (1976).

ALEXANDER, J.C., SILVERMAN, N.A., CHRETIEN, P.B.: Effect of age and cigarette smoking on carcinoembryonic antigen levels. JAMA 235, 1975 – 1979 (1976).

ALI, S.Y., SAJDERA, S.W., ANDERSON, H.C.: Isolation and character of calcifying matrix vesicles from epiphyseal cartilage. Proc. Natl. Acad. Sci. 67, 1513 – 1520 (1970).

ALTMAN, P.L., DITTMAN, D.S. (Eds.). Biology Data Book, 2nd ed. Bethesda, Md.: FASEB, 1974, Vol. III, p. 1847.

ALTSCHUL, R.: Endothelium. New York: Macmillan, 1954, p. 123.

AMATUZIO, D.S., HAY, L.J.: Dietary control of essential hyperlipidemia. A.M.A. Arch. Intern. Med. 102, 173 - 178 (1958).

ANASTASSIADES, T., ANASTASSIADIS, P.A., DENSTEDT, O.F.: Changes in connective tissue of the atherosclerotic intima and media of the aorta. Biochim. Biophys. Acta 261, 418 - 427 (1972).

ANFINSEN, C.B., BOYLE, E., BROWN, R.K.: Science 115, 583 (1952).

ANGELIN, B., EINARSSON, K., HELLSTROM, K.: Abstracts for Fourth International Symposium on Atherosclerosis, Tokyo, Japan. 1976, p. 198.

ANITSCHKOW, N.N.: Über die Rückbildungsvorgänge bei der experimentellen Atherosklerose. Verh. dtsch. Path. Ges. 23, 473 - 478. Zentralbl. Allg. Path. path. Anat., Suppl. to Vol. 43 (1928).

ANITSCHKOW, N.N.: Über die Veränderungen der Kaninchenaorta bei experimenteller Cholesterinsteatose. Beitr. path. Anat. 56, 379 (1913).

ANITSCHKOW, N.N., CHALATOV, S.: Über experimentelle Cholesterinsteatose. Zbl. All. Path. 24, 1 (1913).

APPLEBAUM, D., GOLDBERG, A., GAGNE, C., PYKÄLISTÖ, L., HAZZARD, W.: Effect of estrogen on post-heparin plasma lipolytic activity: selective decline in hepatic triglyceride lipase. Clin. Res. 24, 115A (1976).

ARMITAGE, A.K., DOLLERY, C.T., GEORGE, C.F., HOUSEMAN, T.H., LEQIS, P.J., TURNER, D.M.: Absorption and metabolism of nicotine by man during cigarette smoking. Brit. J. clin. Pharm. 1, 180 P (1974).

ARMSTRONG, M.L.: Atherosclerosis in rhesus and cynomolgus monkeys. Primates in Medicine 9, 16 - 40. Basel: Karger 1976.

ARMSTRONG, M.L.: Regression of atherosclerosis. In: Atherosclerosis Review. PAOLETTI, R., GOTTO, A.M. (eds.). New York: Raven Press, 1976, p. 137.

ARMSTRONG, M.L., MEGAN, M.B.: Arterial fibrous proteins in cynomolgus monkeys after atherogenic and regression diets. Circ. Res. 256 - 261 (1975).

ARMSTRONG, M.L., MEGAN, M.B.: Arterial fibrous proteins in cynomolgus monkeys after atherogenic and regression regimens. Circulation 48, Suppl. 4, 41 (1973).

ARMSTRONG, M.L., MEGAN, M.B.: Dietary disaccharides and experimental atherosclerosis in rhesus monkeys. Circulation 50, Suppl. II, 94 (1974a).

ARMSTRONG, M.L., MEGAN, M.B.: Lipid depletion in atheromatous coronary arteries in rhesus monkeys after regression diets. Circ. Res. 30, 675 - 680 (1972).

ARMSTRONG, M.L., MEGAN, M.B.: Response of two macaque species to atherogenic diet and its withdrawal. In: Atherosclerosis III, Proceedings of Third International Symposium. SCHETTLER, G., WEIZEL, A. (eds.). New York: Springer-Verlag, 1974b, pp. 336 - 338.

ARMSTRONG, M.L., MEGAN, M.B., CHENG, F.H., WARNER, E.D.: Dietary disaccharides in experimental atherosclerosis in rhesus monkeys. Exper. Molec. Path. 24, 302 - 319 (1976).

ARMSTRONG, M.L., WARNER, E.D.: Morphology and distribution of diet-induced atherosclerosis in rhesus monkeys. Arch. Pathol. 92, 395 (1971).

ARMSTRONG, M.L., WARNER, E.D., CONNOR, W.E.: Regression of coronary atheromatosis in rhesus monkeys. Circulat. Res. 27, 59 - 67 (1970).

ARONOW, W.S.: Smoking, carbon monoxide, and coronary heart disease. Circulation 48, 1169 (1973).

ARONOW, W.S., GOLDSMITH, J.R., KERN, J.C., CASSIDY, J., NELSON, W.H., JOHNSON, L.L., ADAMS, W.: Effect of smoking cigarettes on cardiovascular hemodynamics. Arch. Environ Health 28, 330 (1974).

ASCHOFF, L.: Lectures in Pathology. New York: Hoeber, 1924.

ASHBY, P.: Smoking and platelet stickiness. Lancet (1965) II, 158 - 159.

ASSMANN, G.: Structure-function relationships of lipoproteins in Tangier disease. In: Lipoprotein Metabolism. GRETEN, H. (ed.). Berlin: Springer-Verlag, 1976, p. 106.

ASSMANN, G., BREWER, H.B.,Jr.: A molecular model of high density lipoproteins. Proc. Natl. Acad. Sci. US 71, 1534 - 1538 (1974).

ASSMANN, G., HERBERT, P.N., FREDRICKSON, D.S., FORTE, T.: Isolation and characterization of an abnormal high density lipoprotein in Tangier disease. J. Clin. Invest. 60, 242 (1977).

ASSMANN, G., HIGHET, R.J., SOKOLOSKI, E.A., BREWER, H.B., Jr.: ^{13}C nuclear magnetic resonance spectroscopy of native and recombind lipoproteins. Proc. Natl. Acad. Sci. US 71, 3701 - 3705 (1974).

ASSMANN, G., KRAUSS, R.M., FREDRICKSON, D.S., LEVY, R.I.: Characterization, subcellular localization, and partial purification of a heparin-released triglyceride lipase from rat liver. J. Biol. Chem. 248, 1992 - 1999 (1973).

ASSMANN, G., SMOOTZ, E., ADLER, K., CAPURSO, A., OETTE, K.: The lipoprotein abnormality in Tangier disease. Quantitation of A apoprotein. J. Clin. Invest. 59, 565 (1977).

ASTRUP, P.: Carbon monoxide, smoking and atherosclerosis. Postgrad. Med. J. 49, 697 (1973).

ASTRUP, P.: Tobacco smoking and coronary disease. Acta Cardiologica (Suppl. XX), 105 - 117 (1974).

ASTRUP, P.: Some physiological and pathological effects of moderate carbon monoxide exposure. Brit. med. J. 4, 447 - 452 (1972).

ASTRUP, P., KJELDSEN, K.: Carbon monoxide, smoking, and atherosclerosis. Med. Clin. N. Amer. 58, 323 - 350 (1974).

ASTRUP, P., KJELDSEN, K., WANSTRUP, P.: Enhancing influence of carbon monoxide on the development of atheromatosis in cholesterol-fed rabbits. J. Atheroscler. Res. 7, 343 - 354 (1967).

ASTRUP, P., TROLLE, D., OLSEN, H.M., KJELDSEN, K.: Effect of moderate carbon-monoxide exposure on fetal development. Lancet (1972) II, 1220 - 1222.

ATSUMI, T., HONDA, Y., MATSUDA, M.: Follow up study on patients suffering from arteriosclerosis obliterans under pyridinolcarbamate treatment and other treatment. J. Jap. Coll. Angiol. (1974).

AUERBACH, O., HAMMOND, E.C., GARDINKEL, L.: Smoking in relation to atherosclerosis of the coronary arteries. N. Engl. J. Med. 273, 775 - 779 (1965).

AUGUSTIN, J., BOBERG, J., TEJADA, P., BROWN, W.V.: Circulation 50 (Suppl. III), 259 (1974).

AUGUSTIN, J., FREEZE, H., BOBERG, J., BROWN, W.V.: Lipoprotein Metabolism. GRETEN, H. (ed.). Berlin-Heidelberg-New York: Springer 1976, p.7.

AUGUSTIN, J., FREEZE, H., BROWN, W.V.: Comparison of hepatic triglyceride lipase and lipoprotein lipase from human postheparin plasma. Circulation 51-52, II-83 (1975).

AUGUSTIN, J., WIELAND, H., PUHL, W., GRETEN, H.: Circulation 54 (Suppl. II), 25 (1976).

AVIGAN, J.: A method for incorporating cholesterol and other lipids into serum lipoproteins in vitro. J. Biol. Chem. 234, 787 (1959).

AVIGAN, J., BHATHENA, S.J., SCHREINER, M.E.: Control of sterol synthesis and of hydroxymethylglutaryl CoA reductase in skin fibroblasts grown from patients with homozygous type II hyperlipoproteinemia. J. Lipid Res. 16, 151 - 154, (1975).

AVOGARO, P., CAZZOLATO, G.: Changes in the composition and physico-chemical characteristics of serum lipoproteins during ethanol-induced lipaemia in alcoholic subjects. Metabolism 24, 1231 - 1242 (1975).

BACHORIK, P.S., LIVINGSTON, J.N., COOKE, J., KWITEROVICH, P.O.: The binding of low density lipoprotein by liver membranes in the pig. Biochem. Biophys. Res. Comm. 69, 927 - 935 (1976).

BAGDADE, J.D., BIERMANN, E.L., PORTE, D., Jr.: Diabetic lipemia: a form of acquired fat-induced lipemia. N. Engl. J. Med. 276, 427 (1967).

BAGDADE, J., WILSON, D., SHAFRIR, E.: Metabolism of hyperlipidemia in chronic uremia. Clin. Res. 24, 455A (1976).

BAILEY, J.M.: Lipid metabolism in cultured cells. VI. Lipid biosynthesis in serum and synthetic growth media. Biochim. Biophys. Acta 125, 226 - 236 (1966).

BAILEY, J.M., BUTLER, J.: Influence of anti-inflammatory agents on experimental atherosclerosis. Nature 212, 731 - 732 (1966).

BAKER, H., DELAHUNTY, T., GOTTO, A.J.,Jr., JACKSON, R.L.: The primary structure of high density apolipoprotein-glutamine-I. Proc. Natl. Acad. Sci. US 71, 3631 - 3634 (1974).

BAKER, H., GOTTO, A.M., JACKSON, R.L.: The primary structure of human plasma density apolipoprotein glutamine I (apoA-I). The amino acid sequence and alignment of cyanogen fragments IV, III and I. J. Biol. Chem. 250, 2725 (1975).

BALFOUR, J.F., KIM, R.: Homozygous type II hyperlipoproteinemia treatment, partial ileal bypass in two children. J.A.M.A. 227, 1145 (1974).

BÁLINT, A., VEREES, B., JELLINEK, H.: Modifications of surface coat of aortic endothelial cells in hyperlipemic rats. Path. Europ. 9, 105 - 108 (1974).

BALTAXE, H., AMPLATZ, K., VARCO, R.L., BUCHWALD, H.: Coronary arteriography in hypercholesterolemic patients. Am. J. Roentg. 105, 784 (1969).

BARAONA, E., LIEBER, CS.: Effects of chronic ethanol feeding on serum lipoprotein metabolism in the rat. J. Clin. Invest. 49, 769 - 778 (1970).

BARAONA, E., PIROLA, R.C., LIEBER, C.S.: Pathogenesis of postprandial hyperlipemia in rats fed ethanol-containing diets. J. Clin. Invest. 52, 296 - 303 (1973).

BARNARD, P.J.: Experimental fibrin thromboembolism of the lungs. J. Path. Bact. 65, 129 (1953).

BARNDT, R., Jr., BLANKENHORN, D.H., CRAWFORD, D.W., BROOKS, S.H.: Regression and progression of early femoral atherosclerosis in treated hyperlipoproteinemic patients. Ann. Int. Med. 86, 139 (1977).

BARNES, E.M., WAKIL, S.J.: Studies on the mechanism of fatty acid synthesis. XIX. Preparation and general properties of palmityl thioesterase. J. Biol. Chem. 243, 2955 - 2962 (1968).

BAR-ON, H., ROHEIM, P.S., EDER, H.A.: Serum lipoproteins and apoproteins in rats with streptozotocin-induced diabetes. J. Clin. Invest. 57, 714 (1976).

BARTER, P.J., NESTEL, P.J.: Precursor-product relationship between pools of very low density lipoprotein triglyceride. J. Clin. Invest. 51, 174 - 180 (1972).

BARTLETT, G.R.: Phosphorus assay in column chromatography. J. Biol. Chem. 234, 466 - 468 (1959).

BAUER, W., CLARK, W.S., KULKA, J.R.: Aortitis and aortic endocarditis, an unrecognized manifestation of rheumatoid arthritis. Ann. Rheum. Dis. 10, 470 (1951).

BAUMGARTNER, H.R.: Eine neue Methode zur Erzeugung von Thromben durch gezielte Überdehnung der Gefäßwand. Z. Gesamte Exp. Med. 137, 227 (1963).

BAUMGARTNER, H.R.: The role of blood flow in platelet adhesion, fibrin deposition, and formation of mural thrombi. Microvascular Res. 5, 167 (1973).

BAUMGARTNER, H.R.: The subendothelial surface and thrombosis. Thrombos. diath. Haemorrh. (Suppl.) 59, 91 (1974).

BAUMGARTNER, H.R., LEJNIEKS, I., SPAET, R.H.: Incorporation of ^{3}H-thymidine in arteries after removal of endothelium. Experientia 27, 17 (1971).

BAUMGARTNER, H.R., STUDER, A.: Folgen des Gefäßkatheterismus am normo- und hypercholesterolinaemischen Kaninchen. Pathol. Microbiol. 29, 393 - 405 (1966).

BAUMGARTNER, H.R., STUDER, A.: Smooth muscle cell proliferation and migration after removal of arterial endothelium in rabbits. In: Atherosclerosis - Is it Reversible? SCHETTLER, G. (ed.). (1976)(in press).

BAUMGARTNER, H.R., TRANZER, J.P., STUDER, A.: An electron microscopic study of platelet thrombus formation in the rabbit with particular regard to 5-hydroxytryptamine release. Thromb. Diath. Haemorrh. 18, 592 (1967).

BEAUMONT, J.L.: Auto-immune hyperlipidemia. An atherogenic metabolic disease of immune origin. Rev. Europ. Etudes Clin. Biol. 15, 1037 (1970).

BEAUMONT, J.L.: Gamma-globulines et hyperlipidémie. L'hyperlipidémie par autoanticorps. Ann. Biol. Clin. 27, 611 (1969).

BEAUMONT, J.L.: Les facteurs de risque et la pathogénie de l'athérosclérose. Triangle 14, 9 (1975).

BEAUMONT, J.L.: Lipides et athérosclérose. Rev. Franç. Etudes Clin. Biol. 9, 1031 (1964).

BEAUMONT, J.L.: L'hyperlipidémie par auto-anticorps anti-beta-lipoprotéines. Une nouvelle entité pathologique. C.R. Acad. Sci. Paris, Série D 261, 4563 (1965).

BEAUMONT, J.L., ANTONUCCI, M., BERARD, M.: Autoimmune hyperlipidemia in the nephrotic syndrome. In: Proceedings of the International Workshop-Conference on Atherosclerosis. MANNING, G.W., HAUST, M.D. (eds.). New York: Plenum Press, 1976 (in press).

BEAUMONT, J.L., ANTONUCCI, M., LAGRUE, G., GUEDON, J., PEROL, R.: Nephrotic syndrome, monoclonal gammopathy and autoimmune hyperlipidemia. Clin. Exper. Immunol. 18, 225 (1974).

BEAUMONT, J.L., BEAUMONT, V.: Immunological factors of atherosclerosis. In: Atherosclerosis III. SCHETTLER, G., WEIZEL, A. (eds.). Berlin: Springer-Verlag, 1974a, p. 579.

BEAUMONT, J.L., BEAUMONT, V., ANTONUCCI, M.: Présence d'un auto-anticorps anti-beta-lipoprotéines dans le sérum d'un lapin ayant une hyperlipidémie par immunisation (L'hyperlipidémie par auto-anticorps expérimentale). C.R. Acad. Sci. Paris, Série D 268, 1830 (1969).

BEAUMONT, J.L., BEAUMONT, V., LEMORT, N., ANTONUCCI, M.: Les auto-anticorps anti-lipoprotéines de myélome. Etude comparée de deux types: l'IgA anti-Lp P.G. et l'IgG anti-Lp A.S. Ann. Biol. Clin. 28, 387 (1970).

BEAUMONT, J.L., CARLSON, L.A., COOPER, G.R., FEJFAR, Z., FREDRICKSON, D.S., STRASSER, T.: Classification of hyperlipidaemias and hyperlipoproteinaemias. WHO Bulletin 43, 891- 908 (1970).

BEAUMONT, J.L., JACOTOT, B., BEAUMONT, V.: L'hyperlipidémie par auto-anticorps. Une cause d'athérosclérose. Presse Med. 75, 2315 (1967).

BEAUMONT, J.L., LEMORT, N.: Oral contraceptive, pulmonary artery thrombosis and anti-ethinyl-oestradiol monoclonal IgG. Clin. Exper. Immunol. 24, 455 (1976).

BEAUMONT, J.L., LEMORT, N.: Une immunoglobuline anti-héparine dans un sérum hyperlipidémique. (Une nouvelle variété d'hyperlipidémie par auto-anticorps.) C.R. Acad. Sci. Paris, Série D 271, 2452 (1970).

BEAUMONT, J.L., LORENZELLI, L.: Le phénomène d'agglutination des particules lipidiques. Son intérêt en séro-immunologie. Pathol. Biol. 20, 357 (1972).

BEAUMONT, V., BEAUMONT, J.L.: Atherosclerosis and immunology. In: Proceedings of the International Symposium on Atherosclerosis. WILLOUGHBY, D.A., DEROM, F., CICALA, E., MALAN, E. (eds.). Milan: Carlo Erby Foundation 1973, pp.153-157.

BEAUMONT, V., BEAUMONT, J.L.: Hyperlipidemia and tumors: the hyperlipidemia of lymphoma-bearing hamsters. Biomedicine 20, 68 (1974b).

BEAUMONT, V., BEAUMONT, J.L.: L'hyperlipidémie expérimentale par immunisation chez le lapin. Pathol. Biol. 16, 869 (1968).

BECKENBACH, E.S., SELZER, R.H., CRAWFORD, D.W., BROOKS, S.H., BLANKENHORN, D.H.: Computer tracking and measurement of blood vessel shadows from arteriograms. Med. Instrument. 8, 308 - 310 (1974).

BECKER, C.G., DUBIN, T., WIEDEMAN, H.P.: Hypersensitivity to tobacco antigen. Proc. Natl. Acad. Sci. 73, 1712 - 1716 (1976).

BECKER, C.G., MURPHY, G.E.: Demonstration of contractile protein in endothelium and cells of the heart valves, endocardium, intima, arteriosclerotic plaques, and aschoff bodies of rheumatic heart disease. Amer. J. Pathol. 55, 1 (1969).

BEHER, W.T., CASAZZA, K.K., BEHER, M.E., FILUS, A.M., BERTASIUS, J.: Effect of cholesterol on bile acid metabolism in the rats. Proc. Soc. Exper. Biol. Med. 134, 595 - 601 (1970).

BEITZKE, H.: Zur Entstehung der Atherosklerose. Virchows Arch. f. path. Anat. 267, 625 (1928).

BEKHEIT, S., FLETCHER, E.: The effect of smoking on myocardial conduction in the human heart. Am. Heart J. 91, 712 - 720 (1976).

BELL, F.P., ADAMSON, I.L., SCHWARTZ, C.J.: Aortic endothelial permeability of albumin: focal and regional patterns of uptake and transmural distribution of ^{131}I-albumin in the young pig. Exp. Molec. Pathol. 20, 57 (1974a).

BELL, F.P., GALLUS, A.S., SCHWARTZ, C.J.: Focal and regional patterns of uptake and the transmural distribution of ^{131}I-fibrinogen in the pig aorta in vivo. Exp. Molec. Pathol. 20, 281 (1974b).

BELL, F.P., SOMER, J.B., CRAIG, I.H., SCHWARTZ, C.J.: Patterns of aortic Evans Blue uptake in vivo and in vitro. Atherosclerosis 16, 369 (1972).

BEMIS, C.E., GORLIN, R., KEMP, H.G., HERMAN, M.V.: Progression of coronary artery disease. A clinical arteriographic study. Circ. 47, 455 - 464 (1973).

BENDITT, E.P.: Evidence for a monoclonal origin of human atherosclerotic plaques and some implications. Circulation 50, 650 - 652 (1974).

BENDITT, E.P., BENDITT, J.M.: Evidence for a monoclonal origin of human athero-sclerotic plaques (glucose-6-phosphate dehydrogenase/heterozygotic females/aorta). Proc. Nat. Acad. Sci. U.S.A. 70, 1753 - 1756 (1973).

BENSADOUN, A., EHNHOLM, C., STEINBERG, D., BROWN, W.V.: J. Biol. Chem. 249, 2220 (1974).

BERENSON, G.S., FISHKIN, A.F.: Isolation of a glycoprotein from bovine aorta. Arch. Biochem. 97, 18 (1962).

BERENSON, G.S., RADHAKRISHNAMURTHY, B., DALFERES, E.R., Jr., SRINIVASAN, S.R.: Carbohydrate macromolecules and atherosclerosis. Human Pathol. 2, 57 - 79 (1971).

BERENSON, G.S., RADHAKRISHNAMURPHY, B., FISHKIN, A.F., DESSAUER, H., ARQUEM-BOURG, P.: Individuality of glycoproteins in human aorta. J. Atheroscler. Res. 6, 214 - 223 (1966).

BERENSON, G.S., SRINIVASAN, S.R., DOLAN, P.J., RADHAKRISHNAMURTHY, B.: Lipopro-tein and mucopolysaccharide complexes from fatty streaks of human aorta. Circulation 44, II-6 (1971).

BERGSTRÖM, J.: Muscle electrolytes in man. Scand. J. clin. Lab. Invest. (Suppl. 68), (1962).

BERLEPSCH, K., von, STUDER, A.: Acid mucopolysaccharides after over-dilatation of the aortic wall in rabbit. Angiologia 6, 105 - 110 (1969).

BERNARD, C.: An introduction to the study of experimental medicine. New York: Dover Publication, Inc., 1957.

BERSOT, T.P., BROWN, W.V., LEVY, R.I., WINDMUELLER, H.G., FREDRICKSON, D.S., LeQUIRE, V.S.: Further characterization of the apolipoproteins of rat plasma lipoproteins. Biochemistry 9, 3427 (1970).

BERSOT, T.P., MAHLEY, R.W., BROWN, M.S., GOLDSTEIN, J.L.: Interaction of swine lipoproteins with the low density lipoprotein receptor in human fibroblasts. J. Biol. Chem. 251, 2395 (1976).

BEVANS, M., DAVIDSON, J.D., KENDALL, F.E.: Regression of lesions in canine atherosclerosis. Arch. Pathol. 51, 288 - 292 (1951).

BEZMAN, A., FELTS, J.M., HAVEL, R.J.: Relation between incorporation of tri-glyceride fatty acids and heparin-released lipoprotein lipase from adipose tissue slices. J. Lipid Res. 3, 427 - 431 (1962).

BIALE, Y., SHAFRIR, E.: Lipolytic activity toward tri- and monoglycerides in postheparin plasma. Clin. Chim. Acta 23, 413 - 419 (1969).

BIERENBAUM, M.I., FLEISCHMAN, A.I., RAICHELSON, R.I.: Long term human studies on the lipid effects of oral calcium. Lipids 7, 202 (1972).

BIERMAN, E.L.: Insulin and hypertriglyceridemia. Isr. J. Med. Sci. 8, 303 (1972).

BIERMAN, E.L., ALBERS, J.J.: Lipoprotein uptake by cultured human arterial smooth muscle cells. Biochimica et Biophysica Acta 388, 198 (1975).

BIERMAN, E.L., BRUNZELL, J.D., BAGDADE, J.D., LERNER, R.L., HAZZARD, W.R., PORTE, D., Jr.: On the mechanism of action of Atromid-S on triglyceride transport in man. Trans. Assoc. Amer. Phys. 83, 211 - 224 (1970).

BIERMAN, E.L., EISENBERG, S., STEIN, O., STEIN, Y.: Very low density lipoprotein "remnant" particles; uptake by aortic smooth muscle cells in culture. Bio-chim. Biophys. Acta 329, 163 - 169 (1973).

BIERMAN, E.L., STEIN, O., STEIN, Y.: Lipoprotein uptake and metabolism by rat aortic smooth muscle cells in tissue culture. Circ. Res. 35, 136 - 150 (1974).

BIHARI-VARGA, M., VEGH, M.: Quantitative studies on the complexes formed between aortic mucopolysaccharides and serum lipoproteins. Biochim. Biophys. Acta 144, 202 - 210 (1967).

BILHEIMER, D.W., EISENBERG, S., LEVY, R.I.: The metabolism of very low density lipoprotein proteins. I. Preliminary in vitro and in vivo observations. Biochim. Biophys. Acta 260, 212 - 221 (1972).

BILHEIMER, D.W. GOLDSTEIN, J.L., GRUNDY, S.M., BROWN, M.S.: Reduction in chol-esterol and low density lipoprotein synthesis after portacaval shunt surgery in a patient with homozygous familial hypercholesterolemia. J. Clin. Invest. 56, 1420 (1975).

BILLIMORIA, J.D., POZNER, H., METSELAAR, B., BEST, F.W., JAMES, D.C.O.: Effect of cigarette smoking on lipids, lipoproteins, blood coagulation, fibrinolysis and cellular components of human blood. Atherosclerosis 21, 61 - 76 (1975).

BIÖRCK, G.: Contrasting concepts of ischaemic heart disease. Stockholm: Almqvist and Wiksell International, 1975.

BJARTVEIT, K.: Cardiovascular disease study in Norwegian counties. Abstract Book I, Seventh European Congress of Cardiology. Amsterdam: 1976, p. 79.

BJONDERS, G.: Cholesterol accumulation and removal in normal and atherosclerotic arterial tissue. In: Blood and Arterial Wall in Atherogenesis and Arterial Thrombosis. IFMA Scientific Symposia Nr. 4. HAUTVAST, HERMUS, VAN DER HAAR (eds.) Leiden: E.J. Brill, 1975.

BJÖRKERUD, S.: Atherosclerosis initiated by mechanical trauma in normolipidemic rabbits. J. Atheroscler. Res. 9, 209 (1969).

BJÖRKERUD, S., BONDJERS, G.: Arterial repair and atherosclerosis after mechanical injury. Part 1. Permeability and light microscopic characteristics of endothelium in non-atherosclerotic and atherosclerotic lesions. Atherosclerosis 13, 355 (1971a).

BJÖRKERRUD, S., BONDJERS, G.: Arterial repair and atherosclerosis after mechanical injury. Part 2. Tissue response after induction of a total local necrosis (deep longitudinal injury). Atherosclerosis 14, 259 (1971b).

BJÖRKERUD, S., BONDJERS, G.: Arterial repair and atherosclerosis after mechanical injury. Part 5. Tissue response after induction of a large superficial transverse injury. Atherosclerosis 18, 235 (1973).

BLACKBURN, H.: Ischaemic heart disease. The challenge, the controversy and the potential of prevention. Arch. mal du coeur 68 (numéro spécial), 81 - 100 (1976).

BLANCHETTE-MACKIE, E.J., SCOW, R.O.: Sites of lipoprotein lipase activity in adipose tissue perfused with chylomicrons. Electron microscopic cytochemical study. J. Cell Biol. 51, 1 - 25 (1971).

BLANKENHORN, D.H.: Diagnostic methods for the study of human atherosclerosis. In: Diet and Atherosclerosis. SIRTORI, C., RICCI, G., GORINI, S. (eds.). New York: Plenum Publishing Corporation, 1975, pp. 119 - 124.

BLANKENHORN, D.H.: Studies of regression/progression of atherosclerosis in man. In: Proceedings of the International Workshop Conference on Atherosclerosis. London, Ontario: 1975 (in press).

BLANKENHORN, D.H.: Studies of regression/progression of atherosclerosis in man. In: Proceedings of the International Workshop Conference on Atherosclerosis. Manning, G.W., HAUST, M.D. (eds.). New York: Plenum Publishing Co., 1976 (in press).

BLATON, V., SOETEWEY, F., VANDAMME, D., DECLERCQ, B., PEETERS, B.: Effect of polyunsaturated phosphatidylcholine in human types II and IV hyperlipoproteinemias. Artery 2, 309 (1976).

BLIEDEN, L.C., DESNICK, R.J., CARTER, J.B., KRIVIT, W., MOLLER, J.H., SHARP, H.L.: Cardiac involvement in Sandhoff's disease: an inborn error of metabolism. Am. J. Cardiol. 34, 83 (1974).

BLIEDEN, L.C., MOLLER, J.H.: Cardiac involvement in inherited disorders of metabolism. Progr. Cardiov. Dis. 16, 615 (1974).

BLIEDEN, L.C., TSACKRACKLIDES, V., EDWARDS, J.E.: Myocardial infarction associated with systemic lupus erythematosus (Abstract). Proc. Minn. Med. Soc. 16 (1973).

BLIGH, E.G., DYER, W.J.: A rapid method of total lipid extraction and purificytion. Can. J. Biochem. Physiol. 37, 911 - 917 (1959).

BLOCK, W.D., JARRETT, K.J., LEVINE, J.B.: An improved automated determination of serum total cholesterol with a single color reagent. Clin. Chem. 12, 681 - 689 (1966).

BLOCK, W.D., JARRETT, K.J., LEVINE, B.: Use of a single color reagent to improve the automated determination of serum total cholesterol. In: Automation in Analytical Chemistry. SKEGGS, L.T. (ed.). New York: Mediad Inc., 1965, Vol. I, p. 345.

BLOSE, S.H., CHACKO, S.: In vitro behaviour of guinea pig arterial and venous endothelial cells. Devel. Growth and Diff. 17, 153 (1975).

BLUM, C.B., LEVY, R.I.: Interconversions of apolipoprotein fragments. Ann. Revs. Med. 26, 365 (1975).

BOBERG, J., AUGUSTIN, J., BAGINSKY, M., TEJADA, P., BROWN, W.V.: Quantitative determination of hepatic and lipoprotein lipase activities from human postheparin plasma. Abstracts of the 47th Scientific Session of the American Heart Association. Circulation 49 - 50 (Suppl. III), III - 21 (1975a).

BOBERG, J., BOBERG, M., GROSS, R., GRUNDY, S., AUGUSTIN, J., BROWN, W.V.: The effect of clofibrate treatment on hepatic triglyceride lipase and lipoprotein lipase activities of postheparin plasma. Abstracts of the papers of the 9th Annual Meeting of European Society for Clinical Investigation, April 24 - 26. Rotterdam (1975b).

BOBERG, J., CARLSON, L.A., GREYSCHUSS, V., LASSESS, B.W., WAHLQUIST, M.L.: Splanchnic secretion rates of plasma triglycerides and total splanchnic turnover of plasma free fatty acids in man with normo- and hypertriglyceridemia. Europ. J. Clin. Invest. 2, 454 - 466 (1972).

BOBERG, J., CARLSON, L.A., HALLBERG, D.: Application of a new intravenous fat tolerance test in the study of hypertriglyceridemia in man. J. Atheroscler. Res. 9, 159 - 169 (1969).

BOLZANO, K., KREMLER, F., Sandhofer, F.: "Hepatic" and "extrahepatic" triglyceride lipase activity in postheparin plasma of normals and patients with cirrhosis of the liver. Horm. Metab. Res. 7, 238 - 241 (1975).

BOND, M.G., BULLOCK, B.C., CLARKSON, T.B., LEHNER, N.D.M.: The effect of plasma cholesterol concentrations on "regression" of primate atherosclerosis. Am. J. Path. 82, (2) 59a (Abstract)(1976).

BOOYSE, F.M., SEDLAK, B.J., RAFELSON, M.E.: Culture of arterial endothelial cells. Thrombosis, Diathesis Hemorr. 34, 825 (1974).

BORGSTROM, B.: Quantification of cholesterol absorption in man by fecal analysis after feeding of a single isotope-labeled meal. J. Lipid. Res. 10, 331 - 337 (1969).

BORTZ, W.M.: Reversibility of atherosclerosis in cholesterol fed rabbits. Circ. Res. 22, 135 - 139 (1968).

BOWYER, D.E., DUNN, D., GRESHAM, G.A.: Production of advanced atheromatous lesions in an allografted segment of aorta in a normocholesterolaemic rabbit. In: Atherosclerosis III. SCHETTLER, G., WEIZEL, A. (eds.). Berlin: Springer-Verlag, 1974, p. 348.

BRAND, R.I., ROSENMAN, R.H., SHOLTZ, R.I., FRIEDMAN, M.: Multivariate prediction of coronary heart disease in the Western Collaborative Group Study compared to the findings of the Framingham Study. Circulation 53, 348 - 355 (1976).

BRECHER, P.I., CHOBANIAN, A.V.: Cholesteryl ester synthesis in normal and atherosclerotic aortas of rabbits and rhesus monkeys. Circ. Res. 35, 692 - 701 (1974).

BRECKENRIDGE, W.C., LITTLE, J.A., STEINER, G., CHOW, A., POAPST, M.: Hyperlipoproteinemia associated with an absence of CII apoprotein in plasma lipoproteins. Circulation October, 1976 (in press).

BREDT, H.: Morphology. In: Atherosclerosis. SCHETTLER, G., BOYD, G.S. (eds.). Amsterdam: Elsevier, 1969, Chap. 1.

BRESLOW, J.L., SPAULDING, D.R., LOTHROP, P.A., CLOWES, A.W.: Effect of lipoproteins on 3-hydroxy-3-methylglutaryl coenzime A (HMG-CoA) reductase activity in rat liver cell culture: specific suppressant effect of a lipoprotein isolated from hypercholesterolemic rat plasma. Biochem. Res. Comm. 67, 119 (1975).

BRESLOW, J.L., SPAULDING, D.R., LUX, S.E., LEVY, R.I., LEES, R.S.: Homozygous familial hypercholesterolemia: a possible biochemical explanation of clinical heterogeneity; heterogeneity in homozygous familial hypercholesterolemia. New Engl. J. Med. 293, 900 - 902 (1975).

BREWER, H.B., Jr., LUX, S.E., RONAN, R., JOHN, K.M.: Amino acid sequence of human apoLP-Gln-II (apoA-II), an apolipoprotein isolated from the high-density lipoprotein complex. Proc. Natl. Acad. Sci. US 69, 1304 - 1308 (1972).

BREWER, H.B., Jr., SHULMAN, R., HERBERT, P., RONAN, R., WEHRLY, K.: The complete amino acid sequence of alanine apolipoprotein (apoC-III), an apolipoprotein from human plasma very low density lipoproteins. J. Biol. Chem. 249, 4975 - 4984 (1974).

BRICKER, L.A., WEIS, H.J., SIPERSTEIN, M.D.: In vivo demonstration of the cholesterol feedback system by means of a desmosterol suppression technique. J. Clin. Invest. 51, 197 - 205 (1972).

BRIGDEN, W., BYNATERS, E.G.L., LESSOF, M.H. et al.: The heart in systemic lupus erythematosus. Brit. Heart J. 22, 1 (1960).

BROOKS, B.R., SODE, J., ENGEL, W.K., SHIMAMOTO, T.: Cyclic nucleotide metabolism in motor neuron disease (ALS complex). Abstract of American Academy of Neurology.

BROOKS, H., HOLLAND, R., AL-SADIR, J.: Right ventricular performance during myocardial infarction: an anatomic and hemodynamic analysis in the porcine heart. Circulation (1976) (in press).

BROWN, C.E., HUANG, T.C., BORTZ, E.L., McCAY, C.M.: Observations on blood vessels and exercise. J. Geront. 11, 292 (1956).

BROWN, H.B., GREEN, J.G.: Diets suitable for reduction of serum cholesterol levels. The Cleveland Clinic Dietary Research Project. Cleveland Clin. Q. 29, 101 (1962).

BROWN, J.T.: Structural origins of mammalian albumin. Fed. Proc. 35, 2141 - 2144 (1976).

BROWN, M.S., BRANNAN, P.G., BOHMFALK, H.A., BRUNSCHEDE, G.Y., DANA, S.E., HELGESON, J., GOLDSTEIN, J.L.: Use of mutant fibroblasts in the analysis of the regulation of cholesterol matabolism in human cells. J. Cell. Physiol. 85, 425 - 436 (1975).

BROWN, M.S., DANA, S.E., GOLDSTEIN, J.L.: Cholesterol ester formation in cultured human fibroblasts: stimulation by oxygenated sterols. J. Biol. Chem. 250, 4025 - 4027 (1975).

BROWN, M.S., GOLDSTEIN, J.L.: Receptor-mediated control of cholesterol metabolism. Science 191, 150 - 154 (1976).

BROWN, M.S., GOLDSTEIN, J.L.: Suppression of 3-hydroxy-3-methylglutaryl co-enzyme A reductase activity and inhibition of growth of human fibroblasts by 7-ketocholesterol. J. Biol. Chem. 249, 7306 - 7314 (1974).

BROWN, W.V., BAGINSKY, M.L.: Some functional aspects of apolipoproteins: ApoLp-Ala inhibition of lipoprotein lipase and deinhibition by monoolein. In: Lipid Metabolism, Obesity and Diabetes Mellitus. GRETEN, H., LEVINE, R., PFEIFFER, E.F., RENOLD, A.E. (eds.). Stuttgart: Georg Thieme, 1974, p. 11-16.

BROWN, W.V., LEVY, R.I., FREDRICKSON, D.S.: Studies of the proteins in human plasma very low density lipoproteins. J. Biol. Chem. 244, 5687 (1969).

BROWN, W.V., SHAW, W., BAGINSKY, M., BOBERG, J., AUGUSTIN, J.: Lipoprotein Metabolism. GRETEN, H. (ed.). Berlin-Heidelberg-New York: Springer 1976, p. 2.

BROZEK, J. WELLS, S., KEYS, A.: Medical aspects of semi-starvation in Leningrad (Siege 1941-1942). Am. Rev. Soviet Med. 4, 70 (1946).

BRUDERLEIN, H., ROBINSON, W.T., KRAML, M., DVORNIK, D.: A gas liquid chromatographic determination of p-chlorophenoxy-isobutyric acid and its comparison to an ultra-violet method. Clin. Biochem. 8, 261 - 272 (1975).

BRUNS, R.R., PALADE, G.E.: Studies on blood capillaries. II. Transport of ferritin molecules across the wall of muscle capillaries. J. Cell. Biol. 37, 277 (1968).

BRUNZELL, J., ALBERS, J., HOLMES, L., AGADOA, L., SHERRARD, D.: Prevalence and interaction of plasma lipid abnormalities in chronic dialysis. Kidney International 8, 408 (1975).

BRUNZELL, J.D., CHAIT, A., ALBERS, J.: Abstracts of the Fourth International Symposium on Atherosclerosis, Tokyo, Japan, 1976, p.33.

BRUNZELL, J.D., HAZZARD, W.R., PATE, D., Jr., BIERMAN, E.L.: Evidence for a common saturable triglyceride removal mechanism for chylomicrons and very low density lipoproteins in man. J. Clin. Invest. 52, 1578 - 1585 (1973).

BUCHWALD, H.: Alterations in the cutaneous lesions of the hyperlipidemias following partial ileal bypass. Derm. Dig. 9, 65 (1970).

BUCHWALD, H.: The development of the sub-total ileal bypass operation as a therapeutic approach to hypercholesterolemia and atherosclerosis: a review. Diseases Chest 51, 459 (1967).

BUCHWALD, H.: Vitamin B_{12} absorption deficiency following bypass of the ileum. Am. J. Dig. Dis. 9, 755 (1964).

BUCHWALD, H., MOORE, R.B.. LEE, G.B., FRANTZ, I.D., Jr., VARCO, R.L.: Combined dietary, surgical, and bile salt binding resin therapy in the treatment of hypercholesterolemia. Arch. Surg. 97, 275 (1968).

BUCHWALD, H., MOORE, R.B., VARCO, R.L.: Partial ileal bypass operation for control of hyperlipidemia and atherosclerosis. In: Gibbon's Surgery of the Chest, 3rd. ed. SABISON, D.C., SPENCER, F.C. (eds.). Symposia Specialists, 1975a.

BUCHWALD, H., MOORE, R.B., VARCO, R.L.: Surgical treatment of hyperlipidemia. Circulation (Suppl. I), 49, 1 (1974a).

BUCHWALD, H., MOORE, R.B., VARCO, R.L.: Ten years clinical experience with partial ileal bypass in management of the hyperlipidemias. Ann. Surg. 180, 384 (1974).

BUCHWALD, H., MOORE, R.B., VARCO, R.L.: The partial ileal bypass operation in treatment of the hyperlipidemias. In: Lipids, Lipoproteins, and Drugs. KRITCHEVSKY, D., PAOLETTI, R., HOLMES, W.L. (eds.). New York: Plenum Press, 1974, p. 221.

BUCHWALD, H., VARCO, R.L., MOORE, R.B., SCHWARTZ, M.Z.: Intestinal bypass procedures. Curr. Probl. in Surg.(April, 1975b). The Kroc Foundation: Jejuno-ileostomy for Obesity (Symposium). J. Clin. Nutr. (to be published).

BUDDEKE, E.: Chemical changes in the ground substance of the vessel wall in arteriosclerosis. J. Atheroscler. Res. 2, 32 - 46 (1962).

BUDDECKE, E., KRESSE, H.: Metabolic heterogeneity of arterial tissue glycosaminoglycans and proteoglycans. In: VOGEL, H.G. et al. (eds.).Connective Tissue and Ageing. Amsterdam: Excerpta Medica, 1973.

BULLOCK, B.C., CLARKSON, T.B., LEHNER, N.D.M., LOFLAND, H.B., Jr., St.CLAIR, R. W.: Atherosclerosis in Cebus albifrons monkeys. III. Clinical and pathologic studies. Exptl. Mol. Pathol. 10, 39 - 62 (1969).

BULLOCK, B.C., LEHNER, N.D.M., CLARKSON, T.B., FELDNER, M.A., WAGNER, W.D., LOFLAND, H.B., Jr.: Comparative primate atherosclerosis. I. Tissue cholesterol concentration and pathologic anatomy. Exptl. Mol. Pathol. 22, 151 - 175 (1975).

BUONASSISI, V.: Sulfated mucopolysaccharide and secretion in endothelial cell cultures. Exp. Cell. Res. 76, 363 (1973).

BUONASSISI, V., ROOT, M.: Enzymatic degradation of heparin-related mucopolysaccharides from the surface of endothelial cell cultures. B.B. Acta 385, 1 (1975).

BURNSTOCK, G.: Structure of smooth muscle and its innervation. In: Smooth Muscle. BÜLBRING et al. (eds.). Edward Arnold, 170, pp. 4 - 66.

BUSCH, C., WASTESON, A., WESTERMARK, B.: Release of a cell growth promoting factor from human platelets. Thromb. Res. 8, 493 (1976).

BUTCHER, R.W., BAIRD, C.E., SUTHERLAND, E.W.: Effect of lipolytic and antilipolytic substances on adenosine 3',5'-monophosphate levels in isolated fat cells. J. Biol. Chem. 243, 1705 (1968).

BYWATERS, E.G.L.: Peripheral vascular obstruction in rheumatoid arthritis and its relationship to other vascular lesions. Ann. Rheum. Dis. 16, 84 (1957).

CAMEJO, G., BOSCH, V., ARREAZA, C., MENDEZ, H.C.: Early changes in plasma lipoprotein structure and biosynthesis in cholesterol-fed rabbits. J. Lipid. Res. 14, 61 - 68 (1973).

CAMEJO, G., LOPEZ, A., VEGAS, H., PAOLI, H.: The participation of aortic protein in the formation of complexes between low density lipoproteins and intima-media extracts. Atherosclerosis 21, 77 (1975).

CAMEJO, G., MATEU, L., LALAGUNA, F., PADROH, F., WAICH, S., ACQUATELLA, M., VEGA, M.: Structural individuality of human serum LDL associated with a differential affinity of a macromolecular component of the arterial wall. Artery 2, 79 (1976).

CAMPBELL, P.N.: The biosynthesis of serum albumin. FEBS Lett. 54, 119 (1975).

CAPLAN, B.A., SCHWARTZ, C.J.: Increased endothelial cell turnover in areas of in vivo Evans blue uptake in the pig aorta. Atherosclerosis 17, 401 (1973).

CAREW, T.E., KOSCHINSKY, T.K., HAYES, S., STEINBERG, D.: A mechanism by which high density lipoproteins may slow the atherogenic process. Lancet (1976) I, 1315.

CAREW, T.E., SAIK, R.P., JOHANSEN, K.H., DENNIS, C.A., STEINBERG, D.: Turnover of lipoprotein proteins after portacaval shunt in swine. Curculation 50, (Suppl. III), 48 (1974).

CARLSON, K.: Lipoprotein fractionation, J. Clin Path. (Ass. Clin. Path.) 5, (Suppl. 26), 32 (1973).

CARLSON, L.A.: Lipid metabolism and muscular work. Fed. Proc. 26, 1755 (1967).

CARLSON, L.A.: Plasma or patient, paper-electrophoresis of physician? The four-P problem in classification of hyperlipidaemia. Atherosclerosis, Editorial. 12, 181 (1970).

CARLSON, L.A., BALLANTYNE, D.: Changing relative proportions of apolipoproteins CII and CIII of very low density lipoproteins in hypertriglyceridemia. Atherosclerosis 23, 563 - 568 (1976).

CARLSON, L.A., ERICSON, M.: Quantitative and qualitative serum lipoprotein analysis. Atherosclerosis 1, 417 - 433 (1975).

CARLSON, L.A., ERICSON, M.: Quantitative and qualitative serum lipoprotein analysis. Part I.: Studies in healthy man and women. Atherosclerosis 21, 417 - 423 (1975).

CARLSON, L.A., OLSSON, A.G., ORÖ, L., RÖSSNER, S., WALLDIUS, G.: Effects of hypolipidemic regimen on serum lipoproteins. In: Atherosclerosis III. SCHETTLER, G., WEIZEL, A., (eds.). Berlin: Springer-Verlag, 1974, pp. 768 - 781.

CARROLL, K.K., HAMILTON, R.M.G.: Effects of dietary protein and carbohydrate on plasma cholesterol levels in relation to atherosclerosis. J. Food Sci. 40, 18 - 23 (1975).

CARVALHO, A.C.A., COLMAN, R.W., LEES, R.S.: Platelet function in hyperlipoproteinemia. N. Engl. J. Med. 290, 434 (1974).

CAYEN, M.N., DUBUC, J., DVORNIK, D.: Hypolipidemic activity of 2,8-Dibenzyl-ciclooctanone in rats. Biochem. Pharmacol. 25, 1537 (1976).

CHILVERS, A.S., THOMAS, M.L., BROWSE, N.L.: The progression of arteriosclerosis. A radiological study. Circ. 50, 402 - 408 (1974).

CHIN, H.P., BLANKENHORN, D.H.: Separation and quantitative analysis of serum lipoproteins by means of electrophoresis on cellulose acetate. Clin. Chim. Acta 20, 305 - 314 (1968).

CHISOLM, G.M., GAINER, J.L.: Oxygen diffusion and atherosclerosis. Atherosclerosis 19, 135 (1974).

CHISOLM, G.M., Terrado, E.N., GAINER, J.L.: Physiological transport in relationship to ageing. Nature 230, 390 (1971).

CLARKE, N., COLLINS, M.: Immediate fibrinolytic effect of components from the interior of human cells. Brit. J. exp. Path. 50, 153 (1969).

CLARKSON, T.B., KING, J.S., LOFLAND, H.B., FELDNER, M.A.: Changes in pathologic characteristics and composition of plaques during regression. Circulation 44, (Suppl. II), II-48 (1971).

CLARKSON, T.B., KING, J.S., LOFLAND, H.B., FELDNER, M.A., BULLOCK, B.D.: Pathologic characteristics and composition of diet-aggravated atherosclerotic plaques during "regression." Exp. Mol. Path. 19, 267 - 283 (1973).

CLARKSON, T.B., LOFLAND, H.B.: Effects of cholesterol-fat diets on pigeons susceptible and resistant to atherosclerosis. Circ. Res. 3, 106 (1961).

CLARKSON, T.B., PRICHARD, R.W., NETSKY, M.G. LOFLAND, H.B.: Atherosclerosis in pigeons. Its spontaneous occurrence and resemblance to human atherosclerosis. Arch. Pathol. 68, 143 (1959).

CLIFTON-BLIGH, P., MILLER, N.E., NESTEL, R.J.: Increased plasma cholesterol esterifying activity during cholestipol resin therapy in man. Metabolism 23, 437 - 444 (1974).

CLOT, J.P., ROUFFY, J., LOEPER, J., MERCADIER, M.: Derivation ileale, therapeutique, chirurgicale des hypercholesterolemies pures majeures (à propos de deux observations). Chirurgie 97, 57 (1971).

COCHRANE, C.G.: The role of immune complexes and complement in tissue injury. J. Allergy 42, 113 (1968).

COHEN, Y., COSTEROUSSE, O.: Etude autoradiographique chez le Souris d'un anti-diabètique oral: le NN-diméthylbiquanide marqué au carbon 14. Thérapie 16, 109 (1961).

COHN, K., SAKAI, F.J., LANGSTON, M.R., Jr.: Effect of Clofibrate on progression of coronary disease: a prospective angiographic study in man. Am. Heart J. 89, 591 - 598 (1975).

COLON, A.A., GARCIA-PALMIERI, M.R., NAZARIO, E.: Methods and quality control of laboratory determinations in a prospective study of ischemic heart disease. Bol. Asoc. Med. P. Rico. 61, 198 - 201 (1969).

CONNOR, W.E., ARMSTRONG, M.L., JACKSON, C., ALI, A.M.: Persistence of cholesterol $4C^{14}$ in atherosclerotic aortas of animals treated with a diet high in polyunsaturated fat (Abstract). J. Clin. Invest. 45, 997 (1966).

CONNOR, W.E., CONNOR, S.L.: The key role of nutritional factors in the prevention of coronary heart disease. Prev. Med. 1, 49 - 83 (1972).

CONSTANTINIDES, P.: Experimental Atherosclerosis. Amsterdam: Elsevier Publishers, 1965, p. 42.

CONSTANTINIDES, P., BOOTH, J., CARLSON, G.: Production of advanced cholesterol atherosclerosis in the rabbit. Arch. Pathol. 70, 712 (1960).

CONSTANTINIDES, P., ROBINSON, M.: Ultrastuctural injury of arterial endothelium. I. Effects of pH, osmolarity, anoxia, and temperature. Arch. Path. 88, 99 - 105 (1969a).

CONSTANTINIDES, P., Ultrastructural injury of arterial endothelium. II. Effects of vasoactive amines. Arch. Path. 88, 106 (1969b).

CONTI, F., SIRTORI, M., GIANFRANCESCHI, G., TREMOLI, E., SIRTORI, C.R.: Impiego della Metformina nel trattamento delle arteriopatie arteriosclerotiche degli arti inferiori. Giorn. Arterioscl. 1, 53 (1976).

CORAN, A.G., WARREN, R.: Arteriographic changes in femoropopliteal arteriosclerosis obliterans. A five-year follow-up study. The New Eng. J. Med. 274, 643 - 647 (1966).

CORNFIELD, J.: Joint dependence of risk of coronary heart disease on serum cholesterol and systolic blood pressure: discriminant function analysis. Fed. Proc. 21, 58 (1962).

CORNWELL, D.G., KRUGER, F.A.: Molecular complexes in the isolation and characterization of plasma lipoproteins. J. Lipid Res. 2, 110 (1961).

CORONARY DRUG PROJECT: Clofibrate and niacin in coronary heart disease. J. Amer. med. Ass. 231, 360 (1975).

CORONARY DRUG PROJECT RESEARCH GROUP: Clofibrate and niacin in coronary heart disease. J. Amer. med. Ass. 27, 360 - 381 (1975).

CORONARY DRUG PROJECT. Special Communication. Findings leading to further modifications of its protocol with respect to d-thyroxine. J. Amer. med. Ass. 220, 996 (1972).

CORONARY DRUG PROJECT. Special Communication. Initial findings leading to modifications of its research protocol. J. Amer. med. Ass. 214, 1303 (1970).

CORRE, F., LELLOUCH, J., SCHWARTZ, D.: Smoking and leucocyte-counts. Results of an epidemiological survey. Lancet (1971) II, 632 - 634.

COTRAN, R.S., KARNOVSKY, M.J.: Ultrastructural studies on the permeability of the mesothelium to horseradish peroxidase. J. Cell. Biol. 37, 123 (1968).

COTRAN, R.S., KARNOVSKY, M.J.: Vascular leakage induced by horseradish peroxidase in the rat. Proc. Soc. Exp. Biol. Med. 126, 557 (1967).

COYLE, J.J., SCHWARTZ, M.Z., MARUBBIO, A.T., VARCO, R.L., BUCHWALD, H.: The effect of portacaval shunt on plasma lipids and tissue cholesterol synthesis in the dog. Surgery 80, 54 (1976).

COYLE, J.J., VARCO, R.L., BUCHWALD, H.: Vitamin B_{12} absorption following human intestinal bypass surgery. (submitted for publication).

CRAVEN, B., de TITTA, G.: Cholesteryl myristate: structures of the crystalline and mesophases. J. Chem. Soc. Perkin Trans. II, 814 - 822 (1976).

CRAWFORD, D.W., BECKENBACH, E.S., BLANKENHORN, D.H., SELZER, R.H., BROOKS, S.H.: Grading of coronary atherosclerosis. Comparison of a modified IAP visual grading method and a new quantitative angiographic technique. Atherosclerosis 19, 231 - 241 (1974).

CRAWFORD, D.W., BROOKS, S.H., SELZER, R.H., BARNDT, R., Jr., BECKENBACH, E.S., BLANKENHORN, D.H.: Computer densitometry for angiographic assessment of arterial cholesterol content and gross pathology in human atherosclerosis. J. Lab. Clin. Med. (1977) (in press).

CREPALDI, G., FEDELE, D., FELLIN, R., BRIANI, G.: Long-term clofibrate treatment in familial hyperlipoproteinemias. In: Atherosclerosis III. Proceedings of the Third International Symposium. SCHETTLER, G., WEIZEL, A. (eds.). New York: Springer-Verlag, 1974, pp. 812 - 815.

CREPALDI, G., FELLIN, R., BRIANI, G., BAGGIO, G., MANZATO, E., BAIOCCHI, M., BALDO, G.: Risk of atherosclerosis in different types of familial hyperlipoproteinemia. Seventh European Congress of Cardiology. (Abstract) 253 (1976).

CRYER, A., DAVIES, P., ROBINSON, D.S.: The control of lipoprotein lipase. The Hague: Proc. IFMA Symposium, 1974, p. 102.

CRYER, A., RILEY, S.E., WILLIAMS, E.R., ROBINSON, D.S.: Effect of nutritional status on rat adipose tissue, muscle and postheparin clearing factor lipase activities: their relationship to triglyceride fatty acid uptake by fat cells and to plasma insulin concentrations. Clin. Sci. Molec. Med. 50, 213 - 221 (1976).

CURRAN, R.C., CRANE, W.A.J.: Mucopolysaccharides in the atherosclerotic aorta. J. Path. Bact. 84, 405 - 409 (1962).

CURRY, M.D., ALAUPOVIC, P., SUENRAM, C.A.: Determination of apolipoprotein A and its constitutive A-I and A-II polypeptides by separate electroimmunoassays. Clin. Chem. 22, 315 (1976a).

CURRY, M.D., McCONATHY, J.W., ALAUPOVIC, P.: Quantitative determination of human apolipoprotein D by electroimmunoassay and radial immunodiffusion. Biochim. Biophys. Acta (1977)(in press).

CURRY, M.D., McCONATHY, J.W., ALAUPOVIC, P., LEDFORD, J.H., POPOVIC, M.: Determination of human apolipoprotein E by electroimmunoassay. Biochim. Biophys. Acta 439, 413 (1976b).

CYWES, S., DAVIES, M.R.Q., LOUW, J.H., BERGER, G.M.B., BONNICI, F., JOFFE, H.S.: Portacaval shunt in two patients with homozygous type II hyperlipoprotein-aemia. S.A. Med. J. (1976) I, 239.

DALES, L.G., FRIEDMAN, G.D., SIEGELAUB, A.B., SELTZER, C.C.: Cigarette smoking and serum chemistry tests. J. Chronic Dis. 27, 293 - 307 (1974).

DALLOCHIO, M., CROCKETT, R., RAZAKA, G., GANDJI, F.A., BRICAUD, H., PAUTZIZEL, R., BROUSTET, P.: Anticorps anti-aorte et lésions aortique par injections répétées de broyats aortiques (Etude chez le lapin). Arch. Mal. Coeur et Vaiss., Rév. Athérosc1. 3, 44 (1968).

DANIELSSON, B., EKMAN, R., PETERSSON, B.-G.: An abnormal high density lipoprotein in cholestatic plasma isolated by zonal ultrazentrifugation. FEBS Lett. 50, 180 (1975).

DAOUD, A.S.: Effects of homologous and heterologous sera on explants of swine aortic media. In: Proceedings of the Third International Symposium on Athero-sclerosis. Atherosclerosis III. SCHETTLER, G., WEIZEL, A. (eds.). New York-Heidelberg-Berlin: Springer-Verlag, 1974, pp. 169 - 172.

DAOUD, A.S. et al.: Regression of advanced atherosclerosis in swine. Arch. Path. Lab. Med. 100, 372 (1976).

DAOUD, A.S., FRITZ, K.E., JARMOLYCH, J., AUGUSTYN, J.M.: Use of aortic medial explants in the study of atherosclerosis. Exp. Molec. Path. 18, 177 - 189 (1973).

DAOUD, A.S., JARMOLYCH, J., AUGUSTYN, J.M., FRITZ, K.E., SINGH, J.K., KYER, T.L.: Regression of advanced atherosclerosis in swine. Arch. Path. Lab. Med. 100, 372 - 379 (1976).

DAOUD, A.S., JARMOLYCH, J., AUGUSTYN, J.M., FRITZ, K.E., SINGH, J.K., LEE, K.T.: Regression of advanced atherosclerosis in swine. Arch. Path. Lab. Med. 100, 372 (1976).

DAOUD, A.S., JARMOLYCH, J., FRITZ, K., AUGUSTYN, J.: Regression of advanced atherosclerosis in swine. Circulation 50, Suppl. 3, 92 (1974).

DAVIDSON, R.G., NITOWSKY, H.M., CHILDS, B.: Demonstration of two populations of cells in the female heterozygous for glucose-6-phosphate dehydrogenase variants. Proc. Natl. Acad. Sci. U.S.A. 50, 481 - 485 (1963).

DAVIGNON, J., AUBRY, F., NOEL, C., LAPIERRE, Y., LAFORTUNE, M.: Heterogeneity of familial hyperlipoproteinemia type II on the basis of the fasting plasma tri-glyceride/cholesterol ratio and plasma cholesterol response to chlorophenoxy-isobutyrate. Rev. Canada Biol. 30, 307 - 318 (1971).

DAVIGNON, J., LANGELIER, M.: Electrophorèse et ultracentrifugation combinées dans le diagnostic des hyperlipidémies primaires. Union Med. Can. 100, 2120 - 2128 (1971).DAY, A.J., BELL, F.P., MOORE, S., FRIEDMAN, R.: Lipid composition and metabolism of thromboatherosclerotic lesions produced by continued endo-thelial damage in normal rabbits. Circulation Res. 34, 467 (1974).

DAY, C.E., LEVY, R.S.: Control of the precipitation reaction between low density lipoproteins and polyions. Artery 1, 150 (1975).

DAY, C.E., POWELL, J.R., LEVY, R.S.: Sulfated polysaccharide inhibition of aortic uptake of low density lipoproteins. Artery 1, 126 (1975).

DAY, C.E., SHURR, P.E., HEYD, W.E., LEDNICER, D.: Biological activity of a hypo-betalipoproteinemic agent. Adv. Exp. Med. Biol. 67, 231 (1976).

723

DAYTON, S.: Nutrition and atherosclerosis. Progress in Food and Nutrition Science 1, 191 - 206 (1975).

DAYTON, S., PEARCE, M.L.: Prevention of coronary heart disease and other complications of atherosclerosis by modified diet. Amer. J. Med. 46, 751 - 762 (1969).

DAYTON, S., PEARCE, M.L., HASHIMOTO, S., DIXON, W.J., TOMIYASU, U.: A controlled clinical trial of a diet high in unsaturated fat. American Heart Association, Monograph Number 25, 1969.

DECKELBAUM, R.J., SHIPLEY, G.G., SMALL, D.M.: Structure and interactions in human plasma low density lipoproteins. J. Biol. Chem. (1977) (in press).

DECKELBAUM, R.J., SHIPLEY, G.G., SMALL, D.M., LEES, R.S., GEORGE, P.K.: Thermal transitions in human plasma low density lipoproteins. Science 190, 392 - 394 (1975).

DELL, R.B., SMITH, F.R., RAMAKRISHNAN, R., GOODMAN, DeW.S.: Optimal sampling strategy for determining the parameters of cholesterol kinetics. Circulation 50 (Suppl. III), III-262 (1974).

DEMPSTER, W.J.: Atheroma in a transplanted heart. Lancet (1969)II, 1247.

DEMPSTER, W.J., HARRISON, C.A., SHAKMAN, R.: Rejection process in human homo-transplanted. Brit. Med. J. 2, 969 (1964).

De PALMA, R.G., HUBAY, C.A., INSULL, W.,Jr., ROBINSON, A.V., HARTMAN, P.H.: Progression and regression of experimental atherosclerosis. Surg. Gyn. & Ob. 131, 633 - 647 (1970).

De PALMA, R.G., HUBAY, C.A., VOGT, C.J., INSULL, W., HARTMAN, P.H., ROBINSON, A.V.: Regression and prevention of experimental atherosclerosis: effects of diet and bile diversion in the dog. Surg. Forum 19, 308 (1968).

De PALMA, R.G., INSULL, W., BELLON, E.M., ROTH, T.W., ROBINSON, A.V.: Animal models for the study of progression and regression of atherosclerosis. Surgery 72, 268 - 278 (1972).

DHEW Publication 75-628. Manual of Laboratory Operations, Lipid Research Clinics Program, Vol. 1, Lipid and Lipoprotein Analysis. National Heart and Lung Institute (1974).

DIDISHEIM, P., MABASHAN, R.S.: Activation of Hageman factor (factor XII) by long chain saturated fatty acids. Thromb. Diath. Haemorrh. 9, 346 (1963).

DIETSCHY, J.M., WILSON, J.D.: Regulation of cholesterol metabolism. Part I. New Engl. J. Med. 282, 1128 - 1138 (1970).

DÖRNER, G.: Environment-dependent brain differentiation and fundamental processes in life. Acta biol. med. germ. 33, 129 - 148 (1974).

DÖRNER, G., MOHNIKE, A.: Zur möglichen Bedeutung der prä- und/oder frühpostnatalen Ernährung für die Pathogenese des Diabetes mellitus. Acta biol. med. germ. 31, K7 - K10 (1973).

DOERR, W.: Arteriosclerose. In: Allgemeine Pathologie der Organe des Kreislaufs. New York: Springer-Verlag, 1970, p. 568.

DOERR, W.: Perfusionstheorie der Arteriosklerose. In: Zwanglose Abhandlungen aus dem Gebiet der Normalen und Pathologischen Anatomie. BARGMANN, E., DOERR, W. (eds.). Stuttgart: Georg Thieme-Verlag, 1963, Vol.XIII.

DOYLE, J.T., DAWBER, T.R., KANNEL, W.B., KINCH, S.H., KAHN, H.A.: The relationship of smoking to coronary heart disease. JAMA 190, 886 (1964).

DUBLIN, L.I., MARKS, H.H.: Mortality among insured overweights in recent years. In: Transactions of the Association of Life Insurance Medical Directors of America: Sixtieth Annual Meeting. New York: Press of Recording and Statistical Corporation, 1951, Vol. 35, p. 235.

DUFF, G.L., McMILLAN, G.C.: Pathology of atherosclerosis. Amer. J. Med. 11, 92 - 108 (1951).

DUGAN, F.A., RADHAKRISHNAMURTHY, B., BERENSON, G.S.: Enzymograms of glycoprotein preparations from connective tissue. Enzymologia 33, 215 (1967).

DUGUID, J.B.: Mural thrombosis in arteries. Brit. Med. Bull. 2, 36 (1955).

DUGUID, J.B.: Pathogenesis of atherosclerosis. Lancet (1949)II, 925.

DUGUID, J.B.: Thrombosis as a factor in the pathogenesis of coronary atherosclerosis. J. Path. Bact. 58, 207 (1946).

DUSTAN, H.P.: Evaluation and therapy of hypertension - 1976. Mod. Concepts Cardiovasc. Dis. 45, 97 (1976).

DUSTIN, P.,Jr.: Arteriolar hyalinosis. Int. Rev. exp. Path. 1, 73 (1962).

DZOGA, K., WISSLER, R.W., VESSELINOVITCH, D.: The effect of normal and hyperlipemic low density lipoprotein fractions on aortic tissue culture cells. Circulation (Suppl. II), 43-44, (Abstract 17), 6 (1971).

EDWARDS, P.A., GOULD, R.G.: Dependence of the circadian rhythm of hepatic β-hydroxy-β-methylglutaryl coenzyme A reductase on ribonucleic acid synthesis. J. Biol. Chem. 249, 2891 - 2896 (1974).

EGELRUD, R., OLIVECRONA, T.: J. Biol. Chem. 247, 6212 (1972).

EGELRUD, T.: Reversible binding of lipoprotein lipase from hen adipose tissue to insolubilized heparin. Biochim. Biophas. Acta 296, 124 (1973).

EGELRUD, T., OLIVECRONA, T.: Purified bovine milk (lipoprotein) lipase: activity against lipid substrates in the absence of exogenous serum factors. Biochim. Biophys. Acta 306, 115 (1973).

EGGEN, D.A.: Cholesterol metabolism in groups of rhesus monkeys with high or low response of serum cholesterol to an atherogenic diet. J. Lipid Res. 17, 663 - 673 (1976).

EGGEN, D.A.: Cholesterol metabolism in nonhuman primates. In: Atherosclerosis in Primates. STRONG, J.P. (ed.). Basel: Karger, 1976, Vol. IX, pp. 267 - 299.

EGGEN, D.A., SOLBERG, L.A.: Variation of atherosclerosis with age. Lab. Invest. 18, 571 - 579 (1968).

EGGEN, D.A., STRONG, J.P., NEWMAN, W.P., CATSULIS, C., MALCOM, G.T., KOKATNUR, M.G.: Regression of diet-induced fatty streaks in rhesus monkeys. Lab. Investigation 31, 294 - 301 (1974).

EGGSTEIN, M.: Eine neue Bestimmung der Neutralfette im Blutserum und Gewebe. II. Mitteilung, Zuverlässigkeit der Methode, andere Neutralfettbestimmungen, Normalwerte für Triglyceride und Glycerin im menschlichen Blut. Klin. Wschr. 44, 267 - 273 (1966).

EGGSTEIN, M., SCHETTLER, G.: The effect of feeding various fats on the level of blood lipids. In: Essential Fatty Acids. SINCLAIR, H.M. (ed.). London: Butterworths Scientific Publications, 1958.

EHNHOLM, C., BENSADOUN, A., BROWN, W.V.: J. clin Invest. 52, 26a (1973).

EHNHOLM, C., GRETEN, H., BROWN, W.V.: A comparative study of postheparin lipolytic activity and a purified human triglyceride lipase. Biochim. Biophys. Acta 360, 68 - 77 (1974a).

EHNHOLM, C., HUTTUNEN, J.K., KINNUNEN, P.K.J., MIETTINEN, T.A., NIKKILÄ, E.A.: Effect of oxandrolone treatment on the activity of lipoprotein lipase, hepatic lipase and phospholipase A₁ of human postheparin plasma. New Engl. J. Med. 292, 1314 - 1317 (1975a).

EHNHOLM, C., KINNUNEN, P.K., HUTTUNEN, J.K.: FEBS Letters 52, 191 (1975).

EHNHOLM, C., SHAW, W., HARLAN, W., BROWN, W.V.: Circulation 48 (Suppl. IV), 112 (1973).

EHNHOLM, C., SHAW, W., GRETEN, H., BROWN, W.V.: Purification from human plasma of a heparin-released lipase with activity against triglyceride and phospholipids. J. Biol. Chem. 250, 6756 - 6761 (1975b).

EHNHOLM, C., SHAW, C., GRETEN, H., LENGFELDER, W., BROWN, W.V.: Separation and characterization of two triglyceride lipase activities from human postheparin plasma. In: Atherosclerosis III. Proc. III. Int. Symp. Atherosclerosis. SCHETTLER, G., WEIZEL, A. (eds.). Berlin-Heidelberg-New York: Springer-Verlag, 1974, pp. 557 - 560.

EHRLICH, K., RADHAKRISHNAMURTHY, B., BERENSON, G.S.: Isolation of a chondroitin sulfate-dermatan sulfate proteoglycan from bovine aorta. Arch. Biochem. Biophys. 171, 361 (1975).

EINARSSON, K., HELLSTROM, K.: The formation of bile acids in patients with three types of hyperlipoproteinemias. Europ. J. Clin. Invest. 2, 225 (1972).

EISEN, M.E., HAMMOND, E.C.: The effect of smoking on packed cell volume, red blood cell counts, haemoglobin and platelet counts. Can. Med. Assoc. J. 75, 520 - 523 (1956).

EISENBERG, S.: Lipoprotein metabolism and hyperlipemia. In: Atherosclerosis Reviews. PAOLETTI, R., GOTTO, A.M. (eds.). New York: Raven Press, 1976, pp. 23-60.

EISENBERG, S: Metabolism of very low density lipoproteins. In: Lipoprotein Metabolism. GRETEN, H. (ed.). Heidelberg-New York: Springer-Verlag, 1976b, pp. 32-
   43.
EISENBERG, S.: Phospholipid hydrolysis during degradation of rat plasma very low
   density lipoprotein (VLDL). Circulation 51-52, II-17 (1975).
EISENBERG, S., BILHEIMER, D!W., LEVEY, R.I.: The metabolism of very low density
   lipoprotein proteins. II. Studies on the transfer of apoproteins between
   plasma lipoproteins. Biochim. Biophys. Acta 280, 94 (1972a).
EISENBERG, S., BILHEIMER, D.W., LINDGREN, F.T., LEVY, R.I.: On the apoprotein
   composition of human plasma very low density lipoprotein subfractions.
   Biochim. Biophas. Acta 260, 329 (1972b).
EISENBERG, S., BILHEIMER, D.W., LINDGREN, T.F., LEVY, R.I.: On the metabolic conversion of human plasma very low density lipoprotein to low density lipoprotein. Biochim. Biophys. Acta 326, 361 (1973).
EISENBERG, S., LEVY, R.I.: Lipoprotein metabolism. Advan. Lipid Res. 13, 1 - 89
   (1975).
EISENBERG, S., LEVY,R.I.: Lipoproteins and lipoprotein metabolism. In: Hypolipid-
   emic Agents. KRITCHEVSKY, D. (ed.). Berlin-Heidelberg-New York: Springer-
   Verlag, 1975, pp. 191 - 213.
EISENBERG, S., RACHMILEWITZ, D.: Metabolism of rat plasma very low density lipo-
   protein. I. Fate in circulation of the whole lipoprotein. Biochim. Biophys.
   Acta 326, 378 (1973a).
EISENBERG, S., RACHMILEWITZ, D.: The interaction of rat plasma very low density
   lipoprotein with lipoprotein lipase rich (post-heparin) plasma. J. Lipid.
   Res. 16, 451 (1975).
EISENBERG, S., SCHURR, D.: Phospholipid hydrolysis during interaction of rat
   plasma very low density lipoprotein with lipoprotein lipase rich (post heparin) plasma. J. Lipid Res. 17, 578 (1976).
EISENBERG, S., STEIN, Y., STEIN, O.: Phospholipases in arterial tissue. II. Phos-
   phatide acyl-hydrolase and lysophosphatide acylhydrolase activity in human
   and rat arteries. Biochim. Biophys. Acta 164, 205 (1968).
EISENSTEIN, R., KUETTNER, K.: The ground substance of the arterial wall, part 2
   (electron-microscopic studies). Atherosclerosis 24 (1-2), 37 - 46 (1976).
EISENSTEIN, R., LARSSON, S.-E., KUETTNER, K.E., SORGENTE, R., HASCALL, V.C.:
   The ground substance of the arterial wall, part 1. Extractability of glycosaminoglycans and the isolation of a proteoglycan from bovine aorta. Atherosclerosis 22, 1-17 (1975).
ELEMER, G., KERENYI, T., JELLINEK, H.: Effect of temporary hypoxia on the permeability of the rat aorta. Path. Europ. 10, 123- 128 (1975).
ELLIS, E.F., OELZ, O., ROBERT, L.J., PAYNE, N.A., SWEETMAN, B.J., NIES, A.S.,
   OATES, J.A.: Coronary arterial smooth muscle contraction by a substance re-
   leased from platelets: evidence that it is thromboxane A2. Science 193, 1135 -
   1137 (1976).
ENGEL, U.R.: Glycosaminoglycans in the aorta of six animal species. A chemical
   and morphological comparison of their topographical distribution. Atherosclerosis 13, 45 - 60 (1971).
ENOS, W.F. Jr., BEYER, J.C., HOLMES, R.H.: Pathogenesis of coronary disease in
   American soldiers killed in Korea. JAMA 158, 912 (1955).
EPSTEIN, F.H.: Glucose intolerance and the rist of coronary heart disease. Arch.
   mal.du coeur 68 (numéro spécial), 51 - 56 (1976).
EPSTEIN, L., MILLER, G.J., STITT, F.W., MORRIS, I.N.: Vigorous exercise in leisure time, coronary risk factors and resting electrocardiogram in middle-
   aged male civil servants. Brit. Heart J. 38, 403 - 409 (1976).
EPSTEIN, F.H., OSTRANDER, L.D., JOHNSON, B.C., PAYNE, M.W., HAYNER, N.S., KEL-
   LER, J.B., FRANCIS, T.: Epidemiological studies of cardiovascular disease in
   a total community - Tecumseh, Michigan. Ann. Intern. Med. 62, 1170 - 1187
   (1965).
ERNÄHRUNGSBERICHT 1976. Herausgeber: Deutsche Gesellschaft für Ernährung, Frank-
   furt, 1976
ETO, T., YAMAMOTO, T., OMAE, T.: An electron microscope study on permeability in
   cerebral venules in the rats with hypertensive encephalopathy. Arch. histol.
   japon. 38, 299 - 306 (1975).

EUROPEAN SOCIETY OF CARDIOLOGY: Preventing Coronary Heart Disease - a Guide to the Practicing Physician. (in preparation).

EVERED, D.C., ORMSTON, B.J., SMITH, P.A., HALL, R., BIRD, T.: Grades of hypothyroidism. Br. Med. J. 1, 657 - 662 (1973).

FABIEN, H.D., DAVIGNON, J., MARCEL, Y.L.: Plasma cholesterol esterification in normal and hyperlipoproteinemic subjects. Canad. J. Biochem. 51, 550 - 555 (1973).

FAERGEMAN, O., SATA, T., KANE, J.P., HAVEL, J.R.: Metabolism of apoprotein B of plasma very low density lipoproteins in the rat. J. Clin. Invest. 56, 1396 (1975).

FAINARU, M., GLANGEAUD, M.C., EISENBERG, S.: Radioimmunoassay of human high density lipoprotein apoprotein A-I. Biochem. Biophys. Acta 336, 432 (1975).

FAINARU, M., HAVEL, R.J., FELKER, T.E.: Radioimmunoassay of apolipoprotein A-I of rat serum. Biochim. Biophys. Acta (1976a) (in press).

FAINARU, M., HAVEL, R.J., IMAIZUMI, K.: Radioimmunoassay of arginine-rich apolipoprotein of rat serum. (1976b) (submitted for publication).

FALCK, G.: Observations on the possibilities of cellular localization of monoamines by fluorescence method. Acta Physiol. Scand. 56 (Suppl. 197) (1962).

FALLOT, R.W., GLUECK, C.J.: Familial and acquired type V hyperlipoproteinemia. Atherosclerosis 23, 41 - 62 (1976).

FARQUHAR, H.W., GROSS, R.C., WAGNER, R.M., REAVEN, G.M.: Validation of an incompletely coupled two compartment nonrecycling catenary model for turnover of liver and plasma triglyceride in man. J. Lipid Res. 6, 119 - 132 (1965).

FARQUHAR, J., MACCOBY, N., WOOD, P., BROWN, B.: Results of a two-year health education campaign on cardiovascular risk. Stanford three community study. Circulation 52, II, 117 (1975).

FEINLEIB, M.: Twin Studies. In: Task Force on Genetic Factors in Atherosclerotic Disease. DHEW Publication No. (NIH) 76-922, Washington, D.C. (1975).

FELDMAN, H.A., SINGER, I.: Endocrinology and metabolism in uremia and dialysis: a clinical review. Medicine 54, 345 - 376 (1974).

FELKER, T.E., FAINARU, M., HAMILTON, R.L., HAVEL, R.J.: Secretion of apolipoproteins (A-I and ARP) by the isolated perfused rat liver. Circulation (1976) (in press).

FELTS, J.M., RUDEL, L.L.: Mechanism of hyperlipidemia. In: Hypolipidemic Agents. KRITCHEVSKY, D. (ed.). Berlin-Heidelberg-New York: Springer-Verlag, 1975, pp. 151 - 189.

FIDGE, N.H., FOXMAN, C.J.: In vivo transformation of rat plasma very low density lipoprotein into higher density lipoproteins. Aust. J. Exp. Biol. Med. Sci. 49, 581 (1971).

FIDGE, N.H., POULIS, P.: Studies on the metabolism of rat serum very low density lipoproteins. J. Lipid Res. 16, 367 (1975).

FIELDING, C.J.: Further characterisation of lipoprotein lipase and hepatic postheparin lipase from rat plasma. Biochim. Biophys. Acta 280, 569 (1972).

FIELDING, C.J.: Human lipoprotein lipase. I. Purification and substrate specifity. Biochim. Biophys. Acta 206, 109 (1970).

FIELDING, C.J., FIELDING, P.E.: Mechanism of salt-mediated inhibition of lipoprotein lipase. J. Lipid Res. 17, 248 (1976).

FIELDING, C.J., SHORE, V.G., FIELDING, P.E.: A protein cofactor of lecithin: cholesterol acyltransferase. Biochem. Biophys. Res. Commun. 46, 1493 - 1498 (1972).

FIELDING, P.E., SHORE, V.G., FIELDING, C.J.: Biochemistry 13, 4318 (1974).

FILLIOS, L.C., ANDRUS, S.B., NAITO, C.: Coronary lipid deposition during chronic anemia or high altitude exposure. J. appl. Physiol. 16, 103 - 106 (1961).

FINER, E.G., HENRY, R., LESLIE, R.B., ROBERTSON, R.N.: NMR studies of pig low- and high-density serum lipoproteins. Molecular motions and morphology. Biochim. Biophys. Acta 380, 320 - 337 (1975).

FISHER, E.R., FISHER, B.: Effect of induced atherosclerosis on fresh and lyophilised aortic homografts in rabbits. Surgery 40, 530 (1956).

FISHER, E.R., ROTHSTEIN, R., WHOLEY, M.H., NELSON, R.: Influence of nicotine on experimental atherosclerosis and its determinants. Arch. Pathol. 96, 298 - 304 (1973).

FISHER-DZOGA, K., CHEN, R., WISSLER, R.W.: Effects of serum lipoproteins on the morphology, growth and metabolism of arterial smooth muscle cells. Adv. Exp. Med. Biol. 43, 299 (1974).

FISCHER-DZOGA, K., JONES, R.M., VESSELINOVITCH, D., WISSLER, R.W.: Increased mitotic activity in primary cultures of aortic medial smooth muscle cells after exposure to hyperlipemic serum. In: Atherosclerosis III. Proceedings of the Third International Symposium. SCHETTLER, G., WEIZEL, A. (eds.). Berlin: Springer-Verlag, 1974, pp. 193 - 195.

FISCHER-DZOGA, K., JONES, R.M., VESSELINOVITCH, D., WISSLER, R.W.: Ultrastructural and immunohistochemical studies of primary cultures of aortic medial cells. Exp. Mol. Path. 18, 162 - 176 (1973).

FISCHER-DZOGA, K., WISSLER, R.W.: Studies of the stimulation of arterial smooth muscle cell proliferation induced in stationary primary cultures of monkey aortas. II. Effect of varying densities of hyperlipemic sera of low density lipoproteins of varying dietary fat origins. Atherosclerosis 24, 515 (1976).

FISKE, C.H., SUBARROW, Y.: The colorimetric determination of phosphorus. J. Biol. Chem. 66, 375 (1925).

FLORENTIN, R.A., NAM, S.C.: Dietary-induced atherosclerosis in miniature swine. I. Gross and light microscopy observations: time of development and morphologic characteristics of lesions. Exp. and Molec. Path. 8, 263 - 301 (1968).

FLORENTIN, R.A., NAM, S.C.: Gross and light microscopy observations: time of development and morphologic characteristics of lesions. Exp. Molec. Path. 8, 263 (1968).

FLORENTIN, R.A., NAM, S.C., LEE, K.T., LEE, K.J., THOMAS, W.A.: Increased mitotic activity in aortas of swine. After three days of cholesterol feeding. Arch. Path. 88, 463 - 469 (1969).

FLOREY, H.W., GREER, S.J., KISER, J., POOLE, J.C.F., TELANDER, R., WERTHESSEN, N.T.: The development of the pseudointima lining fabric grafts of the aorta. Brit. J. exp. Path. 43, 655 (1962).

FLOREY, H.W., GREER, S.J., POOLE, J.C.F., WERTHESSEN, N.T.: The pseudointima lining fabric grafts of the aorta. Brit. J. exp. Path. 42, 236 (1961).

FLOREY, H.W., SHEPPARD, B.L.: The permeability of arterial endothelium to horseradish peroxidase. Proc. Roy. Soc., London (B) 174, 435 (1970).

FOGELMAN, A.M., EDMOND, J., POLITO, A., POPJAK, G.: Control of lipid metabolism in human leukocytes. J. Biol. Chem. 248, 6928 - 6929 (1973).

FOGELMAN, A.M., EDMOND, J., SAEGER, J., POPJAK, G.: Abnormal induction of 3-hydroxy-3-methylglutaryl co-enzyme A reductase in leukocytes from subjects with heterozygous familial hypercholesterolemia. J. Biol. Chem. 250, 2045 - 2055 (1975).

FOLCH, J., ASCOLI, I., LEES, M., MEATH, J.A., LeBARON, F.N.: Preparation of lipid extracts from brain tissue. J. Biol. Chem. 191, 833 - 841 (1951).

FOLCH, J., LEES, M., STANLEY, G.H.: A simple method for the isolation and purification of total lipids from animal tissues. J. Biol. Chem. 226, 497 - 509 (1957).

FORTE, T., NICHOLS, A.V.: Application of electron microscopy to the study of plasma lipoprotein structure. Advan. Lipid Res. 10, 1 - 41 (1972).

FORTE, T., NICHOLS, A., Glomset, J., NORUM, K.: The ultrastructure of plasma lipoproteins in lecithin:cholesterol acyltransferase deficiency. Scand. J. clin. Lab. Invest. 33, Suppl. 137, 121 (1974).

FORTE, T., NORUM, K.R., GLOMSET, J.A., NICHOLS, A.V.: Plasma lipoproteins in familial lecithin:cholesterol acyltransferase deficiency: structure of low and high density lipoproteins as revealed by electron microscopy. J. Clin. Invest. 50, 1141 (1971).

FOSTER, J.A., MECHAM, R.P., FRANZBLAU, C.: Biochem. Biophys. Res. Commun., submitted for publication (1976).

FRANTZ, I.D., Jr., DAWSON, E.A., BREWER, E.R., GATEWOOD, L.C., BARTSCH, G.E.: The Minnesota Coronary Survey: effect of diet on cardiovascular events and deaths. Circulation 51 and 52,(Suppl. II)(1975).

FRANTZBLAU, C., FARIS, B., KAGAN, H.M., SCHMID, K.: Interaction of glycoprotein with collagen. Circulation 48,(Suppl. IV), 79 (1973).

FRANTZBLAU, D., LENT, R.W.: In: Structure, Function, and Evolution in Proteins. Upton, N.Y.: Brookhaven Symposia in Biology Nr. 21, 2/69 - 300, 1968, pp. 358 - 377.

FREDRICKSON, D.S., GOTTO, A.M., Jr., LEVY, R.I.: Familial lipoprotein deficiency (abetalipoproteinemia, hypobetalipoproteinemia, and Tangier disease). In: The Metabolic Basis of Inherited Disease. 3rd ed. STANBURY, J.B., WYNGAARDEN, J.B., FREDRICKSON, D.S. (eds.). New York: McGraw-Hill, 1972, Chap. 26, p.493.

FREDRICKSON, D.S., LEES, R.S.: Familial hyperlipoproteinemia. In: The Metabolic Basis of Inherited Disease. STANBURY, J.B., WYNGAARDEN, J.B., FREDRICKSON,D. S. (eds.). New York: McGraw-Hill Book Company, 1966, pp. 429 - 485.

FREDRICKSON, D.S., LEVY, R.I.: Familial hyperlipoproteinemia. In: The Metabolic Basis of Inherited Disease. STANBURY, J.B., WYNGAARDEN, J.B., FREDRICKSON,D. S. (eds.). New York: McGraw-Hill Book Company, 1972, p. 545.

FREDRICKSON, D.S., LEVY, R.I., LEES, R.S.: Fat transport in lipoproteins - an integrated approach to mechanism and disorders. New Engl. J. Med. $\underline{276}$, 34 - 44, 94 - 103, 148 - 156, 215 - 225, 273 - 281 (1967).

FREDRICKSON, D.S., MORGANROTH, I., LEVY, R.I.: Type III hyperlipoproteinemia - an analysis of two contemporary definitions. Annals of Int. Med. $\underline{82}$, 150 - 157 (1975).

FREDRICKSON, D.S., ONO, K., DAVIS, L.L.: Lipolytic activity of post heparin plasma in hyperglyceridemia. J. Lipid. Res. $\underline{4}$, 24 - 33 (1963).

FREINKEL, N., SINGER, D.L., ARKY, R.A., BLEICHER, S.J., ANDERSON, J.B., SILBERT, C.K.: Alcohol hypoglycemia. I. Carbohydrate metabolism of patients with clinical alcohol hypoglycemia and the experimental reproduction of the syndrome with pure alcohol reproduction of the syndrome with pure alcohol. J. Clin. Invest. $\underline{42}$, 1112 - 1133 (1963).

FRENCH, J.E.: Atherosclerosis in relation to the structure and function of the arterial intima, with special reference to the endothelium. Int. Rev. Exp. Path. $\underline{5}$, 253 - 353 (1966).

FRENCH, J.E,, MacFARLANE, R.G., SANDERS, A.G.: The structure of haemostatic plugs and experimental thrombi in small arteries. Brit. J. Exp. Pathol. $\underline{45}$, 467 (1964).

FRIEDMAN, G.D., SIEGELAUB, A.B., SELTZER, C.C., FELDMAN, R., COLLEN, M.F.: Smoking habits and the leukocyte count. Arch. Environ. Health $\underline{26}$, 137 - 143 (1973).

FRIEDMAN, H.: Pathogenesis of coronary thrombosis, intramural and intraluminal hemorrhage. In: Thrombosis and Coronary Heart Disease. HALONEN, LOUHIJA, A. (eds.). Basel: Karger, 1970, Vol. IV, p. 3.

FRIEDMAN, M., BYERS, S.O.: Observations concerning the evolution of atherosclerosis in the rabbit after cessation of cholesterol feeding. Am. J. Pathol. $\underline{43}$, 349 - 354 (1963).

FRIEDMAN, M., BYERS, S.O., ROSENMAN, R.H.: Effect of glucagon on blood-cholesterol levels in rats. Lancet (1971) II, 464.

FRIEDMAN, R.J. MOORE, S., SINGAL, D.P., Gent, M.: Regression of injury induced atheromatous lesions in rabbits. Arch. Pathol. Lab. Med. $\underline{100}$, 189 (1976a).

FRIEDMAN, R.J., MOORE, S., SINGAL, D.P., GENT, M.: Repeated endothelial injury and induction of atherosclerosis in normolipemic rabbits by human serum. Lab. Invest. $\underline{30}$, 404 (1975).

FRIEDMAN, J.R., STEMERMAN, M.B., SPAET, T.H., MOORE, S., GAULDIE, J.: The effect of thrombocytopenia on arteriosclerotic plaque formation. Fed. Proc. $\underline{35}$, 207 (1976b).

FRITZ, K.E. et al.: Regression of advanced atherosclerosis in swine. Arch. Path. Lab. Med. $\underline{100}$, 380 (1976).

FRITZ, K.E., AUGUSTYN, J.M., JARMOLYCH, J., DAOUD, A.S., LEE, K.T.: Regression of advanced atherosclerosis in swine. Chemical studies. Arch. Pathol. Lab. Med. $\underline{100}$, 380 (1976).

FRITZ, S.H., WALKER, W.J.: Ileal bypass in the control of intractable hypercholesterolemia. Am. Surg. $\underline{32}$, 691 (1966).

FROST, H.: Endothelschädigungen und Abscheidungen von Elementen des strömenden Blutes als initiales Geschehen in der Pathogenese der Arteriosklerose. Verh. dtsch. Ges. Inn. Med. $\underline{78}$, 1139 - 1145 (1972).

FURLOW, Jr., R.W., BASS, N.H.: Stroke in rats produced by carotid injection of sodium arachidonate. Science 187, 658 - 660 (1975).

GAINER, J.L., CHISOLM, G.M.: Altering diffusion rates. In: Oxygen Transport to Tissue - Pharmacology, Mathematical Studies and Neonatology. BRULEY, D.F., BICHER, H.I. (eds.). New York: Plenum Press, 1973, pp. 729 - 733.

GAINER, J.L., JONES, J.R.: The use of crocetin in experimental atherosclerosis. Experientia 31, 548 (1975).

GAN, J.C., MARASCHIME, P.V., NICHOLS, C.W., CHAIKOFF, I.L.: Mucosubstances in the chicken aorta. 1. Changes with age in acid mucopolysaccharides, glycoproteins, collagen, and elastin. J. Atheroscl. Res. 7, 629 (1967).

GANESAN, D., BRADFORD, R.H., GANESÁN, G., McCONATHY, W.J., ALAUPOVIC, P., BASS, H.B.: Purified postheparin plasma lipoprotein lipase in primary hyperlipo-proteinemia. J. Appl. Physiol. 39, 1022 - 1033 (1975).

GARBORSCH, C., MATHIESSEN, M.C., HELIN, P., LORENZEN, I.: Arteriosclerosis and hypoxia. Part 1. (Gross and microscopic changes in rabbit aorta, induced by systemic hypoxia. Histochemical studies). J. Athero Res. 9, 283 (1969).

GARCIA-PALMIERI, M.R., COSTAS, R., CRUZ-VIDAL, M., CORTÉS-ALICEA, M., COLÓN, A.A., FELIBERTI, M., AYALA, A.M., PATTERNE, D., SOBRINO, R., TORRES, R., NAZARIO, E.: Risk factors and prevalence of coronary heart disease in Puerto Rico. Circulation 42, 541 - 549 (1970).

GARDNER, D.L., MATTHEWS, M.A.: Ultrastructure of the wall of small arteries in early experimental rat hypertension. J. Path. 97, 51 - 62 (1969).

GARFIELD, R.E., CHACKO, S., BLOSE, S.: Phagocytosis by muscle cells. Lab. Invest. 33, 418 - 427 (1975).

GARFINKEL, A.S., NILSSON-EHLE, P., SCHOTZ, M.C.: Regulation of lipoprotein lipase induction by insulin. Biochim. Biophys. Acta 424, 264 - 273 (1976).

GARTLER, S.M., LINDER, D.: Selection in mammalian mosaic cell populations. Symposia on Quantitative Biology 29, 253 - 260 (1964).

GAUTHERON, P., RENAUD, S.: Hyperlipemia induced hypercoagulable state in rat. Role of an increased activity of platelet phosphatidyl serine in response to certain dietary fatty acids. Thromb. Res. 1, 353 (1972).

GAYNOR, E., BOUVIER, C.A., SPAET, T.H.: Circulating endothelial cells in endo-toxin-treated rabbits. Clin. Res. 16, 535 (1968).

GEERTINGER, P., SORENSEN, H.: Complement as a factor in atherosclerosis. Arch. Pathol. Microbiol. Scandinav. A 78, 284 (1970).

GENSINI, G.G., ESENTE, P., KELLY, A.: Natural history of coronary disease in patients with and without coronary bypass graft surgery. Circ. 49, 50 (Suppl. II), II-98-II-102 (1974).

GENTON, E., WEILLY, H.S., STEELE, P.P.: Platelets, thrombosis and coronary artery disease. In: Myocardial Infarction: A New Look at an Old Subject. VOGEL, J.H.K. (ed.). Basel: Karger, 1973, Vol. IX, p. 29.

GERMUTH, F.G., SENTERFIT, L.B., POLLACK, A.D.: Immune complex disease. I. Experimental acute and chronic glomerulonephritis. Johns Hopkins Med. J. 120, 225 (1967).

GERRITY, R.G., RICHARDSON, M., BELL, F.P., SOMER, J.B., SCHWARTZ, C.J.: Endo-thelial cell morphology in areas of in vivo Evans Blue uptake in the young pig aorta. II. Ultrastructure of the intima in areas of differing permeability to proteins. Exp. Molec. Pathol. (1976) (in press).

GHIDONI, J.J., LIOTTA, D., HALL, C.W., ADAMS, J.G., LECHTER, A., BARRIONUEVA, M., O'NEAL, R.M., De BAKEY, M.E.: Healing of pseudointimas in velour-lined im-permeable arterial prosthese. Amer. J. Path. 53, 375 (1968).

GIACOMELLI, F., WIENER, J.: Regional variations in the permeability of the rat thoracic aorta. Am. J. Path. 75, 513 (1974).

GIESE, J.: Deposition of serum proteins in vascular walls during acute hyper-tension. Acta Path. Microbiol. Scand. 53, 167 - 172 (1961).

GILLMAN, T.: On some aspects of collagen formation in localized repair and in diffuse fibrotic reactions to injury. In: Treatise on Collagen. GOULD, B.S. (ed.). New York: Academic Press, 1968, Vol. II, Part B, pp. 331 - 407.

GIMBRONE, M.A., ALEXANDER, R.W.: Angiotensin II. Stimulation of prostaglandin production in cultured human vascular endothelium. Science 189, 219 (1975).

GIMBRONE, M.A., COTRAN, R.S., FOLKMAN, J.: Human vascular endothelial cells in culture. J. Cell. Biol. 60, 673 (1974).

GINSBERG, H., OLEFSKY, J.M., KIMMERLING, G., CRAPO, Ph., REAVEN, G.M.: Induction of hypertriglyceridemia by a low-fat diet. J. of Clin. Endocrinology and Metabolism 42, 729 (1976).

GLAGOV, S.: Hemodynamic risk factors: mechanical stress, mural architecture, medial nutrition, and the vulnerability of arteries to atherosclerosis. In: The Pathogenesis of Atherosclerosis. WISSLER, R.W., GEER, J.E. (eds). Baltimore: Williams and Wilkens, 1972, p. 164.

GLANGEAUD, M.C., EISENBERG, S., OLIVECRONA, T.: Very low density lipoprotein. Dissociation of apolipoprotein C during lipoprotein lipase induced lipolysis. Biochim. Biophys. Acta. (1976) (in press).

GLICKMAN, R.M., KIRSCH, K.: Lymph chylomicron formation during the inhibition of protein synthesis. J. Clin. Invest. 52, 2910 (1973).

GLOMSET, J.A.: Recent studies on the role of the lecithin-cholesterol acyl-transferase reaction in plasma lipoproteins metabolism. In: Lipoprotein Metabolism. GRETEN, H. (ed.). Berlin: Springer-Verlag, 1976, pp. 28-30.

GLOMSET, J.A., NONEM, K.R.: The metabolic role of lecithin: cholesterol acyltransferase: perspectives from pathology. Advanc. Lipid. Res. 11, 1-65 (1973).

GLUECK, C.J., BROWN, W.V., LEVY, R.I., GRETEN, H., FREDRICKSON, D.S.: Amelioration of hypertriglyceridemia by pregestational drugs in familial type V hyperlipoproteinemia. Lancet (1969) I, 1290.

GLUECK, C.J., LEVY, R.I., GLUECK, H.I., GRALNICK, H.R., GRETEN, H., FREDRICKSON, D.S.: Am. J. Med. 47, 318 (1969).

GLUECK, C.I., MacKENZIE, M.R., GLUECK, C.J.: Crystalline IgG protein in multiple myeloma: identification effects on coagulation and on lipcprotein metabolism. J. Lab. Clin. Med. 79, 731 (1972).

GLYNN, M.F., MUSTARD, J.F., BUCHANAN, M.R., MURPHY, E.A.: Cigarette smoking and platelet aggregation. Can. Med. Assoc. J. 95, 549-553 (1966).

GOFMAN, J.W., JONES, H.B., STRISOWER, B., TAMPLIN, A.R.: Evaluation of serum lipoproteins and cholesterol measurements as predictors of clinical complications of atherosclerosis. Report of a cooperative study of lipoproteins and atherosclerosis. Appendix A. Circulation 14, 725-731 (1956).

GOH, E.H., HEIMBERG, M.: Stimulation of hepatic cholesterol biosynthesis by deic acid. Biochem. Biophys. Res. Commun. 55, 382-388 (1973).

GOLDBERG, A.P., SHERRARD, D.J., BRUNZELL, J.D.: Hypertriglyceridemia in hemodialysis patients: dual defect of adipose tissue lipoprotein lipase. Clin. Res. 24, 361A (1976).

GOLDBOURT, U., MEDALIE, J.H., NEUFELD, H.N.: Clinical myocardial infarction over a five-year period - III. A multivariate analysis of incidence. The Israel Ischaemic Heart Disease Study. J. Chron. Diseases 28, 217-237 (1975).

GOLDFISCHER, S., SCHILLER, B., WOLINSKY, H.: Lipid accumulation in smooth muscle cell lyosomes in primate atherosclerosis. Am. J. Pathol. 78, 497 (1975).

GOLDRICK, R.B.: Morphological changes in the adipocyte during fat deposition and mobilization. Am. J. Physiol. 212, 777-782 (1967).

GOLDSMITH, H.L.: The flow of model particles and blood cells and its relation to thrombogenesis. In: Progress in Hemostasis and Thrombosis. SPAET, T.H. (ed.). 1972, Vol. I, pp. 97-139.

GOLDSTEIN, J.L., BASU, S.K., BRUNSCHEDE, G.Y., BROWN, M.S.: Release of low density lipoprotein from its cell surface receptor by sulfated glycosaminoglycans. Cell 7, 85 (1976).

GOLDSTEIN, J.L., BROWN, M.S.: Binding and degradation of low density lipoproteins by cultured human fibroblasts. J. Biol. Chem. 249, 5153 (1974).

GOLDSTEIN, J.L., BROWN, M.S.: A genetic regulatory defect in cholesterol metabolism. Am. J. Med. 58, 147-150 (1975).

GOLDSTEIN, J.L., BROWN, M.S.: Lipoprotein receptors, cholesterol metabolism and atherosclerosis. Arch. Pathol. 99, 181 (1975).

GOLDSTEIN, J.L., DANA, S.E., BROWN, M.S.: Esterification of Low Density Lipoprotein Cholesterol in Human Fibroblasts and Its Absence in Homozygous Familial Hypercholesterolemia. Proc. Nat. Acad. Sci. U.S.A. 71, 4288-4292 (1974).

GOLDSTEIN, J.L., DANA, S.E., BRUNSCHEDE, G.Y., BROWN, M.S.: Genetic heterogeneity in familial hypercholesterolemia: evidence for two different mutations affecting functions of low-density lipoprotein receptor. Proc. Natl. Acad. Sci. USA 72, 1092-1096 (1975).

GOLDSTEIN, J.L., FREDRICKSON, D.S., BROWN, M.S.: Familial hyperlipoproteinemia. In: The Metabolic Basis of Inherited Disease. STANBURY, J.B., WYNGAARDEN, J.B., FREDRICKSON, D.S. (eds.). New York: McGraw-Hill Book Company, 1976 (in press).

GOLDSTEIN, J.L., HAZZARD, W.R., SCHROTT, H.G., BIERMAN, E.L., MOTULSKI, A.G.: Hyperlipidemia in coronary heart disease. J. Clin. Invest. 52, 1533-1543 (1973a).

GOLDSTEIN, J.L., SCHROTT, H.G., HAZZARD, W.R., BIERMAN, E.L., MOTULSKI, A.G.: Hyperlipidemia in coronary heart disease. Genetic analysis of lipid levels in 176 families and delineation of new inherited disorder, combined hyperlipidemia. J. Clin. Invest. 52, 1544-1568 (1973b).

GOODMAN, D.S., DEYKIN, D., SHIRATORI, T.: The Formation of Cholesterol Esters with Rat Liver Enzymes. J. Biol. Chem. 239, 1335-1345 (1964).

GOODMAN, D.S., NOBLE, R.P.: Turnover of plasma cholesterol in man. J. Clin. Invest. 47, 231-241 (1968).

GOODMAN, D.S., NOBLE, R.P., DELL, R.B.: Three-pool model of the long term turnover of plasma cholesterol in man. J. Lipid Res. 14, 178-188 (1973).

GORDIN, A., SAARINEN, P., PELKONEN, R.: Serum thyrotrophin and the response to thyrotrophin releasing hormone in symptomless autoimmune thyroiditis and in borderline and overt hypothyroidism. Acta Endocrinol. (Kbh) 75, 274-285 (1974).

GORDON, E.R.: Effect of an intoxicating dose of ethanol on lipid metabolism in an isolated perfused rat liver. Biochem. Pharmacol. 21, 2991-3004 (1972).

GORDON, T.: Mortality experience among Japanese in the United States, Hawaii and Japan. Public Health Rep. 72, 543 (1957).

GORDON, T., GARCIA-PALMIERI, M.R., KAGAN, A., KANNEL, W.B., SCHIFFMAN, J.: Differences in coronary heart disease in Framingham, Honolulu and Puerto Rico. J. Chron. Dis. 27, 329-344 (1974).

GORDON, T., KANNEL, W.B.: Predisposition to atherosclerosis in the head, heart, and legs. The Framingham study. J. Amer. Med. Ass. 221, 661 (1972).

GORDON, T., THOM, T.: The recent decrease in CHD mortality. Preventive Med. 4, 115-125 (1975).

GORDON, T., VERTER, J.: The Framingham study, section 23. Serum cholesterol, systolic blood pressure, and the Framingham relative weight as discriminators of cardiovascular disease. National Institutes of Health, Bethesda, Maryland,

GORE, I., HIRST, A.E., TANAKA, K.: Myocardial infarction and thromboembolism. Arch. Intern. Med. 113, 323 (1964).

GOTTO, A.M., Jr.: Hyperlipoproteinemia, method of. In: Current Therapy. COHN, H.F. (ed.). Philadelphia: W.B. Saunders Company, 1974, pp. 418-427.

GOTTO, A.M., Jr., DeBAKEY, M.E., FOREYT, J.P., SCOTT, L.W., THORNBY, J.I.: Dietary treatment of type IV hyperlipoproteinemia. J. Am. Med. Assoc. (1976b) (submitted for publication).

GOTTO, A.M., GORRY, G.A., THOMPSON, J.R., COLE, J.S., TROST, J.R., YESHURUN, D., DeBAKEY, M.E.: Relationship between plasma lipid concentrations and coronary artery disease in 496 patients. Circulation (1976a) (submitted for publication).

GOTTO, A.M., Jr., JACKSON, R.L., MORRISETT, J.D., POWNALL, H.J., SPARROW, J.T.: Molecular association of lipids and proteins in the plasma lipoproteins: a review. In: Lipoprotein Metabolism. GRETEN, H. (ed.). Berlin: Springer-Verlag, 1976, p. 152.

GOULD, S.E., HAYASHI, T., TASHIRO, T., TANIMURA, A., NAKASHIMA, T., SOHOJI, T., ASHLEY, F.W.: Coronary heart disease and stroke: atherosclerosis in Japanese men living in Hiroshima, Japan and Honolulu, Hawaii. Arch. Path. 93, 98 (1972).

GRANT, M.E., PROCKOP, D.J.: The biosynthesis of collagen I. New Engl. J. Med. 286, 194-199 (1972).

GRESHAM, G.A.: Is atheroma a reversible lesion? Atherosclerosis 23, 379 (1976).

GRESHAM, G.A., HOWARD, A.N.: The independent production of atherosclerosis and thrombosis in the rat. Brit. J. Exp. Path. 41, 395-402 (1960).

GRETEN, H., DeGRELLA, R., KLOSE, G., RASCHER, W., de GENNES, J.L., GJONE, E.: Measurement of two plasma triglyceride lipases by an immunochemical method: studies in patients with hypertriglyceridemia. J. Lipid. Res. 17, 203-210 (1976).

GRETEN, H., SNIDERMAN, A.D., CHANDLER, J.G., STEINBERG, D., BROWN, W.V.: Evidence for the hepatic origin of a canine postheparin plasma triglyceride lipase. FEBS Letters 42, 157-160 (1974).

GRETEN, H., WALTER, B., BROWN, W.V.: Purification of a human post-heparin plasma triglyceride lipase. FEBS Letters 27, 306-310 (1972).

GRIEBSCH, A., ZÖLLNER, N.: Normalwerte der Plasmaharnsäure in Süddeutschland. Z. Klin. Chem. Klin. Biochem. 11, 348 (1973).

GRINNA, L.S.: Effect of dietary α-tocopherol on liver microsomes and Mitochondria of Aging Rats. J. Nutr. 106, 918-929 (1976).

GROSGOGEAT, Y., ANGUERA, G., LELLOUCH, J., JACOTOT, B., BEAUMONT, J.-L.: L'intoxication chronique par la nicotine chez le lapin nourri au cholesterol. J. Atheroscler. Res. 5, 291-301 (1965).

GRUNDMAN, E.: Histologische Untersuchungen über die Wirkungen experimentellen Sauerstoffmangels auf das Katzenherz. Beitr. path. Anat. 111, 36-76 (1951).

GRUNDY, S.M.: Effects of polyunsaturated fats on lipid metabolism in patients with hypertriglyceridemia. J. Clin. Invest. 55, 269-282 (1975).

GRUNDY, S.M., AHRENS, E.H., Jr., MIETTINEN, T.A.: Quantitative isolation and gas-liquid chromatographic analysis of total fecal bile acids. J. Lipid. Res. 6, 397-410 (1965).

GRUNDY, S.M., AHRENS, E.H., Jr., SALEN, G.: Interruption of enterohepatic circulation of bile acids in man: comparative effects of cholestyramine and ideal exclusion on cholesterol metabolism. J. Labs. Clin. Med. 78, 97-121 (1971).

GRUNDY, S.M., NESTEL, P.J., MONELL, R., MOK, H., von BERGMANN, K., STEINBERG, D.: Kinetics of very low density lipoprotein triglycerides (VLDL=TG) following radioglycerol (G*). Circulation 52, (Suppl. II), 39 (1975).

GUTSTEIN, W.H., FARREL, G.A., ARMELLINI, C.: Blood flow disturbances and endothelial injury in pre-atherosclerotic swine. Lab. Invest. 29, 134 (1973).

GUTSTEIN, W.H., ROBERTSON-LAZZARINI, A., LaTAILLADE, J.N.: The role of local arterial irritability in the development of arterio-atherosclerosis. Am. J. Pathol. 42, 61 (1963).

GUY-GRAND, B., BIGORIE, B.: Effects of fat cell size, restructive diet and diabetes on lipoprotein lipase release by human adipose tissue. Horm. Metab. Res. 7, 471-475 (1975).

GUZMAN, M.A., McMAHAN, C.A., McGILL, H.C., Jr., STRONG, J.P., TEJADA, C., RESTREPO, C., EGGEN, D.A., ROBERTSON, W.B., SOLBERG, L.A.: Selected methodologic aspects of the International Atherosclerosis Project. Lab. Invest. 18, 479-497 (1968).

HADJIISKY, P., SCEBAT, L., RENAIS, J., CACHERA, J.P., DUBOST, C., LENEGRE, J.: Altérations morphologiques des vaisseaux coronaires de deux homotransplants cardiaques de longe durée chez l'homme. Rev. Europ. Etudes clin. Biol. 16, 596 (1971).

HAGENFELDT, L., WAHREN, J.: Human forearm muscle metabolism during exercise. VII. FFA uptake and oxidation at different work intensities. Scand. J. clin. Lab. Invest. 30, 429 - 436 (1972).

HAGENFELDT, L., WAHREN, J., PERNOW, B., CRONESTRAND, R., EKESTROM, S.: Free fatty acid metabolism of the leg muscles during exercise in patients with obliterative iliac and femoral artery disease before and after reconstructive surgery. J. clin. Invest. 51, 3061 - 3071 (1972).

HALL, R.: The immunoassay of thyroid-stimulating hormone and its clinical applications. Clin. Endocrinol. 1, 115 - 125 (1972).

HAMBERG, M., SVENSSON, J., SAMUELSSON, B.: Thromboxanes. A new group of biologically active compounds derived from prostaglandin endoperoxides. Proc. Natl. Acad. Sci. U.S.A. 72, 2994 - 2998 (1975).

HAMBURGER, J., DORMOT, J.: Functional and morphological alterations in long-term kidney transplants. In: Human Transplantation. RAPAPORT, H., DAUSSET, J. (eds.). New York: Grune and Stratton, 1968, p. 201.

HAMILTON, J.A., TALKOWSKI, C., CHILDERS, R.F., WILLIAMS, E., ALLERHAND, A., CORDES, E.H.: Rotational and segmental motions in the lipids of human plasma lipoproteins. J. Biol. Chem. 249, 4872 - 4878 (1974).

HAMILTON, R.L., Jr.: Postheparin Plasma Lipase From the Hepatic Circulation. Ann Arbor, Mich.: University Microfilms, 1964.

HAMILTON, R.L., HAVEL, R.J., KANE, J.P., BLAUROCK, E.A., SATA, T.: Cholestasis: lamellar structure of the abnormal human serum lipoprotein. Science (Wash. C.D.) <u>172</u>, 475 - 478 (1971).

HAMILTON, R.L., HAVEL, R.J., WILLIAMS, M.C.: Lipid bilayer structure of plasma lipoproteins in cholestasis. Fed. Proc. <u>33</u>, 351 (1974).

HAMILTON, R.L., KAYDEN, H.J.: The liver and the formation of normal and abnormal plasma lipoproteins. In: The Liver: Normal and Abnormal Functions, Part A. BECKER, F.F. (ed.). New York: Marcel Dekker, 1974, p. 531.

HAMILTON, R.L., WILLIAMS, M.C., FIELDING, C.J., HAVEL, R.J.: Discoidal bilayer structure of nascent high density lipoproteins from perfused rat liver. J. Clin. Invest. <u>58</u>, 667 (1976).

HAMILTON, R.M.G., CARROLL, K.K.: Effects of dietary protein on plasma cholesterol levels in rabbits fed cholesterol-free semisynthetic diets. In: Atherosclerosis III. SCHETTLER, G., WEIZEL, A. (eds.). Berlin: Springer-Verlag, 1974, pp. 406 - 409.

HAMILTON, R.M.G., CARROLL, K.K.: Plasma cholesterol levels in rabbits fed low fat, low cholesterol diets. Effects of dietary proteins, carbohydrates and fibre from different sources. Atherosclerosis <u>24</u>, 47 - 62 (1976).

HAMMOND, E.C., GARFINKEL, L.: Coronary heart disease, stroke, and aortic aneurysm. Factors in the etiology. Arch. Environ. Health <u>19</u>, 167 - 182 (1969).

HAMOSH, M., HAMOSH, P.: Effect of estrogen on lipoprotein lipase activity of rat adipose tissue. J. Clin. Invest. <u>55</u>, 1132 - 1135 (1975).

HANEFELD, M., HALLER, H., LEONHARDT, W., MOSER, W.: Häufigkeit und Interrelationen metabolischer Risikofaktoren: Die Dresdner Studie. Dtsch. Ges.-wesen <u>28</u>, 1498, 1538, 1585 (1973).

HARDIN, N.J., MINICK, C.R., MURPHY, G.E.: Experimental induction of athero-arteriosclerosis by the synergy of allergic injury to arteries and lipid-rich diet. III. The role of earlier acquired fibromuscular intimal thickening in the pathogenesis of later developing atherosclerosis. Amer. J. Pathol. <u>73</u>, 301. (1973).

HARDING, D.R.K., BATTERSBY, J.E., HUSBANDS, D.R., HANCOCK, W.S.: Synthesis of a protein with the properties of the apolipoprotein C-I (apoLP-Ser). J. Amer. Chem. Soc. <u>98</u>, 2664 - 2665 (1976).

HARKER, L.A., SLICHTER, S.J., SCOTT, C.R., ROSS, R.: Homocystinemia: vascular injury and arterial thrombosis. New Eng. J. Med. <u>291</u>, 537 (1974).

HARLAN, W.R., OBERMAN, A., MITCHELL, R.E., GRAYBIEL, A.: A 30-year study of blood pressure in a white male cohort. In: Hypertension: Mechanisms and Management. ONESTI, G., KIM, K.E., MOYER, J.H. (eds.). New York: Grune and Stratton, 1973, pp. 85 - 91.

HARLAN, W.R., WINESETT, P.S., WASSERMAN, A.J.: Tissue lipoprotein lipase in normal individuals and in individuals with exogenous hypertriglyceridemia and the relationship of this enzyme to assimilation of fat. J. Clin. Invest. <u>46</u>, 239 - 247 (1962).

HARRIS, K.L., HARRIS, P.A.: Kinetics of chylomicron triglyceride removal from plasma in rats: effect of dose on the volume of distribution. Biochim. Biophys. Acta <u>326</u>, 12 (1973).

HARRIS, P.: Some observations on the biochemistry of the myocardium at high altitude. In: High Altitude Physiology. Ciba Foundation Symposium. PORTER, R., KNIGHT, J. (eds.). Edinburgh - London: Churchill Livingstone, 1971.

HARRISON, C.V.: Experimental pulmonary arteriosclerosis. J. Path. Bact. <u>60</u>, 289 (1948).

HART, P., FARRELL, G.C., COOKSLEY, W.G.E., POWELL, L.W.: Enhanced drug metabolism in cigarette smokers. Br. Med. J. <u>2</u>, 147 - 149 (1976).

HARTMANN, G.: Zur Epidemiologie von Hyperlipoproteinämien. In: Symposium über Lipidstoffwechselerkrankungen vom 27. bis 29.9.1973 in Dresden. HALLER, H., HANEFELD, M., JAROSS, W. (Hrsg.) 124 - 136. Berlin, 1974.

HASCALL, V.C., HEINEGARD, D.: Aggregation of cartilage proteoglycans. II. Oligosaccharide competitors of the proteoglycans-hyaluronic acid interaction. J. Biol. Chem. <u>249</u>, 4242 (1974).

HASHIMOTO, S., DAYTON, S.: Influence of Microsomal Cholesterol Concentrations on the Cholesterol-Esterifing Activity of Normal and Atherosclerotic Aortas. Artery <u>1</u>, 308-318 (1975).

HASHIMOTO, S., DAYTON, S., ALFIN-SLATER, R.B., BUI, P.T., BAKER, N., WILSON, L.: Characteristics of the Cholesterol-Esterifying Activity in Normal and Atherosclerotic Rabbit Aortas. Circ. Res. 34, 176 - 183 (1974).

HATCH, F.T., LEES, R.S.: Practical methods of plasma lipoprotein analysis. Adv. Lipid Res. 6, 1 - 68 (1968).

HAUSER, H., HENRY, R., LESLIE, R.B., STUBBS, J.M.: The interaction of apoprotein from porcine high-density lipoprotein with dimyristoyl phosphatidylcholine. Eur. J. Biochem. 48, 583 (1974).

HAUSS, W.H.: Role of Arterial Wall Cells in Sclerogenesis. Annals of the New York Academy of Sciences, 1976b. Vol. 215, p. 286.

HAUSS, W.H.: The Role of the Mesenchymal Cells in Arteriosclerosis. Front. Matrix Biology. Basel: Karger Verlag, 1976a, Vol. II, pp. 89 - 124.

HAUSS, W.H.: Über die Rolle des Mesenchyms in der Genese der Arteriosklerose. Virchows Archiv Abt. A Path. Anat. 359, 135 - 156 (1973).

HAUSS, W.H., GERLACH, U., JUNGE-HÜLSING, G., THEMANN, H., WIRTH, W.: Studies of the monospecific mesenchymal reaction and the transit zone in myocardial lesions and atherosclerosis. Ann. N.Y. Acad. Sci. 156, 207 (1969).

HAUSS, W.H., JUNGE-HÜLSING, G., GERLACH, U.: Die unspezifische Mesenchymreaktion. Stuttgart: Thieme Verlag, 1968.

HAUSS, W.H., JUNGE-HÜLSING, G., MEY, J., WAGNER, H., OBERWITTLER, W.: Untersuchungen über den Einfluß von Training auf die Reaktionsfähigkeit des Mesenchyms. Med. Welt. Stuttgart: F.K. Schattauer Verlag, 1969.

HAUST, M.D.: Arteriosclerosis in concepts of disease. BRUNSON, J.G., GALL, E.A. (eds.). New York - London - Toronto: The Macmillan Co., 1971.

HAUST, M.D.: Fine fibrils of extracellular space (microfibrils). Their structure and role in connective tissue organization. Amer. J. Pathol. 47, 1113 - 1138 (1965).

HAUST, M.D.: The genetic mucopolysaccharidoses (GMS). Intern. Rev. Exp. Pathol. 12, 251 - 314 (1973).

HAUST, M.D.: Platelets, thrombosis and atherosclerosis. In: Platelets, Drugs and Thrombosis. HIRSCH, J. (ed.). Basel: S. Karger, 1975, pp. 94 - 110.

HAUST, M.D., GEER, J.C.: Mechanism of calcification in spontaneous aortic arteriosclerotic lesions of the rabbit. An electron microscopic study. Amer. J. Pathol. 60, 329 - 346 (1970).

HAUST, M.D., MORE, R.H.: Development of modern theories on the pathogenesis of atherosclerosis. In: The Pathogenesis of Atherosclerosis. WISSLER, R.W., GEER, J.C. (eds.). Baltimore: Williams and Wilkins Co., 1972, pp. 1 - 19.

HAUST, M.D., MORE, R.H.: In: Evolution of the Atherosclerotic Plaque. JONES, R. (ed.). Chicago: University of Chicago Press, 1963, pp. 51 - 63.

HAUST, M.D., MORE, R.H.: Mechanism of fibrosis in white atherosclerotic plaques of human aorta: an electron microscopic study (P). Circulation 34 (Suppl. III), 14 (1966).

HAUST, M.D., MORE, R.H.: New functional aspects of smooth muscle cells. Fed. Proc. 17, 440 (1958).

HAUST, M.D., MORE, R.H., BENCOSME, S.A., BALIS, J.U.: Elastogenesis in human aorta: an electron microscopic study. Exp. Molec. Pathol. 4, 508 - 524 (1965).

HAUST, M.D., MORE, R.H., MOVAT, H.Z.: The mechanism of fibrosis in arteriosclerosis. Amer. J. Path. 35, 265 (1959).

HAUST, M.D., MORE, R.H., MOVAT, H.Z.: The role of smooth muscle cells in the fibrogenesis of atherosclerosis. Am. J. Pathol. 37, 377 - 389 (1960).

HAUST, M.D., MOVAT, H.Z., MORE, R.H.: Organization by smooth muscle cells. Amer. J. Pathol. 33, 626 - 627 (1957).

HAVEL, R.J.: Lipoproteins and lipid transport. In: Lipids, Lipoproteins and Drugs (Adv. Exp. Med. Biol.). KRITCHEVSKY, D., PAOLETTI, R., HOLMES, W.L. (eds.). New York: Plenum Press, 1975, p. 37.

HAVEL, R.J., EDER, H.A., BRAGDON, J.H.: The distribution and chemical composition of ultracentrifugally separated lipoproteins in human serum. J. Clin. Invest. 34, 1345 - 1353 (1955).

HAVEL, R.J., FIELDING, C.J., OLIVECRONA, T., SHORE, V.G., FIELDING, P.E., EGELRUD, R.: Cofactor activity of protein components of human very low density lipoproteins in the hydrolysis of triglycerides by lipoprotein lipase from different sources. Biochem. 12, 1828 - 1833 (1973).

HAVEL, R.J., GORDON, R.S.: Idiopathic hyperlipemia: metabolic studies in an affected family. J. Clin. Invest. 39, 1777 - 1790 (1960).
HAVEL, R.J., KANE, J.P.: Primary dysbetalipoproteinemia: predominance of a specific apoprotein species in triglyceride-rich lipoproteins. Proc. Natl. Acad. Sci. U.S. 70, 2015 - 2019 (1973).
HAVEL, R.J., KANE, J.P., BALASSE, E.O., SEGEL, N., BASSO, L.V.: Splanclinic metabolism of free fatty acids and production of triglycerides of very low density lipoproteins in normotriglyceridemic and hypertriglyceridemic humans. J. Clin. Invest. 49, 2017 - 2035 (1970).
HAVEL, R.J., KANE, J.P., KASHYAP, M.L.: Interchange of apolipoproteins between chylomicrons and high density lipoproteins during alimentary lipemia in man. J. Clin. Invest. 52, 32 (1973).
HAWKINS, R.I.: Smoking, platelets and thrombosis. Nature 236, 450 - 452 (1972).
HAZZARD, W.R., PORTE, D., BIERMAN, E.L.: Abnormal lipid composition of very low density lipoproteins in diagnosis of Broad Beta Disease (type III hyperlipoproteinemia). Metabolism 21, 1009 - 1019 (1972).
HEAF, D., KAIJSER, L., EKLUND, B., CARLSON, L.A.: Difference in heparin released lipolytic activity in the superficial and deep veins of the human forearm. Europ. J. Clin. Invest. 7, 195 (1977).
HEARD, B.E.: An experimental study of thickening of the pulmonary arteries of rabbits produced by the organization of fibrin. J. Path. Bact. 64, 13 (1952).
HEATH, D., WOOD, E.H., DUSHANE, J.W., EDWARDS, J.E.: The relation of age and blood pressure to atheroma in the pulmonary arteries and thoracic aorta in congenital heart disease. Lab. Invest. 9, 259 (1960).
HELIN, G., HELIN, P., LORENZEN, I.: The aortic glycosaminoglycans in arteriosclerosis induced by systemic hypoxia. Atherosclerosis 12, 235 - 240 (1970).
HELIN, P., LORENZEN, I.: Arteriosclerosis in rabbit aorta induced by systemic hypoxia: biochemical and morphologic studies. Angiology 20, 1 - 12 (1969).
HELIN, P., LORENZEN, I.: Seasonal variations in the susceptibility of the aortic wall to arteriosclerosis - biochemical studies of glycosaminoglycans and collagen of rabbit aorta. Atherosclerosis 24(1 - 2), 259 - 266 (1976).
HELLMAN, L., ROSENFELD, R.S., INSULL, W., Jr., AHRENS, E.H., Jr.: Intestinal excretion of cholesterol: a mechanism for regulating plasma levels. J. Clin. Invest. 36, 838 (1957).
HELLSTRÖM, K., EINARSSON, K.: Bile acid metabolism in hyperlipoproteinaemia. In: Clinics in Gastroenterology. PAUMGARTNER, G. (ed.). London - Philadelphia - Toronto: W.B. Saunders Co. Ltd., 1976 (in press).
HELLSTRÖM, K.H., SIPERSTEIN, M.D., BRICKER, L.A., LUBY, L.J.: Studies of the in vivo metabolism of mevalonic acid in the normal rat. J. Clin. Invest. 52, 1303 - 1313 (1973).
HELSINGER, N., Jr., ROOTWELT, K.: Partial ileal bypass for surgical treatment of hypercholesterolemia. Nord. Med. 82, 1409 (1969).
HENDERSON, R.R., ROWE, G.G.: The progression of coronary atherosclerotic disease as assessed by cine-coronary arteriography. Am. Heart J. 86, 165 - 172 (1973).
HENNIGAR, G.R., KATZ, H.P.: Effect of i.v. glucosamine-HCl on the aortas of normal and diabetic rabbits. Fed. Proc. 20, 92 (1961).
HEPTINSTALL, R.H.: Experimental pulmonary atheroma. J. Path. Bact. 77, 535 (1959).
HERBERTSON, B.M., KELLAWAY, T.D.: Arterial necrosis in the rat produced by methoxamine. J. Path. Bact. 80, 87 (1960).
HEYDEN, S.: Risikofaktoren für das Herz, 2. Mannheim: Boehringer Mannheim GmbH, 1975.
HEYDEN, S., DURHAM, N.C.: Atherosklerotische Herzerkrankungen und Ernährung. In: Ernährungslehre und Diätetik. HOLTMEIER, H.J. (ed.). Stuttgart: Georg Thieme Verlag, 1972, Vol. II, Part 2, p. 1.
HIGGINS, M.W., KJELSBERG, M.: Characteristics of smokers and of nonsmokers in Tecumseh, Michigan. II. The distribution of selected physical measurements and physiologic variables and the prevalence of certain diseases in smokers and nonsmokers. Am. J. Epidemiol. 86, 60 - 77 (1967).
HIRSCH, J., KNITTLE, J., SALANS, L.: Cell lipid content and cell number in obese and non-obese human adipose tissue. J. Clin. Invest. 45, 1023 (1966).
HIRST, A.E., HADLEY, G.G., GORE, I.: The effect of chronic alcoholism and cirrhosis of the liver on atherosclerosis. Amer. J. Med. Sc. 45, 143 - 149 (1965).

HIRZ, R., SCANU, A.M.: Reassembly in vitro of a serum high-density lipoprotein. Biochim. Biophys. Acta 207, 364 - 367 (1967).

HOFF, H.F., JACKSON, R.L., GOTTO, A.M., Jr.: Apolipoprotein localization in human atherosclerotic arteries. Adv. Exp. Med. Biol. 67, 109 (1976).

HOLLANDER, W., COLOMBO, M.A., KRAMSCH, D.M., KIRKPATRICK, B.: Immunological aspects of atherosclerosis. Adv. Cardiol. 13, 192 - 207 (1974).

HOLLANDER, W., KRAMSCH, D.M., FRANZBLAU, C., PADDOCK, J., COLOMBO, M.A.: Suppression of atheromatous fibrous plaque formation by antiproliferative and anti-inflammatory drugs. Circ. Res. Suppl. 34/35 I, 131 - 141 (1974).

HOLLIS, T.M., ROSEN, L.A.: Histidine decarboxylase activity of bovine aortic endothelium and intima-media. Proc. Soc. Exp. Biol. 141, 978 (1972).

HOLLOSZY, J.O., SKINNER, J.S., TORO, G., CURETON, T.K.: Effects of a six month program of endurance exercises on the serum lipids of middle-aged men. Amer. J. Cardiol. 14, 753 (1964).

HOLMAN, R.L., McGILL, H.C., Jr., STRONG, J.P., GEER, J.C.: The natural history of atherosclerosis: the early aortic lesions as seen in New Orleans in the middle of the 20th century. Am. J. Pathol. 34, 209 (1958).

HOLMSEN, H., DAY, H.J., STORMORKEN, H.: The blood platelet release reaction. Scand. J. Haemat. Suppl. 8, 1 (1969).

HOOVER, J., WAHL, P.W. HAZZARD, W.R., ALBERS, J.: Lipid levels in women: relation to age, education, occupation and hormone use. Proceedings of the Fourth International Symposium on Atherosclerosis, Tokyo, August 26, 1976.

HORLICK, L., KATZ, L.N.: Retrogression of atherosclerotic lesions on cessation of cholesterol feeding in the chick. J. Lab. Clin. Med. 34, 1427 - 1442 (1949).

HORNSTRA, G.: Dietary fats and arterial thrombosis. In: Dietary fats and thrombosis. Haemostasis 2, 21 (1973/74).

HOWARD, A.N.: Hypolipaemic drugs and coronary heart disease. J. Clin. Path. 28, (Suppl. 9), (Roy. Coll. Path.), 106 (1975).

HOWARD, A.N., COURTENAY EVANS, R.J., TOMLINSON, S.: (1977), (in preparation).

HOWARD, A.N., GHOSH, P.: Gemfibrozil treatment: a comparison with clofibrate. Proc. Roy. Soc. Med. (1977), (in press).

HOWARD, A.N., HYAMS, D.E.: Combined use of clofibrate and cholestyramine or DEAE Sephadex in hypercholesterolaemia. Brit. Med. J. 3, 25 (1971).

HOWARD, B.V., MACARAK, E.J., GUNSON, D., KEFALIDES, N.A.: Characterization of the collagen synthesized by endothelial cells in culture. Proc. Natl Acad. Sci. 73, 2361 (1976).

HOWELL, R.W.: Smoking habits and laboratory tests. Lancet (1970) II, 152.

HUEPER, W.C.: Arteriosclerosis. The anoxemia theory. Arch. Path. 38, 162, 245, 350 (1944).

HÜTTNER, I., BOUTET, M, MORE, R.H.: Gap junctions in arterial endothelium. J. Cell. Biol. 57, 247 (1973a).

HÜTTNER, I., BOUTET, M., MORE, R.H.: Studies on protein passage through arterial endothelium. I. Structural correlates of permeability in rat arterial endothelium. Lab. Invest. 28, 672 (1973b).

HÜTTNER, I., JELLINEK, H., KERÉNYI, T.: Fibrin formation in vascular fibrinoid change in experimental hypertension: an electron microscopic study. Exp. Molec. Path. 9, 309 - 321 (1968).

HÜTTNER, I., MORE, R.H., RONA, G.: Fine structural evidence of specific mechanism for increased endothelial permeability in experimental hypertension. Amer. J. Pathol. 61, 395 (1970).

HÜTTNER, I., MORE, R.H., RONA, G., JELLINEK, H.: Diversity of fibrin ultrastructure in experimental vascular fibrinoid. Lab. Invest. (Abstract) 20, 288 (1969a).

HÜTTNER, I., MORE, R.H., RONA, G., JELLINEK, H.: Mechanism of increased transport in arterial endothelium during experimental hypertension. 8th International Congress of the International Academy of Pathology, Mexico City, 1970.

HÜTTNER, I., RONA, G., JELLINEK, H., MORE, R.H.: Atherosclerosis as a healing process of fibrinoid vascular change. An ultrastructural study. 2nd International Symposium on Atherosclerosis. (Abstract) 25. Nov. Chicago (1969b).

HÜTTNER, I., RONA, G., JELLINEK, H., MORE, R.H.: Fibrine se présentant sous la forme particuliere de cristeaux dans les lesions fibrinoides vasculaires. (Abstract). 24e Congr. de l'Assoc. des Méd. de Lab. de la Provence de Quebec. Sherbrooke, 18 - 19, Juin, 1969c.

HUFELAND, Ch.W.: Die Kunst das manschliche Leben zu verlängern. "Makrobiotik". Stuttgart: Hippokrates Verlag, 1958.

HURME, V.O.: Estimation of monkey age by dental formula. Ann. N.Y. Acad. Sci. 85, 795 - 799 (1960).

HUTTUNEN, J.K., EHNHOLM, C., KEKKI, M., NIKKILÄ, E.A.: Postheparin plasma lipoprotein plasma lipase and hepatic lipase in normal subjects and in patients with hypertriglyceridemia: correlations to sex, age and various parameters of triglyceride metabolism. Clin. Sci. Mol. Med. 50, 249 - 260 (1976a).

HUTTUNEN, J.K., EHNHOLM, C., KINNUNEN, P.K.J., NIKKILÄ, E.A.: An immunochemical method for the selective measurement of two triglyceride lipase in human postheparin plasma. Clin. Chim. Acta 63, 335 - 347 (1975a).

HUTTUNEN, J.K., EHNHOLM, C., NIKKILÄ, E.A., OHTA, M.: Effects of fasting on postheparin plasma triglyceride lipases and triglyceride removal. Eur. J. Clin. Invest. 5, 435 - 445 (1975b).

HUTTUNEN, J.K., PASTERNACK, A., EHNHOLM, C., VÄNTTINEN, T.: Lipoprotein metabolism in patients with chronic uremia before and after treatment with hemodialysis. Proceedings of the 2nd Dresdner Lipid Symposium. Dresden (1976b).

IGNATOWSKI, A.: Über die Wirkung des tierischen Eiweisses auf die Aorta und die parenchymatösen Organe der Kaninchen. Virchow's Arch. f. Pathol. Anat. Physiol. u. Klin. Med. 198, 248 - 270 (1909).

IMAI, H., LEE, S.K., PASTORI, S.J., THOMAS, W.A.: Degeneration of arterial smooth muscle cells: ultrastructural study of smooth muscle cell death in control and cholesterol-fed animals. Virchows Arch. Abt. A. Path. Anat 350, 183 - 204 (1970).

IAMI, H., WERTHESSEN, N.T., TAYLOR, C.B., LEE, K.T.: Angiotoxicity and arteriosclerosis due to conteminants of USP grade cholesterol. Arch. Path. (1976) (in press).

IMAIZUMI, K., FAINARU, M., HAVEL, R.J.: Transfer of apolipoproteins (A-I and ARP) between rat mesenteric lymph chylomicrons and serum lipoproteins. Circulation (1976) (in press).

IMMUNOLOGICAL START TO ATHEROSCLEROSIS. Editorial. Lancet (1975) I, 208.

ISAAC, P.F., RAND, M.J.: Cigarette smoking and plasma levels of nicotine. Nature 236, 308 (1972).

ISAGER, H., HAGERUP, L.: Relationship between cigarette smoking and high packed cell volume and haemoglobin levels. Scand. J. Haematol. 8, 241 - 244 (1971).

IVERIUS, P.-H.: Coupling of glycosaminoglycans to agarose beads (Sepharose 4B). Biochem. J. 124, 677 - 683 (1971).

IVERIUS, P.-H.: The interaction between human plasma lipoproteins and connective tissue glycosaminoglycans. J. Biol. Chem. 247, 2607 (1972).

IVERIUS, P.-H.: Possible role of the glycosaminoglycans in the genesis of atherosclerosis. In: Atherosclerosis: Initiating Factors (Ciba Foundation Symposia, New Series No. 12). Amsterdam: Excerpta Medica, 1973, p. 185.

IVERIUS, P.-H., OSTLUND LUNDQUIST, A.M.: J. Biol. Chem. 251, 7791 (1976).

JACKSON, D.S.: Connective tissue growth stimulated by carrageenin. The formation and removal of collagen. Biochem. J. 65, 277 - 284 (1957).

JACKSON, R.L., MORRISETT, J.D., GOTTO, A.M., Jr.: Lipoprotein structure and metabolism. Physiol. Rev. 56, 259 - 316 (1976).

JACKSON, R.L., MORRISETT, J.D., GOTTO, A.M., Jr., SEGREST, J.P.: The mechanism of lipid.binding by plasma lipoproteins. Mol. Cell. Biochem. 6, 43 - 50 (1975).

JACKSON, R.L., MORRISETT, J.D., SPARROW, J.T., SEGREST, J.P., POWNALL, H.J., SMITH, L.C., HOFF, H.F., GOTTO, A.M., Jr.: The interaction of apolipoprotein-serine with phosphatidylcholine. J. Biol. Chem. 249, 5314 - 5320 (1974a).

JACKSON, R.L., SPARROW, J.T., BAKER, H.N., MORRISETT, J.D., TAUNTON, O.D., GOTTO, A.M., Jr.: The primary structure of apolipoprotein-serine. J. Biol. Chem. 249, 5308 - 5313 (1974b).

JACKSON, R.L., STEIN, O., GLANGEAUD, M.C., FAINARU, M., GOTTO, A.M., Jr., STEIN, Y.: The removal of lipids from Landschütz ascites cells and smooth-muscle cells in culture. Adv. Exp. Med. Biol. 67, 453 (1976).

JACQUES, P.J.: Endocytosis. In: Lysosomes in Biology and Pathology. DINGLE, J.T., FELL, H.B. (eds.). Amsterdam: North Holland Publishing Co., 1969, Vol. II, p. 395.

JAFFE, E.A., HOYER, L.W., NACHMAN, R.L.: Synthesis of antihemophilic factor antigen by cultured human endothelial cells. J. Clin. Invest. 52, 2757 (1973a).

JAFFE, E.A., NACHMAN, R.L., BECKER, C.G., MINICK, C.R.: Culture of human endothelial cells derived from umbilical veins. J. Clin. Invest. 52, 2745 (1973).

JAFFEE, E.A., ADELMAN, B., MINICK, C.R., BECKER, C.G., NACHMAN, R.: Synthesis of basement membrane in cultured endothelial cells. J. Exper. Med. (1976) (in press).

JAGANNATHAN, S.N., CONNOR, W.E., BAKER, W.H., BHATTACHARYYA, A.K.: The turnover of cholesterol in human atherosclerotic arteries. J. Clin. Invest. 54, 366 (1974a).

JAGANNATHAN, S.N., CONNOR, W.E., LEWIS, L.J.: Accumulation of esterified cholesterol from plasma low density lipoproteins by human endothelial cells in culture and its effect on biosynthesis of cholesterol. Submitted for publication (1976b).

JAGANNATHAN, S.N., CONNOR, W.E., LEWIS, L.J.: Cholesterol metabolism in human endothelial cells in culture. In: Atherosclerosis: Metabolic, Morphologic and Clinical Aspects. MANNING, G.W., HAUST, M.D. (eds.). Plenum Press, 1976a.

JAGANNATHAN, S.N., LEWIS, L.J., CONNOR, W.E.: The accumulation of free and esterified cholesterol by human endothelial cells cultured with various plasma lipoproteins. Circulation 50, 69, 1974b. Abstract.

JARMOLYCH, J., DAOUD, A.S., LANDAU, J., FRITZ, K.E., McELVENE, E.: Aortic medial explants. Cell proliferation and production of mucopolysaccharides, collagen and elastic tissue. Exp. and Molec. Path. 9, 171 - 188 (1968).

JELLINEK, H.: Arterial lesions and arteriosclerosis. London - New York: Plenum Press, 1974.

JELLINEK, H., HÜTTNER, I., KÁDÁR, A., KERÉNYI, T., VERESS, B.: Vergleichende histologische und elektronenmikroskopische Untersuchungen von Gefäßveränderungen verschiedenen Ursprungs. Verh. Dtsch. Ges. Path. 51, 243 - 247 (1967).

JELLINEK, H., NAGY, Z., HÜTTNER, I., BÁLINT, A., KÓCZÉ, A., KERÉNYI, T.: Investigation of the permeability changes of the vascular wall in malignant hypertension by means of colloidal iron preparation. Brit. J. exp. Path. 50, 13 (1969).

JELLINEK, H., VERESS, B., BÁLINT, A., NAGY, Z.: Lymph vessels to rat aorta and their changes in experimental atherosclerosis. An electron microscopic study. Exp. Molec. Path. 13, 370 (1970).

JELLINEK, H., VERESS, B., HÜTTNER, I., KERÉNYI, T.: Über die Morphologie der lymphstauungsbedingten Koronarveränderungen. Frankf. Z. Path. 75, 331 (1966).

JENKINS, D.J.A., LEEDS, A.R., NEWTON, C., CUMMINGS, J.H.: Effect of pectin, guar gum and wheat fibre on serum cholesterol. Lancet (1975) I, 1116 - 1117.

JENSEN, J.: The kinetics of the in vitro cholesterol uptake at the endothelial cell surface of the rabbit aorta. Biochim. Biophys. Acta 135, 544 (1967).

JENSEN, J., BLANKENHORN, O., KORNERUP, V.: Coronary disease in familial hypercholesterolemia. Circulation 36, 77 (1967).

JOHANSSON, H.G., LAURELL, C.B.: Disorders of serum α-lipoprotein after alcoholic intoxication. Scandin. J. Clin. Invest. 23, 231 - 233 (1969).

JOHNSON, K.G., YANO, K., KATO, H.: Coronary heart disease in Hiroshima: report of a six-year period of surveillance, 1958-1964. Am. J. Public Health 58, 1355 (1968).

JOHNSON, T.F., WONG, H.Y.C.: Effect of exercise on plasma cholesterol and phospholipids in college swimmers. Res. Quart. 32, 514 (1961).

JONAS, A, SEIDEL, D.: Properties of the abnormal plasma lipoprotein (LP-X) characteristic of cholestasis after chemical modification with succinic anhydrid. Archiv of Biochem. and Biophys. 163, 200 - 210 (1974).

JONES, H.B., GOFMAN, J.W., LINDGREN, F.T., LYON, T.P., GRAHAM, D.M., STRISOWER, B., NICHOLS, A.V.: Lipoproteins in atherosclerosis. Am. J. Med. 11, 358 - 380 (1951).

JONES, P.D., LOSOWSKY, M.S., DAVIDSON, C.S., LIEBER, C.S.: Effects of ethanol on plasma lipids in man. J. Lab. Clin. Med. 62, 675 - 682 (1963).

JORDAN, R.E., HEWITT, N., LEWIS, W., KAGAN, H., FRANZBLAU, C.: Regulation of elastase-catalyzed hydrolysis of insoluble elastin by synthetic and naturally occurring hydrophobic ligands. Biochemistry 13, 3497 – 3503 (1974).

JØRGENSEN, L., PACKHAM, M.A., ROWSELL, H.C., MUSTARD, J.F.: Deposition of formed elements of blood on the intima and signs of intimal injury in the aorta of rabbit, pig and man. Lab. Invest. 27, 341 (1972).

JORIS, I., MAJNO, G., RYAN, G.B.: Endothelial contraction in vivo: a study of the rat mesentery. Virch. Arch. Abt. B. Zellpath. 12, 73 (1972).

KADER, M.M.A., HAMMAN, S., HAY, A.A., KAMEL, G., et al.: Die Wirkung von Insulin und Adrenalin auf den Fettstoffwechsel bei Patienten mit Hepatosplenomegalie vor und nach portakavaler Anastomose. Zschr. inn. Med. 14, 421 (1973).

KADER, M.M.A., HAMMAN, S., HAY, A.A., KAMEL, G., AZIZ, M.T.A., FAYTEK, K.: Effect of portacaval anastomosis on lipid metabolism. Acta biol. med. germ. 27, 317 – 326 (1971).

KAGAN, A., HARRIS, B.R., WINKELSTEIN, W., JOHNSON, K.G., KATO, H.: Epidemiologic studies of coronary heart disease and stroke in Japanese men living in Japan, Hawaii and California: demographic, physical, dietary and biochemical characteristics. J. Chron. Dis. 27, 345 (1974).

KAGAN, A., STERNBY, N.H., UEMURA, K., VANECEK, R., VIHERT, A.M.: Atherosclerosis in five European towns. (in press).

KAIJSER, L., ERICSSON, M., EKLUND, B.: Substrate extraction by the human heart during angina pectoris induced by atrial pacing: extraction, release and oxidation of fatty acids. Fyris Tryck AB (Uppsala) (1976).

KALANT, H., KHANNA, J.M.: In: Biochemical and Clinical Aspects of Alcohol Metabolism. SARDESAI, V.M. (ed.). Springfield, Ill.: C.C. Thomas, 1969, pp. 47 – 57.

KAMEYAMA, M.: Basic problems in cerebrovascular diseases in the aged: clinical and pathological considerations. Tokyo Metropolitan Institute of Gerontology and Tokyo Metropolitan Geriatric Hospital. Collected papers No. 3, 253 – 267 (1974). (in Japanese).

KANDUTSCH, A.A., CHEN, H.W.: Inhibition of sterol synthesis in cultured mouse cells by cholesterol derivatives oxygenated in the side chain. J. Biol. Chem. 249, 6057 – 6061 (1974).

KANDUTSCH, A.A., CHEN, H.W.: Inhibition of sterol synthesis in cultured mouse cells by 7-α-hydroxycholesterol, 7-ß-hydroxycholesterol, and 7-ketocholesterol. J. Biol. Chem. 248, 8404 – 8417 (1973).

KANE, J.P.: A rapid electrophoretic technique for identification of subunit species of apoproteins in serum lipoproteins. An. Bioch. 53, 350 – 364 (1973).

KANE, J.P., SATA, T., HAMILTON, R.L., HAVEL, R.J.: Apoprotein composition of very low density lipoproteins of human serum. J. Clin. Invest. 56, 1622 – 1634 (1975).

KANNEL, W.B.: Some lessons in cardiovascular epidemiology from Framingham. Am. J. Cardiol. 37, 269 – 282 (1976).

KANNEL, W.B., CASTELLI, W.P., GORDON, T., McNAMARA, P.M.: Serum cholesterol, lipoproteins, and the risk of coronary heart disease: the Framingham study. Ann. Intern. Med. 74, 1 (1971).

KANNEL, W.B., GARCIA, M.J., McNAMARA, P.M., PEARSON, G.: Serum lipid precursors of coronary heart disease. Hum. Pathol. 2, 129 (1971).

KANNEL, W.B., SORLIE, P.: Hypertension in Framingham. In: Epidemiology and Control of Hypertension. PAUL, O. (ed.). New York – London: Stratton Intercontinental Medical Book Corp., 1975, pp. 553 – 592.

KARLIN, J.B., JOHN, D.J., STARR, J.I., SCANU, A.M., RUBENSTEIN, A.H.: Measurement of human high density lipoprotein apolipoprotein A-I in serum by radioimmunoassay. J. Lipid Res. 17, 30 (1976).

KARLSSON, J., DIAMANT, B., SALTIN, B.: Muscle metabolites during submaximal and maximal exercise in man. Scand. J. clin. Lab. Invest. 26, 385 – 394 (1970).

KARNOVSKY, M.J.: Morphology of capillaries with special reference to muscle capillaries. In: Capillary Permeability. Alfred Benzon Symposium II. CRONE, C.H., LASSEN, N.A. (eds.). New York: Academic Press Inc., 1970, p. 341.

KARNOVSKY, M.J.: The ultrastructural basis of capillary permeability studied with peroxidase as a tracer. J. Cell. Biol. 35, 213 (1967).

KATO, M., GOTO, Y., MIYAZAKI, K., HIRAI, S., SHIGENO, K.: A study on a long term pyridinolcarbamate treatment of postapoplectic patients — In its reference to the prevention of the recurrence of stroke —. Geriatric Med. 13, 301 - 310 (1975).

KATOCS, A.S., LARGAS, E.E., WILL, L.W., McCLINTOCK, D.K., RIGGI, S.J.: Sterol deposition in the aortae of normal cholesterolemic and hypercholesterolemic rabbits subjected to aortic de-endothelialization. Artery 2, 38 - 52 (1976).

KATZ, L.N., STAMLER, J.: Experimental atherosclerosis. Springfield, Ill.: C.C. Thomas, 1963, p 136.

KAUFMANN, R.L., SOELDNER, J.S., WILMSHURST, E.G., LEMAIRE, J.R., GLEASON, R.E., WHITE, P.: Plasma lipid levels in diabetic children, effect of diet restricted in cholesterol and saturated fats. Diabetes 24, 672 - 679 (1975).

KAYDEN, H.J., SENIOR, J.R., MATTSON, F.H.: The monoglyceride pathway of fat absorption in man. J. Clin. Invest. 46, 1695 - 1703 (1967).

KAYE, J.P., GALTON, D.J.: Triglyceride production rates in patients with Type IV hypertriglyceridemia. Lancet (1975) I, 1005 - 1007.

KEELEY, F.W., PARTRIDGE, S.M.: Amino acid composition and calcification of human aortic elastin. Atherosclerosis 19, 287 - 296 (1974).

KEFALIDES, N.A., DENDUCHIS, B.: Structural components of epithelial and endothelial basement membranes. Biochem. J. 8, 4613 - 4621 (1969).

KEKKI, M., MIETTINEN, T.A., WAHLSTRÖM, B.: Measurement of cholesterol synthesis in kinetically defined pools using fecal steroid analysis and double-labeling technique in man. J. Lipid Res. (1977) (in press).

KEKKI, M., NIKKILA, E.A.: Turnover of plasma total and very low density lipoprotein triglyceride in man. Scand. J. Clin. Lab. Invest. 35, 171 - 179 (1975).

KERENYI, T., HORVÁTH, Z., DETRE, Z., KURUNCZI, S., JELLINEK, H.: Permeability of the post-ischemic rat aorta. Acta morph. Acad. Sci. hung. 23, 83-93 (1975).

KERENYI, T., HÜTTNER, I., JELLINEK, H.: Über die Entwicklung der periodischen Struktur in subendothelialen Fibrinoid. Z. Mier Anat. Forsch. 74, 121 - 131 (1966).

KERENYI, T., JELLINEK, H.: Fibrin deposition in smooth muscle cells of muscular type small arteries under temporary conditions of hypoxia. Exp. Molec. Path. 17, 1 - 5 (1972).

KESSLER, G., LEDERER, H.: Fluorimetric measurements of triglycerides. In: Automation in Analytical Chemistry. SKEGGS, L.T. (ed.). New York: Mediad Inc., 1965, Vol. I, p. 341.

KEYS, A.: Coronary heart disease - the global picture. Atherosclerosis 22, 149 - 192 (1975).

KEYS, A.: Coronary heart disease in seven countries. Circulation 41 - 42, (Suppl. 1), I-1-I-211 (1970).

KEYS, A.: Serum Cholesterol and the question of "normal". In: Multiple Laboratory Screening. BENSON, E.S., STANDFORD, P.E. (eds.). New York 1969.

KEYS, A., ANDERSON, J.T., GRANDE, F.: Serum cholesterol response to changes in the diet. I. Iodine value of dietary fat versus 2S-P. Metabolism 14, 747 - 758 (1965a).

KEYS, A., ANDERSON, J.T., GRANDE, F.: Serum cholesterol response to changes in the diet. II. The effect of cholesterol in the diet. Metabolism 14, 759 - 765 (1965b).

KEYS, A., ARAVANIS, C., BLACKBURN, H.W., Van BUCHEM, F.S.P., BUZINA, R., DJORDJEVIC, B.S., DONTAS, A.S., FIDANZA, F., KARVONEN, M., KIMURA, N., LEKOS, D., MONTI, M., PUDDU, V., TAYLOR, H.L.: Epidemiological studies related to coronary heart disease; characteristics of men aged 40 - 59 in seven countries. Acta Medica Scandinavica Suppl. 460 (1967).

KEYS, A., ARAVANIS, C., BLACKBURN, H., Van BUCHEM, F.S.P., BUZINA, R., DJORDJEVIC, B.S., FIDANZA, F., KARVONEN, M.J., MENOTTI, A., PUDDU, V., TAYLOR, H.L.: Probability of middle-aged men developing coronary heart disease in five years. Circulation 45, 815 - 828 (1972).

KHAIRALLAH, P.A., ROBERTSON, A.L., DAVILA, D.: Effects of angiotensin II on DNA, RNA and protein synthesis. In: Hypertension 1972. GENEST, J., KOIW, E. (eds.). Berlin: Springer - Verlag, 1972, p 212.

KIM, D.N., LEE, K.T., REINER, J.M., THOMAS, W.A.: Effect of combined clofibrate-cholestyramine treatment on serum and tissue cholesterol pools and on cholesterol synthesis in hypercholesterolemic swine. Experimental and Molecular Pathology 23, 83 - 95 (1975).

KIM, K.M.: Calcification of matrix vesicles in human aorta valve and aortic media. Fed. Proc. 35, 156 - 162 (1976).

KIMBIRIS, D., LAVINE, P., Van Den BROEK, H., NAJMI, M., LIKOFF, W.: Devolutionary pattern of coronary atherosclerosis in patients with angina pectoris. Coronary arteriographic studies. Am. J. Card. 33, 7 - 11 (1974).

KIMURA, N.: Analysis of 10000 postmortem examinations in Japan. In: World Trends in Cardiology I, Cardiovascular Epedemiology. KEYS, A., WHITE, P.D. (eds.). New York: Hoeber-Harper, 1956, pp. 22 - 23.

KIMURA, N.: A population survey on cerebrovascular and cardiovascular diseases in Kyushu, Japan, Singapore Medical Journal 14, 230 - 233 (1973).

KIMURA, N., et al.: The studies for genesis of ischemic heart disease in Japan. J. Jpn. Soc. Intern. Med. 63, 29 (1974).

KIMURA, N., FURUKAWA, I., et al.: Sogorinsho 8, 564 - 578 (1959). (in Japanese).

KIMURA, N., NANBU, S.: The pattern of hyperlipoproteinemia. Aspect of plasma lipoprotein metabolism. Jap. J. Clin. Med. 33, 3147 - 3156 (1975).

KIMURA, N., TOSHIMA, H., NAKAYAMA, J., MIZUGOCH, T., TAKAYAMA, K., YOSHINAG, M., FUKAMI, T., TASHIRO, H., KATAYAMA, F., ABE, K.: Population survey on cerebrovascular and cardiovascular diseases. The ten years experience in the farming village of Tanushimaru and fishing village of Ushibuka. Jap. Heart J. 13, 118 - 127 (1972).

KIRKPATRICK, J.B.: Pathogenesis of foam cell lesions in irradiated arteries. Am. J. Pathol. 50, 291 - 310 (1967).

KIRSTEN, E.S., WATSON, J.A.: Regulation of 3-hydroxy-3-methylglutaryl coenzyme A reductase in hepatoma tissue culture cells by serum lipoproteins. J. Biol. Cehm. 249, 6104 - 6109 (1974).

KISSEBAH, A.H., ADAMS, P.W., WYNN, V.: Plasma free fatty acids and triglyceride transport kinetics in man. Clin. Sci. Mol. Med. 47, 259 - 278 (1974).

KJELDSEN, K.: Smoking and Atherosclerosis. Copenhagen: Munksgaard, 1969.

KJELDSEN, K., ASTRUP, P., WANSTRUP, J.: Reversal of rabbot atheromatosis by hyperoxia. J. Atheroscler. Res. 10, 173 - 178 (1969).

KJELDSEN, K., KLEM THOMSEN, H.: The effect of hypoxia on the fine structure of the aortic intima of rabbits. Lab. Invest. 33, 533 - 543 (1975).

KJELDSEN, K., WANSTRUP, J., ASTRUP, P.: Enhancing influence of arterial hypoxia on the development of atheromatosis in cholesterol-fed rabbits. J. Atheroscler. Res. 8, 835 - 845 (1968).

KLATSKY, A.L., FRIEDMAN, G.D., SIEGELAUB, B.: Alcohol consumption before myocardial infarction. Ann. Int. Med. 81, 294 - 301 (1974).

KLEINBAUM, D.G., KUPPER, L.L., CASSEL, J.C., TYROLER, H.A.: Multivariate analysis of risk of coronary heart disease in Evans County, Georgia. Arch. Int. Med. 128, 943 - 948 (1971).

KLYNSTRA, F.B.: On the passage-restricting role of acid mucopolysaccharides in the endothelium of pig aortas. Atherosclerosis 19, 215 - 220 (1974).

KLYNSTRA, F.B., BÖTTCHER, C.J.F., VAN MELSEN, J.A., VAN DER LAAN, E.J.: Distribution and composition of acid mucopolysaccharides in normal and atherosclerotic human aortas. J. Atheroscler. Res. 7, 301 - 309 (1967).

KNIGHT, L., SCHEIBEL, R., AMPLATZ, K., VARCO, R.L., BUCHWALD, H.: Radiographic appraisal of the Minnesota partial ileal bypass study. Surg. Forum 23, 141 (1972).

KNIKER, W.I., COCHRANE, C.G.: Pathogenic factors in vascular lesions of experimental serum sickness. J. Exper. Med. 122, 83 (1965).

KOBERNICK, S.D., NIWAYAMA, G., ZUCHLEWSKI, A.C.: Effect of physical activity on cholesterol atherosclerosis in rabbits. Proc. Soc. Exp. Biol. and Med. 98, 623 (1953).

KOGA, S., BOLIS, L., SCANU, A.M.: Isolation and characterization of subunit polypeptides from apoproteins of rat serum lipoprotein. Biochim. Biophys. Acta 236, 416 (1971).

KOKATNUR, M.G., MALCOM, G.T., EGGEN, D.A., STRONG, J.P.: Depletion of aortic free and ester cholesterol by dietary means in rhesus monkeys with fatty streaks. Atherosclerosis 21, 195 - 203 (1975).

KOLATA, G.B.: Thromboxanes: the power behind the prostaglandins? Science 190, 770 - 812 (1975).

KONG, T.Q., KELLUM, R.E., HAZERICK, J.R.: Clinical diagnosis of cardiac involvement in systemic lupus erythematosus: a correlation of clinical and autopsy findings in thirty patients. Circulation 26, 7 (1962).

KONTTINEN, A.: Cigarette smoking and serum lipids in young men. Br. Med. J. 1, 1115 - 1116 (1962).

KONTTINEN, A., NIKKILA, E.A.: Effect of acute exercise on serum triglycerides and free fatty acids. Proc. Symp. Phys. Activity Heart, Helsinki, 208 - 215 (1964).

KONTTINEN, A., RAJASALMI, M.: Effect of heavy cigarette smoking on postprandial triglycerides, free fatty acids, and cholesterol. Br. Med. J. 1, 850 - 851 (1963).

KONYAR, E., KERÉNYI, T., VERESS, B., BÁLINT, A., KOLONICS, I., JELLINEK, H.: Study of experimental hypertensive vascular lesions by ruthenium red staining technique. Path. Europ. 9, 167-175 (1974).

KORN, E.D.: J. biol. Chem. 215, 15 (1955).

KORN, E.D.: The assay of lipoprotein lipase in vivo and in vitro. Methods Biochem. Anal. 7, 145 - 192 (1959).

KORN, E.D., QUIGLEY, T.W.: Lipoprotein lipase of chicken adipose tissue. J. Biol. Chem. 226, 833 (1957).

KOSEK, J.C., BIEBLER, C.H.: Atheroma in a transplanted heart. Lancet (1970) I, p. 563.

KOSTNER, G., HOLASEK, A.: Characterization and quantitation of the apolipoprotein from human chyle chylomicrons. Biochemistry 11, 1217 (1972).

KOSTNER, G.M., PATSCH, J.R., SAILER, S., BRAUNSTEINER, H., HOLASEK, A.: Polypeptide distribution of the main lipoprotein density classes separated from human plasma by rate zonal ultracentrifugation. Eur. J. Biochem. 45, 611 - 621 (1974).

KOTTKE, B.A.: Differences in bile acid excretion. Primary hypercholesterolemia compared to combined hypocholesterolemia and hypertriglyceridemia. Circulation 40, 13 - 20 (1969).

KOURY, S.D., HODGES, R.E.: Soybean proteins for human diets. J. Am. Diet. Ass. 52, 480 - 484 (1968).

KRAKOW, W., ANDRESS, G.F., SIEGEL, B.M., SCHERAGA, H.A.: An EM investigation of the polymerisation of vin fibrin. J. Mol. Biol. 71, 95 (1972).

KRAMSCH, D.M., CHAN, T.C.: Effects of ethane-hydroxy-diphosphonate (EHDP) and N-actyl-N-methyl-colchicine (Colcemid) on progression and regression of experimental atherosclerosis. Federation Proceedings (1975).

KRAMSCH, D.M., FRANZBLAU, C.: In: Atherosclerosis: Metabolic, Morphologic and Clinical Aspects. MANNING, G.W., HAUST, M.D. (eds.). New York: Plenum Press, 1976 (in press).

KRAMSCH, D.M., FRANZBLAU, C., HOLLANDER, W.: Components of the protein-lipid complex of arterial elastin: their role in the retention of lipid in atherosclerotic lesions. In: Arterial Mesenchyme and Arteriosclerosis. WAGNER, W.D., CLARKSON, T. (eds.). New York: Plenum Press, 1974, pp. 193 - 210.

KRAMSCH, D.M., FRANZBLAU, C., HOLLANDER, W.: The protein and lipid composition of arterial elastin and its relationship to lipid accumulation in the atherosclerotis plaque. J. Clin. Invest. 50, 1666 - 1677 (1971).

KRAMSCH, D.M., HOLLANDER, W.: The interaction of serum and arterial lipoproteins with elastin of the arterial intima and its role in the lipid accumulation in atherosclerotic plaques. J. Clin. Invest. 52, 236 - 247 (1973a).

KRAMSCH, D.M., HOLLANDER, W., RENAUD, S.: Induction of fibrous plaques versus foam cell lesions in Macaca fascicularis by varying composition of dietary fats. Circulation 58, (Suppl. IV), 41 (1973b).

KRAUSS, R.M., HERBERT, P.N., LEVY, R.I., FREDRICKSON, D.S.: Further observations on the activation and inhibition of lipoprotein lipase by apolipoproteins. Circ. Res. 33, 403 (1973a).

KRAUSS, R.M., LEVY, R.I., FREDRICKSON, D.S.: Selective measurement of two lipase activities in post-heparin plasma from normal subjects and patients with hyperlipoproteinamia. J. Clin. Invest. 54, 1107 - 1124 (1974).

KRAUSS, R.M., WINDMULLER, H.G., LEVY, R.I., FREDRICKSON, D.S.: Selective measurement of two different triglyceride lipase activities in rat postheparin plasma. J. Lipid Red. 14, 286 - 295 (1973).

KRESSE, H., FRIESE, W., BUDDECKE, E.: Altersveränderungen biogener Makromoleküle des Arteriengewebes. In: PLATT, D. (ed.): Altern. pp. 11 - 21.Stuttgart/New York: Schattauer, 1974.

KRITCHEVSKY, D., DAVIDSON, L.M., SHAPIRO, I.L., KIM, H.K., KITAGAWA, M., MALHOTRA, S., NAIR, P.P., CLARKSON, T.B., BERSOHN, I., WINTER, P.A.D.: Lipid metabolism and experimental atherosclerosis in baboons: influence of cholesterol-free, semi-synthetic diets. Am. J. Clin. Nutr. 27, 29 - 50 (1974a).

KRITCHEVSKY, D., DAVIDSON, L.M., VAN DER WATT, J.J., WINTER, P.A.D., BERSOHN, I.: Hypercholesterolaemia and atherosclerosis induced in vervet monkeys by cholesterol-free, semi-synthetic diets. S. Afr. Med. J. 48, 2413 - 2414 (1974b).

KRITCHEVSKY, D., MOYER, A.W., TESAR, W.C., McCANDLESS, R.F.J., LOGAN, J.B., BROWN, R.A., ENGLERT, M.: Cholesterol vehicle in experimental atherosclerosis. II. Effect of unsaturation. Amer. J. Physiol. 185, 279 - 280 (1956).

KRITCHEVSKY, D., SALLATA, P., TEPPER, S.A.: Experimental atherosclerosis in rabbits fed cholesterol-free diets. 2. Influence of various carbohydrates. J. Atheroscler. Res. 8, 697 - 703 (1968).

KRITCHEVSKY, D., TEPPER, S.A.: Cholesterol vehicle in experimental atherosclerosis. VII. Influence of naturally occurring saturated fats. Med. Pharmacol. Exp. 12, 315 - 320 (1965).

KRITCHEVSKY, D., TEPPER, S.A.: Experimental atherosclerosis in rabbits fed cholesterol-free diets: influence of chow components. J. Atheroscler. Res. 8, 357 - 369 (1968).

KRITCHEVSKY, D., TEPPER, S.A.: Influence of pyridinolcarbamate on oxidation of cholesterol by rat liver mitochondria. Arzneimittel-Forschung, (Drug Res.) 21, 146 - 147 (1971).

KRITCHEVSKY, D., TEPPER, S.A., GENZANO, J.C., KOTHARI, H.V.: Aortic Cholesterol Esterase in Rabbits: Effect of Duration of Cholesterol Feeding. Atherosclerosis 19, 459 - 462 (1974).

KRITCHEVSKY, D., TEPPER, S.A., KITAGAWA, M.: Experimental atherosclerosis in rabbits fed cholesterol-free diets. 3. Comparison of fructose and lactose with other carbohydrates. Nutr. Reports Int. 7, 193 - 202 (1973b).

KRITCHEVSKY, D., TEPPER, S.A., VESSELINOVITCH, D., WISSLER, R.W.: Cholesterol vehicle in experimental atherosclerosis. 11. Peanut oil. Atherosclerosis 14, 53 - 64 (1971).

KRITCHEVSKY, D., TEPPER, S.A., VESSELINOVITCH, D., WISSLER, R.W.: Cholesterol vehicle in experimental atherosclerosis. 13. Randomized peanut oil. Atherosclerosis 17, 225 - 243 (1973a).

KUDCHODKAR, B.J., SODHI, H.S.: Turnover of plasma cholesteryl esters and its relationship to other parameters of lipid metabolism in man. Europ. J. Clin. Invest. 6, 285 - 298 (1976).

KUMAR, V., BERENSON, G.S., RUIZ, H., DALFERES, E.R., Jr., STRONG, J.P.: Acid mucopolysaccharides of human aorta. Part 2. Variations with atherosclerotic involvement. J. Atheroscler. Res. 7, 583 - 590 (1967).

KUTHAN, F., BURKHALTER, A., BAITSCH, R., LUDIN, H., WIDMER, L.K.: Development of occlusive arterial disease in lower limbs. Angiographic follow-up of 705 medical patients. Arch. Surg. 103, 545 - 547 (1971).

KWAK, Y.S., LEE, K.T., KIM, D.N.: Study of drugs affecting cholesterol-induced atherosclerosis in rabbits. In: Atherosclerosis Drug Discovery. DAY, C.E. (ed.). New York: Plenum Publishing Co., 1976, pp. 149 - 167.

LAGGNER, P., DEGOVICS, G., MILLER, K., KRATKY, O., KOSTNER, G., HOLASEK, A.: Molecular packing and fluidity of lipids in human serum low density lipoproteins. Proc. Natl. Acad. Sci. US (1976) (in press).

LAMBERT, G.F., MILLER, J.P., OLSEN, R.T., FROST, D.V.: Hypercholesteremia and atherosclerosis induced in rabbits by purified high fat rations devoid of cholesterol. Proc. Soc. Exp. Biol. Med. 97, 544 - 549 (1958).

LANDIS, E.M.: Micro-injection studies of capillary permeability. II. The relation between capillary pressure and the rate at which fluid passes through the walls of single capillaries. Amer. J. Physiol. 27, 217 (1927).

LANDIS, E.M., PAPPENHEIMER, J.R.: Exchange of substances through the capillary walls. In: Handbook of Physiology. HAMILTON, W.F., DOW, P. (eds.). Washington, D.C.: American Physiol. Soc. 1963, Vol. II, Sect. 2, pp. 961 - 1034.

LANGER, T., STROBERG, W.T., LEVY, R.I.: The metabolism of low density lipoprotein in familial type II hyperproteinemia. J. Clin. Invest. 51, 1528 - 1536 (1972).

LANGNER, R.O., MODRAK, J.B.: Hypercholesterolemia and aortic collagen synthesis in rabbit aortas. Atherosclerosis 24 (1-2), 149 - 153 (1976).

LANGONE, J.J., GJIKA, H.B., VAN VUNAKIS, H.: Nicotine and its metabolites. Radioimmunoassays for nictotine and cotinine. Biochem. 12, 5025 (1973).

LaROSA, J.C., LEVY, R.I., BROWN, W.V., FREDRICKSON, D.S.: Changes in high density lipoprotein protein composition after heparin-induced lipolysis. Am. J. Physiol. 220, 785 (1971).

LaROSA, J.C., LEVY, R.I., HERBERT, R., LUX, S.E., FREDRICKSON, D.S.: A specific apoprotein activator for lipoprotein lipase. Biochem. Biophys. Res. Commun. 41, 57 - 62 (1970).

LaROSA, J.C., LEVY, R.J., WINDMUELLER, H.G., FREDRICKSON, D.S.: Comparison of the triglyceride lipase of liver, adipose tissue and postheparin plasma. J. Lipid Res. 13, 356 - 363 (1972).

LAURENT, T.C., BJÖRK, I., PIETRUSZKIEWICZ, A., PERSSON, H.: The transport of globular particles through hyaluronic acid solutions. Biochim. Biophys. Acta 78, 351 (1963).

LEDET, T., FISCHER-Dzoga, K., WISSLER, R.W.: Growth of rabbot aortic smooth muscle cells cultured in media containing diabetic and hyperlipemic serum. Diab. 25, 207 - 215 (1976).

LEE, K.T., JARMOLYCH, J., KIM, D.N., GRANT, C., KRASNEY, J.A., THOMAS, W.A., BRUNO, A.M.: Production of advanced coronary atherosclerosis, myocardial infarction and "sudden death" in swine. Exp. Mol. Path. 15, 170 - 190 (1971).

LEE, W.M., LEE, K.T.: Advanced coronary atherosclerosis in swine produced by combination of balloon-catheter injury and cholesterol feeding. Exp. Mol. Path. 23, 491 - 499 (1975).

LEE, W.M., SCOTT, R.F., MORRISON, E.S.: Effects of prednisolone and colchicine on the swine atherosclerosis. Atherosclerosis. (1976) (in press).

LEES, R.S., HATCH, F.T.: Sharper separation of lipoprotein species by paper electrophoresis in albumin-containing buffer. J. Lab. clin. Med. 61, 518 (1963).

LENDRUM, A.C.: Deposition of plastic substances in vessel walls. Path. Microbiol. 30, 681 (1967).

LENDRUM, A.C.: The hypertensive diabetic kidney as a model of the so-called collagen diseases. Canad. med. Ass. 88, 442 (1963).

LENZI, S., DESCOVICH, G.: unpublished data, 1976.

LEREN, P.: Dietary treatment of post-myocardial infarction patients. Lipid metabolism and atherosclerosis. Excerpta Medica, Amsterdam 57, (1973).

LEREN, P.: The effect of plasma cholesterol lowering diet in male survivors of myocardial infarction. Acta Medica Scandinavica, (Suppl. 466), (1966).

LEREN, P.: The Oslo diet-heart study. Eleven-year report. Circulation 42, 935 - 942 (1970)

LEREN, P., ASKEVOLD, E.M., FOSS, O.P., FROLI, A., GRYMYR, D., HELGELAND, A., HJERMANN, I., HOLME, I., LUND-LARSEN, P.G., NORUM, K.R.: The Oslo Study. Cardiovascular disease in middle and young Oslo men. Acta Medica Scandinavica, (Suppl. 588), (1975).

LEVINE, P.H.: An acute effect of cigarette smoking on platelet function. A possible link between smoking and arterial thrombosis. Circulation 48, 619 - 623 (1973).

LEVY, L.: A form of immunological atherosclerosis. In: The Reticuloendothelial System and Atherosclerosis. DI LUZZIO, PAOLETTI (eds.). New York: Plenum Press, 1967, p. 431.

LEVY, R.I., BLUM, C.B., SCHAEFER, E.J.: The composition, structure and metabolism of high density lipoprotein. In: Lipoprotein Metabolism. GRETEN, H. (ed.). Berlin: Springer-Verlag, 1976, p. 56.

LEVY, R.I., FREDRICKSON, D.S., SHULMAN, R., BILHEIMER, D.W., BRESLOW, J.L., STONE, N.J., LUX, S.E., SLOAN, H.R., KRAUSS, R.M., HERBERT, P.N.: Dietary and drug treatment of primary hyperlipoproteinemia - NIH Conference. Ann. Intern. Med. 77, 267 - 294 (1972).

LEVY, R., LANGER, T.: Hypolipidemic drugs and lipoprotein metabolism. Pharm. Control. Lipid Metab. 28, 155 (1973).

LEVY, R.I., STONE, N.J.: Atherosclerosis: role of lipoproteins. In: The Pathogenesis of Atherosclerosis. WISSLER, R.W., GEER, J.C. (eds.). Baltimore: Williams & Wilkins Co., 1974, pp. 227 - 238.

LEWIS, B., OUITIRI, A.C., WOOTTON, I.D.P., CHAIT, A., SIGURDSSON, G., OAKLEY, C.M.: Intravenous fat tolerance test in ischemic heart disease and peripheral vascular disease. Clin. Science. (1976) (submitted).

LEWIS, L.A., BROWN, H.B., PAGE, I.H.: Ten year's dietary treatment of primary hyperlipidemia. Geriatrics 25, 64 - 81 (1970).

LEWIS, L.A., BROWN, H.B., PAGE, I.H.: Ten year's treatment of hyperlipidemia. Circulation 38, (Suppl. VI), 128 (1968).

LEWIS, L.A., DE WOLFE, V.G., BUTKUS, A., PAGE, I.H.: Autoimmune hyperlipidemia in a patient. Atherosclerotic course and changing immunoglobulin pattern during 21 years of study. Amer. J. Med. 59, 208 (1975).

LEWIS, L.A., LAZZARINI-ROBERTSON, A., Jr.: Hyperimmuno-globulinemialipoproteinemia and atherogenesis. In: Atherosclerosis III. SCHETTLER, G., WEIZEL, A. (eds.). Berlin: Springer-Verlag, 1974, p. 595.

LEWIS, L.A., OLMSTED, F., PAGE, I.H., LAWRY, E.Y., MANN, G.V., STARE, F.J., HANIG, M., LAUFFER, M.A.: Evaluation of serum lipoprotein and cholesterol measurements as predictors of clinical complications of atherosclerosis. Report of a cooperative study of lipoproteins and atherosclerosis. Appenxid B. Circulation 14, 731 (1956).

LEWIS, L.A., PAGE, I.H., BATTLE, J.D., DE WOLFE, V.G.: How should hyperlipoproteiniemia-hypergammaglobulinemia manifestating of an antilipoprotein autoantibody be treated? Internat. Res. Commun. System 1, 40 (1973).

LEWIS, L.J., HOAK, J.C., MACA, R.D., FRY, G.L.: Replication of human endothelial cells in culture. Science 181, 453 (1973).

LIEBER, C.S., JONES, D.P., DeCARLI, L.M.: Effects of prolonged ethanol intake: production of fatty liver despite adequate diets. J. Clin. Invest. 44, 1009 - 1021 (1965).

LIEBER, C.S., LEEVY, C.M., STEIN, S.W., GEORGE, W.S., CHERRICK, C.R., ABELMANN, W.M., DAVIDSON, C.S.: Effect of ethanol on plasma free fatty acids in man. J. Lab. Clin. Med. 59, 826 - 832 (1962).

LIEBERMAN, N.S., BUCHARD, H.: In: Technician Symposia. LEVINE, R., MORGENSTERN, S., VLASTELICA, D. (eds.). New York: Medical Inc., 1967, p. 25.

LIEPKALNS, V., MEGAN, M., ARMSTRONG, M., LEWIS, J.: Synthesis of fibrous protein by cultured endothelial cells. Circulation 52, (Suppl. II), 61 (1975).

LINDBOM, A.: Arteriosclerosis and arterial thrombosis in the lower limb. Acta Radiol. (Suppl.) 80, 1 - 80 (1950).

LINDNER, J.: What is the morphological and (physico-) chemical evidence that connective tissue in lesions are indeed altered? In: Atherosclerosis III. Proceedings of Third International Symposium. SCHETTLER, G., WEIZEL, A. (eds.). New York: Springer-Verlag, 1974, pp. 218 - 228.

LINDNER, J.: Altern des Bindegewebes. In: ALTMANN, H.-W., et al. (eds.): Handbuch der allgemeinen Pathologie, Vol. VI/4. pp. 245 - 368. Berlin/Heidelberg/New York: Springer-Verlag, 1972a.

LINDNER, J.: Histochemie der Arterienwand. In: HEBERER, G., et al. (eds.): Angiologie, 2. Auflage. pp. 103 - 123. Stuttgart: Thieme Verlag, 1974.

LINDNER, J.: Zur Physiologie und Pathologie der Schleimbildung des Darmes. Verh. dtsch. Ges. Path. 53, 111 - 153 (1969).

LINDNER, J.: Die posttraumatische Entzündung und Wundheilung. In: GOHRBANDT, E., et al. (eds.): Handbuch der plastischen Chirurgie, Vol. I/6. pp. 1 - 153. Berlin/New York: de Gruyter 1972b.

LINDNER, J., GRIES, G., FREYTAG, G., KIND, J.: Stoffwechseluntersuchungen an der atherosklerotischen Gefäßwand. Verh. dtsch. Ges. Path. 51, 228 - 236 (1967).

LINDNER, J., GRIES, G., GRASEDYCK, K., UEBERBERG, H.: Apolar angreifende Kollagenpeptidasen verschiedener Kaninchenorgane und deren Beeinflussung durch Thymektomie und experimentelle Arthritis. Z. Rheumaforsch. 30, 86 - 91 (1971).

LINDSTEDT, S.: The turnover of cholic acid in man. Acta Physiol. Scand. 40, 1 (1957).

LINK, R.P., PEDERSOLI, W.M., SATAMOE, A.H.: Effect of exercise on development of atherosclerosis in swine. Atherosclerosis 15, 107 (1972).

LITTLE, J.A.: Fat in adult nutrition. Can. J. Pub. Health 62, 27 - 35 (1971).

LITTLE, J.A., WHAYNE, T.E., BHAGWAT, A.G., BUCKLEY, G.C., KALLOS, A.: A case of type I hyperliporpoteinemia unusually sensitive to dietary alcohol and fat with induction of lipemia. Clin. Res. 18, 736 (1970).

LIU, G.C.K., AHRENS, E.H., Jr., SCHREIBMAN, P.H., CROUSE, J.R.: Measurement of squalene in human tissues and plasma - validation and application. J. Lipid Res. 17, 38 - 45 (1976).

LOFLAND, H.B., CLARKSON, T.B., RHYNE, L., GOODMAN, H.O.: Interrelated effects of dietary fats and proteins on atherosclerosis in the pigeon. J. Atheroscler. Res. 6, 395 - 403 (1966).

LOFLAND, H.B., Jr., ST. CLAIR, R.W., CLARKSON, T.B., BULLOCK, B.C., LEHNER, N.D.M.: Atherosclerosis in cebus monkeys. II. Arterial Metabolism. Exptl Mol. Pathol. 9, 57 - 70 (1968).

LONDON, J.W., ROSENBERG, S.E., DRAPER, J.W., ALMY, T.P.: The effect of estrogens on atherosclerosis. Am. J. of Int. Med. 55, 63 (1961).

LOSOWSKY, W.S., JONES, D.P., DAVIDSON, C.S., LIEBER, C.S.: Studies of alcoholic hyperlipemia and its mechanism. Am. J. Med. 35, 794 - 803 (1963).

LOSSOW, W.J., LINDGREN, F.T., MURCHIO, J.C., STEVENS, G.R., JENSEN, L.C.: Particle size and protein content of six fractions of Sf 20 plasma lipoproteins isolated by density gradient centrifugation. J. Lipid Res. 10, 68 - 76 (1969).

LOVELL, R.R.H., SHAPER, A.G.: Atherosclerosis - hypertension interrelationships. Workshop. In: Atherosclerosis III - Proceedings of the Third International Symposium. SCHETTLER, G., WEIZEL, A. (eds.). Berlin-Heidelberg-New York: Springer-Verlag, 1974, pp. 608 - 612.

LOWER, R.R., SHUMWAY, N.E.: Studies on orthotopic homotransplantation of the canine heart. Surg. Forum 11, 176 (1970).

LOWRY, O.H., PASSONNEAU, J.V.: The relationships between substrates and enzymes of glycolysis in brain. J. Biol. Chem. 239, 31 - 41 (1964).

LOWRY, O.H., ROSEBROUGH, N.J., FARR, A.L., RANDALL, R.J.: Protein Measurement with the Folin Phenol Reagent. J. Biol. Chem. 193, 265 - 275 (1951).

LUFT, J.H.: Ruthenium red and violet. I. Chemistry, purification, methods of use for electron microscopy and mechanism of action. Anat. Rec. 171, 347 (1971).

LUNA, L. (ed.): Histological staining method of Armed Forces Institute of Pathology. New York: McGraw Hill, 1968, p. 140.

LUX, S.E., JOHN, K.M., BREWER, H.B., Jr.: Isolation and characterization of apo Lp-Gln II (apo A-II), a plasma high density apolipoprotein containing two identical polypeptide chains. J. Biol. Chem. 247, 7510 - 7518 (1972).

LUX, S.E., LEVY, R.I., GOTTO, A.M., Jr., FREDRICKSON, D.S.: Studies on the protein defect in Tangier disease. Isolation and characterization of an abnormal high density lipoprotein. J. Clin. Invest. 51, 2505 (1972).

LUZZATI, V.: X-ray diffraction studies of lipid-water systems. In: Biological Membranes. CHAPMAN, D. (ed.). New York: Academic Press, 1968, pp. 71 - 123.

MACHEBOEUF, M.A.: Recherches sur les phosphoaminolipides et les stérides du sérum et du plasma sanguins; entraînement des phospholipides, des stérols et des stérides par les diverses fractions au cours du fractionnement des protéides du sérum. Bull. Soc. Chim. Biol. 11, 268 - 293 (1929).

MAHADEVAN, V., SINGH, H., LUNDBERG, W.D.: Effect of saturated and unsaturated fatty acids on blood platelet aggregation in vitro. Proc. Soc. Exper. Biol. Med. 121, 82 (1966).

MAHLEY, R.W.: Lipoproteins and arterial smooth muscle cells: regulation of cellular metabolism by swine lipoproteins. In: International Workshop Conference on Atherosclerosis, London, Canada. New York: Plenum Press, 1976 (in press).

MAHLEY, R.W., WEISGRABER, K.H.: Canine lipoproteins and atherosclerosis. Circ. Res. 35, 713 (1974a).

MAHLEY, R.W., WEISGRABER, K.H., INNERARITY, T.: Canine lipoproteins and atherosclerosis. 2. Characterization of the plasma lipoproteins associated with atherogenic and nonatherogenic hyperlipidemia. Circ. Res. 35, 722 (1974).

MAHLEY, R.W., WEISGRABER, K.H., INNERARITY, T., BREWER, H.B., ASSMAN, G.: Swine lipoproteins in atherosclerosis: changes in the plasma lipoproteins and apoproteins induced by cholesterol feeding. Biochemistry 14, 2817 (1975).

MAJERUS, P.W.: Why aspirin? Circulation 54, 357 - 359 (1976).

MAJNO, G.: Ultrastructure of the vascular membrane. In: Handbook of Physiology, Circulation. HAMILTON, W.F., DOW, P. (eds.). Washington, D.C.: Amer. Physiol. Soc., 1965, Sect. 2, p. 2293.

MAJNO, G., SHEA, S.M., LEVENTHAL, M.: Endothelial contraction induced by histamine-type mediators. An electron microscopic study. J. Cell. Biol. 42, 647 (1969).

MALINOW, M.R., McLAUGHLIN, P., DHINDSA, D.S., METCALFE, J., OCHSNER, A.J., HILL, J., McNULTY, W.P.: Failure of carbon monoxide to induce myocardial infarction in cholesterol-fed cynomolgus monkeys (Macaca fascicularis). Cardiovasc. Res. 10, 100 - 108 (1976).

MALMROS, H.: The relation of nutrition to health. A statistical study of the effect of the war-time on arteriosclerosis, cardiosclerosis, tuberculosis and diabetes. Acta Med. Scand. Suppl. 246, 137 - 153 (1950).

MALMROS, H., WIGAND, G.: Atherosclerosis and deficiency of essential fatty acids. Lancet (1959) II, 749 - 751.

MANN, G.V., TEEL, K., HAYES, O., McHAILEY, A., BRUNO, D.: Exercise in the deposition of dietary calories. The New Eng. J. of Med. 253, 349 (1955).

MANZATO, E., FELLIN, R., BAGGIO, G., WALCH, S., NEUBECK, W., SEIDEL, D.: Formation of Lipoprotein-X: its relationship to bile compounds. J. Clin. Invest. 57, 1248 - 1260 (1976).

MAO, S.J.T., GOTTO, A.M., Jr., JACKSON, R.L.: Immunochemistry of human plasma high density lipoproteins. Radioimmunoassay of apolipoprotein A-II. Biochemistry 14, 4127 (1975).

MARKLE, R.A., HOLLIS, T.M.: Rabbit aortic endothelial and medial histamine synthesis following short-term cholesterol feeding. Exp. Molec. Path. 23, 417 (1975).

MARQUIÉ, G., AGID, R.: Effects inhibiteurs d'un biguanide antidiabétique, le NN-diméthylbiguanide, sur les perturbations entraînées par l'administration de cholesterol chez le lapin. Cr. Soc. Biol. 162, 563 (1968).

MARSH, J.B.: Apoproteins of the lipoproteins in a nonrecirculating perfusate of rat liver. J. Lipid REs. 17, 85 (1976).

MARSH, J.B.: The incorporation of amino acids into soluble lipoproteins by cell-free preparations from rat liver. J. Biol. Chem. 238, 1752 (1963).

MARTIN, G.M., SPRAGUE, C.A., NORWOOD, T.H., PENDERGRASS, W.R.: Clonal selection, attenuation and differentiation in an in vitro model of hyperplasia. Am. J. Path. 74 (1), 137 - 150 (1974).

MARUFFO, C.A., PORTMAN, O.W.: Nutritional control of coronary atherosclerosis in the squirrel monkey. J. Atheroscl. Res. 8, 237 - 247 (1968).

MARX, J.L.: Computers: helping to study nerve cell structure. Science. 193, 565 - 609 (1976).

MATHEWS, M.B., LOZAITYTE, I.: Sodium chondroitin sulfate-protein complexes of cartilage. I. Molecular weight and shape. Arch. Biochem. Biophys. 74, 158 (1958).

MATSUNAGA, M., YAMAMOTO, J., HARA, A., OGINO, K., YAMORI, Y., OKAMOTO, K.: Plasma renin and hypertensive vascular complications. An observation in the stroke-prone spontaneously hypertensive rats. Jap. Chirc. J. 39, 1305 - 1311 (1975).

MATTHEWS, J.D.: Ischaemic heart-disease: possible genetic markers. Lancet (1975) II, 681 - 682.

MAY, J.F., PAULE, W.J., ROUNDS, D.E., BLANKENHORN, D.H., ZEMPLENYI, T.: The induction of atherosclerotic plaque-like mounds in cultures of aortic muscle cells. Virchows Arch. B Cell Pathol. 18, 205 - 211 (1975).

McALLISTER, F.F., BERTSCH, R., D'ALESSIO, G.: Experimental atherosclerosis and portacaval shunt. Arch. Surg. 82, 66 (1961).

McALLISTER, F.F., BERTSCH, R., JACOBSON, J.: The accelerating effect of muscular exercise on experimental atherosclerosis. Arch Surg. 80, 54 (1959).

McCONATHY, J.W., ALAUPOVIC, P.: Studies on the isolation and partial characterization of apolipoprotein D and lipoprotein D of human plasma. Biochemistry 15, 515 (1976).

McCULLAGH, K.G., BALIAN, G.: Collagen characterisation and cell transformation in human atherosclerosis. Nature 258, 73 - 75 (1975).

McCULLAGH, K.G., EHRHART, L.A.: Increased arterial collagen synthesis in experimantal canine atherosclerosis. Atherosclerosis 19, 13 - 28 (1974).

McFARLANE, A.S.: Efficient trace-labelling of proteins with iodine. Nature 182, 53 (1958).

McGILL, H.C., Jr. (ed.): The geographic pathology of atherosclerosis. Lab. Invest. 18, 465 (1968).

McGILL, H.C.: The lesion. In: Atherosclerosis III. SCHETTLER, G., WEIZEL, A. (eds.). Berlin-Heidelberg-New York: Springer-Verlag, 1974, p. 27.

McGILL, H.C., GEER, J.C., HOLMAN, R.L.: Sites of vascular vulnerability in dogs demonstrated by Evans Blue. A.M.A. Arch. Pathol. 64, 303 (1957).

McMAHAN, C.A.: Autopsied cases by age, sex, and race. Lab. Invest. 18, 468 (1968).

McMAHAN, C.A., RICHARDS, M.L., STRONG, J.P.: Individual cigarette usage. Self-reported data as a function of respondent-reported data. Atherosclerosis 23, 477 - 488 (1976).

McMILLAN, G.C.: Development of atherosclerosis. Am. J. Cardiol. 31, 542 (1973).

McMILLAN, G.C., DUFF, G.L.: Mitotic activity in the aortic lesions of experimental atherosclerosis in rabbits. Arch. Path. 46, 179 (1948).

McMILLAN, G.C., HOUGH, A.: A survey of research objectives in arteriosclerosis. Circulation 40 (Suppl. III), 18 (1969).

McMILLAN, G.C., STARY, H.C.: Radioautographic observations on DNA synthesis in the cells of arteriosclerotic lesions of cholesterol-fed rabbits. In: Progress Biochemical Pharmacology. MIRAS, C.C., HOWARD, A.N., PAOLETTI, R. (eds.). New York: Karger, 1968, pp. 202 - 281.

MEAD, M.G., DANGERFIELD, W.G.: The investigation of "mid-band" lipoproteins using polyacrylamide gel electrophoresis. Clin. Chem. Acta 51, 173 - 182 (1974).

MEADE, T.W.: Prospective study of the role of platelets and fibrinolytic activity and clotting factor levels in the onset of clinically manifest arterial disease. CVD Epidemiology Newsletter, Am. Heart Ass. 21, 34 (1976).

MECHAM, R.P., FOSTER, J.A., FRANZBLAU, C.: Biochim. Biophys. Acta (1976) (in press).

MEDALIE, J.H., PAPIER, C.M., GOLDBOURT, U., HERMAN, J.B.: Major factors in the development of diabetes mellitus in 10,000 men. Arch. Intern. Med. 135, 811 - 817 (1975).

MEEKER, D.R., KESTEN, H.D.: Experimental atherosclerosis and high protein diets. Proc. Soc. Exp. Biol. Med. 45, 543 - 545 (1940).

MELLER, J., CONDE, C.A., DEPPISCH, L.M., DONOSO, E., DACK, S.: Myocardial infarction due to coronary atherosclerosis in three young adults with systemic lupus erythematosus. Amer. J. Cardiol. 35, 309 (1975).

MENOTTI, A.: unpublished data, 1976.

MIETTINEN, T.A.: Cholesterol and squalene in human adipose tissue. Eur. J. clin. Invest. (Abstract No. 48) 6, 317 (1976).

MIETTINEN, T.A.: Cholesterol metabolism in patients with coronary heart disease. Ann. Clin. Res. 3, 313 - 322 (1971a).

MIETTINEN, T.A.: Cholesterol production in obesity. Circulation 44, 842 - 850 (1971b).

MIETTINEN, T.A.: Clinical implications of bile acid metabolism in man. In: Chemistry, Physiology and Metabolism. NAIR, P.P., KRITCHEVSKY, D. (eds.). New York-London: Plenum Press, 1973, pp. 191 - 247.

MIETTINEN, T.A.: Commentary. In: Proceedings of the Second International Symposium on Atherosclerosis. JONES, R.J. (ed.). New York: Springer-Verlag, 1970, p. 304.

MIETTINEN, T.A., AHRENS, E.H., Jr., GRUNDY, S.M.: Quantitative isolation and gas-liquid chromatographic analysis of total dietary and fecal neutral steroids. J. Lipid Res. 6, 411 - 424 (1965).

MIETTINEN, M., TURPEINEN, O., KARVONEN, M.J., ELOSUO, R., PAAVILAINEN, E.: Effect of cholesterol-lowering diet on mortality from coronary heart disease and other causes. Lancet (1972) II, 835 - 838.

MILLER, E.J., MATUKAS, V.J.: Biosynthesis of collagen. The biochemist's view. Fed. Proc. 33(1), 1197 - 1204 (1974).

MILLER, G.J.: Plasma high-density lipoproteins and coronary heart disease. CVD Epidemiology Newsletter, Am. Heart Ass. 21, 36 (1976).

MILLER, G.J., MILLER, N.E.: Plasma high density-lipoprotein concentration and development of ischemic heart disease. Lancet (1975) I, 16.

MILLER, N.E., CLIFTON-BLIGH, P., NESTEL, P.J.: Effect of cholestipol: a new bile acid-sequestering resin on cholesterol metabolism in man. J. Lab. Clin. Med. 82, 876 (1973).

MILLER, N.E., MILLER, G.J.: High density lipoprotein and atherosclerosis. Lancet (1975) I, 1033.

MILLER, N.E., NESTEL, D.J., CLIFTON-BLIGH, P.: Relationships between plasma lipoprotein and cholesterol concentrations and the pool size and metabolism of cholesterol in man. Atherosclerosis 23, 535 - 547 (1976).

MILLS, G.L., SEIDEL, D., ALAUPOVIC, P.: Ultracentrifugal characterization of a lipoprotein occurring in obstructive jaundice. Clin. Chim. Acta 26, 239 - 244 (1969).

MINICK, C.R., MURPHY, G.E.: Experimantel induction of athero-atheriosclerosis by the synergy of allergic injury to arteries and lipid-rich diet. II. Effect of repeatedly injected foreign protein in rabbits fed a lipid-rich, cholesterol-poor diet. Amer. J. Pathol. 73, 265 (1973).

MINNICK, C.R., MURPHY, G.E.: Immunologic injury and atherosclerosis. In: Arterial Mesenchyme and Arteriosclerosis. WAGNER, W.D., CLARKSON, T.B. (eds.). New York and London: Plenum Press, 1974, pp. 355 - 375.

MISHIMA, Y., KAMIYA, K., SAKAGUCHI, S., KUSABA, A., SAKUMA, A.: A multi-clinical double blind trial on pyridinolcarbamate and inositol niacinate in the ischemic ulcer due to chronic arterial occlusion. Angiology (in press).

MISTILIS, S.P., OCKNER, R.K.: Effects of ethanol on endogenous lipid and lipoprotein metabolism in small intestine. J. Lab. Clin. Med. 80, 34 - 46 (1972).

MITROPOULUS, K.A., MYANT, N., GIBBSON, G., BALASUBRAMANIAM, S., REEVES, B.: Cholesterol precursor pools for the synthesis of cholic and chenodeoxycholic acids in rats. J. Biol. Chem. 249, 6052 (1974).

MIZUHIRA, T.: A new technique for proof of electrolytes in the tissue. Igakuno-Ayumi 76, 349 - 361 (1971)(in Japanese).

MJØS, O.D., PAERGEMAN, O., HAMILTON, R.L., HAVEL, R.J.: Characterization of remnants produced during the metabolism of triglyceride rich lipoproteins of blood plasma and intestinal lymph in the rat. J. Clin. Invest. 56, 603 (1975).

MONTOYE, H.J., VAN HUSS, W.D., BREWER, W.D., JONES, E.M., OHLSON, M.A., MAHONEY, E., OLSON, H.W.: The effects of exercise on blood cholesterol in middle-age men. Am. J. Clin. Nutr. 7, 139 (1959).

MOON, H.D., RINEHART, J.F.: Histogenesis of coronary arteriosclerosis. Circulation 6, 481 - 488 (1952).

MOORE, J.H.: The effect of the type of roughage in the diet on plasma cholesterol levels and aortic atherosis in rabbits. Brit. J. Nutr. 21, 207 - 215 (1967).

MOORE, M.C., GUZMÁN, M.A., SCHILLING, P.E., STRONG, J.P.: Dietary-atherosclerosis study on deceased persons. J. Am. Diet. Assoc. 68, 216 - 223 (1976).

MOORE, M.C., JUDLIN, B.C., KENNEMUR, McA.: Using graduate food models in taking dietary histories. J. Am. Diet. Assoc. 51, 5, 447 - 450 (1967).

MOORE, M.C., MOORE, E.M., BEASLEY, C. deH., HANKINS, G.J., JUDLIN, B.C.: Dietary-atherosclerosis study on deceased persons. Methodology. J. Am. Diet. Assoc. 56, 13 (1970).

MOORE, S., FRIEDMAN, R.J., SINGAL, D.P., GAULDIE, J., BLAJEKMAN, M.A., ROBERTS, R.S.: Inhibition of injury induced thromboatherosclerotic lesions by anti-platelet serum in rabbits. Thrombos. Haemostas. 35, 70 (1976).

MORE, R.H.: In: Atherosclerosis: Metabolic, Morphology and Clinical Aspects. MANNING, G.W., HAUST, M.D. (eds.). New York: Plenum Press, 1976 (in press).

MORE, R.H., HAUST, M.D.: Atherogenesis and plasma constituents. Amer. J. Path. 38, 527 (1961).

MOORE, S.: Atherosclerosis. In: Animal Models of Thrombosis and Haemorrhagic Disease. U.S. Dept. of Health, Education and Welfare Publication No. (N.I.H.) 76-982, 1971, p.132.

MOORE, S.: Thromboatherosclerosis in normolipemic rabbits. A result of continued endothelial damage. Lab. Invest. 29, 478 (1973).

MOORE, S., FRIEDMAN, R.J., SINGAL, D.P., GAULDIE, J., BLAJCHMAN, M.A., ROBERTS, R.S.: Inhibition of injury induces thromboatherosclerotic lesions by anti-platelet serum in rabbits. Thrombos. Haemostas. 35, 70 (1971).

MORRIS, J.N., HEADY, J.A., RAFFLE, P.A.B.: Coronary heart disease and physical activity of work. Lancet (1953) II, 265.

MORRISETT, J.D., JACKSON, R.L., GOTTO, A.M.: Lipid-protein interactions in the plasma lipoproteins. Rev. Biomembranes, Biochim. Biophys. Acta (1977) (in press).

MORRISETT, J.D., JACKSON, R.L., GOTTO, A.M.: Lipoproteins: structure and function. Ann. Rev. Biochem. 44, 183 - 207 (1975a).

MORRISETT, J.D., POWNALL, H.J., JACKSON, R.L., SEGURA, R., GOTTO, A.M.,Jr., TAUNTON, O.D.: Effects of polyunsaturated and saturated fat diets on the chemical composition and thermotropic properties of human plasma lipoproteins. In: The Chemistry and Biochemistry of Polyunsaturated Fatty Acids. HOLMAN, R. T., KUNAU, W.H. (eds.). 1976 (in press).

MORRISETT, J.D., POWNALL, H.J., SPARROW, J.T., JACKSON, R.L., GOTTO, A.M.,Jr.: The interaction of apolipoprotein-alanine (apoC-III) with lipids: study of structural features required for binding. In: Lipids, Lipoproteins and Drugs. KRITCHEVSKY, D., PAOLETTI, R., HOLMES, W.L. (eds.). New York: Plenum Publ. Corp., 1975b, pp. 7 - 35.

MORRISON, L.M., BAJWA, G.S., ALFIN-SLATER, R.B., ERSHOFF, B.H.: Prevention of vascular lesions by chondroitin sulfate A in the coronary artery and aorta of rats induced by a hypervitaminosis D., cholesterol-containing diet. Atherosclerosis 16, 105 - 118 (1972).

MÜLLER, O.: Arterienverkalkung. Vortrag v.d. Dt. Frauenverein für Krankenpflege in den Kolonien. Stuttgart (1909).

MURATA, K.: Infra-red spectroscopic evidence of chondroitin polysulphate and its relation to anticoagulant activity. Nature (London) 193, 578 - 579 (1962b).

MURATA, K.: Inhibitory effects of chondroitin polysulphate on lipemia and atherosclerosis in connection with its anticoagulant activity. Naturwissenschaften 49, 39 - 40 (1962a).

MURATA, K.: Suppression of lipid synthesis in cultured aortic cells by laminaran sulfate. J. Atheroscler. Res. 10, 371 - 378 (1969).

MURATA, K. et al.: Correlation of blood pressure and total serum cholesterol to severity of atherosclerosis in the aorta, the coronary and the cerebral arteries. Jap. J. Geriatrics 8, 323 - 328 (1971) (in Japanese with English abstract).

MURATA, K., IZUKA, K., FURUHASHI, T.: Effects of chondroitin polysulfate on thrombus formation and serum lipid levels. Experientia (Basel) 25, 611 - 612 (1969).

MURATA, K., NAKAZAWA, K., HAMAI, A.: Distribution of acidic glycosaminoglycans in the intima, media and adventitia of bovine aorta and their anticoagulant properties. Atherosclerosis 21, 93 - 103 (1975).

MURATA, K., QUILLIGAN, J.J.,Jr., MORRISON, L.M.: Growth of chick aortic endothelial cells: incorporation of tritiated uridine and thymidine. Experientia (Basel) 21, 637 - 638 (1965).

MURATA, K., QUILLIGAN, J.J., Jr., MORRISON, L.M.: Suppressing effect of histamine on lipid synthesis in chick aortic cells. Nature (London) 213, 1030 - 1031 (1967).

MURPHY, E.A., MUSTARD, J.F.: Tobacco and thrombosis. Am. J. Public Health 56, 1061 - 1073 (1966).

MUSTARD, J.F., MURPHY, E.A.: Effect of smoking on blood coagulation and platelet survival in man. Br. Med. J. 1, 846 - 849 (1963).

MUSTARD, J.F., PACKHAM, M.A.: Platelets, thrombosis and drugs. Drugs 9, 19 (1975).

MUSTARD, J.F., PACKHAM, M.A., MOORE, S., KINLOUGH-RATHBONE, R.L.: Thrombosis and atherosclerosis. In: Atherosclerosis III - Proceedings of the Third International Symposium. SCHETTLER, G., WEIZEL, A.(eds.). Berlin-Heidelberg-New York: Springer-Verlag, 1974, pp. 253 - 267.

MYASNIKOV, A.L.: Influence of some factors on development of experimental cholesterol atherosclerosis. Circulation 17, 99 (1958).

NAKAMURA, T., TOKITA, K., TATENO, S., KOTOKU, T., OHBA, T.: Human aortic acid mucopolysaccharides and glycoproteins. Changes during ageing and in atherosclerosis. J. Atheroscler. Res. 8, 891 - 902 (1968).

NAKASHIMA, Y., DI FERRANTE, N., JACKSON, R.L., POWNALL, H.J.: The interaction of human glycosaminoglycans with plasma lipoproteins. J. Biol. Chem. 250, 5386 (1975).

NAKAZAWA, K., MURATA, K.: Acidic glycosaminoglycans in three layers of human aorta: their different constitution and anticoagulant function. Arterial Wall 2, 203 - 211 (1975).

NAMM, S.C., LEE, W.M., JARMOLYCH, J., LEE, K.T., THOMAS, W.A.: Rapid production of advanced atherosclerosis in swine by a combination of endothelial injury and cholesterol feeding. Exp. Mol. Path. 18, 369 - 379 (1973).

NANBU, S., GOHDA, H., AGETA, M., YAMASAKI, S.: Significance of plasma lipids - from aspects of plasma lipoproteins. Clinical Pathology 23, 167 - 173 (1975).

NANBU, S., KIMURA, N., GOHDA, H.: Effects of low carbohydrate diet on plasma lipoproteins. Conference on Serum Lipoproteins, 1973, Graz, Austria.

NASH, D.T., CALDWELL, N., ANCONA, D.: Accelerated coronary artery disease arteriographically proved: analysis of risk factors. Ny J. Med. 74, 947 - 950 (1974).

NAVARI, R.M., HALL, K.R., GAINER, J.L.: Effect of plasma proteins on diffusion. In: Blood Oxygenation. HERSHEY, D.(ed.). New York: Plenum Press, 1970, pp. 243 ff.

NAZIR, D.J., HORLICK, L., KUDCHODKAR, B.J., SODHI, H.S.: Mechanisms of action of cholestyramine in the treatment of hypercholesterolemia. Circulation 46, 95 - 102 (1972).

NEELDEMAN, P., MONCADA, S., BUNTING, S., VANE, J.R., HAMBERG, M., SAMUELSSON, B.: Identification of enzyme in platelet microsomes which generates thromboxane A2 from prostaglandin endoperoxides. Nature 261, 558 - 560 (1976).

NELSON, E., SUNAGA, T., SHIMAMOTO, T., KAWAMURA, T., NELLES, M.L., HEBEL, R.: Ischemic carotid endothelium. Arch. Path. 99, 125 - 132 (1975).

NEMERSON, Y., MAYNARD, J., PITLICK, F.A.: Activation of blood coagulation by tissue factor. N.Y. Heart Assoc. Symposium on the Intima. Waldorf Astoria Hotel, 1975.

NESTEL, P.J.: Abstracts of the Fourth International Symposium on Atherosclerosis, Tokyo, Japan, 1976, p. 56 (see now page 559).

NESTEL, P.J.: Metabolic studies in hyperlipidaemia. In: Atherosclerosis Proceedings of the Third International Symposium. SCHETTLER, G., WEIZEL, A. (eds.). Berlin-Heidelberg-New York: Springer-Verlag, 1974.

NESTEL, P.J.: Turnover of plasma esterified cholesterol. Influence of dietary fat and carbohydrate and relation to plasma lipids and body weight. Clin. Sci. 38, 593 - 600 (1970).

NESTEL, P.J., HIRSCH, E.Z.: Mechanism of alcohol-induced hypertriglyceridemia. J. Lab. Clin. Med. 3, 357 - 365 (1965).

NESTEL, P.J., HUNTER, J.D.: Differences in bile acid excretion in subjects with hypercholesterolemia, hypertriglyceridemia and overweight. Aust. Nz. J. Med. 4, 491 - 496 (1974).

NESTEL, P.J., MILLER, N.E., CLIFTON-BLIGH, P.: Plasma cholesterol esterification in vivo in man. Scand. J. clin. Lab. Invest. 33 (Suppl. 137), 157 (1974).

NESTEL, P.J., MONGER, E.A.: Turnover of plasma esterified cholesterol in normocholesterolemic and hypercholesterolemic subjects and its relation to body build. J. Clin. Invest. 46, 967 - 974 (1967).

NESTEL, P.J., POYSER, A.: Changes in cholesterol synthesis and excretion when cholesterol intake is increased. Metabolism, 1976.

NESTEL, P.J., SCHREIBMAN, P.H., AHRENS, E.J.,Jr.: Cholesterol metabolism in human obesity. J. Clin. Invest. 52, 2389 - 2394 (1973).

NESTEL, P.J., WHYTE, H.M.: Plasma free fatty acids and triglyceride turnover in obesity. Metabolism 14, 1122 - 1128 (1968).

NESTEL, P.J., WHYTE, H.M., GOODMAN, D.S.: Distribution and turnover of cholesterol in humans. J. Clin. Invest. 48, 982 - 991 (1969).

NEUFELD, H.N.: Mannheimer lecture: studies of the coronary arteries in children and their relevance to coronary heart disease. XI Annual Meeting of European Pediatric Cardiologists, Rhodes, May 2, 1973. Europ. J. Cardiol. 1, 479 (1974).

NEUFELD, H.N., VLODAVER, Z.: Structural changes of coronary arteries in young age groups. Int. Cardiol. 3, 56 (1971).

NEUFELD, H.N., WAGENVOORT, C.A., ONGLEY, P.A., EDWARDS, J.E.: Hypoplasia of ascending aorta. An unusual form of supryvalvular aortic stenosis with apecial reference to localized coronary arterial hypertension. Amer. J. Cardiol. 10, 746 (1962).

NEW, M.I., ROBERTS, T.N., BIERMAN, E.I., READES, G.G.: The significance of blood lipid alterations in diabetes mellitus. Diabetes 12, 208 - 212 (1963).

NICHOLS, A.V., STRISOWER, E.H., LINDGREN, F.T., ADAMSON, G.L., COGGIOLA, E.L.: Analysis of change in ultracentrifugal lipoprotein profiles following heparin and ethyl-p-chlorophenoxyisobutyrate administration. Clin. Chim. Acta 20, 277 - 283 (1968).

NICOLL, A., SIGURDSSON, G., MARSH, A., LEWIS, B.: Intravenous fat tolerance: correlation with very low density lipoprotein apoprotein B kinetics in man. Atherosclerosis (1976)(in press).

NIJKAMP, F.P., FLOWER, R.J., MONCADA, S., VANE, J.R.: Partial purification of rabbit aorta contracting substance-releasing factor and inhibition of its activity by anti-inflammatory steroids. Nature 263, 479 - 482 (1976).

NIKKARI, T., HEIKKINEN, E.: The lipids of collagen preparations. Acta Chem. Scand. 22, 3047 - 3049 (1968).

NIKKILÄ, E.A.: Plasma triglycerides in human diabetes. Proc. Roy. Soc. Med. 67, 662 - 665 (1974).

NIKKILÄ, E.A., H TTUNEN, J.K., EHNHOLM, C.: Effect of clofibrate on postheparin plasma triglyceride lipase activities in patients with hypertriglyceridemia. Metabolism (1976a) (in press).

NIKKILÄ, E.A., HUTTUNEN, J.K., EHNHOLM, C.: Low postheparin plasma hepatic lipase activity in familial Type IIa hyperlipoproteinemia. Ann. Clin. Res. 8, 63 - 67 (1976c).

NIKKILÄ, E.A., HUTTUNEN, J.K., EHNHOLM, C.: Postheparin plasma lipoprotein lipase and hepatic lipase in diabetes mellitus. Relationship to plasma triglyceride metabolism. Diabetes (1976b) (in press).

NIKKILÄ, E.A., KEKKI, M.: Measurement of plasma triglyceride turnover in the study of hypertriglyceridemia. Scand. J. Clin. Invest. 27, 97 - 104 (1971).

NIKKILÄ, E.A., KEKKI, M.: Polymorphism of plasma triglyceride kinetics in normal human adult subjects. Acta Med. Scand. 190, 49 - 59 (1971).

NILSSON, A.: Increased cholesterol-ester formation during forced cholesterol synthesis in rat hepatocytes. Eur. J. Biochem. 51, 337 - 342 (1975).

NILSSON-EHLE, P.: Human lipoprotein lipase activity: comparison of assay methods. Clin. Chem. Acta 20, 283 - 291 (1974).

NILSSON-EHLE, P., BELFRAGE, P.: A monoglyceride hydrolyzing enzyme in human postheparin plasma. Biochim. Biophys. Acta 270, 60 - 64 (1972).

NILSSON-EHLE, P., GARFINKEL, A.S., SCHOTZ, M.C.: Intra- and extracellular forms of lipoprotein lipase in adipose tissue. Biochim. Biophys. Acta 431, 147 - 156 (1976).

NISHIDA, T., COGAN, U.: Nature of the interaction of dextran sulfate with low density lipoproteins of plasma. J. Biol. Chem. 245, 4689 (1970).

NISHIMOTO, A., NISHIMOTO, M.: Methodical study for the measurement of triglyceride in serum (Japanese). Clinical Pathology 13, 479 - 481 (1965).

NOMA, A., KITA, M.: Purification of monoacylglycerol hydrolase from human postheparin plasma. FEBS Lett. 61, 42 - 45 (1976).

NOMA, A., OKABE, H., SAKURADA, T., KITA, M., MIZUNO, K.: Determination and properties of monoglyceride hydrolase in human post-heparin plasma. Clin. Chim. Acta 54, 177 - 183 (1974).

NORUM, K.R., GLOMSET, J.A., NICHOLS, A.V., FORTE, T., ALBERS, J.J., KING, W.C., MITCHELL, C.D., APPLEGATE, K.R., GONG, E.L., CABANA, V., GJONE, E.: Plasma lipoproteins in familial lecithin:cholesterol acyltransferase deficiency: effects of incubation with lecithin:cholesterol acyltransferase in vitro. Scand. J. clin. Lab. Invest. Suppl. 142, 31 (1975).

NOVIKOFF, A.B.: Lysosomes: A personal account. In: Lysosomes and Storage Diseases. HERS, H.G., Van HOOF, F. (eds.). New York: Academic Press, 1973, pp. 1 - 41.

NUMANO, F. et al.: Comparative studies on the preventive effect of pydirinol-carbamate and estrogen against aortic and coronary atherosclerosis of cholesterol fed rabbits. Acta Path. Jap. 21, 177 (1971).

NUMANO, F. et al.: Microassay of cyclic nucleotides in vessel wall. Part I. Cyclic AMP. Exp. Mol. Path. 25, 172 (1976).

NUMANO, F. et al.: Microassay of cyclic nucleotides in vessel wall. Part II. Cyclic AMP phosphodiesterase. Microvascular Research (1977)(in press).

NUMANO, F., MAEZAWA, H., SHIMAMOTO, T., ADACHI, K.: Changes of cyclic AMP and cyclic GMP phosphodiesterase in the progression and regression of experimental atherosclerosis. Ann. N.Y. Acad. Sci. 275, 311 (1976).

NUMANO, F., YAMASAWA, S., TAKANO, T., SHIMAMOTO, T.: On the mechanism of anti-atherosclerotic agents: microchemical studies on the in vitro effects of pyridinol carbamate and estrogen (Premarin) on phosphofructokinase and malate dehydrogenase in the arterial wall. Mech. Age. Devel. 2, 43 - 53 (1973).

NUMANO, F., TAKENOBU, M., SAGARA, A., KOBAYASHI, M., MORIYA, K., KUROIWA, T., YAMAZAWA, S., SHIMAMOTO, T., HIDAKA, J., MOHRI, K.: The search for antiatherosclerotic agents. Histological and biochemical analysis of the preventive effect of estrogen, progesterone and pyridinolcarbamate on experimentally induced atherosclerosis. In: Atherogenesis II. SHIMAMOTO, T., NUMANO, F., ADDISON, G.M. (eds.). Amsterdam: Excerpta Medica, 1972, pp. 98 - 112.

NÜSSEL, E., BUCHHOLZ, L.: Modellstudie zur Früherkennung von Risikofaktoren des Herzinfarktes. Med. Technik 96, 60 - 62 (1976).

NÜSSEL, E., SCOLA, R.: Coronary heart disease, epidemiological aspects. In: Coronary Heart Disease - Novel Antiangional Therapy. Leverkusen: Bayer AG, 1975, pp. 101 - 108.

NÜSSEL, E., WILCKE, S.: Risk factors in myocardial infarction patients. Results from the HNO-Register Study. In: Psychological Approach to the Rehabilitation of Coronary Patients. STOCKSMEIER, U. (ed.). Berlin-Heidelberg-New York: Springer-Verlag, 1976, pp. 173 - 180.

NYGAARD, K., HELSINGER, N., ROOTWELT, K.: Adaptation of vitamin B_{12} absorption after ileal bypass. Scand. J. Gast. 5, 349 (1970).

OALMANN, M.C., PALMER, R.W., STARY, H.C., TRACY, R.E., ROCK, W.A., STRONG, J.P.: Atherosclerosis, coronary heart disease, serum cholesterol, and fatty acids in men 25-44 years. Circulation 48 (Suppl. IV), 9 (Abstract)(1973).

OCKNER, R.K., HUGHES, F.B., ISSELBACHER, K.J.: Very low density lipoproteins in intestinal lymph: origin, composition and role in lipid transport in the fasting state. J. Clin. Invest. 48, 2079 - 2088 (1969).

O'CONNELL, T.X., MOWBRAY, J.F.: Effects of humoral transplantation antibody on the arterial intima of rabbits. Surgery 74, 145 (1973).

OGDEN, J.A.: Congenital anomalies of the coronary arteries. Amer. J. Cardiol. 25, 474 (1970).

OKAMOTO, K.: In: Proceedings of the Second International Congress of Endocrinology, London 1964. Amsterdam: Exc. Med. Found., 1965, p. 1018.

OKAMOTO, K., AOKI, K.: Development of a strain of spontaneous hypertensive rates. Jap. Circ. J. 27, 282 - 293 (1963).

OKAMOTO, K., YAMORI, Y., NAGAOKA, A.: Establishment of the stroke-prone spontaneously hypertensive rat (SHR). Circ.Res. 34-35 (Suppl. I), 143 - 153 (1974).

OKUMA, M., YAMORI, Y.: Platelet survival studies in the stroke-prone spontaneously hypertensive rats (SHRSP). Stroke 6, 60 - 64 (1975).

OLEFSKY, J., REAVEN, C.M., FARQUHAR, J.W.: Effects of weight reduction on obesity - studies of lipid and carbohydrate metabolism in normal and hyperlipoproteinemic subjects. J. Clin. Invest. 53, 64 - 76 (1974).

OLIVECRONA, T., BELFRAGE, P.: Mechanisms of removal of chyle triglyceride from the circulating blood as studied with (^{14}C) glycerol and (^{3}H) palmitic acid labeled chyle. Biochim. Biophys. Acta 98, 81 (1965).

OLIVECRONA, T., BENGTSSON, G., HÖÖK, M., LINDAHL, U.: Physiological implications of the interaction between lipoprotein lipase and some sulfated glycosaminoglycans. In: Lipoprotein Metabolism. GRETEN, H. (ed.). Heidelberg: Springer, 1976, p. 13.

OLIVECRONA, T., BENGTSSON, G., MARKLUND, S.-E., LINDAHL, U., HÖÖK, M.: Heparin-lipoprotein lipase interactions. Fed. Proc. 36, 60 (1977).

OLIVER, M.T., NIMMO, I.A., COOKE, M., CARLSON, L.A., OLSSON, A.G.: Ischaemic heart disease and associated risk factors in 40 year old men in Edinburgh and Stockholm. Europ. J. clin. Invest. 5, 507 - 514 (1975).

OLSSON, A.G., CARLSON, L.: Studies in asymptomatic primary hyperlipidaemia. I. Types of hyperlipoproteinaemias and serum lipoprotein concentrations compositions and interrelations. Acta Med. Scand. Suppl. 580 (1975).

OLSSON, A.G., ORÖ, L., ROSSNER, S.: Dose response effect of single and combined clofibrate (atromidin) and niceritrol (perycit) treatment on serum lipids and lipoproteins in type II hyperlipoproteinemia. Atherosclerosis 22, 91 - 101 (1975).

ONCLEY, J.L.: Lipid protein interactions. In: Brain Lipids and Lipoproteins, and the Leucodystrophies. FOLCHI-Pi, J., BAUER, H. (eds.). Amsterdam: Elsevier Publishing Company, 1963, pp. 1 - 17.

O'NEAL,R.M., JORDAN, G.L., RABIN, R., De BAKEY, M.E., HALPERT, B.: Cells grown on isolated intravascular Dacron hub: an electron microscopic study. Exp. molec. Path. 3, 403 (1964).

ONOYAMA, K., TANAKA, K.: Fibrinolytic activity of the arterial wall. Thrombos. Diathes. Haemorrh. 21, 1 - 11 (1969).

OONEDA, G., OOYAMA, Y., MATSUYAMA, K., TAKATAMA, M., YOSHIDA, Y., SEKIGUCHI, M., ARAI, I.: Electron microscopic studies on the morphogenesis of fibrinoid degeneration in the mesenteric arteries of hypertensive rats. Angiology 16, 8 - 17 (1965).

OONEDA, G., YOSHIDA, Y., SUZUKI, K.: Morphogenesis of arteriosclerosis: proliferation and insudation. Jap. J. Atheroscler. 1, 3 - 13 (1973a).

OONEDA, G., YOSHIDA, Y., SUZUKI, K., SEKIGUCHI, T.: Morphogenesis of plasmatic arterionecrosis as the cause of hypertensive intracerebral hemorrhage. Virchows Arch. Abt. A. Path. Anat. 361, 31 - 38 (1973b).

OPIE, L.H.: Metabolic regulation in ischemia and hypoxia. Effect of regional ischemia on metabolism of glucose and fatty acids. Circ. Res. 38, (Suppl. I), 52 - 74 (1976).

ORIMILIKWE, S.O., WONG, H.Y.C., DAVID, S.N., REINSHAGEN, J.A.: Effect of exercise and guanethidine on plasma cholesterol and aortic atherogenic-fed cockerels. (1977)(in press).

ORMA, E.J.: Effect of physical activity on atherogenesis. Acta Physiol. Scand. 41, (Suppl. 143), 1 - 75 (1957).

OSCAI, C., BABIRAK, S., DUBACH, F., McGARR, J., SPIRAKIS, C.: Exercise or food restriction: effect on adipose tissue cellularity. Am. J. Physiol. 227, 901 - 904 (1974).

OSTWALD, R., GUO, L.S.S.: Changes in the high density (HDL)-apoproteins of guinea pigs (G-P) in response to dietary cholesterol (C). Fed. Proc. 34, 499 (1975).

OTWAY, S., ROBINSON, D.S.: A non-ionic detergent (Triton WR 1339) to determine rates of triglyceride entry into the circulation of the rat under different physiological conditions. J. Physiol. 190, 321 - 332 (1967).

OUZILOU, J., ROBERT, A.M., ROBERT, L., BOUISSOU, H., PIERAGGI, M.T.: Etude sur la composition de la paroi aortique normale et atheroscléreuse. Paroi Arterielle 1, 105 - 116 (1973).

PACKHAM, M.A., ROWSELL, H.C., JØRGENSEN, L., MUSTARD, J.F.: Localized protein accumulation in the wall of the aorta. Exp. Molec. Pathol. 7, 214 (1967).

PAGE, I.H.: Atherosclerosis, a personal overview. Circulation 38, 1164 - 1172 (1968).

PALADE, G.E.: The fine structure of blood capillaries. J. appl. Phys. 24, 1424 (1953).

PAPADOPOULOS, N.M., BLOOR, C.M., STANDETER, J.C.: Effects of exercise and training on plasma lipids and lipoproteins in rat. J. Appl. Physiol. 26, 760 (1969).

PAPPENHEIMER, J.R.: Passage of molecules through capillary walls. Physiol. Rev. 33, 387 (1953).

PARIS, A.W., BROWNING, F.M., IBACH, J.D.: The effect of physical training upon total serum cholesterol levels and arterial distensibility of male white rats. J. Sports Med. 11, 24 (1971).

PARVING, H.-H.: The effect of hypoxia and carbon monoxide exposure on plasma volume and capillary permeability to albumin. Scand. J. clin. Lab. Invest. 30, 49 - 56 (1972).

PARVING, H.-H., OHLSSON, K., BUCHARDT HANSEN, H.J., RØRTH, M.: Effect of carbon monoxide exposure on capillary permeability to albumin and α_2-macroglobulin. Scand. J. clin. Lab. Invest. 29, 381 - 388 (1972).

PATELSKI, J.: Participation of phospholipids in arterial metabolism of cholesterol esters. In: Proceedings of the 1975 International Workshop Conference on Atherosclerosis, London, Canada. New York: Plenum Press, 1976 (in press).

PATELSKI, J., BOWYER, D.E., HOWARD, A.N., GRESHAM, G.A.: Changes in phospholipase A, lipase and cholesterol esterase activity in the aorta in experimental atherosclerosis in the rabbit and rat. J. Atheroscler. Res. 8, 221 (1968).

PATELSKI, J., BOWYER, D.E., HOWARD, A.N., JENNINGS, I.W., THRONE, C.J.R., GRESHAM, G.A.: Modification of enzyme activities in experimental atherosclerosis in the rabbit. Atherosclerosis 12, 41 (1970).

PATELSKI, J., PIORUNSKA, M.: Cholesterol ester:lysolecithin acyltransferase activity of the aorta. In: Proceedings of the 1975 International Workshop Conference on Atherosclerosis, London, Canada. New York: Plenum Press, 1976 (in press).

PATELSKI, J., PNIEWSKA, B., PIORUNSKA, M., OBREBSKA, M.: The arterial acyl-CoA: cholesterol acyltransferase and cholesterol ester hydrolase activities. In vitro effect of substrates with fatty acid of different chain length and saturation. Atherosclerosis 22, 287 (1975).

PATELSKI, J., TORLINSKA, T.: Lecithin: cholesterol acyltransferase and phospholipase A activities of the aortic wall. In: Proceedings of the 1972 International Symposium on Phospholipids. SAMOCHOWIEC, L., WOJCICKI, J. (eds.). Szczecin: Internat. Soc. Biochem. Pharmacol. and Polish Pharmacol. Soc., 1973, p. 91.

PATELSKI, J., WALIGORA, Z., SZULC, S.: Demonstration and some properties of the phospholipase A, lipase and cholesterol esterase from the aortic wall. J. Atheroscler. Res. 7, 458 (1967).

PATRASSI, G., CREPALDI, G.: Hyperlipoproteinemia. Fifty-second Congress of the Italian Society of Internal Medicine, Pozzi, Rome, 1971.

PATSCH, J.R., SAILER, S., BRAUNSTEINER, H.: Lipoprotein of the density 1.006 - 1.020 in the plasma of patients with type III hyperlipoproteinemia in the postabsorptive state. Europ. J. Clin. Invest. 5, 45 - 55 (1975).

PATSCH, J.R., SAILER, S., BRAUNSTEINER, H., FORTE, T.: Electron microscopic characterization of lipoproteins from patients with familial type III hyperlipoproteinemia. Europ. J. Clin. Invest. 6, 307 - 310 (1976).

PATSCH, J.R., SAILER, S., KOSTNER, G., SANDHOFER, F., HOLASEK, A., BRAUNSTEINER, H.: Separation of the main lipoprotein density classes from human plasma by rate zonal ultracentrifugation. J. Lipid. Res. 15, 356 - 366 (1974).

PAUIT, I., HUDRY-CLERGEON, G., SUSCILLON, M.: EM study on the various stages of fibrin formation. Thr. Dieth. Hemorrh. 27, 559 (1972); Biochim. Biophys. Acta 317, 99 (1973).

PAULE, W.J., ZEMPLENYI, T., ROUNDS, D.E., BLANKENHORN, D.H.: Light and electron microscopic characteristics of arterial smooth muscle cell cultures subjected to hypoxia or carbon monoxide. Atherosclerosis (1977) (in press).

PEARSON, T.A., WANG, A., SOLEZ, K., HEPTINSTALL, R.H.: Clonal characteristics of fibrous plaques and fatty streaks from human aortas. Am. J. Path. 81, 379 - 387 (1975).

PEETERS, H., SOETEWEY, F., LIEVENS, J., ROSSENEU, M.: Localization of the lipid-binding units in the plasma apolipoproteins. III. Identification of the lipid-binding units in apoA-III, apoC-I, apoC-III lipoproteins. IRCS 4, 279 (1976).

PENTTILÄ, I.M., MIETTINEN, T.A.: Incorporation of ^{14}C-acetate, ^{3}H-leucine and ^{3}H-mevalonate into plasma and tissue cholesterol of control and cholesterol fed rats. Scand. J. clin. Invest. 21, (Suppl. 101), 20 (1968).

PEREZ-TAMAYA, R.: Collagen resorption in carrageenin granulomas. Collagenolytic activity in "in vitro" explants. Lab. Invest. 22, 137 - 159 (1970).

PERNIS, B., CLERICI, E.: Carbohydrates, collagen and elastin of the normal aortic wall and atherosclerotic hyaline plaques. Experientia 13, 351 - 353 (1957).

PERNOW, B., SALTIN, B., WAHREN, J., CRONESTRAND, R., EKESTRÖM, S.: Leg blood flow and muscle metabolism in occlusive arterial disease of the leg before and after reconstructive surgery. Clin. Sci. & Mol. Med. 49, 265 - 275 (1975).

PERSSON, B.: Lipoprotein lipase activity of human adipose tissue in different types of hyperlipidemia. Acta Med. Scand. 193, 447 - 456 (1973a).

PERSSON, B.: Lipoprotein lipase activity of human adipose tissue in health and in some diseases with hyperlipidemia as a common feature. Acta Med. Scand. 193, 457 - 462 (1973b).

PERTSEMLIDIS, D., PANVELIWALLA, D., AHRENS, E.H.: Effects of clofibrate and of an estrogen-progestin combination on fasting biliary lipids and cholic acid kinetics in man. Gastroenterology 66, 565 (1974).

PETERS, T.J., TAKANU, T., DUVE, C. de: Subcellular fractionation studies on the cells isolated from normal and atherosclerotic aorta. In: Atherogenesis. Initiating factors, Ciba Foundation Symposium No. 12 (new series). PORTER, R., KNIGHT, J. (eds.). Amsterdam-London-New York: Associated Scientific Publishers, 1973, pp. 197 - 222.

PHAIR, R.D., HAMMOND, M.G., BOWDEN, J.A., FISHER, W.R., FRIED, M., BERMAN, M.: A preliminary model for human lipoprotein metabolism in hyperlipoproteinemia. Federation Proc. 34, 2263 (1975).

PHELPS, P.C., LUFT, J.H.: Electron microscopical study of relaxation and constriction in frog arterioles. Amer. J. Anat. 125, 399 (1969).

PICARD, J., VEISSIERE, D.: Separation des lipoprotéines sériques anormales dans la cholestase. C.R. Acad. Sci. (Paris) Ser. D. 270, 1845 - 1848 (1970).

PICARD, J., VEISSIERE, F., VOYER, F., BEREZIAT, G.: Composition en acides gras des phospholipides dans les lipoprotéines sériques anormales de la cholestase. Clin. Chim. Acta 36, 247 - 250 (1972).

PICK, R., STAMLER, J., RODBARD, S., KATZ, L.N.: Estrogen induced regression of coronary atherosclerosis in cholesterol fed chicks. Circulation 6, 858 - 861 (1952).

PIPER, P.J., VANE, J.R.: Release of additional factors in anaphylaxis and its antagonism by anti-inflammatory drugs. Nature 223, 29 - 35 (1969).

POHNDORF, R.H.: Improvement in physical fitness of two middle-age adults. Dissertation (Abstract) 17, 2493 (1957).

POOL, J.D., GAINER, J.L., CHISOLM, G.M.: Oxygen diffusion and atherosclerosis. Adv. Expt'l. Med. Biol. 67, 205 (1976).

POOLE, J.C.F.: Endothelial regeneration. Advanc. exp. Med. Biol. 57, 237 (1975).

POOLE, J.C.F.: The regeneration of aortic tissues in fabric grafts of the aorta. Symp. zool. Soc. Lond. 11, 131 (1964)

POOLE, J.C.F., CROMWELL, S.B., BENDITT, E.P.: Behavior of smooth muscle cells and formation of extracellular structures in the reaction of arterial walls to injury. Amer. J. Path. 62, 391 (1971).

POOLE, J.C.F., SABISTON, D.C., FLOREY, H.W., ALLISON, P.R.: Growth of endothelium in arterial prosthetic grafts and following endarterectomy. Surg. Forum 13, 225 (1962).

POOLE, J.C.F., SANDERS, A.G., FLOREY, H.W.: Further observations on the regeneration of aortic endothelium in the rabbit. J. Path. Bact. 77, 637 (1959).

POOLE, J.C.F., SANDERS, A.G., FLOREY, H.W.: The regeneration of aortic endothelium. J. Path. Bact. 75, 133 (1958).

POPPER, H.: Cholestasis. Annu. Rev. Med. 19, 39 - 55 (1968).

PORTE, D., Jr., BIERMAN, E.L.: The effect of heparin infusion on plasma triglyceride in vivo and in vitro with a method for calculating triglyceride turnover. J. Lab. Clin. Med. 73, 631 - 648 (1969).

POSNER, I.: Abnormal fat absorption and utilization in rats bearing Walker carcinoma. Cancer Res. 20, 551 (1960).

POSTON, R.N., DAVIES, D.F.: Immunity and inflammation in the pathogenesis of atherosclerosis. Atherosclerosis 19, 353 (1974).

POTTER, J.M., NESTEL, P.J.: Greater bile acid excretion with soy bean than with cow milk in infants. Am. J. Clin. Nutr. 29, 546 - 551 (1976b).

POTTER, J.M., NESTEL, P.J.: The effects of dietary fatty acids and cholesterol on the milk lipids of lactating women and the plasma cholesterol of breast-fed infants. Am. J. Clin. Nutr. 29, 54 - 60 (1976a).

PRIOR, J.T., ZIEGLER, D.D.: Regression of experimental atherosclerosis. Arch. Pathol. 80, 50 - 57 (1965).

PROSSER, C.L., BURNSTOCK, G., KAHN, J.: Conduction in smooth muscle. Comparative structural properties. Am. J. Physiol. 199, 545 - 552 (1960).

PUCAK, G.J., LEHNER, N.D.M., CLARKSON, T.B., BULLOK, B.C., LOFLAND, H.B.,Jr.: Spider monkeys (Ateles sp.) as animal models for atherosclerosis research. Exptl. Mol. Pathol. 18, 32 - 49 (1973).

PUGATCH, E.M.J., FOSTER, E.A., MACFARLANTE, D.E., POOLE, J.C.F.: The extraction and separation of activators and inhibotors of fibrinolysis from bovine endothelium and mesothelium. Brit. J. Haematol. 18, 669 (1970).

PYKÄLISTÖ, O.: Regulation of adipose tissue lipoprotein lipase by free fatty acids. Doctorate Thesis, University of Helsinki, Helsinki, Finland, 1970.

PYKÄLISTÖ, O., GOLDBERG, A.P., BRUNZELL, J.D.: Reversal of decreased human adipose tissue lipoprotein lipase and hypertriglyderidemia after treatment of hypothyroidism. J. Clin. Endo. Metab. 43, 549 - 558 (1976) (in press).

PYKÄLISTÖ, O.J., SMITH, P.J., BRUNZELL, J.D.: Determinants of human adipose tissue lipoprotein lipase: effect of diabetes and obesity on basal- and diet-induced activity. J. Clin. Invest. 56, 1108 - 1117 (1975b).

PYKÄLISTÖ, O.J., SMITH, P.J., BRUNZELL, J.D.: Human adipose tissue lipoprotein lipase: comparison of assay methods and expressions of assay methods and expression of activity. Proc. Soc. Exp. Biol. Med. 148, 297 - 300 (1975a).

PYKÄLISTÖ, O.J., VOGEL, W.C., BIERMAN, E.L.: The tissue distribution of triacylglycerol lipase, monoacylglycerol lipase and phospholipase A in fed and fasted rats. Biochim. Biophys. Acta 396, 254 - 263 (1974).

QUARFORDT, S.H., FRANK, A., SHAMES, D.H., BERMAN, M., STEINBERG, D.: Very low density lipoprotein triglyceride transport in type IV hyperlipoproteinemia and the effects of carbohydrate rich diet. J. Clin. Invest. 49, 2281 - 2297 (1970).

QUARFORDT, S.H., GOODMAN, D.S.: Heterogeneity in the rate of plasma clearance of chylomicrons of different size. Biochim. Biophys. Acta 116, 382 - 385 (1966).

QUIGLEY, T.W.C., ROE, C.E., PALLANSCH, M.T.: Fed. Proc. 17, 292 (1958).

QUINTAO, E., GRUNDY, S.M., AHRENS, E.H.,Jr.: An evaluation of four methods for measuring cholesterol absorption by the intestine in man. J. Lipid Res. 12, 221 - 232 (1971).

RACHMILEWITZ, D., STEIN, O., ROHEIM, P.S., STEIN, Y.: Metabolism of iodinated high density lipoproteins in the rat. II. Autoradiographic localization in the liver. Biochim. Biophys. Acta 270, 414 - 425 (1972).

RADHAKRISHNAMURTHY, B., BERENSON, G.S.: Glycopeptides from bovine aorta glycoprotein. J. Biol. Chem. 241, 2106 (1966).

RADHAKRISHNAMURTHY, B., BERENSON, G.S.: Structures of glycopeptides from a glycoprotein from bovine aorta. J. Biol. Chem. 248, 2000 (1973).

RADHAKRISHNAMURTHY, B., EGGEN, D.A., KOKATNUR, M., JIRGE, S., STRONG, J.P, BERENSON, G.S.: Composition of connective tissue in aortas from rhesus menkeys during regression of diet-induced fatty streaks. Lab. Invest. 33, 136 - 140 (1975).

RADHAKRISHNAMURTHY, B., FISHKIN, A.F., HUBBELL, G.J., BERENSON, G.S.: Further studies of glycoproteins from cardiovascular connective tissue. Arch. Biochem. Biophys. 104, 19 (1964).

RAFSKY, H.A., BRILL, A.A., STERN, K.G., CORAY, H.: Amer. J. Med. Sci. 224, 522 (1952).

REARDON, M.F., FIDGE, N., NESTEL, P.J.: Very low density apolipoprotein B catabolism in man (1976) (in press).

REAVEN, G.M., HILL, D.B., CROSS, R.C., FARQUHAR, J.W.: Kinetics of triglyceride turnover of very low density lipoproteins of human plasma. J. Clin. Invest. 44, 1826 - 1833 (1965).

REAVEN, G.M., JAVORSKY, W.C., REAVEN, E.P.: Diabetic hypertriglyceridemia. Am. J. Med. Sci. 269, 382 - 389 (1975).

REDGRAVE, T.G.: Formation of cholesteryl ester-rich particulate lipid during metabolism of chylomicrons. J. Clin. Invest. 49, 465 (1970).

REESE, T.S., KARNOVSKY, M.J.: Fine structural localization of a blood-brain barrier to exogenous peroxidase. J. Cell. Biol. 34, 207 (1967).

REID, D.D.: International studies in epidemiology. Am. J. of Epidem. 102, 469 - 477 (1975).

RENAUD, S. et al.: Circulat. Res. 26, 553 (1970).

RENAUD, S., GAUTHERON, P.: Influence of dietary fats on atherosclerosis, coagulation and platelet phospholipids in rabbit. Atherosclerosis 21, 115 (1974).

RENAUD, S., KUBA, K., GOULET, C., LEMIRE, Y., ALLARD, C.: Relationship between fatty acid composition of platelet and platelet aggregation in rat and man. Relation to thrombosis. Circulat. Res. 26, 553 (1970).

RENAUD, S., LECOMTE, F.: Hypercoagulability induced by hyperlipemia in rat, rabbit and man. Role of platelet factor 3. Circulat. Res. 27, 1003 (1970).

REPORT of a Joint Working Party of the Royal College of Physicians of London and the British Cardiac Society, 1976.

RHEE, C.Y., SPAET, T.H., GAYNOR, E., LAJAM, F., SHIANG, H.H., KARUSO, E., LITWAK, R.S.: Suppression of surgically induced vascular intimal hypertrophy by estrogen. Circ. $\underline{50}$, III-92 (1974).

RHOADS, G.G., GULBRANDSEN, C.L., KAGAN, A.: Serum lipoproteins and coronary heart disease in a population study of Hawaiian Japanese men. New Eng. J. Med. $\underline{294}$, 293 - 298 (1976).

RHODIN, J.: An Atlas of Histology. New York: Oxford University Press, 1975.

RIBBERT, H.: Über die Genese der Arteriosklerosen. Veränderungen der Intima. Verh. Deutsch. Ges. Path. $\underline{8}$, 168 (1904).

RICH, A.R., GREGORY, J.E.: Experimental anaphylactic lesions of the coronary arteries of the "sclerotic" type, commonly associated with rheumatic fever and dissiminated lupus erythematosus. Bull. Johns Hopkins Hosp. $\underline{81}$, 312 (1947).

RICHARDSON, J.B., BEALNES, A.: The cellular site of action of angiotensin. J. Cell. Biol. $\underline{51}$, 419 (1971).

RITTER, M.C., SCANU, A.M.: The role of apolipoprotein A-I in the structure of human serum high density lipoproteins: reconstitution studies. Manuscript in preparation.

RIVIN, A.U., DIMITROFF, S.P.: The incidence and severity of atherosclerosis in estrogen-treated males, and in females with a hypoestrogenic or a hyperestrogenic state. Circulation $\underline{9}$, 533 (1954).

ROBERT, B., SZIGETI, M., DEROUETTE, J.C., ROBERT,L., BOUISSOU, H., FABRE, M.R.: Studies on the nature of the "microfibrillar" component of elastic fibres. Europ. J. Biochem. $\underline{21}$, 507 - 516 (1971).

ROBERT, L.: In: The Smooth Muscle of the Artery. Advances in Experimental Medicine and Biology. WOLF, S., WERTHESSEN, N.T. (eds.). New York: Plenum Press, 1975, Vol. LVII, pp. 110 - 119, 131 - 133, 163 - 165.

ROBERT, L., DISCHE, Z.: Analysis of a sulfated sialofucoglucosamino-galactommano-glycan from corneal stroma. Biochem. Biophys. Res. Comm. $\underline{10}$, 209 - 214 (1963).

ROBERT, L., KADAR, A., ROBERT, B.: The macromolecules of the intercellular matrix of the arterial wall: collagen, elastin, proteoglycans, and glycoproteins. In: Arterial Mesenchyme and Arteriosclerosis. WAGNER, W.D., CLARKSON, T.B. (eds.). New York: Plenum Press, 1974, pp. 85 - 124.

ROBERT, L., ROBERT, A.M.: In: Atherosclerosis: Metabolic, Morphologic and Clinical Aspects. MANNING, G.W., HAUST, M.D. (eds.). New York: Plenum Press, 1976 (in press.)

ROBERT, L., ROBERT, B., ROBERT, A.M.: Molecular biology of elastin as related to aging and atherosclerosis. Exper. Gerontol. $\underline{5}$, 339 (1970).

ROBERT, L., STEIN, F., PEZESS, M.P., POULLAIN, N.: Propriétés immunochimiques de l'élastine. Leur importance dans l'athéromatose. Arch. Mal. Coeur et Vaiss., Rév. Atheroscl. $\underline{1}$, 233 (1967).

ROBERTSON, A.L., Jr.: Functional characterization of arterial cells involved in spontaneous atheroma. In: Atherosclerosis III. SCHETTLER, G., WEIZEL, A. (eds.). Proceedings of the Third International Symposium. Berlin: Springer-Verlag, 1974, p. 175.

ROBERTSON, A.L., Jr.: Oxygen requirements of the human arterial intima in atherogenesis. Prog. Biochem. Pharmacol. $\underline{4}$, 305 (1968).

ROBERTSON, A.L.: Regional variations of human arterial endothelium on atherogenesis. Circulation (Abstract)(Suppl. II), $\underline{54}$, 217 (1976).

ROBERTSON, A.L., Jr., KHAIRALLAH, P.A.: Arterial endothelial permeability and vascular disease. The "trap door" effect. Exp. Mol. Pathol. $\underline{18}$, 241 (1973).

ROBERTSON, A.L., KHAIRALLAH, P.A.: Effects of angiotensin II and some analogues on vascular permeability in the rabbit. Circ. Res. $\underline{31}$, 923 (1972).

ROBERTSON, A.L., McKALEN, A.: Tissue processing of mammalian vascular endothelium for scanning or scanning-transmission electron microscopy. 33rd Ann. Proc. Electron Microscopy Soc. of America. BAILEY, G.W. (ed.), 1975, p. 632.

ROBERTSON, A.L., ROSEN, L.A.: The arterial endothelium. Characteristics and function of the endothelial lining of large arteries in health and disease. Microcirculation (1977)(in press).

ROBERTSON, R.P., GARARESKI, D.J., HENDERSON, J.D., PATE, D.,Jr., BIERMAN, E.L.: Accelerated triglyceride secretion - a metabolic consequence of obesity. J. Clin. Invest. $\underline{52}$, 1620 - 1626 (1973).

ROBERTSON, van B., SCHWARTZ,B.: Ascorbid acid and the formation of collagen. J. Biol. Chem. <u>201</u>, 689 - 696 (1953).

ROBERTSON, W.B., STRONG, J.P.: Atherosclerosis in persons with hypertension and diabetes mellitus. Lab. Invest. <u>18</u>, 538 - 551 (1968).

ROBINSON, D.S.: The clearing factor lipase and its action in the transport of fatty acids between the blood and the tissues. Adv. Lipid Res. <u>1</u>, 133 - 182 (1963).

ROBINSON, D.S.: Comprehensive Biochemistry, Vol. XVIII. FLORKIN, M., STOTZ, E.H. (eds.) New York: Elsevier, 1970, pp. 51 - 116.

ROBINSON, D.S.: The function of the plasma triglyceride in fatty acid transport. In: Comprehensive Biochemistry. FLORKIN, M., STOTZ, E.M. (eds.). Amsterdam: Elsevier, 1970, Vol. XVIII, pp. 81 - 116.

RODBARD, S.: Biophysical factors in vascular structure and caliber. In: Atherosclerosis III, Proceedings of Third International Symposium. SCHETTLER, G., WEIZEL, A. (eds.). New York: Springer-Verlag, 1974, pp. 46 - 63.

RODRIGUEZ, J.L., CATAPANO, A., GHISELLI, G.C., SIRTORI, C.R.: Aortic uptake of very low density lipoproteins (VLDL) as a model for testing antiatherosclerotic compounds. Adv. Exp. Med. Biol. <u>67</u>, 169 (1976b).

RODRIGUEZ, J.L., CATAPANO, A., GHISELLI, G.C., SIRTORI, C.R.: Very low density lipoprotein in normal and cholesterol-fed rabbits: lipid and protein composition and metabolism. 2. Metabolism of very low density lipoproteins in rabbits. Atherosclerosis <u>23</u>, 85 (1976a).

RÖNNEMAA, T., PELLINIEMI, T.-T., KULONEN, E.: Factors stimulating collagen synthesis from the livers of hypercholesterolemic rats.Atherosclerosis <u>24</u>, 311 - 321 (1976).

RÖSSLE, R.: Über die serösen Entzündungen der Organe. Virchow Arch. Pathol. Anat. <u>311</u>, 252 (1944).

RÖSSNER, S.: Studies on an intravenous fat tolerance test. Methodological, experimental and clinical experiences with Intralipid®. Acta Med. Scand. Suppl. 564 (1974).

RÖSSNER, S., BOBERG, J., CARLSON, L.A., FREYSCHUSS, U., LASSERS, G.W.: Comparison between fractional turnover rate of endogenous plasma triglycerides and of Intralipid (intravenous fat tolerance test) in man. Europ. J. Clin. Invest. <u>4</u>, 109 (1974).

RÖSSNER, S., LARSSON-COHN, U., CARLSON, L.A.: Effects of an oral intravenous fat tolerance and the post-heparin lipoprotein lipase activity. Acta Med. Scand. <u>190</u>, 301 - 305 (1971).

ROGERS, W.A., DONOVAN, E.F., KOCIBA, G.J.: Lipids and lipoproteins in normal dogs with secondary hyperlipoproteinemia. J. Am. Vet. Assoc. <u>166</u>, 1092 (1975).

ROGOT, E.: Smoking and mortality among U.S. veterans. J. Chronic Dis. <u>27</u>, 189 - 203 (1974).

ROHEIM, P.S., EDELSTEIN, D., SEGAL, P.: The effect of clofibrate on serum apolipoproteins in sucrose induced hyperlipoproteinemia. Circulation (Suppl. III) 270 (1974).

ROHEIM, P.S., RACHMILEWITZ, D., STEIN, O., STEIN, Y.: Metabolism of iodinated high density lipoproteins in the rat. 1. Half-life in the circulation and uptake by organs. Biochim. Biophys. Acta <u>248</u>, 315 - 329 (1971).

ROKITANSKY, C. von: A manual of pathological anatomy. DAY, G.E.(trans.). London: The Sydenham Society, 1852, Vol. IV.

ROSCH, J., ANTONOVIC, R., RAHIMTOOLA, S.H., DOTTER, C.: Prediction of progression of coronary arterial lesions from coronary arteriograms. (Abstract). Circ. 49, <u>50</u>, (Suppl. III), III-51 (1974).

ROSE, G.: The epidemiology of coronary heart disease in Europe. In: Chronic Diseases. Copenhagen: Regional Office for Europe, World Health Organization, 1973, pp. 48 - 58.

ROSE, G. (chairman): World Health Organization European collaborative group: an international controlled trial in the multifactorial prevention of coronary heart disease. Internat. J. Epidemiol. <u>3</u>, 219 - 224 (1974).

ROSEN, N., GATON, E.: Takayasu's arteritis of coronary arteries. Arch. Pathol. <u>94</u>, 225 (1972).

ROSS, R.: The smooth muscle cell. II. Growth of smooth muscle in culture and formation of elastic fibres. J. Cell. Biol. 50, 172 - 186 (1971).

ROSS, R.: The smooth muscle of the artery. Adv. Exp. Med. Biol. 57, 65 (1975).

ROSS, R., BORNSTEIN, P.: Studies of the components of the elastic fiber. In: Chemistry and Molecular Biology of the Intercellular Matrix. BALAZS, E.A. (ed.). New York: Academic Press, 1970, Vol. I., pp. 641 - 656.

ROSS, R., GLOMSET, J.A.: Atherosclerosis and the arterial smooth muscle cell. Science 180, 1332 - 1339 (1973).

ROSS, R., GLOMSET, J.A.: The pathogenesis of atherosclerosis. N. Eng. J. Med. 295, 369 - 376 (1976).

ROSS, R., GLOMSET, J., KARIYA, B., HARKER, L.: A platelet-dependent serum factor that stimulates the proliferation of arterial smooth muscle cells in vitro. Pros. Nat. Acad. Sci. 71, 1207 - 1210 (1974).

ROSS, R., HARKER, L.: Hyperlipidemia and atherosclerosis. Science 193, 1094 (1976).

ROSSENEU, M., MIDDLEHOFF, G., PEETERS, H., BROWN, W.V.: Study of the lipid binding characteristics of the apolipoproteins from human high density lipoproteins. II. Calorimetry of the binding of apoA-I and apoA-II with phospholipids. Biochim. Biophys. Acta 441, 68 (1976).

ROSSENEU, M., SOETEWEY, F., BLATON,V, LIEVENS, J., PEETERS, H.: Application of microcalorimetry to the study of lipid-protein interaction. Chem. Phys. Lipids 17, 38 (1976).

ROSSENEU, M., SOETEWEY, F., BLATON, V., LIEVENS, J., PEETERS, H.: Microcalorimetric study of phospholipid binding to human apoHDL. Chem. Phys. Lipids. 13, 203 (1974).

ROSSENEU, M., SOETEWEY, F., LIEVENS, J., PEETERS, H.: Localization of the lipid-binding units in the plasma apolipoproteins. I. Calorimetric and potentiometric titration of native apoA-I and of the apoA-I DMPC complex. IRCS 4, 276 (1976).

ROTHBLAT, G.H.: The effect of serum components on sterol biosynthesis in L cells. J. Cell Physiol. 74, 163 - 170 (1969).

ROTHBLAT, G.H.: Cholesteryl ester metabolism in tissue culture cells. I. Accumulation in Fu5AH rat hepatoma cells. Lipids 9, 526 - 535 (1974).

ROTHBLAT, G.H., ARBOGAST, L., KRITCHEVSKY, D., NAFTULIN, M.: Cholesteryl ester metabolism in tissue culture cells. II. Source of accumulated esterified cholesterol in Fu5AG rat hepatoma cells. Lipids 11, 97 - 108 (1976).

ROTHWELL-JACKSON, R.L.: Budd-Chiari syndrome after oral contraceptives. Brit. med. J. 1, 252 (1968).

ROWE, G.G., YOUNG, W.P., WASSERBURGER, R.H.: The effect of reduced serum cholesterol on human coronary atherosclerosis. Circulation 40, (Suppl. III), 22, (1969).

ROWSELL, J.C., MURPHY, E.A., MUSTARD, J.F.: Heparin dosage and atherogenesis in the rabbits. Arch. Path. 80, 63 - 69 (1965).

RUSS, E.M., RAYMUNT, J., BARR, D.P.: Lipoproteins in primary biliary cirrhosis. J. Clin. Invest. 35, 133 - 144 (1956).

RUTHERFORD, R.B., ROSS, R.: Platelet factors stimulate fibroblasts and smooth muscle cells quiescent in plasma serum to proliferate. J. Cell Ciol. 69, 196 (1976).

RYAN, W.G., SCHWARTZ, T.B.: Dynamics of plasma triglyceride turnover in man. Metabolism 14, 1243 - 1254 (1965).

SABA, S.R., MASON, R.G.: Studies of an activity from endothelial cells that inhibits platelet aggragation, serotonin release, and clot retraction. Thrombosis Res. 5, 747 (1974).

SACKETT, D.L., EPID, M.S., GIBSON, R.W., BROSS, D.J., PICKREN, J.W.: Relation between aortic atherosclerosis and the use of cigarettes and alcohol: an autopsy study. New Eng. J. Med. 279, 1413 - 1420 (1968).

SACKETT, D.L., WINKELSTEIN, R.,Jr.: The relationship between cigarette usage and aortic atherosclerosis. Am. J. Epidemiol. 86, 264 - 270 (1967).

SACKS, F., CASTELLI, W.P., DONNER, A., KASS, E.H.: Plasma lipids and lipoproteins in vegetarians and controls. N. Engl. J. Med. 292, 1148 - 1151 (1975).

SAJDERA, S.W., HASCALL, V.C.: Proteinpolysaccharide complex from bovine nasal cartilage. J. Biol. Chem. 244, 77 (1969).

SALTYKOW, S.: Zur Kenntnis der alimentären Krankheiten der Versuchstiere. Virchow. Arch., Path. Anat. 213, 8 (1913).

SAMUEL, P., PERL., W.: Long-term decay of serum cholesterol radioactivity: body
cholesterol metabolism in normals and in patients with hyperlipoproteinemia
and atherosclerosis. J. Clin. Invest. 49, 346 - 357 (1970).

SAMUEL, P., PERL, W., HOLTZMAN, C.M., ROCHMAN, N.D., Lieberman, S.: Long-term
kinetics of serum and xanthoma cholesterol radioactivity in patients with
hypercholesterolemia. J. Clin. Invest. 51, 266 - 278 (1972).

SANMARCO, M.E., SELVESTER, R.H., BROOKS, S.H., BLANKENHORN, D.H.: Risk factors
reduction and changes in coronary arteriography.(Abstract). Circ. 53, 54,
(Suppl. II), II-140 (1976).

SAPHIR, O., STRYZAK, D., OHRINGER, L.: Hypersensitivity changes in coronary arteries of rabbits and their relationship to atherosclerosis. Lab. Invest. 7,
434 (1958).

SARDET, C., HANSMA, H., OSTWALD, R.: Characterization of guinea pig plasma lipoproteins: the appearance of new lipoproteins in response to dietary cholesterol. J. Lipid. Res. 13, 624 (1972).

SARMA, J.S.M., TILLMANNS, H., IDEKA, S., BING, R.J.: The effect of carbon monoxide on lipid metabolism of human coronary arteries. Atherosclerosis 22,
193 - 198 (1975).

SATA, T., HAVEL, R.J., JONES, A.L.: Characterization of subfractions of triglyceride-rich lipoproteins separated by gel chromatography from blood plasma
of normolipemic and hyperlipemic humans. J. Lipid. Res. 13, 757 (1972).

SAUAR, J. BLOMHOFF, J.P., GJONE, E.: Triglyceride lipases in acute hepatitis.
Clin. Chim. Acta 71, 403 (1976).

SAXENA, I.D., NAGCHAUDHURI, J.: A study of the acid mucopolysaccharides of the
rabbit aorta during cholesterol-induced atherosclerosis. Indian J. Med. Res.
57, 1 - 7 (1969).

SCANU, A.: Forms of human serum high density lipoprotein protein. J. Lipid. Res.
7, 295 - 306 (1966).

SCANU, A., EDELSTEIN, C.: Solubility in aqueous solutions of ethanol of the small
molecular weight peptides of the serum very low density and high density lipoproteins: relevance to the recovery problem during delipidation of serum lipoproteins. Anal. Biochem. 44, 576 - 588 (1971).

SCANU, A., READER, W., EDELSTEIN, C.: Biochem. Biophys. Acta 160, 32 - 45 (1968).

SCANU, A., TOTH, J., EDELSTEIN, C., KOGA, S., STILLER, E.: Fractionation of human
serum high density lipoprotein in urea solutions. Evidence for polypeptide
heterogeneity. Biochemistry 8, 3309 - 3316 (1969).

SCANU, A.M.: Human plasma high density lipoproteins. In: Plasma Lipoproteins.
SMELLIE, R.M.S. (ed.). New York: Academic Press, 1971, pp. 29 - 45.

SCANU, A.M., EDELSTEIN, C., KEIN, P.: Serum lipoproteins. In: The Plasma Proteins:
Structure, Function, and Genetic Control. 2nd ed. PUTNAM, F.E. (ed.). New
York: Academic Press, 1975, Vol. I, pp. 317 - 391.

SCEBAT, L., RENAIS, J., GROULT, N.: Pouvoir immunogène et pathogène de la paroi
artérielle. Arch. Mal. Coeur et Vaiss., Rev. Atheroscl. 3, 50 (1967).

SCEBAT, L., RENAIS, J., GROULT, N., IRIS, L., LENEGRE, J.: Lésions artérielles
produites chez le lapin par des injections de broyats d'aorte de rat. Rev.
Franç. Etudes Clin. Biol. 11, 806 (1966).

SCHAPIRO, R.H., SCHEIG, R.L., DRUMMEY, G.D., MANDERSON, J.H., ISSELBACHER, K.J.:
Effect of prolonged ethanol ingestion on the transport and metabolism of
lipids in man. N. Engl. J. Med. 25, 610 - 615 (1965).

SCHETTLER, G.: Arteriosklerose - Ätiologie, Pathologie, Klinik und Therapie.
Stuttgart: Georg Thieme Verlag, 1961.

SCHIEVELBEIN, H., GRUNDKE, K.: Gas-chromatographische Methode zur Bestimmung von
Nicotin in Blut und Geweben. Z. Anal. Chem. 237, 1 (1968).

SCHIEVELBEIN, H., LONDONG, V., LONDONG, W., GRUMBACH, H., REMPLIK, V.: Nicotine
and arteriosclerosis. An experimental contribution to the influence of nicotine on fat metabolism. Z. klin. Chem. u. klin. Biochem. 8, 190 (1970).

SCHIEVELBEIN, H., LONGDON, V., LONGDON, W., et al.: Nicotine and arteriosclerosis.
Z. klin. Chem. 8, 190 - 196 (1970).

SCHLESSINGER, B.S.: Influence of exercise and diet on the blood lipids of a
military population. Journal of the Association of Military Surgeons of the
U.S. 123, 277 (1958).

SCHLIERF, G., OSTER, P., RAETZER, H., SCHELLENBERG, B., HEUCK, C.C., EDLICH, S., SCHILLING, I., WILLENBERG, A.: Acute dietary effects on diurnal plasma lipids in normal subjects. Atherosclerosis 26, 525 (1977).

SCHNATZ, J.D., WILLIAMS, R.H.: The effect of acute insulin deficiency in the rat on adipose tissue lipoprotein lipase activity and plasma lipids. Diabetes 12, 174 - 178 (1963).

SCHONFELD, G., PFLEGER, B.: The structure of human high density lipoprotein and the levels of apolipoprotein A-I in plasma as determined by radioimmunoassay. J. Clin. Invest. 54, 236 (1974).

SCHOTZ, M.C., GARFINKEL, A.S., HUEBOTTER, R.J., STEWART, J.E.: A rapid assay for lipoprotein lipase. J. Lipid Res. 11, 68 - 69 (1970).

SCHREIBMAN, P.H., DELL, R.B.: Human adipocyte cholesterol. Concentration, localization, synthesis, and turnover. J. Clin. Invest. 55, 986 - 993 (1975).

SCHUMAKER, V.N., ADAMS, G.H.: Curculating lipoproteins. Annu. Rev. Biochem. 38, 113 (1969).

SCHWARTZ, S.M., BENDITT, E.P.: Studies on aortic intima. I. Structure and permeability of rat thoracic aortic intima. Amer. J. Pathol. 66, 241 (1972).

SCHWARTZ, S.M., STEMERMAN, M.B., BENDITT, E.P.: The aortic intima. II. Repair of the aortic lining after mechanical denudation. Amer. J. Pathol. 81, 15 (1975).

SCOTT, P.J., HURLEY, P.J.: Incorporation of radio-iodinated serum albumin and low density lipoprotein into human thrombi in vivo. J. Pathol. 97, 603 (1969).

SCOTT, R.F., DAOUD, A.S., FLORENTIN, R.A.: Animal models in atherosclerosis. In: The Pathogenesis of Atherosclerosis. WISSLER, R.W., GEER, J.C. (eds.). Baltimore: Williams and Wilkins, 1972, p. 120.

SCOW, R.O., BLANCHETTE-MACKIE, E.J., SMITH, L.C.: Role of capillary endothelium in the clearance of chylomicrons from blood: a model for lipid transport by lateral diffusion in cell membranes. Circulation Res. 39, 149 (1976).

SCOW, R.O., EGELRUD, T.: Hydrolysis of chylomicron phosphatidyl choline in vitro by lipoprotein lipase, phospholipase A$_2$ and phospholipase C. Biochim. Biophys. Acta 431, 538 (1976).

SEETHANATHAN, P., KURUP, P.A.: Changes in tissue glycosaminoglycans in rats fed a hypercholesterolemic diet. Atherosclerosis 14, 65 - 77 (1971).

SEGREST, J.P., JACKSON, R.L., MORRISETT, J.D., GOTTO, A.M.,Jr.: A molecular theory of lipid-protein interactions in the plasma lipoproteins. FEBS Letters 38, 247 - 253 (1974).

SEIDEL, D.: Hyperlipoproteinämie bei Erkrankungen der Leber. In: Handbuch der Inneren Medizin. Heidelberg: Springer-Verlag, 1977

SEIDEL, D.: Improved techniques for assessment of plasma lipoprotein patterns. I. Precipitation in gels after electrophoresis with polyanionic compounds. Clin. Chem. 19, 737 - 739 (1973).

SEIDEL, D., AGOSTINI, B., MÜLLER, P.: Structure of an abnormal plasma lipoprotein (Lp-X) characterizing obstructive jaundice. Biochim. Biophys. Acta 260, 146 - 152 (1972a).

SEIDEL, D., ALAUPOVIC, P., FURMAN, R.H.: A lipoprotein characterizing obstruction jaundice. I. Method for quantitative separation and identification of lipoproteins in jaundiced subjects. J. Clin. Invest. 48, 1211 - 1223 (1969).

SEIDEL, D., ALAUPOVIC, P., FURMAN, R.H., McCONATHY, W.J.: A lipoprotein characterizing obstructive jaundice. II. Isolation and partial characterization of the protein moieties of low density lipoproteins. J. Clin. Invest. 49, 2396 - 2407 (1970).

SEIDEL, D., GRETEN, H., GEISEN, H.P., WENGELER, H., WIELAND, H.: Further aspects on the characterization of high and very low density lipoproteins in liver disease. Europ. J. Clin. Invest. 2, 359 - 364 (1972b).

SENIOR, J.R., ISSELBACHER, K.J.: Direct esterification of monoglycerides with palmityl coenzym A by intestinal epithelial subcellular fractions. J. Biol. Chem. 237, 1454 - 1459 (1962).

SHAFRIR, E., BIALE, Y.: Lipoprotein lipase activity in some rat tissues as influenced by various metabolic situations and by nicotinic acid. In: Metabolic Effects of Nicotinic Acid and Its Derivatives. GEY, K.F., CARLSON, L.A. (eds.). Vienna: Hans Huber, 1971, p. 515.

SHAINOFF, J.R., LAHIRI, B., PAGE, I.H.: Deposition on modified fibrinogen within the aortic intima. Atherosclerosis 16, 287 (1972).

SHAPER, G. (chairman): Prevention of coronary heart disease. Report of a joint
working party of the Royal College of Physicians of London and the British
Cardiac Society. J. Roy. Coll. Phycns 10, 214 - 275 (1976).
SHELBURNE, F.A., QUARFORDT, S.J.: A new apoprotein of human plasma very low
density lipoproteins. J. Biol. Chem. 249, 1428 (1974).
SHEPPARD, B.L.: Platelet adhesion in the rabbit abdominal aorta following the
removal of endothelium with EDTA. Proc. Roy. Soc., B 182, 103 (1972).
SHEPPARD, B.L., FRENCH, J.E.: Platelet adhesion in the rabbit abdominal aorta
following the removal of the endothelium: a scanning and transmission elec-
tron microscopical study. Proc. Roy. Soc., B 176, 427 (1971).
SHEPRO, D., BATBOUTA, J.C., ROBBLEE, L.S., CARSON, M.P., BELAMARICH, F.A.:
Serotonin transport by cultured bovine aortic endothelium. Circul. Res. 36,
799 (1975).
SHERF, L., NEUFELD, H.N.: The ultrastructure of the coronary microcirculation.
(1977) (in press).
SHIGIYA, R. et al.: Rep. Res. Minist. Educ. Med. 1972 (in Japanese).
SHIMAMOTO, T.: Contracting and swallowing activity of arterial, endothelial
cells induced by cholesterol or epinephrine or angiotensin II or bradykinin. An electron microscopic study. J. Japan Atheroscler. Soc. 1, 29 - 56
(1973).
SHIMAMOTO, T.: Contraction of endothelial cells as a key mechanism in atherosclerosis with endothelial cell relaxants. In: Atherosclerosis III. Proceedings of Third International Symposium. SCHETTLER, G., WEIZEL, A. (eds.).
New York: Springer-Verlag, 1974, pp. 64 - 82.
SHIMAMOTO, T. et al.: Cyclic AMP phosphodiesterase inhibitors in the treatment
of senile mental deterioration cerebellar ataxia and thrombotic and athero-
sclerotic disorders. Frontiers of Int. Med., 1974. 12th Int. Cong. Int. Med.,
Tel Aviv, 1974. Basel: Karger, 1975, p. 110.
SHIMAMOTO, T.: Drugs and foods on contraction of endothelial cells as a key
mechanism in atherogenesis and treatment of atherosclerosis with endothelial
cell relaxants (cyclic AMP phosphodiesterase inhibitors). In: Diet and
Atherosclerosis. SIRTORI, C., RICCI, G., GORINI, S.(eds.). New York: Plenum
Publishing Corporation, 1975a, pp. 77 - 105.
SHIMAMOTO, T.: Experimental study on atherosclerosis. An attempt at its preven-
tion and treatment. Acta Path. Jap. 19, 15 - 43 (1969).
SHIMAMOTO, T.: Hyperreactive arterial endothelial cells in atherogenesis and
cyclic AMP phosphodiesterase inhibitor in prevention and treatment of athero-
sclerotic disorders. Jap. H. J. 16, 76 - 97 (1975b).
SHIMAMOTO, T.: New concept on atherogenesis and treatment of atherosclerotic
diseases. Jap. Heart J. 13, 537 - 562 (1972).
SHIMAMOTO, T.: New treatment of atherosclerosis and its basic background. A review article. Asian Med. J. 18, 355 - 366 (1975c).
SHIMAMOTO, T.: The relationship of edematous reaction in arteries to atherosclerosis and thrombosis. J. Atheroscler. Res. 3, 87 (1963).
SHIMAMOTO, T., ATSUMI, T., NUMANO, F., FUJITA, T.: Treatment of atherosclerosis
with pyridinolcarbamate. In: Progr. Biochem. Pharmacol. MIRAS, C.J., HOWARD,
A.H., PAOLETTI, R. (eds.). Basel-New York: S. Karger, 1968, Vol. IV, pp.
597 - 610.
SHIMAMOTO, T., ATSUMI, T., YAMASHITA, S., MOTOMIYA, T., ISOKANE, N., ISHIOKA, T.,
SAKUMA, A.: Clinical pharmacologic evaluation of the antiatherosclerotic
agent, pyridinolcarbamate. A double-blind crossover trial in the treatment
of atherosclerosis obliterans. Amer. Heart J. 79, 5 - 19 (1970).
SHIMAMOTO, T., KOBAYASHI, M., MORIYA, K., MATSUZAKI, M.: Coexistence of anti-
thrombotic and antihemorrhagic effect in phthalazinol, a competitive cyclic
AMP phosphodiesterase inhibitor. J. Jap. Atheroscler. Soc. 3, 437 - 446
(1975).
SHIMAMOTO, T., MURASE, H., NUMANO, F.: Treatment of senile dementia and cerebellar disorders with phthalazinol. Cyclic AMP-increasing agent, phthalazinol,
in therapeutic trials in hitherto incurable morbid conditions (1). Mech.
Ageing Develop. 5, 241 - 250 (1976).
SHIMAMOTO, T., NUMANO, F.: Atherogenesis I. Proceedings of the First Internatio-
nal Symposium on Atherogenesis, Thrombosis and Pyridinolcarbamate Treatment.
Amsterdam: Excerpta Medica, 1969.

SHIMAMOTO, T., NUMANO, F.: Beta-lipoprotein entry into the arterial wall and its prevention. In: Atherosclerosis III. SCHETTLER, G., WEIZEL, A. (eds.). Berlin-Heidelberg-New York: Springer-Verlag, 1974, pp. 89 - 92.

SHIMAMOTO, T., NUMANO, F., ADDISON, G.M.: Atherogenesis II. Proceedings of the Second International Symposium on Atherogenesis, Thrombosis and Pyridinol-carbamate Treatment. Amsterdam: Excerpta Medica, 1972.

SHIMAMOTO, T., SUNAGA, T.: The contraction and bleeding of endothelial cells accompanied by acute infiltration of plasma substances into the vessel wall and their prevention. In: Atherogenesis II. SHIMAMOTO, T. (ed.). Amsterdam: Excerpta Medica, 1972, pp. 3 - 32.

SHIMAMOTO, T., YAMASHITA, Y., SUNAGA, T.: Scanning electron microscopic observations of endothelial surface of heart and blood vessels. The discovery of intracellular bridges of vascular endothelium. Proc. Jap. Acad. 45, 507 - 511 (1969).

SHINKAI, H., YOSHIDA, Y., OONEDA, G.: An electron microscopic study of plasmatic arterionecrosis in the human cerebral arteries. Virchows Arch. A. Path. and Histol. 369, 181 - 190 (1976).

SHORE, B., SHORE, V.: Isolation and characterization of polypeptides of human serum lipoproteins. Biochemistry 8, 4510 (1969).

SHORE, B., SHORE, V., SALEL, A., MASON, D., ZELIS, R.: An apolipoprotein preferentially enriched in cholesteryl ester-rich very low density lipoproteins. Biochem. Biophys. Res. Commun. 58, 1 (1974a).

SHORE, V.G., SHORE, B.: Heterogeneity of human plasma low density lipoproteins. Separation of species differing in protein components. Biochemistry 12, 502 - 507 (1973).

SHORE, V.G., SHORE, B., HART, R.G.: Changes in apolipoproteins and properties of rabbit very low density lipoproteins on induction of cholesteremia. Biochemistry 13, 1579 - 1585 (1974).

SHULMAN, R.S., HERBERT, P.N., WEHRLY, K., FREDRICKSON, D.S.: The complete amino acid sequence of C-I (apoLP-Ser), an apolipoprotein from human very low density lipoprotein. J. Biol. Chem. 250, 182 - 190 (1975).

SHURR, P.E., SCHULTZ, J.R., DAY, C.E.: High volume screening procedures for hypobetalipoproteinemic activity in rats. Adv. Exp. Med. Biol. 67, 215 (1976).

SIESJÖ, B.K., NORBERG, K., LJUNGGREN, B., SALFORD, L.G.: Hypoxia and cerebral metabolism. In: A Basis and Practice of Neroanaesthesia. GORDON, E. (ed.). Amsterdam: Excerpta Medica, 1976, pp. 47 - 82.

SIGLER, G.F., SOUTAR, A.K., SMITH, L.C., GOTTO, A.M.,Jr., SPARROW, J.T.: The solid phase synthesis of a protein activator for lecithin-cholesterol acyl-transferase corresponding to human plasma apoC-I. Proc. Natl. Acad. Sci. US 73, 1422 - 1426 (1976).

SIGURDSSON, G., NICOLI, A., LEWIS, B.: Conversion of very low density lipoprotein to low density lipoprotein: a metabolic study of apolipoprotein B kinetics in human subjects. Eur. J. Clin. Invest. 56, 1481 (1975).

SIGURDSSON, G., NICOLL, A., LEWIS, B.: The metabolism of low density lipoprotein in endogenous hypertriglyceridaemia. Europ. J. Clin. Invest. 6, 151 (1976).

SIGURDSSON, A., NICELL, A., LEWIS, B.: Metabolism of very low density lipoproteins in hyperlipidemia. Studies of apoprotein B in kinetics in man. Europ. J. Clin. Invest. 6, 167 - 177 (1976).

SILBERBERG, R., STAMP, W.S., LESKER, P.A., HASLER, M.: Aging changes in ultrastructure and enzymatic activity of articular cartilage of guinea pigs. J. Geront. 25, 184 - 199 (1970).

SIMIONESCU, N., SIMIONESCU, M., PALADE, G.E.: Permeability of muscle capillaries to exogenous myoglobin. J. Cell. Biol. 57, 424 (1973).

SIMIONESCU, N., SIMIONESCU, M., PAPADE, G.E.: Permeability of muscle capillaries to small heme-peptides. Evidence for the existence of patent transendothelial channels. J. Cell. Biol. 64, 586 (1975).

SIMMONS, L.A., MYANT, N.B.: Cholesterol metabolism in hypertriglyceridemia and the effects of treatment. Clin. Chim. Acta 65, 117 - 129 (1975).

SIMONS, K., EHNHOLM, C., RENKONEN, O., BLOTH, B.: Characterization of the Lp(a) lipoprotein in human plasma. Acta Pathol. Microbiol. Scand. Sect. B 78, 459 - 466 (1970).

SIMONS, L.A., MYANT, N.B.: A comparison of the effects of polydexide and cholestyramine on the metabolism of cholesterol in man. Artery 2, 129 (1976).

SIMONS, L.A., WILLIAMS, P.F.: The biochemical composition and metabolism of lipoproteins in type V hyperlipoproteinemia. Clinica Chimica Acta 61, 341 - 352
(1975).

SIRTORI, C.R., BIASI, G., VARCELLIO, G., AGRADI, E., MALAN, E.: Diet, lipids and
lipoproteins in patients with peripheral vascular disease. Am. J. Med. Sc.
268, 325 - 332 (1974).

SIRTORI, C.R., CATAPANO, A., GHISELLI, G.C., INNOCENTI, A.L., RODRIGUEZ, J.:
Metformin: an antiatherosclerotic agent modifying very low density lipoproteins in rabbits. Atherosclerosis (1977c) (in press).

SIRTORI, C.R., CATAPANO, A., GHISELLI, G.C., MALINOW, R.: In vivo and in vitro
effect of a sulfated mucopolysaccharide (3GS) on the aortic uptake of a
cholesterol-rich VLDL in rabbits. Artery (1977b) (in press).

SIRTORI, C.R., CATAPANO, A., PAOLETTI, R.: Therapeutic significance of hypolipidemic and antiatherosclerotic drugs. In: Atherosclerosis Reviews. PAOLETTI, R.,
GOTTO, A.M.,Jr. (eds.). New York: Raven Press, 1977a, pp. 113 - 153.

SIRTORI, C.R., TREMOLI, E., SIRTORI, M., CONTI, F., PAOLETTI, R.: Treatment of
hypertriglyceridemia with metformin: effectiveness and analysis of results.
Atherosclerosis (1977d) (in press).

SKIPSKI, V.P., BARCLAY, M., BARCLAY, R.K., FETZER, V.A., GOOD, J.J., ARCHIBALD,
F.M.: Lipid composition of human serum lipoproteins. Biochem. J. 104, 340 -
352 (1967).

SLACK, H.G.B.: Metabolism of elastin in the adult rat. Nature 174, 512 - 513
(1954).

SLACK, J.: Risks of ischaemic heart disease in familial hyperlipoproteinemia
states. Lancet (1969) II, 1380.

SLATER, D.N., SLOAN, J.M.: The porcine endothelial cell in tissue culture.
Atherosclerosis 21, 259 (1975).

SMITH, E.B.: The influence of age and atherosclerosis on the chemistry of the
aortic intima. Part 1 and 2. J. Atheroscler. Res. 5, 224 (1965).

SMITH, E.B., ALEXANDER, K.A., MASSIE, I.B.: Insoluble "fibrin" in human aortic
intima - quantitative studies on the relationship between insoluble "fibrin",
soluble fibrinogen and low density lipoprotein. Atherosclerosis 23, 19
(1976a).

SMITH, E.B., CROTHERS, D.C.: Interaction between plasma proteins and the intercellular matrix in human aortic intima. In: Protides of the Biological
Fluids. PEETERS, H. (ed.). Oxford: Pergamon Press, 1975, Vol. XXII, p. 315.

SMITH, E.B., MASSIE, I.B., ALEXANDER, K.A.: The release of an immobilized lipoprotein fraction from atherosclerotic lesions by incubation with plasmin.
Atherosclerosis (1976b) (in press).

SMITH, E.B., SLATER, R.S.: Lipids and low density lipoproteins in intima in
relation to its morphological characteristics. In: Atherogenesis: Initiati-
ing Factors (Ciba Foundation Symposia, New Series, No. 12). Amsterdam:
Excerpta Medica, 1973, p.39.

SMITH, E.B., SLATER, R.S.: Relationship between low density lipoprotein in aortic
intima and serum lipid levels. Lancet (1972) I, 463.

SMITH, E.B., SMITH, R.H.: Early changes in aortic intima. Atherosclerosis Rev. 1,
119 (1976).

SMITH, F.R., DELL, R.B., NOBLE, R.P., GOODMAN, DeW.S.: Parameters of the three-
pool model of the turnover of plasma cholesterol in normal and hyperlipidemic humans. J. Clin. Invest. 57, 137 - 148 (1976).

SNIDERMAN, A.D., CAREW, T.E., CHANDLER, J.G., STEINBERG, D.: Paradoxical increase in rate of catabolism of low-density lipoproteins after hepatectomy.
Science 183, 526 - 528 (1974).

SOBEL, A.T., ANTONUCCI, M., INTRATOR, L., BERNARD, D., BEAUMONT, J.L., LAGRUE,
G.: Gammapathie monoclonale, glomérulopathie chronique et hyperlipidémie
auto-immune. (Evolutions sous traitement). Nouv. Presse Med. (1976)(in press).

SODAL, G., GJERTSEN, K.T., SCHRUMPF, A.: Surgical treatment of hypercholesterolemia. Acta Chir. Scandinav. 136, 671 (1970).

SODHI, H.S.: Cholesterol metabolism in man. In: Hypolipidemic Agents. KRITCHEV-
SKY, D. (ed.). Berlin-Heidelberg-New York: Springer-Verlag, 1975, pp. 29 -
107.

SODHI, H.S.: A new perspective on cholesterol metabolism in man. Perspect. Biol.
Med. 18, 477 - 485 (1975).

SODHI, H.S., KUDCHODKAR, B.J.: Catabolism of cholesterol in hypercholesterolemia
and its relationship to plasma triglycerides. Clin. Chim. Acta 46, 161 - 171
(1973b).

SODHI, H.S., KUDCHODKAR, B.J.: Cholesterol metabolism in hyperlipoproteinemias.
In: Proceedings of the Third International Symposium on Atherosclerosis.
SCHETTLER, G., WEIZEL, A., (eds.). New York: Springer-Verlag, 1974b, p. 516.

SODHI, H.S., KUDCHODKAR, B.J.: Correlating metabolism of plasma and tissue cholesterol with that of plasma lipoproteins. Lancet (1973c) I, 513 - 519.

SODHI, H.S., KUDCHODKAR, B.J.: Effects of caloric restriction on cholesterol
metabolism in hyperlipidemid obese subjects. In: International Workshop-
Conference on Atherosclerosis, London, Ontario, Canada. HAUST, D. (ed.).
New York: Plenum Press, 1975 (in press).

SODHI, H.S., KUDCHODKAR, B.J.: The relationship of esterification of plasma
cholesterol to hypertriglyceridemia in man. In: Proceedings of the Third
International Symposium on Atherosclerosis. SCHETTLER, G., WEIZEL, A. (eds.).
New York: Springer-Verlag, 1974a, pp. 516 - 519.

SODHI, H.S., KUDCHODKAR, B.J.: Synthesis of cholesterol in hypercholesterolemia
and its relationship to plasma triglycerides. Metabolism 22, 895 - 912
(1973a).

SODHI, H.S., KURCHODKAR, B.J., HORLICK, L.: Hypocholesterolemic agents and mobilization of tissue cholesterol in man. Atherosclerosis 17, 1 - 19 (1973).

SODHI, H.S., KUDCHODKAR, B.J., HORLICK, L., WEDER, C.H.: Effects of chlorophenoxy-
isobutyrate on the synthesis and metabolism of cholesterol in man. Metabolism 20, 348 - 359 (1971).

SOETEWEY, F., ROSSENEU, M., PEETERS, H.: Localization of the lipid-binding units
in the plasma apolipoproteins. II. Identification of the lipid-binding units
in the apoA-I lipoprotein. IRCS 4, 277 (1976).

SOMER, J.B., EVANS, G., SCHWARTZ, C.J.: Influence of experimental coarctation on
the pattern of aortic Evans Blue uptake in vivo. Atherosclerosis 16, 127
(1972).

SOMLYO, A.P.: Ultrastructure and function of vascular smooth muscle. Advanc. exp.
Med. Biol. 57, 1 (1975).

SOMLYO, A.P., SOMLYO, A.V.: Vascular smooth muscle. L. Normal structure, pathology, Biochemistry and biophysics. Pharmacol. Rev. 20, 197 - 272 (1968).

SOUTAR, A., GARNER, C., BAKER, H.N., SPARROW, J.T., JACKSON, R.L., GOTTO, A.M.,
SMITH, L.C.: The effects of plasma apolipoproteins on lecithin:cholesterol
acyltransferase. Biochemistry 14, 3057 - 3064 (1975).

SPAET, T.H., STEMERMAN, M.B., VEITH, F.J., LEJNIEKS: Intimal injury and regrowth
in rabbit aorta, medial smooth muscle cells as a source of neo intima. Circulation Research 36, 58 - 70 (1975).

SPAIN, D.M., BRADESS, V.A.: Sudden death from coronary atherosclerosis. A.M.A.
Arch. Int. Med. 100, 228 - 231 (1957).

SPARROW, J.T., GOTTO, A.M.,Jr., MORRISETT, J.D.: Chemical synthesis and biochemical properties of peptide fragments of apolipoprotein-alanine. Proc.
Natl. Acad. Sci. US 70, 2124 - 2128 (1973).

SPARROW, J.T., MORRISETT, J.D., POWNALL, H.J., JACKSON, R.L., GOTTO, A.M.,Jr.:
The mechanism of lipid binding by the plasma lipoproteins: synthesis of model
peptides. In: Peptides: Chemistry, Structure and Biology. WALTER, R., MEIEN-
HOFER, J. (eds.). Michigan: Ann Arbor Science, 1975, pp. 597 - 602.

SPITZER, J.J., NAKAMURA, H., HORI, S., GOLD, M.: Hepatic and splanchnic uptake
and oxidation of free fatty acids. Proc. Soc. Exp. Biology Med. 132, 281 -
286 (1969).

SPRARAGEN, S.C., BOND, V.P., DAHL, L.K.: Role of hyperplasia in vascular lesions
of cholesterol-fed rabbits studied with thymidine-H3 autoradiography. Circ.
Res. XI, 329 - 339 (1962).

SRINIVASAN, S.R., DOLAN, P., RADHAKRISHNAMURTHY, B., BERENSON, G.S.: Isolation of lipoprotein and mucopolysaccharide complexes from fatty streaks of human aortas. Atherosclerosis 16, 95 (1972).

SRINIVASAN, S.R., DOLAN, P., RADHAKRISHNAMURTHY, B., PARGAONKAR, P.S., BERENSON, G.S.: Lipoprotein-acid mucopolysaccharide complexes of human atherosclerotic lesions. Biochim. Biophys. Acta 388, 58 (1975).

SRINIVASAN, S.R., LOPEZ-S.A., RADHAKRISHNAMURTHY, B., BERENSON, G.S.: Complexing of serum β-lipoproteins and acid mucopolysaccharides. Atherosclerosis 12, 321 (1970).

SRINIVASAN, S.R., LOPEZ-S.A., RADHAKRISHNAMURTHY, B., BERENSON, G.S.: A simplified technique for semi-quantitative, clinical estimation of serum β- and pre-β-lipoproteins. Angiologica 7, 344 (1970).

SRINIVASAN, S.R., RADHAKRISHNAMURTHY, B., PARGAONKAR, P.S., BERENSON, G.S.: Glycoproteins from the connective tissue of twins. Nature 229, 58 (1971).

STAFFORT, W.W., DAY, C.E.: Regression of atherosclerosis effected by intravenous phospholipid. Artery 1, 106 (1975).

STAMLER, J.: The Coronary Drug Project (clofibrate and niacin in coronary heart disease). JAMA 231, 360 - 381 (1975).

STAMLER, J.: Lectures on preventive cardiology. New York: Grune and Stratton, 1967.

STAMLER, J.: Prevenzione primaria e secondaria delle malattie aterosclerotiche. In: Arteriosclerosi. PAOLETTI, R., SIRTORI, C.R. (eds.). Milano: Casa Ed. Ambrosiana, 1977 (in press).

STAMLER, J.: Primary prevention of sudden coronary death. Circulation 52, III 258 - 274 (1975).

STAMLER, J., BERKSON, D.M., LINDBERG, H.A.: Risk factors: their role in the etiology and pathogenesis of the atherosclerotic diseases. In: The Pathogenesis of Atherosclerosis. WISSLER, R.W., GEER, J.C. (eds.). Baltimore: Williams & Wilkins Co., 1974, pp. 41 - 119.

STARR, J.I., IUHN, D.J., MAKO, M.E.: Circulating high density lipoprotein (HDL): measurement of an apoprotein component by radioimmunoassay. J. Clin. Invest. 52, 81a (1973).

STARY, H.C.: Cell proliferation and ultrastructural changes in regressing atherosclerotic lesions after reduction of serum cholesterol. In: Atherosclerosis III. SCHETTLER, G., WEIZEL, A. (eds.). Berlin: Springer-Verlag, 1974b, pp. 187 - 190.

STARY, H.C.: Coronary artery fine structure in rhesus monkeys: the early atherosclerotic lesion and its progression. Primates in Medicine. Basel: Karger, 1976, Vol. IX, pp. 359 - 395.

STARY, H.C.: Proliferation of arterial cells in atherosclerosis. In: Arterial Mesenchyme and Arteriosclerosis. WAGNER, W.D., CLARKSON, B. (eds.). New York: Plenum Press, 1974, pp. 59 - 84.

STARY, H.C.: Progression and regression of experimental atherosclerosis in rhesus monkeys. In: Medical Primatology. GOLDSMITH, E.I., MOOR-JANKOWSKI, J. (eds.). Basel: Karger, 1972, pp. 356 - 367.

STARY, H.C., McMILLAN, G.C.: Kinetics of cellular proliferation in experimental atherosclerosis. Arch. Path. 89, 173 - 183 (1970).

STARY, H.C., STRONG, J.P.: Coronary artery fine structure in rhesus monkeys: nonatherosclerotic intimal thickening. Primates in Medicine. Basel: Karger, 1976a, Vol. IX, pp. 321 - 358.

STARY, H.C., STRONG, J.P.: The fine structure of nonatherosclerotic intimal thickening, of developing, and of regressing atherosclerotic lesions at the bifurcation of the left coronary artery. Adv. Exp. Med. Biol. 67, 89 - 108. New York: Plenum Press, 1976b.

STARZL, T.E., CHASE, H.P., PUTNAM, C.W., PORTER, K.A.: Portacaval shunt in hyperlipoproteinaemia. Lancet (1973) II, 940.

STARZL, T.E., LEE, I.Y.: The influence of portal blood upon lipid metabolism in normal and diabetic dogs and baboons. S.G. & O. 140, 381)1975).

STARZL, T.E., PUTNAM, C.W., CHASE, H.P., PORTER, K.A.: Portocaval shunt in hyperlipoproteinemia. Lancet (1973) II, 940 - 944.

STARZL, Th., CHASE, H.P., PUTNAM, Ch.W., NORA, J.J.: Follow-up of patients with portacaval shunt for the treatment of hyperlipidemia. Lancet (1974) II,714-715.

STATISTICS CANADA, 1970. Causes of death: provinces by sex and Canada by sex and age. Vital Statistics Section, Health and Welfare Division, Ottawa.

ST. CLAIR, R.W.: Metabolism of the arterial wall and atherosclerosis. In: Atherosclerosis Reviews. PAOLETTI, R., GOTTO, A.M.,Jr. (eds.). New York: Raven Press, 1976, p. 61 - 117.

ST. CLAIR, R.W., CLARKSON, T.B., LOFLAND, H.B.: Effects of regression of atherosclerotic lesions on the content and esterification of cholesterol by cell-free preparations of pigeon aorta. Circ. Res. 31, 664 - 671 (1972).

ST. CLAIR, R.W., LOFLAND, H.B., CLARKSON, T.B.: Influence of duration of cholesterol feeding on esterification of fatty acids by cell-free preparations of pigeon aorta. Circ. Res. 27, 213 - 225 (1970).

ST. CLAIR, R.W., TOMA, J.J., LOFLAND, H.B.: Proline hydroxylase activity and collagen content of pigeon aortas with naturally-occurring and cholesterol aggravated atherosclerosis. Atherosclerosis 21, 155 - 165 (1975).

STEFANOVICH, V., GORE, I.: Cholesterol diet and permeability of rabbit aorta. Exp. Molec. Pathol. 14, 20 (1971).

STEHBENS, W.E.: Endothelial cell mitosis and permeability. Quart. J. Exp. Physiol. 50, 90 (1965).

STEIN, E.A., MIENY, C., SPITZ, L., SAARON, I. et al.: Portacaval shunt in four patients with homozygous hypercholesterolaemia. Lancet (1975) I, 832.

STEIN, F., PEZESS, M.P., POULLAIN, N., ROBERT, L.: Anti-elastin antibodies in normal and pathological human sera. Nature 207, 312 (1965).

STEIN, O., RACHMILEWITZ, D., SANGER, L., EISENBERG, S., STEIN, Y.: Metabolism of iodinated very low density lipoprotein in the rat: autoradiographic localization in the liver. Biochim. Biophys. Acta 360, 205 (1974).

STEIN, O., STEIN, Y.: Comparative uptake of rat and human serum low-density and high-density lipoproteins by rat aortic smooth muscle cells in culture. Circulation Res. 36, 436 - 443 (1975).

STEIN, O., STEIN, Y.: An electron microscopic study of the transport of peroxidase on the endothelium of the mouse aorta. Z. Zellforsch. 133, 211 (1972).

STEIN, O., STEIN, Y.: High density lipoproteins reduce the uptake of low density lipoproteins by human endothelial cells in culture. Biochim. Biophys. Acta 431, 363 (1976).

STEIN, O., STEIN, Y.: The removal of cholesterol from Landschutz ascites cells by high density apolipoprotein. Biochim. Biophys. Acta 326, 232 - 244 (1973).

STEIN, O., STEIN, Y.: Surface binding and interiorization of homologous and heterologous serum lipoproteins by rat aortic smooth muscle cells in culture. Biochim. Biophys. Acta 398, 377 - 384 (1975b).

STEIN, O., STEIN, Y., EISENBERG, S.: A radioautographic study of the transport of 125_I-labeled serum lipoproteins in rat aorta. Z. Zellforsch. 138, 223 (1973).

STEIN, O., STEIN, Y., FIDGE, A., GOODMAN, D.S.: J. Cell Biol. 43, 410 (1969).

STEIN, O., VANDERHOEK, J., STEIN, Y.: Cholesterol content and sterol synthesis in human skin fibroblasts and rat aortic smooth muscle cells exposed to lipoprotein depleted serum and high density apolipoprotein-phospholipid mixtures. Biochim. Biophys. Acta 431, 347 - 358 (1976).

STEIN, O., WEINSTEIN, D.B., STEIN, Y., Steinberg, D.: Binding, internalization, and degradation of low density lipoprotein by normal human fibroblasts and by fibroblasts from a case of homozygous familial hypercholesterolemia. Proc. Natl. Acad.Sci. US 73, 14 - 18 (1976).

STEIN, O., STEIN, Y.: The removal of cholesterol from Landschütz ascites cells by high-density apolipoprotein. Biochim. Biophys. Acta 325, 232 (1973).

STEIN, Y., GLANGEAUD, M.C., FAINARU, M., STEIN, O.: The removal of cholesterol from aortic smooth muscle cells in culture and Landschütz ascites cells by fractions of human high density apolipoprotein. Biochim. Biophys. Acta 380, 106 - 118 (1975).

STEIN, Y., STEIN, O.: Lipid synthesis and degradation and lipoprotein transport in mammalian aorta. In: Atherogenesis: Initiating Factors (Ciba Foundation Symposia, New Series No. 12). Amsterdam: Excerpta Medica, 1973, p. 165.

STEIN, Y., STEIN, O.: Lipoprotein synthesis, intracellular transport and secretion in liver. In: Atherosclerosis III. SCHETTLER, G., WEIZEL, A. (eds.). Berlin: Springer-Verlag, 1974, p. 652.

STEIN, Y., STEIN, O.: Transport of lipids in the arterial wall. A biochemical and radioautographic study. In: Exposés Annuels de Biochimie Médicale, 31e série. Paris: Masson, 1972, p. 98.

STEIN, Y., STEIN, O.: Turnover of phospholipids in rat aortic smooth muscle cells in culture. Amer. J. Cardiol. 35, 572 - 578 (1975c).

STEINBACH, J.H., BLACKSHEAR, P.L., Jr., VARCO, R.L., BUCHWALD, H.: High blood cholesterol reduces in-vitro blood oxygen delivery. J. Surg. Res. 16, 134 (1974).

STEINER, G., MURASE, R.: Triglyceride turnover: a comparison of simultaneous determinations using the radioglyceride and the lipolytic rate procedures. Fed. Proc. 34, 2258 - 2262 (1975).

STEINER, G., POAPST, M., DAVIDSON, J.K.: Production of chylomicron-like lipoproteins from endogenous lipid by the intestine and liver of diabetic dogs. Diabetes 24, 263 - 271 (1975).

STEMERMAN, M.B.: Thrombogenesis of the rabbit arterial plaque. Amer. J. Pathol. 73, 7 (1973).

STEMERMAN, M.D., ROSS, R.: Experimental arteriosclerosis. I. Fibrous plaque formation in primates, an electron microscopy study. J. Exper. Med. 136, 769 (1972).

STEMMERMANN, G.N., STEER, A., RHOADS, G.G., LEE, K., HAYASHI, T., NAKASHIMA, T., KEEHN, R.: A comparative pathology study of myocardial lesions and atherosclerosis in Japanese men living in Hiroshima. Japan and Honolulu, Hawaii. Lab. Invest. 34, 592 (1976).

STENDER, S., ASTRUP, P., KJELDSEN, K.: Hyperoxia-induced decrease in aortic accumulation of cholesterol in rabbits previously fed a cholesterol-enriched diet. Exp. molec. Path (1976) (in print).

STERN, M.P., HASKELL, W.L., WOOD, P.D.S., OSANN, K.E., KING, A.B., FARQUHAR, J.W.: Affluence and cardiovascular risk factors in Mexican Americans and other Whites in three Northern California Communities. J. Chronic Dis. 28, 623 - 636 (1975).

STERNBY, N.H.: Atherosclerosis in a defined population: an autopsy survey in Malmö, Sweden. Acta path. Microbiol. Scand. (Suppl. 195), (1968).

STERNE, J.: The present state of knowledge on the mode of action of the anti-diabetic diguanides. Metabolism 13, 791 (1964).

STEVENS, R.L., COLOMBO, M., GONZALES, J.J., HOLLANDER, W., SCHMID, K.: The glycosaminoglycans of the human artery and their changes in atherosclerosis. J. Clin. Invest. 58, 470 - 481 (1976).

STEWART, C.D., HENDRY, E.B.: Phospholipids of blood. J. Biol. Chem. 29, 1683 (1935).

STILL, W.J.S.: The early effect of hypertension on the aortic intima of the rat: an electron microscopic study. Amer. J. Path. 51, 721 - 734 (1967).

STOFFEL, W.: Carbon 13 NMR-spectroscopic studies on liposomes and human high density lipoproteins. In: Lipoprotein Metabolism. GRETEN, H. (ed.). Berlin: Springer-Verlag, 1976, p. 132.

STOFFEL, W., DARR, W.: Human high density apolipoprotein A-I-lysolecithin-lecithin and sphingomyelin complexes. Hoppe-Seyler's Z. Physiol. Chem. 357, 127 (1976).

STOFFEL, W., ZIERENBERG, O., TUNGGAL, B., SCHREIBER, E.: ^{13}C nuclear magnetic resonance spectroscopic evidence for hydrophobic lipid-protein interactions in human high-density lipoproteins. Proc. Natl. Acad Sci. US 71, 3696 - 3700 (1974).

STONE, N.J., LEVY, R.I., FREDRICKSON, D.S., VERTER, J.: Coronary artery disease in 116 kindred with familial Type II hyperlipoproteinemia. Circulation 49, 476 (1974).

STONE, W.L., REYNOLDS, J.A.: The self-association of the apo-Gln-I and apo-Gln-II polypeptides of human serum lipoproteins. J. Biol. Chem. 250, 8045 - 8048 (1975).

STORMOKEN, H.: In: Dietary Fats and Thrombosis. Basel: Karger, 1974, p. 1.

STORMOKEN, H.: Epidemiological studies. Relation between dietary fat and arterial and venous thrombosis. In: Dietary Fats and Thrombosis. Haemostasis 2, 1 (1974/74).

STORY, J.A., TEPPER, S.A., KRITCHEVSKY, D.: Atherosclerosis in rabbits fed cholesterol-free diets: effect of protein and fiber. Fed. Proc. (Abstract) 35, 294 (1976).

STOUT, R.W., BUCHANAN, K.D., VALLANCE-OWEN, J.: The relationship of arterial disease and glucagon metabolism in insulintreated chicken. Atherosclerosis 18, 153 (1973).

STRØM, A., JENSEN, R.A.: Mortality from circulatory diseases in Norway 1940 - 1945. Lancet (1951) I, 126.

STRISOWER, E.H., KRADJIAN, R., NICHOLS, A.V., COGGIOLA, E., TSAI, J.: Effect of ileal bypass on serum lipoproteins in essential hypercholesterolemia. J. Atheroscler. Res. 8, 525 (1968).

STRONG, J.P.: Unexplained variability in extent of atherosclerosis in homogeneous human populations. Fourth International Symposium on Atherosclerosis, Tokyo (1976).

STRONG, J.P.: Workshop on epidemiology of atherosclerosis including geographical differences of risk factors. Proceedings of Fourth International Symposium on Atherosclerosis, Tokyo (1976).

STRONG, J.P., EGGEN, D.A.: Risk factors and atherosclerotic lesions. Atherosclerosis: Proceedings of the Second International Symposium. JONES, R.J. (ed.). New York: Springer-Verlag, 1970, pp. 355 - 364.

STRONG, J.P., EGGEN, D.A., OALMANN, M.C.: The natural history, geographic pathology and epidemiology of atherosclerosis. In: The Pathogenesis of Atherosclerosis. WISSLER, R.W., GEER, J.C. (eds.). Baltimore: Williams & Wilkins, 1972, p. 20.

STRONG, J.P., EGGEN, D.A., STARY, H.C.: Reversibility of fatty streaks in rhesus monkeys. Primates in Medicine 9, 299 - 320. Basel: Karger, 1976.

STRONG, J.P., McGILL, H.C.,Jr.: Diet and experimental atherosclerosis in baboons. Am. J. Pathol. 50, 669 - 690 (1967).

STRONG, J.P., RICHARDS, M.L.: Cigarette smoking and atherosclerosis in autopsied men. Atherosclerosis 23, 451 - 476 (1976).

STRONG, J.P., RICHARDS, M.L., McGILL, H.C.,Jr., EGGEN, D.A., McMURRY, M.T.: On the association of cigarette smoking with coronary and aortic atherosclerosis. J. Atheroscl. Res. 10, 303 - 317 (1969).

STUHRMANN, H.B., TARDIEU, A., MATEU, L., SARDET, C., LUZZATI, V., AGGERBECK, L., SCANU, A.M.: Neutron scattering study of human serum low density lipoprotein. Proc. Natl. Acad. Sci. US 72, 2270 - 2273 (1975).

SUMIYOSHI, A.: Experimental atherosclerosis and thrombosis. J. Japan Atherosclerosis Soc. 3, 407 (1976).

SUMIYOSHI, A., MORE, R.H., WEIGENSBERG, B.I.: Aortic fibrofatty type atherosclerosis from thrombus in normolipidemic rabbits. Atherosclerosis 18, 43 (1973).

SUMIYOSHI, A., TANAKA, K.: Endothelial damage and thrombosis: a scanning and transmission electron microscopic study. Thrombosis Research 8, (Suppl. II), 277 - 286 (1976).

SUTHERLAND, E.W.: Cyclic AMP and hormone action. In: Cyclic AMP. ROBISON, G.A., BUTCHER, R.W., SUTHERLAND, E.W. (eds.). New York: Academic Press, 1971, p.17.

SVENDSEN, E., JØRGENSEN, L.: Loss of endothelial cells in rabbit aorta following short term cholesterol feeding. The Fourth International Symposium on Atherosclerosis. (Abst. F-81) Tokyo, Japan. Aug. 24 - 28, 1976.

SWAN, D.M., McGOWAN, J.M.: Ileal bypass in hypercholesterolemia associated with heart disease. Am. J. Surg. 116, 81 (1968).

SWITZER, S.: Plasma lipoproteins in liver disease. I. Immunologically distinct low-density lipoproteins in patients with biliary obstruction. J. Clin. Invest. 46, 1855 - 1866 (1967).

SZANTO, S.: Smoking and atherosclerosis. Br. Med. J. 3, 178 (1967).

SZIGETTI, I., ORMOS, J., JAKO, J., TOSKEGI, A.: The atherogenic effect of immunization with homologous complex great vessel wall in rabbit. Acta Allergol. (Suppl. 7), 374 (1960).

TAKEUCHI, N., ITO, M., MASUNO, T., YAMAMURA, Y., KATAYAMA, Y., OGAWA, Z., UCHIDA, K.: Cholesterol metabolism and aging. Proc. Japan. Conf. Biochem. Lipid 17, 89 - 92 (1975).

TAKEUCHI, N., ITO, M., YAMAMURA, Y.: Cholesterol metabolism in rats sensitive to
high cholesterol diet. Adv. Exper. Med. Biol. 67, 267 - 288 (1976a).

TAKEUCHI, N., ITO, M., YAMAMURA, Y.: Regulation of cholesterol 7 α-hydroxylation
by cholesterol synthesis in rat liver. Atherosclerosis 20, 481 - 494 (1974).

TAKEUCHI, N., MATSUMIYA, K., TAKAHASHI, Y., HIGASHINO, K., TANAKA, F., KATAYAMA,
Y.: Tiobarbituric acid reactive substances and lipid metabolism in α-tocopherol deficient rats. Exper. Gerontol. (1976b)(in press).

TAKEUCHI, N., TANAKA, F., KATAYAMA, Y., MATSUMIYA, K., YAMARURA, Y.: Effect of
α-tocopherol on thiobarbituric acid reactive substances in serum and hepatic
subcellular organelles and lipid metabolism (1976c)(in press).

TAKEUCHI, N., YAMAMURA, Y., KATAYAMA, Y., HAYASHI, C., UCHIDA, K.: Impairment
of feed back control and induction of cholesterol synthesis in aged rats.
Exper. Gerontol. 11, 121 - 126 (1976d).

TAKEUCHI, T.: Morphology of renal arterial vasospasm and alteration of intrarenal
hemodynamics. Trans. Soc. Path. Jap. 63, 63 - 89 (1974)(in Japanese).

TAKEUCHI, T., MORI, Y., OZAWA, U.: On the morphological analysis of renal arterial
vasospasm and alteration of hemodynamics in the kidney, I, II and III reports.
The Nihon University Jour. of Med. 15, 193, 409 (1973); 15, 81 (1974).

TALL, A., SHIPLEY, G.G., SMALL, D.M.: Thermal behaviour of the human apoA-I proteins. J. Biol. Chem., 251, 37-49 (1976).

TALL, A., SMALL, D.M., SHIPLEY, G.G., LEES, R.M.: Apoprotein stability and lipid-
protein interactions in human plasma high-density lipoproteins. Proc. Nat.
Acad. Sci. US 72, 494 (1975).

TANAKA, K.: Pathology of hemorrhage and thrombosis. Jap. J. Clin. Med. 31, 743
(1974)(in Japanese).

TANASE, H., SUZUKI, Y., OOSHIMA, A., YAMORI, Y., OKAMOTO, K.: Genetic analysis of
blood pressure in spontaneously hypertensive rats. Jap. Circ. J. 34, 1197 -
1212 (1970).

TAYLOR, C.B.: Experimentally induced arteriosclerosis in nonhuman primates. In:
Comparative Atherosclerosis. ROBERTS, J.C.,STRAUS, R. (eds.). New York:
Harper and Row, 1965, pp. 215 - 243.

TAYLOR, C.B., COX, G.E., MANALO-ESTRELLA, P., SOUTHWORTH, J.: Atherosclerosis in
rhesus monkeys. II. Arterial lesions associated with hypercholesteremia induced by dietary fat and cholesterol. Arch. Pathol. 74, 16 (1962).

TAYLOR, C.B., PATTON, D.E., COX, G.E.: Atherosclerosis in rhesus monkeys. V.
Marked diet-induced hypercholesteremia with xanthomatosis and severe atherosclerosis. Arch. Pathol. 76, 239 (1963a).

TAYLOR, C.B., PATTON, D.E., COX, G.E.: Atherosclerosis in rhesus monkeys. VI.
Fatal myocardial infarction in a monkey fed fat and cholesterol. Arch. Pathol.
76, 404 (1963b).

TEJADA, C., STRONG, J.P., MONTENEGRO, M.M., RESTREPO, C., SOLBERG, L.A.: Distribution of coronary and aortic atherosclerosis by geographic location, race and
sex. Lab. Invest. 18, 509 - 526 (1968).

TERRY, E.N., ROUEN, L.R., CLAUSS, R.H., KATZ, M.C., REDISCH, M.: Attempts to de-
ley progression in occlusive atherosclerosis. Ann. N.Y. Acad. Sci.(1975).

THILLY, C., KORNITZER, M., RAMIOUL, L., WILMET, M., de BACKER, G., ROSE, G.: Prediction of coronary risk in middle aged man. Arch. mal. du coeur 68 (numéro
spécial), 101 - 107 (1975).

THOMAS, W.A., DAVIES, J.N.P., O'NEAL, R.M., DIMAKULANGAN, A.A.: Incidence of myocardial infarction correlated with venous and pulmonary thrombosis and embolism. Amer. J. Cardiol. 5, 41 (1960).

THOMAS, W.A., FLORENTIN, R.A., NAM, S.C., KIM, D.N., JONES, R.M., LEE, K.T.:
Preproliferative phase of atherosclerosis in swine fed cholesterol. Arch.
Path. 86, 621 - 643 (1968).

THOMAS, W.A., FLORENTIN, R.A., NAM, S.C., REINER, J.M., LEE, K.T.: Alterations
in population dynamics of arterial smooth muscle cells during atherogenesis.
I. Activation of interphase cells in cholesterol-fed swine prior to gross
atherosclerosis demonstrated by "postpulse salvage labelling". Exp. and Molec.
Path. 15, 245 - 267 (1971).

THOMAS, W.A., FLORENTIN, J.M., REINER, J.M., LEE, LEE, W.M., LEE, K.T.: Alterations in population dynamics of arterial smooth muscle cells during athero-

genesis. IV. Evidence for a polyclonal origin of hypercholesterolemic diet-induced atherosclerotic lesions in young swine. Exp. and Molec. Path. 24, 244 - 260 (1976).

THOMAS, W.A., REINER, J.M., FLORENTIN, R.A., LEE, K.T., LEE, W.M.: Population dynamics of arterial smooth muscle cells. V. Cell proliferation and cell death during initial 3 months in atherosclerotic lesions induced in swine by hypercholesterolemic diet and intimal trauma. Exp. and Molec. Path. 24, 360 - 374 (1976).

THOMPSON, G.R., BARROWMAN, J., GUTIERREZ, DOWLING, R.H.: Action of neomycin on the intraluminal phase of lipid absorption. J. clin.Invest. 50, 319 (1971).

THOMSEN, H.K.: Carbon monoxide-induced atherosclerosis in primates. An electron microscopic sutdy on the coronary arteries of Macaca Irus monkeys. Atheroscl. 20, 233 (1974).

THOMSEN, H.K., KJELDSEN, K.: Threshold limit for carbon monoxide-induced myocardial damage. Arch. Environm. Hlth. 29, 73 - 78 (1974).

THOMSON, J.G.: Atheroma in a transplanted heart. Lancet(1969) I, 1297.

TILLGREN, C.: Obliterative arterial disease of the lower limbs. III. Prognostic influence of concomitant coronary heart disease. Acta Med. Scand. 178, 121 - 128 (1965).

TIMM, J.: Trendanalysen zum Problem des Verbrauchers an Nikotin und Rauchkondensat in der Bundesrepublik Deutschland für die Jahre 1961 bis 1972. Beiträge zur Tabakforschung 7, 206 (1974).

TODD, A.S.: The histological localisation of fibrinolysin activator. J. Path. Bact. 78, 281 (1959).

TORSVIK, H., SOLAAS, M.H., GJONE, E.: Serum lipoproteins in plasma lecithin :cholesterol acyltransferase deficiency, studied by electron microscopy. Clin. Genet. 1, 139 (1970).

TRILLO, A., RANAUD, S., HAUST, M.D.: Ultrastructure of aortic lesions in normotensive and hypertensive hyperlipemic rats. Fed. Proc. (Abstract) 29, 487 (1970).

TRUETT, J., CORNFIELD, J., KANNEL, W.: A multivariate analysis of the risk of coronary heart disease in Framingham. J. Chronic Dis. 20, 511 - 524 (1967).

TRUSWELL, A.S., KAY, R.M.: Bran and blood lipids. Lancet (1975) I, 367.

TSKRALIDES, V.G., BLIEDEN, L.C., EDWARDS, J.E.: Coronary atherosclerosis and myocardial infarction associated with systemic lupus erythematosus. Amer. Heart J. 87, 637 (1974).

TUCKER, C.F., CATSULIS, C., STRONG, J.P., EGGEN, D.A.: Regression of early cholesterol-induced aortic lesions in rhesus monkeys. Amer. J. Pathol. 65, 493 - 514 (1971).

TURITTO, V.T., BAUMGARTNER, H.R.: Platelet deposition on subendothelium exposed to flowing blood: mathematical analysis of physical parameters. Trans. Amer. Soc. Artif. Int. Organs 21, 593 (1975).

TURPEINEN, O., MIETTINEN, M., KARVONEN, M., ROINE, P., PEKKARINEN, M., LEHTOSUD, E.J., ALIVIRTA, P.: Dietary prevention of coronary heart disease: long-term experiment. I - Observations on male subjects. Am J. Clin. Nutr. 21, 255 (1968).

TURPIN, G., TRUFFERT, J., SALMON, D., de GENNES, J.L.: Etude de la distribution des valeurs lipidiques (cholestérol total et triglycérides) normales et pathologiques dans une population présumée saine. Ann. Biol. Clin. 31, 359 - 367 (1973).

TWU, J.S., NILSSON-EHLE, P., SCHOTZ, M.C.: Hydrolysis of tri- and monoacylglycerol by lipoprotein-lipase: evidence for a common active site. Biochemistry 15, 1904 (1976).

TYROLER, H.A., HAMES, C.G., KRISHAN, I., HEYDEN, S., COOPER, G., CASSEL, J.C.: Black-white differences in serum lipids and lipoproteins in evans county. Prevent. Med. 4, 541 - 550 (1975).

TYROLER, H.A., HEYDEN, S., SNEIDERMAN, C., HEISS, G., HAMES, C.: 16-year follow-up of blood pressure in young adult residents of Evans County. Pittsburgh: Medical Horizons Symposium on Hypertension in Childhood and Adolescence, 1976.

TYSZKA, C. von: Ernährung und Lebenshaltung des deutschen Volkes. Berlin: Springer, 1934.

UCHIDA, K., TAKEUCHI, N., YAMAMURA, Y.: Effect of glucose administration on cholesterol and bile acid metabolism. Lipids 10, 473 - 477 (1975).

URRY, D.W.: Neutral sites for calcium ion binding to elastin and collagen: a charge neutralization theory for calcification and its relationship to atherosclerosis. Proc. Natl. Acad. Sci. 68, 810 - 814 (1971).

U.S. DEPARTMENT OF HEALTH, EDUCATION, AND WELFARE: Arteriosclerosis: a report by the National Heart and Lung Institute task force on arteriosclerosis. Publication No. (NIH) 72-137, June 1971.

U.S. DEPARTMENT OF HEALTH, EDUCATION, AND WELFARE: The health consequences of smoking. 1974. Report of a WHO Expert Committee: Smoking and its effects on health. Geneva: WHO, 1975.

U.S. DEPARTMENT OF HEALTH, EDUCATION, AND WELFARE: Task force on genetic factors in atherosclerotic disease. DHEW Publication No. (NIH) 76-922, Washington, D.C. (1975).

U.S. PUBLIC HEALTH SERVICE. The health consequences of smoking. 1971.

UTERMANN, G., JAESCKLE, M., MENZEL, E.: Familial hyperlipoproteinemia type III: deficiency of a specific apolipoprotein (ApoE-III) in the very low density lipoproteins. FEBS Letters 56, 352 - 355 (1975).

UTERMANN, G., MENZEL, H.J., LANGER, K.H.: On the polypeptide composition of an abnormal high density lipoprotein (LP-E) occurring in LCAT-deficient plasma. FEBS Letters 45, 29 - 32 (1974).

UTERMANN, G., MENZEL, H.J., LANGER, K.H., DIEKER, P.: Lipoproteins in lecithin-cholesterol acyltransferase (LCAT)- deficiency. II. Further studies on the abnormal high-density-lipoproteins. Humangenetik 27, 185 (1975).

VAN HANDEL, E., ZILVERSMIT, D.B.: Micromethod for the direct determination of serum triglycerides. J. Lab. Clin. Med. 50, 152 (1957).

VARTIAINEN, I., KANERVA, K.: Arteriosclerosis and war-time. Ann. med. int. Fenniae 36, 748 (1947).

VERDY, M., ORSETTI, A., BALDET, L., PUECH-CATHALA, A.: Effet de la cigarette sur les taux sériques d'hormone de croissance et de tsh dans la diabète. L'Union Médicale Du Canada 104, 1356 - 1359 (1975).

VERESS, B., BÁLINT, A., KÓCZÉ, A., NAGY, Z., JELLINEK, H.: Increasing aortic permeability by atherogenic diet. J. Atheroscler. Res. 11, 369 (1970).

VERESS, B., JELLINEK, H..,HÜTTNER, I., KERÉNYI, T., SOLTI, F., ISKUM, M., HARTAI, A., NAGY, J.: Über die Morphologie der lymphstauungsbedingten Koronarveränderungen. Frankf. Z. Path. 75, 331 (1966a).

VERESS, B., KÓCZÉ, A., JELLINEK, H.: Morphology of early large vessel lesions in experimental hypertension. Brit. J. exp. Path. 50, 600 (1969d).

VERGER, R., de HAAS, G.H.: Interfacial enzyme kinetics of lipolysis. Annu. Rev. Biophys. Bioeng. 5, 77, 1976.

VERGER, R., MIERAS, M.C.E., de HAAS, G.H.: Action of phospholipase A at interfaces. J. Biol. Chem. 248, 4023 (1973).

VESSELINOVITCH, G., GETZ, G.S., HUGHES, R.H., WISSLER, R.W.: Atherosclerosis in the Rhesus monkey fed three food fats. Atherosclerosis 20, 303 - 321 (1974).

VESSELINOVITCH, D., WISSLER, R.W.: Experimental atherosclerosis in rabbits: the effect of oxygen and/or cholestyramine on its reversibility. Circulation 38, VI-198 (1968).

VESSELINOVITCH, D., WISSLER, R.W., DOULL, J.: Experimental production of atherosclerosis in mice. Part 1. Effect of various synthetic diets and radiation on survival time, food consumption and body weight in mice. J. Atheroscler. Res. 8, 483 - 495 (1968).

VESSELINOVITCH, D., WISSLER, R.W., DZOGA, K., HUGHES, R.H., DUBIEN, L.: Regression of atherosclerosis in rabbits. Part 1. Treatment with low-fat diet, hyperoxia and hypolipidemic agents. Atherosclerosis 19, 259 - 275 (1974).

VESSELINOVITCH, D., HUGHES, R., FRAZIER, L., WISSLER, R.W.: Studies of the reversal of advanced atherosclerosis in the rhesus monkey (Abstract). Am. J. Pathol. 70, 41 (1973).

VESSELINOVITCH, D., WISSLER, R.W. HUGHES, R., BORENSZTAJN, J.: Reversal advanced atherosclerosis in rhesus monkeys. Part 1. Light microscopic studies. Atherosclerosis 23, 155 - 176 (1976).

VIEL, B., DONOSO, S., SALCEDO, D.: Coronary atherosclerosis in persons dying violently. Arch. Intern. Med. 122, 97 - 103 (1968).

VIEL, B., DONOSO, S., SALCEDO, D., ROJAS, P., VARELA, A., ALESSANDRI, R.: Alcoholism and socioeconomic status, hepatic damage and arteriosclerosis. Arch. Intern. Med. 117, 84 - 91 (1966).

VIJAYAKUMAR, S.T., KURUP, P.A.: Metabolism of glycosaminoglycans in atheromatous rats. Enzymes concerned with synthesis, degradation and sulphation of glycosaminoglycans. Atherosclerosis 21, 245 - 258 (1975).

VIJAYAKUMAR, S.T., LEELAMMA, S., KURUP, P.A.: Changes in aortic glycosaminoglycans and lipoprotein lipase activity in rats with age and atheroma. Atherosclerosis 21, 1 - 14 (1975).

VIRCHOW, R.: Gesammelte Abhandlungen zur wissenschaftlichen Medizin. Frankfurt/a.M.: Medinger Sohn & Co., 1856.

VITAL STATISTICS, 1975. Japan Health and Welfare Statistics Association, Tokyo. OMAE, T., TAKESHITA, M.: Saisin Igaku 27, 2333 - 2340 (1972)(in Japanese).

VITELLO, L.B., RITTER, M.C., SCANU, A.M.: Self-association of human apolipoprotein A-I in solution: effect on re-lipidation. Fed. Proc. 34, 499 (1975).

VITELLO, L.B., SCANU, A.M.: Studies on human serum high density lipoproteins. Self-association of apolipoprotein A-I in aqueous solutions. J. Biol. Chem. 251, 1131 - 1136 (1976).

VLODAVER, Z., NEUFELD, H.N.: The coronary arteries in coarctation of the aorta. Circulation 37, 449 (1968).

VOGEL, W.C., BRUNZELL, J.D., BIERMAN, E.L.: A comparison of triglyceride, monoglyceride, and phospholipid substrates for post-heparin lipolytic activities from normal and hypertriglyceridemic subjects. Lipids 11, 805 - 814 (1971).

VRACKO, R., BENDITT, E.P.: Capillary basal lamina thickening. Its relationship to endothelial cell death and replacement. J. Cell Biol. 47, 281 - 285 (1970).

WADD, W.: Cursory Remarks on Corpulence; or Obesity Considered as a Disease: With a Critical Examination of Ancient and Modern Opinions, Relative to its Causes and Cure: Containing a Reference to the Most Remarkable Cases that Have Occurred in This Country, 3rd ed. London: J. Callow, 1816.

WADDELL, W.R., HURLEY, N.: Reduction of serum lipids following portacaval transposition in diabetic dogs. Metabolism 13, 562 (1964).

WAGH, P.V.: In: Heparin, Structure, Function and Clinical Implications. BRADSHAW, R.A., WESSLER, S. (eds.). New York: Plenum Press, 1974, pp. 281 - 287.

WAGH, P.V., ROBERTS, B.I., WHITE, H.J., REED, R.C.: Changes in the content of human aortic glycoproteins and acid mucopolysaccharides in atherosclerosis. Atherosclerosis 18, 83 - 91 (1973).

WAGNER, W.D., CLARKSON, T.B. (eds.): Arterial Mesenchyme and Arterosclerosis. New York: Plenum Publishing Corp., 1973.

WAGNER, W.D., CLARKSON, T.B.: Comparative primate atherosclerosis. II. A biochemical study of lipids, calcium, and collagen in atherosclerotic arteries. Exptl. Mol. Pathol. 23, 96 - 121 (1975).

WAGNER, W.D., CLARKSON, T.B.: Slowly miscible cholesterol pools in progressing and regressing atherosclerotic aortas. Soc. Exper. Biol. Med. 143, 804 - 809 (1973).

WAHLBERG, F.: Intravenous glucose tolerance in myocardial infarction, angina pectoris, and intermittent claudication. Acta Med. Scand. (Suppl.), 453, 7 - 93 (1966).

WAHREN, J., JORFELDT, L.: Determination of leg blood flow during exercise in man: an indicator-dilution technique based on femoral venous dye infusion. Clin. Sci. & Mol. Med. 45, 135 - 146 (1973).

WALFORD, R.L., KICKHÖFEN, B.: Selective inhibition of elastolytic and proteolytic properties of elastase. Arch. Biochem. Biophys. 98, 191 (1962).

WALLDIUS, G.: Fatty acid incorporation into human adipose tissue (FIAT) in hypertriglyceridaemia. Methodological, clinical and experimental studies. Acta Med. Scand. (Suppl.) 591 (1976).

WALLENTIN, L.: Abstracts of the Fourth International Symposium on Atherosclerosis, Tokyo, Japan, 1971, p. 122.

WALTON, K.W., CRAIG, G.M., PRIOR, P., WATERHOUSE, J.A.H., SKILTON, J.: A doubleblind crossover clinical trial of pyridinolcarbamate in peripheral arterial disease (arteriosclerosis obliterans). In: Atherogenesis II. SHIMAMOTO, T.,

NUMANO, F., ADDISON, G.M. (eds.). Amsterdam: Excerpta Medica, 1973, pp. 301 - 310.

WALTON, K.W.: Atherosclerosis of heart valves and the formation of the corneal arcus as models for the study of atherosclerosis. Nutrit. Metabol. 15, 37 (1973).

WARNOCK, N.H., CLARKSON, T.B., STEVENSON, R.: Effect of exercise on blood coagulation time and atherosclerosis in cholesterol-fed cockerels. Circulation Res. 5, 478 (1957).

WARREN, B.A., KHAN, S.: The ultrastructure of the lysis of fibrin by endothelium in vitro. Brit. J. Exp. Path. 55, 138 (1974).

WARTMAN, A., LAMPE, T.L., McCANN, D.S., BOYLE, A.J.: Plaque reversal with Mg EDTA in experimental atherosclerosis: elastin and collagen metabolism. J. Atheroscler. Res. 7, 331 - 341 (1967).

WEBER, G., FABBRINI, P., CAPACCIOLI, E., RESI, L.: Repair of early cholesterol-induced aortic lesions in rabbits after withdrawal from short-term atherogenic diet. Scanning electron-microscopical (SEM) and transmission electron-microscopical (TEM) observations. Atherosclerosis 22, 565 (1975).

WEBER, G., FABRINI, P., RESI, L.: On the presence of a Concanavalin-A reactive coat over the endothelial aortic surface and its modifications during early early experimental cholesterol atherogenesis in rabbits. Virch. Arch. Abt. A Path. Anat. 359, 299 - 307 (1973).

WEBER, G., FABRINI, P., RESI, L.: Scanning and transmission electron microscopy observations on the surface lining of aortic intimal plaques in rabbits on a hypercholesterolic diet. Virch. Arch. A. Path. and Histol. 364, 325 - 331 (1974).

WEBSTER, W.S., CLARKSON, T.B., LOFLAND, H.B.: Carbon monoxide-aggravated atherosclerosis in the squirrel monkey. Exp. molec. Path. 13, 36 - 50 (1970).

WEHNER, A.P., OLSON, R.J., BUSCH, R.H.: Increased life span and decreased weights in hamsters exposed to cigarette smoke. Arch. Environ. Health 31, 146 - 153 (1976).

WEINSTEIN, D.B., CAREW, T.W., STEINBERG, D.: Uptake and degradation of low density lipoprotein by swine arterial smooth muscle cells with inhibition of cholesterol biosynthesis. Biochim. Biophys. Acta 424, 404 - 421 (1976).

WELSH, M.J., LEWIS, L.J., HOAK, J.C.: Phagocytosis by cultured human endothelial cells. Fed. Proc. 33, 632 (1974).

WENZEL, D.G., BECKLOFF, G.L.: The effect of nicotine on experimental hypercholesterolemia in the rabbit. J. Amer. pharm. Assoc. 47, 338 (1958).

WERKÖ, L.: Risk factors and coronary heart disease - facts or fancy? Am. Heart J. 91, 87 - 98 (1976).

WERLE, E., SCHIEVELBEIN, H.: Activity of nicotine and inactivity of kallidin in aggregation of blood platelets. Nature 207, 871 (1965).

WESSLER, S.: Clinical implications of heparin. Adv. Exp. Med. Biol. 52, 309 (1974).

WESTERMAN, M.P., WIGGINS, R.G., MAO, R.: Anemia and hypercholesterolemia in cholesterol-fed rabbits. J. Lab. Clin. Med. 75, 893 (1970).

WESTLUND, K., NICOLAYSEN, R.: Ten-year mortality and morbidity related to serum cholesterol. Scand. J. Clin. Lab. Invest, Suppl. 127 (1972).

WHYTE, H.M., NESTEL, P.J., MACGREGOR, A.: Cholesterol metabolism in Papua New Guineans. Europ. J. Clin. Invest (1977) (in press).

WIELAND, H., SEIDEL, D.: Improved techniques for assessment of serum lipoprotein patterns. II. Rapid method for diagnosis of type III hyperlipoproteinemia without ultracentrifugation. Clin. Chem. 19, 1139 - 1141 (1973).

WIENER, J., LATTES, R.G., MELTZER, B.G., SPIRO, D.: The cellular pathology of experimental hypertension. IV. Evidence for increased vascular permeability. Amer. J. Path. 54, 187 - 207 (1969).

WIENER, J., SPIRO, D., LATTES, R.G.: The cellular pathology of experimental hypertension. II. Arteriolar hyalinosis and fibrinoid change. Amer. J. Path. 47, 457 - 485 (1965).

WIGHT, T.N., ROSS, R.: Proteoglycans in primate arteries: 1. Ultrastructural localization and distribution in the intima. J. Cell Biol. 67, 660 - 674 (1975a).

WIGHT, T.N., ROSS, R.: Proteoglycans in primate arteries: II. Synthesis and secretion of glycosaminoglycans by arterial smooth muscle cells in culture. J. Cell Biol. 67, 675 - 686 (1975b).

WIKLUND, O., GUSTAFSON, A., WILHELMSEN, L.: α-lipoprotein cholesterol in men after myocardial infarction compared with a population sample. Artery 1, 399 (1975).

WILCKE, S., KURZ, O.: Ein Testsystem von 25 Persönlichkeitsskalen in der epidemiologischen Anwendung. Med. Technik 95, 118 - 120 (1975).

WILENS, S.L.: The absorption of arterial atheromatous deposits in wasting disease. Am. J. Path. 23, 793 (1947).

WILENS, S.L.: Enhancement of serum sickness lesions in rabbits with pressor agents. Arch. Pathol. 80, 590 (1965).

WILENS, S.L., PLAIR, C.M.: Cigarette smoking and arteriosclerosis. Science 138, 975 - 977 (1962).

WILHELMSEN, L., WEDEL, H., TIBBLIN, G.: Multivariate analysis of risk factors for coronary heart disease. Circulation 48, 950 - 958 (1973).

WILHELMSEN, L., WEDEL, H., TIBBLIN, G.: World Health Organization: myocardial infarction community registers. Copenhagen: Regional Office for Europe, WHO, 1976 (in press).

WILLIAMS, D.C., AVIGNAN, J.: In vitro effects of serum proteins and lipids on lipid synthesis in human skin fibroblasts and leukocytes grown in culture. Biochim. Biophys. Acta 260, 413 - 423 (1972).

WILLS, E.D.: Effects of lipid peroxidation on membrane-bound enzymes of the endoplasmic reticulum. Biochem. J. 123, 983 - 991 (1971).

WILSON, D.E., LEES, R.S.: Metabolic relationships among the plasma lipoproteins. J. Clin. Invest. 51, 1051 (1972).

WILSON, D.E., SCHREINMAN, P.H., BREWSTER, A.C., ARKY, R.A.: The enhancement of alimentary lipemia by ethanol in man. J. Lab. Clin. Med. 75, 264 - 274 (1970).

WINDMUELLER, H.G., HERBERT, P.N., LEVY, R.I.: Biosynthesis of lymph and plasma lipoprotein apoproteins by isolated perfused rat liver and intestine. J. Lipid Res. 14, 215 (1973).

WINTER, I.C., VanDOLAH, J.E., CRANDALL, L.A.Jr.: Lowered serum lipid levels in the Eck fistula dog. Am. J. Physiol. 133, 566 (1941).

WISSLER, R.W.: Coronary atherosclerosis and ischemic heart disease. In: Proceedings of the Third Köln Symposium on Cerebral and Coronary Vascular Disorders and Infarcts. Cologne, West Germany, 1976 (in press).

WISSLER, R.W.: Development of the atherosclerotic plaque. In: The Myocardium: Failure and Infarction. BRAUNWALD, E. (ed.). New York: H.P. Publishing Co., 1974, pp. 155 - 166.

WISSLER, R.W., FRAZIER, L.E., HUGHES, R.H., RASMUSSEN, R.A.: Atherogenesis in the cebus monkey. 1. A comparison of three food fats under controlled dietary conditions. Arch. Path. 74, 312 - 323 (1962).

WISSLER, R.W., VESSELINOVITCH, D.: Studies of regression of advanced atherosclerosis in experimental animals and man. Ann. N.Y. Acad. Sci. 275, 363 - 378 (1976).

WISSLER, R.W., VESSELINOVITCH, D., BORENSZTAJN, J., HUGHES, R.: Regression of severe atherosclerosis in cholestyramine-treated rhesus monkeys with or without a low-fat, low-cholesterol diet. Circulation 52, Suppl. 2, 16 (1975).

WISSLER, R.W., VESSELINOVITCH, D., BORENSZTAJN, J., SCHAFFNER, R., HUGHES, R.: Effect of various dietary responses on progression of atherosclerosis in rhesus monkeys. Fed. Proc. 35, 294 (1976).

WISSLER, R.W., VESSELINOVITCH, D., GETZ, G.S.: Abnormalities of the arterial wall and its metabolism in atherogenesis. Progress in Cardiovascular Diseases, XVIII 5, 341 - 369 (1976).

WOERMANN, E.: Europäische Nahrungswirtschaft. Nova Acta Leopoldina. N.F. 14, 3 - 23 (1944). Z. Sächs. Statist. Landesamtes 66/67 (1920/21).

WOLINSKY, H.: Effects of estrogen and progesterone treatment on the response of the aorta of male rats to hypertension. Circ. Res. 30, 341 - 349 (1972).

WONG, H.Y.C., DAVID, S.N., ORIMILIKWE, S.O., JOHNSON, F.B.: The effects of physical exercise in reversing experimental atherosclerosis. In: Diet and Atherosclerosis. SITORI, C., RICCI, G., GORINI, S. (eds.). Adv. Exp. Med. Biol. 6, 33 - 56 (1973).

WONG, H.Y.C., MENDEZ, H.C., WALTERS, C.S., ORVIS, H.H.: A revised method for determination of total plasma cholesterol in blood. Life Sci. 4, 431 (1965).

WONG, H.Y.C., ORIMILIKWE, S.O., BHIDE, M.G., FLETCHER, A.D.: Influence of exercise and partial occlusion of abdominal aorta on plasma cholesterol and aortic atherosclerosis of cholesterol-fed cockerels. Fed. Proc. 31, (Suppl. II), 344 (1972).

WONG, H.Y.C., SIMMONS, R., KIM, J., LIU, D., HAWTHORNE, E.W.: Hypocholesterolizing effect of exercise on cholesterol-fed cockerels. Fed. Proc. 16, 138 (1957).

WORLD HEALTH ORGANIZATION: Classification of hyperlipidemias and hyperlipoproteinemias. Circulation 45, 501 (1972).

WORTH, R.M., KATO, H., RHOADS, G.G., KAGAN, A., SYME, S.L.: Epidemiologic studies of coronary heart disease and stroke in Japanese men living in Japan, Hawaii and California: mortality. Am. J. Epidemiol. 102 - 481 (1975).

WRIGHT, H.P.: Mitosis patterns in aortic endothelium. Atherosclerosis 15, 93 (1972).

WRIGHT, H.P., GIACONCETTI, N.J.: Circulating endothelial cells and arterial endothelial mitosis in anaphylactic shock. Brit. J. exp. Path. 53, 1 (1972).

WU, K.K., ARMSTRONG, M.L., HOAK, J.C.. MEGAN, M.B.: Platelet aggregates in hypercholesterolemic rhesus monkeys. Thrombos. Res. 7, 917 (1975).

WUSTERMAN, F.S., GOLD, C., WAGNER, J.C.: Glycosaminoglycans and calcification in the lesions of progressive massive fibrosis and in pleural plaques. Amer. Rev. Resp. Dis. 106, 116 - 118 (1972).

YAMANOUCHI, H.: Über die zirkulären Gefäßnähte und Arterien-Venen-Anastomosen, sowie über Gefäßtransplantationen. Deut. Zeit. Chirurg. 112, 1 (1911).

YAMORI, Y.: Contribution of cardiovascular factors to the development of hypertension in spontaneously hypertensive rats. Jap. Heart J. 15, 194 - 196 (1974).

YAMORI, A.: Hypertensive strains of rat. In: Gene-Environment Interaction in Common Diseases. INOUE, E., HIGURE, M. (eds.). Tokyo: Univ. of Tokyo Press, 1976a (in press).

YAMORI, Y.: Interaction of neural and nonneural factors in the pathogenesis of spontaneous hypertension. In: The Nervous System in Arterial Hypertension. JULIUS, S., ESLER, M. (eds.). Springfield: C.C. Thomas, 1976b, pp. 17 - 43.

YAMORI, Y.: Neurogenic mechanism of spontaneous hypertension. In: Regulation of Blood Pressure by the Central Nervous System. ONESTI, F., FERNANDES, M., KIM, K.D. (eds.). New York-San Francisco-London: Grune and Stratton, 1976c, pp. 65 - 76.

YAMORI, Y.: Selection of arteriolipidosis-prone rats (ALR). Jap. Heart J. 18 (1977) (in press).

YAMORI, Y.: Vascular protein metabolism in the pathogenesis of hypertension. Jap. Circ. J. 40, 879 - 886 (1976d).

YAMORI, Y., HAMASHIMA, Y., HORIE, R., HANDA, H., SATO, M.: Pathology of acute arterial fat deposition in spontaneously hypertensive rats. Jap. Circ. J. 39, 593 - 600 (1975a).

YAMORI, Y., HORIE, R., AKIGUCHI, I., NARA, Y., OHTAKA, M., FUKASE, M.: Pathogenic mechanisms of stroke in stroke-prone SHR. In: Hypertension and Brain Mechanisms. DE JONG (ed.). Amsterdam: ASP Biological and Medical Press, 1976a (in press).

YAMORI, Y., HORIE, R., AKIGUCHI, I., OHTAKA, M., NARA, Y., FUKASE, M.: New models of SHR for studies on stroke and atherogenesis. Clin. Exp. Pharmacol. Physiol. (1977) (in press).

YAMORI, Y., HORIE, R., OHTAKA, M., NARA, Y., OHTA, K., OKAMOTO, K., HANDA, H., FUKASE, M.: Pathogenic approach to the prophylaxis of stroke and atherogenesis in SHR. In: Spontaneous Hypertension II. KOLETSKY, S. (ed.). Washington, D.C.: U.S. Government Press, 176b (in press).

YAMORI, Y., HORIE, R., SATO, M.: Hypertension as an important factor for cerebrovascular atherogenesis in rats. Stroke 7, 120 - 125 (1976c).

YAMORI, Y., HORIE, R., SATO., M., FUKASE, M.: Hemodynamic derangement for the induction of cerebrovascular fat deposition in normotensive rats on a hyper-cholesterolemic diet. Stroke 7, 385 - 389 (1976d).

YAMORI, Y., HORIE, R., SATO, M., HANDA, H.: Pathogenetic similarity of stroke in stroke-prone SHR and humans. Stroke 7, 46 - 53 (1976e).

YAMORI, Y., HORIE, R., SATO, M., HANDA, H.: Regional cerebral blood flow in stroke-prone SHR: a preliminary report. Jap. Heart J. 17, (Suppl. III), 384 - 386 (1976f).

YAMORI, Y., HORIE, R., SATO, M., SASAGAWA, S., OKAMOTO, K.: Experimental studies on the pathogenesis and prophylaxis of stroke in stroke-prone spontaneously hypertensive rats (SHR). (1) Quantitative estimation of cerebrovascular per-meability. Jap. Circ. J. 39, 611 - 615 (1975b).

YAMORI, Y., MATSUMOTO, M., YAMABE, H., OKAMOTO,K.: Augmentation of spontaneous hypertension by chronic stress in rats. Jap. Circ. J. 33, 399 - 409 (1969).

YAMORI, Y., NAGAOKA, A., OKAMOTO, K.: Importance of genetic factors in hyper-tensive cerebrovascular lesions, an evidence obtained by successive selective breeding of stroke-prone and -resistant SHR. Jap. Circ. J. 38, 1095 - 1106 (1974).

YAMORI, Y., OKAMOTO, K.: Spontaneous hypertension in the rats, a model of human "essential" hypertension. Proc. 80th Cong., Germ. Soc. Int. Med. 168 - 170 (1974). Institue of Laboratory Animal Resources, National Academy of Sciences, Washington, D.C.. Committee on care and use of spontaneously hypertensive (SHR) rats: guide for the care and use of spontaneously hypertensive (SHR) rats in biomedical research. (1976).

YAMORI, Y., SASAGAWA, S.: Physico-morphological characteristics of aorta in stroke-prone and -resistant spontaneously hypertensive rats. Jap. Heart J. 16, 296 - 298 (1975).

YANO, J., GOHDA, H., YAMASAKI, S., NANBU, S.: Study of the classification for hyperlipidemia (Comparison of paper electrophoresis and disc electrophoresis). The Physico-chemical Biology 18, 43 - 44 (1974).

YU, S.Y.: Calcification processes in atherosclerosis. In: Arterial Mesenchyme and Arteriosclerosis. WAGNER, W.D., CLARKSON, T.B. (eds.). New York: Plenum Press, 1974, pp. 403 - 425.

YUDKIN, J.: Diet and coronary thrombosis. Hypothesis and fact. Lancet (1957) II, 155 - 162.

ZELDIS, S.M., NEMERSON, Y., PUTLICK, F.A.: Tissue factor (thromboplastin) local-ization to plasma membranes by peroxidase-conjugated antibodies. Science 175, 766 (1972).

ZELIS, R., MASON, D.T., BRAUNWALD, E., LEVY, R.I.: Effects of hyperlipoprotein-emias and their treatment on peripheral circulation. J. Clin. Invest. 49, 1007 (1970).

ZEMPLENYI, T., ROSENSTEIN, A.J.: Arterial enzymes and their relation to athero-sclerosis in pigeons. Exp. Mol. Pathol. 22, 225 - 241 (1975).

ZIEGELMAYER, W.: Die Ernährung des deutsches Volkes. 5. Aufl. Dresden: Stein-kopff, 1947.

ZIEVE, F.S., ZIEVE, L.: Post-heparin phospholipase and post-heparin lipase have different tissue origins. Biochem. Biophys. Res. Commun. 47, 1480 (1972).

ZILVERSMIT, D.B.: The design and analysis of isotope experiments. Am. J. Med. 29, 832 - 848 (1960).

ZILVERSMIT, D.B.: Mechanism of cholesterol accumulation in the arterial wall. Am. J. Cardiol. 35, 559 (1975).

ZILVERSMIT, D.B.: A proposal linking atherogenesis to the interaction of lipo-protein lipase with triglyceride rich lipoproteins. Circ. Res. 33, 633 (1973).

ZILVERSMIT, D.B., NEWMAN, H.A.I.: Does a metabolic barrier to circulating choles-terol protect the arterial wall? Circulat. 33, 7 (1966).

ZINDER, O., MENDELSON, C.R., BLANCHETTE-MACKIE, E.J., SCOW, O.: Lipoprotein lipase and uptake of chylomicron triarylglycerol and cholesterol by perfused mammary tissue. Biochim. Biophys. Acta 431, 526 (1976).

ZINNER, S.H., MARTIN, L.F., SACKS, F., ROSNER, B., KASS, E.H.: A longitudinal study of blood pressure in childhood. Am. J. Epidemiol. 100, 437 (1975).

ZOPPI, S., FRATERIGO, L., GATTI, E.: Ricette per l'impiego aspedaliero di una dieta a base di proteine di soja. Min. Dietol. (1976) (in press).

AUTHOR INDEX (ABSTRACTS)

Abe, K. 699
Abe, M. 172,372
Abrahams, P.H. 506
Acquatella, H. 70
Adachi, K. 693
Adler, K. 319
Ageta, M. 321
Ahmad, M.S. 698
Aihara, K. 69
Aizawa, Y. 172, 372
Akanuma, Y. 317,318
Akcasu, A. 547
Akuda, F. 252
Alaupovic, P. 147,247,249,250
Alavi, M. 454
Allam, S.S. 368,648
Altman, S. 479
Amaducci, B. 701
Ando, K. 556
Angelin, B. 146,553
Applebaum, D. 345
Arai, C. 172,372
Arakawa, D. 321
Arisue, K. 704
Arntzenius, A.C. 694
Arreaza-Plaza, C. 703
Asano, E. 547
Assmann, G. 317,319
Ast, E. 319
Astrup, P. 287
Audebert, A. 127
Augustin, J. 347,348
Auogaro, P. 258

Bac, C. de 548
Backwinkel, K.P. 88
Badimon, L. 662
Baggio, G. 253,254,547,553,556,589
Bahler, R.C. 247,545
Baiocchi, M.R. 553,556,589
Balestrieri, P. 553,556,589
Balleisen, L. 366
Barboriak, J.J. 699
Barter, P. 255
Barth, P. 617
Bass, H.B. 344,348
Batayias, G.E. 699
Bates, S.R. 649
Bauer, O. 621
Bayardo, J.R. 699
Baylock, A. 786
Belussi, F. 258
Benvegnù, D. 290
Berchtold, P. 128
Berenson, G.S. 370,483

Berg, K. 256
Berger, H. 128
Berkarda, B. 547
Bermudez, D. 346
Bertoli, E. 549
Bihari-Varga, M. 550
Bing, R.J. 69
Bird, B. 128
Björkerud, S. 70,286,697
Björnheden, T. 697
Blacket, R. 125,455
Blaton, V. 251
Boarato, E. 290
Boberg, J. 347,454,592
Boberg, M. 454
Bondjers, G. 69,70,286,697
Bosanquet, A.G. 257
Bosch, V. 703
Brattsand, R. 551,697,786
Braun, A. 699
Brechemier, D. 645
Brecher, P. 67
Breddin, K. 621,709
Brehmer, U. 648
Bretherton, K.N. 88
Briani, G. 553,556,589
Brita, G. 548
Brown, B. 148
Brozovic, M. 619
Brunner, D. 125,455,479
Buchholz, L. 484
Buchmann, P. 590
Buddecke, E. 647
Burns, T.S. 618
Butkus, A. 703

Camejo, G. 70
Caparrotta, L. 290,702
Caramia, F.G. 548
Carlson, L.A. 554
Caruzzo, C. 707
Catapano, A. 248
Cazzolato, G. 258
Ceccarelli, G. 548
Cerutti, R. 507
Chakrabarti, R. 619
Chan, C.T. 456
Chan, S.W. 366
Chad, Y.-S. 320
Chaplain, R.A. 548
Chapman, K.P. 288
Chatelet, F. 693
Chen, C.-M. 125
Chen, J. 456
Chen, J.-S. 125

781

Schellenberg, B. 550,552
Scherstén, T. 69
Schlicht, I. 700
Schlierf, I. 253,550,552
Schmid-Schönbein, H. 710
Schmidt, C.M. 288
Schmitt, G. 88
Schmitz, G. 317,319
Schneider, F. 291,693
Schneider, J. 557
Schönborn, J. 555
Schrott, H.G. 128,506
Schubotz, R. 557
Schurr, P.E. 288,701
Schwartz, S. 455,479
Schwartzkopff, W. 64,700
Schweppe, J.S. 71
Seban, C. 693
Sebestyén, G. 287
Seepers, J. 171
Segal, P. 257
Seidel, D. 253,254,547
Seki, T. 258
Sekiguchi, M. 706
Servelle, M. 709
Sheers, M. 646
Shibata, N. 65
Shibutani, K. 369
Shigematsu, H. 69
Shimamoto, T. 618,701
Shimizu, T. 71
Shinkai, H. 67
Shio, H. 620
Shkhvatsabaya, I.K. 694
Sibinga, C.T.S. 288,617,618
Simon, B. 553
Simon-Crisan, G. 553
Sirô, I. 705
Sirtori, C. 248,549,701
Sjöström, L. 69
Skinner, S.L. 88
Slack, J. 506, 590,619
Sluyter, D.P. 694
Snoek, J. 706
Sodhi, H.S. 315,318,319
Soetewey, F. 251
Sohn, E. 481
Solberg, L.A. 90,91
Soloway, H. 695
Spadaro, R. 548
Spaet, T.H. 645
Srinivasan, S.R. 483
Stähelin, H.B. 256,479,590
Stafford, W.W. 288
Stănescu, C. 482
Stange, E.F. 454
Steinbach, M. 482
Steiner, G. 128,146,592
Stender, S. 287,289
Stirling, Y. 619
Stolberg, H. 128
Stolze, T. 128

Stone, M. 703
Stork, H. 547
Stout, C. 66
Straja, D. 146
Strub, P. 590
Styblo, K. 694
Subramanyam, V. 695
Suciu, A. 482
Sudo, H. 480
Suenram, A. 249
Sugano, M. 292
Sugawara, H. 171
Sugita, K. 320
Sumiyoshi, A. 619
Suzuki, M. 699
Suzuki, S. 292,507

Takahashi, S. 700
Takamatsu, S. 171
Takano, T. 701
Takeda, R. 373
Takeno, K. 701
Tamura, G. 556
Tan, E. 703
Tanaka, K. 64,619
Tănăsescu, C. 482
Taroni, G.C. 258
Taylor, G.W. 127
Teodorescu, S. 482
Teramoto, T. 346,675
Terata, T. 369
Terpstra, J. 171
Thayer, R. 147
Theodorini, S. 482
Thiel, G. 590
Thomsen, H.K. 66,371
Thorp, J. 703
Thurnherr, N. 256
Timmer, W.G. 287
Titus, J.L. 699
Toffano, G. 290,702
Tokita, K. 372
Tomaszewski, J.J. 371
Tomomatsu, T. 481
Toshima, H. 321
Toyama, S. 65
Truffert, J. 554
Tsai, K.-F. 456
Tseng, W.-P. 125
Tsuchida, T. 547
Tsuji, E. 507
Tsuji, T. 507
Tsushima, M. 547
Tsuchida, T. 700
Tsuzuku, A. 372
Turner, D.M. 695
Turpin, G. 554

Udenfriend, S. 368
Ueda, K. 373
Urbinati, G. 480
Uzawa, H. 479

delta 8-dihydroabietamide 557
deoxycholic acid 303
dermatan sulphate 32, 354
diabetes mellitus 568
-- as factor 473
diabetic angiopathies 170
1,3-diaryloxipropanol-(2) derivative
    546
diet and atherosclerosis 95, 386
-, coronary heart disease 514, 676
- induced atherosclerosis, cholesterol
    feeding 278
--- in nonhuman primates 278, 280
-, influence of nutritions 437
-, -on lipoprotein composition 439
-, -on plasma lipids 439
dietary fats, thrombogenic and
    atherogenic effects 609
- management 511
- modification of plasma cholesterol in
    children 444
-- of plasma cholesterol in adults 444
diets, effect on plasma lipids 514
differential scanning calorimetry 222
3,7-dimethyl-1-C S-oxohexyl)-xanthine
    (BL 191) 698
dipyridamole 609
domains 180
drugs and atherosclerosis 517
-, interaction of lipoproteins 521
-, lipoprotein structure 522
-, modifying lipoprotein distribution
    519
D-thyroxine 286, 576
-, regression of atherosclerosis 286

edematous plaques 601
elastase 34, 372, 373
elastic tissue in atherosclerosis 34
-- in normal arteries 33
elastin 34, 350, 366, 371
-, regression changes 408, 409
elimination of cholesterol, high den-
    sity lipoprotein (HDL) dependent 70
endogenous VLDL-TG catabolism 139
endothelial cells 47
-, contraction 3
-, glycocalyx 2
-, growth, dynamics 274
-, histamine 2
-, injury 4, 601ff
-, integrity 12
-, permeability in hypercholesterolemia
    4
-, prostaglandin 2
-, regeneration 274
endothelium
-, capillary 12
-, cholesterol content 286
-, defective 286

-, gross mechanical injury 13, 386
-, properties 1
-, regeneration 12, 13
-, uptake of ferritin 6
energy dispersive analysis 9
enthalpy change on binding DMPC 234
epidemiology of atherosclerosis 92
epinephrine 47
EPL 148
essential fatty acid deficiency 703
estrogens 569
ethanol-lipemia 658
evans blue model 4
experimental animals 511
- atherosclerosis, autoimmune theory
    65
--, dogs 286
--, prevention 65
--, rabbit 287, 288
- models, atherogenesis 79
--, hypertension 79
--, stroke 79
eye ground changes in hyperlipemia
    456

Fabry's disease 504
familial broad-β disease 215
- combined hyperlipidemia 214
- hypercholesterolemia 214
--, genetic heterogenety 590
- hypertriglyceridemia 216
- lipoprotein lipase deficiency 214
- type V hyperlipoproteinemia 217
fat intake in Japan 462
- loading, experimental atheroscle-
    rosis 276
- tolerance test, portocaval shunt
    137, 139, 140, 700
fatty acid synthesis in dog aortas 68
- streaks 17, 260, 601
-- in abdominal and thoracic aorta 279
--, composition 283
--, distribution 283
-- in monkeys 278
ferritin 2
fetal aorta, ultrastructural studies
    371
fiat 139, 147
fibrin 75, 76
fibrinogen in normal intima 26
fibrinolytic system, hyperlipemia 620
fibroblast 30
-, binding 52
-, cell surface receptors 52
-, lipid metabolism 647
fibrous plaques 17, 66, 601
--, composition 283
--, mineralization 283
-- in monkeys 278
filaments 14

Related Titles

H. BEGEMANN, J. RASTETTER
Atlas der klinischen Hämatologie

Begründet von L. Heilmeyer, H. Begemann. Mit einem Anhang über
tropische Krankheiten von W. Mohr
2., völlig neu bearbeitete Auflage
208 Abbildungen (davon 191 farbig). XVI, 324 Seiten. 1972
ISBN 3-540-05604-1
Vertriebsrechte für Japan: Maruzen Co. Ltd., Tokyo

Brain and Heart Infarct

Proceedings of the Third Cologne Symposium, June 16–19, 1976
Edited by K. J. Zülch, W. Kaufmann, K.-A. Hossmann, V. Hossmann
155 figures, 14 tables. XX, 351 pages. 1977
ISBN 3-540-08270-0

L. DEMLING, M. CLASSEN, P. FRÜHMORGEN
Atlas of Enteroscopy

Endoscopy of the Small and Large Bowel; Retrograde Cholangio-Pan-
creatography. With the Collaboration of H. Koch, H. Bauerle.
Translated from the German and Adapted by K. H. Soergel with the
Assistance of H. Pease.
286 figures, most in color. XI, 246 pages. 1975
ISBN 3-540-07292-6

Diagnose und Therapie in der Praxis

Nach der amerikanischen Ausgabe von M. A. Krupp, M. J. Chatton.
Bearbeitet, ergänzt und herausgegeben von K. Huhnstock, W. Kutscha.
Unter Mitarbeit von H. Dehmel, G.-W. Schmidt.
4., neubearbeitete und erweiterte Auflage.
29 Abbildungen. XVI, 1403 Seiten. 1976
ISBN 3-540-07781-2

H. G. FASSBENDER
Pathology of Rheumatic Diseases

Translated from the German Edition by G. Loewi
444 figures. XI, 353 pages. 1975
ISBN 3-540-07289-6
Distribution rights for Japan: Igaku Shoin Ltd., Tokyo

FRANZ BÜCHNER
Hypoxie

Beiträge von Franz Büchner aus den Jahren 1932-1972. Anläßlich sei-
nes 80. Geburtstages im Auftrag seiner Schüler herausgegeben von
E. Grundmann.
128 Abbildungen. VI, 472 Seiten. 1975
ISBN 3-540-07078-8

Pathology of the Gastro-Intestinal Tract

Editor: B. C. Morson
155 figures. VI, 356 pages. 1976.
(Current Topics in Pathology, Volume 63)
ISBN 3-540-07927-0

The Genetics of Diabetes Mellitus

Editors: W. Creutzfeldt, J. Köbberling, J. V. Neel
In cooperation with numerous experts.
64 figures, 74 tables. IX, 248 pages. 1976
ISBN 3-540-07651-4

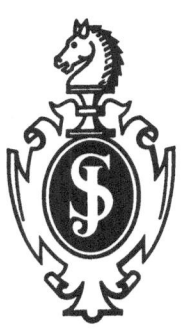

Springer-Verlag
Berlin
Heidelberg
New York

Handbuch der allgemeinen Pathologie

Herausgeber: H.-W. Altmann, F. Büchner, H. Cottier, E. Grundmann,
G. Holle, E. Letterer, W. Masshoff, H. Meessen, F. Roulet, G. Seifert,
G. Siebert
Band 3
Zwischensubstanzen, Gewebe, Organe
Teil 7
Mikrozirkulation/Microcirculation
Redigiert von H. Meessen
Etwa 260 Abbildungen. Etwa 1090 Seiten. (Etwa 360 Seiten in Eng-
lisch). 1977
ISBN 3-540-07750-2

A. LABHART

Clinical Endocrinology

Theory and Practice
With a Foreword by G. W. Thorn. In collaboration with numerous ex-
perts.
Translators: A. Trachsler, J. Dodsworth-Philips
400 figures. XXXII, 1092 pages. 1974
ISBN 3-540-06307-2
Distribution rights for Japan: Igaku Shoin Ltd., Tokyo

W. A. McALPIN

Heart and Coronary Arteries

An Anatomical Atlas for Clinical Diagnosis, Radiological Investigation
and Surgical Treatment
1098 figures, mostly in color. XVI, 224 pages. 1975
ISBN 3-540-06985-2
Distribution rights for Japan: Igaku Shoin Ltd., Tokyo

P. OTTO, K. EWE

Atlas der Rectoskopie und Coloskopie

31 Schwarzweißabbildungen, 115 farbige Abbildungen auf 21 Tafeln,
1 Tabelle. IX, 96 Seiten. 1976
ISBN 3-540-07489-9

M.R. PARWARESCH

The Human Blood Basophil

Morphology, Orgin, Kinetics, Function, and Pathology
With a Foreword by K. Lennert
58 figures, some in color. XI, 235 pages. 1976
ISBN 3-540-07649-2

K. SIGG

Varizen
Ulcus cruris und Thrombose

Mit Beiträgen von C. C. Arnoldi, E. Imhoff, R. Kressig, H. J. Leu,
C. Montigel, T. Wuppermann
4., neubearbeitete und erweiterte Auflage.
130 farbige und 411 Schwarzweiß-Abbildungen. XV, 403 Seiten. 1976
ISBN 3-540-07373-6

Atherosclerosis 3

Proceedings of the Third International Symposium, 24-28 Oct., 1973
Editors: G. Schettler, A. Weizel
349 figures, 222 tables. XXXV, 1034 pages. 1974
ISBN 3-540-06909-7
Distribution rights for Japan:
Maruzen Co. Ltd., Tokyo

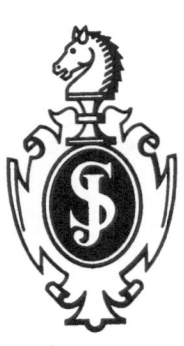

Springer-Verlag
Berlin
Heidelberg
New York